Handbook of Hematologic Pathology

DIAGNOSTIC PATHOLOGY

1. *Diagnostic Neuropathology*, Harry V. Vinters, Michael A. Farrell, Paul S. Mischel, and Karl H. Anders
2. *Handbook of Hematologic Pathology,* edited by Harold R. Schumacher, William A. Rock, Jr., and Sanford A. Stass

ADDITIONAL VOLUMES IN PREPARATION

Handbook of Hematologic Pathology

edited by

HAROLD R. SCHUMACHER
University of Cincinnati Medical Center
Cincinnati, Ohio

WILLIAM A. ROCK, JR.
University of Mississippi Medical Center
Jackson, Mississippi

SANFORD A. STASS
University of Maryland School of Medicine
Baltimore, Maryland

MARCEL DEKKER, INC. NEW YORK • BASEL

ISBN: 0-8247-0170-4

This book is printed on acid-free paper.

Headquarters
Marcel Dekker, Inc.
270 Madison Avenue, New York, NY 10016
tel: 212-696-9000; fax: 212-685-4540

Eastern Hemisphere Distribution
Marcel Dekker AG
Hutgasse 4, Postfach 812, CH-4001 Basel, Switzerland
tel: 41-61-261-8482; fax: 41-61-261-8896

World Wide Web
http://www.dekker.com

The publisher offers discounts on this book when ordered in bulk quantities. For more information, write to Special Sales/Professional Marketing at the headquarters address above.

Current printing (last digit):
10 9 8 7 6 5 4 3 2 1

PRINTED IN THE UNITED STATES OF AMERICA

In loving memory of my parents, Catherine and Philip

Harold R. Schumacher

To Vannie, William, and Megan,
whose patience and acceptance of the time to write these pages
will forever be appreciated.

William A. Rock, Jr.

To my wife, Ann, and in loving memory of my father, Morris

Sanford A. Stass

Preface

This book should capture the interest of a large audience engaged in or dependent on laboratory hematology, including medical technologists, medical students, hematologists, and hematopathologists. It should be helpful to those preparing for boards related to hematology. In addition, it offers a source of rapid review for individuals who have been working outside hematology for a while and who wish to return to the field with up-to-date knowledge. Furthermore, the book provides an expeditious source of cross-training that will be especially valuable to medical technologists who are required to be competent in various areas of the laboratory.

This book was written by authors who apply every day what they write about in their chapters. Theory is fine and needs to be understood, but learning and knowing how to apply the information to the patient's situation is one of the major goals of this text. This goal is achieved through direct discussion of the issues and theory and application of the information by using case histories. The approach is not to solve all the reader's problems, but rather to show how to gather information about a problem and how to deal with it. Individual variations in approaches are expected, since everyone will have different experiences and new methods and technologies become available every day. What this book is designed to achieve is to help the reader develop a method to look at a problem and to think about diagnosing and fixing what can be fixed.

We have stressed certain basic approaches or themes throughout the book that should appeal to a wide segment of the medical community. These include the simplicity of style, ease of readability, current information, ready application of the information to a working laboratory, and other practical applications. To further emphasize applications some case studies are offered at the end of each chapter to allow the reader to become involved in the pragmatic use of the new knowledge acquired.

This book reflects the varied backgrounds of the editors. Dr. Schumacher began his career in clinical hematology/oncology with a special interest in leukemias and ultimately migrated to laboratory hematology. Dr. Rock began his career in morphologic atherosclerosis and found a home as a clinical pathologist and developing practical experience and knowledge in the field of applied coagulation. Dr. Stass began his career in bone marrow pathology and the study of hematology and malignancies and eventually emerged as a cancer center director. As editors, we selected a group of authors who are experts in their fields. The editors thank them for a job well done.

The editors have directed their efforts toward the diagnosis and management of hematological problems, utilizing practical, current, and relevant laboratory investigative procedures. However, we have also emphasized pertinent clinical information in those areas where such knowledge is a necessary adjunct to diagnosis.

The book further directs medical technologists, hematopathologists, and hematologists on how to utilize blood, plasma, serum, instrumentation, bone marrow, lymph nodes, and splenic tissue to establish a diagnosis.

Finally, the book emphasizes practical technical information to aid in the operation of an efficient hematology laboratory involved in hematological procedures. The editors anticipate the reader will enjoy a book directed toward a practical and useful source of laboratory hematological information.

Harold R. Schumacher
William A. Rock, Jr.
Sanford A. Stass

Acknowledgments

We are indebted to a number of people who through their efforts, support, and cooperation made this book possible.

Harold R. Schumacher would like to give a very special thanks to our secretaries Pat Hathaway and Roland Randolph, and Pauline Harris, administrative coordinator, who communicated with many of the contributors, the editor, and the staff.

Special thanks to our fellows in hematopathology, Fermina Mazzella and Carmelita Alvares, who helped us read and edit many of the chapters.

Further thanks to the pathology residents at our institutions who provided new information and procedures that were important to our presenting a timely content.

In addition, our gratitude is extended to Dr. Paul Steele, who gave advice and counsel in molecular hematology; Dr. Ruth Blough, in cytogenetics; and Dr. Paul Hurtubise, in flow cytometric analysis.

William A. Rock, Jr., would like to thank the medical technologists (particularly Dan Haun and Pam Moore) in the Hematology and Coagulation Laboratories at Charity Hospital, New Orleans, Louisiana, and University Hospital, Jackson, Mississippi, who were eager to push the envelope in developing new procedures in coagulation and assuring that they worked consistently. He is also grateful to the Pathology Residents at Charity Hospital, New Orleans, Louisiana, and University Hospital, Jackson, Mississippi, who struggled tirelessly to implement the new approaches and procedures for bleeding and clotting problems.

Finally, Dr. Rock thanks Dr. Alain Marengo-Rowe, whose encouragement and conviction were an inspiration to aggressively assault the coagulation problem, to learn about it, and to struggle with the difficult cases, as well as Dr. Frederick G. Schechter, who first opened for me the door to the direct laboratory application of coagulation theory to the more complex patient coagulophathies; Dr. Douglas Triplett, whose thoughtful support was an inspiration to continue writing, and Dr. Jack Perry Strong, for without his confidence and trust none of this would have happened.

Lastly, a very special thanks to Elizabeth Curione, production editor at Marcel Dekker, Inc., for her tenacity of purpose and encouragement. We all enjoyed working with her.

Contents

Contributors

Lynne V. Abruzzo, M.D., Ph.D. Department of Pathology, University of Texas M.D. Anderson Cancer Center, Houston, Texas

William F. Baker, Jr., M.D., F.A.C.P. Department of Medicine, U.C.L.A. Center for Health Sciences, Los Angeles, California

Robert F. Baugh, Ph.D. Department of Research, Medtronic Blood Management, Parker, Colorado

Mark D. Brissette, M.D. Division of Hematology/Flow Cytometry, Department of Pathology, Madigan Army Medical Center, Tacoma, Washington

Bradley E. Copeland, M.D.* Department of Pathology and Laboratory Medicine, University of Cincinnati Medical Center, Cincinnati, Ohio

James W. Cook, M.D. Departments of Pathology and Family Medicine, University of Mississippi Medical Center, Jackson, Mississippi

James D. Cotelingam, M.D. Department of Pathology, Louisiana State University Medical Center, Shreveport, Louisiana

Hernani D. Cualing, M.D. Department of Pathology and Laboratory Medicine, University of Cincinnati Medical Center, Cincinnati, Ohio

Kojo S. J. Elenitoba-Johnson, M.D. Department of Pathology, University of Utah Health Sciences Center, Salt Lake City, Utah

Robert B. Fairweather, M.D., Ph.D. Department of Pathology, Dartmouth Hitchcock Medical Center, Lebanon, New Hampshire

Louis M. Fink, M.D. Department of Pathology, University of Arkansas for Medical Sciences and Little Rock Veterans Administration Medical Center, Little Rock, Arkansas

---

*Former Chairman of the Commission on World Standards, World Association of Pathologists

David F. Garvin, M.D. Department of Pathology, Georgetown University Medical Center, Washington, D.C.

Zoran Gatalica, M.D., D.Sc. Departments of Pathology and Hematology, Jefferson Medical College, Thomas Jefferson University, Philadelphia, Pennsylvania

Scott J. Graham, M.D. Department of Pathology, Naval Medical Center, Portsmouth, Virginia

Gene L. Gulati, Ph.D., SH (ASCP), DLM Department of Pathology, Anatomy, and Cell Biology, Jefferson Medical College, Thomas Jefferson University, Philadelphia, Pennsylvania

Robert J. Hartsock, M.D. Department of Laboratory Medicine, Allegheny General Hospital, Pittsburgh, Pennsylvania

Bong H. Hyun, M.D., D.Sc. Department of Laboratory Medicine, Ajou University School of Medicine, Suwon City, Korea, and Jefferson Medical College, Thomas Jefferson University, Philadelphia, Pennsylvania

Lawrence Kass, M.S., M.D. Department of Pathology and Medicine, Case Western Reserve University School of Medicine, and Metro Health Medicine Center, Cleveland, Ohio

Aubrey A. Lurie, M.D. Department of Pathology, Louisiana State University Medical Center, and Department of Pathology and Laboratory Medicine Service, Overton Brooks VA Medical Center, Shreveport, Louisiana

Nicole A. Massoll, M.D. Department of Pathology, University of Arkansas for Medical Sciences, Little Rock, Arkansas

Fermina Maria Mazzella, M.D. Department of Pathology and Laboratory Medicine, The Guthrie Clinic, Sayre, Pennsylvania

Robert T. Means, Jr., M.D. Hematology-Oncology Division, Department of Medicine, Medical University of South Carolina and R. H. Johnson VA Medical Center, Charleston, South Carolina

L. Jeffrey Medeiros, M.D. Department of Pathology, University of Texas M.D. Anderson Cancer Center, Houston, Texas

Anwar Mikhael, M.D., Ph.D. Department of Pathology and Laboratory Medicine, University of Cincinnati Medical Center, Cincinnati, Ohio

Jonathan L. Miller, M.D., Ph.D. Department of Pathology, State University of New York Health Science Center at Syracuse, Syracuse, New York

Ronald L. Nagel, M.D. Albert Einstein College of Medicine, Bronx, New York

James R. Newland, M.D. Department of Pathology and Microbiology, University of Nebraska College of Medicine, Omaha, Nebraska

Alex A. Pappas, M.D. Departments of Pathology and Laboratory Medicine, University of Arkansas for Medical Sciences, Little Rock, Arkansas

Gerardo Perrotta, M.P.A., M.T.(A.S.C.P.)S.H. Department of Pathology and Laboratory Medicine, University of Cincinnati Medical Center, Cincinnati, Ohio

LoAnn C. Peterson, M.D. Department of Pathology, Northwestern University Medical Center, Chicago, Illinois

Powers Peterson, M.D. Department of Pathology, Sentara Norfolk General Hospital, Norfolk, Virginia

William A. Rock, Jr., M.D. Division of Clinical Pathology, Department of Pathology, University of Mississippi Medical Center, Jackson, Mississippi

Francis R. Rodwig, Jr., M.D., M.P.H. Blood Bank, Ochsner Medical Institutions, New Orleans, Louisiana

Donald L. Rucknagel, M.D., Ph.D. Department of Pediatrics and Internal Medicine, University of Cincinnati College of Medicine, and Hemoglobin Diagnostic Laboratory, Cincinnati Comprehensive Sickle Cell Center, Children's Hospital Medical Center, Cincinnati, Ohio

Ronald A. Sacher, M.D., F.R.C.P.C. Department of Laboratory Medicine, Georgetown University Medical Center, Washington, D.C.

Abdus Saleem, M.D. Department of Pathology, Baylor College of Medicine, Houston, Texas

Harold R. Schumacher, M.D. Department of Pathology and Laboratory Medicine, University of Cincinnati Medical Center, Cincinnati, Ohio

Salwa Shabbir Sheikh, M.D. Department of Pathology, Georgetown University Medical Center, Washington, D.C.

Donald P. Skoog, M.D. Department of Pathology and Microbiology, University of Nebraska College of Medicine, Omaha, Nebraska

Sanford A. Stass, M.D. Department of Pathology and Program in Oncology, University of Maryland School of Medicine, Baltimore, Maryland

Sue D. Walker, M.D. Department of Pathology, Hattiesburg Clinic, Hattiesburg, Mississippi

John C. Winkelmann, M.D., F.A.C.P. Division of Hematology-Oncology, University of Cincinnati College of Medicine, Cincinnati, Ohio

Joseph P. Yoe, M.D. Division of Hematology/Oncology, Department of Medicine, North General Hospital, New York, New York

1

Peripheral Blood and Bone Marrow

Fermina Maria Mazzella
The Guthrie Clinic, Sayre, Pennsylvania

Gerardo Perrotta
University of Cincinnati Medical Center, Cincinnati, Ohio

I. PERIPHERAL BLOOD

A properly prepared and stained peripheral blood smear remains an essential component in the practice of laboratory hematology. Although many automated hematology instruments have lessened the need for peripheral blood smear (PBS) review, none has been able to totally replace human evaluation. The slide, then, augments the quantitative analysis of sophisticated instruments with the qualitative assessment made by the pathologist and/or technologist in cases requiring interpretive and diagnostic findings not currently detected by automated instruments.

A. Preparation of Smear

There are two common methods for preparation of peripheral blood films:

1. Preparation on glass slides (push or spinner)
2. Preparation on coverslips

The glass slide method is shown in Fig. 1. Blood from a fingerstick is preferable, although ethylenediaminetetraacetic acid (EDTA)-anticoagulated blood is used more frequently. Glass slides have the advantages of

1. Ease of handling and labeling
2. Ease of smear production and staining
3. Lack of fragility—easy to store and transport

The major disadvantage of a glass slide is the irregular distribution of cells, which may cause difficulty in evaluating platelets and leukocytes. Slides made from a fingerstick may invalidate platelet estimates, in that their distribution is characteristically clumped or clustered.

The coverslip technique is more difficult to master. A small drop of either EDTA-anticoagulated blood or blood from a fingerstick is placed in the center of a coverslip. A second

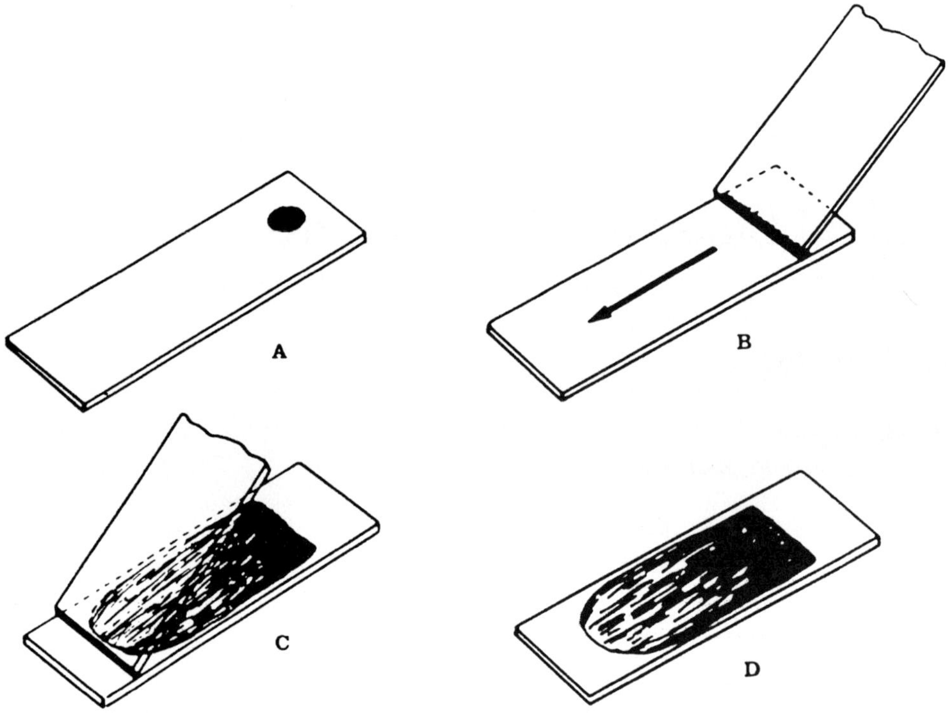

Figure 1 Glass slide method for preparation of peripheral blood smear: A, slide with small drop of blood; B, spreader slide is pulled back over drop of blood; C, spreader slide is advanced in smooth motion; D, completed slide. (From Schumacher et al., 1984.)

coverslip is placed over the one containing the drop. The blood spreads between the coverslip by capillary action. Then the two coverslips are separated with a steady, firm, quick, gentle pulling motion in appropriate directions (Fig. 2). The major advantage to this method is the uniform distribution of platelets and leukocytes over the entire coverslip. The disadvantages, as mentioned previously, are mainly in the handling and labeling.

Automated slide-smearing processors have been developed for producing uniform smears. These instruments usually spread cells either by mechanical means or by centrifugation. Smears prepared manually by an experienced technologist are preferred over those made by a mechanical slide maker. The centrifugation method has the obvious disadvantage of being time consuming for preparation of routine slides.

Under special circumstances when body fluids other than blood are being examined, a cytocentrifuge is necessary to concentrate the small numbers of cells to be identified. A monolayer of cells is concentrated on a small circular area of a glass slide.

In general, an acceptable blood smear will cover one-half to two-thirds of the glass slide, with the feathered end producing a rainbowlike effect when held to the light.

B. Staining of Smear

Blood smears are usually stained with either Wright's or May-Grunwald-Giemsa stains, which are modifications of the original Romanowsky techniques. These are polychrome stains, formu-

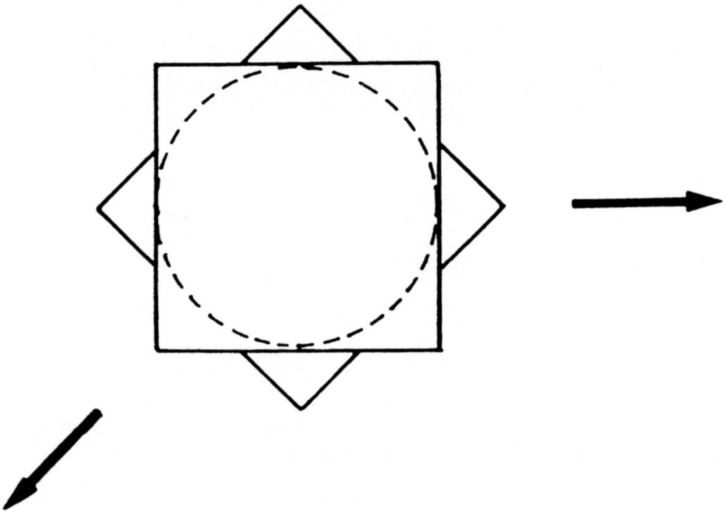

Figure 2 Coverslip method for preparing peripheral blood smears. Coverslips are pulled in directions of arrows. (From Schumacher et al., 1984.)

lated from methylene blue and eosin, which color the cell constituents at the appropriate pH of 6.4–6.8. Wright's stain uses sodium bicarbonate to convert methylene blue to the active forms (methylene azures). Giemsa stains add acid biochromate-converted azure compounds. Most Romanowsky stains are of no value when water is present in the alcohol, since neutral dyes are precipitated from the solution. Acetone in the alcohol creates a similar problem. The active forms of methylene blue are basic dyes which impart a violet-blue color to nucleic acids and nucleoproteins. Eosin is an acidic compound which stains pink-orange-red the basic components of the cell, such as hemoglobin and eosinophilic granules.

Although manual staining procedures are no longer used in most automated laboratories, understanding of ideal staining conditions for manual methods enhances an appreciation of evolving automated staining instruments. The slides or coverslip preparations may be fixed with anhydrous methyl alcohol or air dried. For Wright's stain, the material on the glass surface is covered with dye for 2–3 min. Then an equal volume of phosphate buffer is added and mixed by blowing on the surface or drawing the mixture up and down gently in an eyedropper. A greenish metallic sheen should appear on the surface of the stains, indicating optimal pH. The buffer–stain mixture is incubated for approximately 3 min, but this time varies from batch to batch of reagents. The smear is washed by adding drops of distilled water to the horizontal slide or coverslip. This process allows the precipitated stain to float off the surface. The slide is then washed vigorously, air dried, and mounted. Macroscopically, a good stain appears salmon-pink. The nuclei of leukocytes appear purplish blue; erythrocytes stain pink. Eosinophilic granules should be orange-red. There should be no background stain or debris in the area between the cells.

Excessive blueness of the smear may be related to one of these factors:

1. Thick smear (due to high white blood cell count, protein abnormality, etc.)
2. Prolonged staining

3. Insufficient washing with buffer
4. Excessive alkalinity of stain, buffer, or water (pH >6.8)

Such blueness may be improved by decreasing the staining time or increasing the washing time. Alternatively, less stain and more diluent may be used. If these alterations do not correct the problem, the buffer may be too alkaline. A new mixture of buffer should be prepared.

If the whole stain is too red, the coloration is usually due to

1. Excessive acidity of the buffer, or water (pH <6.4)
2. Short staining time
3. Excessive washing
4. Very thin smears

To correct excessive acidity, it is usually necessary to use a fresh batch of stain and/or buffer. Also, substituting alkaline tap water for distilled water in washing may be beneficial.

If nuclei, eosinophilic granules, and erythrocytes are pale, the washing time should be decreased and the staining time should be increased.

Serum or precipitated stain between the cells is related to

1. Faulty washing
2. Unclean coverslip
3. Dust on the smear
4. Talc from gloves

These problems can be eliminated by holding the slide horizontally during washing, using clean coverslips, and keeping smears clean during preparation and staining.

A number of commercially prepared stains are available. Most utilize a modified Wright-Giemsa technique requiring much less time than the procedure described above. Some stains are "quick" stains and can impart colors within 10 sec. In general, the results from these stains are acceptable. Care must be exercised in keeping the stain and rinse solution clean.

The previously described techniques outline a *manual method* for staining slides and coverslips with Wright stain. Modern, high-volume laboratories utilize *automated slide stainers*, which can handle a large volume of slides. Some stainers convey separate slides face down over a precision-formed flat area, where exact amounts of stain, buffer, and rinse are applied. The solutions are delivered into a capillary space between the slide and the flat surface of the instrument. After the first slide, this type of instrument can stain one slide per minute. Other automated stainers use the *dip method* of staining and can handle up to 50 slides at one time. These can be stained and dried in about 10 min.

Whatever method is used, the resulting stained slide appears pinkish-gray to the naked eye. If not, they can be rinsed with methanol and restained, even after a long period of time has elapsed.

After staining, the smear should be examined first under a low-power lens to determine overall distribution of the cells. If this distribution is satisfactory, an ideal area is then selected for evaluation (Fig. 3). A systematic approach should be used to evaluate every peripheral smear. The order in which the elements are examined is inconsequential, provided that all cellular constituents are included. Leukocytes are evaluated as to number, differential count, and morphologic abnormalities. Platelets are evaluated as to number and abnormal morphology. Erythrocytes are evaluated as to size, shape, color, and inclusions.

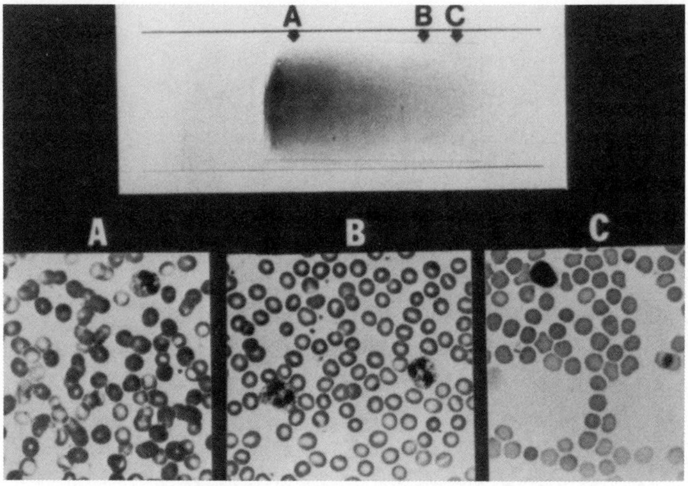

Figure 3 Peripheral blood smear: A, thick area with clumped RBCs and rouleaux; B, ideal area with RBCs just touching; C, feather edge with cobblestone appearance. (From Schumacher et al., 1984.)

C. Morphology of Erythrocytes

The qualitative assessment must correlate with quantitative factors [red blood cell (RBC) count, hemoglobin (Hb), hematocrit (Hct), mean corpuscular volume (MCV), red cell distribution width (RDW)] and must explain flags generated by the automated cell-counting instruments.

It is very important to evaluate the size of RBCs on the peripheral smear, since size may be the first clue to the cause of an anemia. The erythrocytes are macrocytic (large), normocytic (normal), or microcytic (small) when compared to the nucleus of the mature lymphocyte. Variation in size (anisocytosis) is estimated and recorded on a 0 to 4-plus scale or simply as present or increased.

The presence of abnormally shaped cells such as teardrops, sickle cells, spur cells (long irregular points), schistocytes (RBC fragments), and ovalocytes must be noted, since these cells have diagnostic significance (Fig. 4). The degree of variation in shape (poikilocytosis) should be evaluated and recorded on a 0 to 4-plus scale or as present or increased.

The intensity of color in erythrocytes is extremely important, since it can be used to estimate the mean corpuscular hemoglobin concentration fairly accurately. Variation in color (anisochromia) between erythrocytes may be associated with transfused blood or sideroblastic anemia. Hypochromia, when present, should be scored 1 to 4-plus or present or increased.

Inclusions such as basophilic stippling (small, diffuse particles, composed of RNA), Howell-Jolly bodies (larger spherical particles, usually single, composed of DNA), precipitated hemoglobin (HbC), and nucleated and parasitized RBCs are noted (Fig. 5). The number of nucleated RBCs is usually expressed per 100 leukocytes in the differential count.

D. Platelets (Thrombocytes)

The qualitative assessment must correlate with quantitative factors [platelet count, mean platelet volume (MPV), and platelet distribution width (PDW)] and must explain flags generated by the automated cell-counting systems.

The platelet count is estimated roughly by evaluating 10 oil-immersion fields, calculating

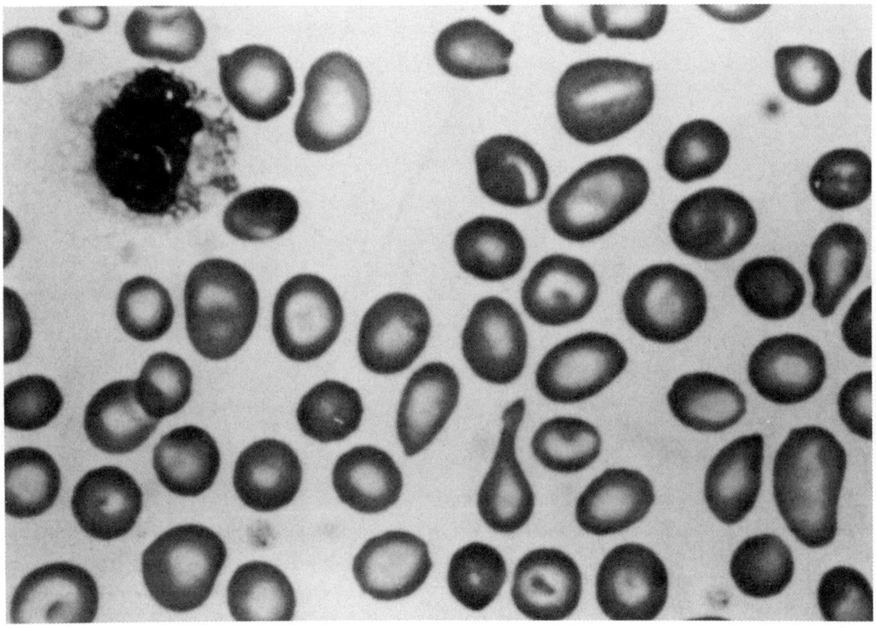

Figure 4 Teardrops in peripheral blood smear of patient with myelofibrosis. (From Schumacher et al., 1984.)

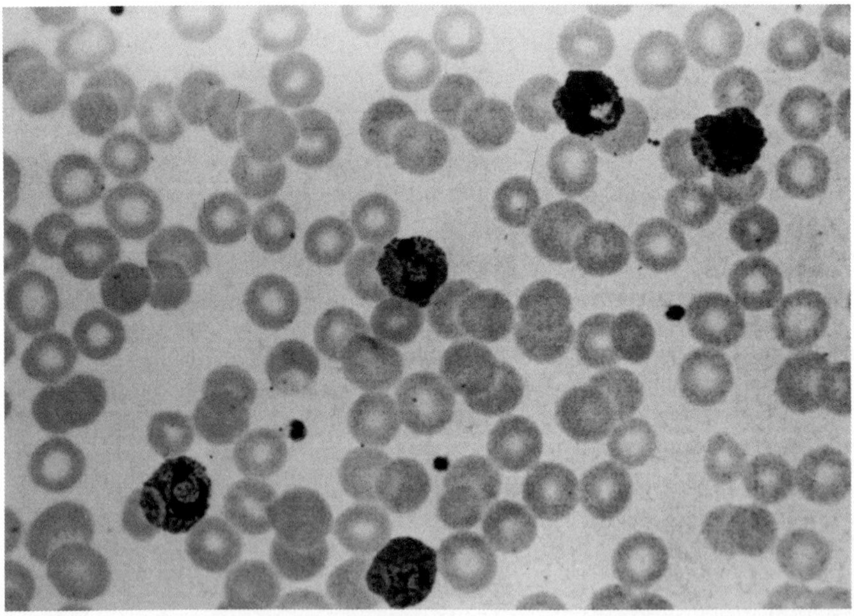

Figure 5 Peripheral blood smear showing malaria inclusions (trophozoites, schizonts, and Schüffner's dots). (From Schumacher et al., 1984.)

an average number of platelets per field, and multiplying by 15,000. The platelets should be evenly distributed on the slide when making such an evaluation. Platelets cluster on slides prepared from fingersticks and render estimates difficult. No report should go out as "no platelets seen" until the entire slide has been reviewed. The size and morphology of platelets may vary in disease. Usually, platelets have a central granular area, granulomere, surrounded by a hyalomere and measure 1–3 μm in diameter. In disease they may become extremely large and bizarre, as in myeloproliferative disorders. In some disorders the platelets may be quite small, as in iron deficiency. All morphologic variants should be included in the report.

E. Leukocytes

The qualitative assessment must correlate with quantitative factors (WBC, relative and absolute counts) and must resolve flags generated by the automated cell-counting system.

The leukocytes are evaluated as to number, type, and morphology. An estimate of the white blood count is made by observing the number of leukocytes per high-power field. Leukocytes are usually classified by an oil-immersion lens (50× or 100×). One hundred sequential cells are counted (differential count), and a percentage is determined for each population of cells. The absolute numbers of a particulate cell type are calculated by multiplying the total leukocyte count by the percentage obtained in the differential count. It is as important to note if certain types of cells are excessive (small lymphocytes, monocytes, granulocytes) or absent (granulocytes) as it is to look for immature white cell elements. All of these morphologic abnormalities have diagnostic significance: toxic granulation (large basophilic granules), bilobed neutrophils, multisegmented neutrophils (over five lobes), Döhle bodies (light blue bodies of endoplasmic reticulum in the cytoplasm, Fig. 6), and degeneration and vacuolization of the nucleus and cytoplasm. All such findings should be evaluated in light of the clinical picture and other laboratory parameters.

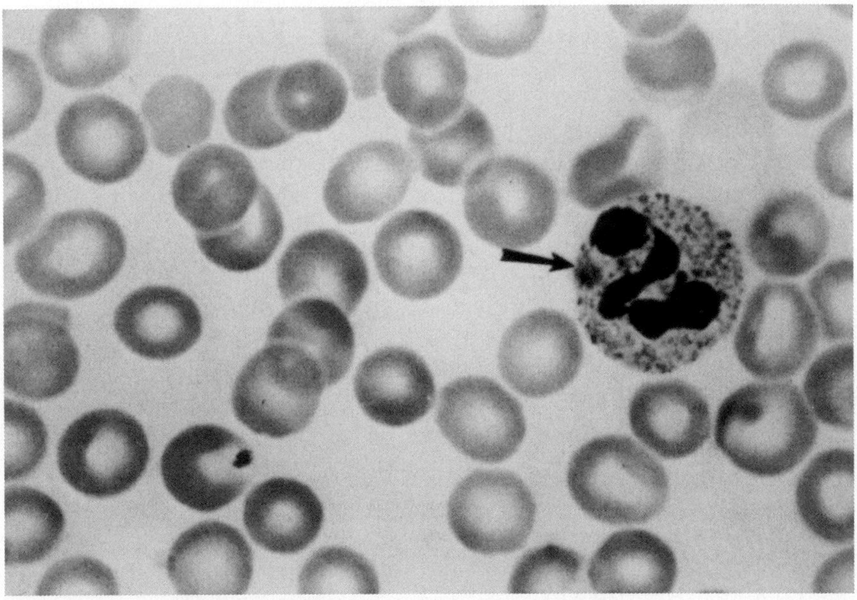

Figure 6 Neutrophil with toxic granulation and Döhle body (arrow). (From Schumacher et al., 1984.)

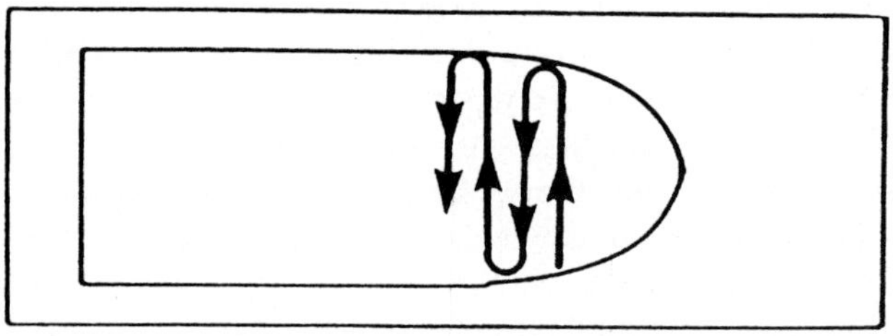

Figure 7 Method for scanning a peripheral blood smear for a leukocyte differential count and RBC and platelet morphology. (From Schumacher et al., 1984.)

F. Differential Count

The manual differential count is performed under oil immersion with a mechanical stage. Usually 100 cells are counted, but some laboratories count 200 cells. The count is made in a well-spread area of the slide (Fig. 3). The area should be about 1–2 cm back from the tip of the feathered portion of the slide. A common method for counting is to move across the slide, perpendicular to the smear (Fig. 7).

Normal values for adults are shown in Table 1. At birth, the neutrophil–lymphocyte ratio is similar to that of the adult. The ratio shows lymphocyte predominance from shortly thereafter until 4 years of age, when the two cellular elements are equal. The ratio then rises to adult levels by 6 years, where it remains.

The leukocytes observed in a normal differential are shown in Fig. 8. They are as follows.

1. The segmented neutrophil has a nucleus separated into definite lobes only by narrow filaments. The cytoplasm is light pink and small, with evenly distributed light pink to bluish-purple granules scattered throughout the cytoplasm.
2. The neutrophilic band often contains a C-shaped nucleus which is characteristically nonfilamented, degenerative, and pyknotic at areas of future lobe formation. The cytoplasmic granules are similar to those of the neutrophil.
3. The eosinophil is about the size of a neutrophil and usually has a bandlike or two-lobed nucleus. The cytoplasmic granules are spherical, uniform in size, and usually evenly distributed throughout the cell. They stain bright reddish-orange with brownish tints.

Table 1 Normal Values for Differential White Count in Adults

Cell	Percent	Absolute ($\times 10^3$ cum)
Neutrophils	40–80	1.5–8.0
Bands	[a]	
Lymphocytes	15–45	1.0–4.8
Monocytes	0–12	0–1.0
Eosinophils	0–10	0–0.7
Basophils	0–4	1–0.2

[a]Included in the neutrophil percentage.

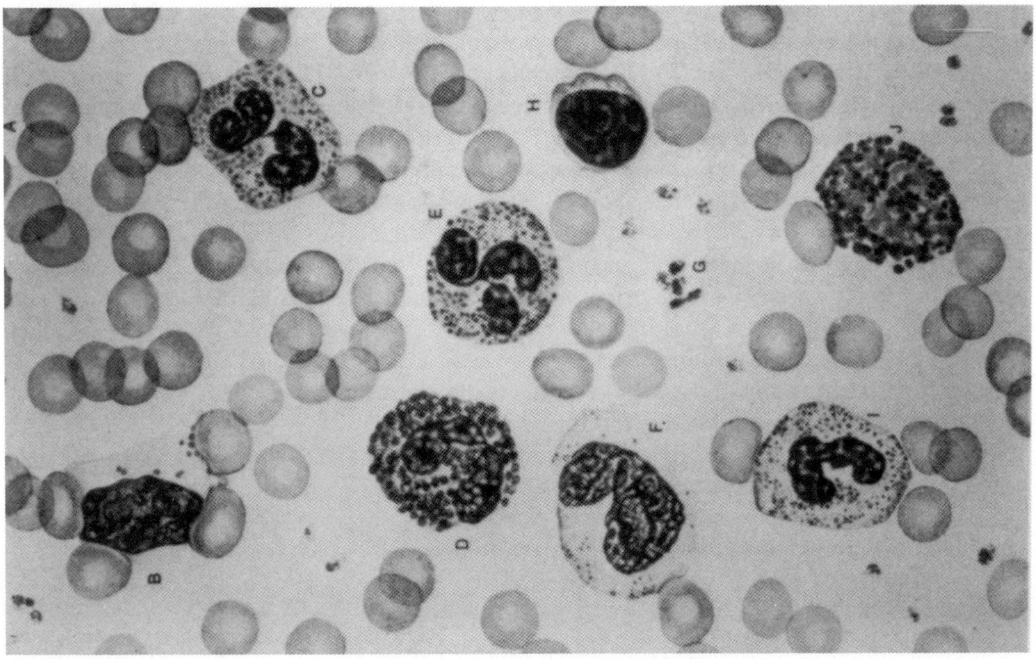

Figure 8 Cells observed in normal peripheral blood smear: A, erythrocytes; B, large lymphocyte with azurophilic granules and deeply indented by adjacent erythrocytes; C, segmented neutrophil; D, eosinophil; E, segmented neutrophil; F, monocyte with ground glass cytoplasm, coarse linear chromatin, and blunt pseudopods; G, thrombocytes; H, lymphocyte; I, band neutrophil; J, basophil. (From Schumacher et al., 1984.)

4. The basophil has a round, indented band or tabulated nucleus. The cytoplasm contains dark granules that are usually visible above, below, and lateral to the relatively light nucleus.
5. The monocyte is larger than the neutrophil and varies in shape from round to oval. The nucleus is usually round, centriform, or kidney shaped, but may be deeply indented or have two or more lobes separated by narrow filaments. The cytoplasm of monocytes is dull gray-blue, and the cytoplasmic granules are usually fine, stained lightly bluish-gray, numerous, and evenly distributed.
6. The lymphocytes in the peripheral blood vary in size from small (7–10 μm) through intermediate, to large, which are comparable in size to the granulocytes and monocytes. The nucleus of the lymphocyte is usually round, but may be slightly indented. The cytoplasm stains light to dark blue. Although most lymphocytes do not have true granules, a few unevenly distributed, well-defined granules (lysosomes) may be noted. These lysosomes are called azurophilic granules because they stained sky blue with the original azure stains. However, with the current polychrome stains, the granules are predominantly red.

Automated white cell differential counts are performed by pattern recognition or flow-through cytochemical instruments. Pattern recognition uses image processing techniques and evaluates numerous morphologic measurements. Some instruments employ high-resolution color video scanning systems, which allow additional color analysis of the slide.

Early digital image processors analyzed blood smears placed on an automated microscope stage. Automatic scanning began in a region of the smear where morphology was of good quality. With some instruments, 100–1000 cells could be counted. Automatic focusing made the necessary adjustments while the instrument scanned the slide. Cells not recognized by the instruments were flagged for review by the technologist. All data, including red cell morphology, platelet estimate, and differential count, were presented on a summary data printout. The printout was used by the technologist to review data prior to printing on the patient's ticket. All data was checked prior to transmission to the central laboratory computer.

Today, a fully automated "walk away" image analyzer has reentered the automated PBS arena. The MicroSystem 21 uses a neural network technology to scan a PBS and store all cells seen (Fig. 9). Cells that do not meet criteria are reviewed on-screen by a technologist. Unlike some predecessors, this new image analyzer now can also store several fields for RBC morphology, which can facilitate the technologist's complete review of a PBS.

The pattern recognition process has the advantages of

1. Ability to screen large numbers of slides
2. Accuracy and precision for routine smears
3. Lack of error secondary to technologist fatigue

Its disadvantages are

1. Need for precise wedge or spun smears
2. Reduced efficiency when many abnormal smears are introduced into the system

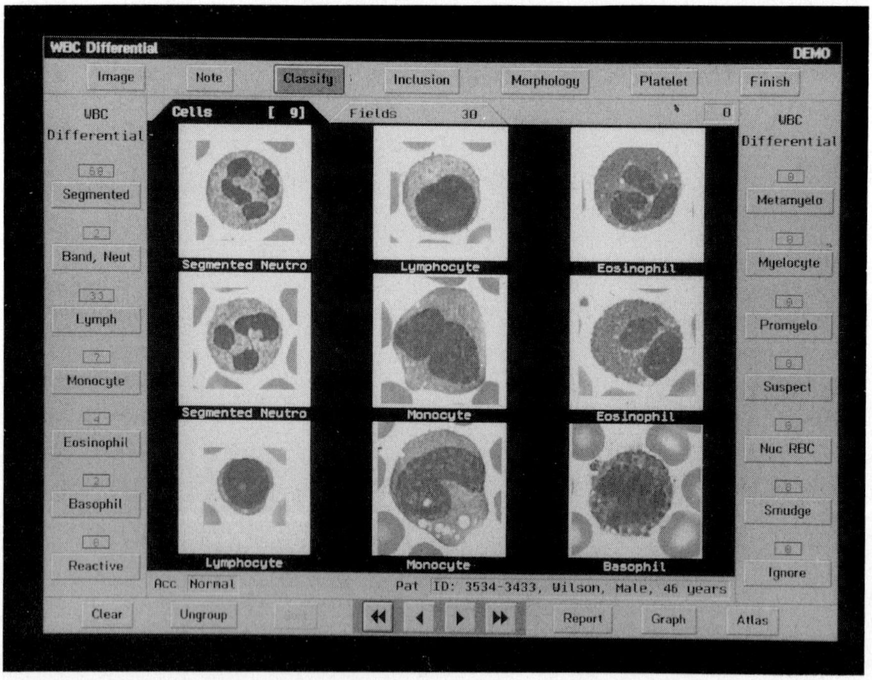

Figure 9 MicroSystem 21, showing a WBC differential screen. Cells are classified by computer and can be edited by a technologist. (From Intelligent Medical Imaging, with permission.)

Bayer : peroxidase and basophil channels	Abbott: MAPPS, low and high angle; polarized and depolarized light.
Coulter: VCS; impedance , conductivity, scatter	Sysmex: Direct current and radiofrequency
Roche: impedance and light absorption	

Figure 10 Automated leukocyte classification cytogram schema.

3. High cost, requiring a high-volume laboratory to make such an instrument cost effective
4. May require use of proprietary stain

The flow-through cytochemical instruments produce leukocyte differentials based on cytochemistry, light scatter, and conductivity (Fig. 10). Bayer H1,H2 systems (formerly Technicon) use myeloperoxidase (MPO) and basophil/lobularity (nuclear) analysis to enumerate and classify WBCs. Abbott Cell Dyn produces differentials by multiangle light scatter and a 90°-depolarized scatter to separate eosinophils. This technology is known as multiangle polarized scatter separation (MAPSS). Coulter uses volume, conductivity, and scatter (VCS) technology to differentiate WBC populations. Sysmex systems differentiate WBCs by using direct current (DC) and radiofrequency (RF). The Roche Cobas Argos 5 Diff uses impedance and light absorption.

The flow-through cytochemical instrument has the advantages of

1. Increased precision, especially on leukopenic samples
2. Utilization of EDTA-anticoagulated blood
3. Ability to process large numbers of samples
4. Ability to count large numbers of cells in a short time period
5. Provides graphic representation of cell population

Its disadvantages are

1. Lack of recall of abnormal cells
2. Constant replacement of stain packs
3. Expense

These instruments are evolving into sophisticated analyzers combining the best flow cytometry with expanded capabilities in precision and reproducibility, especially in the area of blast identification.

All automated white cell differential counting instruments generate a large amount of data which may be unnecessary. However, in large-volume laboratories, such instruments provide the necessary screening for good patient care.

II. BONE MARROW

A. Introduction

Examination of the bone marrow by needle aspiration had been available since 1929, but it was of limited value in assessing cellularity, topography, and focal disease. Bone marrow biopsy was originally attempted by open surgery, in the form of a wedge biopsy. The technique of needle biopsy of the bone marrow was first described in the late 1950s using Vim-Silverman needles, commonly used for liver biopsies. Subsequent modifications by Jamshidi, Islam, and others improved the quality of the sample obtained. Currently, the J-type needle, a modification of Jamshidi's design, is most commonly used to obtain all the material needed for an accurate evaluation of the bone marrow.

The manner in which bone marrow is obtained and processed is critical to the evaluation of the specimen. A major emphasis in bone marrow pathology is the study of cytologic detail. This can be accomplished only with optimal histopathologic processing of the specimen. Improper handling may lead to serious difficulties in interpretation and, possibly, erroneous conclusions.

Erroneous conclusions may also be reached by "fuzzy logic." A bone marrow evaluation and interpretation, even in the best of all possible worlds, is meaningless without clinical correlation. All biopsy conclusions must always be drawn in association with a complete history and physical examination. Many findings have drastically different interpretations in different clinical settings. For example, blasts in the peripheral blood may be seen in a patient with acute leukemia, but may also be identified in a patient on G-CSF therapy. An absolute lymphocytosis, composed of small lymphocytes, is typical of chronic lymphocytic leukemia (CLL), but is also characteristic of an acute pertussis infection.

B. Indications

Indications for bone marrow examination are many and varied, but in practically all situations they are related to an abnormality in the peripheral blood that cannot be accounted for by any preexisting medical condition. These abnormalities include anemia, thrombocytosis, leukocytosis, cytopenia, peripheral dysplasia, and abnormal cells found within the peripheral blood. The finding of a monoclonal spike on serum or urine protein electrophoresis, with or without radiographic lytic lesions of bone, may indicate a bone marrow evaluation for workup of multiple myeloma. Bone marrow aspiration and biopsy may also be useful in the investigation of storage diseases, such as Gaucher's disease and Niemann-Pick disease, and in the identification of malarial parasites, when the organisms are not identified in the peripheral blood.

Staging of patients with extramedullary disease processes is a further indication for bone marrow examination. Neoplasias necessitating staging bone marrow biopsy include lymphomas, particularly Hodgkin's disease, and carcinomas. Special mention must be made at this point of small cell carcinoma of the lung, as this particular tumor tends to disseminate early in its course, with a high propensity for bone marrow. At the time of diagnosis, approximately 70% of patients with small cell carcinoma have evidence of metastatic disease. In these cases, marrow evaluation in addition to bone scan has been found to be far superior to either technique alone, as bone scan evaluates cortical bone and bone marrow biopsy samples the medullary cavity.

Certain disease processes, although traditionally subject to marrow examination, are no longer considered indications for bone marrow biopsy. These include adult-onset idiopathic thrombocytopenia purpura (ITP), iron deficiency anemia, B_{12} and/or folate deficiency, polycythemia vera, and infectious mononucleosis. It is believed that these diagnoses can be made on clinical grounds, with appropriate confirmatory laboratory studies.

Actual contraindications to bone marrow aspiration and biopsy are practically nonexistent. The only causes of mortality reported from bone marrow needle aspiration and biopsy are due to puncture of cardiac or vascular structures during a sternal approach. In neutropenic patients, serious infection may occur at the biopsy site, although rarely. The formation of a localized hematoma is also rare, even in thrombocytopenic patients, provided sustained pressure is applied after the procedure.

C. Procedure

As for any other consulting specialist, the first step in the performance of bone marrow aspiration and biopsy is contact with the primary care physician. An open working relationship with the clinician is vital, as a set of glass slides is not to be considered an inanimate "case," but a patient waiting for potential treatment. Once a differential diagnosis has begun to take shape, a full chart review is indispensable. Particular attention should be given to the patient's medical history, any related conditions, medications, pertinent surgical and/or cytologic specimens, and previous bone marrow biopsies with any available cytogenetic analyses. Finally, a recent complete blood count (CBC) should be reviewed.

Preparation for any ancillary studies should be made in advance of the actual biopsy procedure. Depending on the differential diagnosis, the patient may need any, or all, of the ancillary studies outlined at the end of this chapter. The appropriate departments should be contacted, in order to assure that they are aware a specimen is in transit, and also to find out how much aspirated marrow is needed and how it is to be handled.

The most widely used instrument available for obtaining bone marrow biopsies, the J-type needle, is patterned on the 1971 design by Jamshidi and Swaim (Fig. 11). These needles are available in a variety of adult and pediatric sizes, and yield high-quality specimens with a wide margin of safety. Used correctly, biopsy should involve only minor discomfort to the patient.

In general, bone marrow aspirate alone is taken from infants and children, as well as the sternal site in adults. Bone marrow aspirate combined with biopsy is recommended for the remainder of the population. The site chosen also depends on the age of the patient (Fig. 12). In children less than 1 year of age, the anteromedial surface of the tibia is the preferred location. On occasion, in older children and adults, the sternum, anterior iliac crest, or spinous processes of the L1 or L2 vertebrae may be required. However, the great majority of marrow aspirates and biopsies are obtained from the posterior superior iliac crest. This site provides a large surface area for placement of the needle. The posterior superior iliac crest is remote from vital organs, thereby minimizing the potential for complications.

Once the site has been selected, sterile technique must be observed. The skin over the puncture site is shaved if necessary, and cleansed with a disinfectant solution. Then the skin, subcutaneous tissue, and periosteum are infiltrated with a local anesthetic, such as 1% lidocaine. The patient may experience a burning sensation or discomfort during infiltration. After about 5 min, when the anesthetic has taken effect, the actual procedure may commence.

Although the general practice has been the reverse, current literature recommends that the core biopsy always be obtained before marrow aspiration. Aspirating marrow with the biopsy needle and then advancing the needle for biopsy may result in hemorrhage into the area of the biopsy site, "aspiration artifact," leading to difficulties in interpretation and possibly erroneous conclusions.

The bone marrow needle is inserted through the skin, subcutaneous tissue, and bony cor-

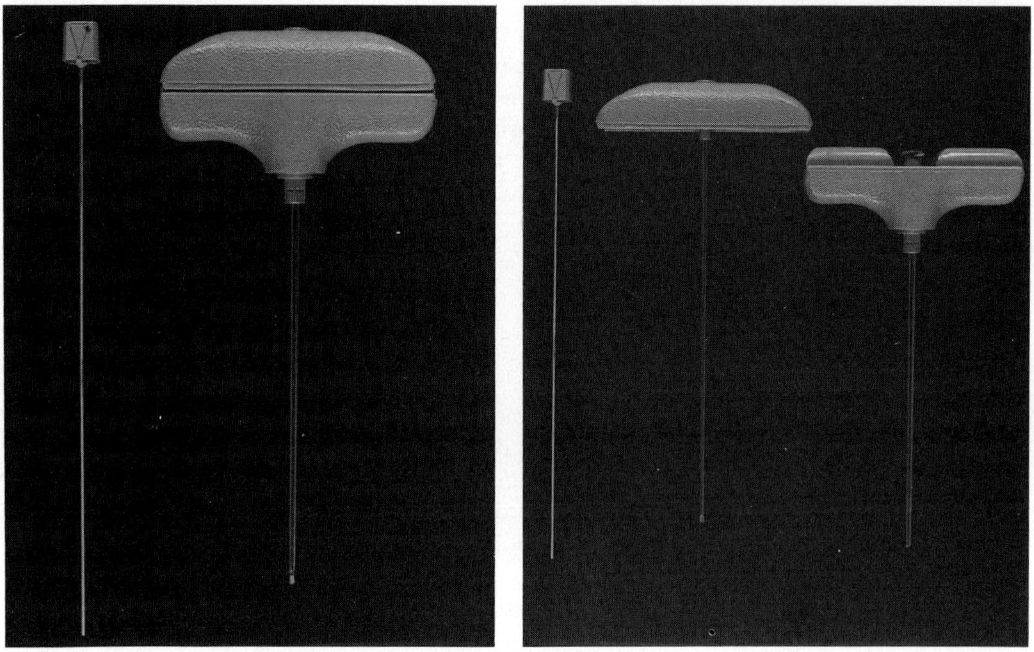

Figure 11 J-type bone marrow biopsy needle with stylet: *left*, biopsy needle with inserted obturator; *right*, biopsy needle with obturator removed. Left to right: stylet, obturator, needle.

tex. Penetration of the cortex can be sensed by a sudden ease in advancing the needle. The obturator of the needle is removed, and the needle is advanced. By gently replacing the obturator, an estimate of the biopsy size may be made. Review of published findings suggests that the minimum adequate length of the biopsy material is in the range of 1.5–2 cm before tissue processing. The needle is rocked to and fro, and then pulled back slightly, to be reinserted at a slightly different angle, in order to detach the biopsy from the underlying bone. As the needle is tapered at the distal end, the biopsy is removed by inserting the stylet into the distal end and allowing the biopsy to exit from the hub.

Before placing the biopsy into fixative, up to 10 touch imprint preparations should be made for routine Wright-Giemsa staining and possible other procedures, such as cytochemical studies. Less damage to the biopsy specimen will result if the imprints are made by gently touching a glass slide to the specimen rather than by squeezing the specimen with a forceps and touching it to a slide. The touch preparations are allowed to air dry.

After obtaining the core biopsy, aspiration is performed by inserting the same or a smaller needle through the same skin incision used for the biopsy, but placed on the periosteal surface at a distance of approximately 1.0 cm from the biopsy site. Once the needle is within the marrow cavity, the obturator is removed and a 10-mL syringe is attached to the hub. Approximately 1.0 mL of fluid should be aspirated for morphologic studies. Increasingly larger quantities of aspirated material obtained contain logarithmically larger amounts of peripheral blood. If more material is required, the needle should be repositioned. Smears should be made at the bedside, using freshly obtained marrow (see "Preparation of Material"). These smears result in better preservation of cellular detail than when the specimen is placed into anticoagulant. Additional material for ancillary studies should be placed into the appropriate transport medium.

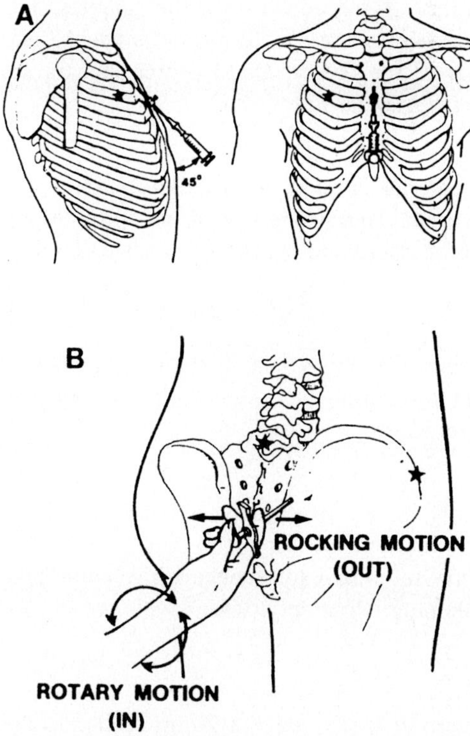

Figure 12 Schematic diagram of bone marrow biopsy sites indicated by needle tips and stars. (From Ref. 23.) Reproduced by permission of Alan Liss, Inc.

In cases of staging bone marrow biopsies, where staging is central to the clinical assessment of the condition and therapeutic decision making depends on whether or not the bone marrow is involved, it is highly recommended that bilateral biopsies be performed. Recent studies have shown that the performance of bilateral biopsies increased the yield of positive bone marrows by 26%.

Occasionally, no marrow can be obtained upon aspiration. Some cases may be due to faulty technique, but extensive marrow fibrosis and/or hypercellularity are also mechanisms for the inability to withdraw marrow by aspiration. The conditions most commonly associated with a "dry tap" include leukemias, particularly chronic myelogenous leukemia (CML) and hairy cell leukemia, metastatic tumors, and myelofibrosis. In these cases, the collection of any material in the needle following the first aspiration pull should be sent for cytogenetic analysis. A 2-mm section is cut off the distal end of the biopsy and submitted fresh for collagenase digestion to obtain cells.

D. Preparation of Material

1. Aspirate

As mentioned in the "Procedure" section, aspirate smears should be made at the bedside. The aspirate is placed into a petri dish. Spicules are selected and placed onto each of eight or nine slides. A clean glass slide, deemed the "spreader slide," is placed flat over the spicules. The smears are made by using a "push–pull" technique, whereby the spreader slide is pushed and then pulled over the spicules. The smears are allowed to air dry. One to three smears are subsequently stained with Wright-Giemsa, according to standard procedure.

2. Clot

After the aspirate smears are prepared, and after material is taken for ancillary studies, the remaining material is allowed to clot within the syringe. The clot is placed into filter paper, and then into fixative for standard histopathologic processing and hematoxylin-eosin staining. Routinely, three levels are cut for case review.

3. Touch Preparations

As mentioned in the "Procedure" section, touch imprints should be made at the bedside, before the bone marrow biopsy is placed into fixative. One to three of these slides may be subjected to Wright-Giemsa staining, according to standard procedure.

4. Biopsy

Once the touch imprints are made, the bone marrow biopsy may be placed into a fixative solution, such as formalin or, preferably, B5, for a minimum of 3 hr. It is then subjected to decalcification in 7% nitric acid for 1–2 hr and then submitted for standard histopathologic tissue processing, followed by hematoxylin-eosin staining. Routinely, three levels are cut for case review.

5. "Dry Tap" Specimen

As mentioned in the "Procedure" section, in the event of a "dry tap," a 2-mm section is cut from the biopsy and submitted fresh for digestion with collagenase, as reported by Maung et al. The liberated cells are resuspended in phosphate-buffered saline (PBS), and are then suitable for flow cytometry and, after cytocentrifugation, for Wright-Giemsa staining and a wide range of cytochemical studies.

At the time of sign-out, a routine bone marrow "case" consists of a peripheral blood smear from the day of the biopsy, one to three Wright-Giemsa-stained bone marrow aspirate smears, one to three touch imprints, three levels of the bone marrow biopsy and bone marrow clot, a Prussian blue-stained bone marrow aspirate smear (iron stain), and a periodic acid Schiff (PAS)-stained bone marrow biopsy and clot section. In special situations, such as immunosuppressed or AIDS patients, stains for acid fast bacilli and fungi are performed automatically, as these patients are often incapable of forming the tell-tale granulomata. Also, silver stain for reticulin fibers is routinely performed, as in this patient population the reticular network is invariably increased.

When looking for tumor infiltration, all of the biopsy touch imprints should be stained and examined. Features that are not readily apparent on the aspirate smear, such as metastatic nonhematologic tumor, are better seen on biopsy imprints.

E. Review of the Case

1. Ancillary Material

As with anything else, a patient's medical condition is an ever-evolving, ever-changing phenomenon. It cannot be assessed adequately by review of a bone marrow biopsy. Any attempt to do so is simply an attempt to reconstruct a series of events by observing a single moment in time. Therefore, review of the bone marrow "case" must include review of the clinical situation, as outlined in the "Procedure" section. Recent serum or urine protein electrophoreses, immunofixation assay, and blood chemistries, including serum iron and B_{12} levels, red cell folate levels, as well as liver function tests and a renal profile should also be assessed. If any ancillary studies were performed on the current bone marrow aspirate material, follow-up as to any results is also helpful.

2. *Peripheral Blood*

Review of the peripheral blood begins with evaluation of the data from the automated hematologic cell analyzer. This is followed by, and compared to, examination of the peripheral blood smear. Each cell series is assessed individually, for morphology, maturation, intracellular inclusions, and any abnormal cells present, as elucidated in the "Peripheral Blood" section.

3. *Aspirate Smears/Touch Imprints*

Examination of the aspirate smears begins with a gross examination to detect the presence of marrow spicules. These appear as darkly stained blue to purple irregular areas on the film, contrasting with the violet or pink background. The presence of spicules is confirmatory of the fact that bone marrow itself is being evaluated.

The marrow film and touch imprints should first be examined under low-power magnification to assess the hematopoietic cells and the number of megakaryocytes, plasma cells, and mast cells present. Low-power examination will also permit detection of osteoclasts and osteoblasts, groups of malignant cells, and Gaucher cells. These cells are larger than normal cells and are usually found around the periphery of the slide. The entire film should be examined, including the spicules, and higher magnification should be employed to study any abnormalities discovered.

As the primary purpose of aspirate smear examination is to evaluate the cells cytologically, once the slide has been screened under low power, a good area is selected for detailed examination under oil immersion (Fig. 13). Each cell line is evaluated for morphology, maturation, and dysplastic change. Morphology of the predominant cells observed in the bone marrow is demonstrated schematically in Fig. 14.

Under certain circumstances, such as a leukemic process, a differential count may be desirable. This count should be done on a total of 300–500 cells over several well-spread areas of the slide. Each cell type is recorded as a percentage of the total. Normal values for the cells present vary in different studies. This variation may be attributed to differences in the morphologic definition of cells, variations in the degree of contamination by peripheral blood, the inclusion of areas with ruptured cells and stripped nuclei, and inclusion of sick patients with "normal blood." Also, the normal cell range changes with different age groups (Table 2).

The myeloid-to-erythroid (M : E) ratio is the relationship of the proportion of granulocytes to the proportion of erythrocytes. The normal adult range varies from 1.5 : 1 to 3.5 : 1. Inferences concerning this ratio depend on the assumption that the mass of one of these series is normal. If both systems are judged to be abnormal, no estimate of either system is valid.

4. *Biopsy/Clot Section*

Marrow sections are particularly valuable for estimating marrow cellularity and detecting myelofibrosis, patchy aplasia, and infiltrative diseases, such as granulomata, storage diseases, and infiltration by a nonhematologic tumor. Marrow necrosis and serous atrophy are more readily detected in marrow sections than in aspirate films.

A biopsy specimen may have dense cortical bone at its outer end, but for the most part consists of a meshwork of delicate trabecular bone within which the hemopoietic tissue is suspended. The distribution of the bony trabecula is determined primarily by mechanical aspects of bone function. The trabecular surfaces are covered by a layer of endosteal cells, which

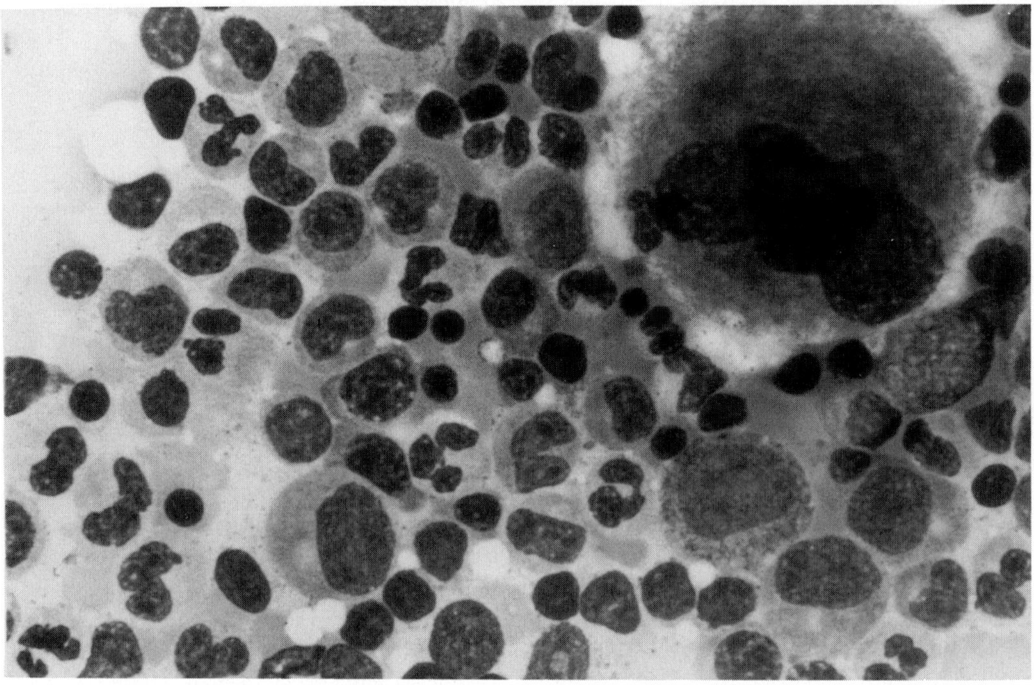

Figure 13 Photomicrograph of well-spread area within bone marrow aspirate smear (Wright-Giemsa, original magnification 1000×, oil immersion).

are usually inconspicuous. Occasional osteoblasts and osteoclasts are also a normal finding, particularly in children.

Support of the hematopoietic precursors is provided by the bone marrow stroma. Arterioles and venules tend to lie toward the center of intertrabecular spaces. Adipocytes are readily apparent, and scattered fibroblasts can usually be discerned. Macrophages appear rarely, usually in association with lymphoid aggregates and erythroid islands.

Marrow cellularity varies with age and is expressed as an estimate of the percentage of the area occupied by hematopoietic cells to the total available space. The normal cellularity decreases with age (Fig. 15). The average adult has a marrow cellularity of 30–70% (Fig. 16). In evaluating cellularity, it must be remembered that marrow spaces directly subjacent to cortical bone are frequently fatty in the elderly and are not representative of the true cellularity.

Once cellularity has been determined, the biopsy and clot sections are then examined for the presence and distribution of megakaryocytes. Mature megakaryocytes can easily be identified in tissue sections because of their large size and voluminous cytoplasm. They are normally scattered singly throughout intertrabecular spaces, except for the immediate paratrabecular zones, which are occupied by early granulocytes. Mature megakaryocytes do not usually occur in groups or lie in contact with each other. Typically, one to two megakaryocytes can be seen on a 40× objective field.

The next step in the evaluation of bone marrow is assessing myeloid and erythroid development, both quantitatively and qualitatively. There should be a normal distribution of all cell types within each of the cell lines, indicating a normal maturational process.

The earliest recognizable granulocytic precursors, the promyelocytes and myelocytes, are

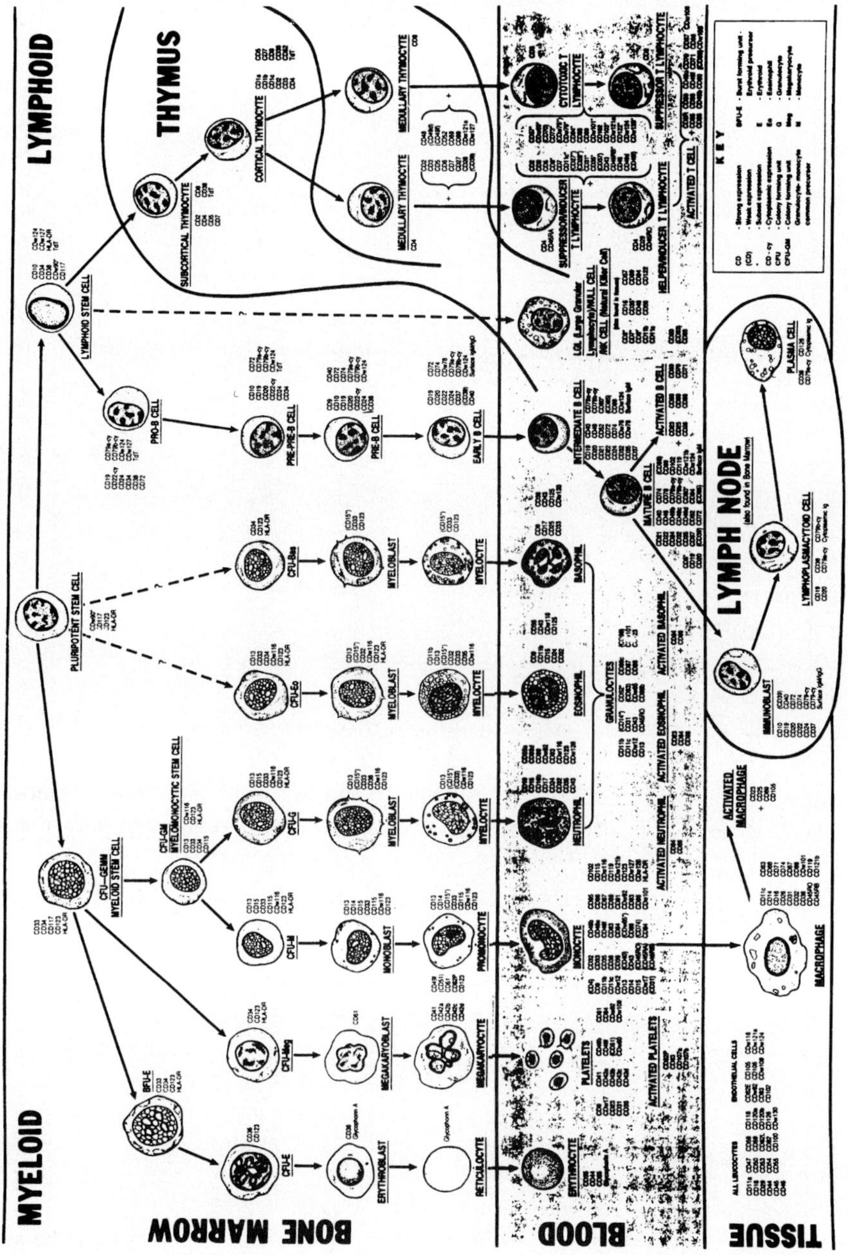

Figure 14 Schematic diagram of hematopoiesis, with CD antigen expression. (Reproduced by permission of Serotec, Ltd.)

Table 2 Normal Values for Marrow Differential Cell Count According to Several Authors

Type of cell	Rosse et al. Infants tibial marrow			Glaser et al. Subjects aged 1–20 sternal marrow, 1mL aspirated	Osgood and Seaman Adult sternal marrow, 0.5–10 mL aspirated	Vaughan and Brockmyre Adult sternal marrow, 3 mL aspirated	Wintrobe Adults
	0 month ($n = 57$)	1 month ($n = 7$)	18 months ($n = 19$)				
Myeloblast	—	—	—	1.2 (0–3)	0.4 (0–1)	1.3 (0–3)	2 (0.3–5)
Promyelocyte	0.79 ± 0.92	0.76 ± 0.65	0.64 ± 0.59	1.8 (0–4)	1.4 (0–3)	—	5 (1–8)
Myelocyte	3.95 ± 2.93	2.50 ± 1.48	2.49 ± 1.39	16.5 (8–25)	4.2 (0–12)	8.9 (3–15)	—
Neutrophilic							12 (5–19)
Eosinophilic							1.5 (0.5–3)
Basophilic							0.3 (0–0.5)
Metamyelocyte	19.37 ± 4.84	11.34 ± 3.59	12.42 ± 4.15	23 (14–34)	6.5 (3–10)	8.8 (4–15)	22 (13–22)
Band form	28.89 ± 7.56	14.10 ± 4.63	14.20 ± 5.63	—	24 (17–33)	23.9 (12–34)	
Segmented							
Neutrophil	7.37 ± 4.64	3.64 ± 2.97	6.31 ± 3.91	12.9 (4.5–29)	15 (5–25)	18.5 (0–32)	20 (7–30)
Eosinophil	2.70 ± 1.27	2.61 ± 1.40	2.70 ± 2.16	—	2 (0–4)	1.9 (0–6)	2 (0.5–4)
Basophil	0.12 ± 0.20	0.07 ± 0.16	0.10 ± 0.12	—	0.2 (0–5)	0.2 (0–1)	0.2 (0–0.7)
Lymphocyte	14.42 ± 5.54	47.05 ± 9.24	43.55 ± 8.56	16 (5–36)	14 (3–25)	16.2 (8–26)	10 (3–17)
Monocyte	0.88 ± 0.85	1.01 ± 0.89	2.12 ± 1.59	—	2 (0–4)	2.4 (0–6)	—
Plasma cell	0.00 ± 0.02	0.02 ± 0.06	0.06 ± 0.08	—	—	0.3 (0–1.5)	0.4 (0–2)
Proerythroblast	0.02 ± 0.06	0.10 ± 0.14	0.08 ± 0.13	0.5 (0–1.5)	0.2 (0–1)	—	4 (1–8)
Erythroblast						9.5 (2–18)	18 (7–32)
Basophilic	0.24 ± 0.25	0.34 ± 0.33	0.50 ± 0.34	1.7 (0–5)	2 (0–4)		
Polychromatophilic	13.06 ± 6.78	6.90 ± 4.45	6.97 ± 3.56	18 (5–34)	6 (4–8)		
Orthochromatic	0.09 ± 0.73	0.54 ± 1.88	0.44 ± 0.49	2.7 (0–8)	3 (1–5)		
Megakaryocyte	0.06 ± 0.15	0.05 ± 0.09	0.07 ± 0.12	—	—	1–38/50 low-power fields	—
Transitional cells[f]	1.18 ± 1.13	1.95 ± 0.94	1.99 ± 1.00	—	—	—	—
Broken cell	5.79 ± 2.78	5.50 ± 2.46	5.05 ± 2.15	—	19 (10–30)	7.9 (2–16)	—
M/E ratio	4.4:1	4.4:1	4.8:1	2.9:1 (1:5:1)	3.6:1 (2:1–8:1)	3.5:1–30:1	3:1–4:1

[f]Transitional cells are intermediate in size between lymphocytes and blast cells. They have fine chromatin and a small amount of basophilic cytoplasm. They are morphologically similar to blast cells. (Reprinted by permission of McGraw-Hill.)

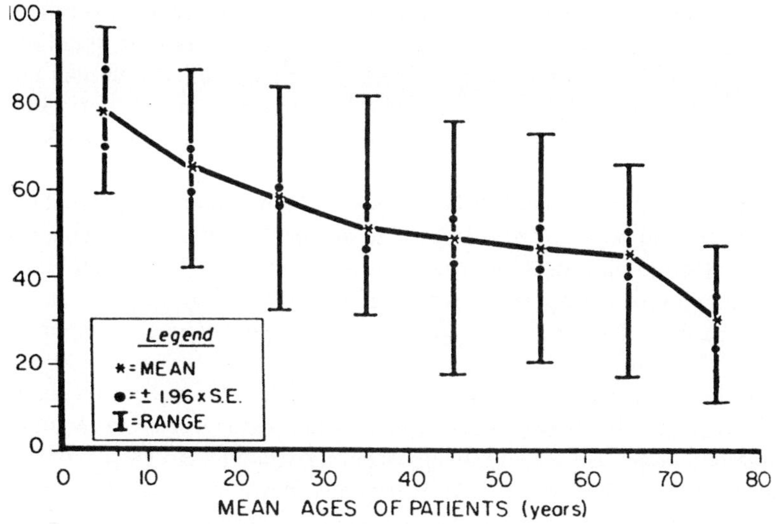

Figure 15 Graphic representation of declining cellularity with increasing age. (From Am J Clin Pathol, 1965; 43(4):326–331. Reproduced by permission of Lippincott-Raven Publishers.)

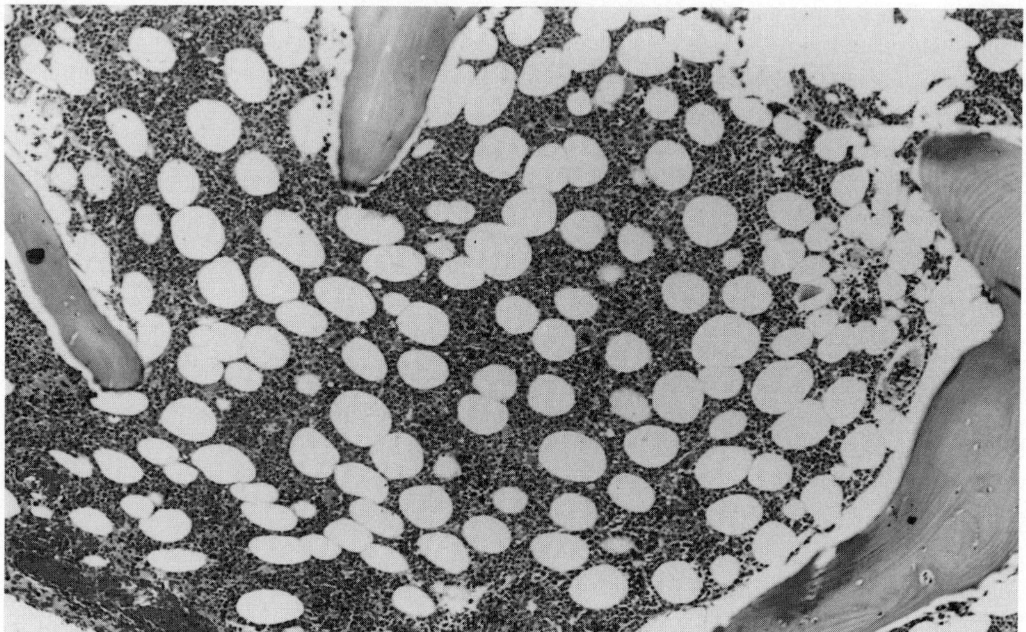

Figure 16 Photomicrograph of normocellular bone marrow biopsy (hematoxylin-eosin, original magnification 200×).

found adjacent to the bony trabecula and the adventitia of blood vessels, with maturation progressing outward, toward the intertrabecular region. In normal marrow, a few small collections of immature cells may appear to be abnormally located, as the plane of section may not include the subjacent endosteal surface or vessel; however, the presence of three or more aggregates per section of these so-called abnormally localized immature precursors (ALIPs) is considered pathologic.

Erythrocytes develop in small aggregations which are dispersed throughout the intertrabecular spaces, extending to the first adipocyte. They tend not to encroach on the zones occupied by the early granulocytes. Erythroid clusters have a radial organization, with pronormoblasts in the center and progressively more mature forms toward the periphery. Associated with many erythroid islands is a macrophage, which is usually located centrally and frequently contains free, stainable iron.

Small lymphocytes are present in low to moderate numbers, scattered throughout the intertrabecular spaces. Clusters of a few lymphocytes, deemed a lymphoid aggregate, and larger collections, termed a lymphoid nodule, are also frequently seen. Lymphoid aggregates increase in number with age, and are frequently seen in elderly patients. However, cases with more than three lymphoid aggregates present, or when the aggregates are in a paratrabecular distribution, are suggestive of a neoplastic rather than a reactive process.

Plasma cells are usually present in small numbers, scattered throughout the intertrabecular spaces and surrounding small blood vessels.

5. Iron Stain

A Prussian blue iron stain of the bone marrow aspirate provides useful information concerning a patient's iron stores. Iron stain of the bone marrow biopsy must be interpreted with caution, as decalcification may cause a false-negative result. Stainable iron is scored as absent stores, trace, and scaled from 1+ to 4+ out of a possible score of 4, with 4+ stores recognized macroscopically; 2+ out of 4 indicates normal deposition. Normally, iron is accumulated within the reticuloendothelial system. Rare deposition of ferric iron within erythrocytes, "sideroblasts" may be seen.

Iron stains should always be evaluated for the presence or absence of ringed sideroblasts. A ringed sideroblast (type III sideroblast) contains abnormal iron deposition, in the form of ferric phosphate, within the mitochondria, surrounding the nucleus in a halo fashion. In the absence of stainable iron, ringed sideroblasts may still be demonstrable by silver stain, as the silver stain detects the phosphate rather than the iron moiety.

6. Periodic Acid Schiff Stain

Periodic acid Schiff stain of the bone marrow biopsy and clot sections allows better differentiation between the erythrocytic series and the lymphocytes. Cells of erythroid lineage appear as round darkly staining nuclei with clear cytoplasm. Lymphocytes display darkly staining nuclei with pink cytoplasm. Megakaryocytes show variation in their staining pattern, with deeper staining associated with advanced maturation.

7. Other Stains

Reticulin stain highlights the reticular fibers, composed of type III collagen. The degree of deposition is scaled as absent, trace, or scored from 1+ to 4+ out of 4, with a score of 4+ representing a pericellular distribution. In normal bone marrow, a reticular network is practically absent.

Trichrome stain is used to determine the amount of type I collagen, that is, fibrosis, that is present. Frank collagen fibrosis is absent in normal bone marrow, and uncommon in hematopoietic disorders. It does, however, occur frequently in the presence of metastatic tumor and certain acute leukemias (FAB-M7).

Suspicion of an infectious etiology may indicate routine diagnostic workup by any number of standard histopathologic special stains.

8. Immunohistochemical Stains

Immunohistochemical stains involve the use of fluorochromes to identify cellular antigens, through the binding of a specific antibody to a particular antigen. A great many monoclonal and polyclonal antibodies are available, for most hematopoietic cells. The precise antibodies will be expounded upon in the appropriate chapters.

9. Cytochemical Stains

Cytochemical stains have proven helpful in the diagnosis of certain hematologic abnormalities. The stains are most useful in the diagnosis of acute leukemias and are therefore discussed in greater detail in the appropriate sections. Table 3 tabulates the most commonly used of these stains, with their predominant staining patterns.

F. Ancillary Studies

1. Cytogenetic Analysis

Because specific chromosomal abnormalities are associated with certain hematologic disorders, such as *t*(15 : 17) for acute promyelocytic leukemia, cytogenetic analysis may aid in the classification these disease processes. Cytogenetic studies can also be used to monitor remissions and relapses, and to distinguish between donor and recipient cells in bone marrow transplantation. New and exciting methods, particularly fluorescent in-situ hybridization (FISH), have been developed which permit chromosomal analysis on either metaphase or interphase cells, as well as paraffin-embedded tissue. Fluorescent-labeled probes unique to many chromosomes and fusion genes, such as *bcr/abl* in chronic myelogenous leukemia (CML), are already available.

2. Flow Cytometry

Flow cytometry is virtually unique in that the laboratory may study several populations of cells within a specimen for multiple features and/or markers. The primary use of cell surface markers in hematopathology is to identify alterations in a particular group of cells that may correlate with a disease state. Flow cytometric assays, however, are by no means limited to immunophenotyping. Assays have been described for the quantitation of DNA for ploidy and proliferation studies, cell surface receptors, carbohydrates, intracellular antigens such as cytoplasmic mu and terminal deoxynucleotidyl transferase (TdT), ion fluxes, and phagocytosis.

3. Molecular Studies

Gene rearrangement studies in diagnostic hematopathology may be utilized either as an indicator of clonality or in the determination of cellular lineage of a neoplastic proliferation. The ability of Southern blot hybridization studies to detect small numbers of clonal cells has enabled evaluation for either minimal or residual disease following therapeutic intervention. The newest methodology adapted for the detection of gene rearrangement is the polymerase chain reaction (PCR). The PCR uses a unique gene sequence to amplify, and semiquantify, small amounts of either DNA or cDNA for a known gene, such as *bcl-2* in follicular center cell lymphoma, thereby enabling the assessment of the presence or absence of disease. This procedure may use either fresh aspirate material or paraffin-embedded tissue. This methodology is further elucidated in the "Molecular Hematology" section.

Table 3 Cytochemical Reactions for Various Hemapoietic Cell Lines[a]

	Granulocytic series			Monocytic series			Erythrocytic series			Megakaryocytes			Lymphocytic series			Plasma cells		
	Normal	Dyspl	Malig	Normal	Dyspl	Malig	Normal	Dyspl	Malig	Normal	Dyspl	Malig	Normal	Dyspl	Malig	Normal	Dyspl	Malig
Fe	–	–	–	+	–	–	–	+/–	+/–	–	–	–	–	–	–	–	–	–
PAS	+	+	+/–	+/–	–	–	–	–	+	+	+	+/–	+	+	+	+/–	+/–	+/–
Perox	+	+	+	+/–	+/–	+/–	–	–	–	–	–	–	–	–	–	–	–	–
CAE	+	+	+	–	–	+/–	–	–	–	–	–	–	–	–	–	–	–	–
A-EST	–	–	+/–	+	+	+	–	–	–	+	+/–	+/–	+	+/–	+/–	+	+/–	+/–
A-EST/FI	–	–	+/–	–	–	–	–	–	–	+	+/–	+/–	+	+/–	+/–	+	+/–	+/–
LAP	+	+/–	+/–	–	–	–	–	–	–	–	–	–	+/–	+/–	+/–	–	–	–
TdT	–	+	+	–	–	+	–	–	–	–	–	–	–	+/–	+	–	–	–
SBB	+	+	+	+/–	+/–	+/–	–	–	+	–	–	–	–	–	+	–	–	–
Ac phos	+/–	+/–	+/–	+	+	+	+/–	+/–	+/–	–	–	–	+	+	+	+/–	+/–	+

[a]Dyspl, dysplastic; Malig, malignant.

Fe, iron; PAS, periodic acid Schiff; Perox, myeloperoxidase; CAE, chloracetate esterase; A-EST, alpha naphthyl acetate esterase; A-EST/FI, alpha naphthyl acetate esterase with sodium fluoride; LAP, leukocyte alkaline phosphatase; TdT, terminal deoxynucleotidyl transferase; SBB, Sudan black B; Ac phos, acid phosphatase.

4. *Electron Microscopy*

The two types of electron microscopic techniques available for diagnostic hematopathology are the transmission electron microscopy (TEM) and scanning electron microscopy (SEM). These techniques are not used with great frequency, although TEM may be helpful in a small number of difficult cases, such as for the classification of undifferentiated blasts (FAB-M0 or FAB-M7) or in the detection of viral particles.

SELECTED READINGS

Peripheral Blood

1. Bauer JD. Classical Laboratory Methods. St. Louis: Mosby, 1982: 27–36.
2. Bessman JD. New parameters on automated hematology instruments. Lab Med 1983; 14:488–491.
3. Bentley SA. Automated differential white cell counts: a critical appraisal. Bailliere's Clin Haematol 1990; 3(4).
4. College of American Pathologists (CAP). Proficiency Testing Program Hematology, Clinical Microscopy and Body Fluid Glossaries. 1996.
5. Föodinger M, Speiser W, Karabentcheva S, et al. Evaluation of a total hematology analysis system (Sysmex HS-430). Am J Clin Pathol 1995; 104(5).
6. Groner W, Simson E. Practical Guide to Modern Hematology Analyzers. Wiley, 1995.
7. Hoyer JD, Fisher CP, Soppa VM, et al. Detection and classification of acute leukemia by the Coulter STKS Hematology Analyzer. Am J Clin Pathol 1996; 106(3).
8. Hyun BH, Gulati GL, Ashton JK. Differential leukocyte count; manual or automated, what should it be? Yonsei Med J 1991; 32(4).
9. Internet sites: Atlas of Hematology, http://pathy.fujita-hu.ac.jp; Normal Peripheral Blood, www.med.nagoya-u.ac.jp (1996).
10. Lacombe F, Cazaux N, Briais A, et al. Evaluation of the leukocyte differential flags on an hematologic analyzer, the Cobas Argos 5 diff. Am J Clin Pathol 1995; 104(5).
11. Schumacher HR, Garvin DF, Triplett DA. Introduction to Laboratory Hematology and Hematopathology. New York: Alan R. Liss, 1984.
12. Simson E, Groner W. The state of the art for the automated WBC differential. Lab Hematol 1995; 1(1).
13. Wintrobe MM. Clinical Hematology. Philadelphia: Lea & Febiger, 1993: 7–37.

Bone Marrow

1. Bishop PW, McNally K, Harris M. Audit of bone marrow trephines. J Clin Pathol 1992; 45:1105–1108.
2. Brown DC, Gatter KC. The bone marrow trephine biopsy: a review of normal histology. Histopathology 1993; 22:411–422.
3. Brunning RD, Bloomfield CD, McKenna RW, Peterson L. Bilateral trephine bone marrow biopsies in lymphoma and other neoplastic diseases. Ann Intern Med 1975; 82:365–366.
4. Brunning RD. Bone marrow specimen processing. In: Knowles DM, ed. Neoplastic Hematopathology. Baltimore: Williams & Wilkins, 1992:1081–1095.
5. Chauvin F, Trillet V, Court-Fortune I, et al. Pretreatment staging evaluation in small cell lung carcinoma. Chest 1992; 102(2):497–502.
6. Dewald GW, Morris MA, Lilla VC. Chromosome studies in neoplastic hematologic disorders. In: McClatchey KD, ed. Clinical Laboratory Medicine. Baltimore: Williams & Wilkins, 1994:703–740.
7. Diggs LW, Sturm D, Bell A. Leukocytes, erythrocytes, thrombocytes. In: The Morphology of Human Blood Cells. 3d ed. North Chicago, IL: Abbott Laboratories, 1975:6, 9, 11–12.
8. Hansen HH, Dombernowsky P, Hirsch FR. Staging procedures and prognostic features in small cell anaplastic bronchogenic carcinoma. Sem Oncol 1978; 5(3):280–287.

9. Hanson CA, Ross CW. Hematopoietic disorders. In: McClatchey KD, ed. Clinical Laboratory Medicine. Baltimore: Williams & Wilkins, 1994:175–209.
10. Hanson CA. Peripheral blood and bone marrow: morphology, counts, and differentials, and reactive disorders. In: McClatchey KD, ed. Clinical Laboratory Medicine. Baltimore: Williams & Wilkins, 1994:827–863.
11. Hartsock RJ, Smith EB, Petty CS. Normal variations with aging of the amount of hematopoietic tissue in bone marrow from the anterior iliac crest. Am J Clin Pathol 1965; 43(4):326–331.
12. Hernandez-Garcia MT, Hernandez-Nieto L, Perez-Gonzalez E, Brito-Barroso M. Bone marrow trephine biopsy: anterior superior iliac spine versus posterior superior iliac spine. Clin Lab Hematol 1993; 15:15–19.
13. Humphries JE. Dry tap bone marrow aspiration: clinical significance. Am J Hematol 1990; 35: 247–250.
14. Krech R, Thiele J. Histopathology of the bone marrow in toxic myelopathy. Virch Arch [Pathol Anat] 1985; 405:225–235.
15. Li CY, Yam LT. Cytochemical, histochemical, and immunohistochemical analysis of the bone marrow. In: Knowles DM, ed. Neoplastic Hematopathology. Baltimore: Williams & Wilkins, 1992: 1097–1134.
16. Maung ZT, Bown NP, Hamilton PJ. Collagenase digestion of bone marrow trephine biopsy specimens: an important adjunct to hematological diagnosis when marrow aspiration fails. J Clin Pathol 1993; 46:576–577.
17. Menon NC, Buchanan JG. Bilateral trephine bone marrow biopsies in Hodgkin's and non-Hodgkin's lymphoma. Pathology 1979; 11:53–57.
18. Pasquale D, Chikkappa G. Comparative evaluation of bone marrow aspirate particle smears, biopsy imprints, and biopsy sections. Am J Hematol 1986; 22:381–389.
19. Rothstein G. Origin and development of the blood and blood-forming tissues. In: Lee GR, Bithell TC, Foerster J, Athens JW, Lukens JN, eds. Wintrobe's Clinical Hematology. 9th ed. Philadelphia: Lea & Febiger, 1993:59–78.
20. Rywlin AM, Ortega RS, Dominguez CJ. Lymphoid nodules of bone marrow: normal and abnormal. Blood 1974; 43(3):389–400.
21. Schmid C, Isaacson PG. Bone marrow trephine biopsy in lymphoproliferative disease. J Clin Pathol 1992; 45:745–750.
22. Schumacher HR, Nand S. Cytochemistry and immunohistochemistry. In: Myelodysplastic Syndromes. New York: Igaku-Shoin, 1995:53–70.
23. Schumacher HR, Garvin DF, Triplett DA. Peripheral blood and bone marrow. In: Introduction to Laboratory Hematology and Hematopathology. New York: Alan R. Liss, 1984:13–28.
24. Wilkins BS. Histology of normal hemopoiesis: bone marrow histology I. J Clin Pathol 1992; 45: 645–649.
25. Williams WJ, Nelson DA. Examination of the marrow. In: Beutler E, Lichtman MA, Coller BS, Kipps TJ, eds. Williams' Hematology. 5th ed. New York: McGraw-Hill, 1995:15–22.
26. Winfield DA, Polacarz SV. Bone marrow histology 3: value of bone marrow core biopsy in acute leukemia, myelodysplastic syndromes, and chronic myeloid leukemia. J Clin Pathol 1992; 45:855–859.

2

Benign Lymph Node Lesions

Robert J. Hartsock
Allegheny General Hospital, Pittsburgh, Pennsylvania

I. INTRODUCTION

This discussion addresses a practical approach to benign lymph node lesions with an emphasis on selected conditions that present diagnostic challenges in both establishing a diagnosis and separating these lesions from other reactive and neoplastic processes. There have been excellent reviews addressing these processes in books, monographs, and articles, so a detailed discussion of the entire spectrum of these entities is unwarranted.

Unexplained enlargement of a single lymph node or multiple lymph nodes demands attention. In difficult clinical cases when a diagnosis is nebulous, one approach is a careful examination of the patient for enlarged lymph nodes; if any are found, biopsy may provide the diagnosis. Unfortunately, lymph nodes are still one of the more difficult diagnostic tissues for surgical pathologists. In the earlier editions of *Ackerman's Surgical Pathology*, it was noted that more diagnostic mistakes are made on lymph nodes than on any other tissue removed from the patient. This probably still holds true today, so it is important to know the major pitfalls in the interpretation of lymph nodes (Table 1). A present-day addition to this list is the misinterpretation of immunohistochemistry, flow cytometry, and other sophisticated biologic techniques used to analyze the cellular changes in lymph nodes. Although these techniques are powerful additions to the armamentarium of surgical pathologists, the results from these studies must be kept in perspective, with their interpretation made in conjunction with the histologic changes. Generally, there is overuse and inappropriate application of these expensive procedures, so judgment is required to utilize these procedures optimally.

It is not mundane to stress the importance of knowing the age, sex, the exact location of the biopsy, and any other relevant information about the patient before analyzing the tissue and rendering a diagnosis. The pathologist is a consultant, and the histologic changes must be evaluated in the context of the appropriate information.

II. LYMPH NODE PROCESSING

Selection of the lymph node to remove is a clinical decision, but it is best to remove the largest node or preferably the two largest nodes, to minimize the chance of obtaining a nondiagnostic

Table 1 Pitfalls in Interpretation of Lymph Nodes

1.	Incomplete clinical information
2.	Inadequate histology
3.	Imprecise diagnostic criteria
4.	Lack of appreciation of the reactive capacity of lymph nodes
5.	Limited differential diagnosis
6.	Failure to use appropriate biologic techniques
7.	Misinterpretation and/or inappropriate use of biologic techniques

specimen. A great deal is made about avoiding the inguinal region as a site for biopsy, but the inguinal region is not an infrequent area of involvement by malignant lymphoma and other processes, and if one maintains appropriate diagnostic criteria, nodes removed from this region should not present any greater diagnostic concern. When a lymph node or lymph nodes are removed, they should be resected with their capsules intact and immediately transported to the laboratory for evaluation. This evaluation should include the preparation of thin slices of tissue to be placed in appropriate fixative such as buffered neutral formalin or other fixatives such as B5. Excellent histologic sections, however, can be prepared from tissue fixed in buffered neutral formalin, and this fixative also has the advantage that many histochemical reactions work well in such tissue. Fresh tissue preparations should be snap-frozen for molecular biologic studies, if they become necessary. The preparation of touch imprints from fresh nodal tissue is also an integral part of the gross evaluation, because correlation of the cytology from these imprints with histology can frequently be invaluable diagnostically. These inexpensive imprints also provide a cellular resource that may be used for both immunohistochemical and histochemical studies. Proper fixation and thin histologic sections prepared at 5 μm are the two most fundamental aspects of obtaining excellent histology. Should the clinical history or gross examination of the lymph nodes suggest an infectious process, portions of tissue can be prepared for inoculation into culture media such as Lowenstein-Jensen, Sabouraud, thioglycolate, or blood agar.

III. SPECTRUM OF HISTOLOGIC CHANGES OF ANTIGENIC STIMULATION

Fundamental to the interpretation of lymph nodes is the appreciation of the histologic spectrum of their reactivity. Once this appreciation is acquired, the interpretation of the malignant lymphomas, benign lesions, and other neoplastic processes become less difficult. The spectrum of reactivity in lymph nodes is best appreciated from a study of the antigenic response of lymph nodes. The histopathology of early antigenic stimulation which one may encounter with infectious mononucleosis, postvaccinial lymphadenitis, herpes zoster, cytomegalovirus infections, autoimmune disorders, bacterial infections, and other stimulants to lymph nodes is foreign to many pathologists because lymph nodes harboring these changes are usually not removed during the early antigenic phase. When these lymph nodes are removed, however, diagnostic mistakes can occur, particularly in those cases in which the immunoblastic response of early antigenic reaction appears to destroy the nodal architecture. Secondary germinal center formation is a late immunologic development that requires time to develop following antigenic stimulation. The primary germinal center consists of nodules of small lymphocytes surrounded by a loose sinusoidal network. One of the first observable changes by light microscopy in the primary germinal center following antigenic challenge is the activation of T lymphocytes with the transformation of these cells into large, noncleaved immunoblasts. Activation of small B lymphocytes with immunoblastic transformation appears to occur concomitantly with the T-cell transformation with resultant expansion of the lymphocytic mass. Cytologically, the immunoblasts, whether T or B, have large, open, round to oval nuclei with distinct nuclear borders surrounded by scant to moderate cytoplasm. The nucleoli of these cells may vary in number from one to usually three. These nucleoli frequently have irregular shapes such as V shapes (Fig. 1). Some of the cells which have two nucleoli are referred to as "snake eye" cells. Reactive immunoblastic cells may be misconstrued as Reed-Sternberg cells or the cells of a large cell lymphoma in certain cases. In contrast to immunoblasts, diagnostic Reed-Sternberg cells have two or more distinct nuclei, each containing a prominent single nucleolus that usually occupies an appreciable volume of the nucleus. The nucleoli of the Reed-Sternberg cell may be surrounded by a perinucleolar halo simulating a viral inclusion. In other Reed-Sternberg cells, a fine filamentous strand may extend from the nucleolus to the nuclear membrane. The cytoplasm of the Reed-Sternberg cell varies from scant to abundant (Fig. 2). A major difficulty is encountered with the distinction between a mononuclear Reed-Sternberg cell and an immunoblast containing a single prominent nucleolus. Because of the cytologic similarity at times between a mononuclear Reed-Sternberg cell and some immunoblasts with a prominent nucleolus, a diagnosis of Hodgkin's disease should be established only with the identification of binucleated and/or multinucleated Reed-Sternberg cells in a proper histologic background.

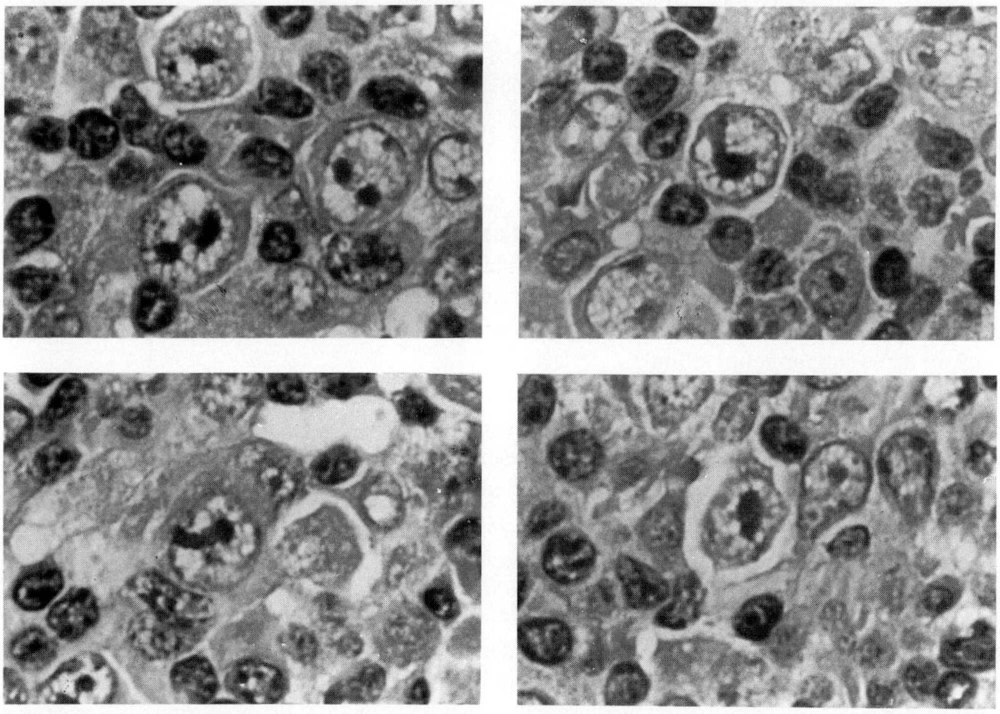

Figure 1 Composite illustrates cytologic variations of immunoblasts found in case of infectious mononucleosis. These cells have scant to moderate cytoplasm, a large open nucleus, and one or more nucleoli. (H & E; ×1200.)

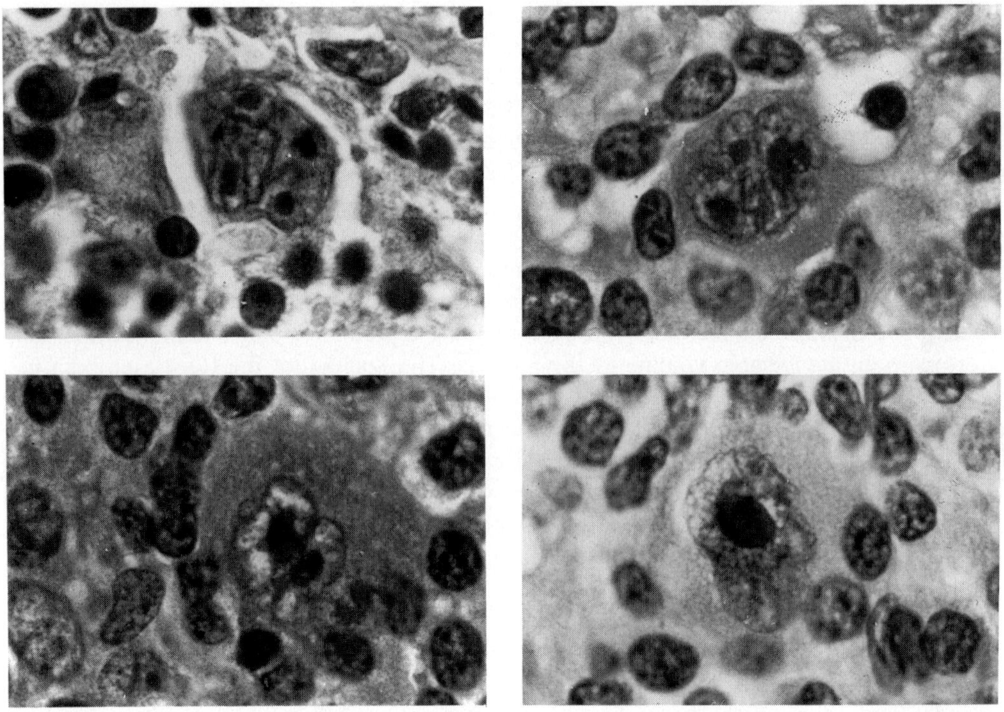

Figure 2 Composite contains various types of Reed-Sternberg cells. Diagnostic Reed-Sternberg cells have two or more nuclei each with an acidophilic nucleolus. The mononuclear R-S cell can sometimes ape the mononuclear immunoblast. (H & E; ×1200.)

It is pertinent to underscore the axiom that a diagnosis of Hodgkin's disease is dependent on the identification of Reed-Sternberg cells in an appropriate histologic background. The mottled pattern of early antigenic stimulation is not the appropriate background for Hodgkin's disease (Fig. 3). This mottled pattern of early antigenic stimulation is nonspecific and can occur following many different antigenic stimuli.

The late immunologic response is characterized histologically by the development of distinct secondary germinal centers (Fig. 4). It is only 15 or 20 days following stimulation of lymph nodes that secondary germinal center formation becomes dominant. Lymph nodes already containing secondary reactive germinal centers will respond to an antigenic stimulus by the outcropping of immunoblasts in the mantle zone.

IV. INFECTIOUS MONONUCLEOSIS

Infectious mononucleosis is the great masquerader of the malignant lymphomas, and the surgical pathologist should keep this diagnostic possibility foremost in mind when dealing with lymph nodes removed from young patients. The spectrum of histologic changes in infectious mononucleosis varies appreciably. These lymph nodes may harbor an apparent nonspecific follicular hyperplasia or exhibit the diffuse hyperplasia of early antigenic change with its mottled pattern imparted by immunoblasts in a background of well differentiated lymphocytes. In

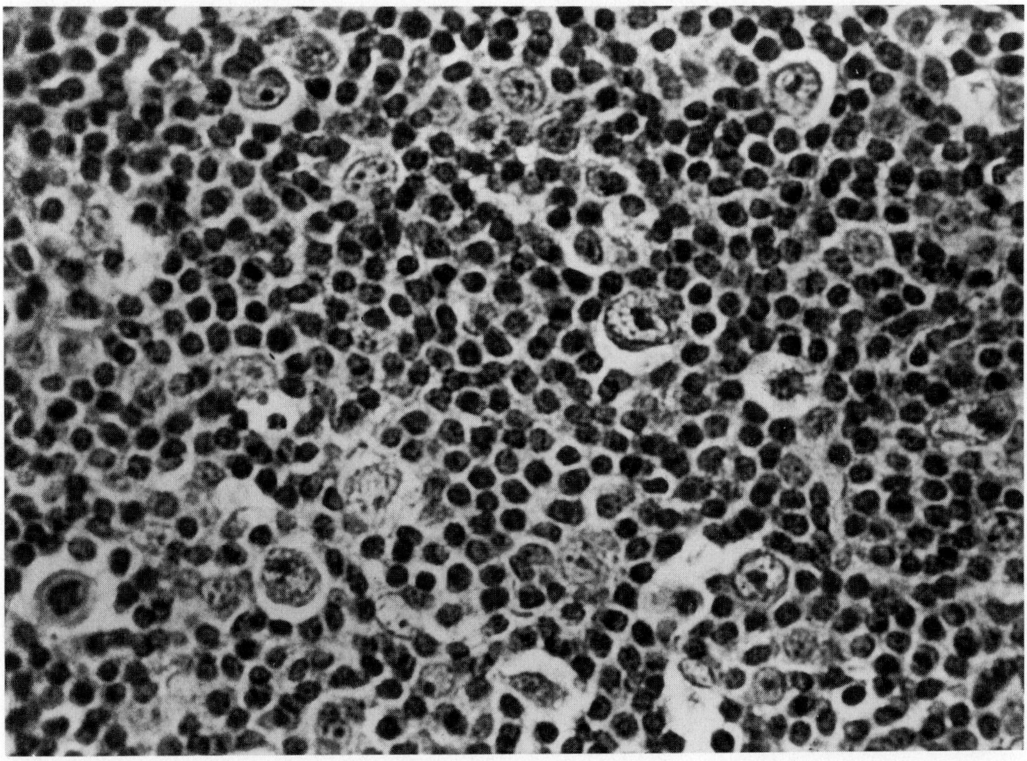

Figure 3 Diffuse hyperplasia of early antigenic stimulation with mottled pattern imparted by immunoblasts in background of small lymphocytes. (H & E; ×400.)

other instances, the architecture of the lymph node will appear to be effaced by a diffuse proliferation of reactive immunoblasts that simulate a large cell lymphoma (Fig. 5).

Unfortunately, one may encounter cells indistinguishable from Reed-Sternberg cells in the histologic changes of infectious mononucleosis (Fig. 6). The nucleoli of these immunoblasts may be either basophilic or eosinophilic, as may the nucleoli of Reed-Sternberg cells in Hodgkin's disease. The tinctorial staining of the nucleoli is a function of processing, and it cannot be used reliably as a feature to discriminate between these two types of cells. The Reed-Sternberg cell in infectious mononucleosis, however, will be typically encountered in lymph nodes exhibiting either a mottled pattern or a florid immunoblastic proliferation, which are histologic backgrounds not in keeping with Hodgkin's disease. To prevent the misinterpretation of the reactive changes of infectious mononucleosis for a malignant lymphoma, it is imperative not to diagnose a large cell lymphoma in the young before excluding infectious mononucleosis or other reactive conditions. Serologic studies for the Epstein-Barr antibodies and the evaluation of the peripheral blood film for reactive lymphocytes (Downey cells) can be crucial.

Occasionally the serologic studies for infectious mononucleosis may be initially negative, so these studies may have to be repeated. In addition, careful examination of the histologic tissue for presence of plasma cells or plasmacytoid cells may alert one to a diagnosis of a benign process. Recuts of the paraffin block to identify areas of more conventional hyperplasia such as the presence of germinal centers can be an important diagnostic maneuver, and immu-

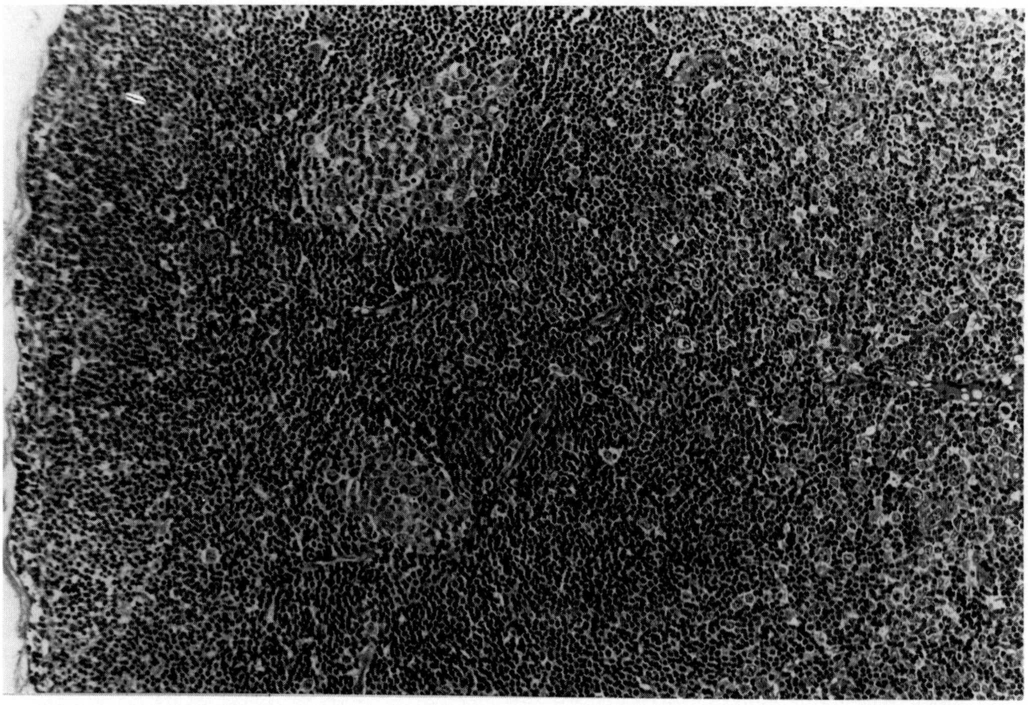

Figure 4 Reactive follicular hyperplasia with outcropping of immunoblasts in mantle zone. (H & E; ×160.)

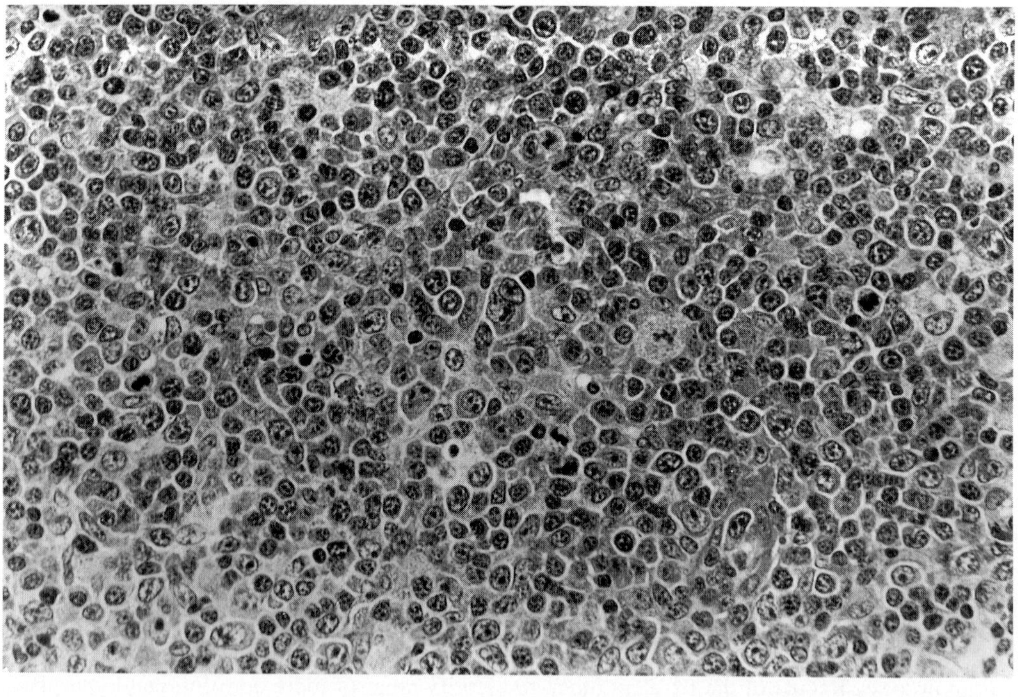

Figure 5 Florid response of immunoblasts in early antigenic stimulation. Infectious mononucleosis. (H & E; ×400.)

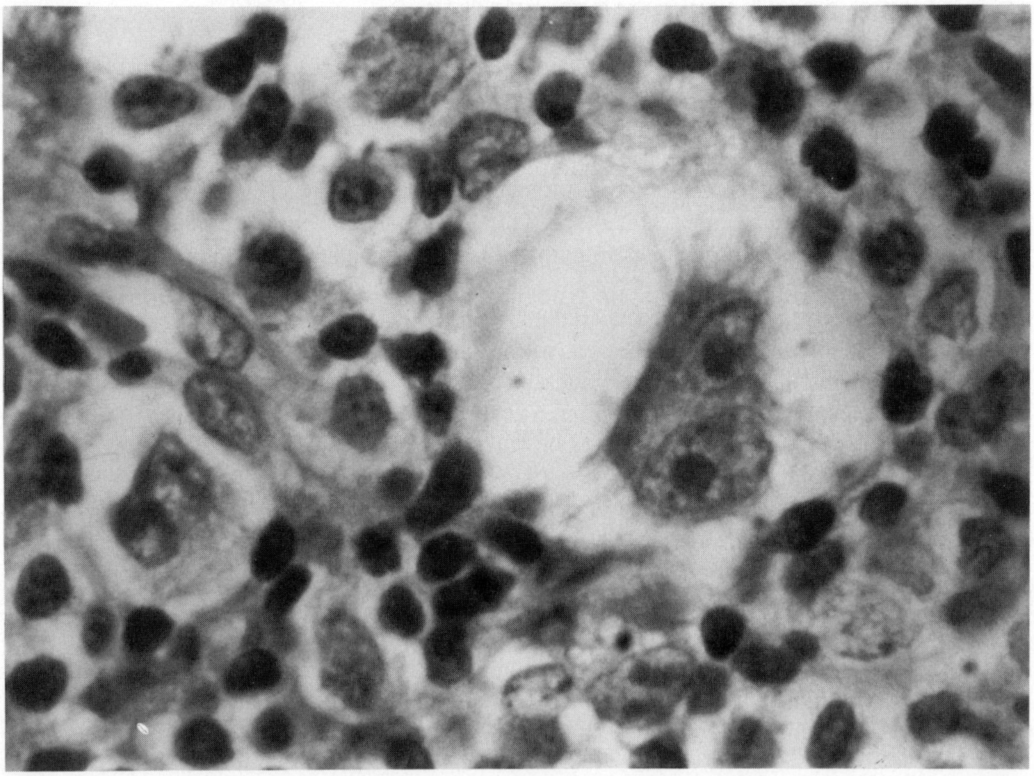

Figure 6 Reed-Sternberg cell in florid immunoblastic stage of infectious mononucleosis. Cervical lymph node, 15-year-old boy. Living and well 22 years later. (H & E; ×1200.)

nohistochemistry reactions for kappa and lambda light chains can be helpful in demonstrating a polyclonal population in infectious mononucleosis.

V. FOLLICULAR HYPERPLASIA "NONSPECIFIC"

Note should be made of the so-called routine follicular hyperplasia of lymph nodes encountered in surgical pathology. These lymph nodes are characterized by follicles that vary in size and shape and have defined secondary germinal centers with phagocytosis. Mantle zones and sinuses surround the germinal centers. This diagnosis must be approached judiciously, because these lymph nodes are responding to an antigenic challenge and it has been demonstrated in a follow-up of a significant number of patients with follicular hyperplasia that approximately one-half of these patients subsequently developed a pathologic process, which usually emerges within 1 year. These processes include such entities as malignant lymphoma, leukemia, infectious diseases, and immune disorders. The clinician should be alert to these possibilities and follow the patient appropriately.

Several diseases manifest a follicular hyperplasia in lymph nodes that causes changes which are suggestive of the disorders. These disorders include toxoplasmic lymphadenopathy, rheumatoid lymphadenopathy, luetic adenopathy, AIDS-associated adenopathy, measles, and Castleman's disease.

VI. TOXOPLASMIC LYMPHADENOPATHY

Toxoplasmic lymphadenopathy is characterized histologically by a follicular hyperplasia with aggregates of epithelioid cells inside and around the germinal center complex. The surrounding epithelioid complexes can distort and partially invade the edges of the germinal centers. Clusters of reactive monocytoid cells in the subcapsular and medullary sinuses occur, and they may be either quite prominent or sparse. Although toxoplasmosis can present with generalized adenopathy, the cervical lymph nodes are typically involved. Diagnostically, therefore, the pathologist dealing with lymph nodes from the cervical or subnuchal regions of a patient should evaluate these nodes carefully for the triad of follicular hyperplasia, epithelioid aggregates in and around germinal centers, and sinusoidal monocytoid B cells. Occasionally only a single germinal center complex will be involved, so the significance of this subtle change should not be overlooked. Sometimes toxoplasmic lymphadenopathy may be accompanied by a significant response of immunoblasts which impart a mottled pattern to the interfollicular nodal architecture. The occurrence of immunoblasts in this setting can be suggestive of interfollicular Hodgkin's disease; in such instances, careful attention to cytologic detail distinguishing immunoblasts from Reed-Sternberg cells is essential. Hodgkin's disease and toxoplasmic lymphadenitis can be confused with each other. It is rare to find the organisms or pseudocysts of *Toxoplasma gondii* in a conventional case, although pseudocysts and individual organisms can be seen in acute necrotizing toxoplasmic lymphadenitis.

The histologic changes associated with toxoplasmic lymphadenopathy are not pathognomonic and may be encountered with a substantial number of entities, including infectious mononucleosis, cytomegalovirus infection, leishmaniasis, and brucellosis. Excellent reviews of the various entities encountered in the differential diagnosis of toxoplasmic lymphadenopathy have been published. Because of the nonspecificity of toxoplasmic lymphadenopathy, the diagnosis of toxoplasmosis must be established serologically. Although the cat is the animal reservoir for *Toxoplasmic gondii*, the patient may have a history of drinking unpasteurized milk or eating poorly cooked meat.

VII. HUMAN IMMUNODEFICIENCY VIRUS LYMPHADENOPATHY

Lymph nodes from patients infected with human immunodeficiency virus (HIV) can present a particularly vexing diagnostic challenge to the surgical pathologist, because these lymph nodes present a spectrum of histologic changes from reactive to neoplastic. In addition, the histologic changes of these lymph nodes are nonspecific, so a diplomatic approach must be used when suggesting serologic studies to confirm a suspected diagnosis of HIV infection from the examination of a lymph node. Early in the course of this viral infection, the nodes may have a florid follicular hyperplasia with large serpiginous germinal centers that lack mantle zones. These germinal centers may be infiltrated by lymphocytes that disrupt their architecture and simulate follicular lymphomas. Foci of hemorrhage and lymphocytic islands may be seen. As the infection evolves, the lymph nodes become depleted of lymphocytes and lose their follicular pattern. Certain stages in the progression to depletion simulate the appearance of angioimmunoblastic lymphadenopathy, and one must be alert not to confuse these two entities. HIV-associated lymph nodes should always be examined for opportunistic infections, Kaposi's sarcoma, and malignant lymphoma. Occasionally an overwhelming infection with *Mycobacterium avium-intracellulare* will simulate Gaucher's disease. It should also be noted that *M. avium-intracellu-*

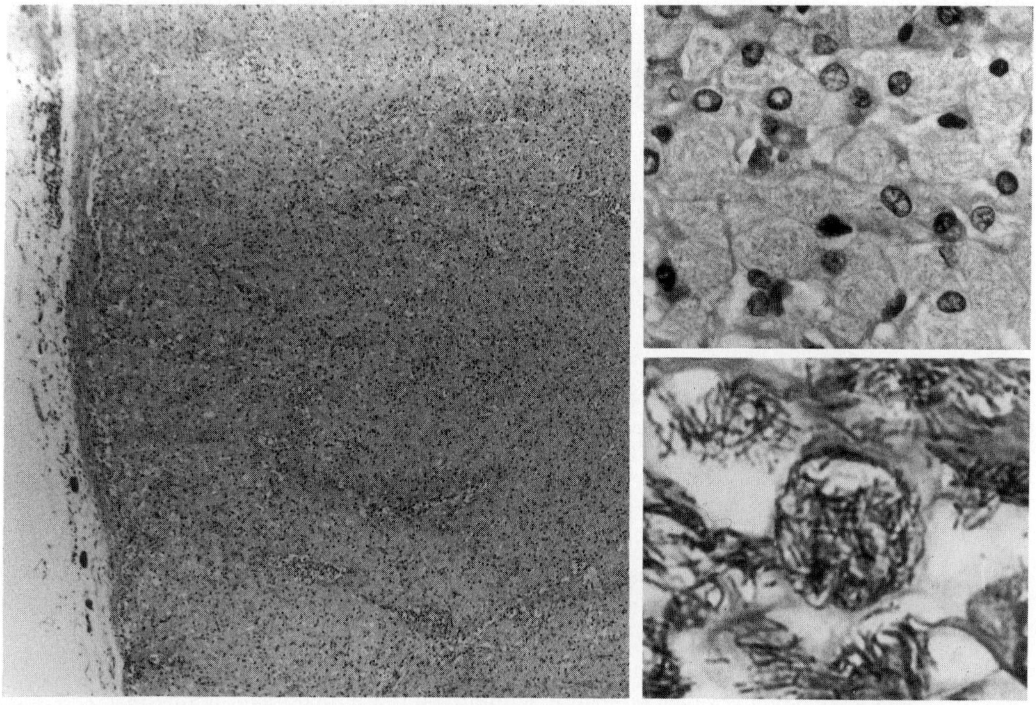

Figure 7 Effacement of the architecture of lymph node by macrophages infected by *M. avium-intracellulare*. (H & E; ×160.) Top insert, macrophages with Gaucher-like streaked cytoplasm. (H & E; ×640.) Bottom insert, PAS-positive sickle-form mycobacteria. (PAS; ×1200.)

lare will stain strongly with the periodic acid Schiff reaction and simulate the sickle-form particles of Whipple's disease (Fig. 7).

VIII. RHEUMATOID LYMPHADENOPATHY

Patients with rheumatoid arthritis can have significant lymphadenopathy. Although the lymph nodes have prominent follicular hyperplasia with a significant interfollicular component of plasma cells and dilated sinuses that may contain neutrophils, the changes are not pathognomonic. In some cases, plasma cells occur within the germinal centers. Occasionally the reactive follicular component of rheumatoid lymphadenopathy can be misinterpreted as follicular lymphoma and the paracortical infiltration and expansion by small abnormal lymphocytes as a T-cell lymphoma. Patients with rheumatoid arthritis, however, have an increased incidence of developing malignant lymphoma, so in difficult diagnostic cases one must utilize immunohistochemical and other biologic techniques appropriately.

IX. LUETIC LYMPHADENOPATHY

The incidence of syphilis is increasing, and usually both clinicians and pathologists are unaware of the underlying infection, since the serologic examination for this infection is no longer mandated. The luetic lymph node usually harbors a significant follicular hyperplasia that can be misinterpreted as a follicular lymphoma, although this hyperplasia is typically accompanied by pericapsular fibrosis, numerous plasma cells both within the capsule and interfollicular areas, and associated vasculitis and endarteritis. These constellation of changes should prompt an examination for spirochetes and appropriate serologic studies, particularly when the lymph node is removed from the inguinal region. Spirochetes have a predilection to localize in and around blood vessels, so it is advantageous to search for the organisms near vessels. A not infrequent clinical presentation of luetic lymphadenopathy is that of a painful mass in the inguinal region that simulates a hernia. Histologic changes that may occur in these lymph nodes are granulomas, pseudosarcoid reactions, abscesses, and bland follicular hyperplasia unassociated with other changes.

X. MEASLES LYMPHADENOPATHY

In evaluating lymph nodes removed from pediatric patients, it is important to examine the germinal centers of these nodes for Warthin-Finkeldey giant cells (polykaryocytes), the presence of which should suggest a diagnosis of measles lymphadenopathy. Usually, measles is not overlooked clinically, but on rare occasions lymph nodes may be removed from these patients because the prodromal phase of measles is characterized by significant hyperplasia of lymphoid tissue. The Warthin-Finkeldey cell (polykaryocytes) are most prominent during this phase of the infection. Polykaryocytes, however, are not pathognomonic for measles, as these cells may also be found in lymph nodes from patients with a wide variety of conditions, including HIV-associated lymphadenopathy, Kimura's disease, malignant lymphoma, and other reactive processes. In addition to their germinal center location, polykaryocytes may also be found in the interfollicular lymphoid tissue, and in this location these cells have a T-cell phenotype.

XI. CASTLEMAN'S DISEASE

Castleman's disease was initially described as mediastinal lymph node hyperplasia that simulated thymomas because of the large size and the presence of small, contracted, sclerotic-appearing germinal centers. Among the various synonyms for this lesion, the term giant lymph node hyperplasia is appropriate. These lesions occur not only in the mediastinum, the most common location, but also in other areas such as the retroperitoneum, cervical, and axillary regions, as well as the abdomen, lungs, and skeletal muscle. Grossly, these lesions range in size from 1.5 to 16 cm, and two histologic forms have been described, a hyaline vascular type and a plasma cell type. The hyaline vascular type is the most common, and these patients are usually asymptomatic, while patients with the plasma cell type are frequently symptomatic and have systemic changes such as fever, hypergammaglobulinemia, and anemia. Microscopically, the hyaline vascular type is characterized by sclerotic follicles and interfollicular vascularity. The follicles are numerous and typically small, with compact germinal centers composed almost exclusively of follicular dendritic cells surrounded by concentric rings of small lymphocytes. Small hyalinized blood vessels penetrate many of these follicles. The presence of multiple small germinal centers in a large lymphoid nodule is highly typical of the hyaline vascular form of Castleman's disease. The interfollicular areas are rich in endothelial venules, small lymphocytes, and clusters of plasmacytoid monocytes. This type of germinal center is not specific for Castleman's disease, as similar follicles may occur in patients with acquired immune deficiency disease (AIDS), AIDS-related complex, angioimmunoblastic lymphadenopathy, and nonspecific reactive nodes. Thus, a histologic diagnosis of Castleman's disease requires the constellation of small sclerotic follicles, interfollicular zones dominated by venules and small lymphocytes, and an enlarged lymph node or lymphoid mass.

In contrast to the hyaline vascular type of Castleman's disease, the plasma cell type is uncommon and not infrequently multifocal. Some cases of the multifocal type are thought to represent systemic Castleman's disease. The histologic changes of the plasma cell type are also not pathognomonic but, in contrast to the hyaline vascular form, the plasma cell type is characterized histologically by sheets of plasma cells between follicles. The follicles in the plasma cell type appear normal. Histologically, similar changes may be seen in HIV-associated lymphadenopathy, rheumatoid arthritis, and lymph nodes draining carcinomas. Some cases of the plasma cell type are associated with Hodgkin's disease, either in the same lymph node or in a subsequent lymph node biopsy. Occasionally some lesions of this entity have a mixed form combining both the features of the hyaline vascular and plasma cell type.

The multicentric type of Castleman's disease is important to recognize because the patient may have a declivitous course. The median survival of patients with the multicentric type is 26 months, with a survival range from 8 to 170 months. In contrast to the localized type of Castleman's disease, the multicentric type tends to occur predominantly in an older age group, although cases have been reported in children. The multicentric type involves multiple peripheral and visceral lymph nodes; histologically these lymph nodes are typically of the plasma cell type, although in the latter stages of the process, hyaline vascular forms occur. Patients with the multicentric form of Castleman's disease may develop malignant lymphoma, Kaposi's sarcoma, plasmacytomas, POEMS syndrome, and glomeruloid hemangiomas.

XII. INFECTIOUS PROCESSES

Although lymph nodes are most often removed diagnostically to evaluate a patient for a malignant process, lymph nodes can be involved with any of the other basic pathologic processes of inflammation, degeneration, disturbance of flow, or congenital defects. Infectious diseases involving lymph nodes are a major diagnostic challenge because of the importance of determining the etiologic agent, so that appropriate therapy may be instituted.

The decision to have microbial cultures performed on lymph nodes frequently resides with the clinician or surgeon who suspects an infectious process. When lymph node cultures are not ordered clinically, there is a tendency to submit the entire lymph node in fixative, thus losing a critical opportunity for diagnostic cultures. This is another important reason to insist that lymph nodes be submitted to surgical pathology unfixed, but this does not occur automatically so one must insist vigilantly on fresh tissue. If the gross or frozen section examination of the lymph node discloses a granuloma or other infectious lesion, a portion of the lymph node can be cultured in appropriate media. Alternatively, a small portion of tissue can be placed in a sterile petri dish for refrigeration until the permanent sections are evaluated the following day.

If the permanent sections disclose an infectious process, refrigerated tissue can be used for culture without significant loss of effectiveness, as the most significant pathogens survive. The basic cultures for identification of an etiologic agent are Lowenstein-Jensen for acid-fast organisms, Sabouraud media for fungi, blood agar for general isolation of organisms, and thioglycolate broth for the anaerobes. Alternatively, a large study evaluating the effectiveness of lymph node cultures indicated that cultures be limited to only those lymph nodes containing granulomas or acute inflammation, and that the media used be limited to those effective for the isolation of fungi and acid-fast organisms when the patient is immunocompetent.

The identification of granulomas in lymph nodes conveys important diagnostic information, but a diagnosis of granulomatous lymphadenitis is nonspecific. A uniform approach is therefore needed to identify an etiologic agent. The following stains are helpful in identifying organisms in granulomas: acid-fast stain for *M. tuberculosis*, atypical mycobacteria, and *Nocardia*; Grocott modification of the methenamine silver technique for fungi; and Brown-Brenn stain for bacteria. Other reactions such as silver stain and periodic acid-Schiff reaction (PAS) can be used selectively. In addition, one may utilize immunofluorescence, immunohistochemistry, DNA in-situ hybridization, and polymerase chain reaction (pcr) techniques when appropriate. It is important to underscore that bacterial cultures frequently identify an etiologic agent when the special stains are unrevealing. Specific note should be made that the identification of acid-fast organisms in tissues is also nonspecific and the growth patterns in the Lowenstein-Jensen media are vital to the identification of *M. tuberculosis* and the various atypical mycobacteria. When acid-fast organisms are identified in tissue, it is good practice to have the organisms verified by a neutral observer.

Noncaseating granulomas are a particularly vexing problem because they may be caused by a wide spectrum of entities including sarcoidosis, tuberculosis, fungal infections, syphilis, pseudosarcoid reactions of neoplastic processes, and Whipple's disease. It is pertinent that the granulomas of sarcoid may exhibit necrosis, while the granulomas of tuberculosis and other infectious diseases may be nonnecrotizing. A diagnosis of Boeck's sarcoid is a clinical pathological undertaking and a diagnosis of exclusion. The designation noncaseating granulomatous disease compatible with sarcoid should be avoided because it can be misleading. All noncaseating granulomas must be evaluated in a manner similar to those used to evaluate caseating granulomas. The granuloma of Boeck's sarcoid usually contains large, multinucleated giant cells and may also contain Schaumann's bodies, calcium oxylate crystals, and asteroid bodies. All these structures are nonspecific. Peculiar small, cigar-shaped amorphous structures which are PAS- and acid-fast-positive may also occur nonspecifically in the lymph node harboring Boeck's sarcoid. These ceroid structures are known as Hamazaki-Wesenberg bodies.

Occasionally the diagnostic biopsy of Hodgkin's disease will contain a significant pseudosarcoid component and simulate the histologic appearance of sarcoidosis, so one must be alert to this diagnostic pitfall and evaluate such nodes carefully for diagnostic areas of Hodgkin's disease (Fig. 8). Pseudosarcoid reactions in lymph nodes can also occur in association with non-Hodgkin's lymphomas and other neoplasms.

A peripheral lymph node may be the first diagnostic tissue removed from a patient with Whipple's disease, and these peripheral lymph nodes frequently harbor a pseudosarcoid reaction that can be misinterpreted as sarcoidosis. In one large series, one-third of the lymph nodes of Whipple's disease patients contained granulomatous lesions. In contrast to the lymph nodes from the abdominal region in Whipple's disease, the peripheral lymph nodes generally lack lipid vacuoles, but instead have sinus histiocytosis and a pseudosarcoid reaction. The granulomas and macrophages in these lymph nodes typically react strongly with the PAS reaction, demonstrating sickle-form structures (Fig. 9). It has been recommended that before making an unequivocal diagnosis of Whipple's disease on a peripheral lymph node, one should demonstrate the organism by electron microscopy or identify the diagnostic lesion of the gastrointestinal tract. Utilizing the polymerase chain reaction, the organism of Whipple's disease is thought to be related to *Actinobacteria* and has been given the name *Tropheryma whippelii*. Whipple's disease presenting with peripheral adenopathy can also be confused with lymphoepithelial cell lymphoma (Lennert's lymphoma) is certain cases, so a recommended approach is to apply the periodic acid-Schiff reaction to both sarcoid-like lesions and lymphoepithelial cell lymphomas.

In immunosuppressed patients, lymph nodes including the peripheral lymph nodes may be involved with *M. avium-intracellulare* and simulate Whipple's disease, both histologically and

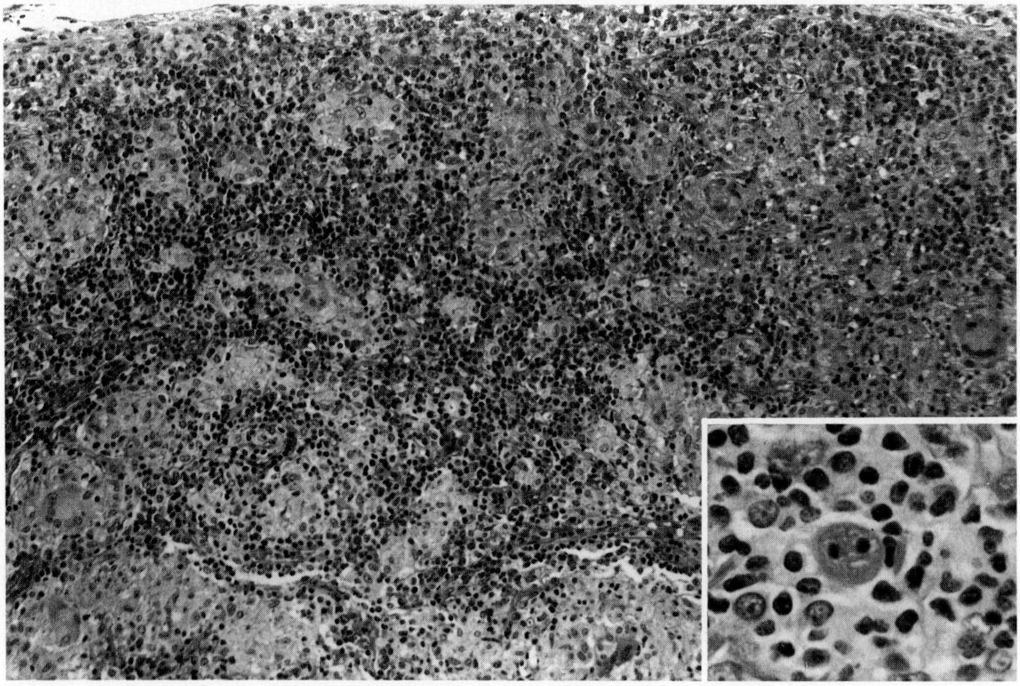

Figure 8 Hodgkin's disease with prominent pseudosarcoid reaction. Initial biopsy from cervical area. (H & E; ×100.) Insert, Reed-Sternberg cell (×640).

cytologically. *M. avium-intracellulare* is strongly PAS positive, and these organisms can assume a sickle-form configuration apeing the sickle-form structures of Whipple's disease.

XIII. SUPPURATIVE NECROTIZING GRANULOMATOUS LYMPHADENITIS

Histologically, suppurative necrotizing granulomatous lymphadenitis typically has geographic granulomas with necrotic centers containing neutrophils and necrotic debris surrounded by palisaded histiocytes and giant cells. A commonly encountered example of this granuloma is cat-scratch disease, but similar granulomas occur with a range of infectious diseases including lymphogranuloma venereum, tularemia, brucellosis, tuberculosis and yersinia, and fungal and atypical mycobacterial infections. These granulomas must be evaluated methodically, just like any other granuloma, in an attempt to identify the etiologic organism.

The organism that causes cat-scratch disease is a coccobacillary pleomorphic extracellular bacterium that can be stained with the Warthin-Starry technique. This organism is place in the class of Proteobacteria and named *Afipia felis*.

The etiologic agent of lymphogranuloma venereum is *Chlamydia trachomatis*, which has been identified in infected tissue utilizing special procedures including the polymerase chain reaction, but this chlamydia cannot be reliably identified on a routine basis so serum antibody studies may be useful in confirming a diagnosis. Although it is uncommon, tularemia is also a disease that can present with geographic necrotizing granulomas. This infection is caused by

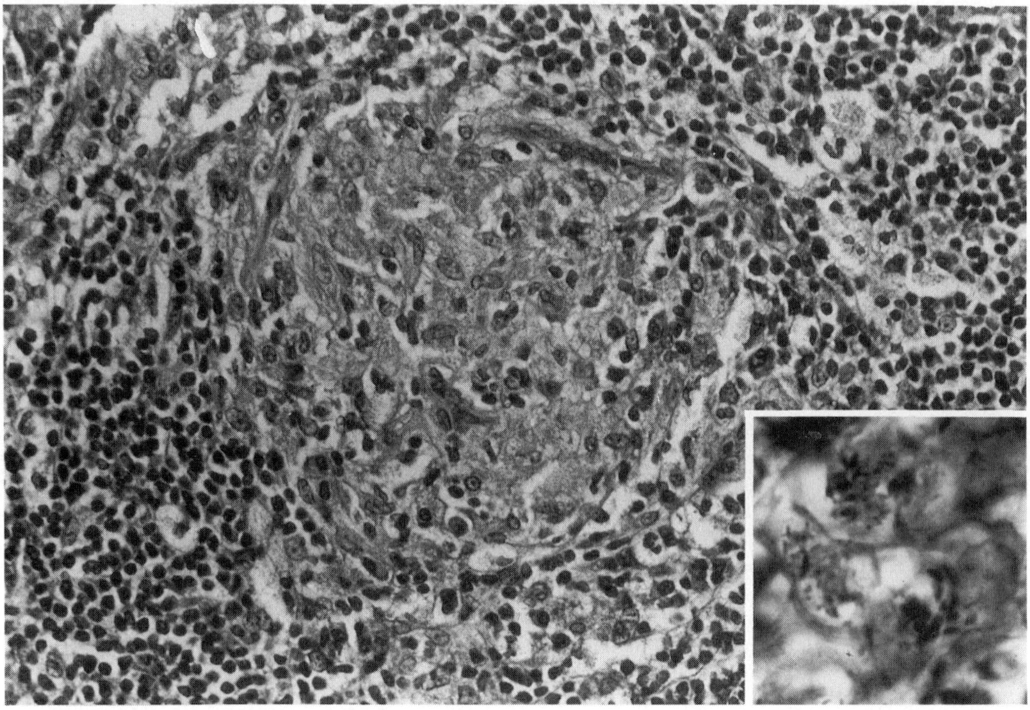

Figure 9 Peripheral lymph node with granuloma of Whipple's disease. (H & E; ×400.) Insert, PAS-positive sickle-form particles in granuloma. (PAS; ×1200.)

an extremely virulent bacterium, *Pasteurella tularensis*, that is hazardous to culture in the laboratory, so special precautions must be taken in handling any such attempt at isolation. Confirmation of a diagnosis of both lymphogranuloma venereum and tularemia is best accomplished serologically. Occasionally the necrosis in Hodgkin's disease may be geographic and resemble the necrosis of cat-scratch disease. Thus, Hodgkin's disease can be misinterpreted as cat-scratch disease if histologic changes of Hodgkin's disease are not appreciated (Fig. 10).

XIV. LANGERHANS' CELL GRANULOMATOSIS/EOSINOPHILIC GRANULOMA OF LYMPH NODES

Eosinophilic granuloma (Langerhans' cell granulomatosis) of the lymph nodes is a distinctive histologic lesion usually characterized by an intact architecture with significant sinusoidal distention by Langerhans' cells associated with a variable number of eosinophils which may be prominent and form eosinophilic microabscesses. The process not infrequently may extend into the perinodal tissue, and the nodal architecture may in advanced cases may be partially or totally destroyed. Bizarre multinucleated giant cells can occur within the sinusoidal areas. The Langerhans' cells have a moderate amount of eosinophilic cytoplasm, rather distinct borders, and a large, round, oval or elongated nucleus which is characteristically folded, grooved, or lobulated and has small nucleoli. Typically, mitoses are sparse, with a median of two per 10 high-magnification fields, but in individual cases the mitoses may range from 0 to 25. The etiology and pathogenesis is unknown, and some maintain that it is a reactive process; however, recent studies have demonstrated eosinophilic granuloma to be a clonal proliferation.

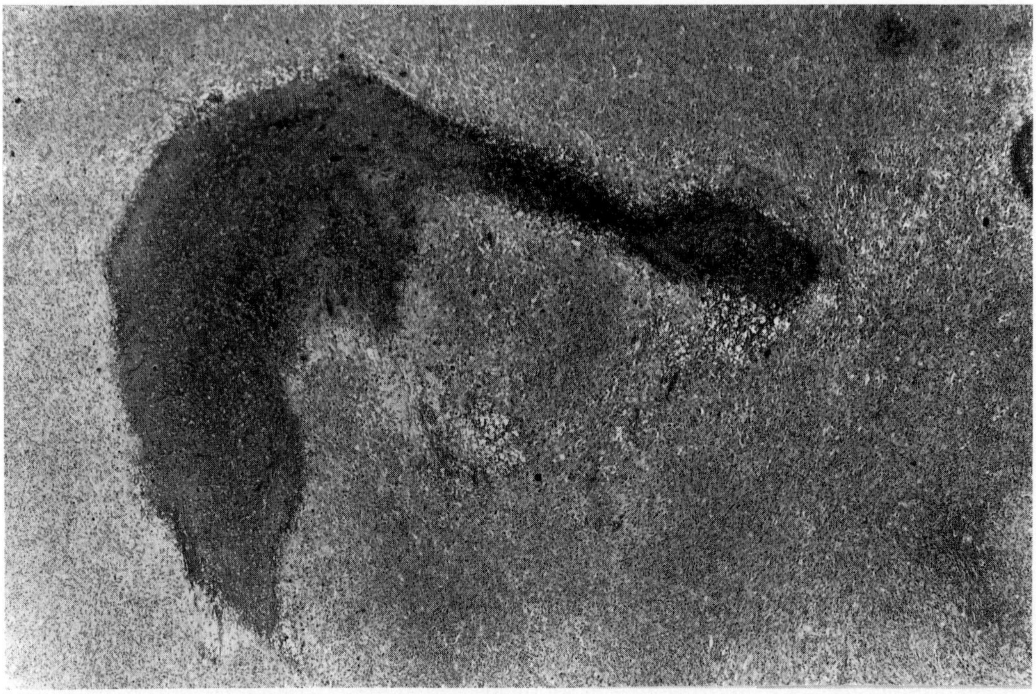

Figure 10 Hodgkin's disease with geographic necrosis simulating cat-scratch disease. (H & E; ×160.)

Lymph nodes harboring eosinophilic granulomas may be isolated lesions or part of a multisystemic disease. When these nodes are associated with eosinophilic granulomas of bone or skin, they are generally smaller in size and have only focal sinusoidal involvement. These granulomas may also be associated with either Hodgkin's disease or non-Hodgkin's lymphoma; when they occur in this setting, the process is typically nonsinusoidal, limited in size, and adjacent to the lymphoma. In paraffin sections, the Langerhans' cell is S100 positive in nearly all instances, and in most cases the vimentin, CD74, and HLA-DR are positive.

Kimura's disease may superficially simulate the histologic changes of Langerhans' granulomatosis in lymph nodes because of a prominent eosinophilic infiltration. The lymph nodes in Kimura's disease, however, are distinctively different and are characterized by a florid, reactive follicular hyperplasia, prominent infiltration of eosinophils, vascularization of germinal centers and paracortical regions, and mantle cell infiltration of the germinal centers. Eosinophils may also infiltrate germinal centers and form abscesses. Kimura's disease is categorized as a chronic allergic inflammatory disease of unknown etiology that afflicts young to middle-aged patients. The process has a predilection for the head and neck regions and may simulate a malignant lymphoma clinically. In most cases there is associated elevation of IgE immune complexes and peripheral blood eosinophilia. Twelve percent of patients with this disease may develop proteinuria and the nephrotic syndrome. Histologically, Kimura's disease can be confused with angiolymphoid hyperplasia with eosinophilia, which is a vascular lesion with a predilection also for the neck region. In angiolymphoid hyperplasia, however, the involved vessels are lined with hobnail-like endothelial cells with abundant, dense eosinophilic cytoplasm, which is in sharp contrast to the thin, scant endothelial cells lining the venules in

Kimura's disease. Not infrequently an adjacent damaged muscular vessel can be identified in angiolymphoid hyperplasia. The distinctive features of Kimura's disease help distinguish it from other lymph nodes infiltrated with significant numbers of eosinophils, such as may occur with allergic reactions, drug sensitivity, Hodgkin's disease, and parasitic infections.

XV. HISTIOCYTIC NECROTIZING LYMPHADENITIS/ KIKUCHI'S LYMPHADENITIS

Histiocytic necrotizing lymphadenitis (Kikuchi-Fujimoto's disease) is an uncommon reactive entity involving lymph nodes that deserves special consideration because the histologic changes may be misinterpreted as a malignant lymphoma. This lesion of unknown etiology is usually a self-limited process, although the disease may occasionally recur and a rare patient die. This lymphadenitis usually presents with painful cervical lymph nodes in young women, and the diagnosis is usually made by biopsy. Histologically, the involved nodes on low magnification usually have multiple, defined, irregular karyorrhectic foci, which may also contain zones of coagulative necrosis. Germinal centers are not prominent, and the cellular composition of the process varies. The earliest developing foci contain sheets of plasmacytoid monocytes with associated nuclear debris and distinctive crescent histiocytes. Other areas contain an admixture of plasmacytoid monocytes, nuclear debris, histiocytes, and immunoblasts. The histiocytes in this disorder have peripherally placed crescent-shaped nuclei and abundant cytoplasm containing phagocytized nuclear debris. Polymorphonuclear leukocytes are either sparse or totally absent, and plasma cells similarly are sparse. Fields rich in plasmacytoid monocytes and immunoblasts can be misinterpreted as malignant lymphoma, particularly as mitoses may not be infrequent. Some lymph nodes will have sweeping zones of necrosis with nuclear debris, mimicking the hematoxylin bodies of lupus erythematosus. Histologically, the spectrum of changes in Kikuchi's lymphadenitis has been subclassified as proliferative, necrotizing, and xanthomatous, depending on the dominant histologic expression. Identical cellular changes may occur in mesenteric lymph nodes in patients with mesenteric lymphadenitis who were thought to have appendicitis. The nodal changes of Kikuchi's lymphadenitis may be indistinguishable from acute lupus erythematosus, and a small percentage of these cases may later evolve with lupus erythematosus or other collagen disorders.

Lymph nodes in Kawasaki's disease may superficially simulate the histologic changes in Kikuchi's disease, but Kawasaki's disease is usually recognized clinically, so lymph nodes are rarely removed. When they are removed, however, these nodes have extensive geographic necrosis, prominent fibrinoid thrombi of blood vessels, and a prominent component of neutrophils. These histologic features are not present in Kikuchi's disease. The distinction between Kawasaki's disease and Kikuchi's disease is important because Kawasaki's disease should be treated immediately with aspirin in order to prevent the development of coronary artery aneurysms.

XVI. SINUS HISTIOCYTOSIS WITH MASSIVE LYMPHADENOPATHY/ROSAI-DORFMAN DISEASE

Sinus histiocytosis with massive lymphadenopathy is a distinctive lesion involving lymph nodes that is better known by its eponym, Rosai-Dorfman disease. Involved lymph nodes are significantly enlarged, with yellowish-white cut surfaces. Microscopically, these lymph nodes have prominent fibrous capsular thickening, but the outstanding and distinctive change is massive expansion of the sinuses, containing numerous histiocytes with abundant cytoplasm and

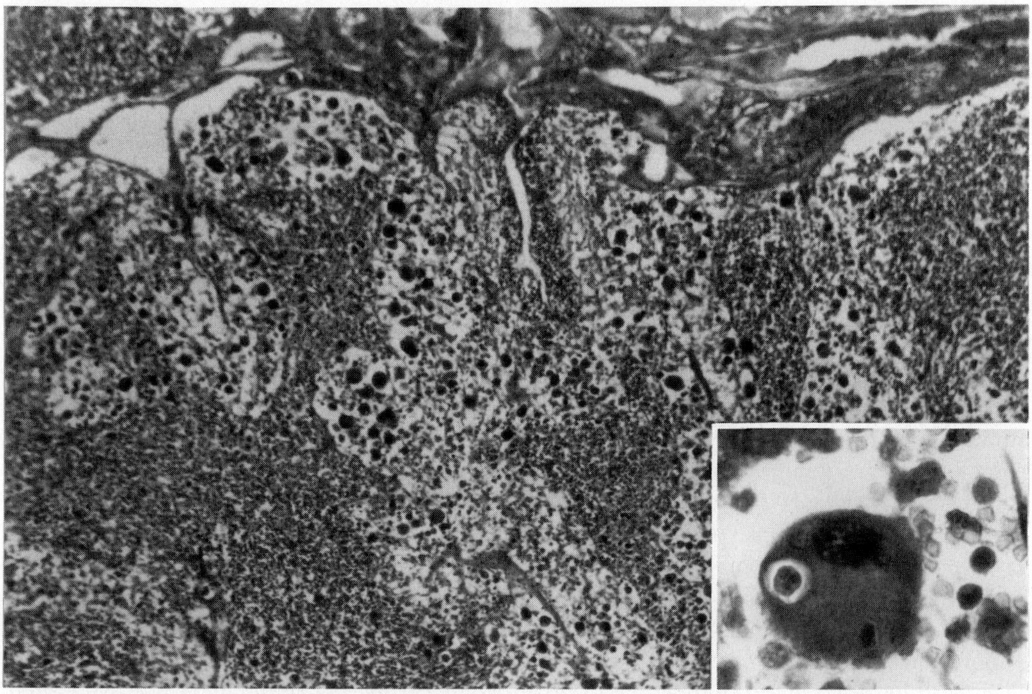

Figure 11 Megakaryocytic myeloid metaplasia simulating Rosai-Dorfman lymphadenopathy. Sinuses filled with megakaryocytes. (H & E; ×160.) Insert, megakaryocytes with lymphocyte in cytoplasm (emperipolesis). (H & E; ×1200.)

centrally placed vesicular nuclei with one or several nucleoli. Nuclear atypia is usually not present. The cytoplasm of the histiocytes characteristically contains numerous intact lymphocytes, but sometimes the cytoplasm will also contain neutrophils, plasma cells, and red blood cells. Plasma cells are prominent in both the sinuses and intrasinusoidal areas. Foamy macrophages may also occur, but eosinophils are absent and germinal centers are usually not prominent. Numerous extranodal sites may also be involved with this process.

Rosai-Dorfman disease most often presents with painless, isolated, massive, bilateral cervical adenopathy that clinically apes malignant lymphoma. Other lymph node groups, however, may be involved, with or without associated cervical involvement. Some patients have no symptoms, but fever, night sweats, weight loss, and arthralgia may be present.

Conditions that may cause diagnostic confusion with sinus histiocytosis with massive adenopathy include florid reactive sinus histiocytosis, Langerhans' cell histiocytosis, metastatic carcinoma and melanoma, and sinusoidal lymphoma. Myeloid metaplasia of the megakaryocytic type in which lymphocytes are present in the cytoplasm of the megakaryocytes (emperipolesis) may also resemble this entity superficially (Fig. 11).

XVII. INFARCTION OF LYMPH NODES

Infarction of lymph nodes is frequently misinterpreted as nonspecific necrosis or occasionally as chronic necrotizing granulomatous inflammation when histiocytes and giant cells organize in response to the injury. Recognition of nodal infarction is important because it usually reflects an underlying process of significance, such as malignant lymphoma, vasculitis or vascular thrombosis, or infections. It also been associated with mechanical pressure and gold therapy.

The important association between malignant lymphoma and nodal infarction is underscored by the results of a multicentric study evaluating this association. Approximately 28% of patients with infarcted lymph nodes had malignant lymphoma at the time of diagnosis, either in the same node or in other lymph nodes. In those patients without obvious lymphoma, about 16% developed malignant lymphoma within 2 years, but after 2 years the risk of developing lymphoma was negligible.

XVIII. INFLAMMATORY PSEUDOTUMOR OF LYMPH NODES

The lymph nodes involved by an inflammatory pseudotumorous reaction may be single or multiple, and they can be massively enlarged, matted, and adherent to adjacent soft tissue structures. This reaction may develop suddenly or gradually, and when it is associated with anorexia, fever, and night sweats, it usually is indicative of systemic involvement. The process may resolve spontaneously or disappear following surgical removal of the involved tissues, but it can persist or relapse. Histologically, the nodal connective tissue is the primary target of involvement, and this involvement may be focal or extensive, with extension into the capsule and pericapsular areas. The affected connective tissue is usually edematous and contains fibroblastic-like cells, polygonal-shaped histiocytes, small blood vessels, and plasma cells admixed with varying proportions of lymphocytes, eosinophils, and neutrophils. Venulitis is a distinctive feature of this process. In addition, the histiocytes and fibroblastic cells can form loose, vesicular or storiform patterns, which may cause confusion with soft tissue tumors. Reactive follicles are typically inconspicuous.

When lymph nodes are involved secondary to an extranodal inflammatory pseudotumor, the involved lymph nodes contain a space-occupying lesion that is distinctively different from the histologic changes of a primary inflammatory pseudotumor of lymph nodes.

XIX. VASCULAR TRANSFORMATION OF LYMPH NODE SINUSES AND PRIMARY VASCULAR TUMORS OF LYMPH NODES

Vascular transformation of lymph node sinuses is important to recognize and appreciate because it can be associated with a regional neoplasm or confused with other entities such as Kaposi's sarcoma, bacillary angiomatosis, nodal hemangiomas, and mycobacterial spindle cell pseudotumors. Any lymph node may be affected by vascular transformation, but usually these lymph nodes are identified as part of a surgical specimen containing another lesion, usually a neoplasm.

There is considerable variation in the extent and type of vascular transformation of sinuses. The transformation may be limited, with preservation of the nodal architecture, or there may be extensive distortion of the architecture. The capsular tissue of the node is spared, and typically the subcapsular, intermediate, and medullary sinuses are affected segmentally or diffusely, with concominant reduction of the lymph node parenchyma. The vascular changes express a range of histologic patterns including small delicate vessels, branching vascular clefts with associated fibrous tissue, cellular endothelial proliferations with a spindle cell pattern, solid nodules composed of plump spindle-shaped cells, and a plexiform variant with a netlike configuration of vessels. Occasionally the cellular variant will form large multiple nodules within the nodal tissue that simulate a metastatic tumor.

In the differential diagnosis of vascular transformation of sinuses, it is important to differentiate bacillary angiomatosis and mycobacterial spindle cell pseudotumors because these entities must be treated. Mycobacterial spindle cell pseudotumors are characterized by multiple large, nodular areas composed of spindle-shaped cells forming fascicles associated with plasma cells. These pseudotumors have a predilection of involve the connective tissue of the lymph node rather than sinuses, and the lesion contains many mycobacteria. The other lesion, bacillary angiomatosis, is purported to be caused by *Rochalimaea quintana*, and the diagnostic histologic triad for this angiomatosis is proliferating blood vessels lined by plump endothelial cells with pale cytoplasm, interstitial amorphous material containing the bacteria, and neutrophils infiltrating the interstitial areas. The *Rochalimeae* organism can be identified with the Warthin-Starry technique. Kaposi's sarcoma involving lymph nodes has prominent capsular and trabecular involvement rather than sinusoidal involvement, and the diagnostic areas of Kaposi's sarcoma are slitlike, poorly formed vessels with a spindle cell component. In addition, the cytoplasm of these spindle cells contains eosinophilic hyaline globules which are PAS positive.

Primary vascular tumors of lymph nodes are rare, but they may be confused with vascular transformation of sinuses. These primary vascular tumors include hemangiomas, angiomyomatous hamartomas, hemangioendotheliomas, polymorphous hemangioendotheliomas, and lymphangiomas. Histologically, these primary vascular tumors are identical to their counterparts which occur elsewhere in the body. The exception is angiomyomatous hamartomas, which are unique lesions and appear to occur exclusively in the inguinal lymph nodes and extensively replace the nodal parenchyma. This hamartoma is composed of smooth muscle and fibrous tissue with progressive loss of identifiable blood vessels.

XX. OTHER DIAGNOSTIC ENTITIES

Space does not permit a discussion of the following processes that may involve lymph nodes and also present diagnostic challenges. These entities include pseudofungi in lymph node sinuses, silicone lymphadenopathy, polyvinylpyrrolidone storage simulating signet ring carcinoma, sinus histiocytosis secondary to prosthetic material, nodal changes in Henoch-Schönlein purpura, dilantin-associated lymphadenopathy, intranodal hemorrhagic spindle cell tumor with amianthoid fibers simulating Kaposi's sarcoma, decidual changes in pelvic lymph nodes, benign lymph node inclusions mimicking metastatic carcinoma, cytomegalovirus, and *Herpes simplex* lymphadenitis, *Pneumocystis carinii* lymphadenitis, lymphangiography-induced lymph node lesions, and iatrogenic lesions of lymph nodes induced by fine needle aspiration.

CASE STUDY

A 52-year-old Caucasian man first noticed a mass in his inguinal region approximately 3 weeks before removal of an enlarged lymph node in this area. The duration of the enlargement was unknown, but when the lymph node failed to respond to antibiotic therapy, it was removed.

On gross examination, the lymph node was firm and 2.5 cm in greatest diameter. Its cut surface was smooth, grayish-white, and glistening. Histologically, the lymph node was replaced by a uniform population of large, round to oval cells with moderate cytoplasm and nuclei that had finely stippled chromatin and indistinct nucleoli that varied from one to three. Some of the nucleoli were in apposition to the nuclear membrane. The nucleoli had a dustlike appearance, and mitoses were numerous (Fig. 12).

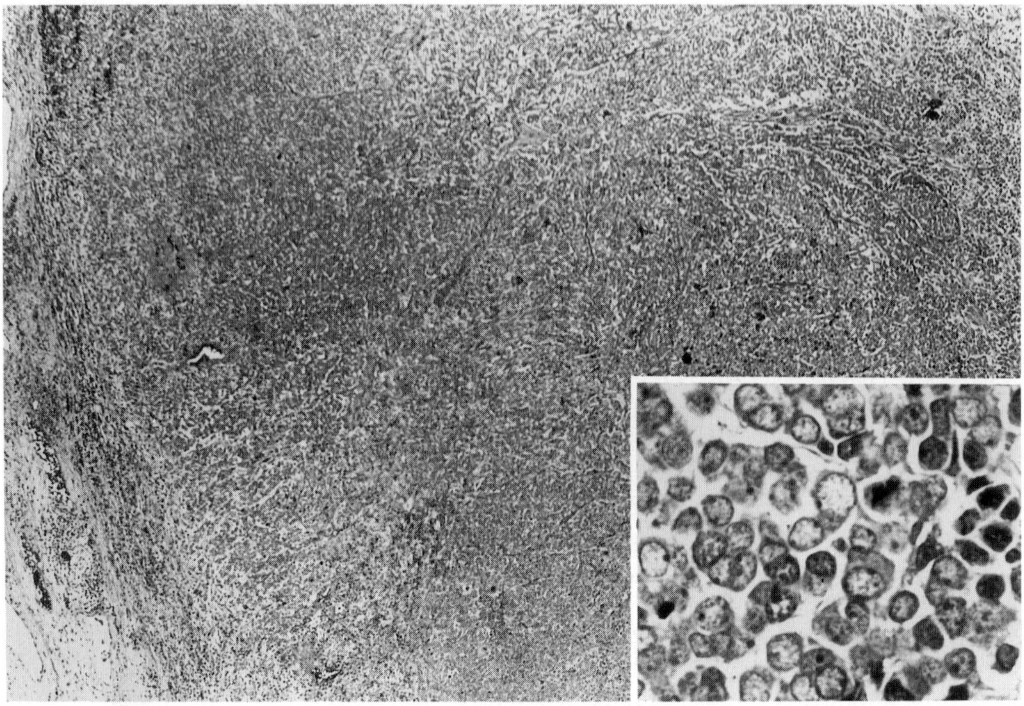

Figure 12 The lymph node is effaced by a uniform population of large cells. (H & E; ×40.) Insert, large cells have dustlike chromatin and indistinct nucleoli. (H & E; ×640.)

Questions

1. What is your differential diagnosis?
2. What additional studies would you request to analyze this tumor?

Discussion

The primary differential diagnosis of this lesion is malignant lymphoma, large cell type, and metastatic neoplasms including undifferentiated carcinoma, Merkel cell carcinoma, adult neuroblastoma, carcinoid tumor, and melanoma. Leukemic involvement also deserves consideration.

The uniform population of cells, the dustlike appearance of the nuclei, and the significant increase in mitotic activity are features, however, that alert one to a diagnosis of Merkel cell carcinoma. Immunohistochemical reactions helpful in solidifying a diagnosis include the leukocyte common antigen, low- and high-molecular-weight keratins, and S100. Additional reactions that can prove helpful in the analysis are neuron specific enolase, chromogranin, and synaptophysin (1). In this neoplasm, the low-molecular-weight keratin was strongly positive with membrane staining and a characteristic punctate highlighting of a paranuclear neurofilaments (Fig. 13). The high-molecular-weight antibody against keratin, however, failed to stain the cell membrane, but it did react with the paranuclear neurofilaments. There was negative staining of the S100 protein and the leukocyte common antigen. The histology, cytology, and immunohistochemical reactions are characteristic of Merkel cell carcinoma. Additional reactions that

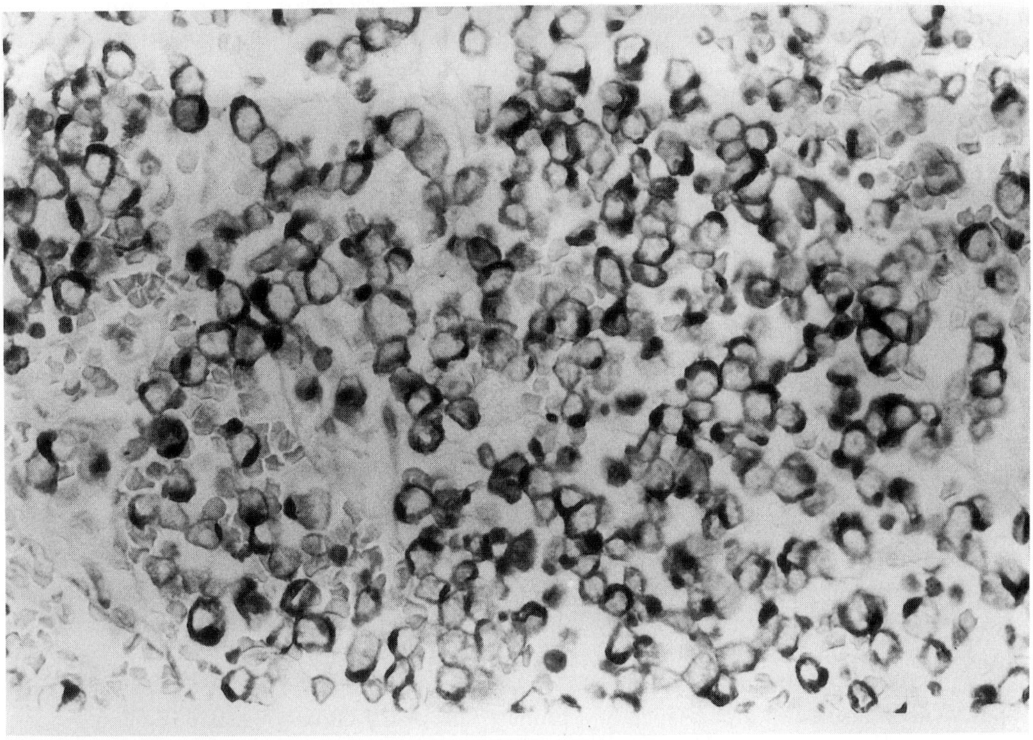

Figure 13 The immunohistochemical reaction with low-molecular-weight keratin discloses strong paranuclear punctate staining and staining of the cytoplasmic membranes. Low-molecular-weight cytokeratin, monoclonal antibody. (×160.)

were strongly positive were the neuron specific enolase, the synaptophysin, and the chromogranin reactions.

Undifferentiated metastatic carcinomas generally have strong cytoplasmic reaction with high-molecular-weight cytokeratin or, in some instances, with low-molecular-weight keratin. Typically, however, carcinomas lack expression of synaptophysin, chromogranin, and neuron specific enolase and do not have punctate staining in the paranuclear region with low-molecular-weight keratin.

Metastatic oat cell carcinoma, adult neuroblastoma, and carcinoid tumors, however, can express both cytokeratin and the neuroendocrine markers (neuron specific enolase, synaptophysin, chromogranin) and thus be potentially confused for Merkel cell carcinoma (1). These neoplasms, however, lack the characteristic punctate paranuclear labeling with the low-molecular-weight cytokeratins. The immunohistochemical reaction patterns are also not in keeping with a metastatic melanoma or malignant lymphoma of large cell type. Melanomas fail to exhibit the characteristic paranuclear punctate labeling with keratin, and usually melanomas possess the S100 protein. Characteristically, most malignant lymphomas react strongly to the leukocyte common antigen and lack the paranuclear punctate labeling with keratin antibodies.

Histologically, it is possible to confuse Merkel cell carcinoma for a leukemic infiltrate, but the labeling of the neoplastic cells with the antibodies against the keratins, chromogranins, and synaptophysin are not in keeping with a leukemic process.

Once the diagnosis of Merkel cell carcinoma was established, it was recommended to thoroughly evaluate the patient for evidence of a primary lesion in the skin. In this case, no lesion was identified. The diagnosis of metastatic Merkel cell carcinoma in a lymph node in the absence of an identifiable primary lesion in the skin is extremely rare and always difficult to explain, but there have been sporadic reports and case presentations of such occurrences. One report included eight patients with Merkel cell carcinoma with involvement of the inguinal lymph nodes (five cases), axillary lymph nodes (two cases), and submandibular lymph nodes (one case) in which no primary skin lesion was found. In all these cases, the patients underwent extensive evaluation, and rigid criteria were followed in making the diagnosis of Merkel cell carcinoma (2).

The patient presented in this case underwent local lymph node dissection, following which he received four courses of cisplatin and etoposide therapy. Three years after he was diagnosed with metastatic Merkel cell carcinoma, he is working full time and free of disease (3).

References

1. Ratner D, Nelson BR, Brown MD, Johnson TM. Merkel cell carcinoma. J Am Acad Dermatol 1993; 29:143–156.
2. Eusubi V, Capella C, Cossu A, Rosai J. Neuroendocrine carcinoma within lymph nodes in the absence of a primary tumor with special reference to Merkel cell carcinoma. Am J Surg Pathol 1992; 16:658–666.
3. Straka JA, Straka MB. A review of Merkel cell carcinoma with emphasis on lymph node disease in the absence of a primary site. Am J Otolaryn 1997; 18:55–65.

ACKNOWLEDGMENTS

The secretarial assistance of Sue Pish is appreciated.

SELECTED READINGS

1. Chan JKC, Tsang WYW. Reactive lymphadenopathies. In: Weiss LM, ed. Pathology of Lymph Nodes. New York: Churchill Livingstone, 1996:81–167.
2. Chan JKC, Tsang WYW. Uncommon syndromes of reactive lymphadenopathy. Semin Oncol 1993; 20:648–657.
3. Schnitzer B. Reactive lymphadenopathies. In: Knowles DM, ed. Neoplastic Hematopathology. Baltimore: Williams & Wilkins, 1992:427–457.
4. Stansfeld AG, d'Ardenne AJ. Lymph Node Biopsy Interpretation. 3d ed. Edinburgh: Churchill Livingston, 1992.
5. Swerdlow SH. Biopsy Interpretation of Lymph Nodes. Biopsy Interpretation Series. New York: Raven Press, 1992.
6. Ioachim HL. Lymph Node Pathology. 2d ed. Philadelphia: Lippincott, 1994.
7. Schnitzer B. Reactive lymphoid hyperplasias. In: Jaffe ES, ed. Surgical Pathology of the Lymph Nodes and Related Organs. 2d ed. Major Problems in Pathology. Vol. 16. Philadelphia: Saunders, 1995:98–132.
8. Burke JS. Reactive lymphadenopathies. Semin Diag Pathol 1988; 5:312–316.
9. Henry K. Lymph nodes. In Henry K, Symmers WStC, eds. Thymus, Lymph Nodes, Spleen and Lymphatics. 3d ed. Systemic Pathology. Vol. 7. Edinburgh: Churchill Livingstone, 1992:141–325.

10. Weiss LM, Arber DA, Chang KL. Lymph nodes and spleen. In: Silverberg SG, ed. Principles and Practice of Surgical Pathology and Cytopathology. 3d ed. New York: Churchill Livingstone, 1997: 675–772.
11. Dorfman RF, Warnke RA. Lymphadenopathy simulating the malignant lymphomas. Hum Pathol 1974; 5:519–550.
12. Hartsock RJ. Reactive lesions in lymph nodes. In: Rebuck J, Berard C, eds. The Reticuloendothelial System. International Academy of Pathology. Monograph 16. Baltimore: Williams & Wilkins, 1975: 152–183.
13. Ackerman LV. Surgical Pathology. St. Louis: Mosby-Year Book, 1959.
14. Custer, RP. Pitfalls in the diagnosis of lymphoma and leukemia from the pathologist's point of view. In: Proceedings of the Second National Cancer Conference, 1952. Vol. 1. New York: American Cancer Society, 1954:554–558.
15. Beard C, Nabers K, Bowling MC, Berard CW. Achieving technical excellence in lymph node specimens. An update. Lab Med 1985; 16:468–475.
16. Banks PM. Technical factors in the preparation and evaluation of lymph node biopsies. In Knowles DM, ed. Neoplastic hematopathology. Baltimore: Williams & Wilkins, 1992:367–384.
17. Collins RD. Lymph node examination. What is an adequate work-up? Arch Pathol Lab Med 1985; 109:796–799.
18. Koneman EW, Allen SD, Janda WM, Schreckenberger PC, Winn WC Jr. Diagnostic Microbiology. A Color Atlas and Textbook. Philadelphia: Lippincott, 92–93.
19. Hartsock RJ. Postvaccinial lymphadenitis. Hyperplasia of lymphoid tissue that simulates malignant lymphoma. Cancer 1966; 21:632–649.
20. van der Valk P, Meijer CJLM. The histology of the reactive lymph node. Histology for pathologists. Am J Surg Pathol 1987; 11:866–882.
21. DeWolf-Peeters C, Delabie J. Anatomy and histophysiology of lymphoid tissue. Semin Oncol 1993; 20:555–569.
22. Salvador AH, Harrison EG, Kyle RA. Infectious mononucleosis. Its confusion with malignant lymphoma. Cancer 1971; 27:1029–1040.
23. Childs CC, Parham DM, Berard CW. Infectious mononucleosis: the spectrum of morphologic changes simulating lymphoma in lymph nodes and tonsils. Am J Surg Pathol 1987; 11:122–132.
24. Tindle BH, Parker JW, Lukes RJ. "Reed-Sternberg cells" in infectious mononucleosis. Am J Clin Pathol 1972; 58:607–617.
25. Moore RD, Weisberger AS, Bowerfind ES Jr. An evaluation of lymphadenopathy in systemic disease. Arch Intern Med 1957; 99:751–759.
26. Saxen L, Saxen E, Tenhunen A. The significance of histological diagnoses in glandular toxoplasmosis. Acta Pathol Microbiol Scand 1962; 56:284–294.
27. Dorfman RF, Remington JS. Value of lymph node biopsy in the diagnosis of acquired toxoplasmosis. N Engl J Med 1973; 289:878–881.
28. Mettinen M. Histologic differential diagnoses between lymph node toxoplasmosis and other benign lymph node hyperplasia. Histopathology 1981; 5:205–216.
29. Mettinen M, Franssila K. Malignant lymphoma simulating lymph node toxoplasmosis. Histopathology 1982; 6:129–140.
30. Meyer PR, Yanagihara ET, Parker JW, Lukes RJ. A distinctive follicular hyperplasia in the acquired immune deficiency syndrome (AIDS) and the AIDS related complex. Hematol Oncol 1984; 2: 319–347.
31. Said JW. AIDS-related lymphadenopathies. Semin Diagn Pathol 1988; 5:365–375.
32. Stanley MW, Frizzera G. Diagnostic specificity of histologic features in lymph node biopsy specimens at risk for the acquired immunodeficiency syndrome. Hum Pathol 1986; 17:1231–1239.
33. O'Murchada MT, Wolf BC, Neiman RS. The histologic features of hyperplastic lymphadenopathy in AIDS-related complex are nonspecific. Am J Surg Pathol 1987; 11:94–99.
34. Nosanchuk JS, Schnitzer B. Follicular hyperplasia in lymph nodes from patients with rheumatoid arthritis, a clinicopathologic study. Cancer 1969; 24:343–354.

35. Cammarata R, Rodnan GP, Jensen WM. Systemic rheumatic disease and malignant lymphoma. Arch Intern Med 1963; 111:112–119.
36. Miller D. The association of immune disease and malignant lymphoma. Ann Intern Med 1967; 66: 507–521.
37. Hartsock RJ, Halling LW, King FM. Luetic lymphadenitis: a clinical and histologic study of 20 cases. Am J Clin Pathol 1970; 53:304–314.
38. Choi YJ, Reiner L. Syphilitic lymphadenitis. Immunofluorescent identification of spirochetes from imprints. Am J Surg Pathol 1979; 3:553–555.
39. Strano AJ. Measles. In Binford CH, Connor DH. Pathology of Tropical and Extraordinary Diseases. Washington, DC: Armed Forces Institute of Pathology, 1976:73–75.
40. Kjeldsberg CR, Kim H. Polykaryocytes resembling Warthin-Finkeldey giant cells in reactive and neoplastic lymphoid disorders. Hum Pathol 1981; 12:267–272.
41. Delsol G, Pradere M, Voigt JJ, Nespoulous M, Gorguet B, Marty C, Fabre J. Warthin-Finkeldey-like cells in benign and malignant lymphoid proliferations. Histopathology 1982; 6:451–465.
42. Keller AR, Hochholzer L, Castleman B. Hyaline-vascular and plasma-cell types of giant lymph node hyperplasia of mediastinum and other locations. Cancer 1972; 29:670–683.
43. Frizzera G, Massarelli G, Banks PM, Rosai J. A systemic lymphoproliferative disorder with morphologic features of Castleman's disease: Pathologic findings in 15 patients. Am J Surg Pathol 1983; 7:211–231.
44. Frizzera G. Castleman's disease and related disorders. Semin Diagn Pathol 1988; 5:346–364.
45. Zarate-Osorno A, Medeiros LJ, Danon AD, Neiman RS. Hodgkin's disease with coexistent Castleman-like histologic features, a report of three cases. Arch Pathol Lab Med 1994; 118:270–274.
46. Weisenburger DD, Nathwani BN, Winberg CD, Rappaport H. Multicentric angiofollicular lymph node hyperplasia: a clinicopathologic study of 16 cases. Hum Pathol 1985; 16:162–172.
47. Roberts FJ, Linsey S. The value of microbial cultures in diagnostic lymph node biopsy. J Infect Dis 1984; 149:162–165.
48. Rosai J. Lymph nodes. In: Rosai J, ed. Ackerman's Surgical Pathology. New York: Mosby, 1996: 1661–1774.
49. Freidig EE, McClure SP, Wilson WR, Banks PM, Washington JA II. Clinical-histologic microbiologic analysis of 419 lymph node biopsy specimens. Rev Infect Dis 1986; 8:322–328.
50. Ioachim HL. Granulomatous lesions of lymph nodes. In: Ioachim HL, ed. Pathology of Granulomas. New York: Raven Press, 1983:151–187.
51. Sacks EL, Donaldson SS, Gordon J, Dorfman RF. Epithelioid granulomas associated with Hodgkin's disease: clinical correlation in 55 previously untreated patients. Cancer 1978; 41:562–567.
52. Dobbins WO. Diagnosis and differential diagnosis. In: Dobbins WO, ed. Whipple's Disease. Springfield, IL: Charles C Thomas, 1989:131–138.
53. Relman DA, Schmidt TM, MacDermott RP, Falkow S. Identification of the uncultured bacillus of Whipple's disease. N Engl J Med 1992; 327:293–301.
54. Kaiserling E, Patsouris E, Muller-Hermelink HK, Wichterich D, Lennert K. Bacterial lymphadenitis with the picture of a lymphoepithelioid cell lymphoma (Lennert's lymphoma). Histopathology 1989; 14:161–178.
55. Evans ME, Gregory DW, Schaffner W, McGee ZA. Tularemia. A 30-year experience with 88 cases. Medicine 1985; 64:251–267.
56. Strickler JG, Warnke RA, Weiss LM. Necrosis in lymph nodes. In: Rosen PP, Fechner RE, eds. Pathology Annual 1987 (Part 2). Norwalk, CT: Appleton and Lange, 1987:253–282.
57. Wear DJ, Hadfield TL, Fisher FW, Schlagel CJ, King FM. Cat-scratch disease. A bacterial infection. Science 1983; 221:1403–1405.
58. Yu X, Raoult D. Monoclonal antibodies to *Afipia felis*—a pulative agent of cat-scratch disease. Am J Clin Pathol 1994; 101:603–606.
59. Hadfield TL, Lamy Y, Wear DJ. Demonstration of *Chlamydia tracomatis* in inguinal lymphadenitis of lymphogranuloma venereum: a light microscopy, electron microscopy and polymerase chain reaction study. Mod Pathol 1995; 8:924–929.

60. Joseph AK, Rosen T. Laboratory techniques used in the diagnosis of chancroid, granuloma inguinale, and lymphogranuloma venereum. Dermatol Clin 1994; 12:1–8.
61. Overholt EL, Tigertt WW, Kadull PJ. Analysis of forty-two cases of laboratory-acquired tularemia: treatment with broad spectrum antibiotics. Am J Med 1961; 30:785–806.
62. Warnke RA, Weiss LM, Chan JKC, Cleary ML, Dorfman RF. Atlas of Tumor Pathology. Third Series, Fascicle 14. Tumors of the Lymph Nodes and Spleen. Washington, DC: Armed Forces Institute of Pathology, 1995:341–349.
63. Hui PK, Chan JKC, Ng CS, Yuen NWF, Kung ITM, Gwi E. Lymphadenopathy of Kimura's disease in Chinese. Histopathology 1989; 15:557–574.
64. Chan JKC, Frizzera G, Fletcher CDM, Rosai J. Primary vascular tumors of lymph nodes other than Kaposi's sarcoma, analysis of 39 cases and delineation of two new entities. Am J Surg Pathol 1992; 16:3335–350.
65. Chamulak GA, Brynes R, Nathwani BN. Kikuchi-Fujimoto disease mimicking malignant lymphoma. Am J Surg Pathol 1990; 14:514–523.
66. Chan JKC, Wong KC, Ng CS. A fatal case of multicentric Kikuchi's histiocytic necrotizing lymphadenitis. Cancer 1989; 63:1856–1862.
67. Dorfman RF, Berry GJ. Kikuchi's histiocytic necrotizing lymphadenitis: an analysis of 108 cases with emphasis on differential diagnosis. Semin Diagn Pathol 1988; 5:329–345.
68. Foucar E, Rosai J, Dorfman RF. Sinus histiocytosis with massive lymphadenopathy (Rosai-Dorfman disease): review of the entity. Semin Diagn Pathol 1990; 7:19–73.
69. Shaw S, Kisilevsky R. Infarction of lymph nodes: a cause of a palisading macrophage reaction mimicking necrotizing granulomas. Hum Pathol 1978; 9:597–599.
70. Maurer R, Schmid U, Davies JD, Mahy NJ, Stansfeld AG, Lukes RJ. Lymph node infarction and malignant lymphoma: a multicenter survey of European, English and American cases. Histopathology 1986; 10:571–588.
71. Rothschild B, Marshall H. Lymphadenopathy and lymph node infarction in the course of gold therapy. Am J Med 1986; 537–540.
72. Perrone T, de Wolf-Peeters C, Frizzera G. Inflammatory pseudotumor of lymph nodes: a distinctive pattern of nodal reaction. Am J Surg Pathol 1988; 12:351–361.
73. Chan JKC, Warnke RA, Dorfman RF. Vascular transformation of sinuses in lymph nodes, a study of its morphological spectrum and distinction from Kaposi's sarcoma. Am J Surg Pathol 1991; 15:732–743.
74. Chen KTK. Mycobacterial spindle cell pseudotumor of lymph nodes. Am J Surg Pathol 1992; 16: 276–281.
75. Chan JKC, Lewin KJ, Lombard CM, Teitelbaum S, Dorfman RF. Histopathology of bacillary angiomatosis of lymph node. Am J Surg Pathol 1991; 15:430–437.
76. Chan JKC, Frizzera G, Fletcher CDM, Rosai J. Primary vascular tumors of lymph nodes other than Kaposi's sarcoma. Am J Surg Pathol 1992; 16:335–350.
77. Teague MD, Tham KT. Hyphalike pseudofungus in a lymph node. Arch Pathol Lab Med 1994; 118:95–96.
78. Lin RP, DiLeonardo M, Jacoby RA. Silicone lymphadenopathy, a case report and review of the literature. Am J Dermatopathol 1993; 15:82–84.
79. Kuo TT, Hsueh S. Mucicarminophilic histiocytosis, a polyvinylpyrrolidone storage disease simulating signet-ring cell carcinoma. Am J Surg Pathol 1984; 8:419–428.
80. Akosa AB, Ali MH. Lymph node pathology in Henoch-Schölein purpura. Histopathology 1989; 15: 297–301.
81. Abbondanzo SL, Irey NS, Frizzera G. Dilantin-associated lymphadenopathy: spectrum of histopathologic patterns. Am J Surg Pathol 1995; 19:675–686.
82. Suster S, Rosai J. Intranodal hemorrhagic spindle-cell tumor with "amianthoid" fibers. Report of six cases of a distinctive mesenchymal neoplasm of the inguinal region that simulates Kaposi's sarcoma. Am J Surg Pathol 1989; 13:347–357.
83. Covell LM, Disciullo AJ, Knapp RC. Decidual changes in pelvic lymph nodes in the presence of cervical squamous cell carcinoma during pregnancy. Am J Obstet Gynecol 1977; 127:674–676.

84. Gaffey MJ, Ben-Ezra JM, Weiss LM. Herpes simplex lymphadenitis. Am J Clin Pathol 1991; 95: 709–714.
85. Barnett RN, Hull JG, Vortel V. Pneumocystis carinii in lymph nodes and spleen. Arch Pathol 1969; 88:175–180.
86. Chan JKC, Tang SK, Tsang WYW, Lee KC, Batsakis JC. Histologic changes induced by fine needle aspiration. Adv Anat Pathol 1996; 3:71–90.

3

Pathology of the Spleen

Hernani D. Cualing
University of Cincinnati Medical Center, Cincinnati, Ohio

I. INTRODUCTION

Disorders affecting the bone marrow and lymph node components of the hematopoietic system frequently involve the spleen. The pathology usually manifests as splenomegaly secondary to an expansion of either the red pulp or the white pulp compartments of the spleen. With few exceptions, red pulp disease is secondary to leukemia and white pulp disease is secondary to lymphoma. Unlike cut surfaces of lymph node and bone marrow, cut surface of the spleen offers clues to the pathology—homogeneous red cut surface when infiltrated by leukemia and prominent Malphigian corpuscles (white pulp nodules) when lymphoma is involved.

II. EMBRYOLOGY

The spleen is first visible in the human embryo by the fifth week of gestation as condensation of the mesogastrium, the mesentery attaching the stomach to the dorsal wall of the abdominal cavity. It is completely derived from the mesoderm, initially recognized as sinuses and cords and eventually complemented by the white pulp by the sixth fetal month. Primitive follicles lacking germinal centers are initially observed. Well-formed germinal centers first appear around the time of birth. Lymphocytes appear early and B cells predominate, but immunoglobulins of the IgM and IgG type are synthesized late in the third trimester.

In lower vertebrates, such as the lamprey, splenic tissue first appeared as a spiral fold of the gut; later in evolution, as in fish, the typical spleen arose from dorsal mesentery of the stomach.

III. ANATOMY

A normal spleen weighs about 150 (±38) g, and this weight decreases after the seventh decade. The spleen has a fibrous capsule, but lacks smooth muscle and contractibility. Splenic afferent and efferent arteries and veins, nerves and efferent lymphatics, and lymph nodes are located in the hilum. The spleen is part of the vascular system and derives its blood supply from the splenic artery. This artery branches to trabecular arteries to become the central arteries of the white pulp. The central arteries terminate as penicilliary arterioles in the white and red pulp.

Blood empties into the cords of Billroth and some directly into the venous sinuses (Fig. 1). The splenic sinuses and veins drain directly into the porto-hepatic venous system.

The spleen is divided into a white pulp and a red pulp compartment owing to the color of these areas on cut section of the gross specimen. Microscopically, there is a marginal zone between the red pulp and the white pulp. This zone, which envelops the B- and T-cell areas, contains marginal-zone lymphocytes, macrophages, and plasma cells and is supplied by terminal branches of the central artery (Fig. 1).

The white pulp is a 1–2 mm white nodule on cut section, uniformly distributed and intimately associated with the arterial network. Depending on the angle of microscopic section, this cuff of white pulp may look round, elliptical, or elongated. Primary lymphoid follicles containing a homogeneous nodule of B lymphocytes branch periodically, and when they are activated by antigen, may display a secondary follicle composed of a germinal center, mantle zone, and marginal zone. Unlike some other animal species, there is no marginal sinus dividing the mantle from the marginal zone. These B-cell compartments (Fig. 2) are easily recognized by their distinct tripartite zonation: The center has germinal center lymphocytes; followed by a mantle zone of small lymphocytes, and a third, outermost rim of polymorphous lymphoid cells with pale, generous monocytoid cytoplasm—the so-called marginal zone lymphocytes. A cuff of lymphocytes, predominantly of T-cell type, envelops the central arteries, sometimes referred to as the periarteriolar lymphoid sheath (PALS).

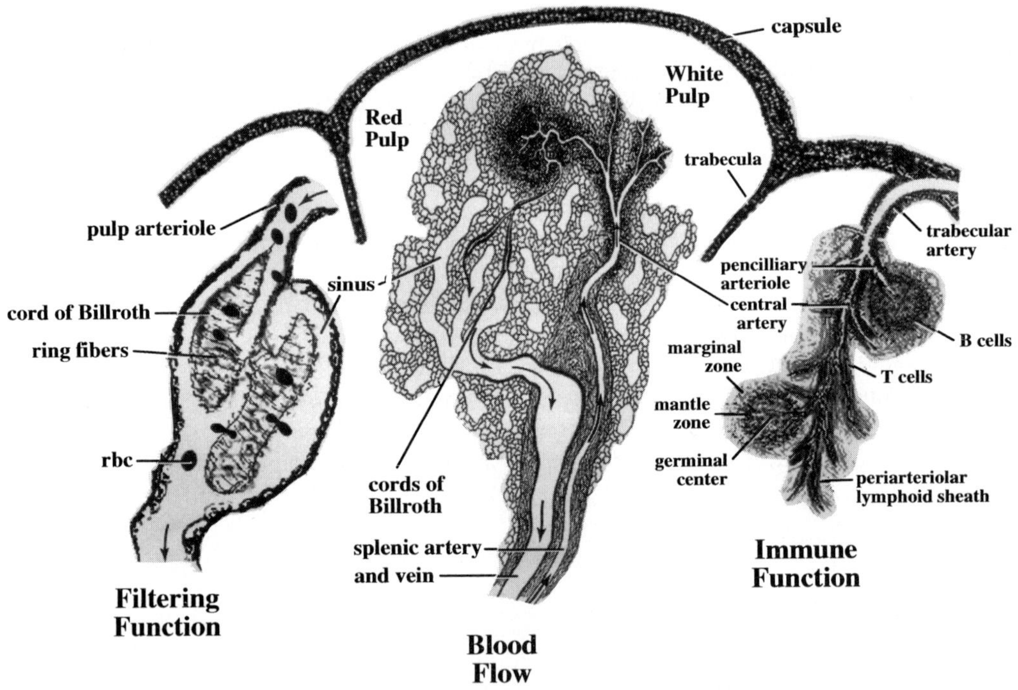

Figure 1 Diagram of the spleen including functional areas and circulation. The left side of the figure depicts microcirculation in the red pulp subserving filtering function, and the right side of the figure depicts lymphoid architecture of the white pulp subserving immune function. The central figure depicts blood flow through the white pulp vessels and into the red pulp sinuses and veins.

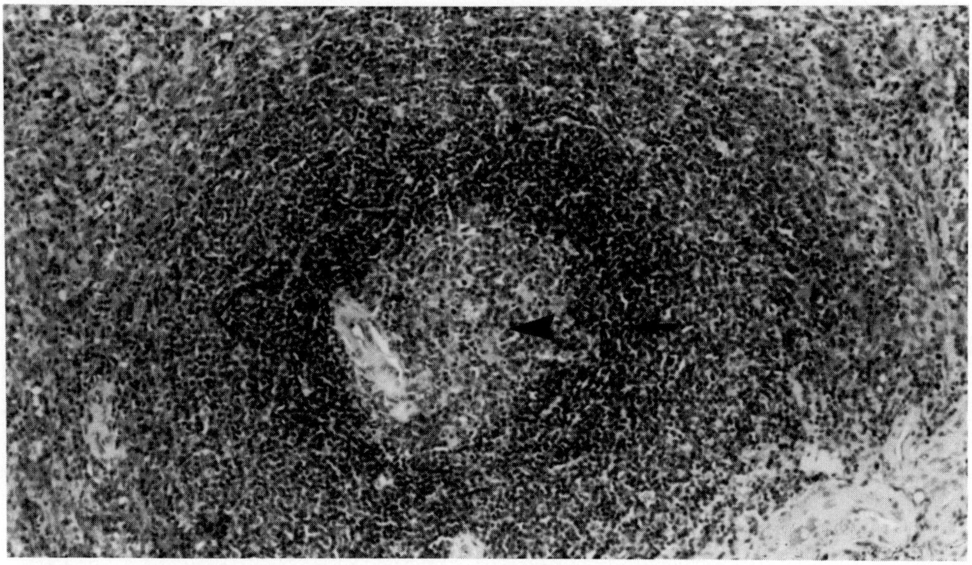

Figure 2 Histoarchitecture of activated follicle in the white pulp. A tripartite zonation is present: The center is composed of the germinal center cells (arrowhead), followed by a cuff of mantle zone cells (broken arrow), and the outermost monocytoid-like cells is the marginal zone cells (open arrow). This area of the white pulp corresponds to the secondary follicle in a lymph node. The cells from these zones are the putative cells of origin of the follicular center cell lymphoma, mantle cell lymphoma, and marginal zone lymphoma, respectively. Although all derives from the B-cell population, subset immunophenotyping allows diagnosis of type of lymphoma. (×200, PAS.)

The red pulp is composed of the sinuses, the cords of Billroth, and terminal arterioles. The structure of the red pulp sinuses, as compared to other organs, is uniquely suited for blood filtration. The sinuses are lined by spindle-shaped endothelial-like cells called littoral cells, which do not possess desmosomes or tight junctions, and which act as a framework structure enclosed by a sieve composed of a specialized basement membrane. These membranes or ring fibers are discontinuous, transversely oriented, and function as a net in the cordal sieve (1). Cordal macrophages attach to the ring fibers. This arrangement allows only pliable, healthy cells to pass from the cordal spaces to the sinuses and further traps abnormal blood elements. Unlike hematoxylin and eosin preparations, only periodic acid Schiff (PAS) or argyrophilic stain highlights the ring fiber filtering architecture of the red pulp.

IV. PHYSIOLOGY

The anatomy serves its filtering and immune function well; progressive branching of arteries helps skim off the plasma from the cells. The soluble antigens are perfused in the marginal zone, where phagocytic macrophages process them and induce antibody production. Cellular elements continue on to the spaces of the cords of Billroth in the red pulp. Blood passes through the pulp cords, where pitting (removal of inclusion bodies from the red cells) and culling (cell destruction) takes place. As a filter, trapping of elements may lead to red pulp-related pathology. If these elements are otherwise altered in their plasticity, opsonized by antibody, or carry aberrant membrane or cytoplasmic biomolecules, the cords and its sievelike architecture will entrap and cull them away from circulation. Senescent red cells as well as other blood elements may be trapped in the spleen. It also functions as a reservoir of freely exchangeable platelets and, to a lesser extent, red cells. The red pulp compartment serves as a filter of blood and the white pulp compartment performs its other major function: primary immune response.

The spleen is the largest lymphoid organ in the body and plays a crucial role in the function of host defense by trapping antibody-coated cells and microbes. The white pulp, which is composed of lymphoid-rich periarteriolar structures, is involved in humoral (antibody) and cell-mediated immunity. As an organ serving immune recognition and function, diseases affecting the lymph nodes may lead to white pulp-related pathology. Similar to the lymph nodes in function and architecture, the "Malphigian corpuscles" swell and atrophy along with lymph node follicles upon activation by particulate antigens, infectious agents, or ingress of neoplastic lymphocytes. Both lymph nodes and spleen contain areas for B- and T-lymphocyte microenvironment. The PALS corresponds to the paracortical area and the white pulp follicle corresponds to the germinal center of lymph nodes.

V. BLOOD FLOW PATHOPHYSIOLOGY

Blood flow abnormality from both the arterial and the venous sides of the circulation may lead to pathology. Infarction (*peliosis lienis*) is secondary to embolization or vascular thrombosis. It is often wedged-shaped, with its base along the capsule.

Because of the spleen's rich vascular and reticular framework, extrasplenic neoplasms that disseminate via the bloodstream can be trapped in the spleen. The most common are metastatic melanoma, breast, and lung carcinoma.

In addition, because of the close continuity of the spleno-portal venous system, portal venous hypertension will lead to congestion of the splenic sinuses. Congestive splenomegaly may be caused by:

Cirrhosis
Budd-Chiari syndrome
Splenic vein thrombosis
Portal vein thrombosis
Banti's syndrome—idiopathic portal hypertension

The fibrocongestive splenomegaly triad includes:

Hemosiderotic nodules (Gamna-Gandy bodies)
Fibrosis of the red pulp
Sinusoidal dilatation

VI. SPLENIC FUNCTION

Hypersplenism and hyposplenism are two major clinicopathologic processes associated with excessive or decreased splenic function, respectively.

A. Hypersplenism

Hypersplenism is characterized by cytopenias, compensatory bone marrow hyperplasia, splenomegaly, and correction of cytopenia after splenectomy. The differential diagnosis of splenomegaly is shown in Table 1. The pathogenesis is attributed to splenic sequestration and destruction of trapped blood elements. Sequestration is caused by abnormalities in the blood cells or of the spleen itself. Abnormalities of red cells are either congenital or acquired. Congenital red cell abnormalities include hereditary spherocytosis, hemoglobinopathies, and hereditary hemolytic anemias. Acquired red cell disorders include malaria and autoimmune hemolytic anemia. Splenic causes of hypersplenism are due to disorders of cordal macrophages or secondary to infiltrative diseases. Disorders of cordal macrophages include the storage diseases, Langerhans cell histiocytosis, and hemophagocytic syndromes. In these disorders, the cords are widened and macrophages are abundant. Infiltrative neoplastic diseases and vascular abnormalities may also cause hypersplenism.

Table 1 Differential Diagnosis of Splenomegaly

- Splenic vein hypertension
  - Cirrhosis, portal or splenic vein thrombosis, hepatic vein occusion, heart failure
- Inflammatory
  - Rheumatoid arthritis, systemic lupus erythematosus, Felty's syndrome, sarcoidosis, amyloidosis
- Hematologic disorders
  - Hemolytic anemias (congenital and acquired): thalassemia major, sickle and spherocytic anemias
- Tumors
  - Benign
    - Hamartoma
    - Cysts
  - Malignant
    - Chronic leukemia—chronic lymphocytic and hairy cell leukemia
    - Myeloproliferative disorders—chronic myeloid leukemia, myelofibrosis with myeloid metaplasia, polycythemia rubra vera, essential thrombocythemia
    - Acute leukemia—granulocytic sarcoma
    - Malignant lymphomas
    - Metastatic solid tumors
    - Sarcomas
- Infectious
  - Acute
    - Viral (infectious mononucleosis, hepatitis, CMV)
    - Bacterial (mycobacterium avium intracellulare, salmonellosis)
  - Subacute and chonic
    - Subacute bacterial endocarditis
    - Tuberculosis
    - Malaria
    - Schistosomiasis
    - Kala-azar (*Leishmania* sp.)
- Storage diseases
  - Gaucher's disease
  - Niemann-Pick's disease
  - Sea-blue histiocyte-associated diseases

B. Hyposplenism

Hyposplenism is characterized by absent or decreased splenic function. Splenectomy, atrophy, infarction, and acquired or congenital immune deficiency may produce hyposplenism. In AIDS patients, lymphoid depletion and overwhelming mycobacteria infection lead to hyposplenism.

Peripheral blood findings in the asplenic or hyposplenic state include erythrocyte inclusions and abnormalities in morphology. These inclusions include Howell Jolly, Pappenheimer, and Heinz bodies (supravital stains). Additional erythrocyte abnormalities in the peripheral blood include target cells, pitted or bitten red cells, or nucleated red cells.

VII. DISEASES OF THE WHITE PULP

A. Introduction

The white pulp does not normally contain germinal centers. Pathology may show as increase or decrease of lymphoid elements. Antigenic stimuli induce reactive germinal centers and plasmacytosis. Certain immunodeficiency syndromes cause lymphoid depletion of the white pulp. Various granulomatous conditions also affect the spleen. The major neoplastic disease of the white pulp is non-Hodgkin's lymphoma, usually secondary to systemic disease. Table 2 shows a list of white pulp pathology.

B. Reactive Lymphoid Hyperplasia

Tripartite white pulp architecture is present. Reactive hyperplasia of the white pulp can be seen in:

- Spleen removed incidentally for traumatic injury
- Children and adolescents
- Acute infections, especially infectious mononucleosis
- Rheumatoid arthritis and other collagen vascular diseases
- Idiopathic thrombocytopenic purpura-detected as PAS-positive foamy histiocytes in the marginal zone
- Graft versus host disease (GVH)

C. Lymphoid Depletion

Lymphoid depletion occurs with:

Table 2 Diseases of the White Pulp

Reactive lymphoid hyperplasia
Lymphoid depletion
Granulomatous processes
Infectious
Noninfectious
Malignant lymphomas
Non-Hodgkin's lymphomas
Hodgkin's disease

Acquired immune deficiency syndrome (AIDS): At autopsy, plasmacytosis and white pulp depletion are common findings (2). Other findings include immunoblast proliferation, microabscesses, fibrosis, congestion of red pulp, erythrophagocytosis, infection [mycobacteria (16%), cytomegalovirus (15%)] and neoplasms [malignant lymphoma (14%), perivascular Kaposi sarcoma (15%)].
Primary immunodeficiency diseases: X-linked agammaglobulinemia of Bruton (B-cell deficiency), DiGeorge thymic hypoplasia syndrome (T-cell depletion), severe combined immunodeficiency (B- and T-cell defect).
Cytotoxic chemotherapy and radiotherapy
Immunosuppressive agents—corticosteroids and antilymphocyte serum

D. Granulomatous Processes

Histologic types of granulomas include:

Lipogranulomas (20% of surgical pathology splenectomy specimens)
Active granulomas with or without necrosis
Small sarcoidal-type epithelioid granulomas
Old, inactive hyalinized granulomas

Etiologically, granulomas are classified as infectious or noninfectious.

1. Infectious Granulomas

Infectious granulomas are uncommon as primary in spleen, but atypical mycobacterium is becoming prevalent in HIV+ patients. Inactive tuberculosis and histoplasmosis are common causes of inactive hyalinized granuloma. Plamodium vivax, syphilis, leprosy, tularemia, and yersinia are unusual.

A rare necrotizing granulomatous splenitis, cause unknown, has been described (3). This perplexing disease uncommonly reveals an associated bacterial infection.

2. Noninfectious Granulomas

Certain noncaseating sarcoid-type splenic granulomas (6% of splenectomy specimens) are significant. They are often associated with central arteries. They are observed in

Hodgkin's disease
Sarcoidosis
Non-Hodgkin's lymphoma
Chronic uremia
IgA deficiency

E. Malignant Lymphoma

Splenectomy is not usually performed in patients with non-Hodgkin's lymphoma (NHL) except when there is hypersplenism or a suspected primary splenic lymphoma. The majority of lymphomas involve the white pulp and form nodules. Hence, it is difficult to classify splenic lesions as nodular or diffuse initially, unless there is massive involvement beyond the white pulp. Grossly, solitary or multiple tumor masses are characteristic of large cell lymphoma or Hodgkin's disease (HD), and miliary tumor nodules are characteristic of small lymphoid neoplasms (Fig. 3). Flow cytometry immunophenotyping and immunohistochemistry are useful

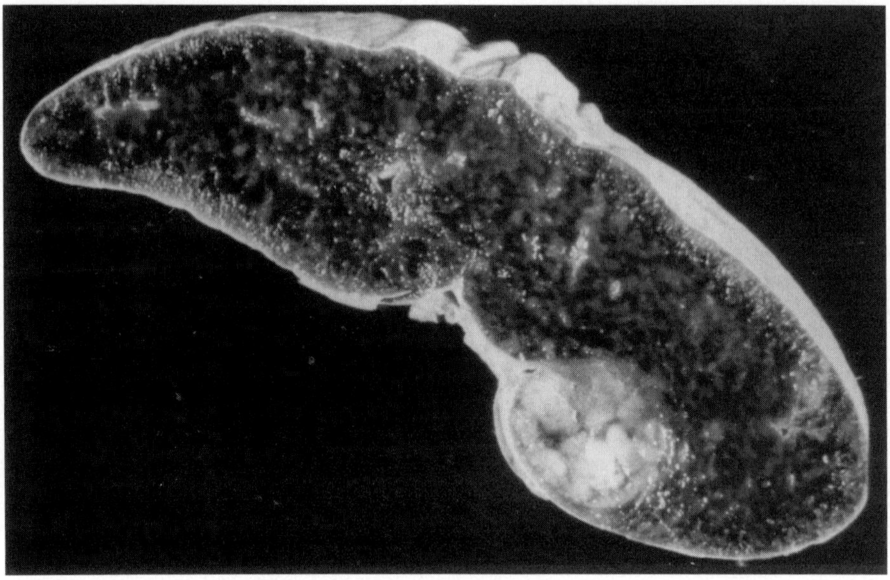

Figure 3 Gross picture of the cut surface of the spleen showing a large, subcapsular, well-delineated tumor mass, a finding often associated with involvement by either Hodgkin's lymphoma or non-Hodgkin's lymphoma of large cell histologic type.

tools in evaluation and diagnosis of malignant lymphomas (see Study Case 1 at the end of the chapter for discussion).

Primary lymphoma of the spleen is rare, accounting for less than 1% of all lymphomas. Most are non-Hodgkin's lymphomas; as primary, splenic Hodgkin's disease is rare. Large cell lymphomas comprise 63% (4), small cell (lymphocytic and cleaved) comprise 32%, and mixed small and large and small noncleaved types are rare. Phenotypically, most are B cell. Other NHLs occurring primarily in the spleen are rare.

Splenic marginal zone lymphoma is a recently described rare primary splenic lymphoma (5). It appears to be a distinct clinicopathologic entity, presents in older women, and is characterized by splenomegaly and associated circulating monocytoid cells or villous lymphocytes (Fig. 4).

Secondary lymphoma of the spleen is more common. This occurs in 25–100% of all NHL patients and 33% of all HD patients. Small lymphocytic lymphoma commonly involves the spleen, whereas large cell lymphoma does so relatively infrequently. The frequency of secondary spleen involvement by types of lymphomas is as follows (4).

1. Non-Hodgkin's Lymphoma

Small lymphocytic, lymphoplasmacytic, mantle cell—most common (60–100%), miliary pattern

Follicular small cleaved—common, 49–61%, monotonous small cleaved, miliary pattern

Follicular, mixed—uncommon, may be mistaken for benign follicles

Large cell—6–38% of cases, tumor mass

Small noncleaved—rare

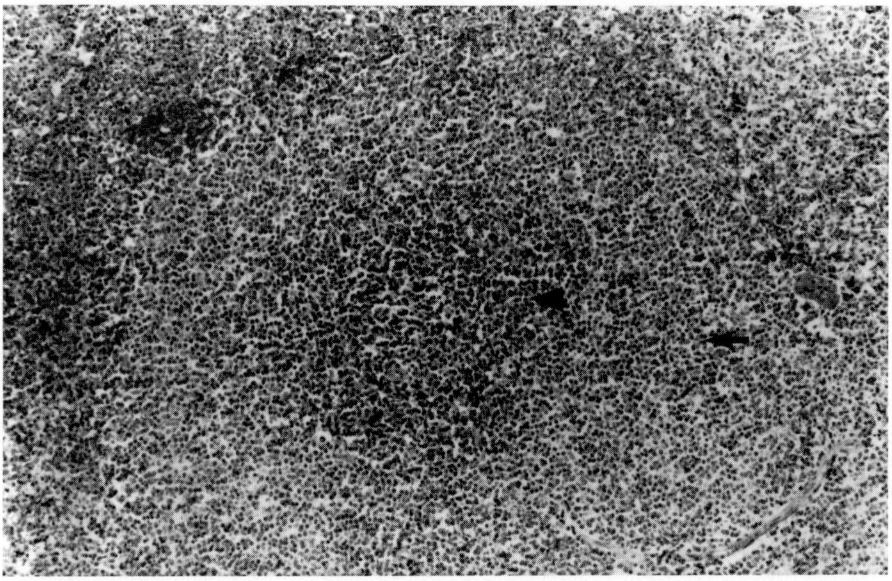

Figure 4 Involvement by marginal zone lymphoma characterized by expansion of the marginal zone (broken arrow) and effacement of germinal center architecture secondary to "colonization" by neoplastic cells (arrowhead). Unlike the normal germinal center shown in Fig. 2, the follicle is infiltrated by a monotonous infiltrate of cells which have round to irregular nuclei, moderately abundant pale cytoplasm, and inconspicuous mitosis. Although a nodular pattern is often observed, areas of diffuse involvement of the red pulp may be present. (×400, PAS.)

T-cell lymphomas—rare, including the recently described hepatosplenomegalic gamma-delta T-cell lymphoma

2. *Hodgkin's Disease*

Hodgkin's disease most commonly involves the spleen extranodally. About one-third of patients who had a staging laparotomy show involvement. Splenic involvement is correlated with bone marrow and liver involvement. Grossly, solitary or multiple tumor masses are commonly seen at presentation, but subtle small lesions are also seen. Microscopically, most are found in the white pulp. Histologic subtyping is better performed using lymph node biopsy.

VIII. DISEASES OF THE RED PULP

A. Introduction

Most of the diseases identifiable in the red pulp are secondary to a systemic disorder. Table 3 shows red pulp-related disorders. Intrinsic lesions are rare and will be discussed later.

B. Congestion of Red Pulp

Sinusoidal dilatation associated with increased portal pressure can lead to congestion of red pulp. This may result in ischemic infarcts, fibrosis, and hemosiderotic nodules. Histologically, the red blood cells are normal and sinuses are dilated.

Cordal space dilatation associated with abnormalities in red cell membrane (i.e., hereditary

Table 3 Diseases of the Red Pulp

Congestion
Infection
Histiocytic disorders
Storage disorders
Hemophagocytic disorders
Langerhan's cell histiocytosis
Foamy histiocytosis
Myeloproliferative disorders and leukemias
Dysproteinemias

spherocytosis) can also cause congestion of splenic pulp. The cords are expanded and sinusoidal spaces are usually compressed. There is a "laking" phenomenon (ghost red cells) better appreciated in cytologic imprints than on histologic preparation. Most of these cases are first diagnosed in children, but the diagnosis of hereditary spherocytosis in adults is not uncommon. Splenectomy for hereditary spherocytosis has been tempered in recent years by reports of fatal sepsis, usually due to *Streptococcus pneumoniae*.

C. Infection

Infectious mononucleosis—important to recognize because it may be histologically mistaken for leukemia (4).

AIDS sepsis—atypical mycobacteria appearing histologically as foamy histiocytosis with AFB-positive intracellular organisms.

D. Histiocytic Disorders

Histiocytic disorders are derived from a common bone marrow mononuclear stem cell. At maturity, these cells perform either a phagocytic or an immune effector role at diverse tissue sites. K. Foucar aptly referred to these cells as belonging to the M-PIRE (mononuclear phagocyte and immunoregulatory effector) system (6).

1. Storage Disorders

The characteristic pathology in storage disorders is red pulp expansion. Microscopically, there is widening of, and sequestration in, the cords of Billroth by inclusion-laden histiocytes. Most are rare genetic disorders producing a specific lysosomal enzyme defect or deficiency that gives rise to storage diseases. There may be certain organ predilection or systemic involvement, but splenomegaly may be a prominent initial presentation. Histiocytes are almost always affected, and Wright-Giemsa (WG) stain preparation may reveal "sea-blue histiocytes" (Fig. 5). Several prototype syndromes are as follows.

a. Lipidosis

Gaucher's cell—crumpled tissue paper-like cytoplasm, clear to pale blue in WG stain.

Niemann-Pick cell—globular lipid inclusions in "foam cell," clear or blue in WG stain. PAS positive, diastase resistant.

Sea-blue histiocyte syndrome—deep blue in WG stain, may be a variant of Niemann-Pick.

Lecithin cholesterol:acyltransferase deficiency (L-CAT)—accumulation of intracytoplas-

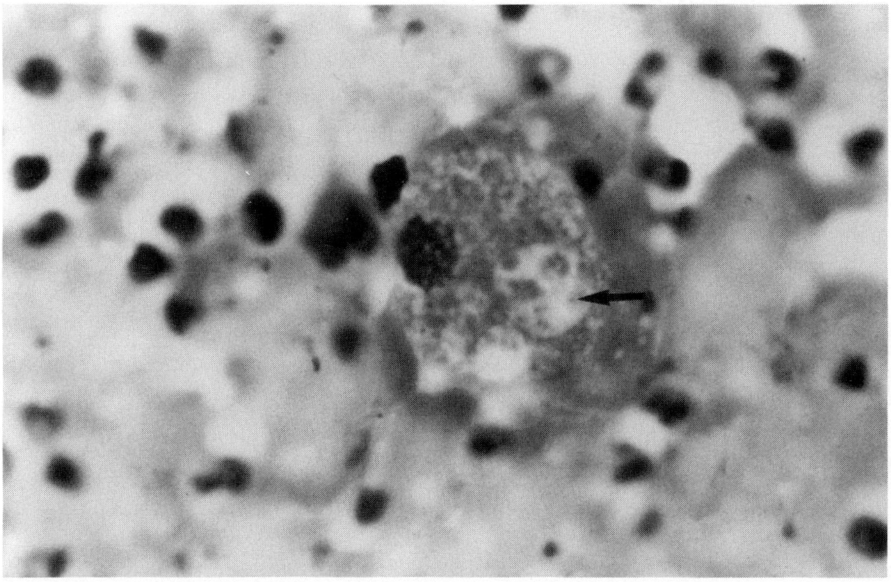

Figure 5 Sea-blue histiocyte is a debris-laden phagocytic macrophase, with plump foamy cytoplasm filled with lipid globules (arrow). The cells are often called "sea blue" because of their distinct color in WG-stained imprints. However, the hematoxylin-and-eosin appearance of the foamy histiocytes is yellowish brown. This type of cell is found in a few storage diseases, a finding that may help in arriving at a correct diagnosis. (Oil immersion, Giemsa.)

mic and extracytoplasmic lipids secondary to inherited deficiency of enzyme normally present in the plasma; manifests in the spleen as splenomegaly and shows in the kidney as glomerular lipid membranous deposition. Spleen is almost always involved, and imprint cytology shows sea-blue histiocytosis in WG stain.

b. *Gangliosidosis*

Tay-Sachs cell—blue in WG stain

c. *Mucopolysaccharidosis*

Hurler and Hunter syndrome—"baloon cells," metachromatic in WG stain, zebra bodies in electron microscopy.

d. *Glycogenoses*

von Gierke's—foamy cells, clear in WG stain, PAS positive, diastase-sensitive inclusions.

2. *Hemophagocytic Syndromes*

Hemophagocytic diseases are often systemic and may show red pulp expansion due to an increase in hemocytophagic histiocytes. The general types identified in the spleen with findings of hemophagocytic cordal macrophages include:

Microorganism-induced: viral, bacterial, or mycoplasma infection
Familial types: rare, fatal, infantile disorders
Neoplasms: mainly NHL of T or NK cell type, may be associated with hemophagocytic syndrome.

3. Langerhans Cell Histiocytosis

Langerhans cell histiocytosis includes a spectrum of "histiocyte-like" disorders with diverse clinical presentation, including Letterer-Siwe disease, Hand-Schuller-Christian disease, and eosinophilic granuloma. Using molecular techniques (HUMARA, human androgen receptor assay), Willman et al. (7) recently reported this disorder as a clonal proliferation of an immune effector—the Langerhans cell. The red pulp is preferentially involved.

4. Disease Associated with Foamy Histiocytosis in Spleen

ITP
Hyperlipidemia
Chronic granulomatous diseases
Gaucher's, Niemann-Pick, Tay-Sachs disease

E. Myeloproliferative Disorders and Leukemias

Chronic myeloproliferative disorders are a group of similar diseases (8) that are clonal, often associated with cytogenetic abnormalities, in which splenomegaly is almost always found. Each syndrome may transform to another. Splenectomy is not usually performed, especially for essential thrombocythemia or polycythemia vera, in which fatal thrombotic complications may be seen. Microscopically, they variably express extramedullary hematopoiesis, immature granulocytes, and megakaryocytes (Fig. 6). These disorders include:

Chronic myeloid leukemia
Polycythemia vera

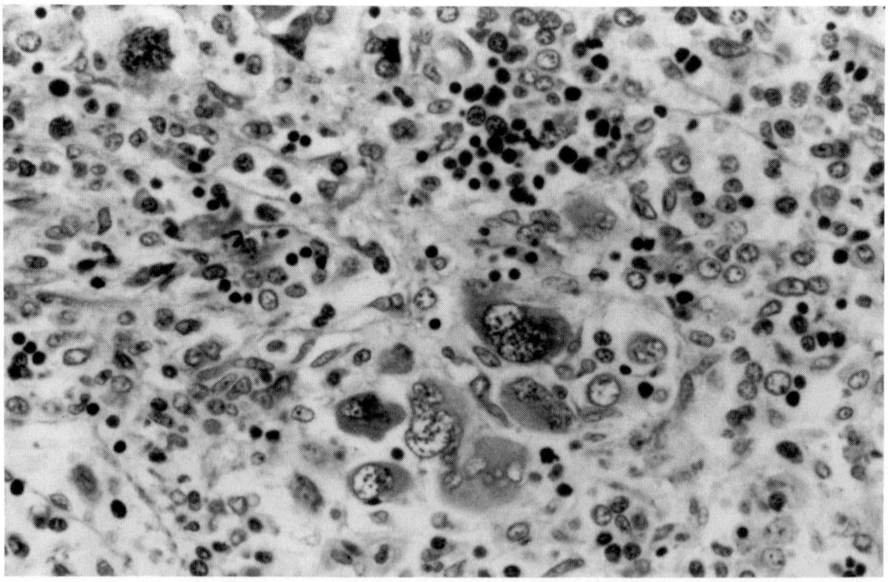

Figure 6 Sinuses and cords infiltrated by clusters of megakaryocytes, immature granulocytes, and erythroid precursors; seen in a number of myeloproliferative syndromes especially those secondary to myelofibrosis with myeloid metaplasia. (×450, PAS.)

Myeloid metaplasia with myelofibrosis
Essential thrombocythemia

Chronic myeloid leukemia (CML) is a clonal Philadelphia translocation (t 9,22)-associated stem cell disorder, which is characterized clinically by a chronic phase followed by either a blastic crisis or accelerated signs of leukemic transformation. Examination of the spleen in the chronic phase reveals an infiltrate of maturing granulocytes. Most of the leukemic process is manifested in the bone marrow, but occasional blast crisis presents in the spleen.

Myeloid metaplasia with myelofibrosis (MMM) denotes a syndrome characterized by maturing extramedullary hematopoiesis resulting in splenomegaly. Although diagnostic features are better appreciated in the bone marrow biopsy, the spleen characteristically is enlarged secondary to the presence of numerous maturing megakaryocytes, red cell and granulocytic precursors in the cords of Billroth and sinuses (Fig. 6).

Polycythemia vera (PV) is a chronic myeloproliferative disorder characterized by splenomegaly and elevated red blood cell mass in the absence of hypoxemia or inappropriate erythropoietin elevation. Splenectomy is contraindicated because it can lead to thrombotic complications. Autopsy findings of the spleen in patients with PV show congestion and minimal extramedullary hematopoiesis.

Essential thrombocythemia (ET) is characterized by persistent thrombocytosis above 1000 $\times 10^9$/L and thromboembolic phenomena. Mild splenomegaly, with platelet trapping in the cords and sinuses, is the usual finding. Splenectomy is contraindicated because of life-threatening thrombotic complications.

Hairy cell leukemia is a B-cell malignancy that manifests characteristics splenic and peripheral blood morphology, cytochemistry, and phenotype. Splenomegaly occurs frequently and demonstrates a leukemic infiltrate involving the red pulp. The cut surface is beefy red, and on microscopic examination reveals infiltration with hairy cells and blood lakes lined by hairy cells. Hairy cells demonstrate strong positivity for acid phosphatase even after treatment with tartrate (tartaric acid-resistant acid phosphatase granules) (TRAP). These cells express monotypic immunoglobulin light chains and coexpress CD11c (myelomonocytic marker) and CD20 (B-cell marker) antigens.

F. Dysproteinemias

Dysproteinemias are abnormal systemic immune reactions which are not self-limited, may be malignant, and may have associated polyclonal or monoclonal gammopathy. Plasmacytosis, lymphoid depletion, prominent red pulp, and peritrabecular fibrosis are observed. Examples are

Angioimmunoblastic lymphadenopathy with dysproteinemia (AILD)
Angiofollicular giant lymph node hyperplasia (Castleman's disease)

IX. CYSTS AND NONHEMATOPOIETIC TUMORS

A. Splenic Cyst

Pseudocyts—about 80% of splenic cysts, so-called false cysts because of the absence of epithelial lining, occur in young adults; there is history of trauma in many patients.
Epithelial—about 20% of splenic cysts, benign, unilocular, mesothelial or squamoid lining,

occur in children and young adults; asymptomatic but may be complicated by rupture or carcinoma.

Parasitic-hydatid cyst or *Echinococcus* cysts—rare except in endemic areas.

B. Benign Splenic Vascular Neoplasms

Hemangioma and *lymphangioma* are the most common of splenic benign tumors, often subcapsular in location. Grossly, hemangioma has bloody cavities and lymphangioma has clear fluid-filled spaces. The vascular channels are lined by flat endothelium.

Littoral cell angioma is very rare but is characterized as distinct vascular lesions composed of anastomosing littoral cell-lined sinuses. The lining cells show histiocytic and endothelial differentiation manifested by phagocytosis and lysozyme and CD68 (KP-1) (histiocyte marker), factor VIII RA (vascular endothelium) positivity.

Splenic hamartoma, also called *splenoma*, is an abnormal tumorlike expansion compressing adjacent normal spleen. It is composed of normal red pulp elements lacking trabeculae or white pulp. It may cause hypersplenism, abdominal discomfort, can even rupture, and may be associated with congenital genetic disease such as tuberous sclerosis. Splenectomy is curative.

Peliosis, characterized by blood-filled cystic spaces, may be associated with peliosis hepatis and an underlying disease such as tuberculosis or carcinomatosis. It may occasionally be seen in patients on anabolic-androgenic steroids.

C. Malignant Vascular Tumors

Hemangioendothelioma—rare vascular tumor of intermediate malignancy.

Angiosarcoma—rare, occurs in older patients, who may have abdominal pain and signs of hypersplenism, it is widely metastatic and fatal within 1 year. Littoral cell angiosarcoma is a variant.

D. Rare Tumors

Metastatic carcinoma—breast, melanoma, and lung cancer account for most cases.

Malignant fibrous histiocytoma—rare, occurs in middle-aged patients, presents with splenomegaly and abdominal pain, is aggressive and widely metastatic

Inflammatory pseudotumor—reactive mass lesion mimicking lymphoma, occurs in middle age as a solitary lesion, microscopically is composed of myofibroblasts and inflammatory cells.

Amyloid tumor or *amyloidoma*—rare, almost always an expression of systemic disease.

Systemic mastocytosis—almost always involves the spleen. Histologically, there is fibrosis and granuloma-like foci around blood vessels composed of mast cells in clusters. Leder's stain (chloroacetate esterase) or toluidine blue for mast cell may help if histology is equivocal.

Follicular dendritic tumor—rare, recently described, multinodular tumor.

Lipoma and myelolipoma—rare.

E. Systemic Vasculitides

Systemic lupus erythematosus may sometimes be associated with fibrinoid necrotizing vasculitis, but typically may produce periarteriolar onion-skin fibrosis. Fibrin thrombi in small vessels in thrombotic thrombocytopenic purpura (TTP) may lead to microangiopathic hemolytic anemia.

Periarteritis nodosa and Churg-Strauss allergic granulomatosis may rarely involve the splenic vessels, characterized by periarteriolar eosinophilia and eosinophilic abscess.

F. Congenital Anomalies

Accessory spleen—10% of normal individuals.
Congenital asplenia—other associated congenital anomalies are seen.
Splenic-gonadal fusion—usually testicular, left sided, may rarely involve the ovary.
Spleno-hepatic or spleno-renal fusion—rare anomalies.

CASE STUDY 1

Patient

Sixty-seven-year-old woman.

Chief Complaint

A left neck "lump" following a bout of flu and common cold.

Medical History

Adult-onset diabetes mellitus and arthritis.

Medications

None.

Physical Examination

Right cervical lymphadenopathy and hepatosplenomegaly and enlarged retroperitoneal lymph nodes. There was a slight papular rash on the patient's neck.

Laboratory Results

Test	Patient result	Reference range
Hemoglobin	11.5 g/dL	14–18 g/dL
Hematocrit	34%	42–52%
WBC count	9500/μL	4,800–10,800/μL
Lymphocytes	56%	20–45%
Platelet count	56,000/μL	150,000–375,000/μL
LDH	700 U/L	30–200 U/L

Cervical lymph node biopsy was performed and diagnosed as low-grade malignant lymphoma. A bone marrow biopsy performed for staging revealed intertrabecular nodules of lymphoma involvement. Peripheral blood smear showed lymphocytosis and Howell-Jolly bodies. The lymphocytes had monocytoid and villous cytoplasm. Due to persistent thrombocytopenia, splenectomy was done. The patient was discharged to home after an unremarkable postoperative recovery.

The spleen weighed 1867 g. The cut surface was firm, red, and showed prominent nodules averaging 0.3 cm in size. Histologically, there was prominent white pulp with confluent and expanded marginal zone surrounding a monotonous nodule of neoplastic cells (see Fig. 4). The red pulp showed infiltrates of monotonous, small to medium-sized lymphocytes with round to irregular nuclear shape and large amounts of pale cytoplasm. Immunophenotypic studies on the cell suspension of the spleen showed a distinct clonal population expressing IgM/D kappa. These cells coexpressed CD19, CD20, and CD22, and lacked CD5, CD10, CD11c, CD23, and CD25. Using touch imprints of the spleen, these cells expressed acid phosphatase and were sensitive to tartrate.

Questions

1. What is the diagnosis?
2. What other splenic lymphomas have to be ruled out?
3. What gene rearrangement result is expected on *bcl-2* and *bcl-1* oncogenes?
4. What is the relationship with low-grade B-cell lymphoma of MALT (mucosa-associated lymphoid tissue lymphoma) and monocytoid B-cell lymphoma? Is splenic B-cell lymphoma with villous lymphocytes synonymous with this condition?

Diagnosis

Splenic marginal zone cell lymphoma (SMZCL).

Discussion

This is a rare disease of elderly women that can be confused with other low-grade lymphomas affecting the spleen. Patients usually present with massive splenomegaly and cytopenias (1). It is generally considered a low-grade lymphoma that corresponds roughly in the Working Formulation with a malignant lymphoma of small lymphocytic type.

At presentation, most patients have bone marrow involvement—described as usually being intertrabecular nodules of small lymphocytes. Staging usually reveals a stage IV disease. There is often lymph node, liver, and peripheral blood involvement, although an absolute lymphocytosis is unusual. The diagnosis is established by a combination of histomorphology, immunophenotype, and gene rearrangement results.

Grossly, the spleen involved by SMZCL is usually large and histologically shows tumor cells concentrically involving the marginal zone, effacing normal germinal centers, and infiltrating the zone around periarteriolar sheath (see Fig. 4). Diffuse red pulp involvement is sometimes present. Immunophenotype shows a monotypic B-cell population lacking CD5, CD23,CD10, and CD11c, markers that tend to rule out small lymphocytic/CLL, mantle cell, follicular center cell lymphoma, and hairy cell leukemia. Gene rearrangement results typically show absence of *bcl-1* or *bcl-2*, oncogenes associated with t(11;14) or t(14;18), respectively.

The differential diagnoses include chronic lymphocytic leukemia/small lymphocytic lymphoma, mantle cell lymphoma, follicular center cell lymphoma, hairy cell leukemia, and prolymphocytic leukemia.

Chronic lymphocytic leukemia/small lymphocytic leukemia is a disease of the elderly. Lymphadenopathy and splenomegaly as well as lymphocytosis (only in CLL) is common. Pseudofollicular center pattern is characteristics of lymph node involvement and cytologically "mature" or well-differentiated lymphocytes are found in the peripheral blood. The spleen shows white pulp replacement by small lymphocytes. The flow cytometry immunophenotype is characteristic: There is dim surface immunoglobulin, and certain markers allow diagnosis (Table 4). A third of the cases show trisomy 12.

Mantle cell lymphoma (MCL) (mantle zone, centrocytic lymphoma, intermediately differentiated lymphocytic lymphoma) is a disease of older adults who often present with generalized

Table 4 Findings in Low-Grade B-Cell Lymphomas/Leukemias That Involve the Spleen

	SMZCL	B-CLL/SL	FCC	MCL	HCL	PLL
CD5	–	+	–	+	–	–
CD10	–	–	+	–/+	–	–
CD11c	–/+	–	–	–	+	–
CD19	+	+	+	+	+	+
CD20	+	+	+	+	+	+
CD23	–	+	–	–	–	–
CD25	–	–	–	–	+	–
IgH	+	+	+	+	+	+
IgL	+	+	+	+	+	+
TcR	–	–	–	–	–	–
bcl-1	–	–	–	+	–	–
bcl-2	–	–	+	–	–	–
Cytogenetics	–	Trisomy 12	t(14;18)	t(11;14)	–	14q+
TRAP	–	–	–	–	+	–

lymphadenopathy. Splenomegaly is common and systemic involvement is seen at presentation in a quarter of the cases. Histologically, the mantle cell lymphocytes show a nodular monotonous effacement of white pulp, and cytologically they show round to irregular and slightly indented nuclear contours and scant cytoplasm. Immunophenotype findings are also characteristic (Table 4). Cytogenetically, a t(11;14)(q13;32) translocation corresponding to overexpression of *bcl-1* oncogene is present in about half to two-thirds of cases.

Follicular center cell lymphoma (follicular lymphoma, nodular poorly differentiated lymphocytic lymphoma, germinal center lymphoma) of small cleaved type is a disease of older adults that typically presents with lymphadenopathy and stage IV disease. The spleen is involved in about half of the cases, and peripheral blood involvement is unusual. Histologically, there is a nodular pattern of white pulp involvement. The nodular pattern of involvement has to be distinguished from other "small cell" lymphomas. Cytologically, tumor cells are small, cleaved predominantly with a mixture of transformed cells. Phenotypically, the neoplastic cells express bright monotypic immunoglobulins, and again show characteristic phenotype (Table 4). The majority of follicular lymphomas have t(14;18)(q32;q21) translocation and overexpress *bcl-2* oncogene. The protein plays a pivotal role in inhibiting apoptosis or programmed cell death.

Prolymphocytic leukemia (PLL) is a malignancy of older male adults characterized by massive splenomegaly and hyperleukocytosis. Absolute lymphocytosis often exceeds 100,000/μL. There is a minimal or absent lymphadenopathy. The spleen shows white pulp involvement by prolymphocytes, which show a prominent nucleolus and generous pale cytoplasm. Phenotypically, by flow cytometry, these cells express bright monotypic immunoglobulin and a set of immunophenotype (Table 4). No characteristic cytogenetic abnormality is seen, but a subset of cases shows 14q+.

Hairy cell leukemia is a disease of older males commonly presenting with splenomegaly. Systemic symptoms are common, and lymphadenopathy is minimal or absent. Pancytopenia is a common laboratory finding. Peripheral blood reveals cells with a generous amount of cytoplasm, some of which show hairy projections on WG stain and phase-contrast microscopy.

Histologically, the spleen shows diffuse red pulp involvement, and blood-filled sinuses. The cytology is often referred to as that of a "fried-egg appearance." Phenotypically, hairy cells express pan-B antigens, with strong expression of surface immunoglobulins, and distinctive phenotype (Table 4). The characteristic cytochemical finding is the presence of abundant cytoplasmic acid phosphatase positive granules that are resistant to tartrate treatment (TRAP positive). Cytogenetic findings are noncontributory.

Splenic marginal zone cell lymphoma (SMZCL) has similarities with monocytoid B-cell lymphoma and low-grade B-cell lymphomas of mucosa-associated lymphoid tissue (MALT), and all are currently regarded as originating from the marginal zone area of the follicles. SMZCL and SLVL are believed to be variants of the same disease (2). Like SMZCL, splenic B-cell lymphoma with circulating villous lymphocytes (SLVL) is a rare disease occurring in the sixth decade, usually affects females, and demonstrates splenomegaly and localized lymphadenopathy. There is often mild lymphocytosis. Cells show a circumferential to relatively polarized villous cytoplasm imparting a villous cytologic appearance. The latter cells are more easily seen on the thicker part of the peripheral blood smear. Histologically, like the SMZCL, the spleen has white pulp involvement of lymphocytes with a moderate amount of clear cytoplasm. The immunophenotype is identical with SMZCL.

References

1. Hammer RD, Glick AD, Greer JP, Collins RD, Cousar JB. Splenic marginal zone lymphoma. Am J Surg Pathol 1996; 20:613–626.
2. Isaacson PG, Matutes E, Burke M, Catovsky D. The histopathology of splenic lymphoma with villous lymphocytes. Blood 1994; 84:3828–3834.

CASE STUDY 2

Patient

Thirty-one-year-old male.

Chief Complaint

Progressive left upper quadrant abdominal pain with radiation toward the left flank.

Medical History

Appendectomy and hernia repair, weight gain of more than 20 lb in the past year.

Family History

The patient has 13 siblings, including one sister with anemia, but none with splenomegaly. His father had "throat cancer" and his mother had colon cancer.

Medications

None.

Physical Examination

No lymphadenopathy. The spleen was palpable three finger-breadths below the left costal margin. The liver was not palpable; there was no jaundice, and neurologic examination was normal.

Courses

An abdominal CT scan demonstrated a homogeneously enlarged spleen. No lymph node enlargement was seen. Bone marrow biopsy showed a hypercellular maturing trilineage hematopoiesis. The patient was discharged, only to come back several days later with severe left upper quadrant pain. Peripheral blood preoperatively showed target cells and mild lymphocytosis. The serum was lipemic. Serum protein electrophoresis demonstrated an albumin at 2.8 g% and all forms of globin at the lower limits of normal. Liver biopsy and laparoscopic splenectomy were performed for a suspected splenic lymphoma. Liver biopsy was normal and the spleen was enlarged 780 g. Cut section show a beefy red appearance, and touch imprint WG showed many sea-blue histiocytes. Flow cytometry of the lymphocytes was not diagnostic for lymphoma. Renal biopsy demonstrated a membranous type of nephropathy with extramembranous and intramembranous deposition of lipids.

Laboratory Results

Test	Patient result	Reference range
Hemoglobin	10.8 g/dL	14–18 g/dL
Hematocrit	31%	42–52%
MCV	82.9 fl	80–94 fl
MCH	29.1 pg	27–31 pg
MCHC	35 g/dl	32–36 g/dl
WBC count	6,200/μL	4,800–10,800/μL
Lymphocytes	56%	20–45%
Platelet count	123,000/μL	150,000–375,000/μL
LDH	152 U/L	30–200 U/L
Urinalysis	300 mg protein, RBCs, WBCs	
BUN	22 mg%	5–20 mg%
Cr	1.3 mg%	0.7–1.4 mg%
Peripheral blood	Target cells	
Lipid profile	Appearance—lipemic	Clear
	Triglycerides 3590 mg/dL	300 mg/dL
	Total cholesterol 610 mg/dL	200 mg/dL
	High-density cholesterol 12 mg%	>35 mg%
	Serum cholesterol ester 16%	60–70%
Special serology	LCAT activity decreased	
Bone marrow	Low iron stores, sea blue histiocytes	

Questions

1. What is the diagnosis?
2. What are sea-blue histiocytes?
3. What is the significance of splenomegaly and lipemia?
4. What is the differential diagnosis?

Diagnosis

Lecithin:cholesterol aceyltransferase deficiency.

Discussion

Lecithin:cholesterol acyltransferase (L-CAT) is a membrane-bound plasma enzyme synthesized in the liver, catalyzing the transfer of a fatty acid from lecithin to cholesterol to form cholesteryl esters and lysolecithin. The absence or deficiency of L-CAT leads to elevation of serum free cholesterol, triglycerides, phospholipids, and a low esterified cholesterol. The deficiency of L-CAT may either be acquired or congenital. Acquired deficiency is secondary to liver disease. The hereditary deficiency is familial, has an autosomal recessive pattern of inheritance, and can be sometimes be traced to families of Scandinavian descent (1).

Hereditary deficiency of L-CAT is rare and appears in about equal frequency in both sexes. Symptoms show toward the second decade of life and progress slowly. Deficiency of this enzyme can result in a rare syndrome that includes diffuse corneal opacities, normocytic normochromic anemia with target cells, sea-blue histiocytosis in the spleen (2), proteinuria, and renal failure. There is heterogeneity in gene mutations as well as the clinical and laboratory presentation. Two distinct phenotypes are observed: the classic L-CAT and "fish eye" disease. Patients with fish eye disease have a selective defect in alpha-L-CAT and a normal cholesterol esterification. In contrast, classic L-CAT patients have abnormal cholesterol esters and increased renal and hematologic abnormalities. The structural gene at chromosome 16q22 usually demonstrates point mutations leading to the production of an abnormal enzyme (3). Diagnosis requires a high index of suspicion and evidence of impairment of enzyme mass or activity (or both) and abnormalities of the lipid profile.

The kidney, the spleen, and to a lesser extent the bone marrow and peripheral blood are affected. The spleen is enlarged in many cases, and sea-blue histiocytosis is a common finding (2). Histologically, there are features found in storage disease: red pulp expansion with cordal accumulation of foamy histiocytes and sea-blue histiocytes. Sea-blue histiocytes are phagocytic histiocytes distended with phospholipid-rich granules and inclusions that have high affinity for the blue dyes of Romanowsky stains (see Fig. 5). In the kidney, foam cells are present and lipid is deposited in subendothelial spaces, mesangium, and glomerular basement membrane under the epithelium as in membranous glomerulonephritis; the latter finding is associated with nephrotic syndrome.

The bone marrow is usually normal but may also show scattered foam cells or sea-blue histiocytes. The peripheral blood shows target cells secondary to an increased content of cholesterol and lecithin in erythrocyte membrane.

Diagnosis can be established using several modalities. Serum is usually lipemic and shows elevated free cholesterol/triglycerides and a low cholesterol ester, as in this case. L-CAT activity is decreased (as in this case) or absent, and the protein is 0–60% of normal (4). Histologically, the clues to the diagnosis include sea-blue histiocytes in the spleen or bone marrow on WG-stained cytologic imprints, target cells in the peripheral blood, and the characteristic splenic and kidney histopathology. Electron microscopy is useful and typically shows dense and myelin bodies—lamellated membranous structures resembling onion rings or rose petals. The kidney biopsy shows foam cells as well as a collection of serpiginous lipid myelin bodies (5).

NOTE ADDED IN PROOFS

Since the manuscript was completed, there has been progress in separating splenic marginal zone lymphoma from extranodal lymphomas of marginal zone origin (low-grade B cell lymphoma of MALT and monocytoid lymphoma) and this entity has been recognized in the progress report of the WHO Classification of Neoplastic Diseases of hematopoietic and lymphoid tissues (9). In addition, blastic transformation of splenic marginal zone lymphoma is documented (10), which suggest that like other low grade lymphomas, rare transformation of this entity is observed.

REFERENCES

1. Hovig T, Gjone E. Familial plasma lecithin:cholesterol acyltransferase (L-CAT) deficiency. Ultrastructural aspects of a new syndrome with particular reference to lesions in the kidneys and the spleen. Acta Pathol Microbiol Scand A, Pathology 1973; 81(5):681–697.
2. Jacobsen CD, Gjone E, Torstein H. Sea-blue histiocytes in familial lecithin:cholesterol acyltransferase deficiency. Scand J Hematol 1972; 9:106–113.
3. Funke H, von Eckardstein A, Pritchard PH, et al. Genetic and phenotypic heterogeneity in familial lecithin:cholesterol acyltransferase (L-CAT) deficiency. Six newly identified defective alleles further contribute to the structural heterogeneity in this disease. J Clin Invest 1993; 91(2):677–683.
4. Taramelli R, Pontoglio M, Candiani G, et al. Lecithin cholesterol acyl transferase deficiency: molecular analysis of a mutated allele. Hum Genet 1990; 85(2):195–199.
5. Faraggiana T, Churg J. Renal lipidoses: a review. Hum Pathol 1987; 18:661–679.

SELECTED READINGS

1. Neiman RS, Wolf BC. Disorders of the Spleen. Philadelphia: Saunders, 1989.
2. Klatt EC, Meyer PR. Pathology of the spleen in the acquired immunodeficiency syndrome. Arch Pathol Lab Med 1987; 111:1050–1053.
3. Collins RD, Neiman RS. Granulomatous diseases of the spleen. In: Ioachim HL, ed. Pathology of Granulomas. New York: Raven Press, 1983:189.
4. Warnke RA, Weiss LM, Chan JKC, Cleary ML, Dorfman RF. Tumors of the lymph nodes and spleen. In: Rosai J, ed. Atlas of Tumor Pathology. Bethesda, MD: Armed Forces Institute of Pathology, 1995:412.
5. Hammer RD, Glick AD, Greer JP, Collins RD, Cousar JB. Splenic marginal zone lymphoma. Am J Surg Pathol 1996; 20:613–626.
6. Foucar K. Bone Marrow Pathology. Chicago: American Society of Clinical Pathologists Press, 1995.
7. Willman C, Busque L, Griffith BB, Favara BF, McClain KL, Duncan MH, Gilliland DG. Langerhans'-cell histiocytosis (histiocytosis-X)—A clonal proliferative disease. N Engl J Med 1994; 331: 154–160.
8. Schumacher HR, Cotelingam JD. Chronic Leukemia: Approach to Diagnosis. Tokyo: Igaku-Shoin, 1993.
9. Jaffe E, Harris N, Diebold J, Muller-Hermelink K. World Health Organization Classification of Neoplastic Diseases of the Hematopoietic and Lymphoid Tissues. Am J Clin Pathol 1999; 111(Suppl. 1) S8–S12.
10. Cualing H, Steele P, Zellner D. Blastic Transformation of Splenic Marginal Zone B-cell Lymphoma. Arch Pathol Lab Medicine 1999. In press.

4

The Non-Hodgkin's Lymphomas and Plasma Cell Dyscrasias

Lynne V. Abruzzo and L. Jeffrey Medeiros
University of Texas M.D. Anderson Cancer Center, Houston, Texas

I. INTRODUCTION

Non-Hodgkin's lymphomas (NHLs) are neoplasms that arise from either B or T lymphocytes, or rarely from cells of the moncyte/histiocyte series. In benign lymph nodes, spleen, and other lymphoid tissues, B and T lymphocytes are localized to different compartments. B cells are concentrated in the follicles and medullary cords of the lymph nodes, and in the follicles of the spleen. They proliferate and form secondary germinal centers in response to antigenic stimulation. Plasma cells secrete immunoglobulin in the medullary cords of the lymph node. T cells are concentrated in the paracortical regions of the lymph nodes, and within the periarterial lymphoid sheaths of the spleen. They are also found in small numbers within lymphoid follicles, where they induce B-cell differentiation. Histiocytes, the tissue counterparts of peripheral blood monocytes, are found preferentially in the subcapsular and medullary sinuses of the lymph nodes, and the cords of Billroth in the splenic red pulp. Most histiocytes are phagocytic; a minority are specialized to present antigen to B and T lymphocytes.

Monoclonal antibodies that are specific for B-cell, T-cell, and histiocyte antigens have become essential to the diagnosis and classification of lymphoid malignancies. Cell lineage and stage of differentiation can be assessed with these antibodies. International workshops for leukocyte typing have developed a standard nomenclature for these monoclonal antibodies. Antibodies that react with the same antigen, or different epitopes of the same antigen, are grouped into the same "cluster of differentiation," or "CD." There are now over 100 CDs reported.

The hallmark of the B lymphocyte is its ability to synthesize immunoglobulin (Ig). Because B lymphocytes express either κ or λ Ig light chain, staining for Ig light chain is used as a marker of clonality. Since a neoplastic clone is derived from a single cell, all of the B cells in a monoclonal population will express the same Ig light chain. In contrast, a polyclonal proliferation of B cells, which is derived from many different precursor cells, will contain a mixture of Igκ and Igλ positive cells. In addition to antibodies that react with immunoglobulins, antibodies that react with pan-B-cell antigens and B-cell-associated antigens have been developed. These antibodies are used to assess the lineage and stage of differentiation of B cells.

Specific monoclonal antibodies also react with T lymphocytes and histiocytes. In contrast to the clonal expression of Ig light chain by malignant B cells, there is no known marker of clonality that is expressed by T cells or histiocytes. However, monoclonal antibodies allow T cells to be separated into subsets, and may demonstrate aberrant T-cell immunophenotypes. Monoclonal antibodies have also shown that histiocytes are a heterogeneous population of cells that contain subpopulations of phagocytic cells and specialized antigen-processing cells.

A small subset of NHLs, designated "null cell" neoplasms, fail to express all lineage-specific markers. The frequency of "null cell" lymphomas is substantially lower (less than 1% of NHLs) than in the past because of the availability of lineage-specific monoclonal antibodies and molecular genetic studies for immunoglobulin and T-cell receptor gene rearrangements.

A. Classification of Non-Hodgkin's Lymphomas

The Rappaport classification of NHL, introduced in 1956, was widely used by pathologists. In this system, non-Hodgkin's lymphomas were first divided by growth pattern, either nodular or diffuse, and then divided by cytology. As knowledge accumulated, additional categories were added to the Rappaport classification (Table 1).

The Rappaport classification was easy to learn, reproducible, and accepted by clinicians. However, as our knowledge of the normal immune system increased, it became apparent that the Rappaport classification was scientifically inaccurate. In an attempt to address the inaccuracies, and to relate lymphoid neoplasms more closely to their normal counterparts, new classification systems were proposed. By the late 1970s, in addition to the classification system of Rappaport, there were the Lukes and Collins, the Kiel, and several other lymphoma classification systems. The resulting situation was one of confusion and controversy.

In an attempt to resolve these differences, the National Cancer Institute funded an international study to test each of the major classification systems on more than 1000 NHLs that had been staged and treated in a relatively consistent manner. The investigators involved in the study jointly developed a Working Formulation of NHL for clinical use (Table 2). They proposed that this formulation be viewed as a common language to be used by investigators to translate one classification scheme into another, rather than as an alternative classification system. It is important to emphasize that the Working Formulation was based purely on histologic data; immunologic and molecular genetic data were not included.

Table 1 Modified Rappaport Classification

Nodular
Lymphocytic, poorly differentiated
Mixed lymphocytic-histiocytic
Histiocytic
Diffuse
Lymphocytic, well differentiated
Lymphocytic, intermediate differentiation
Lymphocytic, poorly differentiated
Mixed lymphocytic-histiocytic
Undifferentiated, Burkitt's type
Undifferentiated, non-Burkitt's type
Histiocytic
Lymphoblastic

Table 2 International Working Formulation

Low grade
A. Malignant lymphoma, small lymphocytic
Consistent with chronic lymphocytic leukemia
Plasmacytoid
B. Malignant lymphoma, follicular, predominantly small cleaved cell
Diffuse areas
Sclerosis
C. Malignant lymphoma, follicular, mixed small cleaved and large cell
Diffuse areas
Sclerosis
Intermediate grade
D. Malignant lymphoma, follicular, predominantly large cell
Diffuse areas
Sclerosis
E. Malignant lymphoma, diffuse, small cleaved cell
Sclerosis
F. Malignant lymphoma, diffuse, mixed small and large cell
Sclerosis
Epithelioid cell component
G. Malignant lymphoma, diffuse, large cell
Cleaved
Noncleaved
High grade
H. Malignant lymphoma, large cell immunoblastic
Plasmacytoid
Clear cell
Polymorphous
Epithelioid cell
I. Malignant lymphoma, lymphoblastic
Convoluted cell
Nonconvoluted cell
J. Malignant lymphoma, small noncleaved
Burkitt's
non-Burkitt's
K. Miscellaneous
Composite
Mycosis fungoides
Histiocytic
Extramedullary plasmacytoma
Unclassifiable

B. The Revised European-American Classification of Lymphoid Neoplasms

Since the International Working Formulation was published in 1982, immunophenotypic and molecular genetic analyses of lymphoid neoplasms have shown that the categories in the Working Formulation are immunologically and molecularly heterogeneous. Recently, a group of hematopathologists, the International Lymphoma Study Group, has proposed a new classification system, the Revised European-American Classification of Lymphoid Neoplasms (REAL) (Table 3). This system incorporates morphologic, immunophenotypic, and molecular genetic data into a provisional classification scheme that attempts to define disease-specific disease entities. Studies are underway to correlate the diagnoses in the Revised European-American Classification with the clinical data.

II. PRECURSOR LYMPHOBLASTIC LYMPHOMA/LEUKEMIA

Lymphoblastic lymphoma (LBL) shares many clinical, histologic, and immunologic features with acute lymphoblastic leukemia (ALL), and these entities appear to represent different clinical manifestations of the same disease. Thus, in the recent proposal by the International Lymphoma Study Group, the term "precursor lymphoblastic leukemia/lymphoma" of either B-cell or T-cell lineage is used to emphasize the close relationship between LBL and ALL. Approxi-

Table 3 Revised European-American Classification of Lymphoid Neoplasms

B-cell lymphoma

I. Precursor B-cell neoplasm: Precursor B-lymphoblastic leukemia/lymphoma

II. Peripheral B-cell lymphomas
  1. B-cell chronic lymphocytic leukemia/small lymphocytic lymphoma
  2. Lymphoplasmacytoid lymphoma/immunocytoma
  3. Mantle cell lymphoma
  4. Follicle center lymphoma
  5. Marginal zone B-cell lymphoma
     Extranodal (MALT type ± monocytoid B cells)
     Provisional subtype: Nodal (± monocytoid B cells)
  6. Provisional entity: Splenic marginal zone lymphoma (±villous lymphocytes)
  7. Hairy cell leukemia
  8. Plasmacytoma/myeloma
  9. B-cell large cell lymphoma
     Subtype: Primary mediastinal (thymic) B-cell lymphoma
  10. Burkitt's lymphoma
  11. Provisional entity: High-grade B-cell lymphoma, Burkitt's-like

T-cell and putative NK-cell lymphomas

I. Precursor T-cell neoplasm: Precursor T-lymphoblastic lymphoma/leukemia

II. Peripheral T-cell and NK-cell neoplasms
  1. T-cell chronic lymphocytic leukemia/prolymphocytic leukemia
  2. Large granular lymphocyte leukemia (LGL).
     T-cell type
     NK-cell type
  3. Mycosis fungoides/Sezary's syndrome
  4. Peripheral T-cell lymphomas, unspecified
     Provisional subtype: Hepatosplenic $\gamma\delta$ T-cell lymphoma
     Provisional subtype: Subcutaneous T-cell lymphoma
  5. Angioimmunoblastic lymphoma
  6. Angiocentric lymphoma
  7. Intestinal T-cell lymphoma (± enteropathy-associated; ITCL)
  8. Adult T-cell lymphoma/leukemia (ATL/L)
  9. Anaplastic large cell lymphoma, CD30+, T- and null-cell types
  10. Provisional entity: Anaplastic large-cell lymphoma, Hodgkin's-like

mately 10–20% of all LBLs, and 80–90% of ALLs, have a precursor B-cell immunophenotype. Approximately 80–90% of LBLs, and 10–20% of ALLs, are of precursor T-cell lineage.

In both precursor B-cell and T-cell lymphoblastic lymphoma/leukemia (LBLL), patients tend to be adolescents and young adults, males outnumber females in a 2:1 ratio, and widespread, supradiaphragmatic lymphadenopathy is common. Patients with precursor B-cell LBLL may present with disease in unusual sites, including subdiaphragmatic lymph nodes, skin and bone. They rarely present with a mediastinal mass. In contrast, precursor T-cell LBLL occurs with a peak incidence in the second decade of life, and most patients present with a mediastinal mass. Peripheral blood involvement is seen in at least one-third of patients with precursor B-cell and T-cell LBLL at presentation, and sometime during the clinical course in most patients who die from the disease. Bone marrow and central nervous system involvement at presentation are adverse prognostic signs. Unless they receive aggressive therapy, patients have a rapidly progressive downhill course with dissemination of tumor to the bone marrow and cerebrospinal fluid. Children and adolescents with LBLL respond favorably to therapeutic regimens designed after those used for ALL, which differ from those used for other clinically high-grade NHL. Adults with precursor LBLL appear to require more aggressive therapy.

The histologic findings in precursor B-cell and T-cell LBLL are identical. The normal lymph node architecture is effaced by a diffuse and relatively monotonous proliferation of small to medium-sized cells that have a tendency to stream out into perinodal tissues. The neoplastic cells have fine nuclear chromatin and scant cytoplasm (Fig. 1). The nuclei may be either convoluted or round. Mitotic figures are numerous, and a "starry sky" pattern, which results from individually necrotic cells having been ingested by macrophages, may be seen. No histologic features correlate with the immunophenotype of the neoplastic cells.

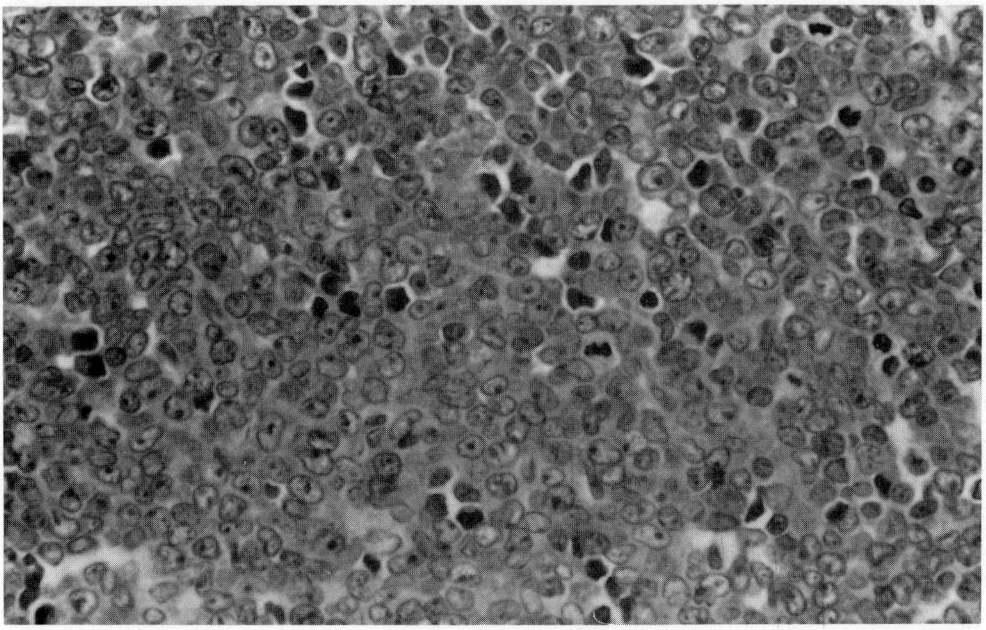

Figure 1 Precursor T-cell lymphoblastic lymphoma. The neoplastic cells are small with blastic chromatin and scant cytoplasm. (Hematoxylin-eosin, 528X.)

The immunophenotypes of precursor LBLL reflect the sequence of antigen expression by non-neoplastic lymphoid cells during development. Precursor B-cell LBLL initially express the CD10 (CALLA; common acute lymphoblastic leukemia antigen) and CD19 antigens on their surfaces, followed by CD22, and then CD20. These antigens are detectable in the cytoplasm before they are expressed on the cell surface. The neoplastic cells do not express surface immunoglobulin.

Precursor T-cell LBLL express T-cell antigens in patterns that correspond closely to the stages of normal thymocyte differentiation. The earliest precursor T-cell LBLLs correspond to the prothymoctye stage. They express the T-cell antigens CD2 and CD7. The CD7 antigen is the earliest T-cell-specific antigen, and is expressed before T-cell receptor β-chain gene rearrangement. The CD2 antigen is the E rosette receptor. They also express the activation antigen CD38 and the proliferation marker CD71, the transferrin receptor. T-cell neoplasms that correspond to the cortical thymocyte stage express the CD1 and CD5 antigens, and are either CD4– CD8– or CD4+ CD8+. At this stage the CD3 antigen is present in the cytoplasm, but may not be expressed on the cell surface. Thus, it may be detected by immunohistochemical stains, but not by flow cytometry. T-cell LBLL of the late cortical or medullary stage of thymic differentiation express surface CD3 antigen, and either a T-helper/inducer (CD4+ CD8–) or T-suppressor/cytotoxic (CD4– CD8+) immunophenotype.

An extremely useful marker in the diagnosis of both precursor B-cell or T-cell LBLL is terminal deoxynucleotidyl transferase (TdT). TdT is a distinct type of DNA polymerase that is normally present only in immature lymphocytes. It is involved in the process of gene rearrangement, and is believed to add extra nucleotide bases between the variable (V), diversity (D), and joining (J) regions of the genes undergoing rearrangement.

Similar to surface antigen expression, the antigen receptor genes appear to rearrange sequentially, with a developmental hierarchy. Ig heavy-chain gene rearrangement is followed by kappa light-chain and then lambda light-chain gene rearrangement, if neither Ig kappa light-chain gene allele is functionally rearranged. Precursor B-cell LBLL always contain Ig heavy-chain gene rearrangements. More mature neoplasms also have Ig light-chain gene rearrangements.

Precursor T-cell LBLL also show patterns of T-cell receptor (TCR) gene rearrangement that correspond to the stages of T-cell differentiation. The TCRδ gene rearranges first, followed by the TCRγ and the TCRβ genes; the TCRα locus rearranges last. In a small subset of cases of T-cell LBLL with an early thymic immunophenotype, only rearrangements of the TCRδ and/or TCRγ genes may be identified. In the remaining T-cell LBLL with early thymic or mid to late thymic immunophenotypes, all of the TCR genes are rearranged.

Lineage infidelity or promiscuity is common in precursor LBLL. Immunoglobulin heavy-chain gene rearrangements occur in approximately 30% of precursor T-cell neoplasms Similarly, TCR gene rearrangements occur in up to 80% of precursor B-cell LBLL.

Many nonrandom chromosomal translocations have been identified in precursor B-cell and T-cell LBLL. These translocations may be divided into two groups. In one group, and oncogene is brought into continuity with an antigen receptor gene locus. This results in deregulated expression of the corresponding protein, but a fusion protein is not created. In the other group, two nonantigen receptor gene loci are joined to form a fusion gene. This results in a chimeric protein that posesses novel structural and functional features. In precursor B-cell neoplasms, the most common translocations are t(9;22), t(1;19), and translocations that involve 11q23. In precursor T-cell neoplasms, the t(1;14)(p32;q11) and del 1p may be most common.

The t(9;22)(q34;q11), also known as the Philadelphia chromosome, is one of the most common chromosomal translocations. It is detected in 5% of children and approximately 20–

25% of adults with precursor B-cell ALL. This translocation joins the *c-abl* gene at chromosome 9q34 with the bcr locus at 22q11. It results in a chimeric mRNA transcript that encodes a fusion protein with increased tyrosine kinase activity.

The t(1;19) is commonly found in precursor B-cell lymphoblastic leukemia of "pre-B cell" (cytoplasmic IgM positive) type. This translocation joins the *E2A* gene on chromosome 1 with the *PbxI* gene on chromosome 19. A chimeric transcription factor is produced that is believed to deregulate genes involved in leukemogenesis. Similarly, translocations that involve 11q23, such as t(4;11), t(9;11), and t(11;19), occur in infants with precursor B-cell lymphoblastic leukemia. This translocation involves the *MLL* gene on chromosome 11q23. These infants present with a high white blood cell count, have an increased frequency of central nervous system involvement, and have a poor prognosis. The t(1;14)(p32;q11) has been described in up to 30% of cases of precursor T-cell lymphoblastic leukemia. In this translocation the *tal-1* gene (also know as *SCL* and *tcl-5*) and the *SIL* gene are joined as a result of illegitimate recombination.

III. NON-HODGKIN'S LYMPHOMAS OF MATURE B-CELL LINEAGE

A. B-Cell Chronic Lymphocytic Leukemia/Small Lymphocytic Lymphoma

Because the malignant cells usually resemble small, mature-appearing lymphocytes, this neoplasm has been classified as well differentiated lymphocytic lymphoma (Rappaport) and malignant lymphoma, small lymphocytic type (Working Formulation). The cytology and immunophenotype of the malignant cells of chronic lymphocytic leukemia (CLL) and nodal-based small lymphocytic lymphoma (SLL) are identical. Although patients with SLL present with lymphadenopathy, subclinical peripheral blood involvement can be found in many cases and progression to CLL occurs frequently. Conversely, many patients with CLL subsequently develop lymph node involvement. They are classified as B-cell chronic lymphocytic leukemia/small lymphocytic lymphoma (B-CLL/SLL) in the Revised European-American classification because they are believed to represent different manifestations of the same disease (See Chapter 9, "Chronic Leukemias").

Lymph nodes involved by CLL/SLL show effacement of the normal lymph node architecture by a proliferation of lymphoid cells with a diffuse growth pattern. Rarely the growth pattern may be vaguely nodular. The neoplastic cells are predominantly small round lymphocytes with inconspicuous nucleoli, clumped chromatin, scant cytoplasm, and infrequent mitotic figures (Fig. 2a). However, slightly larger lymphoid cells with more prominent nucleoli (prolymphocytes) and larger cells with round vesicular nuclei and central nucleoli (paraimmunoblasts) are also found. Prolymphocytes and paraimmunoblasts may be scattered throughout the neoplasm or they may form clusters called "proliferation centers" or "pseudofollicular growth centers" (Fig. 2b). At low power, proliferation centers may impart a vaguely nodular appearance. Although mitotic figures may be seen in proliferation centers, the presence of proliferation centers does not indicate a more aggressive course. However, cases of CLL/SLL with a high mitotic rate (>30 mitotic figures per 20 high-power fields) and necrosis behave more aggressively, and have been designated by some investigators as being in "accelerated phase."

The immunophenotype of CLL/SLL is characteristic. The neoplastic cells express mono-

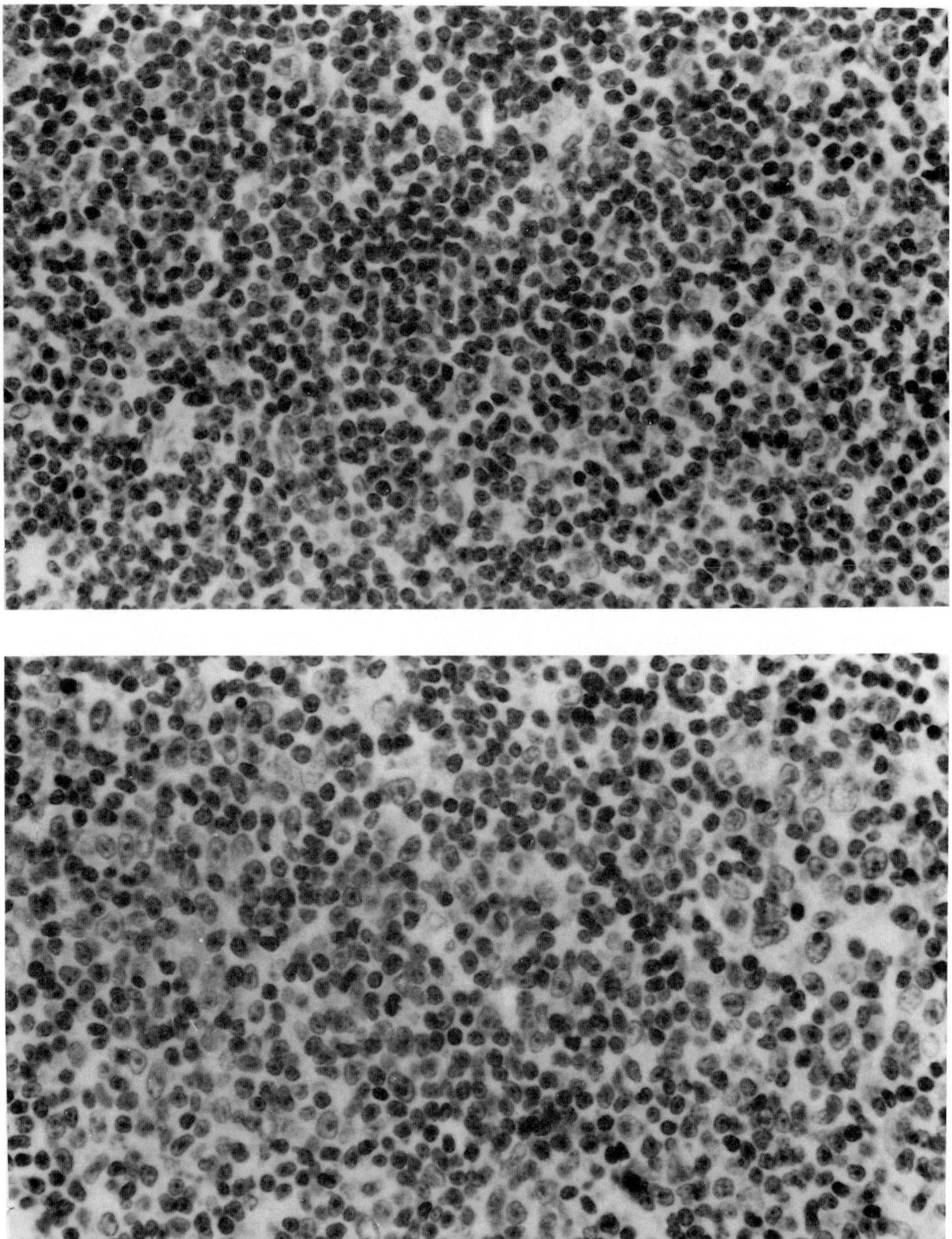

Figure 2 B-cell small lymphocytic lymphoma. (a) The neoplastic cells are small with condensed nuclear chromatin. (b) Proliferation centers with prolymphocytes and paraimmunoblasts help to distinguish B-cell small lymphocytic lymphoma from mantle cell lymphoma. (Hematoxylin-eosin, 528X.)

typic surface IgM (dim) and usually IgD ($\kappa > \lambda$), and the pan-B-cell antigens CD19, CD20 (dim), and CD79a. The B-cell-associated antigens CD21 and CD23 are usually positive, and CD10 (CALLA) is usually negative. The cells express the CD5 antigen, a pan-T-cell antigen that is also expressed on a small subpopulation of normal B-cells. Expression of CD5 is characteristic of CLL/SLL and mantle cell lymphoma. However, CLL/SLL is usually CD23-positive and mantle cell lymphoma is usually CD23-negative.

Molecular genetic studies of the antigen receptor genes in CLL/SLL have demonstrated rearrangement of the Ig heavy and light chain genes. The TCR genes are usually in the germline configuration, although occasional cases may have TCR gene rearrangement, i.e., lineage promiscuity.

Chromosomal abnormalities have been found in CLL/SLL. Trisomy 12 is most common and is seen in approximately one-third of cases. However, chromosomal translocations are unusual. Approximately 5–10% of cases of CLL/SLL contain the t(2;18) or t(18;22). These translocations juxtapose the *bcl-2* oncogene at 18q21 with the kappa (2p13) or lambda (22q11) light chain genes. Rare cases have been reported to contain the t(14;18)(q32;q21), which is characteristic of follicle center cell lymphomas.

Chronic lymphocytic leukemia/small lymphocytic lymphoma may undergo histologic progression to diffuse large cell or large cell immunoblastic lymphoma; this phenomenon has been given the eponym Richter's syndrome. Most cases of large cell NHL that arise in the setting of CLL/SLL have been shown to represent histologic progression of the neoplastic clone. Immunophenotypic and molecular diagnostic studies have demonstrated that both neoplasms express the same immunoglobulin light chain, have the same chromosomal abnormalities, or have an identical pattern of immunoglobulin gene rearrangements. However, in a subset of cases, the large cell NHL and the CLL/SLL have different molecular genetic findings. Although some of these large cell lymphomas may represent transformation, others may have arisen independently. Infrequently, patients with CLL/SLL develop neoplasms that morphologically and immunophenotypically resemble Hodgkin's disease, designated as the Hodgkin's variant of Richter's transformation.

B. Lymphoplasmacytoid Lymphoma/Immunocytoma

These neoplasms have been classified as well-differentiated lymphocytic lymphoma-plasmacytoid (Rappaport) and malignant lymphoma, small lymphocytic, plasmacytoid (Working Formulation). Many different types of NHL may exhibit plasmacytoid differentiation, and previously have been designated lymphoplasmacytoid lymphoma/immunocytoma (LPL/I). However, the Revised European-American classification recommends that the term LPL/I be reserved for those neoplasms that are associated with a monoclonal IgM paraprotein, and often with the syndrome of Waldenstrom's macroglobulinemia. Some observers use the term Waldenstrom's macroglobulinemia as a pathologic diagnosis; we prefer to consider Waldenstrom's macroglobulinemia as a clinical syndrome, usually associated with LPL/I.

Patients with LPL/I may present with a variety of signs and symptoms, including bleeding from mucous membranes, lymphadenopathy, hepatosplenomegaly, peripheral neuropathy, and central nervous system abnormalities. Constitutional symptoms are anemia and more common than in patients with CLL/SLL. Most patients have a monoclonal serum IgM paraprotein, greater than 1 g/dL; one-third of patients develop hyperviscosity and the clinical syndrome of Waldenstrom's macroglobulinemia. Lymphadenopathy is generalized, but is usually modest compared to CLL/SLL. Hepatosplenomegaly is common. Involvement of peripheral blood and extranodal sites is relatively uncommon. Analogous to Richter's syndrome in CLL/SLL, some patients with LPL/I subsequently develop a high-grade NHL.

Lymph nodes involved by LPL/I tend to retain their underlying architecture. The neoplastic cells preferentially involve the medullary cords and paracortex, and spare the sinuses. The cells infiltrate the capsule and extend into the perinodal adipose tissue. The neoplastic cells show a spectrum of differentiation that ranges from small mature-appearing lymphocytes to plasma cells. The extent of plasmacytoid differentiation varies between cases, and may be subtle or marked. The neoplastic cells may contain cytoplasmic globules (Russell bodies) or intranuclear pseudo-inclusions (Dutcher bodies) of IgM. In the bone marrow, the neoplasm may focally or extensively involve the medullary space in a nodular (but not truly follicular) or diffuse pattern. Particularly in the bone marrow, cytologic evidence of plasmacytoid differentiation may not be apparent.

Immunophenotypic studies have shown that LPL/I express monotypic surface IgM ($\kappa > \lambda$) and pan-B-cell antigens such as CD19, CD20, and CD22. They are negative for IgD and T-cell antigens, including CD5. In cases with more extensive plasmacytoid differentiation, the neoplastic cells may lose surface expression of CD20 antigen and immunoglobulin, and may express cytoplasmic immunoglobulin, like normal plasma cells. The cells also express plasma cell-associated antigens, such as CD38.

As expected for a neoplasm of mature B-cells, the Ig heavy and light chain genes show clonal rearrangements, and the TCR genes are usually in the germline configuration. There are no characteristic chromosomal abnormalities, although numerical abnormalities have been reported rarely.

C. Mantle Cell Lymphoma

The term mantle cell lymphoma (MCL) has been suggested recently as the most appropriate name for a neoplasm previously known as malignant lymphoma, intermediate lymphocytic type; lymphocytic lymphoma of intermediate differentiation; centrocytic lymphoma; and mantle zone lymphoma. The majority of these neoplasms would be classified as malignant lymphoma, diffuse small cleaved cell type, in the Working Formulation.

Patients with MCL are usually older adult men with generalized disease. The male-to-female ratio is approximately 3 to 1. Most patients present with stage III or IV disease. Most have generalized lymphadenopathy and bone marrow involvement. The liver and spleen are commonly involved. Peripheral blood involvement is unusual and is associated with a poor prognosis. However, subclinical peripheral blood involvement can be detected frequently with sensitive molecular diagnostic techniques. Extranodal disease may occur, usually in association with lymph node involvement. Patients may present with numerous polyps involving the gastrointestinal tract below the level of the gastrointestinal junction, referred to in the literature as multiple lymphomatous polyposis of the intestine. Although MCL are composed of small, relatively mature-appearing lymphoid cells, they behave aggressively.

The lymph node architecture is effaced by a proliferation of lymphoid cells with a diffuse or vaguely nodular growth pattern. In some cases the malignant cells selectively involve the mantle zones that surround reactive germinal centers, and give the neoplasm a mantle zone pattern. The infiltrate of MCL is composed of a monotonous population of small lymphoid cells with slightly to clearly irregular nuclear contours, clumped chromatin, and scant cytoplasm (Fig. 3). Although MCL show a wide spectrum of nuclear irregularity between cases, in an individual case the neoplastic cells are uniform. In contrast to CLL/SLL, pseudo-follicular growth centers, large transformed-appearing cells, and cells with plasmacytoid differentiation are not seen in MCL.

Unlike CLL/SLL, MCLs do not transform to large cell lymphoma. However, in a subset

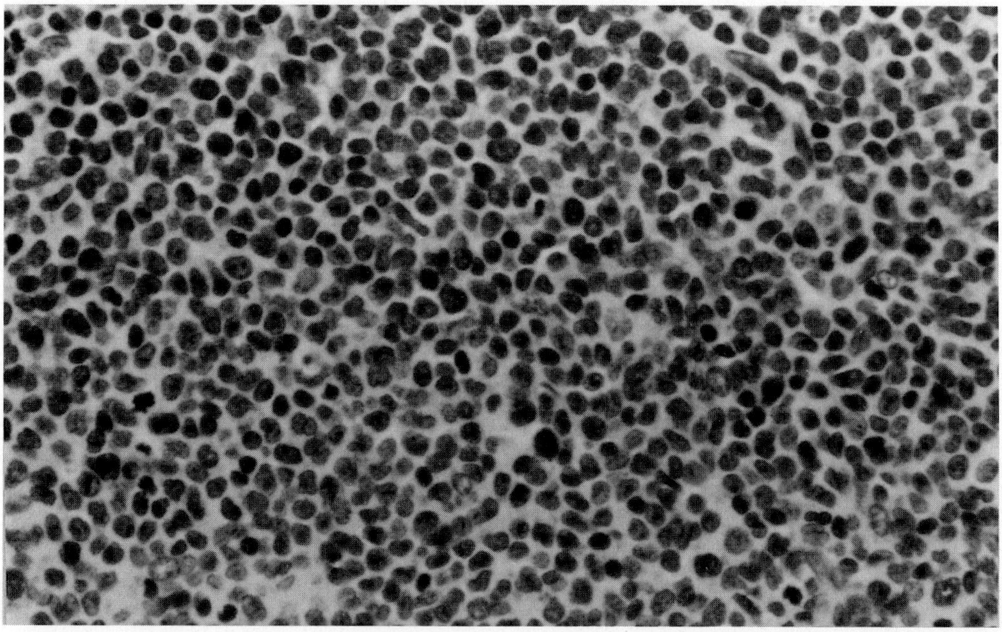

Figure 3 Mantle cell lymphoma. The neoplastic cells are small with condensed nuclear chromatin and slightly irregular nuclear contours. The infiltrate is monotonous. (Hematoxylin-eosin, 528X.)

of MCLs, the neoplastic cells are slightly larger with finely dispersed nuclear chromatin and mitotic figures are numerous. These neoplasms have a more aggressive clinical course, and are designated the blastoid variant of MCL.

Immunophenotypic studies have demonstrated that MCLs express monotypic surface IgM and IgD, and pan-B-cell antigens. In contrast to other B-cell neoplasms, MCLs are more likely to express lambda than kappa immunoglobulin light chains. Like CLL/SLL, the neoplastic cells express the CD5 antigen. However, CLL/SLL is usually CD23-positive and MCL is usually CD23-negative. In addition, the density of CD20 antigen and immunoglobulin on the surface of MCL cells is characteristically dense, or "bright" by flow cytometry.

MCLs have clonal rearrangements of the Ig heavy and light chain genes. The TCR genes are usually in the germline configuration. Most cases of MCL contain evidence of the t(11; 14)(q13;q32), either by conventional cytogenetic analysis or by molecular diagnostic techniques. This translocation juxtaposes the immunoglobulin heavy-chain regulatory region on chromosome 14 with the *bcl-1* gene (also known as PRAD-1) on chromosome 11, and results in overexpression of the corresponding protein, cyclin D1, a cell cycle protein that is not normally expressed by lymphoid cells. It is believed that the cells are unable to exit the cell cycle.

D. Follicle Center Cell Lymphoma, Follicular

Follicle center cell lymphomas have been previously designated as nodular (Rappaport), and follicular (Working Formulation). The natural history of follicle center cell lymphomas is to become diffuse and accumulate large lymphoid cells. The recent Revised European-American

Classification emphasizes that all follicle center cell lymphomas are the same biologic entity, at different stages of disease evolution.

Follicle center lymphoma (FCL) is the most common type of NHL in the United States, and comprises approximately 20% of adults with NHL. These NHL affect primarily older adults, with a peak incidence in the fifth and sixth decades. They are rare in patients under the age of 20 years. Men and women are equally affected. Whites are affected more often than blacks. Most patients have clinical stage III or IV disease at the time of diagnosis. Involvement of the lymph nodes, spleen, liver and bone marrow is common. Some patients with FCL present with or develop clinical evidence of leukemia. The characteristic cell in the peripheral blood has a deeply clefted nucleus and has been referred to as a "buttock cell." Leukemic involvement does not appear to influence prognosis, unless the peripheral white blood cell count is high. Subclinical involvement of the peripheral blood is common when sensitive techniques, such as Southern blot hybridization, are used.

In spite of the presence of widespread disease, patients with FCL composed of predominantly small cleaved lymphoid cells (grade I) have relatively long survival. Progression from a purely follicular to a follicular and diffuse pattern is common, and the presence of a diffuse component without a significant increase of large lymphoid cells does not affect survival. As the number of large lymphoid cells increases, the tumor becomes a mixture of small cleaved and large cells (grade II), and then is composed of predominantly large lymphoid cells (grade III). A diffuse component usually accompanies the increased number of large cells. Patients with mixed FCL also have an indolent clinical course, although their survival is shorter than patients with grade I neoplasms. Patients with grade III FCL clearly have a more aggressive clinical course than patients with other subtypes of FCL, and require aggressive therapy.

The lymph node architecture is partially or completely effaced by neoplastic follicles, with a paucity of interfollicular tissue (Fig. 4). A large absolute number of follicles has been found to be the most reliable criterion of lymphoma. Unlike the lymphoid follicles in reactive follicular hyperplasia, the follicles of follicle center cell lymphoma are of relatively uniform size, lack a well-defined lymphoid cuff, and lack polarization of germinal centers. Tingible body macrophages are usually less frequent in neoplastic follicles than in reactive follicles. Plasmacytoid differentiation is rare in all subtypes of FCL.

The distinction between grade I, II and III FCL is based on arbitrary criteria that are not shared by all pathologists. At the NCI, the distinction between grades has been based on the counting of the number of large noncleaved lymphoid cells present. In grade I, predominantly small cleaved cell subtype, large lymphoid cells are infrequent (Fig. 5). In grade II, mixed small cleaved and large cell subtype, the neoplastic follicles contain > 5 large lymphoid cells per 400× microscopic field. In grade III, the neoplastic follicles are composed predominantly of large noncleaved lymphoid cells. In neoplasms in which the neoplastic follicles contain different mixtures of cells, we grade the neoplasm on the basis of the follicles with the greatest number of large noncleaved lymphoid cells.

Immunophenotypic studies have shown that FCL are neoplasms of mature B-cell lineage. Most grade I and II neoplasms strongly express surface Ig, but up to 50% of grade III neoplasms are Ig-negative. Of the neoplasms that express Ig, most express IgM ($\kappa > \lambda$). However, approximately 25% express IgG or IgA. All FCL strongly express pan-B-cell markers such as CD19, CD20, and CD22, and most are positive for the B-cell-associated antigen CD10 (CALLA). The B-cell antigens CD21 and CD23, and all T-Cell antigens, including CD5, are negative.

Follicle center lymphomas have rearrangements of the Ig heavy and light chain genes. The TCR genes are usually in the germline configuration. The molecular hallmark of FCL is the

Figure 4 Follicle center lymphoma, follicular. The neoplasm has a nodular growth pattern that mimics normal lymphoid follicles. (Hematoxylin-eosin, 53X.)

t(14;18)(q32;q21) chromosomal translocation. Cytogenetic and molecular genetic analyses have demonstrated the t(14;18) in more than 90% of cases. This translocation juxtaposes the *bcl-2* oncogene on chromosome 18q21 with the joining region of the Ig heavy chain gene on chromosome 14q32. It results in the overexpression of bcl-2 protein, which prevents programmed cell death (apoptosis).

E. Marginal Zone B-Cell Lymphoma

This category in the Revised European-American Classification includes low-grade lymphomas that were originally designed as low-grade B-cell lymphoma of the mucosa-associated lymphoid tissue (MALT) and monocytoid B-cell lymphoma. Both MALT-lymphoma and monocytoid B-cell lymphoma are thought to represent different clinical presentations of the same B-cell neoplasm. Splenic marginal zone lymphoma is closely related to these neoplasms. Monocytoid B-cell lymphoma, low-grade B-cell lymphoma of MALT, and splenic marginal zone lymphoma are believed to arise from normal marginal zone B-cells in the lymph node, their extranodal counterparts, or spleen, respectively. A feature shared by all of the marginal zone B-cell lymphomas is that they have distinctive histologic findings that are not easily or reproducibly classified in previously published classification schemes.

1. Low-Grade B-Cell Lymphoma of Mucosa-Associated Lymphoid Tissue (MALT)

Before the advent of immunologic and gene rearrangement techniques, the diagnosis of extranodal low-grade B-cell lymphoma was made infrequently in patients without a history of nodal low-grade NHL. Instead, extranodal infiltrates composed of small round or slightly irregular

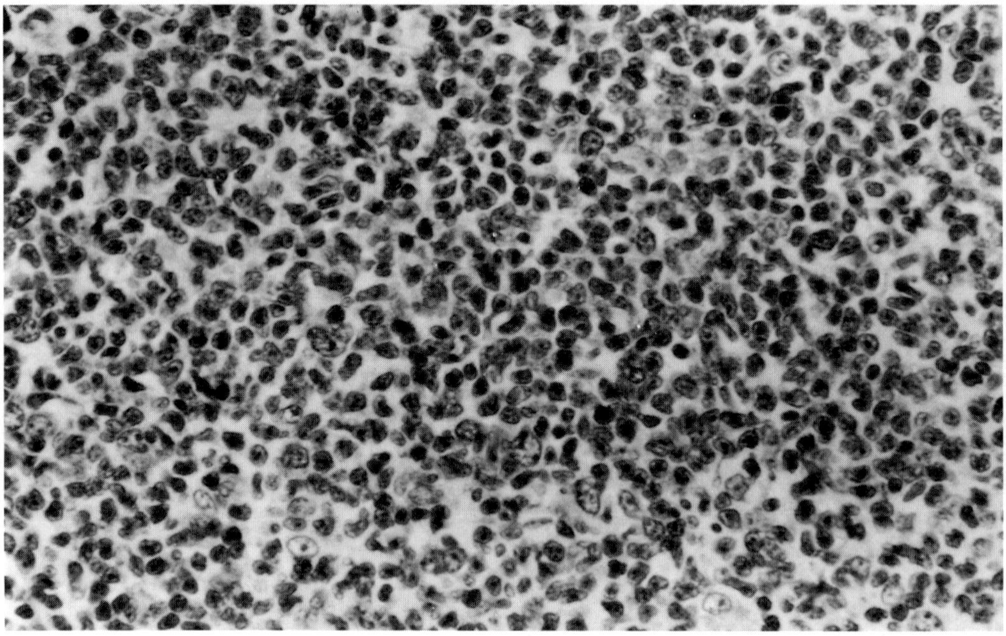

Figure 5 Follicle center lymphoma, follicular, cytologic grade I (predominantly small cell). The cellular composition is monotonous. The neoplasm is composed predominantly of small cleaved cells with occasional large noncleaved cells. (Hematoxylin-eosin, 528X.)

lymphoid cells, often admixed with plasma cells, histiocytes, and lymphoid follicles were classified as "pseudo-lymphomas," since clinical studies showed that these lesions pursued an indolent clinical course. Immunophenotypic and gene rearrangement studies have since shown that most "pseudo-lymphomas" express monotypic Ig light chain and contain clonal Ig gene rearrangements. Thus, these lesions are now classified as low-grade B-cell lymphomas, and most cases represent low-grade B-cell lymphomas of MALT.

Low-grade B-cell lymphomas of MALT were originally recognized by Isaacson and Wright as a subset of gastrointestinal lymphomas in European patients that resembled immunoproliferative small intestinal disease (also know as Mediterranean lymphoma). Isaacson and colleagues then identified similar neoplasms arising in the lung and salivary gland, and suggested that these neoplasms arose from lymphoid tissue associated with mucosal surfaces. However, MALT-lymphomas were identified subsequently in a variety of extranodal sites including the thyroid gland, thymus, breast, conjunctiva, gallbladder, cervix, larnyx, trachea, skin, and kidney, as well as other sites. Thus, the term MALT lymphoma is somewhat misleading, since not all MALT-lymphomas arise in mucosal surfaces. Two common findings in MALT-lymphomas are the presence of glandular epithelium and chronic inflammation, either preceding or accompanying the tumor. For example, Sjögren's syndrome is common in patients with low-grade B-cell lymphoma of salivary gland MALT.

Both low-grade and high-grade lymphomas arising in MALT have been recognized. Since high-grade MALT lymphomas and high-grade nodal lymphomas behave similarly, we will focus this discussion on the distinctive clinical and histologic features of low-grade MALT-lymphomas.

Clinically, low grade B-cell lymphomas of MALT tend to remain localized for prolonged intervals. Patients may present with a long history of clinical findings that may be confused with an inflammatory process. When MALT lymphomas disseminate, they tend to spread to other extranodal sites, unlike nodal low-grade lymphomas. Despite the indolent clinical behavior of localized low-grade B-cell lymphomas of MALT, patients with disseminated MALT-lymphomas behave similarly to patients with disseminated nodal low-grade B-cell lymphomas.

Four histologic findings are present in most low-grade B-cell lymphomas of MALT: a population of centrocyte-like cells, lymphoepithelial lesions, reactive lymphoid follicles, and occasional large lymphoid cells. The neoplastic centrocyte-like (CCL) cells exhibit a range of cytologic appearances: lack of nucleoli, small lymphocytes (which may show plasmacytic differentiantion), monocytoid B cells, and small cleaved lymphocytes. Some of the neoplasms are biphasic, one component of small lymphoid cells with scant cytoplasm and the other component with extension plasmacytoid differentiation.

The CCL cells have a marked tendency to invade epithelium and form small clusters or larger aggregates, called lymphoepithelial (LE) lesions (Fig. 6). In the stomach, LE lesions in small endoscopic biopsy specimens are diagnostically helpful because they usually correlate with malignancy. At other MALT sites, LE lesions may be found in both benign and malignant processes. Reactive lymphoid follicles are usually present in MALT lymphomas, and are usually surrounded by neoplastic CCL cells (Fig. 7). The CCL cells may infiltrate the follicles (referred to as "follicular colonization") and give the neoplasm a nodular appearance on low magnification. However, these neoplasms are not truly of follicle center cell origin.

Although the features described above are common to all low-grade B-cell lymphomas of MALT, there are site-specific differences. For example, lymphoid tissue is not normally pres-

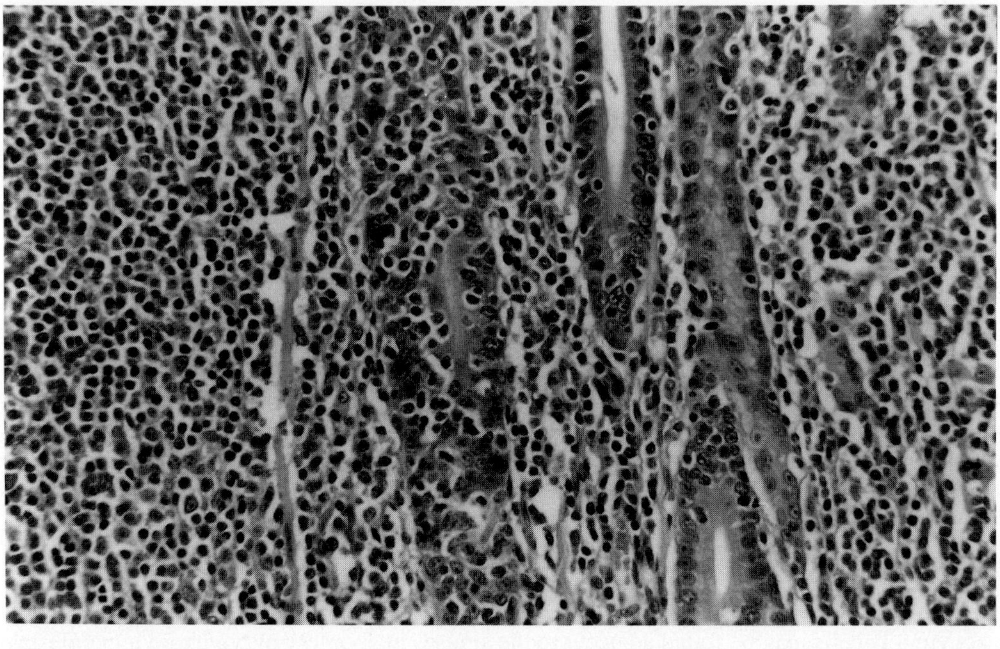

Figure 6 Marginal-zone B-cell lymphoma (low-grade B-cell lymphoma of MALT). The neoplastic cells invade the gastric epithelium to form lymphoepithelial lesions. (Hematoxylin-eosin, 264X.)

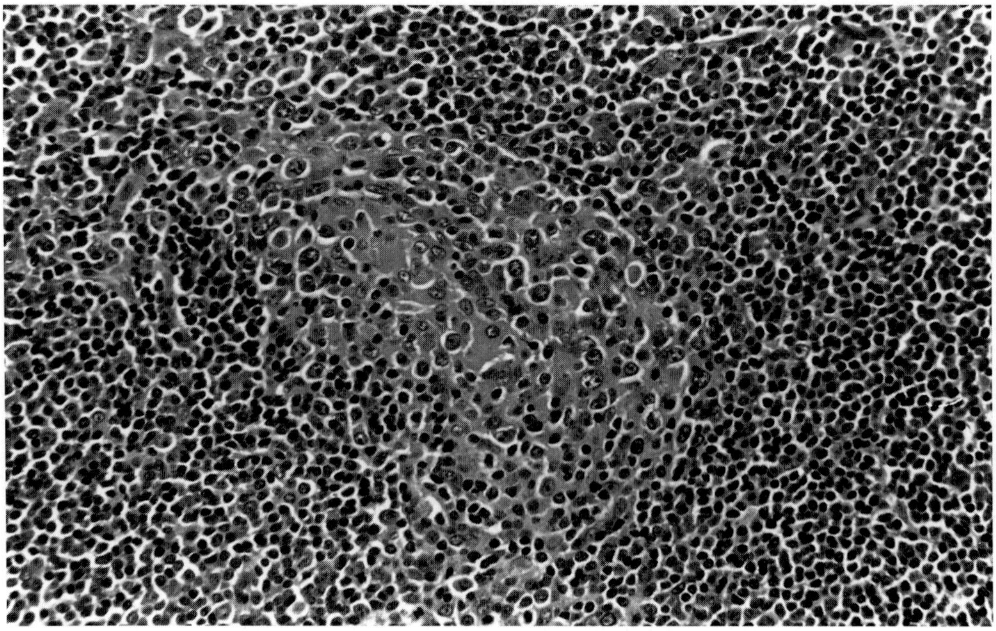

Figure 7 Marginal-zone B-cell lymphoma (low-grade B-cell lymphoma of MALT). The neoplastic cells surround a reactive germinal center. (Hematoxylin-eosin, 264X.)

ent in the stomach. Benign gastric MALT is acquired, probably in response to *Helicobacter pylori* infection. Approximately 30% of cases of *H. Pylori*-induced chronic gastritis are associated with lymphoid follicles. Over 90% of gastric MALT lymphomas are associated with *H. pylori* infection. Recent reports also have shown that benign MALT tissue and low-grade B-cell lymphomas of gastric MALT may regress following antibiotic therapy appropriate for *H pylori*.

In the normal adult lung, MALT tissue is poorly developed, and inflammatory conditions usually precede the development of low-grade B-cell lymphoma of pulmonary MALT. Two inflammatory diseases that are frequently associated with pulmonary MALT lymphoma are Sjögren's syndrome and lymphoid interstitial pneumonia. Similarly, low-grade B-cell MALT lymphomas of the salivary gland are usually associated with Sjögren's syndrome, and Hashimoto's thyroiditis often precedes MALT lymphomas of the thyroid gland.

Immunophenotypic studies have shown that low-grade B-cell lymphomas of MALT express monotypic IgM ($\kappa > \lambda$) and pan-B-cell antigens. They typically do not express IgD, the B-cell-associated antigens CD10, CD21, or CD23, and the T-cell antigens, including CD5.

Low-grade B-cell lymphomas of MALT have clonal Ig heavy- and light-chain gene rearrangements. TCR genes are usually in the germline configuration. There are no known specific chromosomal abnormalities associated with lymphomas. However, trisomy 3 has been identified by FISH in approximately half of low-grade B-cell lymphomas of MALT.

2. *Monocytoid B-Cell Lymphoma*

Monocytoid B-cells may be found adjacent to the sinuses in a variety of lymphoid hyperplasias, most typically in toxoplasma lymphadenitis and AIDS-associated lymphoid hyperplasia. These cells have cytologically bland oval to reniform nuclei and abundant clear cytoplasm with easily appreciated cell membranes. Malignant lymphomas have been recognized that morphologically and immunophenotypically resemble monocytoid B-cells, and have been called "monocytoid B-cell lymphoma" (MBCL) (Fig. 8). These neoplasms are believed to arise from the lymph-node marginal zone, the nodal counterpart of low-grade B-cell lymphomas of MALT.

Patients with MBCL are usually elderly, and women are affected more often than men. Most patients present with lymphadenopathy, usually clinical stage I or II, that involves lymph nodes of the cervical and parotid regions. The parotid gland is involved in 10–20% of patients, and most of these patients have Sjögren's syndrome. In less than one-third of cases, patients present with widespread disease. Liver, spleen, and bone marrow involvement are uncommon, even in patients with disseminated disease. When nodal and extranodal sites are involved concurrently, the neoplasm in extranodal sites closely resembles low-grade B-cell lymphoma of MALT.

Most patients reported with localized MBCL respond well to localized therapy, either surgical excision or local irradiation. Patients with generalized disease respond more poorly to therapy, similar to patients with other types of low-grade nodal NHL. Patients with high clinical stage disease are also at greater risk for transformation to high-grade lymphoma, and patients may develop composite lymphoma (i.e., MBCL coexistent with another type of NHL).

Lymph nodes involved by MBCL have a pale appearance due to the abundant clear cytoplasm of the neoplastic cells. Monocytoid B-cell lymphomas have a propensity to involve the marginal zones and surround the sinuses of the lymph node. In most cases, MBCL either completely efface the lymph node architecture, or involve the marginal zones and perisinusoidal regions, infiltrate the perifollicular compartments of the lymph node, and spare the germinal centers. In a minority of cases, the neoplasm is confined to the perisinusoidal region and is

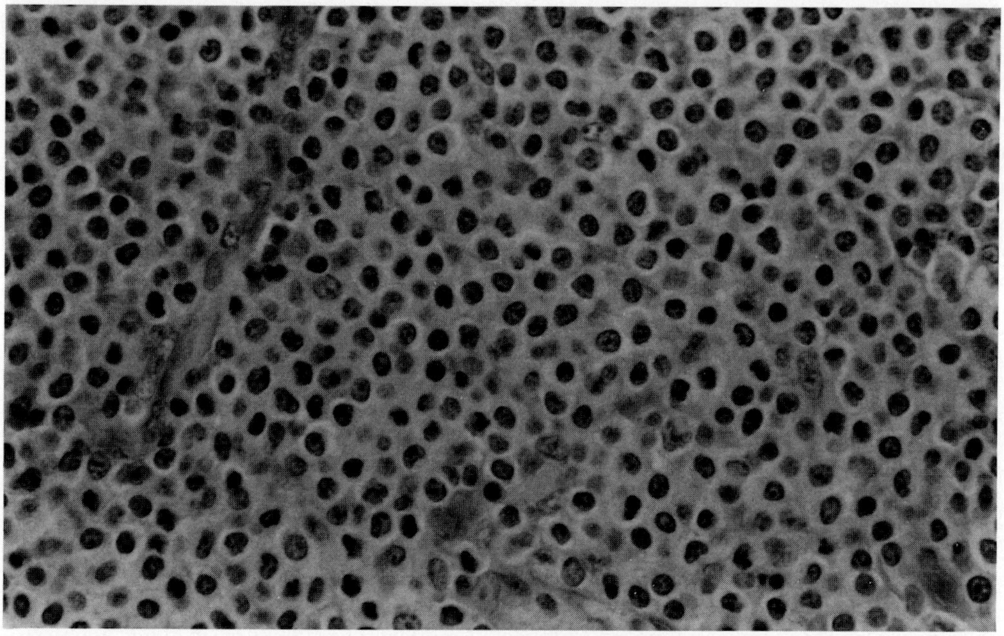

Figure 8 Marginal-zone B-cell lymphoma (monocytoid B-cell lymphoma). The neoplastic cells have small nuclei with round to slightly irregular nuclear contours, condensed chromatin, and abundant clear cytoplasm with discernible cell borders. (Hematoxylin-eosin, 528X.)

difficult to distinguish from reactive monocytoid B-cell hyperplasia without immunophenotypic or gene rearrangement studies.

Immunophenotypic studies have shown that MBCLs are mature B-cell neoplasms that express monotypic Ig ($\kappa > \lambda$), usually IgM, and pan-B-cell antigens. The cells usually do not express IgD or the B-cell-associated antigens CD10, CD21, and CD23. They are negative for pan-T-cell antigens, including CD5.

Monocytoid B-cell lymphomas have clonal Ig heavy- and light-chain gene rearrangements. The TCR genes are usually in the germline configuration. Although conventional cytogenetic studies have identified a variety of abnormalities, no characteristic chromosomal translocations have been described.

3. Splenic Marginal Zone Lymphoma

These neoplasms are believed to arise from splenic marginal-zone B cells, and are closely related to other marginal-zone B-cell lymphomas. Splenic marginal zone lymphoma (SMZL) is currently recognized as a provisional category in the Revised European-American Classification. Cases with prominent peripheral blood involvement also have been called splenic B-cell lymphoma with villous lymphocytes.

Patients with SMZL are usually elderly, and women are affected more commonly than men. Patients usually present with marked splenomegaly, and often have anemia and/or thrombocytopenia. Systemic symptoms are usually absent. Most patients have generalized disease with involvement of lymph nodes, liver, and bone marrow in addition to the spleen. When the peripheral blood is involved, the neoplastic cells often have irregular or villous cytoplasmic projections and resemble hairy-cell leukemia cells. Most patients with SMZL have clinically indolent disease. However, some patients may have a more aggressive course, as is the case for other marginal zone B-cell lymphomas.

In the spleen the neoplastic cells preferentially involve the marginal zones that surround the lymphoid follicles of the white pulp. When the infiltrate is extensive, the cells replace the lymphoid follicles and extend into the red pulp. The neoplastic cells have central round, bland nuclei and relatively abundant clear cytoplasm. Mitotic figures are rare. Occasional large lymphoid cells are always present. SMZL that involves lymph nodes resembles MBCL.

Immunophenotypic studies have shown that SMZCLs are mature B-cell neoplasms. They express monotypic Ig light chain ($\kappa > \lambda$), usually IgM and IgD, and pan-B-cell antigens. A subset express IgG and are IgD negative. The neoplastic cells usually express the B-cell-associated antigen CD21, but usually fail to express the B-cell antigens CD10 and CD23. They are negative for the pan-T-cell antigens, including CD5. Unlike hairy cell leukemia, SMZL are negative for the CD11c and CD25 antigens, and for tartrate resistant acid phosphatase (TRAP).

Relatively few cases of SMZCL have been studied using molecular techniques. Splenic marginal-zone cell lymphomas contain clonal Ig heavy- and light-chain gene rearrangements. The TCR genes are in the germline configuration. There are no known specific chromosomal abnormalities.

F. Diffuse Large B-Cell Lymphoma

1. General Features

This category as defined in the Revised European-American Classification includes neoplasms previously designated as diffuse histiocytic lymphoma (Rappaport), and the categories of diffuse mixed small and large cell, diffuse large cleaved or noncleaved cell, and large cell immunoblastic (Working Formulation).

Diffuse large B-cell lymphomas (DLBCL) are aggressive neoplasms. These neoplasms have a diffuse growth pattern. They are composed of neoplastic cells with nuclei greater in size than the nuclei of benign macrophages, which are always admixed with the neoplastic cells. Mitotic figures are usually numerous. In the Working Formulation, the neoplastic cells are described as large cleaved cells, large noncleaved cells, and immunoblasts Although many neoplastic large B cells fit these cytologic categories, neoplastic large cells exhibit a spectrum of differentiation and often have intermediate cytologic features. Furthermore, diffuse large B-cell lymphomas are commonly composed of a mixture of these cell types. While some clinical studies have suggested a poorer prognosis for immunoblastic lymphomas as compared with large-cell lymphomas, other studies have not found any differences in the clinical features or response to therapy. For these reasons, large cleaved, large noncleaved, and large-cell immunoblastic B-cell lymphomas are combined into one category, diffuse large B-cell lymphoma, in the Revised European-American Classification.

Immunophenotypic studies have shown that DLBCL are neoplasms of mature B-cell lineage. Approximately two-thirds of cases express monotypic Ig ($\kappa > \lambda$), usually IgM. A subset of cases express IgA or IgG; IgD is usually negative. Approximately one-third of DLBCL are surface immunoglobulin-negative. Plasmacytoid lymphomas commonly express monotypic cytoplasmic Ig. DLBCL express pan-B-cell antigens, and a subset are CD10 positive. They are negative for pan-T-cell antigens. Most express activation markers, such as CD25 and CD38, and have a high proliferative rate (Ki-67 and CD71 positive).

Diffuse large B-cell lymphomas have clonal rearrangements of the Ig heavy and light chain genes. The TCR genes are usually in the germline configuration. A subset of cases have the t(14;18) by conventional cytogenetics or rearrangement of the *bcl-2* oncogene by molecular diagnostic techniques. These lymphomas may represent histologic transformation of FCL. Patients with de-novo DLBCL with *bcl-2* rearrangement have an increased tendency to relapse compared to histologically similar tumors without *bcl-2* rearrangement, similar to the behavior of FCL. Another subset of DLBCL have translocations or other abnormalities that involve chromosome 3q27. This locus is the site of the *bcl-6* gene, a zinc finger transcription factor and putative oncogene. The *bcl-6* gene is rearranged in approximately one-third of these neoplasms, more often in those that arise in extranodal sites.

2. Extranodal Diffuse Large B-Cell Lymphomas

Approximately 25–50% of DLBCL arise in extranodal sites. There is evidence to suggest that DLBCL that arise in extranodal sites have a different pathogenesis than histologically similar neoplasms that arise in nodal locations. For example, extranodal DLBCL are commonly localized and may be cured with surgical excision and/or radiation therapy. Nodal DLBCL have a relatively high frequency of t(14;18) or *bcl*-2 gene rearrangement, and rarely have *c-myc* gene rearrangement. In contrast, extranodal DLBCL infrequently have the t(14;18) or *bcl-2* gene rearrangement, and may have *c-myc* rearrangement. There also may be differences between extranodal DLBCL that arise in different extranodal sites.

3. Primary Mediastinal Large B-Cell Lymphoma

The mediastinum contains lymph nodes and the thymus gland. Mediastinal lymphomas may be either primary, localized to the mediastinum, or secondary, as a part of widespread lymph node-based disease. Primary mediastinal large B-cell lymphomas have distinct clinicopathologic and histologic features and, therefore, have been proposed as a provisional category in the Revised European-American Classification.

The median age of affected patients is the fourth decade, and the male-to-female ratio is

1 to 2. Patients typically present with large, bulky masses that cause local symptoms such as cough, chest pain, shortness of breath, or superior vena cava syndrome. Most neoplasms are localized at time of diagnosis. The prognosis is relatively good if patients receive combination chemotherapy and irradiation. Relapses commonly occur at extranodal sites.

Primary mediastinal large B-cell lymphomas have a diffuse growth pattern They are composed of large lymphoid cells that exhibit a spectrum of cytologic appearances: large cleaved, large noncleaved, immunoblasts, and rarely small noncleaved. Sclerosis is common, mitotic figures are usually numerous, and the neoplastic cells often have clear cytoplasm (Fig. 9).

The immunophenotype and molecular genetic features of primary mediastinal large B-cell lymphomas are similar to other nodal diffuse large B-cell lymphomas. They express pan-B-cell antigens, are usually negative for CD10 and CD21, and are often Ig-negative. They have clonal Ig heavy- and light-chain gene rearrangements. The TCR genes are usually in the germline configuration. The *bcl-2* gene is in the germline configuration, and Epstein-Barr virus is not identified.

4. T-Cell-Rich B-Cell Lymphoma

T-cell-rich B-cell lymphomas (TCRBCL) are malignant lymphomas of B-cell origin in which the majority of cells in the biopsy specimen are reactive T cells. The predominance of T cells in these neoplasms may lead to an erroneous assessment of T-cell lineage and, in the past, many of these cases were classified as diffuse mixed small and large lymphomas of T-cell lineage.

The growth pattern of TCRBCL is diffuse. They are composed predominantly of small, cytologically bland T-cells. Numerous benign histiocytes also may be present (Fig. 10a).

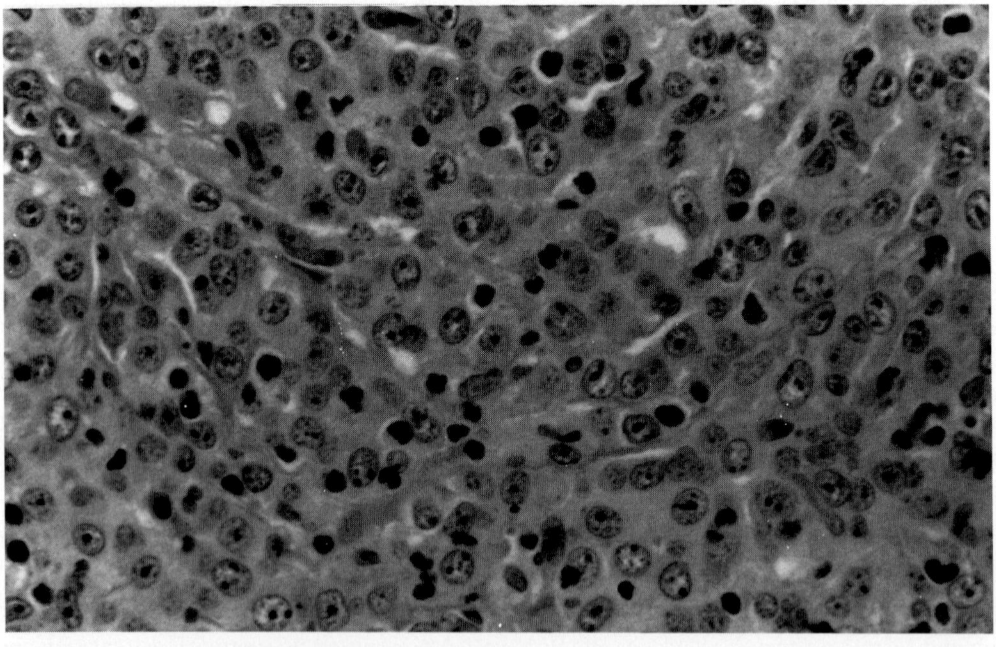

Figure 9 Primary mediastinal B-cell lymphoma. The neoplasm has a diffuse growth pattern with fine sclerosis. The neoplastic cells are large. (Hematoxylin-eosin, 528X.)

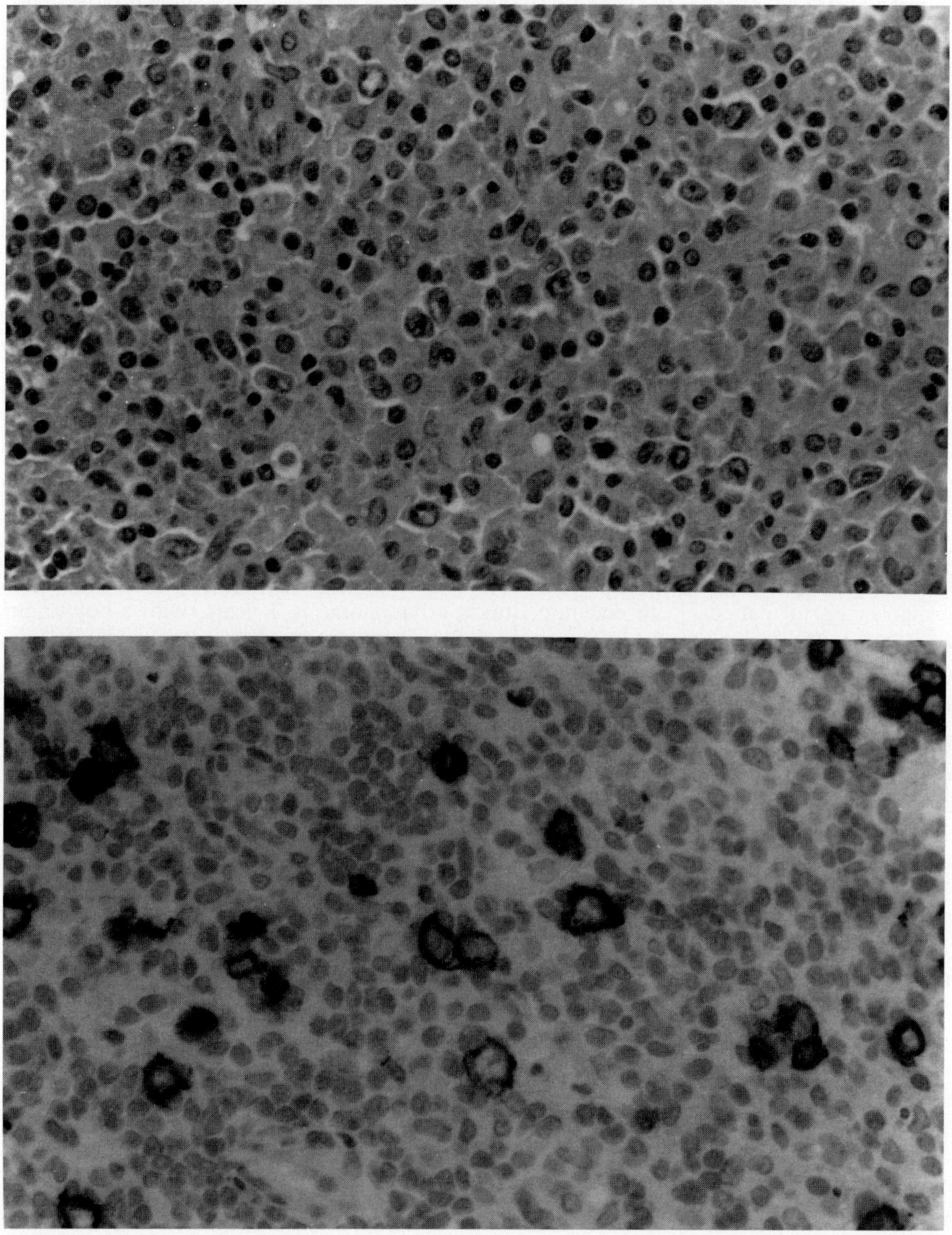

Figure 10 T-cell-rich B-cell lymphoma. (a) The majority of the cells are small reactive T cells and histiocytes. The neoplastic cells are large. (b) Immunohistochemical stain for CD20 accentuates the large neoplastic cells. (a, Hematoxylin-eosin, 528X; b, Immunoperoxidase, 528X.)

Within this infiltrate, often representing less than 5–10% of all cells, are scattered large, cytologically atypical lymphoid cells of B-cell lineage (Fig. 10b).

Because the neoplastic cells are relatively infrequent, it is often difficult to demonstrate monotypic Ig light chain expression. However, the large cells are B cells that express a variety of pan-B-cell antigens. These neoplasms contain clonal Ig heavy- and light-chain gene rearrangements. The TCR genes are usually in the germline configuration. A subset of TCRBCL have the t(14;18) or *bcl-2* gene rearrangements. The presence of the t(14;18) or *bcl-2* gene rearrangement in such a subset supports the opinion that TCRBCL is an unusual histologic manifestation of DLBCL, rather than a distinct clinicopathologic entity.

G. Burkitt's Lymphoma

These neoplasms have been designated previously as undifferentiated, Burkitt's type (Rappaport), or small noncleaved cell, Burkitt's type (Working Formulation). The small noncleaved cell category in the Working Formulation also includes neoplasms of non-Burkitt's type. Small noncleaved cell, non-Burkitt's (Burkitt-like) lymphomas are considered as a separate provisional group in the Revised European-American Classification and will be discussed separately.

Burkitt's lymphoma may be divided into three clinical groups: endemic (African), sporadic (nonendemic), and AIDS-associated. Endemic Burkitt's lymphoma was first described in equatorial Africa. Evidence of Epstein-Barr virus (EBV) infection is present in 95% of patients. The median age of patients with endemic Burkitt's lymphoma is 7 years, with a boy-to-girl ratio of 3 to 1. The jaw, either the maxilla or mandible, is involved in 60% of patients. Patients also may present with large abdominal masses that involve retroperitoneal structures or gastrointestinal tract, or with involvement of the gonads.

Sporadic Burkitt's lymphoma occurs in industrialized nations. EBV infection is present in approximately 25% of patients. Most patients are in the second or third decades of life, with a male-to-female ratio of 3 to 1. Most patients present with large abdominal, frequently ileocecal, masses. Other sites that are commonly involved include abdominal and peripheral lymph nodes, pleura, and pharynx. The jaw is involved infrequently. In patients with either endemic or sporadic Burkitt's lymphoma, bone marrow and central nervous system are uncommonly involved at presentation (approximately 10–20% of cases), but are frequently involved later in the clinical course. AIDS-associated Burkitt's lymphoma occurs in the setting of human immunodeficiency virus-1 (HIV-1) infection. Approximately 50% of cases are EBV-associated. Lymph nodes are extranodal sites are commonly involved.

Because the neoplasm is usually widely distributed at presentation and has an extremely rapid clinical course, aggressive systemic chemotherapy is the treatment of choice. With combination chemotherapy regimens, approximately 80% of patients, including those with high-stage disease, may respond completely and have long-term survival.

The endemic, sporadic, and AIDS-associated types of Burkitt's lymphoma are histologically indistinguishable (Fig. 11). At low power, the neoplasm grows as and expansile mass that diffusely infiltrates contiguous tissues. Tingible-body macrophages are almost always scattered throughout the tumor. The relatively clear cytoplasm of the macrophages in a background of blue neoplastic cells imparts a "starry sky" appearance. The neoplastic cells are round to ovoid, strikingly monotonous, and uniform in shape. The nuclei are the same size or smaller than the nuclei of the benign macrophages. The nuclear membrane is prominent, and the chromatin is coarse with two to five distinct, basophilic nucleoli. Mitotic figures are numerous.

Immunophenotypic studies of endemic, sporadic, and AIDS-associated Burkitt's lymphomas show similar findings. These neoplasms are of mature B-cell lineage. They express mono-

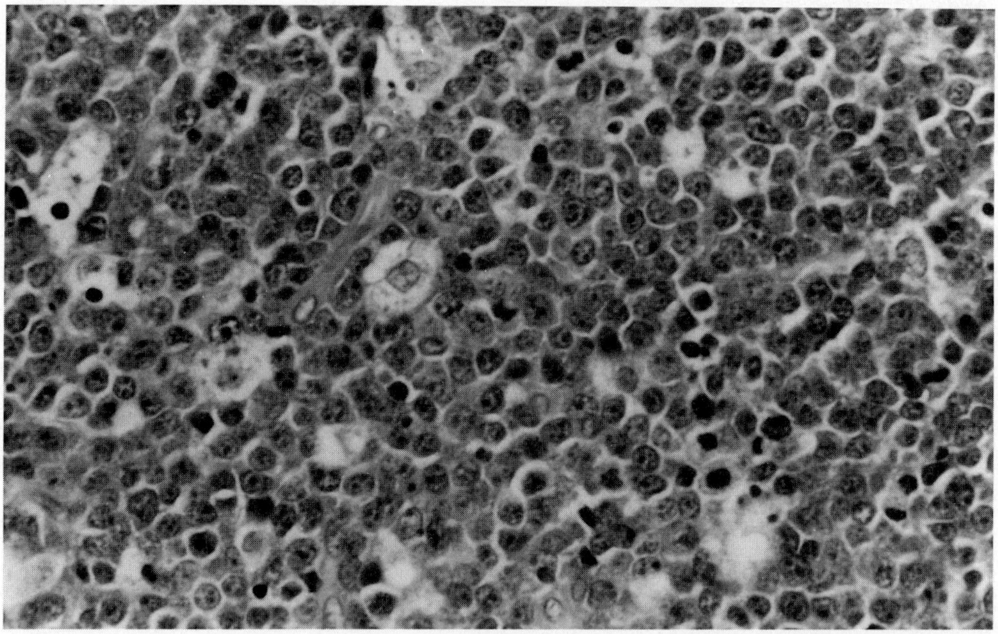

Figure 11 Burkitt's lymphoma. A starry-sky pattern is present. The nuclei of the neoplastic cells are monotonous, contain one to several distinct nucleoli, and are medium-sized, approximately the size of benign histiocyte nuclei. (Hematoxylin-eosin, 528X.)

typic IgM ($\kappa > \lambda$), pan-B-cell antigens, and the CD10 antigen. Virtually all of the neoplastic cells express proliferation markers, such as CD71 and Ki-67. They are negative for pan-T-cell antigens, including CD5.

Burkitt's lymphomas have clonal Ig heavy- and light-chain gene rearrangements. The TCR genes are usually in the germline configuration. Approximately 80% of cases carry the t(8;14)(q24;q32). The remaining cases have one of two variant translocations, either the t(2;8)(p11;q24) or the t(8;22)(q24;q11). These translocations juxtapose the *c-myc* oncogene at 8q24 with either the Ig heavy chain (14q32), κ light chain (2p13), or λ light chain (22q11) genes. The translocation deregulates the *c-myc* oncogene, and results in constitutive production of *c-myc* protein, which drives proliferation.

The t(8;14) chromosomal translocations are distinctive in endemic and sporadic Burkitt's lymphoma. In endemic Burkitt's lymphoma, the breakpoint on chromosome 8 occurs far 5' to the location of the *c-myc* gene. The breakpoint on chromosome 14 usually occurs within the joining region of the Ig heavy chain gene. In contrast, in sporadic Burkitt's lymphoma, the breakpoint on chromosome 8 occurs within the *c-myc* gene, usually in the first exon or in adjacent flanking sequences. The breakpoint on chromosome 14 usually occurs within the Ig heavy-chain switch region. The breakpoints in Burkitt's lymphomas that occur in AIDS patients are similar to sporadic cases.

H. High Grade B-Cell Lymphoma, Burkitt-Like

These lymphomas have been designated as undifferentiated, non-Burkitt's type (Rappaport), and small noncleaved cell, non-Burkitt's type (Working Formulation). In the Revised European-American Classification these tumors are recognized as a provisional category.

Most patients with small noncleaved cell non-Burkitt's (or Burkitt-like) lymphoma are adults, but children may be affected. The male-to-female ratio is approximately 2 to 1. Lymph nodes are involved more often than extranodal sites, but extranodal sites are frequently involved. Involvement of the bone marrow and Waldeyer's ring is more common in patients with Burkitt-like than Burkitt's lymphomas. Burkitt-like lymphoma responds to combination chemotherapy, and is potentially curable.

The histologic features of Burkitt-like lymphoma resemble Burkitt's lymphoma. The cytologic features of the neoplastic cells are intermediate between Burkitt's lymphoma and diffuse large B-cell lymphoma. Like Burkitt's lymphoma, the nuclei of the malignant cells are the same size or smaller than benign macrophages. However, like diffuse large B-cell lymphoma, there is greater nuclear pleomorphism, and the nuclear chromatin is more vesicular with more prominent nucleoli (Fig. 12). In some cases it may not be possible to distinguish between Burkitt-like and diffuse large B-cell lymphoma.

Immunophenotypic studies have demonstrated that Burkitt-like lymphomas are of mature B-cell lineage. They express monotypic IgM ($\kappa > \lambda$), and pan-B-cell antigens. These neoplasms also express activation antigens, such as CD25 and CD38, and proliferation antigens. Molecular genetic studies have shown clonal Ig heavy- and light-chain gene rearrangements. The TCR genes are in the germline configuration in most cases. The *bcl*-2 gene is rearranged in up to 30% of cases, *c-myc* rearrangements are rare, and EBV may be present in a minority of cases. These immunophenotypic and molecular findings are similar to diffuse large B-cell lymphomas.

Because of the clinical, histologic, immunophenotypic, and genetic similarities between

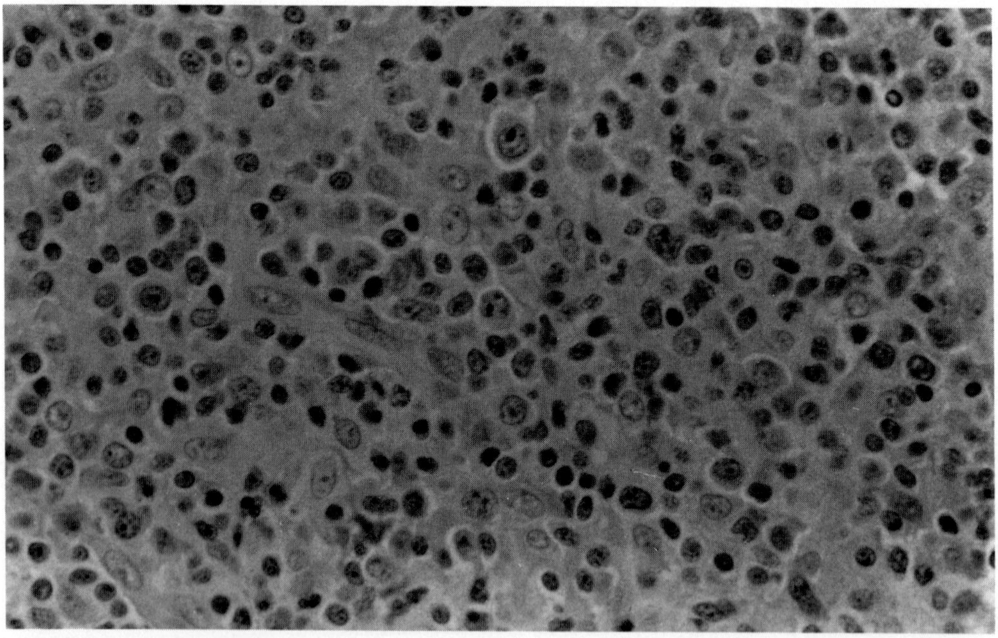

Figure 12 High-grade B-cell lymphoma, Burkitt-like. A starry-sky pattern is present and the tumor cells are medium-sized. Unlike Burkitt's lymphoma, the nuclear size is more variable and the chromatin is more vesicular. (Hematoxylin-eosin, 528X.)

Burkitt-like and diffuse large B-cell lymphoma, the authors of the Revised European-American Classification believe that Burkitt-like lymphoma probably does not represent a true biologic entity, and may not be histologically reproducible. A large subset of these neoplasms may represent the most aggressive end of the spectrum of diffuse large B-cell lymphomas.

IV. NON-HODGKIN'S LYMPHOMAS OF MATURE T-CELL LINEAGE

A. T-Cell Chronic Lymphocytic Leukemia/T-Cell Prolymphocytic Leukemia

This category in the Revised European-American Classification includes neoplasms previously designated as well or poorly differentiated lymphocytic lymphoma (Rappaport), small lymphocytic lymphoma (Working Formulation), and T-cell prolymphocytic leukemia (French-American-British classification). Some authors believe T-CLL = small cell T-PLL. Others think T-CLL a separate entity!

Patients with T-cell chronic lymphocytic leukemia/prolymphocytic leukemia (T-CLL/PLL) present with high white blood cell counts, often greater than 100×10^9/L. Lymph nodes, liver, spleen, bone marrow, skin, and mucosal surfaces may be involved. The median survival is often less than one year.

In blood smears the leukemic cells are small to medium-sized. The nuclei have irregular nuclear contours and a prominent central nucleolus. The cytoplasm is abundant and agranular. In some cases, the nuclei are less irregular, and the cells resemble B-cell CLL. The neoplastic cells involve lymph nodes either in a paracortical distribution or diffuse pattern. Proliferation centers, which are common in B-cell CLL/SLL, are absent. In the liver, T-CLL/PLL often involves the sinusoids. In the spleen, the red pulp is preferentially involved. Skin involvement is characterized by dermal infiltrates without epidermotropism.

Immunophenotypic studies have shown that T-CLL/PLL are neoplasms of mature T-cell lineage. The neoplastic cells express pan-T-cell antigens and the TCRα/β receptor. Aberrant T-cell immunophenotypes may be detected, but are uncommon. Approximately two-thirds of cases are CD4+ CD8-, 20% coexpress CD4 and CD8, and rare cases are CD4- CD8+. Occasional cases express S100 protein. As expected for mature neoplasms, TdT is negative. Immunoglobulins and B-cell antigens are negative.

Molecular genetic studies have shown clonal rearrangements of the TCRβ and TCRγ genes; the TCRδ gene is usually deleted. The Ig heavy and light chain genes are usually in the germline configuration. Approximately two-thirds of cases of T-cell CLL/PLL contain a characteristic chromosomal abnormality, the *inv* (14)(q11;q32). A subset of cases lack the *inv* (14), but have translocations that involving the 14q11 locus.

B. Large Granular Lymphocyte Leukemia

These neoplasms have been designated previously as T-cell CLL (Kiel and French-American-British classification), Tγ lymphoproliferative disease, and T8 lymphocytosis with neutropenia. There are two subtypes of large granular lymphocyte leukemia (LGLL): the T-cell and natural-killer (NK) cell subtypes.

Patients with LGLL are usually adults older than 50 years. Men and women are equally affected. Patients frequently seek medical attention for infections that recur over months to years; others complain of fatigue or bleeding. Patients, particularly those with T-cell LGLL, may have autoimmune phenomena, such as rheumatiod arthritis. The physical examination is usually unimpressive in T-cell LGLL.; lymphadenopathy is minimal, and the liver and spleen are normal or slighly enlarged. Lymphadenopathy is more common in NK-cell LGLL, but otherwise the physical findings are similar. Laboratory studies demonstrate a minimal to marked absolute lymphocytosis. Lymphocytosis is usually higher in NK-LGLL. Neutropenia, anemia, and/or thrombocytopenia are common. The clinical course is usually indolent, but some LGLL may behave aggressively.

The lymphoid cells in blood smears are large, oval or round, and have abundant cytoplasm with scattered granules. The neoplastic cells may involve the sinusoids of the liver and the splenic red pulp. Lymph node biopsy specimens, which are more likely to be obtained from patients with NK-cell LGLL, show diffuse architectural effacement. In the bone marrow, lymphoid infiltrates are usually small and focal, but may be diffuse.

The T-cell and NK-cell subtypes of LGLL are distinguished by immunophenotypic studies. The major difference between these subtypes is that T-cell LGLL express the CD3 antigen and T-cell receptors (usually the α/β TCR, rarely the γ/δ TCR) on their surface. NK-cell LGLL lack CD3 and T-cell receptors. Both subtypes express T-cell antigens, such as CD2, and have a CD4-CD8+ immunophenotype. Natural killer cell-associated antigens, such as CD16 and CD57, may be expressed by both subtypes. NK-cell LGLL also may be CD56-positive. Both subtypes of LGLL are negative for TdT, the CD1 and CD25 antigens, Ig, and B-cell antigens.

Molecular studies have shown that T-cell LGLL have clonal rearrangements of the TCRγ, TCRα, and TCRβ chain genes; the TCRδ chain gene is usually deleted. NK-cell LGLLs lack TCR gene arrangements. In both subtypes of LGLL, the Ig genes are usually in the germline configuration.

C. Peripheral T-Cell Lymphoma, Unspecified

The term "peripheral" T-cell lymphoma (PTCL) is used to describe lympoid neoplasms of mature T-cell lineage, as opposed to neoplasms of thymic or "central" origin. The terms post-thymic and mature T-cell lymphoma also have been used to described these neoplasms. In the Working Formulation, most PTCLs fit within the diffuse mixed small and large cell, diffuse large cell, and large cell immunoblastic categories. These neoplasms are common in Japan, and less common in Europe and the United States.

Most patients with PTCL are adults who present with generalized lymphadenopahty. Extranodal sites are commonly involved, and include skin, liver, Waldeyer's ring, and lung. These neoplasms may be associated with hemophagocytic syndrome. Peripheral T-cell lymphomas are diffuse, aggressive neoplasms that require combination chemotherapy. Although the rates of complete remission are similar for both B-cell and T-cell lymphomas, some studies suggest that peripheral T-cell lymphomas relapse more frequently and have a worse prognosis.

In most cases, PTCL diffusely efface the lymph node architecture. However, in some cases the neoplastic cells have a paracortical distribution, and spare lymphoid follicles. Rarely, the growth pattern is nodular, but not truly follicular. The neoplastic cells often exhibit a range in cell size, from small to large, and may have abundant clear cytoplasm. Large Reed-Sternberg-like cells may be seen. Mitotic figures are usually easily found and are often numerous (Fig. 13). Benign inflammatory cells, such as eosinophils and histiocytes, may be numerous. Cases with numerous epithelioid histiocytes have been referred to as lymphoepithelioid, and have been designated in the literature as Lennert's lymphoma. Blood vessels may be prominent.

Immunophenotypic studies have shown that PTCL are neoplasms of mature T-cell lineage. Thus, the neoplastic cells express pan-T-cell antigens such as CD2, CD3, CD5, and CD7; the

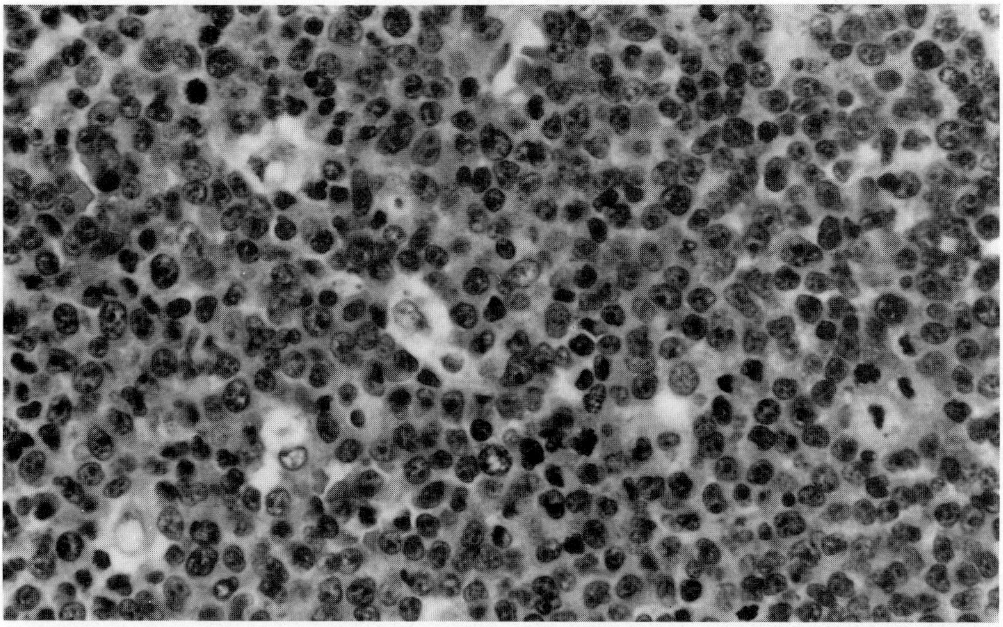

Figure 13 Peripheral T-cell lymphoma, unspecified. In this case the neoplastic cells range in size from small to large, and there are scattered eosinophils. (Hematoxylin-eosin, 528X.)

α/β TCR; and are either CD4 + CD8 - or CD4 - CD8+. They are negative for TdT, Ig, and B-cell antigens. Approximately 75% of cases demonstrate an aberrant T-cell immunophenotype. In other words, the neoplastic cells may inappropriately fail to express one or more pan-T-cell antigens. Alternatively, the cells may either co-express the CD4 and CD8 antigens, or fail to express either of these antigens. The presence of an aberrant T-cell immunophenotype correlates strongly with monoclonality and malignant clinical behavior.

Molecular genetic studies have shown clonal TCRβ and TCRγ gene rearrangements in most cases; the TCRδ gene is usually deleted. The Ig genes are usually in the germline configuration.

D. Peripheral T-Cell Lymphomas, Specific Variants

1. Mycosis Fungoides/Sezary Syndrome

Non-Hodgin's lympomas of either T-cell or B-cell lineage may arise in the skin. A number of different types of T-cell lymphoma may involve the skin, the most common of which is mycosis fungoides/Sezary syndrome. Although the term cutaneous T-cell lympoma has been used as a synonym for mycosis fungoides/Sezary syndrome, cutaneous T-cell lymphomas are a heterogeneous group of disorders. Mycosis fungoides/Sezary syndrome is a distinct clinicopathologic entity.

Many patients with mycosis fungoides (MF) are symptomatic for months to years before the diagnosis of MF can be established histologically. In this early stage, MF may present as small patches or limited plaques. Eventually patients with MF progress to generalized plaques, and then cutaneous tumors. In the late stages of MF, widespread extracutaneous dissemination occurs, similar to other late-stage NHLs. Patients who present with Sezary syndrome have generalized erythroderma and cerebriform lymphoid cells in the peripheral blood (Sezary cells). Mycosis fungoides (MF) and Sezary syndrome (SS) are considered to represent different clinical manifestations of the same disease.

Stage is the most important prognostic variable in patients with MF/SS, and reflects tumor burden and/or biologic behavior. Patients with disease confined to the skin (stage I) have a clinically indolent disease, with long survival (up to 30 years) and the best response to treatment. Survival is much shorter with the presence of lymphadenopathy, even if lymph node biopsy fails to demonstrate involvement (stage II). Patients with histologically proven lymph node involvement (stage III) or visceral disease (stage IV) have the worst survival. A Tumor Nodes Metastasis (TNM) staging system is also used. In addition, patients with the tumor form of disease and those over 50 years of age have poorer survival.

The treatment for MF/SS is different than for other NHL. Topical therapies are used commonly, particularly for patients with limited skin involvement. Common topical treatments include nitrogen mustard, mechlorethamine, PUVA, and electron beam therapy. Topical regimens usually result in a high response rate, but relapse is common. More aggressive regimens that include combination chemotherapy, α-interferon, and monoclonal antibodies have been used in patients with tumor stage and extracutaneous disease.

The histologic findings in MF and SS are identical. The earliest lesions in the patch stage mimic a variety of benign lymphohistiocytic disorders. In the more advanced plaque, tumor, or erythrodermic skin lesions, the findings are more specific, and include acanthosis and parakeratosis of the epidermis, a bandlike infiltrate of atypical lymphoic cells in the papillary dermis, and exocytosis of the atypical lymphoid cells into the epidermis (epidermotropism). The neoplastic cells may aggregate to form Pautrier's microabscesses, which are highly suggestive of MF/SS (Fig. 14).

The neoplastic cells in MF/SS exhibit a spectrum of cell sizes. They may be small, slightly, larger than benign lymphocytes, intermediate, approximately 12 μm, or large. In early lesions, small cells predominate and are mixed with numerous benign inflammatory cells. In more

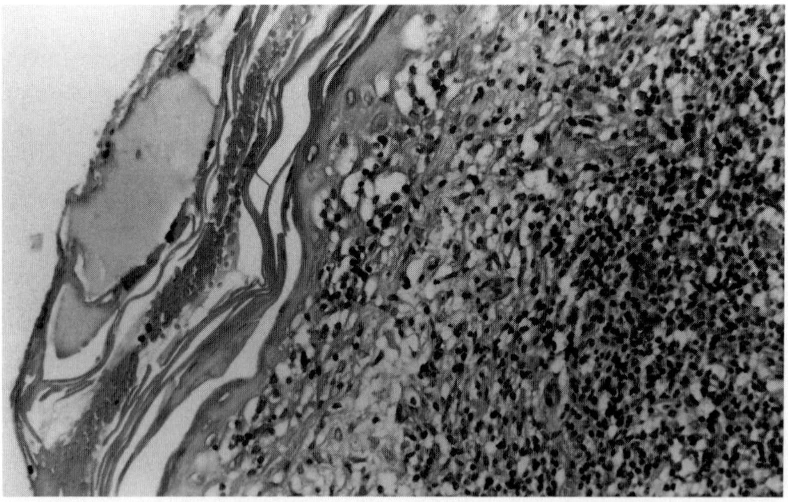

Figure 14 Mycosis fungoides. The neoplastic cells form a bandlike infiltrate in the papillary dermis and infiltrate the epidermis to form Pautrier microabscesses. (Hematoxylin-eosin, 264X.)

advanced lesions, intermediate and large cells are more numerous and inflammatory cells are fewer. In Sezary syndrome, the leukemic phase of MF, the atypical cells in the peripheral blood are of intermediate or large size, with a high nucleus-to-cytoplasm ratio and a lobulated nucleus. Sites of visceral involvement are less distinctive and resemble other types of NHL, most often large cell lymphoma.

Immunophenotypic studies have shown that the neoplastic cells in MF/SS have a mature T-cell immunophenotype; over 95% of cases have a T-helper/inducer cell immunophenotype. Thus, the tumor cells express pan-T-cell antigens such as CD2, CD3, and CD5 and the α/β T-cell receptor; they are CD4-positive and CD8-negative. Cases with a T-cell suppressor/cytotoxic cell immunophenotype (CD4– CD8+) are rare. Pan-B-cell antigens and Ig are negative.

T-cell receptor gene rearrangement analysis has shown that the ability to detect monoclonal TCR gene rearrangements is dependent upon the stage of the disease. Almost all cases of the tumor form and high-clinical-stage MF/SS have clonal rearrangements of the TCRβ and TCRγ chain genes; the TCRδ chain genes are usually deleted. The Ig genes are usually in the germline configuration. In contrast, clonal TCR gene rearrangements may not be detected in biopsies of early (patch or plaque) stage MF/SS. T-cell receptor gene rearrangements in MF/SS are identical in multiple sites of disease obtained from the same patient. This finding indicates that separate lesions arise from the same monoclonal process, despite their different anatomic sites. Gene rearrangement analysis appears to be a better method than morphologic evaluation for assessing peripheral blood involvement, particularly when the number of circulating malignant cells is low.

2. *Angioimmunoblastic T-Cell Lymphoma*

Angioimmunoblastic lymphadenopathy with dysproteinemia (AILD), also called immunoblastic lymphadenopathy and lymphogranulomatosis X, was first described in 1974. Patients with AILD develop acute onset of generalized lymphadenopathy, and often hepatomegaly, splenomegaly, and skin rash. Most patients have constitutional symptoms such as fever, chills, night sweats, and malaise. Laboratory abnormalities include polyclonal hypergammaglobulinemia, anemia (often with a positive direct Coomb's test), and eosinophilia. The median survival for all AILD is 30 months. Infection is the most common cause of death.

Lymph node biopsies show diffuse effacement of the architecture by a polymorphous proliferation of small- and medium-sized lymphocytes, some with clear cytoplasm, plasma cells, eosinophils, and immunoblasts. Normal-sized or hyperplastic lymphoid follicles are absent, and an arborizing proliferation of small blood vessels are seen. Other histologic features that may be found are small, atrophic "burned-out" germinal centers, and intercellular, sludgy, eosinophilic material that is PAS positive.

Shortly after the recognition of AILD, patients with AILD were shown to be at risk for malignant lymphoma, most often of T-cell lineage, but occasionally of B-cell lineage. These lymphomas were composed of large, cytologically atypical lymphoid cells. In addition, de-novo high-grade lymphomas with histologic features similar to lymphomas arising in AILD were described. Since then, antigen receptor gene rearrangement studies have shown that most cases of AILD have clonal T-cell receptor rearrangements. Thus, many investigators believe that AILD is a T-cell lymphoma from its inception, and AILD is included in the category of angioimmunoblastic T-cell lymphoma in the Revised European-American Classification. However, others believe that AILD is a preneoplastic condition.

Immunophenotypic studies of AILD and angioimmunoblastic T-cell lymphoma have shown that these lesions are composed of mature T-cells with relatively few B cells. An aberrant T-cell immunophenotype may be identified. The T-cells are usually of the T-helper/inducer cell subset (CD4 + CD8–). The B cells and plasma cells expressed polytypic Ig light chains.

Gene rearrangement studies have demonstrated that the majority of cases of angioimmunoblastic T-cell lymphoma have clonal rearrangements of the TCRγ and TCRβ chain genes; the TCRδ gene is deleted. Occasional cases have clonal rearrangements of the Ig heavy chain gene. Nonrandom clonal chromosomal abnormalities that involve chromosome 3 or 5 have been identified. Many cases of AILD are Epstein-Barr virus-associated, and it has been suggested that EBV contributes to the pathogenesis of AILD.

3. *Angiocentric Lymphoma*

The term angiocentric lymphoma is recommended in the Revised European-American Classification for a histologically similar group of disorders that were previously called lymphomatoid granulomatosis, when the lower respiratory tract was involved, or polymorphic reticulosis and midline malignant reticulosis, for lesions that involved the nose, nasopharynx, palate, and sinuses. These lesions are predominantly localized processes at onset and may be present for years before diagnosis. The histologic findings, particularly in the early stages of disease, are difficult to interpret and may be misdiagnosed as a benign inflammatory processes. A subset of cases of pulmonary lymphomatoid granulomatosis are of B-cell lineage.

Angiocentric lymphomas have a propensity to involve extranodal sites, most commonly the lung, nasal cavity, and upper respiratory tract. Skin, kidney, and central nervous system are less commonly involved. Lymph node involvement is uncommon. Patient survival is inversely proportional to the number of large lymphoid cells present. However, patients whose lesions contain numerous large cells more often respond to combination chemotherapy. Angiocentric lymphomas are often associated with a hemophagocytic syndrome, characterized clinically by fever, hepatosplenomegaly, pancytopenia, and laboratory evidence of hemolysis.

Angiocentric lymphomas are composed of a mixture of atypical lymphoid cells admixed with benign lymphocytes, plasma cells, and histiocytes. Eosinophils are rare and neutrophils are absent. Angiocentric lymphomas display a marked propensity to invade and destroy blood vessels, which often results in coagulative necrosis. Over time, these lesions tend to accumulate large atypical cells, with relatively fewer inflammatory cells. Thus, a grading scheme has been proposed for these neoplasms: grade I lesions contain relatively few large cells and many inflammatory cells, grade III lesions contain many cytologically atypical small and large cells and few inflammatory cells, and grade II lesions have intermediate features.

Immunophenotypic studies of angiocentric lymphomas may be difficult to interpret, especially grade I lesions, because of the many admixed inflammatory cells. The neoplastic cells in most angiocentric lymphomas express T-cell associated antigens such as CD2 and CD7. Aberrant T-cell immunophenotypes are common, and the T-cell-specific antigen CD3 is often absent. Angiocentric lymphomas also commonly express the natural killer cell-associated antigen CD56. Immunoglobulins and B-cell antigens are negative.

Molecular genetic studies of angiocentric lymphomas have demonstrated an absence of TCR and Ig gene rearrangements in the majority of cases studied. This finding, combined with the frequent CD56+ CD3– immunophenotype, suggests that these neoplasms may arise from natural killer cells. Because Epstein-Barr viral genomes have been identified in the malignant cells by a variety of molecular diagnostic techniques, EBV may be involved in the pathogenesis of angiocentric lymphomas.

4. *Intestinal T-Cell Lymphoma*

These neoplasms were originally designated malignant histiocytosis of the intestine because the neoplastic cells morphologically resembled histiocytes. Subsequent immunophenotypic and genotypic studies demonstrated that these neoplasms are T-cell lymphomas with a mature immunophenotype that may arise from intramucosal T lymphocytes. They have also been called enteropathy-associated T-cell lymphoma.

Patients with intestinal T-cell lymphoma (ITCL) present with abdominal pain or weight loss. Although originally described in patients with a history of gluten-sensitive enteropathy or celiac disease, who are known to have an increased incidence of lymphoma, these neoplasms also frequently arise in patients without this history. The survival of individuals with enteropathy-associated T-cell lymphoma is poor despite therapy, and death is often the result of ulcers and intestinal perforation.

On microscopic examination, the intestine that is not involved by neoplasm may or may not show features of celiac disease. The neoplastic cells are found at the base of the ulcers and within the lamina propria and submucosa. The growth pattern is diffuse. The neoplastic cells are a mixture of small, medium, and large lymphoid cells that may have clear cytoplasm. Karyorrhexis may be prominent and mitotic figures may be numerous.

Immunophenotypic studies have shown that ITCL express pan-T-cell antigens including CD3, and are often CD4-CD8– or CD4-CD8+. They are negative for immunoglobulin and B-cell antigens. Most express CD30 and CD103, an antigen expressed by normal lymphocytes that reside in the intestinal mucosa.

Molecular studies have shown that most cases have clonal rearrangements of the TCRβ and TCRγ chain genes; the TCRδ genes have not been studied. The Ig heavy and light chain genes in the germline configuration.

5. Adult T-Cell Leukemia/Lymphoma

Adult T-cell leukemia/lymphoma (ATLL) is a distinct clinicopathologic entity associated with infection by the human retrovirus, HTLV-1. ATLL accounts for the extraordinarily high incidence of T-cell lymphoma in Japan, particularly on the island of Kyushu, where approximately 15% of normal individuals have serologic evidence of HTLV-1 infection. Clusters of cases also have been reported in Pacific Ocean islands, the Caribbean, and the southeastern United States, predominantly in African-American patients.

Patients with ATLL are usually adults, with a median age of 41 years. They usually present with one of four syndromes. The most common form of the disease is acute ATLL. These patients present with generalized lymphadenopathy, hepatosplenomegaly, skin lesions, peripheral blood involvement, lytic bone lesions, and hypercalcemia, which may develop in the absence of bone lesions. The cerebrospinal fluid is commonly involved. Survival is usually poor. The second most common form of the disease is lymphomatous ATLL. These patients present with lymphadenopathy and organ infiltrates, without hepatosplenomegaly or hypercalcemia. The prognosis is better than for patients with acute ATLL. The third form of the disease is chronic ATLL. These patients have an absolute lymphocytosis and cytologically abnormal cells in the peripheral blood. Skin lesions, lymphadenopathy, and involvement of other viscera may occur. Survival is usually longer than two years. The fourth form is smoldering ATLL. These patients have chronic disease, usually skin lesions, for years. Peripheral blood involvement is minimal and the viscera are usually spared.

The peripheral blood findings are characteristic of ATLL. The circulating neoplastic cells are medium-sized, with basophilic cytoplasm and markedly irregular, multilobated nuclei, including "cover-leaf" shapes. Lymph nodes and viscera that are involved by ATLL are replaced by neoplastic cells that exhibit a range in cell size, from small to large, with relatively round to markedly irregular nuclear contours. Many cases that involve lymph nodes cannot be reliably distinguished from peripheral T-cell lymphomas that are not HTLV-1-associated without serologic or molecular studies. Histologic findings do not correlate with survival.

Immunophenotypic studies have shown that ATLL have a mature T-cell immunophenotype. The tumor cells express pan-T-cell antigens, the TCRα/β receptor, and are CD4 + CD8–. Characteristically, the neoplastic cells intensely express CD25 antigen (interleukin-2 receptor α chain). The tumor cells are negative for Ig and B-cell antigens. They are usually negative for activation antigens.

Antigen reeceptor gene rearrangement studies have shown clonal rearrangements of the TCRβ and TCRγ chain genes. The TCRα chain gene has been rearranged in a small number of cases studied. The TCRδ chain genes are usually deleted. The Ig genes are usually in the germline configuration. Cytogenetic studies commonly show abnormalities in ATLL, including trisomy 12, 6q-, and translocations involving the chromosome 14q11 or 7p14-15 loci.

The hallmark of ATLL is the demonstration of HTLV-1, either by serologic methods to detect serum antibodies, or by molecular genetic methods, such as Southern blot hybridization or polymerase chain reaction, to detect virus. The virus is clonally integrated into the host cell genome, and the integration site of the virus is similar in most cases.

6. Hepatosplenic γ/δ T-Cell Lymphoma

These neoplasms represent a relatively recently recognized type of peripheral T-cell lymphoma that is currently considered as a provisional category in the Revised European-American Classification. The small number of reported cases precludes definitive statements regarding the clinical features of this disease. Most patients have been young adult men. Patients present with marked hepatosplenomegaly and minimal or absent lymphadenopathy. Skin lesions may occur. The clinical course is aggressive, with a high rate of relapse and death.

The neoplastic cells are medium-sized and deceptively bland, with round to slightly irregular nuclear contours, condensed chromatin, and small nucleoli (Fig. 15). In the liver, the neoplastic cells infiltrate sinusoids and spare the portal tracts. In the spleen, the red pulp is involved and the white pulp is spared. The bone marrow, especially sinusoids, may be involved.

Immunophenotypic studies have demonstrated that the neoplastic cells have a mature T-cell immunophenotype. The CD5 antigen is often aberrantly absent. They characteristically express the TCRγ/δ receptor. Immunoglobulin and pan-B-cell antigens are not expressed.

Molecular genetic studies are limited, but most cases show clonal TCRδ-chain gene rearrangements. The TCRβ chain gene also may be rearragned. The Ig genes are in the germline configuration. Although relatively few cases have had cytogenetic analysis, many of the cases that have been studied have contained an isochromosome 7q.

7. Subcutaneous Panniculitic T-Cell Lymphoma

This is another relatively recently recognized group of peripheral T-cell lymphomas that is included in the Revised European-American Classification as a provisional category. Patients are usually adults who present with multiple, usually relatively small, subcutaneous nodules. Approximately one-third of patients present with a hemophagocytic syndrome that causes systemic symptoms. Additional patients will develop a hemophagocytic syndrome during the disease course that is often fatal.

These neoplasms involve the subcutaneous tissue, with minimal involvement of overlying dermis (Fig. 16). The neoplastic cells infiltrate the septae of adipose tissue, and there is often marked coagulative and fat necrosis. Thus, at low power these lesions resemble panniculitis. However, the neoplastic are cytologically atypical, and may be mixture of small and large cells, or predominantly large cells. Large cells accumulate over time. Karyorrhexis is often prominent and mitotic figures are easily found.

Immunophenotypic studies have shown that the neoplastic cells have a mature T-cell im-

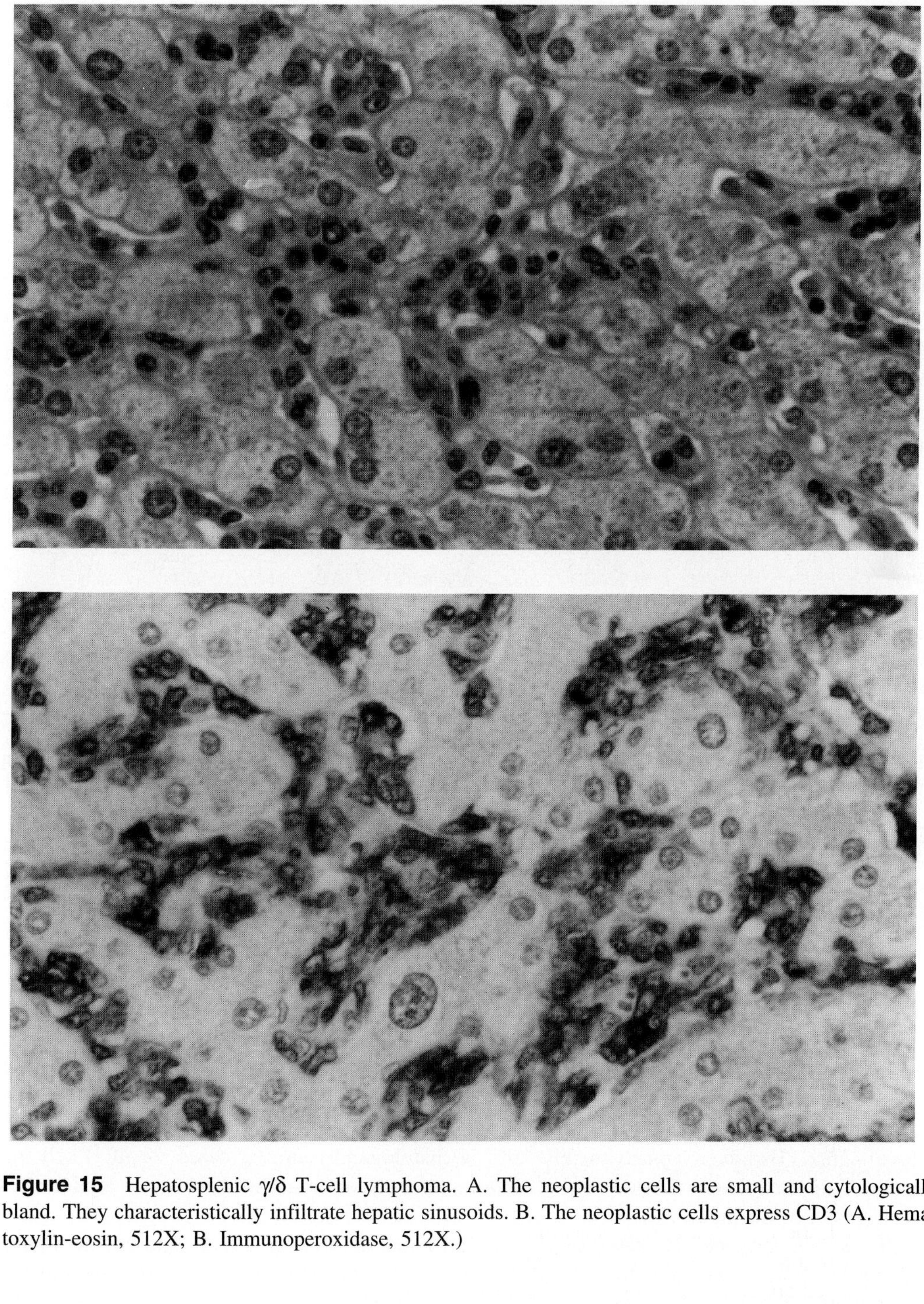

Figure 15 Hepatosplenic γ/δ T-cell lymphoma. A. The neoplastic cells are small and cytologically bland. They characteristically infiltrate hepatic sinusoids. B. The neoplastic cells express CD3 (A. Hematoxylin-eosin, 512X; B. Immunoperoxidase, 512X.)

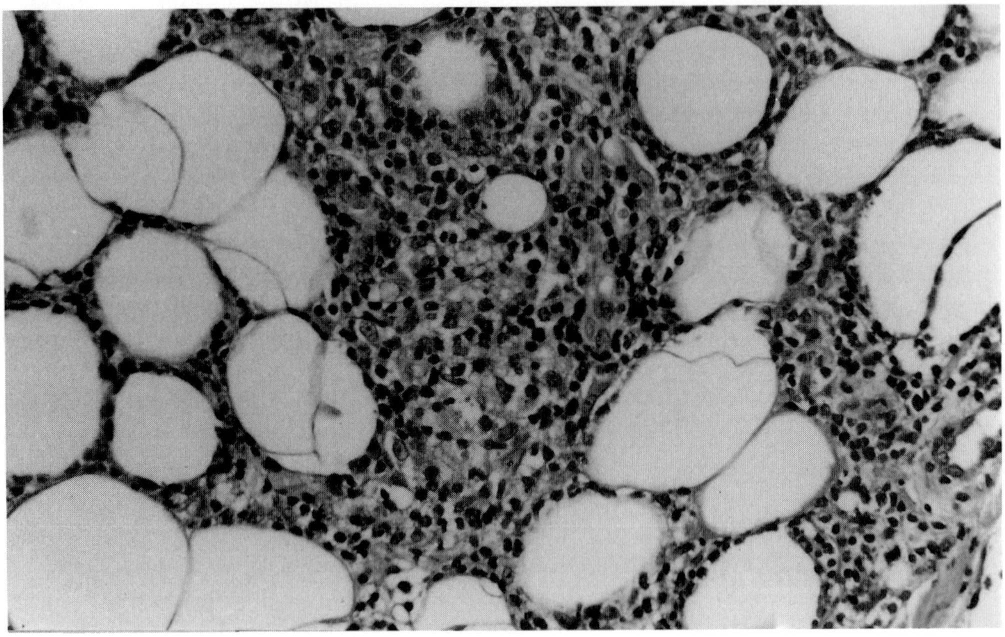

Figure 16 Subcutaneous panniculitic T-cell lymphoma. The neoplastic cells infiltrate the septae between adipocytes and are cytologically atypical. The neoplasm is located primarily in the subcutaneous tissue, and spares the epidermis and dermis. (Hematoxylin-eosin, 264X.)

munophenotype. An aberrant T-cell immunophenotype may be detected, more commonly in lesions composed of many large cells. Immunoglobulins and pan-B-cell antigens are negative.

Molecular genetic studies have demonstrated clonal TCRβ and TCRγ gene rearrangements. The Ig genes are in the germline configuration.

V. LYMPHOID NEOPLASMS OF EITHER T-, B-, OR NULL-CELL LINEAGE

A. Anaplastic Large Cell Lymphoma

Anaplastic large cell lymphoma (ALCL) was originally called Ki-1 lymphoma because the neoplastic cells reacted with the Ki-1 antibody, which recognizes the CD30 antigen. The majority of cases are of T-cell lineage and have distinct clinicopathologic features. Thus, this category is included as one of the specific variants of peripheral T-cell lymphoma in the REAL Classification. However, approximately 20% of histologically similar cases are of B-cell lineage, and approximately 5% lack either immunophenotypic or molecular genetic evidence of T-cell or B-cell lineage.

Anaplastic large cell lymphomas of T-cell and null cell lineage affect children and adults, and may involve nodal or extranodal sites. There appears to be two forms of this disease: systemic and cutaneous. Systemic ALCL affects children and adults. Systemic symptoms are common, and extranodal sites are frequently involved. These neoplasms are clinically aggressive and require combination chemotherapy. The rates of complete remission and survival are similar to other diffuse aggressive lymphomas. Primary cutaneous ALCL affects predominantly adults, usually remains localized to the skin, may undergo spontaneous regression, and has an excellent prognosis. This form of disease is histologically and immunophenotypically similar to the clinicopathologic entity of lymphomatoid papulosis, and may represent one end of the spectrum of this disease.

In lymph nodes, T-cell and null-cell ALCL often localize preferentially to the sinuses, particularly in lymph nodes that are not extensively involved. With greater involvement, the pattern of involvement may be paracortical or diffuse. The neoplastic cells often appear cohesive. Because the neoplastic cells preferentially involve sinuses and appear cohesive, these lymphomas were often misdiagnosed as metastatic carcinoma in the past. The neoplastic cells are anaplastic with very large and bizzare, irregularly-shaped, often polylobated nuclei (Fig. 17A). The nuclear chromatin is vesicular with prominent nucleoli. The cytoplasm is abundant and usually basophilic.

B-cell ALCL are morphologically similar to T-cell and null-cell ALCL, although they less often preferentially involve lymph node sinuses and often are less cytologically bizarre. In addition, they do not have characteristic clinical findings. B-cell ALCLs behave as do other diffuse aggressive lymphomas of B-cell lineage. Thus, it is not clear if these neoplasms represent a distinct clinicopathologic entity.

Immunophenotypic studies have shown that the neoplastic cells express the activation antigen CD30 (Fig. 17B). However, CD30 antigen expression is not specific for ALCL. The majority of ALCL are of mature T-cell lineage. The neoplastic cells express pan-T-cell antigens, and are most often CD4 + CD8−. Abberrant immunophenotypes are common, and a large subset of cases are negative for CD3. They lack immunoglobulin and pan-B-cell antigens. Approximately half of cases lack the pan-leukocyte antigen CD45RB. Most cases express a variety of activation antigens and proliferation antigens. A small subset of cases express cytokeratin. Epithelial membrane antigen is often expressed by the systemic form of ALCL, but is usually negative in the cutaneous primary form. Null-cell ALCL lack immunophenotypic and molecular evidence of lineage. B-cell ALCL express pan-B-cell antigens such as CD20, but lack Ig. They are negative for pan-T-cell antigens.

Gene rearrangement studies have shown a variety of findings in ALCL. T-cell ALCL usually contain clonal rearrangements of the TCR genes. B-cell ALCL usually contain clonal Ig gene rearrangements. There is a high incidence of lineage promiscuity in ALCL, with clonal TCR gene rearrangements in cases of B-cell ALCL, and clonal Ig rearrangements in T-cell ALCL. Approximately one-third of cases, regardless of immunophenotype, lack antigen receptor gene rearrangements.

Chromosomal translocations that involve chromosome 5q35, usually as the t(2;5)(p23; q35), occur in a subset of cases of ALCL. This translocation juxtaposes the anaplastic lymphoma kinase (ALK) gene on chromosome 2p23 with the nucleophosmin (NPM) nucleolar phosphoprotein gene on 5q35. A chimeric transcript and protein results from this translocation, and is believed to be involved in neoplastic transformation. The t(2;5) translocation is usually found in the systemic form of T-cell ALCL, in up to one-half of cases. However, the t(2;5) is not restricted to either ALCL or to T-cell lineage neoplasms.

B. True Histiocytic Lymphoma

True histiocytic lymphomas currently represent less than 1% of all non-Hodgkin's lymphomas. With the development of immunologic and molecular studies, neoplasms once thought to be histiocytic have been proven to be of B-cell or T-cell lineage.

True histiocytic lymphomas are thought to arise from histiocytes normally present in the

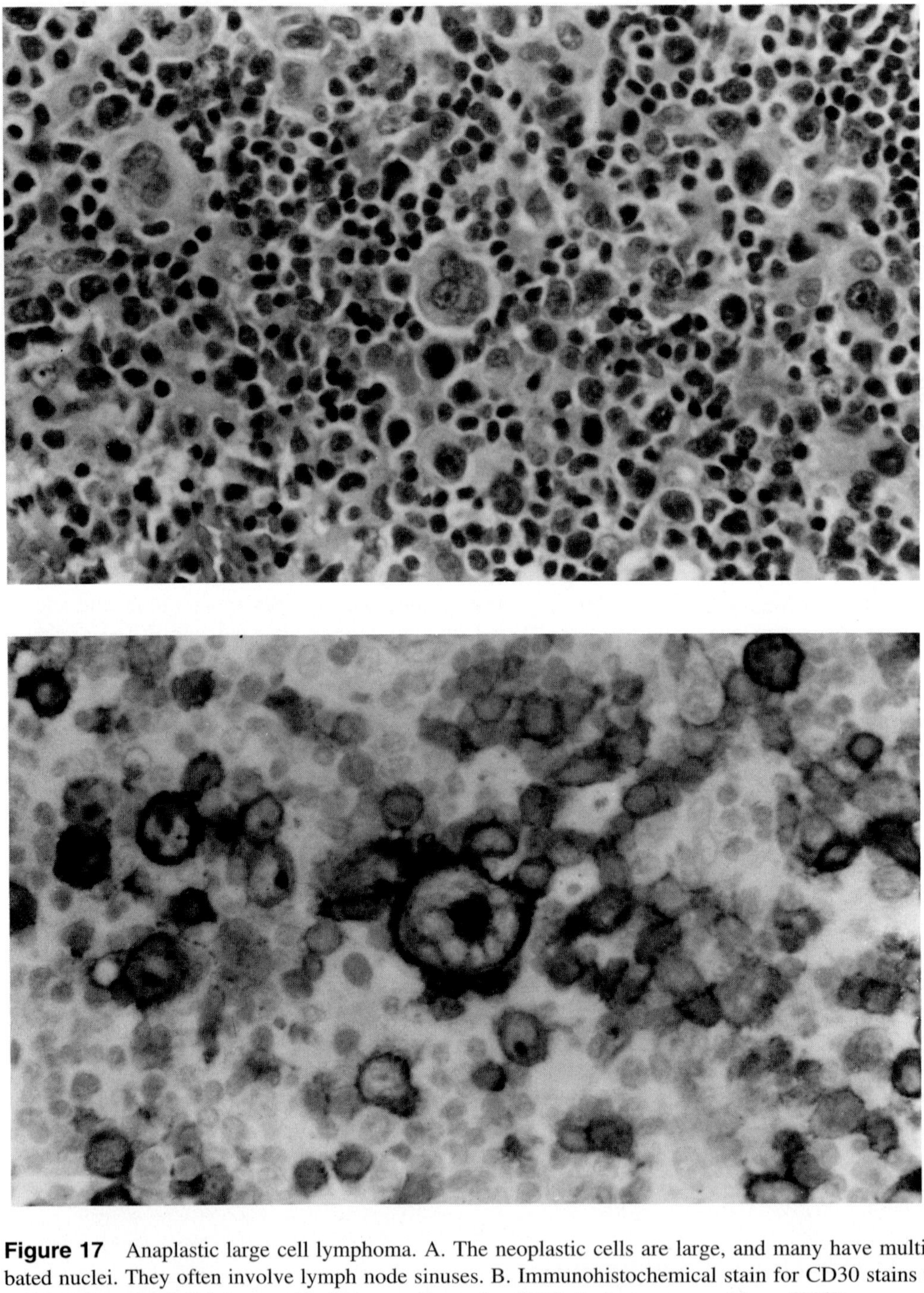

Figure 17 Anaplastic large cell lymphoma. A. The neoplastic cells are large, and many have multilobated nuclei. They often involve lymph node sinuses. B. Immunohistochemical stain for CD30 stains the cell membrane and Golgi zone. (A. Hematoxylin-eosin, 528X; B. Immunoperoxidase, 528X.)

lymph node. These cells include phagocytic sinusoidal histiocytes, follicular dendritic reticulum cells, and interdigitating reticulum cells. Thus, histiocytic neoplasms have been reported in the literature as dendritic reticulum cell sarcoma or interdigitating reticulum cell sarcoma, as well as true histiocytic lymphoma. In addition, some true histiocytic lymphomas may be examples of extramedullary myeloid cell tumors with pure monocytic differentiation.

Histologically, these neoplasms are composed of large cells with abundant cytoplasm and oval or lobulated nuclei. Dendritic and interdigitating cell sarcomas may have spindled nuclei. The histiocytic origin of these tumores, although it may be suspected histologically, cannot be ascertained without cytochemical, immunophenotypic, or genotypic analyses. Cytochemical studies of smears or touch imprint preparations often demonstrate that the neoplastic cells have strong reactivity for nonspecific or butyrate esterases. Immunophenotypic studies show an absence of B-cell or T-cell specific antigens, and expression of histiocyte-associated antigens such as CD1, CD4, CD11c, and CD14. The CD1 antigen and S100 protein are expressed by normal interdigitating reticulum cells and interdigitating reticulum cell sarcomas.

The very small number of these cases precludes definitive statements regarding the clinical course of dendritic and interdigitating cell sarcomas. However, some patients have developed disseminated disease. Patients with extramedullary myeloid cell tumors with monocytic differentiation usually have a history of or concurrent bone marrow disease. However, some patients present with de-novo extramedullary disease and are at risk to develop acute leukemia, usually within months.

VI. PLASMA CELL DYSCRASIAS

A. Plasmacytoma and Plasma Cell Myeloma

Plasmacytoma and plasma cell myeloma are neoplasms that are composed of cells that resemble mature or immature plasma cells, and that secrete abnormal amounts of monoclonal immunoglobulin molecules or immunoglobulin lights chains (monoclonal or M-proteins). Because plasmacytoma and plasma cell myeloma rarely arise in lymph nodes, they were not included in the Rappaport classification or the Working Formulation. However, they are included in the Revised European-American Classification, which seeks to classify nodal and extranodal lymphoid neoplasms.

Plasma cell myeloma affects middle-aged or older adults; the incidence increases with increasing age. The ratio of men to women is 3:2. The most common symptom is bone pain due to lytic lesions or, less often, generalized osteoporosis. Many patients report weakness and malaise, usually due to anemia. They also develop infections, bleeding, and signs and symptoms of renal failure or hypercalcemia later in the disease course. The physical findings are usually nonspecific. Because the disease is initially localized to bone, patients usually do not present with lymphadenopathy, hepatomegaly, or splenomegaly.

A variety of laboratory studies are used to evaluate patients for plasma cell myeloma. These tests include serum and urine protein electrophoresis, urine protein quantitation, serum and urine immunoglobulin quantitation, serum and urine immunoelectrophoresis, radiographic skeletal survey, and bone marrow examination. Patients have monoclonal immunoglobulin in the serum and/or urine, with decreased amounts of normal serum immunoglobulins. Monoclonal proteins usually appear as a "spike" in the gamma globulin region on serum or urine protein electrophoresis. Free light chains may be found in the urine (Bence-Jones proteins) in the absence of a detectable serum monoclonal protein. Thus, in patients suspected of having plasma cell myeloma, both serum and urine should be examined for M-protein. Serum and urine immunoelectrophoresis is one of the most sensitive methods to detect a monoclonal protein, and is used to determine the heavy chain class (IgM, IgG, IgA, IgD, or IgE) and light chain type (kappa or lambda). Because it is sensitive, it may detect a monoclonal protein in the absence of an apparent spike, for example, in patients with small amounts of monoclonal immunoglobulin or light chain myeloma. Plasma cell myelomas most commonly secrete monoclonal IgG (about 50% of cases), followed by IgA (about 20% of cases) or free light chains (about 20% of cases). Plasma cell myelomas that secrete IgD or IgE are unusual. Nonsecretory plasma cell myelomas are rare (fewer than 1% of cases).

Bone marrow examination that includes an aspirate smear and core biopsy is required to make the diagnosis of plasma cell myeloma. Because the infiltrate may be focal, it is difficult to give a specific percent of plasma cells that is diagnostic of plasma cell myeloma. However, most diagnostic systems require more than 10% plasma cells, and more than 3 g/dL of serum M-protein or 1 g/24 hr of light chain in the urine. The diagnosis of plasma cell myeloma can be established solely on bone marrow examination if two of the three following criteria are met: (a) the plasma cells shows marked nuclear atypia, (b) there are large aggregates or solid sheets of plasma cells, and (c) there is a light chain restriction. If the laboratory or radiographic findings support the diagnosis, then only one of the criteria must be met.

Neoplastic plasma cells can show a broad spectrum of morphology. They can vary from mature-appearing plasma cells to blastlike cells or anaplastic cells that are unrecognizable as plasma cells without a high degree of suspicion. In most cases the cells are recognizable as plasma cells, although they appear immature or atypical (Fig. 18). Atypical nuclear features include large size, more open chromatin, and conspicuous nucleoli. Atypical cytoplasmic features include irregular cytoplasmic borders, vacuoles, granules, and hyaline and crystalline inclusions. Cytoplasmic inclusions are found in benign and neoplastic plasma cells. Dutcher

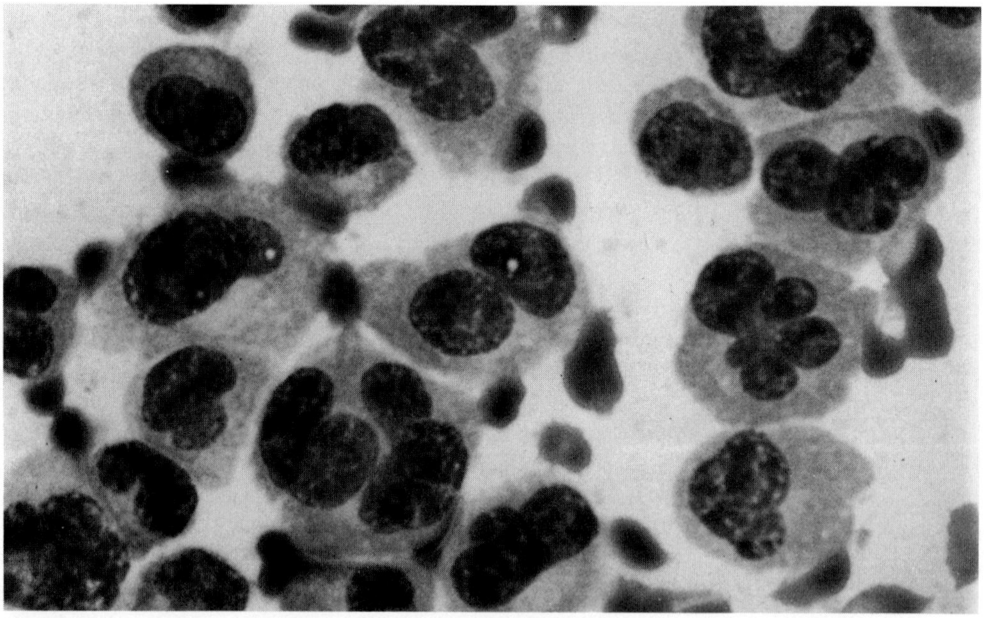

Figure 18 Plasma cell myeloma. In this unusual case many of the malignant plasma cells have lobated nuclei. (Wright-giemsa, 4000X.)

bodies, which resemble nuclear inclusions, are actually invaginations of cytoplasm into the nucleus. Occasional plasma cells with Dutcher bodies may be seen in reactive processes, but large numbers should raise the suspicion of a malignant plasma cell dyscrasia. The presence of immature blastic plasma cells, either plasmablasts or immunoblasts, is associated with a more aggressive disease course. Plasmablasts have a high nuclear/cytoplasmic ratio, fine nuclear chromatin, and variably prominent nucleoli. In core biopsies the pattern of involvement may be interstitial, focal, or diffuse. As the disease progresses, the neoplastic cells replace the hematopoietic cells, the pattern becomes diffuse, and patients develop signs and symptoms of marrow failure. Bony trabeculae may show increased osteoclast activity with resorption of bone and marrow fibrosis. Peripheral blood smears may show rouleaux formation, depending on the amount and type of monoclonal protein. Circulating plasma cells are found infrequently and in low numbers, expect as a terminal event.

POEMS syndrome is a rare variant of plasma cell myeloma that occurs in less than 3% of myeloma patients. The syndrome is characterized by: *p*olyneuropathy, *o*rganomegaly, *e*ndocrine *a*bnormalities, *m*onoclonal spike, and *s*kin changes. Patients with POEMS syndrome differ from patients with typical myeloma in several ways. They are often younger, have osteosclerotic rather than lytic bone lesions, and have an IgA lambda monoclonal protein. The unusual features are believed to result from the abnormal production of cytokines produced by the neoplastic plasma cells.

Solitary plasmacytoma is a monoclonal plasma cell tumor that involves a single site. Patients suspected to have a solitary plasmacytoma must receive a complete evaluation to exclude plasma cell myeloma. Solitary plasmacytomas can arise in soft tissue, particularly in the head and neck (solitary extramedullary plasmacytoma), bone (solitary plasmacytoma of bone), or rarely lymph node. Up to one-half of patients with solitary plasmacytoma have an M-protein in serum (usually less than 2 g/dL) or urine, but other immunoglobulin levels are not decreased. There is no anemia, renal failure, or hypercalcemia. Solitary extramedullary plasmacytomas most commonly arise in the head and neck, particularly in mucous membranes of the upper respiratory tract, but may arise in other sites. Patients with solitary plasmacytoma of bone present with a single bone lesion, most often in a vertebra, the skull, or pelvis. They have no evidence of other bone lesions on radiographic studies, and random bone marrow biopsies fail to demonstrate plasma cell infiltrates.

The immunophenotype of plasma cell myeloma and plasmacytoma is similar to benign plasma cells. Like benign plasma cells, the neoplastic cells express cytoplasmic, but not surface, immunoglobulin. However, unlike reactive process, which contains a mixture of kappa- and lambda-positive plasma cells, neoplastic plasma cells express monoclonal immunoglobulin and show a light chain restriction. A population is said to demonstrate a light chain restriction when the ratio of one light chain type to the other exceeds 16:1. Both benign and malignant plasma cells fail to express most B-cell-associated antigens, such as CD19, CD20, and CD22. However, they express the B-cell-associated antigen CD79a, which is also expressed on plasma cells. Like benign plasma cells, the neoplastic cells are usually negative for CD45 (leukocyte common antigen), positive for CD38 and the mature plasma cell antigens, PC-1, and PCA-1. They also may express epithelial membrane antigen (EMA). Neoplastic plasma cells, but not benign plasma cells, stain with the antibody MB2, and also often epxress CD56, an adhesion molecule that is associated with natural killer cell differentiation. A minority of cases express CD10 (CALLA), and markers of myelomonocytic differentiation, such as CD11b, CD11c, CD13, CD15, and CD33.

Immunohistochemical stains for immunoglobulin light chains performed on core biopsy or clot sections are the single most helpful technique to distinguish malignant from reactive plasma cell proliferations. Because plasma cells fail to express most markers of lymphoid differentiation, and may express EMA, these stains are especially helpful in cases where the malignant cells are anaplastic.

Plasma cell myelomas and plasmacytomas have clonal immunoglobulin heavy- and light-chain gene rearrangements. The TCR genes are usually in the germline configuration. Up to one-half of cases of plasma cell myeloma have chromosomal abnormalities. The abnormalities are variable, and are usually both structural and numerical. However, there are no known characteristic cytogenetic abnormalities.

Patients with solitary plasmacytoma are treated with local irradiation with curative intent. Most patients with solitary extramedullary plasmacytoma (approximately two-thirds) are cured, and do not develop plasma cell myeloma. Most patients with solitary plasmacytoma of bone (approximately two-thirds) eventually develop plasma cell myeloma over a period of years.

Patients with plasma cell myeloma usually are not treated until they become symptomatic or develop evidence of disease progression, such as a significant increase in the amount of M-protein. Standard therapy for plasma cell myeloma consists of an alkylating agent, usually melphalan, and prednisone. This regimen, developed 25 years ago, is used to control symptoms and reduce the tumor burden. It extends survival in about one-half of patients. A newer regimen, VAD (vincristine, adriamycin, dexamethasone) has been used to treat patients who are refractory to standard alkylating agent regimens, or who have relapsed. However, treatment with VAD does not improve the survival of previously untreated patients. Autologous bone marrow and peripheral blood stem cell transplantation significantly extends survival in up to one-half of patients. Autologous transplantation is most effective early in the course of the disease, when complete remissions can still be achieved, and when hematopoietic progenitor cells have not been compromised by prolonged exposure to alkylating agents. Allogeneic transplantation is limited by the age of the patients and availability of donors.

Plasma cell myeloma is a progressive disease with a poor prognosis. The median survival with conventional therapy is approximately 3 years. The length of survival is closely related to the stage of the disease at diagnosis. Patients are monitored with periodic determinations of serum and urine M-protein levels, and serum beta-2 microglobulin levels. Elevated levels of serum beta-2 microglobulin are associated with progressive disease and a worse prognosis. Complete remissions are unusual, and patients die of the disease. Infection is the most common cause of death. Renal failure is a contributing factor in many cases.

B. Heavy Chain Diseases

The heavy chain diseases are a group of rare monoclonal gammopathies that are characterized by the production of free immunoglobulin α, μ, or γ heavy chains. Alpha-chain disease, the most common of the heavy chain diseases, is now termed immunoproliferative small intestinal disease (IPSID). IPSID is a disease of young adults that is most common in the Middle East. Patients present with signs and symptoms of severe malabsorption. The small intenstine and mesenteric lymph nodes are infiltrated by malignant lymphoplasmacytic cells, which generally remain confined to these sites. Patients usually die from malabsorption.

Most patients with μ-chain disease have a history of B-CLL. Hepatosplenomegaly is common, but lymphadenopathy is unusual. The bone marrow shows a lymphocytosis with admixed atypical vacuolated plasma cells. In about one-half of patients, the malignant cells also secrete light chains that do not associate with the heavy chains, and that can be detected in the urine as Bence-Jones proteins.

Patients with γ-chain disease are usually older adults who present with constitutional symptoms. Lymph nodes, liver, spleen, and bone marrow contain malignant lymphoplasmacytic or plasmacytic infiltrates. Waldeyer's ring is typically involved. Patients lack lytic bone lesions and free light chains in the urine.

C. Primary Amyloidosis

There are three types of systemic amyloidosis: primary or light-chain (AL) amyloidosis, secondary (AA) amyloidosis, and familial amyloidosis. Primary amyloidosis is a rare subtype of plasma cell dyscrasia that is characterized by the widespread deposition of amyloid protein composed of free immunoglobulin light chain. The light chains are usually λ, but may be κ. Systemic amyloidosis may also occur in patients with chronic infections or collagen vascular diseases (secondary or AA amyloid), or as a hereditary syndrome. Because the amyloid protein in secondary and familial amyloidosis is neither immunoglobulin nor associated with a plasma cell dyscrasia, these entities will not be discussed further.

Primary amyloidosis is a disease of older adults. Most patients present with vague symptoms, such as fatigue and weight loss. Approximately 20% of patients with primary amyloidosis fulfill the diagnostic criteria for plasma cell myeloma or Waldenstrom's macroglobulinemia. The remaining 80% of patients do not fulfill the criteria, but have a small monoclonal immunoglobulin in the serum or urine. In these patients, the bone marrow contains a slightly increased number of morphologically normal or atypical plasma cells. In most cases immunohistochemical stains demonstrate that the plasma cells are monoclonal. Rouleaux may be seen in the peripheral blood, depending on the amount and type of M-protein.

The clinical manifestations of amyloidosis result from the widespread deposition of amyloid protein that leads to organ dysunction. Renal involvement leads to nephrotic syndrome in approximately one-third of patients. Amyloid deposition in the heart results in congestive heart failure and arrhythmias. Patients may develop malbsorption when the gastrointestinal tract is involved. Involvement of the nervous system is characterized by peripheral neuropathy. Coagulation abnormalities result from acquired factor X deficiency, increased fibrinolysis, and decreased fibrinogen. Amyloid deposition in the liver and spleen leads to hepatomegaly and splenomegaly, but lymphadenopathy is unusual.

The diagnosis of amyloidosis is established by demonstrating amyloid in tissue sections. The most useful test to demonstrate amyloid is the Congo red stain; amyloid is Congo red-positive and shows apple-green birefringence on polarized light. Amyloid can be found in the walls of blood vessels in bone marrow biopsies, in subcutaneous fat aspirates, or in rectal biopsies. Although it also can be found in heart, kidney, liver, and nerve, these organs are sampled less often because of the increased risk of complications. Electron microscopy shows interlacing bundles of parallel fibrils that are 7–10 nm in diameter.

The prognosis for patients with primary amyloidosis is poor, with a median survival of 12 months after diagnosis. Patients are treated with alklyating agents, usually melphalan, and steroids. Treatment with colchicine may inhibit amyloid deposition. In addition, patients receive supportive care for the manifestations of amyloid deposition. Death from cardiac complications is most common, but patients also die from renal failure, infection, hepatic failure, and other complications.

D. Monoclonal Gammopathy of Undetermined Significance

Patients with monoclonal gammopathy of undetermined significance (MGUS) have an M-protein in their serum and/or urine without other evidence of a malignant plasma cell dyscrasia or lymphoproliferative disorder. MGUS is often identified in the course of evaluation for another disorder, such as collagen vascular or heart disease. MGUS is found in approximately 1% of healthy people older than 50 years, and in 3% of healthy people older than 70 years. The incidence increases with increasing age.

Most patients with MGUS have an M-protein on serum electrophoresis that ranges in amount from 0.3 to 3 g/dL, rarely higher. A minority have free light chain in the urine, usually less than 1 g/24 hr. The M-protein is usually IgG, but may be IgM or IgA; the light chain may be either κ or λ. Polyclonal serum immunoglobulins are usually present in normal amounts, but may be decreased in up to one-third of patients. Blood counts are normal, although rouleaux may be seen. About half of patients with MGUS have slightly increased numbers of plasma cells in the bone marrow, less than 10%. The plasma cells are morphologically normal and may be scattered through the marrow or in small clusters, usually adjacent to blood vessels, Immunohistochemical stains show a polyclonal plasmacytosis in most cases; a minority of cases are monoclonal.

The differential diagnosis of MGUS includes other plasma cell dyscrasias, especially plasma cell myeloma. Patients with MGUS lack other clinical and laboratory findings that are associated with a malignant plasma cell dyscrasia, and treatment is unnecessary. However, it may be difficult to distinguish MGUS from early plasma cell myeloma or other plasma cell dyscrasia, especially when the M-protein exceeds 3 g/dL. Because about 20% of patients with MGUS will progress to a malignant process over 15–20 years, they are followed with periodic serum and urine protein electrophoresis. An increase in the amount of the M-protein is the best predictor of progression. In addition, serum beta-2 microglobulin levels are usually normal in patients with MGUS, but elevated in patients with plasma cell myeloma.

CASE STUDY 1

Patient

43-year-old woman

Chief Complaint

Pain in her left knee. No complaints of fever, night sweats, weight loss, or fatigue.

Medical History

Unremarkable.

Physical Examination

Tender left leg just above the knee. No lymphadenopathy or hepatosplenomegaly.

Laboratory Results

Screening procedures:

CBC with differential: All values within normal limits.
x-Ray of the left distal femur: Mixed lytic and blastic lesion with periosteal reaction in the left distal femur.
Bone scan: Increased uptake in the left distal femur.
A bone biopsy was performed.

Questions

1. Based on the clinical presentation and imaging studies, what conditions are in the differential diagnosis?
2. What would be the results of immunohistochemical stains performed on fixed, paraffin-embedded sections?

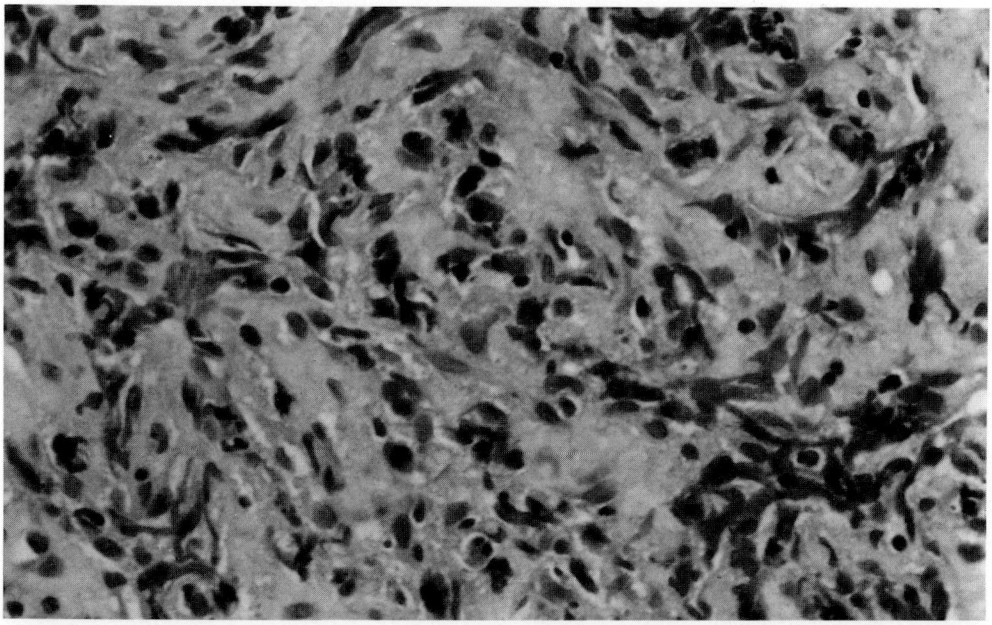

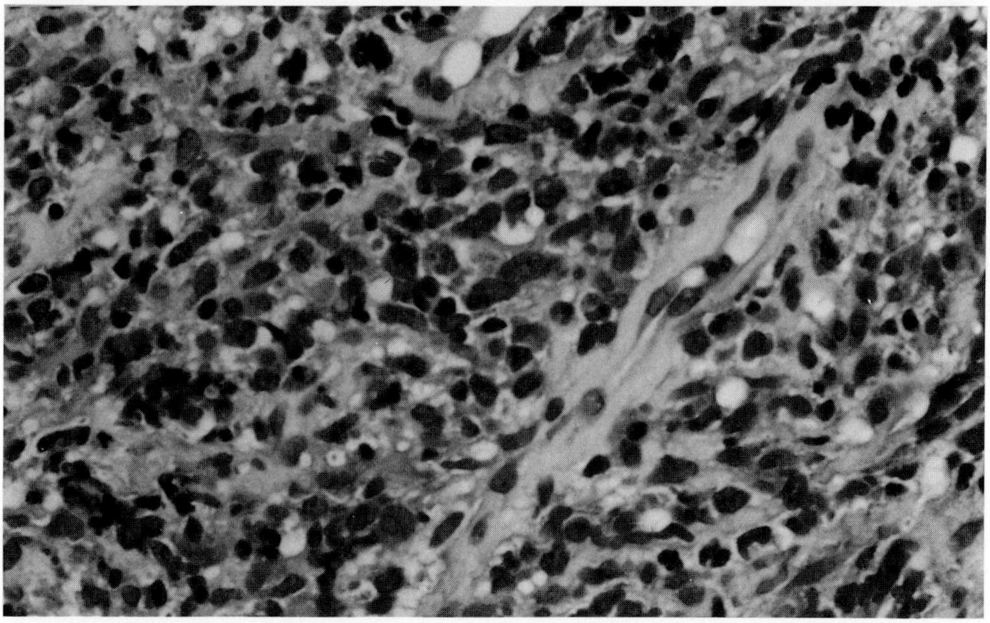

Case Study 1 Diffuse large B-cell lymphoma (primary osseous lymphoma). (Top) In many areas, the cytology of the neoplastic cells is obscured by sclerosis and crush artifact. (Hematoxylin-eosin, 528×.) (Bottom) In better preserved areas, the neoplastic cells are large with cleaved and lobated nuclei. There are admixed reactive small lymphocytes. (Hematoxylin-eosin, 528×.) (Next page) The neoplastic cells express CD20 (L26 antibody), a marker of B-cell differentiation. (Immunoperoxidase, 528×.)

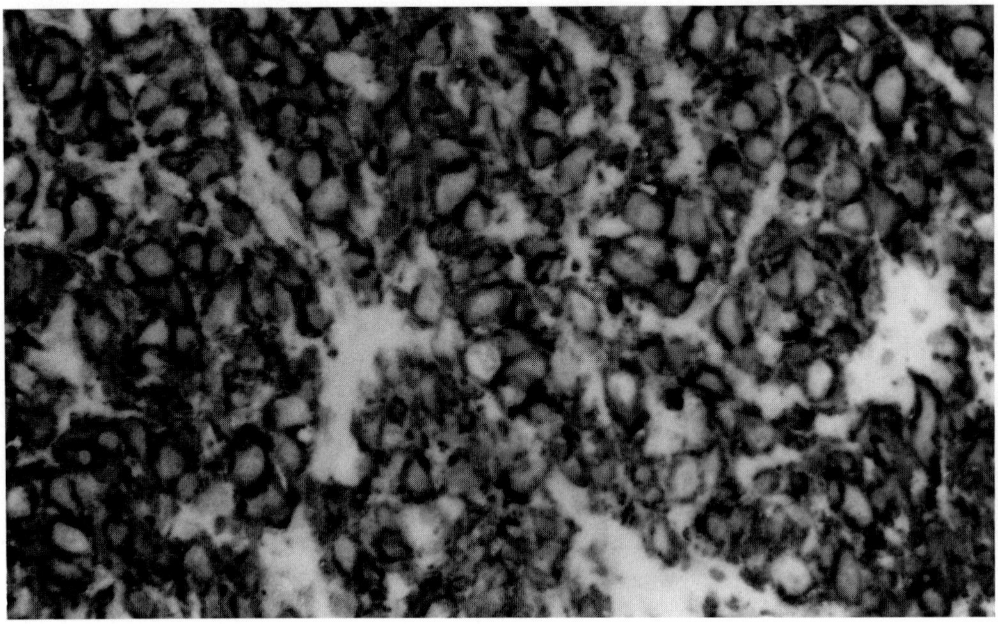

Case Study 1 (Continued)

Additional Laboratory Results

Confirmatory results: A biopsy of the distal left femur demonstrated a diffuse large B-cell lymphoma. There was extensive sclerosis and crush artifact in many of the sections. However, in the better-preserved areas, the neoplastic cells were large, and many had cleaved or lobated nuclear contours. There were numerous admixed small lymphocytes. Immunohistochemical stains were performed on fixed paraffin-embedded sections. The large neoplastic cells expressed CD45RB (leukocyte common antigen), CD20 (L26 antibody), and vimentin. Staining for markers of T-cell differentiation (CD3, CD45RO) accentuated the admixed small reactive T cells. The neoplastic cells did not express cytokeratin.

Diagnosis

Diffuse large B-cell lymphoma (primary osseous lymphoma).

Discussion

Primary osseous lymphoma is defined as a malignant lymphoma that arises within the medullary cavity of a single bone, without concurrent regional lymph node or visceral involvement within a six-month period. Patients are usually adults who present with localized pain, but are otherwise asymptomatic. There is a male predilection, with a male:female ratio of 1.5:1. Bone x-rays demonstrate lytic, blastic, or mixed lytic and blastic lesions. Most primary osseous lymphomas are classifed as diffuse large B-cell lymphomas. The neoplastic cell nuclei are often cleaved or multilobated, and there is often a marked proliferation of fibroblasts with a sclerotic background. Primary osseous lymphoma may be difficult to classify and diagnose for several reasons. First, it is rare; it comprises approximately 3% of all malignant bone tumors. Second, the biopsies may be small, with significant crush or decalcification artifact. Third, the cytology of the neoplastic lymphoid cells may resemble nonhematopoietic neoplasms. The fibroblastic proliferation and sclerosis may give the neoplastic cells a spindled appearance, or they may have clear cytoplasm and form clusters. Thus, primary osseous lymphoma may radiographically and histologically resemble chronic osteomyelitis, Ewing's sarcoma, spindle cell sarcoma, or metastatic carcinoma. In addition, granulocytic sarcoma may present occasionally as a single lytic bone lesion. Immunohistochemical stains are particularly helpful to establish the diagnosis. The malignant cells express CD45RB (leukocyte common antigen) and markers of B-cell differentiation, such as CD20 and CD79a. Immunohistochemical stains for markers of T-cell differentiation demonstrate admixed small, reactive T cells. On frozen section immunohistochemistry the malignant cells often express monotypic IgG. It is important to distinguish between primary osseous lymphoma and non-Hodgkin's lymphoma that has disseminated to bone, because patients with primary osseous lymphoma have a better prognosis. Most patients treated with aggressive multiagent chemotherapy and localized radiation therapy have a favorable outcome.

Reference

Fechner RE, Mills AS. Lesions of hematopoietic, lymphoid, and histiocytic elements. In: Rosai J, Sobin LH, eds. Atlas of Tumor Pathology. Tumors of the Bones and Joints. Fascicle 8, third series. Washington, DC: Armed Forces Institute of Pathology, 1992:211–232.

BIBLIOGRAPHY

1. Alexanian R, Weber D, Liu F. Differential diagnosis of monoclonal gammopathies. Arch Pathol Lab Med 1999; 123:108–113.
2. Chan JKC. Anaplastic large cell lymphoma: redefining its morphologic spectrum and importance of recognition of the ALK-positive subset. Adv Anat Pathol 1998; 5:281–313.
3. Cline MJ. The molecular basis of leukemia. N Engl J Med 1994; 330:328–336.
4. Diamondidou E, Cohen PR, Kurzrock R. Mycosis fungoides and Sezary syndrome. Blood 1996; 88:2385–2409.
5. Farcet J-P, Gaulard P, Marolleau J-P, et al. Hepatosplenic T-cell lymphoma: sinus/sinusoidal localization of malignant cells expressing the T-cell receptor $\gamma\delta$. Blood 1990; 75:2213–2219.
6. Fonseca R, Yamakawa M, Nakamura S, et al. Follicular dendritic cell sarcoma and interdigitating reticulum cell sarcoma: a review. Am J Hematol 1998; 59:161–167.
7. Foucar K. Chronic lymphoid leukemias and lymphoproliferative disorders. Mod Pathol 1998; 12: 141–150.
8. Gonzalez CL, Medeiros LJ, Braziel RM, Jaffe ES. T-cell lymphoma involving subcutaneous tissue: a clinicopathologic entity commonly associated with hemophagocytic syndrome. Am J Surg Pathol 1991; 15:17–27.
9. Guinee D, Jaffe E, Kingma D, et al. Pulmonary lymphomatoid granulomatosis: evidence for a proliferation of Epstein-Barr virus infected B-lymphocytes with a prominent T-cell component and vasculitis. Am J Surg Pathol 1994; 18:753–764.
10. Harris NL, Jaffe ES, Stein H, et al. A revised European-American classification of lymphoid neoplasms: a proposal from the International Lymphoma Study Group. Blood 1994; 84:1361–1392.
11. Isaacson PG. Lymphomas of mucosa-associated lymphoid tissue (MALT). Histopathology 1990; 16:617–619.
12. Jaffe ES. Post-thymic T-cell lymphomas. In: Jaffe ES, ed. Surgical Pathology of Lymph Nodes and Related Organs. Major Problems in Pathology Series, Volume 16. 2d ed. Philadelphia: Saunders, 1994:344–389.
13. Keren DF, Alexanian R, Goeken JA, Gorevic PD, Kyle RA, Tomar RH. Guidelines for clinical and laboratory evaluation of patients with monoclonal gammopathies. Arch Pathol Lab Med 1999; 123: 106–107.

14. Kyle RA. Sequence of testing for monoclonal gammopathies. Arch Pathol Lab Med 1999; 123: 114–118.
15. Lamarre L, Jacobson JO, Aisenberg AC, Harris NL. Primary large cell lymphoma of the mediastinum. A histologic and immunophenotypic study of 29 cases. Am J Surg Pathol 1989; 13:730–739.
16. Lipford EH, Margolick JB, Longo DL, Fauci AS, Jaffe ES. Angiocentric immunoproliferative lesions: a clinicopathologic spectrum of post-thymic T-cell proliferations. Blood 1988; 72:1674–1681.
17. Loughran TP. Clonal diseases of large granular lymphocytes. Blood 1993; 82:1–14.
18. Lukes RJ, Collins RD. Immunological characterization of human malignant lymphomas. Cancer 1974; 34:1488–1503.
19. Macon WR, Williams ME, Greer JP, Stein RS, Collins RD, Cousar JB. T-cell-rich B-cell lymphomas. A clinicopathologic study of 19 cases. Am J Surg Pathol 1992; 16:351–363.
20. Magrath IT. African Burkitt's lymphoma: history, biology, clinical features, and treatment. Am J Pediatr Hematol Oncol 1991; 13:222–246.
21. Matutes E, Brito-Babapulle V, Swansbury J, et al. Clinical and laboratory features of 78 cases of T-prolymphocytic leukemia. Blood 1991; 78:3269–3274.
22. Medeiros LJ, Bagg A, Cossman J. Molecular genetics in the diagnosis and classification of lymphoid neoplasms. In: Jaffe ES, ed. Surgical Pathology of Lymph Nodes and Related Organs. Major Problems in Pathology Series. Volume 16. 2d ed. Philadelphia: Saunders, 1994:58–97.
23. Medeiros LJ, Jaffe ES. Pathology of non-Hodgkin's lymphomas and Hodgkin's disease. In: Wiernik PH, Canellos GP, Dutcher J, Kyle RA, eds. Neoplastic Diseases of the Blood. 3d ed. New York: Churchill Livingstone, 1996:753–805.
24. National Cancer Institute sponsored study of classifications of non-Hodgkin's lymphomas: summary and description of a working formulation for clinical usage. The Non-Hodgkin's Lymphoma Pathologic Classification Project. Cancer 1982; 49:2112–2135.
25. Rappaport H, Winter WJ, Hicks EB. Follicular lymphoma: a reevaluation of its position in the scheme of malignant lymphoma, based on a survey of 253 cases. Cancer 1956; 9:792.
26. Roth MJ, Medeiros LJ, Elenitoba-Johnson K, Kuchnio M, Jaffe ES, Stetler-Stevenson M. Extramedullary myeloid cell tumors: an immunohistochemical study of 29 cases using routinely fixed and processed paraffin-embedded tissue sections. Arch Pathol Lab Med 1995; 119:790–798.
27. Shimoyama M. Diagnostic criteria and classification of clinical subtypes of adult T-cell leukemia/lymphoma. A report from the Lymphoma Study Group. Br J Haematol 1991; 79:428–437.
28. Stansfeld AG, Diebold J, Kapanci Y, et al. Updated Kiel classification for lymphomas. Lancet 1998; 1:292–293.
29. Stetler-Stevenson M, Medeiros LJ, Jaffe ES. Immunophenotypic methods and findings in the diagnosis of lymphoproliferative diseases. In: Jaffe ES, ed. Surgical Pathology of Lymph Nodes and Related Organs. Major Problems in Pathology Series. Volume 16. 2d ed. Philadelphia: Saunders, 1994:22–57.
30. Swerdlow S. Small B-cell lymphomas of the lymph nodes and spleen: practical insights to diagnosis and pathogenesis. Mod Pathol 1998; 12:125–140.
31. Weiss LM, Jaffe E, Liu X, Chen YY, Shibata D, Medeiros LJ. Detection and localization of Epstein-Barr viral genomes in angioimmunoblastic lymphadenopathy and angioimmunoblastic lymphadenopathy-like lymphomas. Blood 1992; 79:1789–1795.
32. Yano T, van Krieken JHJM, Magrath IT, Longo DL, Jaffe ES, Raffeld M. Histogenetic correlations between subcategories of small noncleaved cell lymphomas. Blood 1992; 79:1282–1290.

5

Hodgkin's Disease

Lynne V. Abruzzo and L. Jeffrey Medeiros
University of Texas M.D. Anderson Cancer Center, Houston, Texas

Kojo S. J. Elenitoba-Johnson
University of Utah Health Sciences Center, Salt Lake City, Utah

I. INTRODUCTION

Approximately 75% of patients with Hodgkin's disease (HD) will be cured with appropriate treatment. The major factors that affect response include patient age, presence or absence of systemic or "B" symptoms (fevers, night sweats, weight loss of 10% or more body weight), stage, tumor bulk, and various laboratory abnormalities, such as high serum lactate dehydrogenase or β-2 microglobulin levels. All histologic types of HD are responsive to treatment. Therefore, the pathologist's most important task is to distinguish HD from non-Hodgkin's lymphoma (NHL) and to identify HD in staging specimens. Histologic typing of HD also is of interest and value because these determinations correlate with clinical findings such as sites of involvement, stage at presentation, and systemic symptoms.

In this chapter, first we will review the clinical and histologic findings of HD. Next we will summarize the results of immunologic and molecular studies of HD. These results indicate that HD is heterogeneous, and may represent more than one disease entity that share clinical and histologic findings. In addition, immunohistochemical methods have been tremendously helpful in improving pathologists' ability to differentiate HD from NHL.

II. PATHOLOGIC DEFINITION

HD is defined as a malignant hematopoietic neoplasm composed of diagnostic Reed-Sternberg (RS) cells in an appropriate reactive cellular background. Because RS-like cells can occur in a variety of neoplastic and reactive diseases that involve lymph nodes and other sites, both components are necessary to establish the diagnosis.

The classic RS cell is large, with a large, bilobed nucleus. Each nuclear lobe contains a prominent round eosinophilic nucleolus, surrounded by a clear zone or halo. The nucleoli are about one-quarter the size of the nucleus. The nuclear chromatin is marginated to form a thickened nuclear membrane (Fig. 1). The RS cell often is said to resemble an "owl's eye." The cytoplasm is frequently abundant and stains lightly eosinophilic to amphophilic. RS cells also may have three or four nuclear lobes and corresponding nucleoli. The cellular background

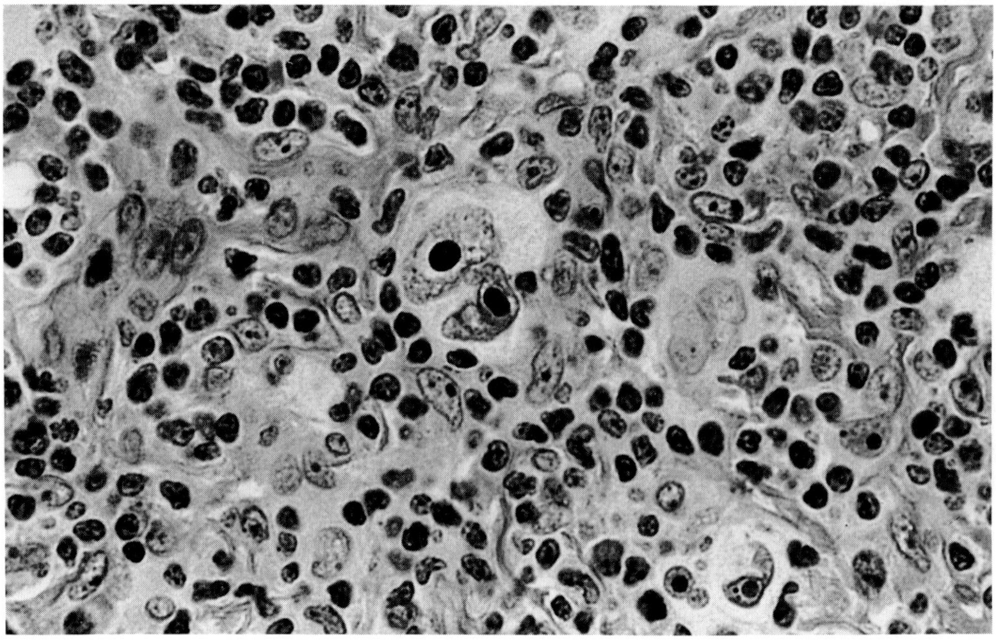

Figure 1 Reed-Sternberg cell. The nucleus is bilobed and each lobe contains a prominent, eosinophilic nucleolus surrounded by a clear zone. (Hematoxylin-cosin, 680×.)

in HD is cytologically benign and composed of a variable mixture of inflammatory cells that includes small lymphocytes, histiocytes, plasma cells, eosinophils, neutrophils, and fibroblasts.

III. HISTOLOGIC CLASSIFICATION

During the past 50 years, three major classification systems have been used to evaluate HD. The first, proposed by Jackson and Parker in 1944, subdivided HD into three categories: paragranuloma, granuloma, and sarcoma. Although this classification system recognized that the prognosis is generally excellent for paragranuloma and poor for sarcoma, it places approximately 90% of HD in the granuloma category, a group with heterogeneous clinical presentations, histologic findings, and prognosis.

In 1966, Lukes and Butler made a major contribution to our understanding of HD. They expanded the Jackson and Parker system to six categories: lymphocytic and/or histiocytic (L& H) nodular, L&H diffuse, mixed cellularity (MC), nodular sclerosis (NS), diffuse fibrosis, and reticular. This classification system recognized the distinctive mononuclear cell variants found in different types of HD, and the differences in the composition of the reactive cell component. It also described two distinct types of connective-tissue proliferation found in NS and diffuse fibrosis. Particularly noteworthy is that this system recognized NSHD as a distinct category (classified as granuloma in the Jackson and Parker scheme), with a predilection for mediastinal involvement in young adults.

At an international symposium in Rye, NY, in 1966, the six categories proposed by Lukes and Butler were consolidated into four: lymphocytic predominance (LP), NS, MC, and lymphocytic depletion(LD). The L&H nodular and diffuse categories were combined to form the LP category; NS and MC were left unchanged; the diffuse fibrosis and reticular categories were combined to form the LD category.

The Rye modification has gained universal acceptance. Pathologists and clinicians find it easy to use, and the different diagnostic categories correlate with clinical parameters such as sites of involvement, stage, and prognosis. However, from a pathologic standpoint, the Lukes and Butler classification is more helpful in understanding histologic findings in HD. Thus, we use the Rye system to describe the pathology of HD and expand the discussion, where appropriate, to include the types specified in the Lukes and Butler classification.

Since these classification systems were proposed, it has become apparent that LPHD is clinically and immunophenotypically distinct from the other categories of HD, collectively referred to as the "classical" subtypes of HD. The Revised European-American Classification of Lymphoid Neoplasms, proposed by the International Lymphoma Study Group, classifies the non-Hodgkin's lymphomas and Hodgkin's disease based on histologic, immunologic, genetic, and clinical features. This system retains the four categories of HD of the Rye system, and has added a provisional entity, lymphocyte-rich classical Hodgkin's disease.

A. Lymphocytic Predominance

About 5% of patients with HD have the LP subtype, which most often is diagnosed as a localized process (clinical stage I or II). Cervical lymph nodes are common initial sites of involvement. Typically, the patient has one or more enlarged lymph nodes that measure up to 3–5 cm. The disease affects patients of all ages, with a male-to-female ratio of approximately 2.5 to 1. The clinical course is usually indolent. From 1978 to 1986, the 5-year survival rate was 83.9%, according to data recently collected by the National Cancer Institute's (NCI) Statistics, Epidemiology, and End Results (SEER) program.

Two subgroups of LPHD are recognized, nodular and diffuse, which correspond to nodular and diffuse L&H disease in the Lukes and Butler system. Nodular LPHD, also known as nodular paragranuloma, is characterized by effacement of nodal architecture by variably sized, poorly defined nodules (Fig. 2A). The nodules are composed of cytologically distinctive L&H cells and rare diagnostic RS cells in a sea of small lymphocytes with scattered histiocytes. The histiocytes occasionally may aggregate to form granulomata. The abnormal, large polyploid L&H cells may be concentrated in the centers of the nodules. The neoplasm may demonstrate uninvolved lymph node at the periphery. Eosinophils and plasma cells are scant or absent, and there usually is no associated fibrosis or necrosis. The capsule typically is intact and not fibrotic.

The L&H cell is a large lymphoid cell characterized by a large vesicular nucleus with delicate nuclear chromatin (Fig. 2B). The nucleus often is polylobated and has an inconspicuous nucleolus, although some of these cells may be relatively round and have small but distinct nucleoli. The cytoplasm is pale and eosinophilic. The polylobated cells have been referred to as "popcorn" cells because they resemble kernels of popped corn.

Nodular LPHD may be associated with an unusual form of follicular hyperplasia, known as progressive transformation of germinal centers (PTGC). PTGC is a reactive process that resembles nodular LPHD. However, unlike nodular LPHD, PTGC does not efface the normal architecture, and L&H cells and RS cells are absent. Some researchers have suggested that PTGC is a premalignant condition that may give rise to nodular LPHD because it is morphologically similar to and frequently occurs in patients with nodular LPHD. However, we disagree with this suggestion because PTGC has been observed in lymph nodes of patients with other types of HD, as well as in patients without evidence of HD. Thus, the presence of PTGC

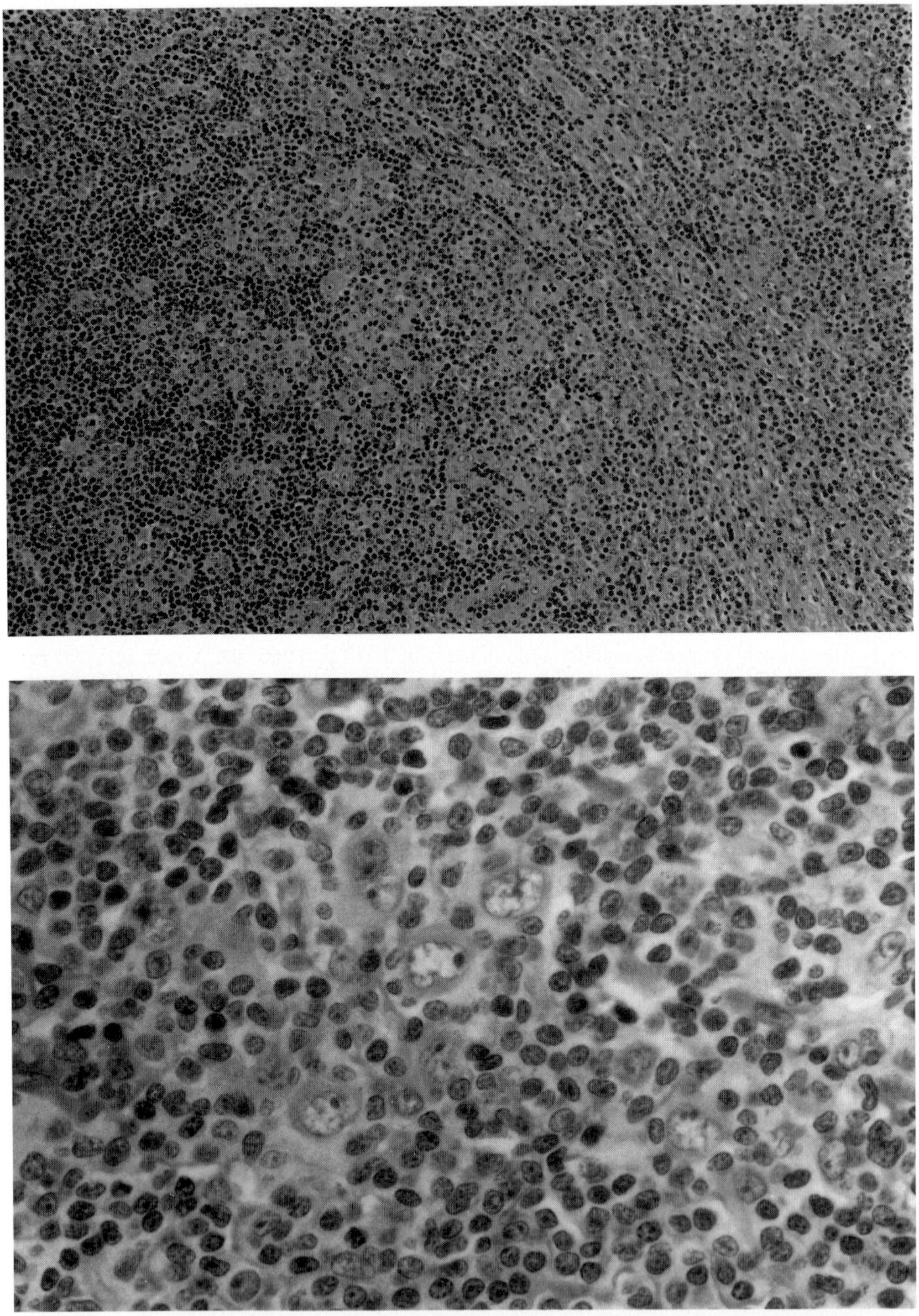

Figure 2 Nodular lymphocytic predominance HD. (A) The neoplasm is vaguely nodular with a mottled apearance as a result of the many reactive small lymphocytes and larger histiocytes. (B) An L&H cell is at the center of the field. L&H cells are large with polylobated nuclei and inconspicuous nucleoli, and resemble popcorn. (Hematoxylin-eosin, A, 50×; B, 630×.)

should not be considered evidence of nodular LPHD. Recent clinical and immunohistochemical studies have suggested that nodular LPHD may be closely related to B-cell NHLs and is distinct from other types of HD.

Diffuse LPHD, also known as diffuse paragranuloma, is characterized histologically by diffuse effacement of the lymph node architecture. Other than its diffuse growth pattern, the neoplasm is cytologically similar to nodular LPHD, with L&H cells, rare RS cells, numerous small lymphocytes, and a variable number of histiocytes. Eosinophils, plasma cells, fibrosis, and necrosis are rare or absent. Capsular fibrosis is absent.

A subset of cases that histologically resemble diffuse LPHD have been shown immunohistochemically to have an immunophenotype similar to other classical types of Hodgkin's disease. These cases have relatively infrequent classic RS cells, may have lacunar cells, and lack L and H cells. The International Lymphoma Study Group has suggested that these tumors be diagnosed as lymphocyte-rich classical Hodgkin's disease.

B. Nodular Sclerosis

NS is the most common subtype of HD. About 60% of all patients with HD have NS, and it is the most common type of HD in those younger than age 50. In contrast to other types of HD, it is equally common in men and women, but whites are affected more often than blacks. The age-adjusted incidence rate is increasing, from 1.1 per 100,000 between 1973 and 1977 to 1.6 per 100,000 between 1983 and 1987. This increase has been greatest in adolescents and young adults ages 15–45, the group with peak incidence.

NSHD has unique clinical features, including a remarkable predilection for involving anterior mediastinal lymph nodes, and lymph nodes in scalene, supraclavicular, and cervical areas. The thymus also may be involved. Patients often are diagnosed with clinical stage I or II disease, which has an excellent prognosis. The 5-year survival rate was 82.2% from 1978 to 1986, according to recent NCI SEER data.

In addition to the presence of RS cells in the appropriate cellular background, three histologic findings are required to establish the diagnosis of NSHD: lacunar cells, nodular architecture, and dense collagen fibrosis. Sclerosis is present as broad bands of collagen that originate from a thickened fibrotic capsule and circumscribe tumor nodules (Fig. 3). The collagen exhibits birefringence when viewed with polarization microscopy. Although this characteristic is helpful, the broad collagen bands are sufficiently well developed in most cases that polarization microscopy is not necessary for diagnosis. In some patients, most of the cellular component is obliterated by fibrosis, thought to represent end-stage NSHD. Fibrosis in NSHD also may increase after therapy.

Lacunar cells are the characteristic cells of NSHD. They are mononuclear variants of RS, with large prominent multilobed nuclei, small to medium-size nucleoli, and abundant pale eosinophilic cytoplasm with well-defined cell borders (Fig. 4). In formalin-fixed tissue, the cytoplasm artifactually retracts leaving the cell within a lacunar-like space, hence the name lacunar cell. Retraction is absent or greatly reduced in B5-fixed tissue.

Tumor nodules are composed of lacunar cells and RS cells, with a variable mixture of small lymphocytes, histiocytes, eosinophils, plasma cells, and neutrophils. Diagnostic RS cells are much less common than lacunar cells and sometimes can be difficult to identify. Typically, lacunar cells are located in the center of the nodules. Large areas of necrosis may be present, and lacunar cells are most abundant in viable tumor surrounding necrotic foci.

Because the reactive-cell population in NSHD varies so greatly, NSHD has sometimes been subdivided according to number and types of reactive cells present. Correlation of these

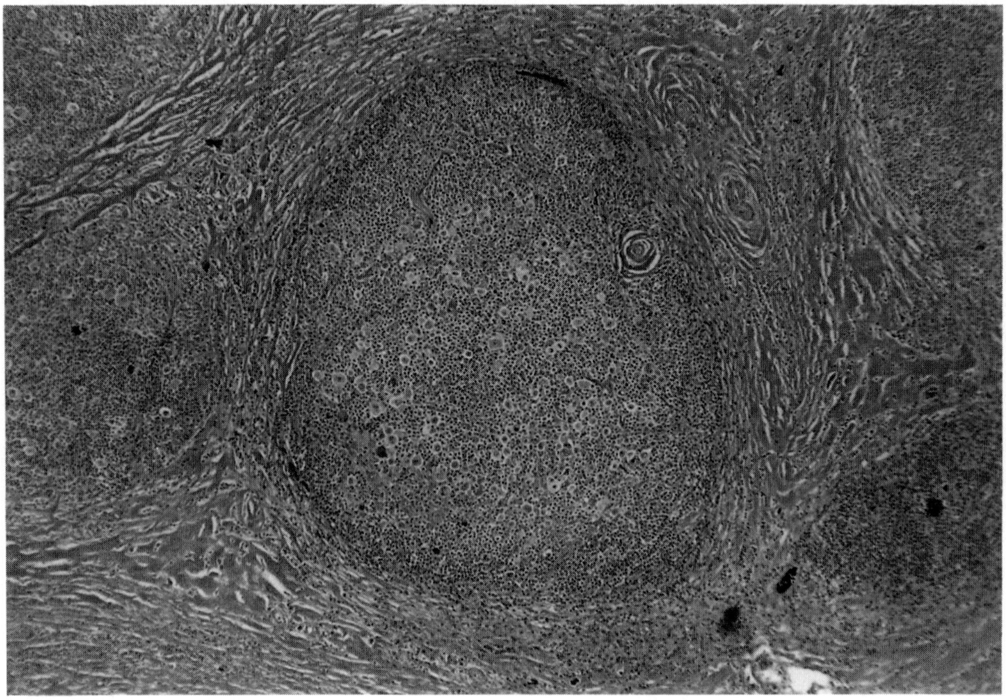

Figure 3 Nodular sclerosis HD. The neoplasm is composed of nodules surrounded by dense collagen bands. (Hematoxylin-eosin, 20×.)

findings with prognosis has been inconsistent. However, most investigators agree that patients with NSHD with extensive lymphocyte depletion and many RS cells have a poorer prognosis.

A "syncytial" variant of NSHD, characterized by large clusters and sheets of lacunar cells that surround necrotic areas, also has been referred to as the lymphocyte-depleted variant of NSHD. This form of NSHD is associated with a poorer prognosis. For example, Kant and colleagues found that patients with the lymphocyte-depleted subtype of NSHD more often have clinical stage III or IV disease and systemic symptoms. In addition to having prognostic significance, the presence of sheets of large atypical cells may result in incorrect diagnosis because these neoplasms may resemble other hematopoietic or nonhematopoietic tumors.

A "fibroblastic" variant of NSHD has been described in which fibroblasts proliferate abundantly, and lymphocytes are relatively depleted. Foci of fibroblastic proliferation with a storiform architectural growth pattern are seen. Because pleomorphic giant lacunar cells also are present, this neoplasm may resemble malignant fibrous histiocytoma. This variant, which is probably related to the lymphocyte-depleted subtype of NSHD and the syncytial form of NSHD, has a poorer prognosis.

A "cellular phase" of NSHD has been described in the literature. The neoplasm has a nodular growth pattern, and the nodules are composed of lacunar cells and RS cells in an appropriate cellular background. However, collagen bands that surround the nodules are scarce or absent. Some observers suggest that at least one sclerotic band is necessary to designate a neoplasm as cellular phase NSHD. When relapse occurs in these patients, the histologic findings are often typical of NSHD, supporting the initial interpretation. However, because diag-

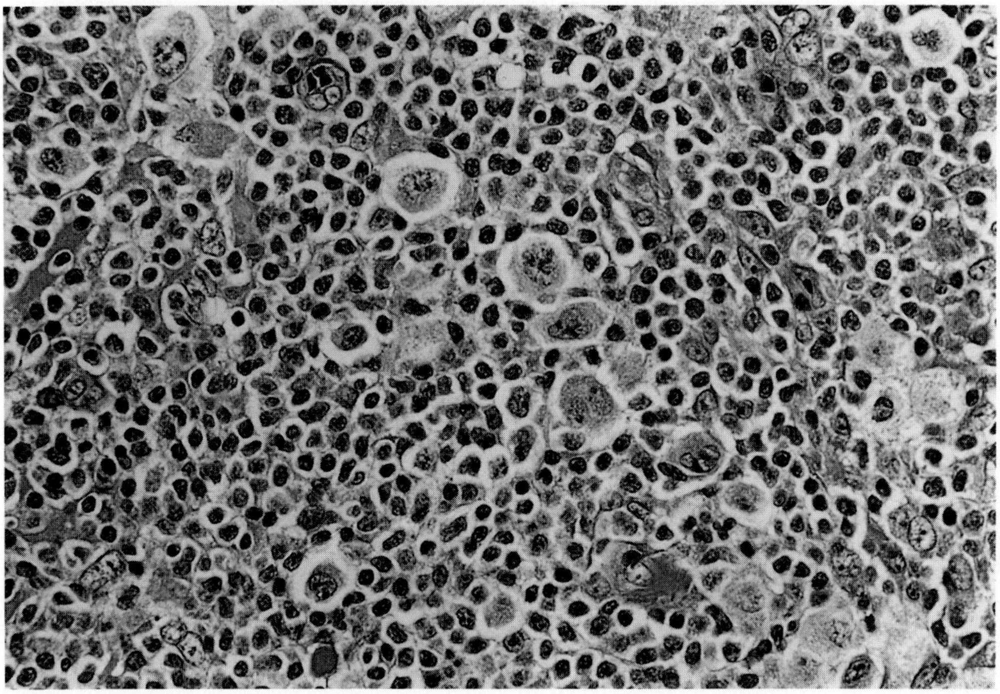

Figure 4 Nodular sclerosis HD. Lacunar cells are large, often multilobated cells. In formalin-fixed tissue sections these cells lie in spaces (lacunae) that result from cytoplasm retraction. Lacunar cells tend to cluster in the center of the nodules. (Hematoxylin-eosin, 425×.)

nostic histologic criteria for cellular-phase NSHD vary, others recommend that these cases be classified as mixed cellularity (MCHD) to ensure diagnostic consistency and high interobserver concordance.

An important feature of the Rye classification system is that NS histology takes precedence over any other HD type present. For example, a neoplasm with foci of both NS and other HD types is classified as NSHD even if the focus of NS represents only a small component of the tumor.

C. Mixed Cellularity

MC is the second most common type of HD, occurring in 24% of patients. MCHD is the most common type of HD in patients older than 50 years. Males are affected more often than females (1.7 to 1). A significant proportion of patients are diagnosed with clinical stage III or IV disease and systemic symptoms. The 5-year survival rate was 68.1% from 1978 to 1986, according to recent NCI SEER data.

A wide spectrum of histologic findings may be seen in MCHD. Lymph node architecture often is completely effaced by a neoplasm that is composed of numerous diagnostic RS cells and mononuclear cell variants, also known as Hodgkin (H) cells. Although similar to classic RS cells, H cells have a unilobed nucleus or one nuclear lobe visible in the plane of section. The reactive cellular background includes numerous eosinophils, plasma cells, and histiocytes in a variable mixture (Fig. 5). Focal necrosis may be present but usually is not marked. Fibrosis

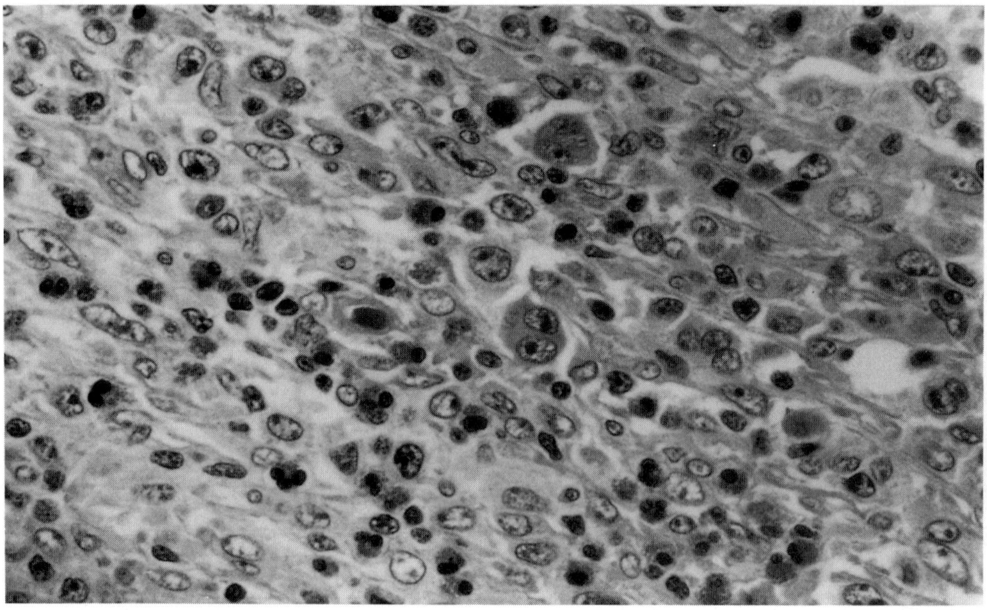

Figure 5 Mixed cellularity HD. The Reed-Sternberg cell (center) is surrounded by numerous inflammatory cells, including neutrophils, eosinophils, histiocytes, and small lymphocytes. (Hematoxylin-eosin, 630×.)

occurs in focal areas, but is not organized into broad fibrous bands that surround nodules. In some cases, epithelioid histiocytes may aggregate to form relatively cohesive clusters or granulomata.

In the literature, some have placed cases of HD that are not readily classifiable into the MC category. The result of this practice is that the MCHD category becomes a pathologic "wastebasket." We and others believe that difficult-to-classify cases should remain unclassified, rather than be forced into the MC category. Thus, we designate a small subset of cases of HD as being unclassified.

D. Lymphocytic Depletion

LD is the least common HD subtype, representing fewer than 5% of cases. Patients with LDHD usually are elderly; the disease is rare in those younger than 40 years. The male-to-female ratio is 1.3 to 1, and whites and blacks are equally affected. Patients most often are diagnosed with advanced stage disease and systemic symptoms. LD is associated with the poorest prognosis of all HD types; from 1978 to 1986, the 5-year survival rate was 36.4% in recent NCI SEER data.

The LD category includes two HD variants recognized by Lukes and Butler, diffuse fibrosis and reticular. Diffuse fibrosis HD is characterized by an extensive proliferation of disordered, nonbirefringent, compact, hypocellular fibrosis (Fig. 6). In some cases, fibroblasts may be abundant. Unlike the fibrosis seen in NSHD, the connective tissue proliferation in diffuse fibrosis HD is irregular, patchy, and nonbirefringent. Diagnostic RS cells usually are numerous, but may be difficult to identify. In contrast, reticular HD is characterized by numerous RS and H cells that may be present in sheets and may easily be mistaken for NHL. Background

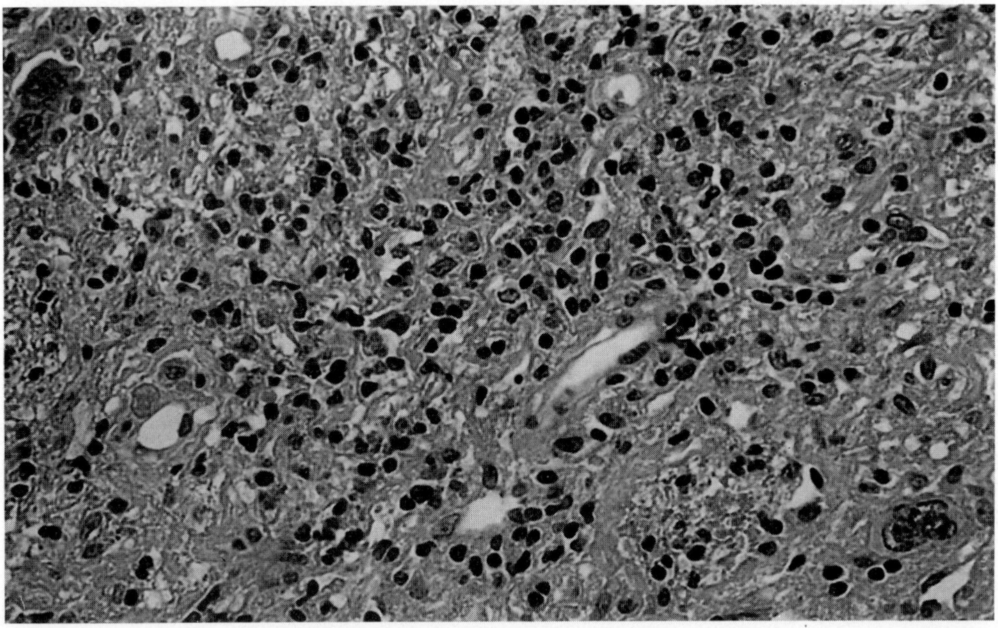

Figure 6 Lymphocyte depletion HD (diffuse fibrosis variant). In this tumor, there is generalized lymphocyte depletion and amorphous, nonbirefringent fibrosis. Large Reed-Sternberg and Hodgkin cells also are visible. (Hematoxylin-eosin, 250×.)

deposits of cellular amorphous fibrous tissue are less extensive than those seen in diffuse fibrosis. Areas of necrosis are common. In a small subset of cases of reticular HD, the RS and H cells appear pleomorphic and bizarre, with marked variation in nuclear shape, huge nucleoli, and many mitotic figures. These cases resemble sarcomas, accounting for their original name of Hodgkin's sarcoma in the Jackson and Parker classification. All patients with LDHD, as defined in the Rye classification, characteristically have numerous malignant cells and a paucity of lymphocytes and other reactive cells relative to other HD types.

Grossly, the tumor in patients with LDHD often is larger than that seen in other HD types, and represents either a large mass of contiguous lymph nodes or diffuse visceral replacement. Patients with the diffuse fibrosis variant often have subdiaphragmatic disease, with abdominal lymph node and visceral involvement. Patients with the reticular variant often have peripheral lymphadenopathy and bone marrow involvement. With appropriate therapy, patients with the diffuse fibrosis variant have longer median survival than those with the reticular variant.

The age-adjusted incidence rate of LDHD was lower from 1983 to 1987 than from 1973 to 1977 in the NCI SEER data. This decrease may be explained, in part, by the recognition by pathologists that many tumors previously classified as LDHD were, in fact, NHLs. Improved classification is a result of immunohistochemical stains and antigen receptor gene rearrangement studies. For example, in one retrospective study, only 23% of cases originally classified as LDHD were still considered to be HD. Reclassification to NHL occurred most often in cases previously classified as the reticular variant of HD. The type of NHL most frequently diagnosed as LDHD in the past was anaplastic large-cell lymphoma (also known as Ki-1 lymphoma).

E. Interfollicular Hodgkin's Disease

In a small subset of patients with HD, the neoplasm may only partially involve the lymph node, typically as a distinct focus within the paracortical region. Within this focus, the histologic findings are typical of HD, and usually resemble MCHD, with diagnostic RS cells, mononuclear variants, and an array of inflammatory cells. In a smaller group of patients, the interfollicular focus of HD may have fibrous bands and resembles NSHD. The HD focus may be quite small and represent less than 5% of the lymph node. The uninvolved lymph node may mimic a reactive process, with marked follicular hyperplasia and plasmacytosis. Although the degree of lymph node involvement may appear small, cases of interfollicular HD behave clinically like cases of HD with more extensive lymph node involvement. Clinical follow-up studies have shown that patients with interfollicular HD may relapse with neoplasms that are histologically more characteristic of either MCHD or NSHD. Thus, the importance of interfollicular HD lies in its unusual histologic findings, which may result in the neoplasm being missed.

IV. DISEASE IN EXTRANODAL SITES

As is the case for HD involving lymph nodes, a primary diagnosis of HD involving an extranodal site requires the presence of diagnostic RS cells within an appropriate cellular background. HD may involve extranodal sites, such as the lung or skin, by direct extension from involved lymph nodes. Patients with HIV-1 infection are at increased risk to present with extranodal involvement. However, extranodal involvement at presentation is unusual in patients who have neither HIV-1 infection nor concurrent disease in lymph nodes; it occurs in fewer than 1% of all patients with HD. Furthermore, a significant number of cases diagnosed previously as primary extranodal HD involving sites such as skin and gastrointestinal tract have been shown since to be aggressive NHL. Thus, a diagnosis of primary extranodal HD in immunocompetent patients should be made cautiously.

V. PATHOLOGIC FINDINGS IN STAGING SPECIMENS

In patients with an established diagnosis of HD (usually by lymph node biopsy), the criteria for diagnosing HD at other sites may be less rigorous. For example, in liver and bone marrow biopsy specimens, only mononuclear cell variants in an appropriate cellular background are required to conclude that the findings are consistent with involvement by HD (Fig. 7). Similarly, diagnostic RS cells may not be identifiable within an extranodal HD site, particularly if involvement is focal. In involved abdominal lymph nodes and spleens obtained at staging laparotomy, diagnostic RS and H cells usually are identified, and there is no need to be less rigorous in establishing the diagnosis of HD. Splenic involvement by HD is characterized grossly by large white-tan or miliary nodules. Detection of five or more nodules of HD on gross examination is associated with a poorer prognosis.

VI. PATHOLOGIC FINDINGS AT RELAPSE

One-third of patients whose disease initially responds completely to therapy later relapse. A smaller subset of patients will relapse after 3 years or longer. Risk of relapse is greatest in those with systemic symptoms and advanced disease at diagnosis. At relapse, the neoplasm may or may not resemble the initial diagnostic biopsy specimen. NS is the type of HD most likely to resemble the initial biopsy specimen. This is particularly true if relapse occurs at a

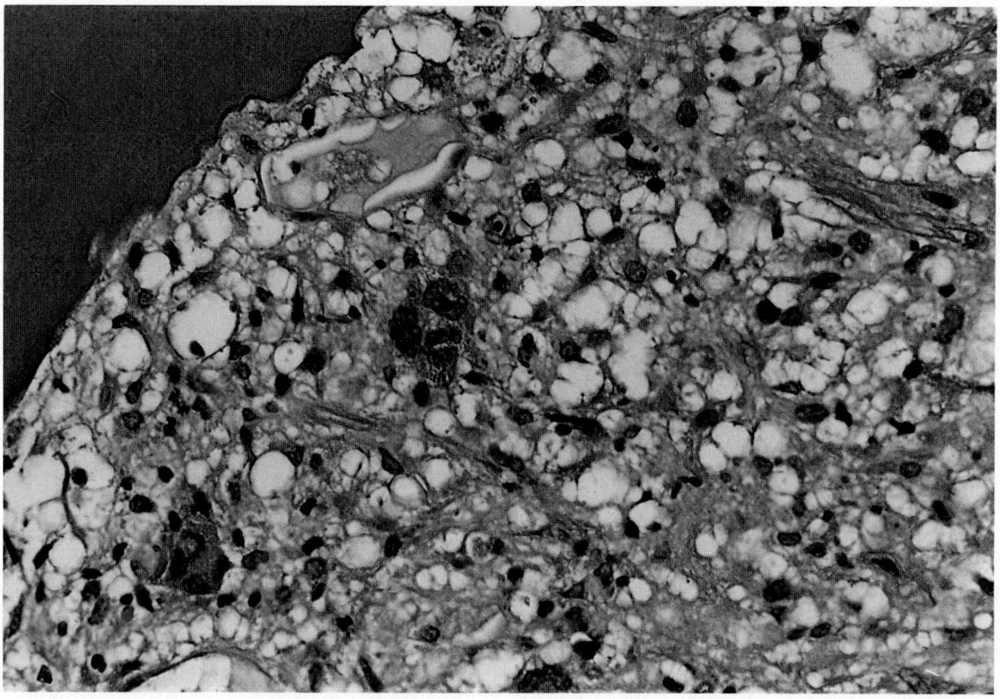

Figure 7 Bone marrow involvement in HD. The malignant cells are found in a background of fibroblasts and inflammatory cells. (Hematoxylin-eosin, 400×.)

site that was not previously irradiated. When histologic findings are not conserved, the tumor generally contains a larger number of RS and H cells, more necrosis, and is depleted of reactive lymphocytes. Thus the pattern of histologic progression suggests that LDHD, particularly the diffuse fibrosis variant, is the common terminal histologic manifestation of HD.

VII. IMMUNOPHENOTYPIC FINDINGS IN HODGKIN'S DISEASE

Immunohistochemical methods have been a tremendous help in improving the pathologist's ability to differentiate HD from NHL. Analysis of cases of HD using immunohistochemical methods allows direct observation of the immunoreactivity of the RS and H cells as well as the reactive cells. Frozen sections have the advantage that many monoclonal antibodies are available for analysis. However, it is often difficult to appreciate cellular detail in frozen sections. Although the number of antibodies that are reactive with fixed, paraffin-embedded sections is somewhat limited, the cytologic detail is more readily appreciated. In general, analysis of cell suspensions of specimens involved by HD using flow cytometry is not helpful. The RS and H cells typically represent fewer than 1% of all cells in an involved lymph node and, thus, are difficult to assess.

In frozen sections, the RS and H cells in cases of classical Hodgkin's disease (types other than LPHD) react with various markers of lymphocyte activation such as CD30 (Ki-1 antigen), CD25 (the interleukin-2 receptor), and HLA-DR. They also react with markers of proliferation, such as CD71 (the transferrin receptor), and with granulocyte-associated antigens, such as CD15 (LeuM1). In some cases, the RS and H cells also express B-cell or T-cell antigens. These results have led some observers to suggest that RS and H cells are of lymphoid origin. It is also conceivable that HD may be heterogeneous and represent both B-cell and T-cell lymphoid neoplasms that share clinical and histologic findings.

The background lymphocytes in HD are reactive and are predominantly T cells with a normal immunophenotype. T-helper/inducer cells outnumber T suppressor/cytotoxic cells in approximately a 3-to-1 ratio. The B cells express polytypic immunoglobulin light chains. Nodular LPHD has a greater percentage of reactive B cells compared to other types of HD.

Immunohistochemical studies have shown that nodular LPHD is distinct from the other types of HD. The L&H cells express the pan-leukocyte marker, leukocyte common antigen (LCA, CD45), immunoglobulin J chain, B-cell antigens, and epithelial membrane antigen (EMA); they are negative for CD30 (Ki-1 antigen) in more than two-thirds of cases, and almost always negative for CD15 (LeuM1) (Fig. 8). The nodules are composed of numerous B cells within an irregular network of dendritic reticulum cells. The internodular areas are composed predominantly of T cells. These results suggest that nodular LPHD is of B-cell lineage.

In contrast, the RS and H cells in NS, MC, and LDHD react with antibodies to CD30 and CD15 (Fig. 9) with a typical membrane and paranuclear dotlike (Golgi) pattern of staining; they are negative for CD45(LCA), EMA, and usually T-cell antigens. The B-cell antigen CD20 is expressed in a subset of cases, approximately 20%.

These findings are of great help in differentiating these subtypes of HD from NHL. Non-Hodgkin's lymphomas usually express pan-leukocyte markers, such as CD45, and either B-cell or T-cell antigens, depending upon the lineage of the neoplasm; they lack CD15. Since

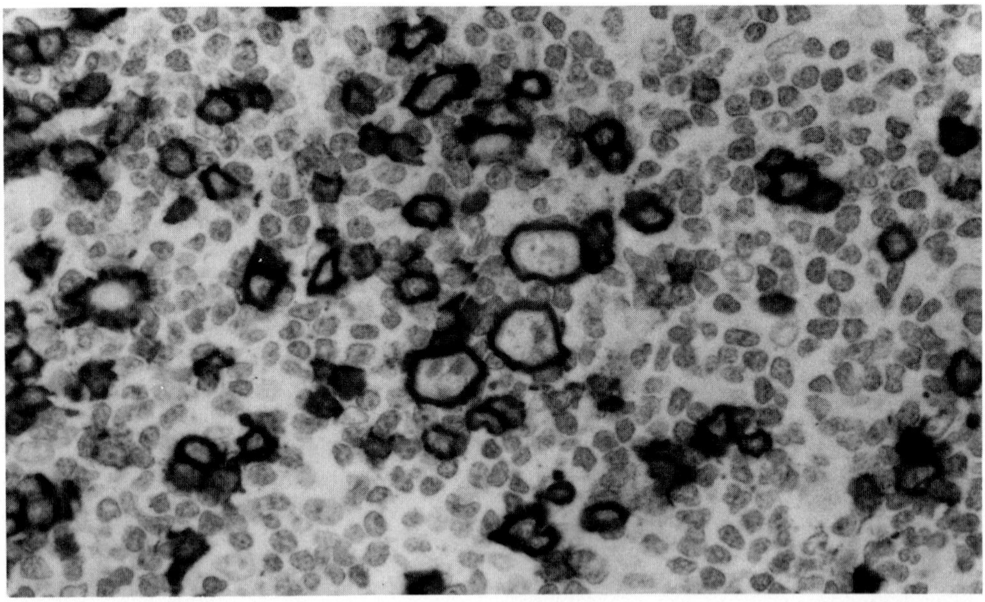

Figure 8 Nodular lymphocytic predominance HD. The L&H cells and small lymphocytes react with B-cell antibodies such as L26 (CD20). They also express epithelial membrane antigen and pan-leukocyte markers such as LCA (CD45RB) (not shown). (Immunoperoxidase, 400×.)

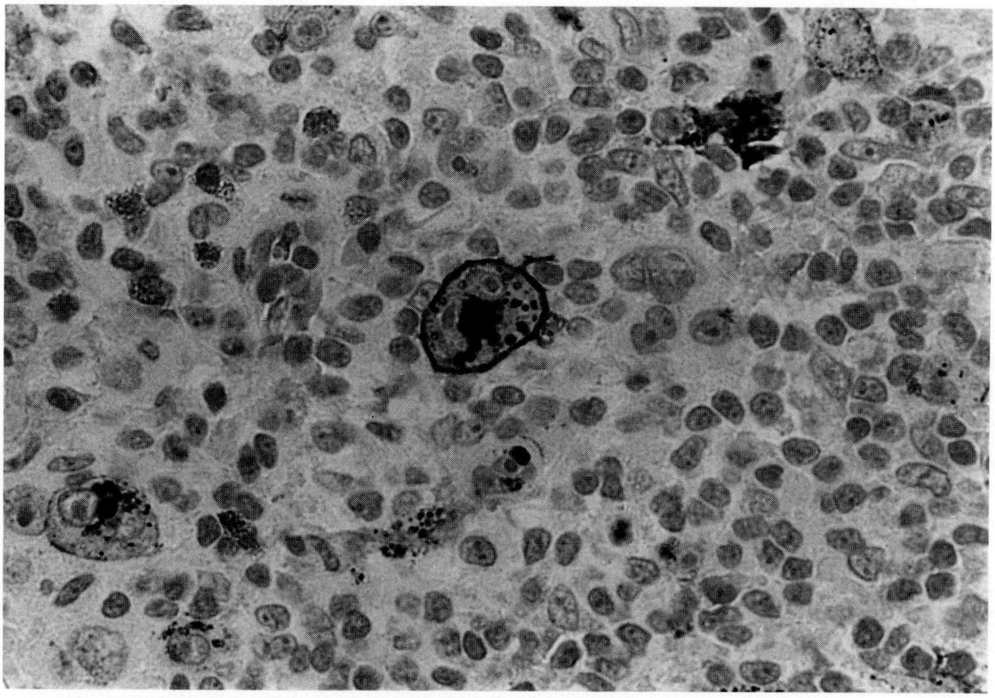

Figure 9 Nodular sclerosis HD. The Reed-Sternberg and lacunar cells express CD15 (LeuM1) and CD30 (not shown). (Immunoperoxidase, 1000×.)

there are exceptions to these general statements, most hematopathologists recommend that a panel of monoclonal antibodies be used to distinguish HD from NHL. Immunohistochemical studies are one of the important factors that has led to the recognition that many cases previously classified as LDHD are, in fact, NHL.

VIII. MOLECULAR GENETIC FINDINGS IN HODGKIN'S DISEASE

Conventional cytogenetic studies of classical HD have revealed nonrandom, often complex abnormalities in up to half of cases. For example, Cabanillas and colleagues have shown chromosomal breakpoints involving 11q32, 14q32, 6q11-21, and 8q22-24. Other reported breakpoint regions include 12p11-13, 13p11-13, 3q26-28, 6q15-16, and 7q31-35. Consistent and specific cytogenetic abnormalities have not been identified in NLPHD.

Initial studies of HD that assessed the antigen receptor genes by Southern blot hybridization demonstrated that they were in the germline configuration in most cases. These results are not surprising, since the RS and H cells usually represent fewer than 1% of the total cell population in involved tissues, and the sensitivity of Southern blot hybridization for detecting monoclonal populations of cells is approximately 1–5%. In approximately 20% of cases of HD, rearrangements of either the immunoglobulin genes or the T-cell receptor genes have been detected. The immunoglobulin genes are rearranged more frequently than the T-cell receptor genes, in a 3-to-1 ratio. The rearranged bands are usually faint and represent only a small percentage of the cell population within the specimen.

In most studies it is not clear which cells within the neoplasm contain the gene rearrangements. However, gene rearrangements have been found more commonly in cases with numerous RS and H cells. These results suggest that the RS and H cells contain the immunoglobulin gene rearrangements. Studies performed using the polymerase chain reaction (PCR) have demonstrated that the majority of cases of classical HD cases that express B-lineage antigens also contain clonal rearrangements of the immunoglobulin heavy-chain gene. However, the results of PCR studies that compare the immunoglobulin heavy-chain gene rearrangement patterns of single cells obtained from cases of HD are more variable. Depending on the study, the RS and H cells have been shown to be polyclonal, monoclonal, or contain no immunoglobulin heavy-chain gene rearrangements. In some cases, single-cell PCR followed by DNA sequence analysis has revealed extensive somatic mutations in the IgH-variable region genes in addition to clonal rearrangements of the IgH in the RS and H cells. Recent studies of NLPHD also have demonstrated clonal and productive rearrangements of the IgH genes, and hypermutated IgH genes, consistent with germinal center derivation. Thus, it is currently believed that the RS and H cells in at least a subset of cases of HD are derived from B cells.

The polymerase chain reaction technique has been used to amplify the t(14;18)(q32;q21) in cases of HD. This translocation occurs in approximately 90% of cases of follicular non-Hodgkin's lymphomas. The t(14;18) may be present in up to one-third of cases of HD of all histologic types. However, presently it is uncertain which cell population in HD contains the translocation, and recent data suggest that the t(14;18) is not present in the RS and H cells.

In summary, the results of molecular studies are consistent with the hypothesis that the RS and H cells are monoclonal, of lymphoid origin, and are most often of B-cell lineage, although some cases may be of T-cell lineage.

IX. EPSTEIN-BARR VIRUS AND HODGKIN'S DISEASE

It has been known for many years that there is an association between Epstein-Barr virus (EBV) and HD, although the role of the virus in the etiology and pathogenesis of HD is unknown. EBV is known to be the cause of infectious mononucleosis, and adolescents who have recovered from infectious mononucleosis have an increased risk of subsequent HD. Patients with HD often have high serum antibodies directed against EBV antigens, such as early antigen and viral capsid antigen. The presence of antibodies against EBV early antigen suggest that the virus is active. Also, Mueller and colleagues have shown using blood donor serum that high titers to EBV antigens may be present before the onset of HD. Subsequent studies using molecular biologic techniques have directly demonstrated the virus within HD. The EBV genome is present in approximately 50% of cases of HD, preferentially within the RS and H cells (Fig. 10), in the monoclonal episomal form. Further, the RS and H cells express virus-associated proteins, such as latent membrane protein-l (LMP-l). These results suggest that RS cells and mononuclear variants are latently infected by EBV, and that the cells were infected before neoplastic transformation. Thus, EBV may be involved in the pathogenesis of at least a subset of HD.

The presence of EBV is correlated with the histologic type of HD. More than two-thirds of cases of MCHD and LDHD, and about one-fourth of cases of NSHD contain EBV. However, EBV is uncommon in LPHD.

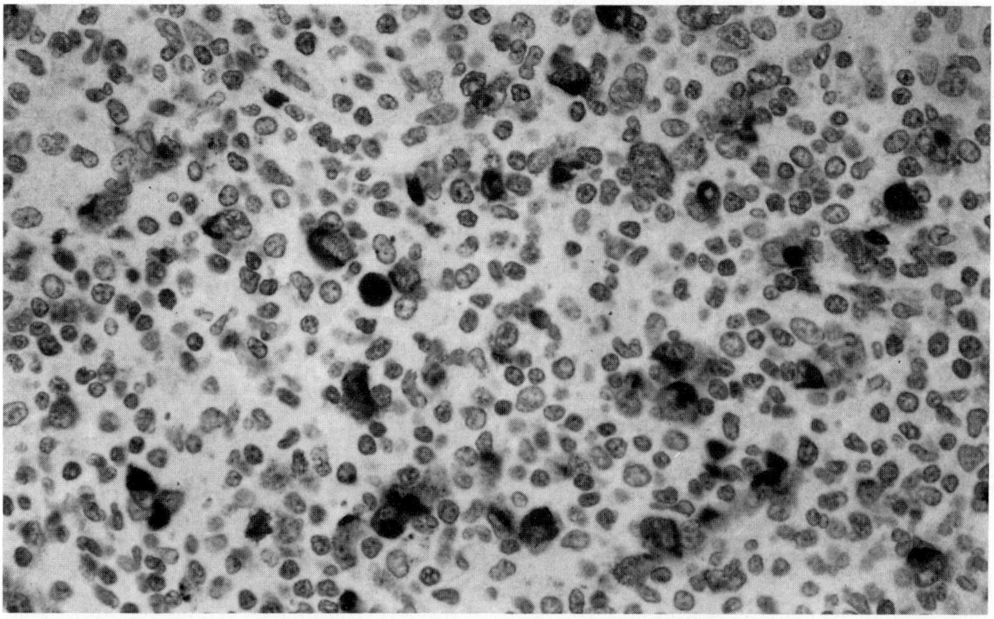

Figure 10 Mixed-cellularity HD. Epstein-Barr virus EBER1 RNA is present predominantly within the Reed-Sternberg and Hodgkin cells. (In-situ hybridization, 630×.)

X. HODGKIN'S DISEASE AND THE TWO-DISEASE HYPOTHESIS

For many years epidemiologists have suggested that HD is heterogeneous and represents more than one disease. The "two-disease hypothesis" considers NSHD and MCHD to be two different diseases. The epidemiologic, clinical, and pathologic findings support this hypothesis. More recent molecular studies also support this hypothesis, and suggest that NSHD, itself, is heterogeneous.

The epidemiological features of NSHD and MCHD are distinct. Nodular sclerosis HD preferentially affects young adults between the ages of 15 and 34 years. Males and females are affected almost equally. Mediastinal lymph node involvement and low clinical stage disease are the rule. The following social factors correlate with an increased risk of NSHD: small family size, early birth order, a single-family home, fewer neighborhood playmates, higher maternal education, and higher paternal social class. These epidemiologic findings suggest that NSHD is the result of relatively late exposure to an infectious agent, analogous to the paralytic polio model. In contrast, MCHD is relatively more common in children and in adults older than 50 years of age. Males are affected more often than females. Mediastinal involvement is relatively uncommon and advanced stage disease is relatively more frequent. Social factors that correlate with increase risk of MCHD are the converse of NSHD: large family size, late birth order, more neighborhood playmates, lower maternal education and lower paternal social class. These findings suggest that early exposure to an infectious agent may play a role in MCHD.

Epstein-Barr virus, commonly identified in MCHD, may explain some of the epidemiologic features of MCHD. Children younger than 5 years of age rarely develop HD. Perhaps children in this age group, especially those living in poor socioeconomic conditions, are exposed to EBV, but a latency period is needed before HD develops as a result of primary infection. Mixed-cellularity HD in the older adult and elderly population may result from reactivation of EBV, perhaps secondary to immunodeficiency that results from aging or other causes. The relatively low prevalence of EBV in NSHD suggests that EBV infection is not necessary for this disease to develop, and that another infectious agent or other factors may be responsible. The marked heterogeneity of the pathologic and clinical findings among patients with NSHD also raises the possibility that this disease may result from more than one infectious agent.

XI. HODGKIN'S DISEASE IN PATIENTS WITH HUMAN IMMUNODEFICIENCY VIRUS-1

Although HD presently is not considered a diagnostic criterion for establishing the diagnosis of acquired immunodeficiency syndrome (AIDS), HD may occur with slightly increased frequency in human immunodeficiency virus-1 (HIV-1)-infected patients. For example, in San Francisco County, where there is a high prevalence of HIV-1 infection in young adult men, the incidence of HD has increased with the onset of the AIDS epidemic. Rubio and colleagues also have suggested that patients who become infected with HIV-1 as the result of intravenous drug use may develop HD more frequently than those who become infected as the result of homosexual practices. Hodgkin's disease in HIV-1-positive patients may occur either before or after the diagnosis of AIDS is established.

Clinically, HD is more aggressive in HIV-1-positive patients than uninfected patients. Patients with HIV-1 are more likely to present with advanced-stage disease, bone marrow involvement, and systemic symptoms. In one collaborative study by Rubio and colleagues of 46 patients with HIV-1 and HD, more than 80% presented with stage III or IV disease and systemic symptoms, and 41% had bone marrow involvement. In the same study fewer than 50% of the patients responded completely to therapy, and 43.5% died of HD.

Histologically, MC is the most frequent type of HD in HIV-1 positive individuals. Nodular sclerosis and LDHD are also common. Lymphocytic predominance HD is rare. The disease also tends to show a faster rate of histologic progression than is usually seen in uninfected patients. For example, at relapse, the neoplasm contains a larger number of RS and H cells, more lymphocyte depletion, and more necrosis than the original biopsy specimen. We have observed HIV-1-positive patients with HD in whom two or three biopsy specimens within a 1- to 2-year period demonstrated dramatic histologic progression from NSHD or MCHD to LDHD.

The immunohistochemical findings are similar in HIV-1-associated and non-HIV-1-associated HD. However, EBV is usually present within the neoplastic cells of HIV-1-associated HD cases.

XII. CYTOKINES IN HODGKIN'S DISEASE

Recent studies have demonstrated the presence of cytokines in HD tissues. Cytokines are low-molecular-weight glycoproteins or proteins that are secreted primarily by histiocytes or activated lymphocytes. Cytokines have a wide variety of functions, including regulating immune responses and hematopoiesis. They also appear to play a role in the histologic findings in HD.

Hsu and colleagues, in a relatively recent review, have summarized the literature pertaining to the role of cytokines in HD. The cytokines identified in HD may be secreted by either the RS and H cells and/or the reactive cells. For example, the numerous T cells found in tissues involved by HD may be recruited by interleukin (IL)-1, IL-6, IL-9, and tumor necrosis factor (TNF) α secreted by the RS and H cells. Further, the reactive cells may respond by secreting other cytokines, such as IL-2 and IL-4, that enhance the T-cell reaction. Interleukin-5 may be responsible for the eosinophil reaction found in a subset of cases of HD. In cases with many plasma cells, IL-6 is likely to be involved. Interleukin-1, IL-6, TNFα, and TNFβ, secreted either by the RS and H cells or by the reactive cells such as eosinophils, can induce fibrosis, as is seen in nodular sclerosis HD.

Reed-Sternberg and H cells also express receptors for cytokines on their surfaces. For example, RS and H cells express the interleukin-2 receptor (CD25). More recently, the CD30 antigen, which reacts with the Ki-1 antibody, has been identified as a member of the TNF receptor family.

XIII. RELATIONSHIP OF HODGKIN'S DISEASE TO NON-HODGKIN'S LYMPHOMA

Hodgkin's disease and non-Hodgkin's lymphoma (NHL) may occur in the same patient, either simultaneously or at different times. Further, this phenomenon occurs more frequently than can be accounted for by coincidence alone.

Approximately 2–3% of patients with LPHD develop diffuse large B-cell lymphoma. The L&H cells in nodular LPHD are of B-cell lineage, and some cases have many L&H cells in sheets that resemble large-cell lymphoma. These findings have led some observers to suggest that nodular LPHD may transform into diffuse large-cell lymphoma, and that these two tumors are clonally related. Patients with large B-cell lymphoma that arises in association with nodular LPHD may have a better response to standard therapy than patients with de-novo large B-cell lymphoma, which suggests that the large-cell lymphoma is related to the nodular LPHD.

Composite lymphoma is defined as two histologically distinct neoplasms, such as HD and NHL, that involve the same lymph node or anatomic site. In such cases, the NHL is usually of B-cell lineage. Follicular lymphoma is the most common type of NHL found. In some of these cases, both the RS and H cells in the HD component, and the large cells in the NHL component, have been positive for EBV. This finding suggests that both neoplasms originated from a common EBV-infected progenitor.

Patients treated successfully for HD may develop non-Hodgkin's lymphomas. The cumulative risk at 10 years for NHL in these patients is approximately 4–5%. These NHLs tend to be diffuse, histologically aggressive, of B-cell lineage, and involve extranodal sites, similar to the NHLs that occur in patients with congenital or acquired immunodeficiency syndromes. Thus, it has been hypothesized that the immunologic deficits that occur with HD, and are known to persist following successful therapy, predispose these patients to an increased risk of subsequent NHL. However, unlike NHLs that develop in acquired immunodeficiency states, such as following organ transplantation, in-situ hybridization studies for EBV have shown that the virus is found infrequently in the NHLs that follow HD.

Hodgkin's disease also may develop following successful treatment of NHL. Patients with NHL are at slightly increased risk to develop HD. In this clinical setting, the HD is similar to de-novo HD in its clinical and pathologic features. In the majority of these cases, the previous

NHL has been of B-cell lineage, and is usually follicular lymphoma. In a recent study, LeBrun and colleagues studied a patient who had follicular lymphoma in 1970, followed by NSHD in 1985. Using a polymerase chain reaction-based method, they detected the t(14;18) in both neoplasms. Further, the fused *bcl*-2/IgH sequences in both tumors were identical. They hypothesized that the HD was genetically related to, and may have evolved from, the follicular lymphoma.

Hodgkin's disease also has been associated with T-cell NHLs. For example, a histogenetic and clinical relationship appears to exist between some cases of HD, usually NSHD, and either mycosis fungoides or lymphomatoid papulosis. Hodgkin's disease may precede, coexist with, or follow either skin disease. One hypothesis to explain this phenomenon is that these three entities may arise from a common activated T-cell precursor cell.

The occurrence of HD and NHL in the same patient is further clinical evidence to suggest that the RS and H cells of HD are of lymphoid origin. The association of HD with B-cell and T-cell NHLs suggests that HD may arise from either a B cell or a T cell, or from an uncommitted lymphoid cell precursor.

CASE STUDY 1

Patient

26-year-old woman.

Chief Complaint

"Lump" in her armpit. No complaints of fever, night sweats, weight loss, or fatigue.

Medical History

Unremarkable.

Physical Examination

Bilateral axillary lymphadenopathy. No other lymphadenopathy or hepatosplenomegaly.

Laboratory Results

Screening procedures:

CBC with differential: All values within normal limits.
Chest x-ray: Anterior mediastinal mass.
An axillary lymph node biopsy was performed.

Questions

1. Based on the clinical presentation, what conditions are in the differential diagnosis?
2. What would be the results of immunohistochemical stains performed on fixed, paraffin-embedded sections for these entities?

Additional Laboratory Results

Confirmatory results: An axillary lymph node biopsy demonstrated Hodgkin's disease, nodular sclerosis subtype. The normal lymph node architecture was effaced and the capsule was thickened by dense collagen. Collagenous bands extended from the capsule into the parenchyma and divided it into large nodules composed of predominantly small lymphocytes with admixed histiocytes, plasma cells, eosinophils, lacunar cells, Hodgkin's cells, and rare classic Reed-Sternberg cells.

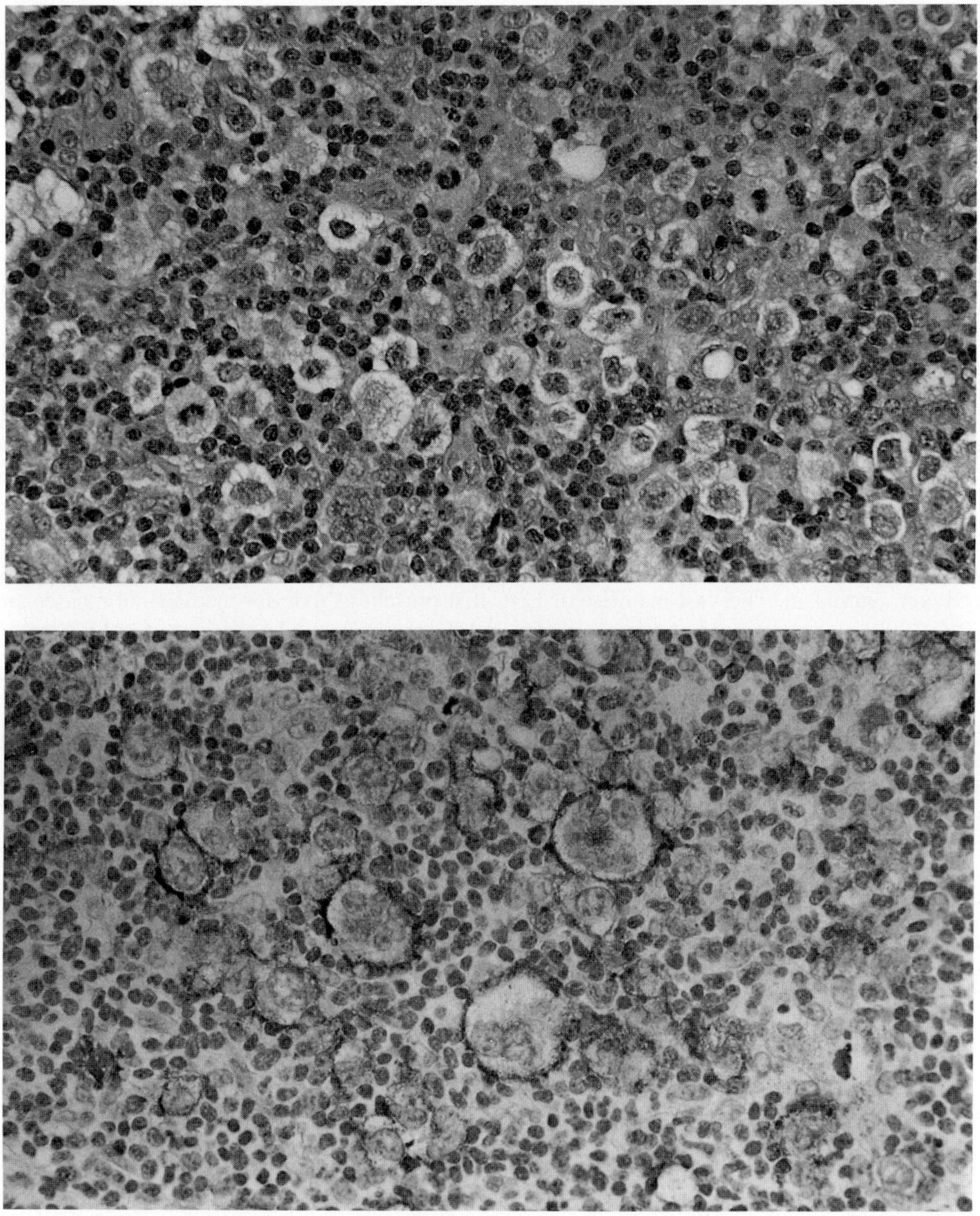

Case Study 1 Lacunar cells in a background of reactive lymphocytes with admixed histiocytes, plasma cells, and eosinophils.

Immunohistochemical stains were performed on fixed paraffin-embedded sections. The malignant cells expressed CD15 (LeuM1 antibody) and CD30 (BerH2 antibody). They did not express CD45 (leukocyte common antigen), or markers of B-cell (CD20, L26 antibody) or T-cell (CD3; CD45RO, UCHL-1 antibody).

Diagnosis

Hodgkin's disease, nodular sclerosis subtype.

Discussion

The differential diagnosis of an anterior mediastinal mass in a young woman includes: NSHD, lymphoblastic lymphoma (LBL), primary mediastinal large B-cell lymphoma (PMLBCL), and a germ cell tumor. In this case, because the patient also had axillary lymphadenopathy, she underwent a lymph node biopsy rather than a biopsy of the mediastinal mass. The distinction between these entities may be difficult in cases where the biopsies are small and fragmented, such as those obtained by mediastinoscopy. Immunohistochemical stains are particularly helpful in this circumstance. Like NSHD, PMLBCL is a disease of young women, and the tumor characteristically is sclerotic. However, the malignant cells in PMLBCL express CD45 and CD20. They are negative for CD15, CD30, and markers of T-cell differentiation. The malignant cells of LBL are small to intermediate in size, with fine chromatin, inconspicuous nucleoli, and scant cytoplasm. The vast majority of LBL that present as anterior mediastinal masses are of T-cell lineage, and would also express terminal deoxynucleotidyl transferase (TdT). Finally, the malignant cells in germ cell tumors express cytokeratin and placental alkaline phosphatase, unlike the other entities, and fail to express CD15, CD30, or markers of lymphoid differentation (CD45, CD20, CD3, CD45RO).

NOTE ADDED IN PROOF

Since this manuscript was prepared, the following information was presented.

Table 7 World Health Organization Classification of Neoplastic Diseases of the Lymphoid Tissues (Proposed)

- B-cell neoplasms
  - Precursor B-cell lymphoblastic leukemia/lymphoma[a]
  - Mature B-cell neoplasms
    - B-cell chronic lymphocytic leukemia/small lymphocytic lymphoma
    - B-cell prolymphocytic leukemia
    - Lymphoplasmacytic lymphoma[b](lymphoplasmacytoid lymphoma)[c]
    - Mantle cell lymphoma[b]
    - Follicular lymphoma[b] (follicle center lymphoma)[c]
    - Cutaneous follicle center lymphoma
    - Marginal zone B-cell lymphoma of mucosa-associated lymphoid tissue type
    - Nodal marginal zone lymphoma +/– monocytoid B-cells
    - Splenic marginal zone B-cell lymphoma
    - Hairy cell leukemia
    - Diffuse large B-cell lymphoma[b]
      - Mediastinal (thymic)
      - Intravascular
      - Primary effusion lymphoma

Burkitt's lymphoma[b]
Plasmacytoma
Plasma cell myeloma[b]
T-cell neoplasms
Precursor T-cell lymphoblastic leukemia/lymphoma[a]
Mature T-cell and natural killer cell neoplasms
T-cell prolymphocytic leukemia
T-cell large granular lymphocytic leukemia
Aggressive natural killer cell leukemia
T/natural killer cell lymphoma, nasal and nasal-type (angiocentric lymphoma)[c]
Mycosis fungoides[b]
Sézary syndrome
Angioimmunoblastic T-cell lymphoma
Peripheral T-cell lymphoma (unspecified)[b]
Adult T-cell leukemia/lymphoma (HTLV1+)[b]
Anaplastic large-cell lymphoma (T- and null-cell types)[b]
Primary cutaneous CD-30 positive T-cell lymphoproliferative disorders[b] (cutaneous anaplastic large cell lymphoma)[v]
Subcutaneous panniculitis-like T-cell lymphoma
Enteropathy-type intestinal T-cell lymphoma
Hepatosplenic γ/δ T-cell lymphoma
Hodgkin's lymphoma (Hodgkin's disease)[c]
Nodular lymphocyte-predominant Hodgkin's lymphoma
Classical Hodgkin's lymphoma
Hodgkin's lymphoma, nodular sclerosis (Grades I and II)
Classical Hodgkin's lymphoma, lymphocyte-rich
Hodgkin's lymphoma, mixed cellularity
Hodgkin's lymphoma, lymphocytic depletion (includes most "Hodgkin's-like anaplastic large-cell-lymphoma")[c]

REAL = Revised European-American Classification of Lymphoid Neoplasms; WHO = World Health Organization.
[a]The classification of acute lymphoid leukemias will expand upon the classification of precursor B-cell and T-cell malignancies, incorporating both immunpphenotypic and genetic features.
[b]Morphologic and/or clinical variants of these diseases are not listed for the prupose of clarity and ease of presentation.
[c]This term represents a term used in the REAL classification but modified in the WHO scheme.

BIBLIOGRAPHY

1. Berard CW, Thomas LB, Axtell LM, Kruse M, Newell G, Kagan R. The relationship of histopathological subtype to clinical stage of Hodgkin's disease at diagnosis. Cancer Res 1971; 31:1776–1785.
2. Cabanillas F. A review and interpretation of cytogenetic abnormalities identified in Hodgkin's disease. Hematol Oncol 1988; 6:271–274.
3. Colby TV, Hoppe RT, Warnke RA. Hodgkin's disease: a clinicopathologic study of 659 cases. Cancer 1981; 49:1848–1858.
4. Colby TV, Warnke RA. The histology of the initial relapse of Hodgkin's disease. Cancer 1980; 45: 289–292.
5. Doggett RS, Colby TV, Dorfman RF. Interfollicular Hodgkin's disease. Am J Surg Pathol 1983; 7: 145–149.
6. Ferry JA, Zukerberg L, Harris NL. Florid progressive transformation of germinal centers: a syn-

drome affecting young men, without early progression nodular lymphocyte predominance Hodgkin's disease. Am J Surg Pathol 1992; 16:252–258.
7. Gonzalez CL, Medeiros LJ, Jaffe ES. Composite lymphoma. A clinicopathologic analysis of nine patients with Hodgkin's disease and B-cell non-Hodgkin's lymphoma. Am J Clin Pathol 1991; 96: 81–89.
8. Greer JP, Kinney MC, Cousar JB, et al. Lymphocyte-depleted Hodgkin's disease. Clinicopathologic review of 25 patients. Am J Med1986; 81:208–214.
9. Grogan TM. Hodgkin's disease. In: Jaffe ES, ed. Surgical Pathology of the Lymph Nodes and Related Organs. 2d ed. Philadelphia: Saunders, 1996:133–192.
10. Harris NL, Jaffe ES, Stein H, et al. A revised European-American Classification of lymphoid neoplasms: A revised European-American Classification of lymphoid neoplasms: A proposal from the International Lymphoma Study Group. Blood 1994; 84:1361–1392.
11. Hoppe RT, Cox RS, Rosenberg SA, Kaplan HS. Prognostic factors in pathologic stage III Hodgkin's disease. Cancer Treat Rep 1982; 66:743–749.
12. Hsu SM, Waldron JW Jr, Hsu PL, Hough AJ Jr. Cytokines in malignant lymphomas: review and prospective evaluation. Hum Pathol 1993; 24:1040–1057.
13. Hummel M, Ziemann K, Lammert H, Pileri S, Sabattini E, Stein H. Hodgkin's disease with monoclonal and polyclonal populations of Reed-Sternberg cells. N Engl J Med 1995; 333:901–906.
14. Jackson H Jr, Parker F Jr. Hodgkin's disease. II. Pathology, N Engl J Med 1944; 231:35–44.
15. Kadin ME. Common activated helper-T-cell origin for lymphomatoid papulosis, mycosis fungoides, and some types of Hodgkin's disease. Lancet 1985; 2:864–865.
16. Kadin ME, Glatstein SS, Dorfman RF. Clinicopathologic studies of 117 untreated patients subjected to laparotomy for the staging of Hodgkin's disease. Cancer 1971; 27:1277–1294.
17. Kamel OW, Chang PP, Hsu FJ, Dolezal MV, Warnke RA, van de Rijn M. Clonal VDJ recombination of the immunoglobulin heavy chain gene by PCR in classical Hodgkin's disease. Am J Clin Pathol 1995; 104:419–423.
18. Kant JA, Hubbard SM, Longo DL, Simon RM, DeVita VT Jr, Jaffe ES. The pathologic and clinical heterogeneity of lymphocyte-depleted Hodgkin's disease. J Clin Oncol 1986; 4:284–294.
19. Kingma DW, Medeiros LJ, Barletta J, et al. Epstein-Barr virus is infrequently identified in non-Hodgkin's lymphomas associated with Hodgkin's disease. Am J Surg Pathol 1994; 18:48–61.
20. Küppers R, Rajewsky K, Zhao M, et al. Hodgkin disease: Hodgkin and Reed-Sternberg cells picked from histologic sections show clonal immunoglobulin gene rearrangements and appear to be derived from B cells at various stages of development. Proc Natl Acad Sci USA 1994; 91:10962–10966.
21. LeBrun DP, Ngan B-Y, Weiss LM, Huie P, Warnke RA, Cleary ML. The bcl-2 oncogene in Hodgkin's disease arising in the setting of follicular non-Hodgkin's lymphoma. Blood 1994; 83:223–230.
22. Lukes RJ. Criteria for involvement of lymph node, bone marrow, spleen, and liver in Hodgkin's disease. Cancer Res 1971; 31:1755–1767.
23. Lukes RJ, Butler JJ. The pathology and nomenclature of Hodgkin's disease. Cancer Res 1966; 26: 1063–1083.
24. Lukes RJ, Craver LF, hall TC, et al. Report of the nomenclature committee. Cancer Res. 1966; 26: 1311.
25. Medeiros LJ, Bagg A, Cossman J. Application of molecular genetics to the diagnosis of hematopoietic neoplasms. In: Knowles DM, ed. Neoplastic Hematopathology, Baltimore: Williams & Wilkins, 1992:263–298.
26. Medeiros LJ, Greiner T. Hodgkin's disease. Cancer 1995 75:357–369.
27. Orazi A, Jiang B, Lee CH, et al. Correlation between presence of clonal rearrangements of immunoglobulin heavy chain genes and B-cell antigen expression in Hodgkin's disease. Am J Clin Pathol 1995; 104:413–418.
28. Poppema S, Kaiserling E, Lennert K. Hodgkin's disease with lymphocytic predominance, nodular type (nodular paragranuloma) and progressively transformed germinal centers—a cytohistological study. Histopathology 1979; 3:295–308.

29. Roth J, Daus H, Trumper L, Gause A, Salamon-Looijen M, Pfreundschuh M. Detection of immunoglobulin gene rearrangements at the single-cell level in malignant lymphomas: no rearrangement is found in Hodgkin and Reed-Sternberg cells. Int J Cancer 1994; 57:799–804.
30. Stein H, Mason DY, Gerdes J, et al. The expression of the Hodgkin's disease associated antigen Ki-1 in reactive and neoplastic lymphoid tissue: evidence that Reed-Sternberg cells and histiocytic malignancies are derived from activated lymphoid cells. Blood 1985; 66:848–858.
31. Strickler JG, Michie SA, Warnke RA, Dorfman RF. The "syncytial variant" of nodular sclerosing Hodgkin's disease. Am J Surg Pathol 1986; 10:460–477.
32. Travis LB, Gonzalez CL, Hankey BF, Jaffe ES. Hodgkin's disease following non-Hodgkin's lymphoma. Cancer 1992; 69:2337–2342.
33. Wood NL, Coltman CA. Localized primary extranodal Hodgkin's disease. Ann Intern Med 1973; 78:113–118.
34. Zarate-Osorno A, Medeiros LJ, Kingma DW, Longo DL, Jaffe ES. Hodgkin's disease following non-Hodgkin's lymphoma. A clinicopathologic and immunophenotypic study of nine cases. Am J Surg Pathol 1993; 17:123–132.
35. Zarate-Osorno A, Medeiros LJ, Longo DL, Jaffe ES. Non-Hodgkin's lymphoma arising in patients successfully treated for Hodgkin's disease. A clinical, histologic, and immunophenotypic study of 14 cases. Am J. Surg Pathol 1992; 16:885–895.

6

Histiocytosis and Lipid Storage Diseases

Salwa Shabbir Sheikh and David F. Garvin
Georgetown University Medical Center, Washington, D.C.

I. HISTIOCYTOSIS

A. Introduction and Historical Background

The term *histiocytosis* was first used to designate large, nonspecific cells with increased amounts of granular cytoplasm, sometimes containing ingested particles, and round to irregular nuclei. These cells were normally found in the spleen and lymph nodes. Later the term was used synonymously with monocyte/macrophage lineage cells. Recently this term has been extended to include Langerhans cells of the skin, interdigitating dendritic cells of the lymph nodes, spleen, and thymus, and dendritic reticulum cells present in the germinal centers of the lymph nodes. Currently, histiocytosis includes both monocyte/macrophage cell lineage as well as Langerhans/dendritic cells. Sometimes this is also referred to as the mononuclear phagocyte and immunoregulatory effector system (M-PIRE).

Histiocytosis
Stem cells
1. Monocytes/macrophages
   (a) Reactive macrophage histiocytosis
   (b) Malignant macrophage histiocytosis
2. Langerhans cells/dendritic cells
   (a) Reactive Langerhans cell histiocytosis
   (b) Malignant Langerhans cell histiocytosis

Very few diseases are as confusing as the histiocytic disorders. In 1893 Alfred Hand, a medical resident, presented a case of "polyuria and tuberculosis" in which he also described the patient as having several cranial bone defects. In 1915 Arthur Schuller and in 1920 Henry Christian described similar cases. In 1924 Eurch Letterer described a case of nonmalignant proliferation of reticuloendothelial cells in a 6-month-old baby, which was presented again 9 years later by Stern Siwe along with two other, similar cases.

Lichtenstein and Jaffe, and Olani and Ehrlich described eosinophilic granuloma simultaneously in 1940. In 1941 Sidney Farber brought pathologists' attention to the close histologic similarities between Hand-Schuller-Christian disease, Letterer-Siwe disease, and eosinophilic granuloma. In 1953 Lichtenstein proposed the term "histiocytosis X" for all these entities, "X" being the unknown etiologic factor. In 1966 Nezeloff and Bassett identified the characteristic cell of histiocytosis X as being the Langerhans cell. All these conditions show roughly similar histopathologic changes:

1. Abnormal proliferation of histiocytes intermingled with eosinophils.
2. Low mitotic rate.
3. Histiocytes may fuse to form giant cells.
4. Variable amount of lymphocytes, plasma cells, necrosis, and fibrosis can be present.

In 1994 Martin Cline proposed a new classification for histiocytosis depending on the histiocytic cell lineage based on ultrastructural and phenotypic markers of the cells. He divided histiocytosis into Langerhans cell histiocytosis and macrophage histiocytosis, and then subdivided each one into a reactive and a malignant process. Cline's classification was as follows.

- I. Reactive macrophage histiocytosis
  - M-1. Storage diseases
    - A. Gaucher's disease
    - B. Niemann-Pick disease
    - C. Sphingomyelinase deficiency, etc.
  - M-2. Benign proliferative macrophage diseases
    - A. Xanthoma disseminata
    - B. Multicentric reticulohistiocytosis
    - C. Juvenile xanthogranuloma
  - M-3. Nonmalignant hemophagocytic macrophage diseases
    - A. Fulminant hemophagocytic syndrome
    - B. Histiocytosis with massive lymphadenopathy (Rosai-Dorfman disease)
- II. Malignant diseases of macrophages
  - M-4. Acute monocytic leukemia
  - M-5. Chronic myelomonocytic leukemia
  - M-6. Malignant 5q35 histiocytosis
- III. Reactive langerhans cell histiocytosis
  - L-1. Benign Langerhans cell histiocytosis
    - A. Eosinophilic granuloma and Hand-Schuller-Christian disease
    - B. Relapsing Langerhans cell histiocytosis
    - C. Self-healing histiocytosis
- IV. Presumptively malignant Langerhans cell histiocytosis
  - L-2. Progressive Langerhans cell histiocytosis (Letterer-Siwe disease)
  - L-3. Langerhans cell lymphoma
  - L-4. Dendritic cell lymphoma

The markers listed in Table 1 are helpful in differentiating between Langerhans cells and macrophages.

Recently, Willman and her colleagues, and Yu et al. reported, consequently, clonality of Langerhans cells in both reactive as well as presumptively malignant Langerhans cell histiocytosis. This indicates that the disease is probably a clonal neoplastic disorder with highly variable biologic behavior. For this reason both reactive and malignant Langerhans cell histiocytosis can be lumped together under the heading of "Langerhans cell neoplasia."

B. Reactive Macrophage Histiocytosis

1. Storage Diseases

These are discussed in Section II.

Table 1 Markers for Differentiating Langerhans Cells and Macrophage

		Macrophage	Langerhans cells	MH[a]	LCH[b]
Antigens	S-100	+/−	++	−	++
	Neuron-specific enolase	−	++	−	++
	CD1a, c	+	++		++
	CD15	++	−	+	−
	CD30 (Ki-1)	+		+/−	−
	CD68 (KP-1)	++	−	+	+/−
Morphology	Birbeck granules	−	++		+
Enzymes	Lysozyme	++	−	+	+/−
	Acid phosphatase	++	+/−	+	−
	Antitrypsin	++	−	+	+/−
	Antichymotrypsin	++	−	+	+/−
	Cathepsin E	−	+		+
Function	Phagocytosis	++	+/−		−
	Antigen presentation	+	++		

[a]MH = multicentric histiocytosis.
[b]LCH = Langerhans cell histiocytosis.
References: Cline M. Histiocytes and histiocytosis. Blood 1994; 84(9):2846–2853.
Kanitakis J, et al. Neuron-specific enolase is a marker of cutaneous Langerhans cell histiocytosis (X). (A comparative study with S-100 protein.) Anticancer Res. 1991; 11(2):635–9.

2. Benign Proliferative Macrophage Diseases

Benign proliferative macrophage diseases include a group of disorders with multiple skin nodules and macrophage infiltration. They are of unknown etiology and have a variable clinical course; the disease spectrum extends from self-limited to an aggressive disease with complications of infection and tissue destruction.

a. Juvenile Xanthogranuloma. Juvenile xanthogranuloma usually presents during infancy, but lesions may be present at birth or may appear during adulthood. There are widespread skin and mucous membrane nodules (Fig. 1) measuring 0.5–1.0 cm in diameter, which are yellow to red in color and most commonly affect the scalp and face, but may involve mesentery and viscera as well. The disease usually involutes spontaneously.

b. Xanthoma Disseminata. Xanthoma disseminata is also characterized by widespread nodules involving the skin and mucous membranes.

c. Multicentric Histiocytosis. Multicentric histiocytosis is a rare multisystem disease affecting mainly adults, with involvement of the viscera, muscle, and destructive synoarthritis of the joints. Few cases are reported associated with tuberculosis or concomitant malignancy. It is not a malignant disease per se, but sometimes chemotherapy is recommended to prevent destructive synoarthritis and disfiguring skin lesions.

3. Nonmalignant Hemophagocytic Macrophage Disease

a. Fulminant Hemophagocytic Syndrome. Fulminant hemophagocytic syndrome is characterized by systemic reactive histiocytic proliferation, usually affecting children. It is an aggressive disease, and is fatal in ~40% of cases. The pathophysiology is poorly understood, but the syndrome usually occurs in patients with an immune deficiency, whether inherited,

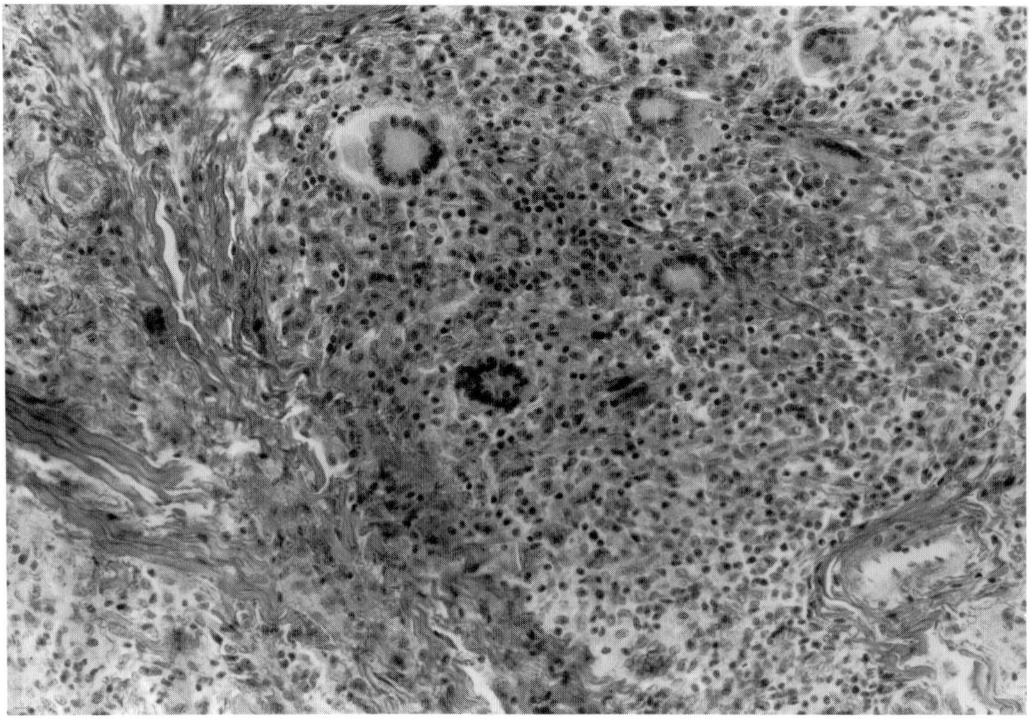

Figure 1 Juvenile xanthogranuloma: skin (surface epithelium not shown in this field) with histiocytic proliferation and multiple "Touton" giant cells. (×40.)

acquired, or iatrogenic due to immunosuppressive drugs, and is thought to be mediated through aberrant release of cytokines (Fig. 2).

i. Viral-Associated Hemophagocytic Syndrome or Infection-Associated Hemophagocytic Syndrome (VAHS or IAHS): Initially, 19 patients were described in 1979 associated with viral infections most commonly herpes group and adenovirus. Later other viral, bacterial, and protozoal infections were also reported to be associated with hemophagocytic syndrome, for example:

Viruses—cytomegalovirus, Epstein-Barr virus, parvovirus B19, measles, rubella, HIV virus, and ECHO virus
Bacteria—typhoid fever, brucellosis, and tuberculosis
Protozoa—leishmania
Drugs—chemotherapy

ii. Immunosuppression: Certain malignancies (T- and B-cell lymphoproliferative disorders), autoimmune diseases, e.g., systemic lupus erythematosus, and accelerated phase of Chediak-Higashi syndrome have been reported associated with fulminant hemophagocytic syndrome.

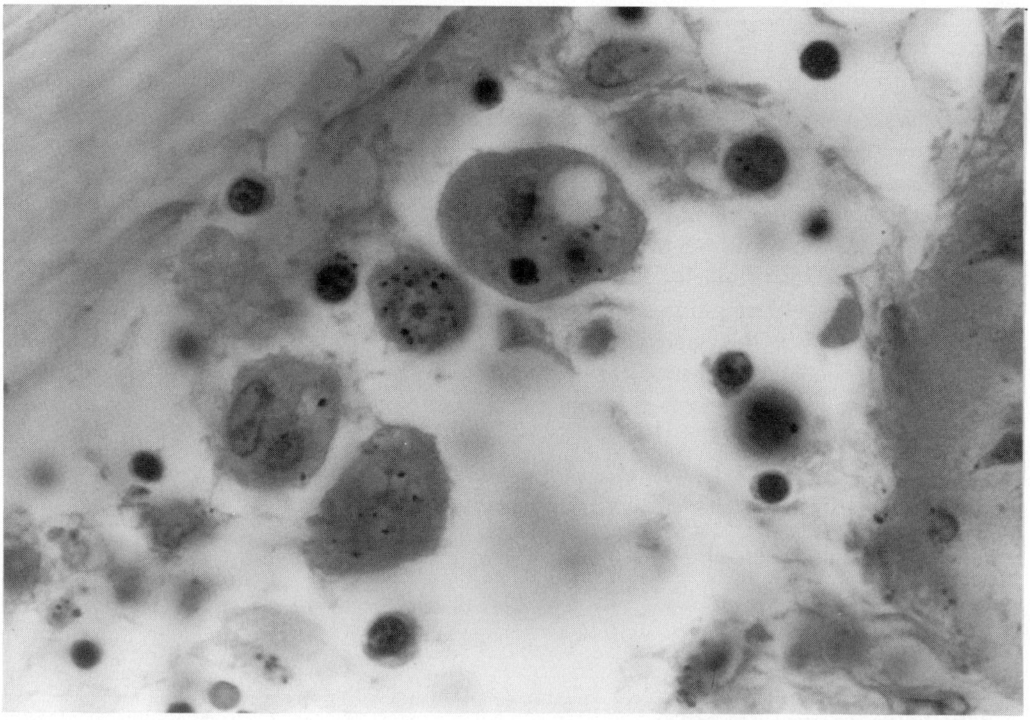

Figure 2 Hemophagocytic syndrome: bone marrow biopsy exhibiting replacement of the marrow by histiocytes engulfing the red and white cells. (×100.)

iii. Fat Overload Syndrome: Hemophagocytic syndrome may occur during prolonged parenteral nutrition.

iv. Multiple Blood Transfusions: Healthy individuals receiving multiple blood transfusions show, within hours, histiocytosis with hemophagocytosis in the bone marrow, lymph nodes, and spleen.

v. Familial Hemophagocytic Lymphohistiocytosis (FHL): Familial forms have been described which are associated with defects in the cellular and humoral immunity. The clinical and histopathologic findings of the familial type are very similar to those of sporadic IAHS. There is an autosomal recessive mode of inheritance, and usually there is a positive family history of FHL in first- or second-degree relatives or evidence of parental consanguity. However, the child may be the first one with FHL, representing a mutation, and obviously may not have any positive family history.

The common denominator in all these clinical conditions with hemophagocytosis is an injury to the lymphocytes with alterations in recognition of certain antigens, including those on red blood cells with expansion of the antigen-presenting cells or histiocytes which lead eventually to hemophagocytosis.

All the following criteria are required to diagnose hemophagocytic lymphohistiocytosis (HLH):

Fever, splenomegaly, cytopenia, hypertriglyceridemia, and/or hypofibrinogenemia
Hemoglobin <9 g/L, platelet $<100 \times 10^9$L, neutrophils $<1.0 \times 10^9$ g/L
Histopathologic criteria—hemophagocytosis in the bone marrow, spleen, or lymph nodes

b. Sinus Histiocytosis with Massive Lymphadenopathy (Rosai-Dorfman Disease). Rosai-Dorfman disease (RDD) was first recognized in 1969 as an uncommon proliferative histiocytic disorder (Fig. 3). It is a benign, self-limiting disorder of unknown etiology. Some cases are associated with Epstein-Barr virus, herpes virus 6 infection, and lymphoma. It usually occurs in the first two decades of life. There is a predilection for children, especially <10 years, with the clinical picture of inflammation, i.e., fever, leukocytosis, high ESR, lymphadenopathy, and systemic symptoms. Significant numbers of cases appear in children with immunologic disorders, e.g., Wiskott-Aldrich syndrome, autoimmune hemolytic disease, and glomerulonephritis. The entity was originally described in lymph nodes, but has been reported to involve almost every organ system. Almost half of patients with RDD have at least one site of extranodal disease. In this hemophagocytic syndrome the internalized lymphocytes are intact, suggesting that they entered the histiocytes by emperipolesis rather than phagocytosis. Usually the course is benign and requires no therapy, but steroids and chemotherapy are used in severe cases.

C. Malignant Diseases of Macrophages

See the chapter on malignant diseases of macrophages.

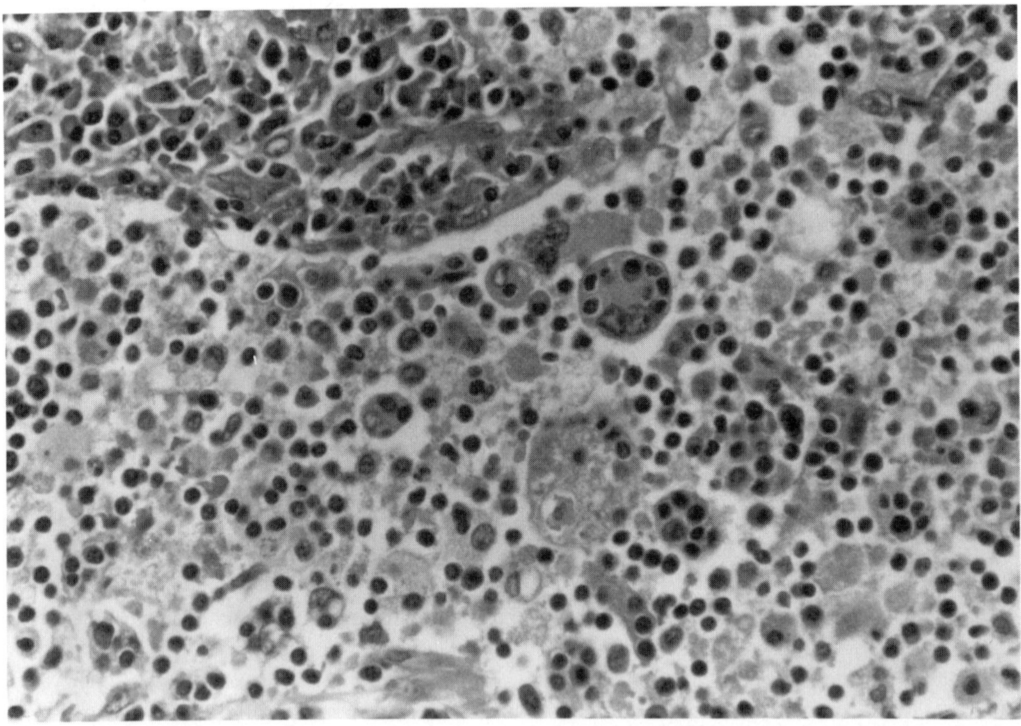

Figure 3 Rosai-Dorfman disease: lymph node with distended sinusoids exhibiting multiple histiocytes with emperipolesis. (×100.)

D. Reactive Langerhans Cell Histiocytosis

1. Benign Langerhans Cell Histiocytosis

There are several nonmalignant diseases of Langerhans cells. With the recent evidence of all Langerhans cells being clonal, even the reactive Langerhans cell histiocytosis should be considered as a neoplastic disorder as opposed to a reactive phenomenon.

a. Eosinophilic Granuloma and Hand-Schuller-Christian Disease.

i. Eosinophilic Granuloma (Fig. 4): Eosinophilic granuloma (EG) usually affects children and adolescents. It has a variable clinical course, from benign to aggressive. Most commonly it starts as a solitary lytic bone lesion with pain and swelling, which if treated appropriately has an excellent prognosis. Multifocal lesions may be present early. The lesions may involve bone or soft tissue. Untreated, the lesions often spread and continue to wax and wane throughout life. Fifty percent of patients have pituitary involvement with diabetes insipidus.

ii. Hand-Schuller-Christian Disease: The distinction between EG and Hand-Schuller-Christian (HSC) disease is often blurred. HSC disease is characterized by polymorphous lesions of the bone and soft tissues, diabetes insipidus, and exophthalmus as frequent findings. Treatment is usually excision of the lesion if possible, or radiation.

b. Relapsing Langerhans Cell Histiocytosis. Relapsing Langerhans cell histiocytosis often starts in adolescence, but continues throughout life. It is characterized by granulomas involving skin, mucous membranes of the female genital tract, occasionally viscera and the pituitary gland. These lesions may be disfiguring, with lung involvement being life threatening.

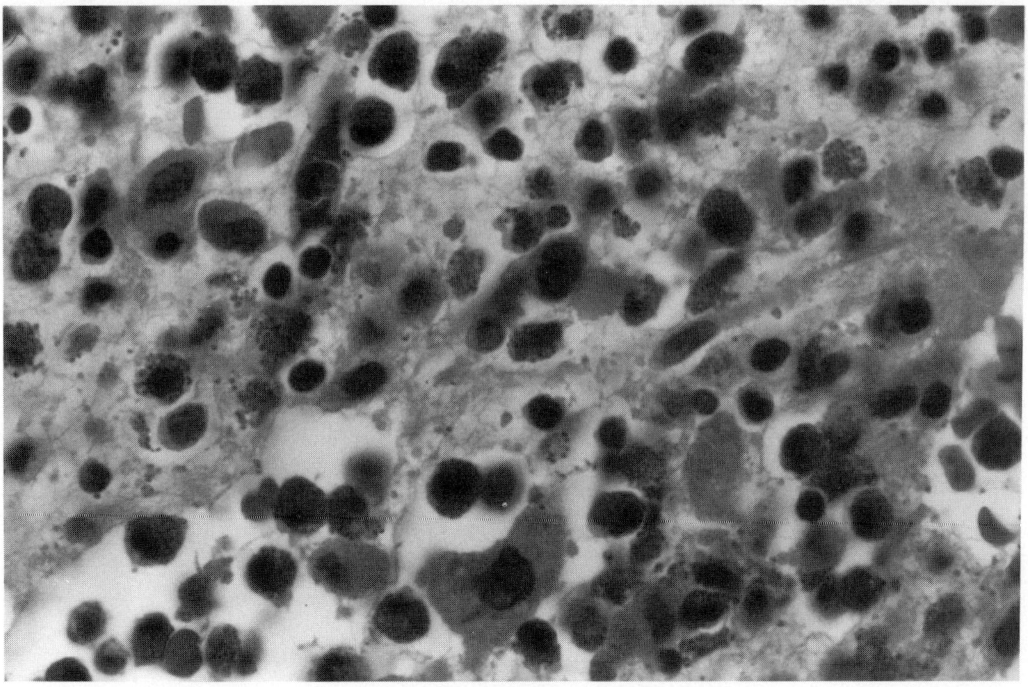

Figure 4 Eosinophilic granuloma: multiple eosinophils, with bilobed nuclei and coarsely granular cytoplasm, and histiocytes with convoluted nuclei. (×100.)

Few cases develop a lymphoproliferative disorder. The treatment for a localized lesion is excision or radiation. For systemic disease, treatment is with chemotherapy, e.g., vinblastine and etoposide, bone marrow or organ transplant.

c. Congenital Self-Healing Histiocytosis. Congenital self-healing histiocytosis is a rare, benign disorder, usually diagnosed at birth, with predominant skin involvement. It is also called "blueberry muffin baby" due to the widespread skin involvement. The condition usually resolves spontaneously, although lung involvement can be life threatening.

E. Presumptively Malignant Langerhans Cell Histiocytosis (LCH)

1. Progressive LCH (Letterer-Siwe Disease)

Progressive LCH primarily affects children but may occur in adults. It has a poor prognosis and is frequently fatal. It is an acute, progressive, and disseminated disease. An abnormality of gene *p53* on chromosome 17p13 is reported. There is infiltration of skin, bone marrow, and viscera. The clinical presentation is usually with a seborrheic dermatitis-like lesion, especially on the back and postauricular area. The bone lesions are lytic, most commonly involving the skull, with proptosis if there is orbital involvement. It commonly involves the pituitary gland but rarely other areas of the central nervous system. There is lymphadenopathy, with lungs often showing honeycombing. Some progress to acute myeloid leukemia (AML). Treatment is with chemotherapy, bone marrow and organ transplant.

2. Langerhans Cell Lymphoma

There is some evidence that a localized form of LCH occurs involving several organs, called Langerhans cell lymphoma. It is an aggressive neoplasm.

3. Dendritic Cell Lymphoma

Dendritic cell lymphoma is usually limited to lymph nodes, with cells exhibiting long interdigitating processes ultrastructurally. They generally lack macrophage markers, but are positive for CR4/23 antibody, a marker specific for dendritic cells.

II. LIPID STORAGE DISEASES

The lipid storage diseases are hereditary disorders with lipid deposition in one or more tissues. The type of lipid and its distribution have a characteristic pattern for each of the different lipid disorders. The various sphingolipids are normally degraded within lysosomes of macrophages in the reticuloendothelial system, particularly in liver, spleen, and bone marrow. Figure 5 summarizes the pathways for catabolism of sphingolipids by lysosomal enzymes. Breakdown of these lipids in visceral organs begins with engulfment of red cell and white cell membranes rich in lactosylceramide (Cer-Glc-Gal) and hematoside (Cer-Glc-Gal-NANA). In the brain, most of the cerebroside-type lipids are gangliosides. There is extensive turnover of the gangliosides in the central nervous system of neonates.

Lipid storage diseases are basically characterized by the following:

1. An enzyme defect in the normal catabolic pathway
2. Accumulation of nondigestible intracellular material in the macrophages
3. Usually considered as inborn errors of metabolism

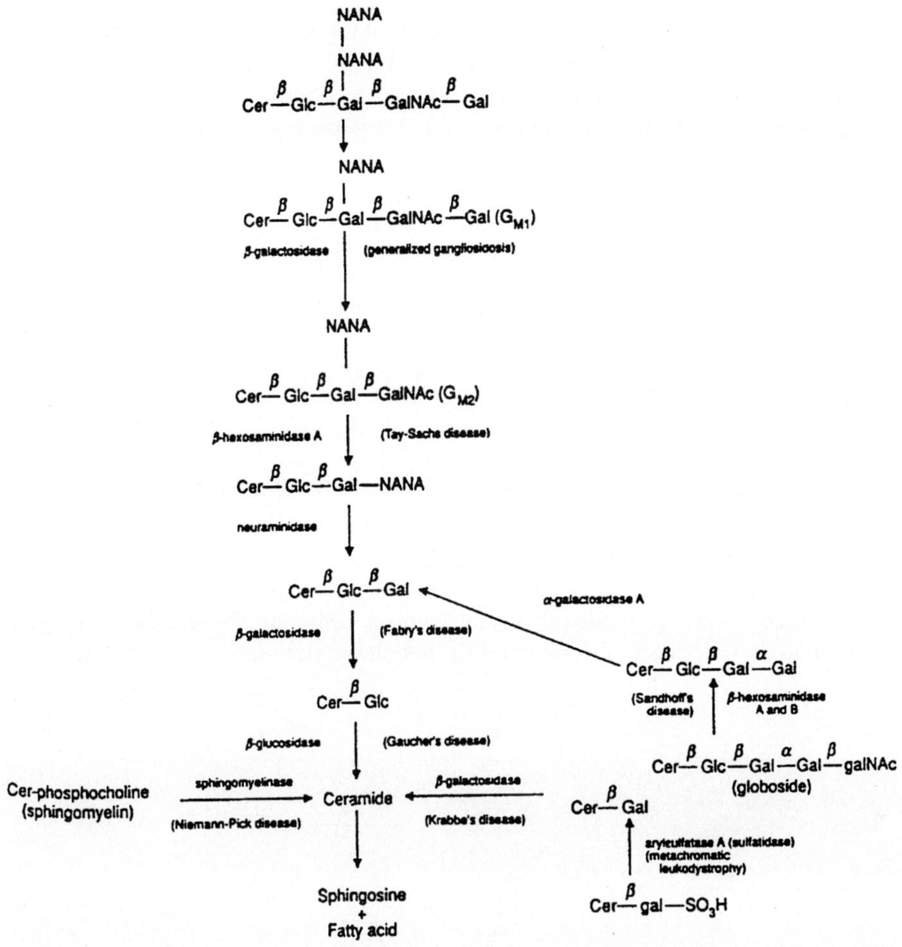

Figure 5 Summary of the pathways for catabolism of sphingolipids by lysosomal enzymes. (From Devlin TM. Lipid metabolism II: pathways of metabolism of special lipids. In: Thomas Devlin, ed. Textbook of Biochemistry with Clinical Correlations. 3d ed. New York: Wiley-Liss, 1992:456–461.)

A. Gaucher's Disease

1. Introduction

Gaucher's disease was the first lysosomal storage disease, described by Phillipe Gaucher in 1882. In 1965 the specific enzyme defect was delineated and it was the first to be successfully treated by enzyme therapy in 1991 and 1992.

Gaucher's disease is the most common lysosomal storage disease, characterized by accumulation of glucocerebroside, leading to organomegaly and lesions in the bone. It is caused by an inherited deficiency of glucocerebrosidase or b-glucosidase enzyme deficiency. Rare examples of mutations at the activator or prosaposin locus lead to Gaucher's disease-like phenotype with accumulation of glycosylceramide. (The saposins activate the enzyme glucocerebrosidase.) Gaucher's is the most prevalent Jewish genetic disease, with an autosomal recessive mode of inheritance resulting almost exclusively from mutations in the gene encoding the enzyme glucocerebrosidase. Many mutations exist, but four of them account for more than 97% of the mutations in Ashkenazi Jews. At least 1 of 50 Jews may be a heterozygote. Both human acid b-glucosidase gene and its nonprocessed pseudogene are located on chromosome 1.

The Gaucher cells (glucocerebroside-laden macrophages) (Fig. 6) are 20–100 μm in size, with a small eccentric nucleus and wrinkled cytoplasm with a crumpled tissue paper appearance. Electron microscopy shows inclusion bodies in the cytoplasm which consist of small tubules.

2. *Classification*

Three major types of Gaucher's disease have been described depending on primary central nervous system involvement (see Table 2).

3. *Clinical Manifestations*

a. Spleen. There may be massive splenomegaly (usually hard in consistency), with splenic sequestration. Nodules appear on the surface in regions of extramedullary hematopoiesis, Gaucher cell accumulations, and fibrotic infarcts.

b. Liver. The hepatomegaly is hard in consistency, with an irregular surface. Jaundice is a poor prognostic factor. Gaucher cells (abnormal Kupffer cells) are almost always evident in the sinusoids on biopsy specimens. Hepatocytes do not show glucocerebroside storage.

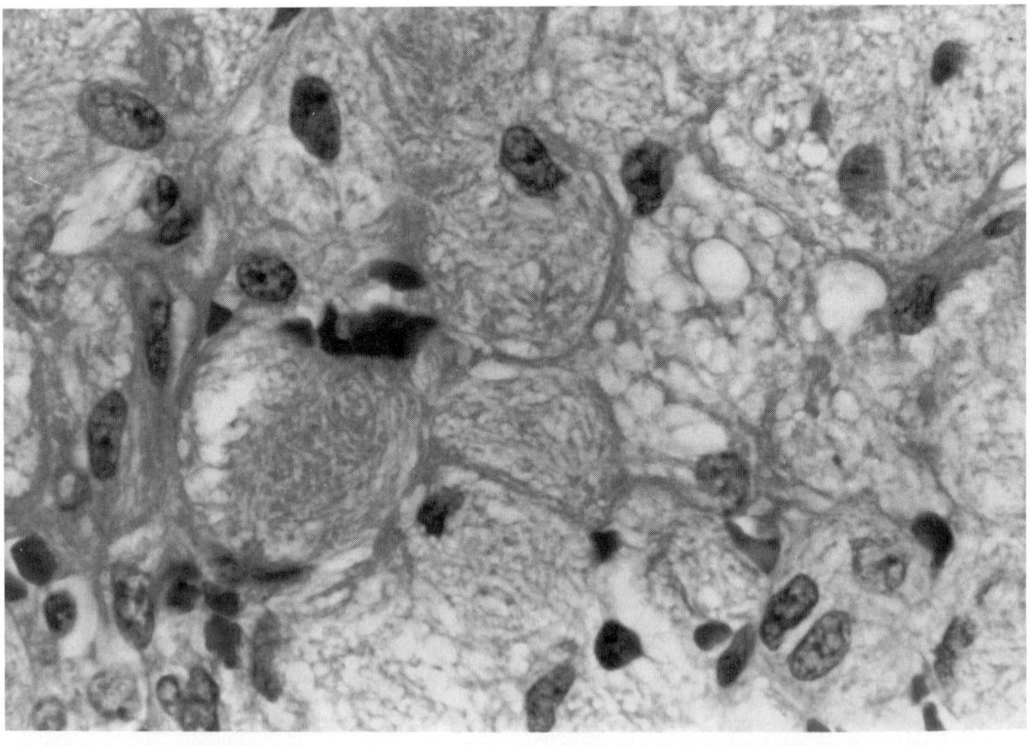

Figure 6 Gaucher's disease: Gaucher cells with characteristic wrinkled tissue paper appearance. (×100.)

Table 2 Gaucher Disease: Clinical Types

Clinical features	Type 1 (adult or nonneuropathic)	Type 2 (infantile or acute neuronopathic)	Type 3 (juvenile or subacute neuronopathic)
Onset	Childhood/adulthood	Infancy	Childhood
Hepatosplenomegaly	+	+	+
Hypersplenism	+	+	+
Bone crises/fractures	+	−	+
Neurodegenerative course	−	+++	++
Survival	6–80+ yr	<2 yr	Second to fourth decade
Ethnic predilection	Ashkenazi Jews	Panethnic	Swedish Norrbottnian
Frequency	1/40,000–1/60,000 1/400–1/600 (Ashkenazi Jews)	<1/100,000	~1/50,000

Source: Harris H, Hirschhorn K. Gaucher disease enzymology, genetics, and treatment. Adv Hum Gene 1993; 21:377–427.

c. Lungs. Lung involvement is uncommon, but when it does occur it is associated with a poor prognosis. Pulmonary disease may be due to Gaucher cell infiltration, or right-to-left intrapulmonary shunting secondary to the liver disease.

d. Bones. Bone lesions may be widespread with fever. Thirty percent have "Erlenmeyer flask" deformity (widening of the distal femur). Destructive lesions of hips are particularly common. Twenty to forty percent develop "bone crises," with severe, deep, dull pain.

e. Nervous System. Gaucher cells are present in perivascular Virchow-Robin spaces in the brain parenchyma. There is widespread neuronal loss; dentate nucleus of cerebellum is almost always involved. Multiple myeloma, chronic lymphocytic leukemia, and amyloidosis are associated with Gaucher's disease more commonly than in the normal population. Pregnancy is not contraindicated, but is considered to be high risk because of thrombocytopenia, and coagulation defects that might lead to bleeding. *Pseudo-Gaucher cells* are morphologically similar to Gaucher cells, but do not contain tubular structures characteristic of the Gaucher cells. These can be seen in various conditions, e.g., acute lymphoblastic leukemia, multiple myeloma, chronic granulocytic leukemia, plasmacytoid lymphoma, Hodgkin's lymphoma, and AIDS with *Mycobacterium avium* infection. Patients with Gaucher's disease receiving alglucerase treatment show a false-positive pregnancy test, as alglucerase is a placenta-derived drug and contains human chorionic gonadotrophin.

4. Diagnosis

Normocytic, normochromic anemia, leukopenia, and thrombocytopenia.

Leukocytes or cultured fibroblasts exhibit deficiency of b-glucosidase. Carrier state can be determined most of the time by finding reduced activity of the enzyme.

Increased serum acid phosphatase.

Factor IX deficiency and other abnormalities of clotting factors.

Glycosylceramide plasma levels are elevated to 2- to 20-fold but do not correlate with the type of Gaucher's disease.

Plasma chitotriosidase activity has been reported to be markedly elevated in most patients with symptomatic Gaucher's disease.
CSF glycosphingolipids can be used for the diagnosis and therapeutic monitoring of patients with neurologic involvement.
DNA analysis. PCR or PCR-based techniques are being done for the different mutations.

5. Treatment

Enzyme replacement therapy.
Splenectomy (partial or total). Cytopenia responds well to splenectomy.
Pain management for bone crises.
Joint replacement.
Alglucerase. It is a form of a placental glucocerebrosidase which improves signs and symptoms of Gaucher's disease.
Bone marrow transplant.

B. Niemann-Pick Disease

1. Introduction

Niemann-Pick disease was first described in 1914 by Niemann. It is characterized by accumulation of sphingomyelin and other lipids in the reticuloendothelial system.

2. Classification

Due to the differences in the clinical manifestations and accumulated lipids, Crocker, in 1961, proposed a classification of four subgroups: type A, acute neuropathic; type B, chronic with visceral involvement but nonneuropathic; type C, subacute with later nervous system involvement; and type D, subacute neuropathic and ancestry from southwestern Nova Scotia. A group E was later added as an intermediate form. Type C is considered to be a cholesterol lipidosis secondary to defective intracellular cholesterol transport. A new classification was later proposed to distinguish two main forms of the disease (see Table 3).

The gene encoding for sphingomyelinase enzyme is on chromosome 11. Recently, type C has been reported to be linked with chromosome 18. Niemann-Pick cells are 20- to 100-μm foamy histiocytes in the reticuloendothelial system (Fig. 7). The cytoplasm in these cells is filled with sphingomyelin, ceroid (brown pigment), and cholesterol. Ultrastructurally, the cells have small eccentric nuclei with cytoplasmic lipid inclusions (lamellar bodies). Wright or Giemsa stain shows blue-green cytoplasmic granules. These cells were previously described as "sea-blue histiocytes," and the patients were characterized by sea-blue histiocyte syndrome. However, sea-blue histiocytes are found in a wide variety of hereditary disorders, including Niemann-Pick disease.

3. Clinical Manifestations

The disease usually manifests during infancy, with developmental delay, poor weight gain, and abdominal enlargement. The infants may be blind, deaf, or have protracted jaundice. In their second year of life they are still flaccid, have enormous hepatosplenomegaly, mild lymphadenopathy, and xanthomatous rash. Bone lesions are present but are less prominent. Type I usually shows absence of CNS involvement.

In type 1a, symptoms usually develop within 6 months, with death occurring by 2–3 years of life; 50% have "cherry red spots." A cherry red spot represents accentuation of the normal color of macular choroid contrasted with the pallor produced by the swollen ganglion cells in the remainder of the retina.

Table 3 Two Distinctive Types of Niemann-Pick Disease

Feature	Type 1	Type 2
	Acid sphingomyelinase deficiency	Primary defect uncertain (some evidence of defects in processing exogenous cholesterol), and secondary sphingomyelin storage
Sphingomyelinase activity	Usually <10%	Normal or minimally reduced
Classification	1a: Acute (A) 1s: Subacute (B) 1c: Chronic (E)	2a: Acute 2s: Subacute (C,D) 2c: Chronic (E)
Accumulated lipids		
Sphingomyelin	Massive	Slight to moderate
Cholesterol	Slight to moderate	Moderate
Bis(MAG)P (Bis-monoacylglycerol phosphate)	Consistently increased	Consistently increased
Genetics	Autosomal recessive mutant sphingomyelinase gene (two mutant genes described) Types 1a and 1s are more frequent among Ashkenazi Jews	Autosomal recessive Panethnic

Source: Weisz B, Spirer Z, Reif S. Neimann-Pick disease. Newer classification based on genetic mutations of the disease. Adv Pediatr 1994; 41:415–426.

Type 1s usually develops during early childhood; hepatosplenomegaly is the prominent feature. However, compared to Gaucher's disease, hepatomegaly is more prominent.

Liver: foamy cells appear both in Kupffer cells and hepatocytes (in contrast with Gaucher's disease).
Spleen: foamy cells are present in the red pulp and particularly around the arteries.
Lungs: histiocytes are present in the alveoli as small white nodules, and are not in the septum.
Foamy histiocytes can also be seen in kidneys, around myocardial fibers, in the gastrointestinal tract, and in the adrenal gland.
Bone lesions: osteoporosis, metaphyseal splaying, and quadrate deformation of the lumbar vertebrae.
Brain: in type 2 the neural cells are swollen and foamy by accumulated phospholipids.
Eye: retinal lipid storage leads to "cherry red spots" in 50% of type 1a patients; type 1s patients usually shows a discrete manifestation of storage retinopathy, "macula-halo syndrome," or in its milder form a grayish discoloration or granular pigmentation around the macula.

4. *Diagnosis*

Hemoglobin—normal or mild anemia.
Lymphocytes contain 1–9 lipid-containing vacuoles.
Marrow shows foamy cells with small droplets.

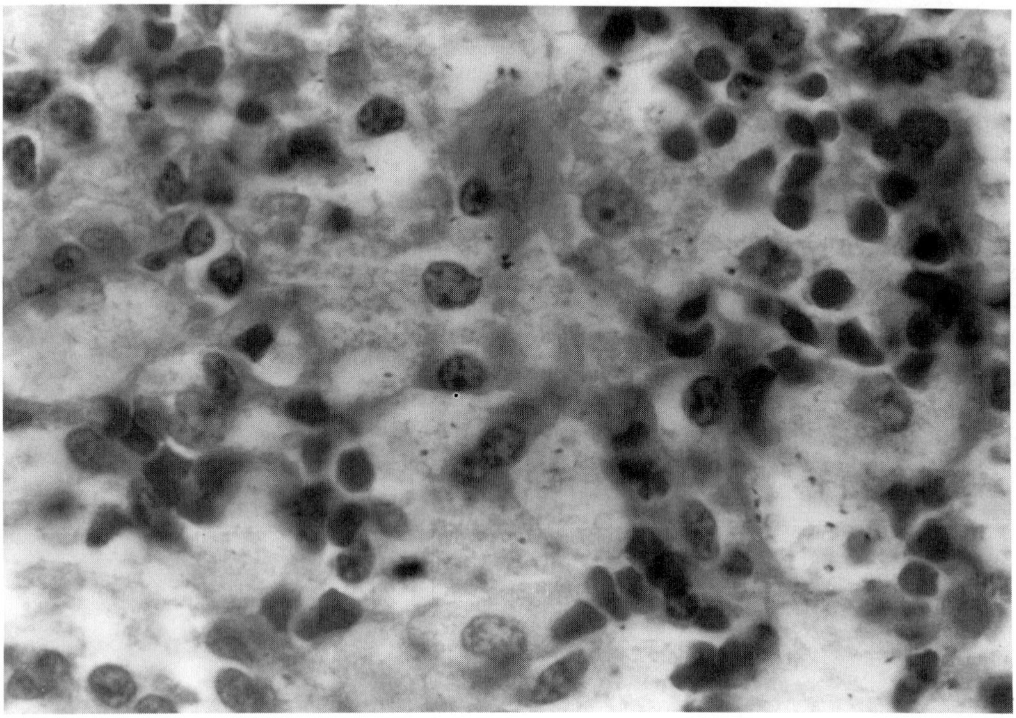

Figure 7 Niemann-Pick disease: infiltration of the spleen by lipid laden histiocytes. (×100.)

Peripheral leukocytes or cultured fibroblasts demonstrate sphingomyelinase deficiency (in types A and B). Heterozygotes may be detected by measuring the enzyme activity.
In type C disease, cholesterol uptake studies by cultured fibroblasts are helpful.
Filipin test (for the diagnosis of type C disease). The test is based on the reaction of unesterified cholesterol with florescent antibiotic filipin, giving a strongly florescent, stable, cholesterol-filipin complex suitable for in-situ detection.
Prenatal diagnosis is possible by amniocentesis.

Prognosis is usually poor, especially for type 1a. Other variants may have a much more favorable outcome.

5. Treatment

Supportive treatment; splenectomy for hypersplenism, and symptomatic treatment for respiratory problems and failure to thrive.
Bone marrow transplant is helpful provided that there is no CNS involvement; recently, liver transplantation has been carried out and shows somewhat encouraging results.
Implantation of amniotic epithelial cells has been reported, with some evidence of improvement.
Gene therapy will probably be developed in the near future.

To conclude, most of the currently available treatment is for nonneuropathic forms of the disease.

C. Tay-Sachs Disease

1. Introduction

GM2 gangliosidosis is a group of neurologic disorders divided into three major types: the B variant (Tay-Sachs disease), the O variant (Sandhoff disease), and the AB variant, caused by genetic abnormalities in the genes coding for b-hexosaminidase alpha or beta subunit, or the GM2 activator protein. Tay-Sachs disease (TSD) is the most common form of GM2 gangliosidosis.

2. Classification

Tay-Sachs is an autosomal recessive disorder characterized by deficiency of b-hexosaminidase. Lysosomal hexosaminidases occur in two forms, hexosaminidase A and B (Hex A and Hex B).

3. Manifestation

Tay-Sachs and Sandhoff are clinically very similar. Both disorders are exclusively an affliction of the nervous system, with progressive developmental failure in the first few months. These children usually die in their third or fourth year of life with decerebrate rigidity. Tay-Sachs disease is associated with a wide variety of expression and age of onset. The classical infantile form is characterized by onset at 3–5 months and leading to death in 3–5 years. The later-onset forms are extremely variable. Patients may present with signs of dementia, seizures, psychosis, cerebellar dysfunction, and atypical spinocerebellar degeneration. There is a high incidence of Tay-Sachs disease in Ashkenazi Jews, attributed predominantly to high frequency of three mutations in the Jewish population, while in non-Jews more than two dozen mutations have been identified. The carrier frequency is estimated at 1 in 25 in Ashkenazi Jews.

The viscera appear normal microscopically, but chemical analysis shows increased concentration of glycosphingolipids.

4. Diagnosis

Enzyme immunoassay of beta-hexosaminidase A and B in serum. It is elevated in TSD patients as well as carriers.

Prenatal diagnosis: amniocentesis, chorionic villi biopsy, and preimplantation genetic diagnosis by polymerase chain reaction and in-situ hybridization are being used for early detection and prevention of this disease.

5. Treatment

Amniotic tissue transplantation has been reported.

D. Fabry's Disease

1. Introduction

Fabry's disease is characterized by deficiency of one of the isoenzymes alpha-galactosidase and alpha-galactosidase A, resulting in accumulation of ceramide trihexoside all over the body. Fabry's disease is an X-linked inborn error of glycosphingolipid catabolism, resulting from mutations in the alpha-galactosidase A gene at Xq22.1. About 49 different mutations have been described. Female heterozygotes usually manifest stigmata of the disease, which may be severe even with relatively high levels of alpha-galactosidase A.

2. Clinical Manifestation

Cutaneous lesions are characteristic; these are small red spots found primarily on the lower abdomen, thighs, and scrotum. Because of these lesions the disease is also referred to as "Angiokeratoma corporis fusum universale." There is recurrent fever, with decreased sweating (anhydrosis) and burning paraesthesia of the extremities. Renal failure usually develops in the third or fourth decade.

3. Diagnosis

Alpha-galactosidase A absence or deficiency in leukocytes, fibroblasts, urine or plasma
Detection of gene rearrangement by polymerase chain reaction
Prenatal diagnosis by amniocentesis

4. Treatment

Partially purified enzyme infusion leads to some improvement. However, heterozygotes with disease manifestations and relatively high levels of the enzyme suggest that the enzyme may not have a role in this disorder.
Symptomatic treatment; diphenylhydantoin and phenoxybenzamine.
Renal transplantation.

E. Metachromatic Leukodystrophy

1. Introduction

Metachromatic leukodystrophy (MLD) is an autosomal recessive disorder having estimated incidence of 1 : 40,000. The lysosomal enzyme deficient in MLD is arylsulfatase A (ASA), resulting in accumulation of cerebroside sulfate.

2. Clinical Manifestation

There are three main clinical forms of this disease.

Late infantile form: This is the most common type and usually presents between 15 months and 2 years. There is loss of acquired motor skills, hypotonia, ataxia, and mental retardation. The disease course is usually short, and most patients die 1–7 years from onset.

Juvenile form: Usually presents between age 4 and 12 years. The clinical presentation is usually progressive mental illness with dementia, psychosis, and emotional disturbances. Walking and speaking difficulties are seen later. The course of the disease is less severe than with the late infantile form. Most patients die, but occasionally the course can last for more than 20 years.

Adult form: The onset may vary from 19 to 46 years of age. The presentation is usually missed early, as most patients present with behavioral changes which are attributed to psychiatric problems. The progress of the disease is slow, and 5- to 10-year survival is quite common.

3. Diagnosis

Measurement of ASA in leukocytes and cultured fibroblasts for postnatal, or amniotic fluid and chorionic villi for prenatal diagnosis
Urinary sulfatide excretion
Measurement of sulfatide degradation by cultured fibroblasts
Molecular techniques, e.g., hybridization and PCR

4. Treatment

Intrauterine bone marrow transplant has been reported.
Studies on gene transfer and germ-line modification are being performed.

F. Krabbe's Disease (Globoid Cell Leukodystrophy)

1. Introduction

Krabbe's disease has an autosomal recessive mode of inheritance and is characterized by deficiency of the enzyme galactocerebroside beta-galactosidase (galactosylceramidase 1).

2. Clinical Manifestation

Clinical onset is usually between 3 and 5 months of age. Few late-onset cases have been reported. Affected infants are usually normal for the first few months. Later they develop intermittent fever, feeding problems, seizures, hyperesthesia, irritability, dementia, peripheral neuropathy, and motor abnormalities. Optic atrophy is common, and frequently the child has a small head. The brain is small, with cerebral atrophy. Death usually occurs by 2 years of age.

3. Diagnosis

There is decreased enzyme activity in serum, leukocytes, and cultured fibroblasts.
CSF protein is usually elevated.
The cDNA for galactocerebrosidase has recently been cloned and expressed, and corresponds to chromosome 14q31.

4. Treatment

Major progress in gene therapy has been made for several inherited diseases, and is in progress for Krabbe's disease.

G. Wolman's Disease

Wolman's disease is a rare disorder, clinically very similar to Niemann-Pick disease, in which death may occur in infancy. Enzyme acid esterase is severely deficient, resulting in accumulation of triglycerides and cholesterol esters in many tissues. X-rays show punctate calcification of the adrenal glands. Foam cells are seen in the bone marrow and almost any other tissue or organ. The changes in the CNS are usually confined to the endothelial cells and are not prominent in the neurons.

H. Tangier Disease

The first reported case of Tangier disease was from Tangier Island in Chesapeake Bay. It is a very rare disease with an autosomal recessive mode of inheritance. There is deficiency of high-density alpha-lipoprotein (HDL), with accumulation of cholesterol esters. Clinically it is characterized by hepatosplenomegaly, lymphadenopathy, mild weakness, and greatly enlarged tonsils with a unique orange band. Plasma cholesterol levels are low, and there is absence of HDL (alpha-lipoprotein) by electrophoresis. The disease usually has a benign course during childhood but is unclear in adulthood, as lip deposition in arteries probably carries risk of coronary occlusion.

I. Hyperlipidemia

Conditions associated with high plasma cholesterol, triglyceride, and phospholipid concentrations may be associated with lipid storage in foam cells in different tissues and may occur in any age group. Diabetes mellitus and type 1 glycogen storage disease usually lead to impressive secondary hyperlipidemia. Some cases of hyperlipidemia are due to a deficiency of lipoprotein lipase, an autosomal recessive disorder. The plasma lipid levels are so high that the plasma usually has a milky appearance. Familial hypercholesterolemia is a disorder secondary to a receptor defect. Homozygotes may show foamy cells with very high cholesterol levels sometimes seen even during childhood.

Sphingolipid storage diseases of humans are summarized in Table 4.

CASE STUDY 1

Patient

Forty-two-year-old male.

Chief Complaint

The patient presented to the hospital with left upper quadrant abdominal pain radiating to his back and left shoulder. There was also accompanying left-side chest pain, minimal shortness of breath, and progressive cough.

Medical History

The patient had had hypertension for the past year. He also underwent T-12 laminectomy 12 years ago.

Medication

Ziac, 5 mg q.d.

Allergies

No known drug allergies.

Physical Examination

The patient was a well-developed male in no apparent distress. His vital signs were stable. His abdomen was soft and mildly distended, with tenderness in the left upper quadrant. There were no peritoneal signs or ecchymosis. The spleen was palpable below the costal margin.

Laboratory Results

4 weeks prior to hospital admission		Reference range
WBC	4.2	3.7–10.5 thousand/mm^3
RBC	5.25	4.1–5.6 million/mm^3

Hgb	15.4	12.5–17.0 g/dL
Hct	45.1	36–50%
McV	86	80–98 μm^3
Plat	158	155–385 thousand/mm^3

On the day of admission his hematocrit was 40, and in 2 days it dropped to 25.7.

A CT scan of the abdomen revealed some splenomegaly with subcapsular hematoma and a rupture with free intraperitoneal blood. There was no splenic vein thrombosis. The patient underwent splenectomy, and his postoperative course was uncomplicated.

Questions

1. What are the findings in this histology section of his spleen (see Fig. 8)?
2. What is the differential diagnosis?
3. What tests would you do to confirm your diagnosis?

Table 4 Sphingolipid Storage Diseases of Humans

Disorder	Principal signs and symptoms	Principal storage substance	Enzyme deficiency
Tay-Sachs disease	Mental retardation, blindness, cherry red spots on macula, death between second and third year	Ganglioside GM2	Hexosaminidase A
Gaucher's disease	Liver and spleen enlargement, erosion of long bones and pelvis, mental retardation in infantile form only	Glucocerebroside	Glucocerebrosidase
Fabry's disease	Skin rash, kidney failure, pains in lower extremities	Ceramide trihexoside	alpha-Galactosidase A
Niemann-Pick disease	Liver and spleen enlargement, mental retardation	Sphingomyelin	Sphingomyelinase
Globoid leukodystrophy (Krabbe's disease)	Mental retardation, absence of myelin	Galactocerebroside	Galactocerebrosidase
Metachromatic leukodystrophy	Mental retardation, nerves stain yellowish brown with cresyl violet dye (metachromasia)	Sulfatide	Arylsulfatase A
Generalized gangliosidosis	Mental retardation, liver enlargement, skeletal involvement	Ganglioside GM1	GM1 ganglioside: beta-galactosidase
Sandhoff-Jatzkewitz disease	Same as Tay-Sachs disease; has more rapidly progressing course	GM2 ganglioside, globoside	Hexosaminidase A and B
Fucosidosis	Cerebral degeneration, muscle spasticity, thick skin	Pentahexosylfucoglycolipid	Alpha-L-fucosidase

Source: Devlin TM. Lipid metabolism II: pathways of metabolism of special lipids. In: Devlin T, ed. Textbook of Biochemistry with Clinical Correlations. 3d ed. New York: Wiley-Liss, 1992:456–461.

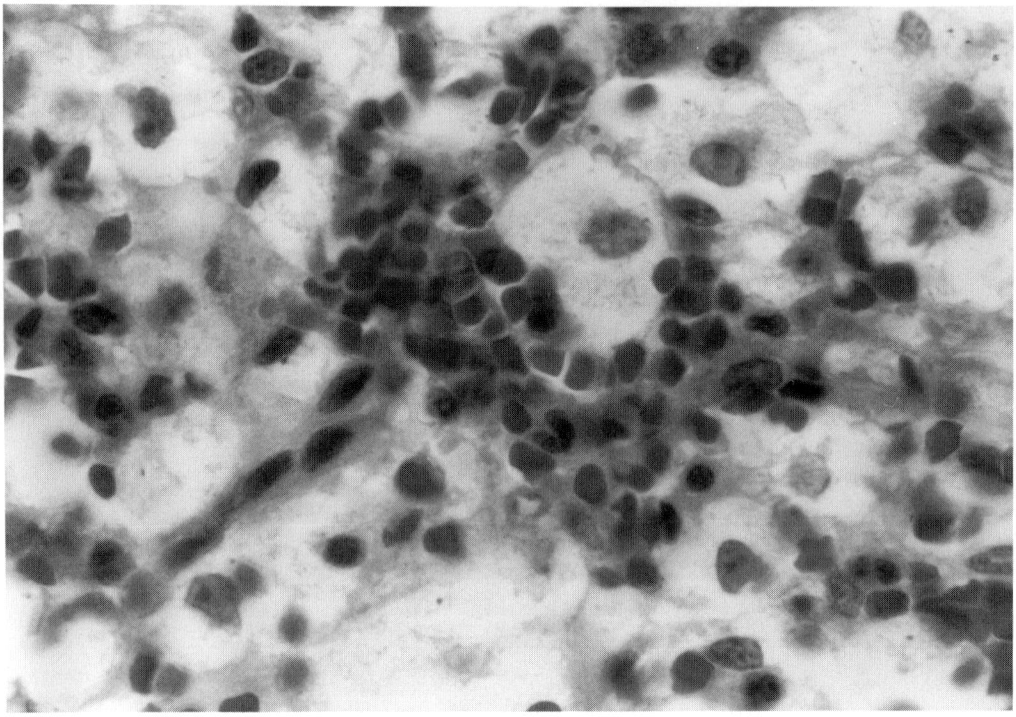

Figure 8 Case Study 1.

Diagnosis

Neimann-Pick disease.

Discussion

The spleen is infiltrated by lipid-laden histiocytes. Among the differential diagnoses of lipid-laden histiocytic infiltration, adult type (type C) Niemann-Pick disease is favored, especially if the patient has been healthy except for splenomegaly. Other possibilities include Gaucher's disease, pseudo-Gaucher cells, and sea-blue histiocytosis. Electron microscopy exhibits histiocytes filled with lamellated myelinosomes, characteristic but not pathognomonic of Niemann-Pick disease. Therefore correlation with clinical findings and histology is always recommended.

Type C Niemann-Pick disease, which is under type 2 in the new classification system, has almost normal sphingomyelinase activity. It is considered to be a cholesterol lipidosis secondary to defective intracellular cholesterol transport and is a quite distinct entity from types A and B. Adult onset with splenomegaly in an otherwise healthy person, as in this case, is not uncommon in type C Niemann-Pick disease. Typical Niemann-Pick disease is an affliction of infancy. These infants during their first months of life gain weight poorly, and have developmental delays. During their second year the child is usually flaccid, with huge hepatosplenomegaly, lymphadenopathy, and skin and bone lesions. The typical disease has been designated as type A.

Bibliography

1. Weisz B, Spier Z, Reif S. Neimann-Pick disease: newer classification based on genetic mutations of the disease. Advances in Pediatrics 1994; 41:415–426.
2. Vanier MT, Penchev P, Rodriguez-Lafrasse C, Rousson R. Niemann-Pick group of disease. Nippon Rinsho 1993; 51(9):2293–2299.
3. Vanier MT, Rodriguez-Lafrasse C, Rousson R, et al. Type C Niemann-Pick disease: biochemical aspects and phenotypic heterogeneity. Dev Neurosci 1991; 13(4–5):307–314.

CASE STUDY 2

Patient

Sixty-four-year-old woman.

Chief Complaint

The patient presented to the hospital with febrile neutropenia 6 months after receiving chemotherapy for large cell lymphoma 2 years prior to her current admission, and Waldenström's macroglobulinemia 10 years ago. She also had hypothyroidism, for which she was on thyroid replacement hormone.

Medication

Synthroid 125 μg q.d.

Allergies

Not known.

Physical Examination

The patient was febrile but not in distress. Her abdomen was soft, with tenderness in the right upper quadrant. The liver was three fingers below the costal margin. The rest of the physical examination was unremarkable.

Laboratory Results

On admission		Reference range
WBC	0.9	4.8–10.8 1000/μ
RBC	3.58	4.2–5.4 10 × 6/μL
Hgb	12.9	12–16 g/dL
Hct	36.8	37–47%
MCV	102.7	81–99 fl
Plat	95	130–400 10 × 9/L

Course

During her hospitalization she continued to have persistent fever and her CD4 counts dropped. She also developed abdominal distension, generalized edema, and abnormal liver, kidney, and coagulation profile tests. A bone marrow biopsy was performed, which showed an increased number of blasts suggestive of lymphoma, and the patient was started on chemotherapy.

Additional Laboratory Results

WBC	0.3	
RBC	3.43	
Hgb	10.5	
Hct	30.7	
MCV	89.4	
Plat	12.	
CD4	14%	
PT	16.3	10.1–12.5 sec
PTT	38.5	24.2–34.0 sec
Fibrinogen	390	150–350 mg/dL

Blood culture: a few colonies of *Candida* spp.
Viral serology for CMV: negative
All viral cultures: negative
Chest x-ray: showed diffuse process with bilateral infiltrates and a small left pleural effusion.

The patient continued to deteriorate, and 2 days after being on chemotherapy, i.e., 25 days after her admission, she died of severe shortness of breath secondary to pulmonary hemorrhage.

Questions

1. What are the findings in the bone marrow biopsy of this patient (see Fig. 9)?
2. What is the diagnosis?
3. What is the prognosis for this condition?

Diagnosis

Hemophagocytic syndrome.

Discussion

The bone marrow biopsy shows entirely packed marrow by benign-appearing histiocytes phagocytosing red and white blood cells (hemophagocytosis). Less than 5% of the marrow showed remaining atypical large cell lymphoma cells (not shown in Fig. 9). The liver, spleen, and lymph nodes also exhibited hemophagocytosis.

Fulminant hemophagocytic syndromes are aggressive and often fatal disorders characterized by fever, systemic symptoms, jaundice, multiple organ failure, hepatosplenomegaly, coagulopathy, hypertriglyceridemia, and/or hypofibrinogenemia and hemophagocytosis. The condition may be fatal in up to 40% of cases. The etiology is usually not known, but some cases appear to be reactive to drugs or infections with viruses, e.g., Epstein-Barr virus, CMV, parvovirus, and bacteria, e.g., brucella, tuberculosis and typhoid. In sporadic cases the clinical setting is often associated with immunodeficiency. A few cases have been associated with T-cell lymphomas. It is uncertain in these cases whether viral infection, e.g., Epstein-Barr virus, is the inciting event to hemophagocytosis or the malignant nature of the process itself.

In this case the patient was admitted with febrile neutropenia and continued to have persistent fever despite antibiotic therapy. She was on chemotherapy for her high-grade lymphoma and was immunocompromised. She had multiple factors which would have predisposed her to this fulminant hemophagocytic syndrome. Her immediate cause of death was bilateral severe pulmonary hemorrhage with entire obliteration of the air spaces.

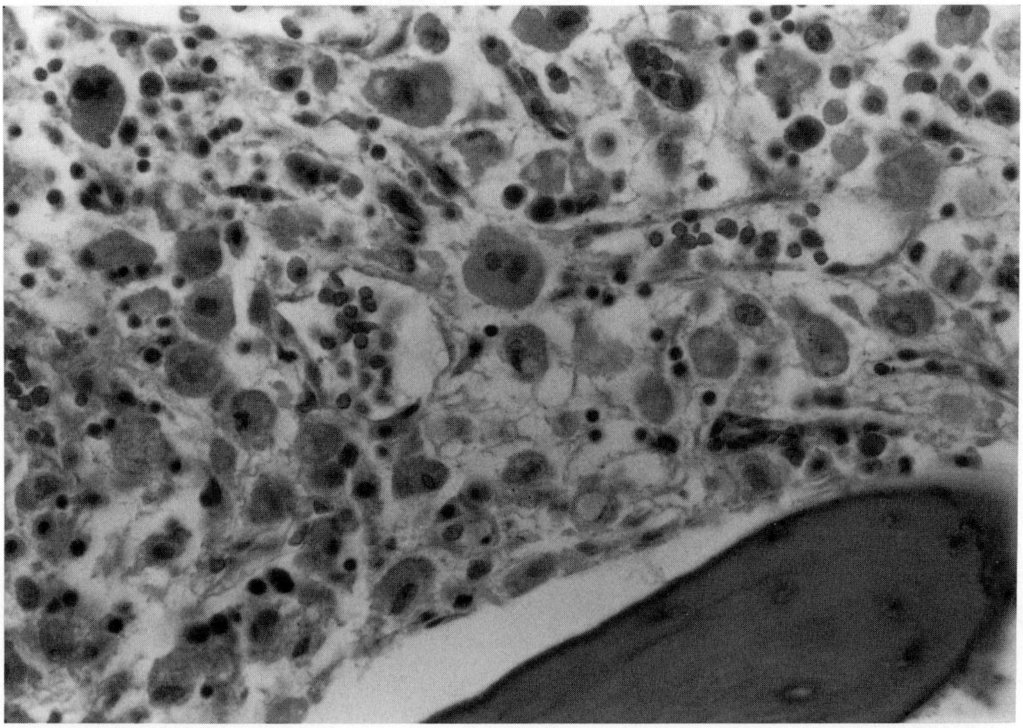

Figure 9 Case Study 2.

Bibliography

1. Cline MJ. Histiocytes and histiocytosis. Blood 1994; 84(9):2840–2853.
2. Henter J-I, Elinder G, Ost A, and FHL Study Group of the Histiocyte Society. Diagnostic Guidelines for Hemophagocytic Lymphohistiocytosis. Semin Oncol 1991; 18(1):29–33.
3. Dehner L. Morphologic findings in the histiocytic syndromes. Semin Oncol 1991; 18(1):8–17.

SUGGESTED READINGS

1. Aicardi J. The inherited leukodystrophies: a clinical overview. J Inherit Metab Dis 1993; 16(4): 773–743.
2. Barth ML, Fensom A, Harris A. The arylsulphatase A gene and molecular genetics of metachromatic leukodystrophy. J Med Genet 1994; 31(9):663–666.
3. Black SH. Preimplantation genetic diagnosis. Curr Opin Pediatr 1994; 6(6):712–716.
4. Bourquelot P, Oksenhendler E, Wolff M, et al. Hemophagocytic syndrome in HIV infection. Presse Med 1993; 22(26):1217–1220.
5. Broadbent V, Egeler RM, Nesbit ME Jr. Langerhans cell histiocytosis—clinical and epidemiological aspects. Br J Cancer 1994; 23:S11–S16.
6. Carrington PA, Stevens RF, Lendon M. Pseudo-Gaucher cells. J Clin Pathol 1992; 45(4):360.

7. Christian HA. Defects in membranous bones, exophthalmus and diabetes insipidus, an unusual syndrome of dyspituitarism. Med Clin N Am 1920; 3:849–71.
8. Chun SI, Song MS. Congenital self-healing histiocytosis—report of a case of the solitary type and review of the literature. Yonsei Med J 1992; 33(2):194–198.
9. Cline ME. Histiocytes and histiocytosis. Blood 1994; 84(9):2840–2853.
10. Dehner LP. Morphologic findings in the histiocytic syndromes. Semin Oncol 1991; 18(1):8–17.
11. Devlin TM. Lipid metabolism II: pathways of metabolism of special lipids. In: Devlin T, ed. Textbook of Biochemistry with Clinical Correlations. 3d ed. New York: Wiley-Liss, 1992:456–461.
12. Dunger DB, Broadbent V, Yeoman E, et al. The frequency and natural history of diabetes insipidus in children with Langerhans-cell histiocytosis. N Engl J Med 1989; 321:1157–1162.
13. Etcheverry R, Daiber A, Boris E, Duran N. Sea-blue histiocyte syndrome. Rev Med Child 1991; 119(9):1008–1015.
14. Hand A Jr. General tuberculosis. Trans Pathol Soc Phila 1893; 16:282–284.
15. Harris H, Hirschhorn K. Gaucher disease enzymology, genetics, and treatment. Adv Hum Genet 1993; 21:377–427.
16. Henter J, Elinder G, Ost A. FHL Study Group of the Histiocyte Society. Diagnostic guidelines for hemophagocytic lymphohistiocytosis. Semin Oncol 1991; 18(1):29–33.
17. Hollak CE, Weely SV, Van Oers MH, Aerts JM. Marked elevation of plasma chitotriosidase activity. A novel hallmark of Gaucher's disease. J Clin Invest 1994; 93:1288–1292.
18. Jimenez SM, Romero CR, Carrasco DF, Herrerias GJM. Gaucher's disease type I, anticoagulant factor and pregnancy. Ann Med Int 1991; 8(6):294–295.
19. Kaur M, Das GP, Verma IC. Sphingomyelinase enzyme assay in Niemann-Pick disease. Indian J Pediatr 1993; 60(4):583–590.
20. Kaye EM, Ullman MD, Kolodny EH, Krivit W, Rischert JC. Possible use of CSF glycosphingolipids for the diagnosis and therapeutic monitoring of lysosomal storage diseases. Neurology 1992; 42:2290–2294.
21. Ladisch S, Gadner H. Treatment of Langerhans cell histiocytosis—evolution and current approaches. Br J Cancer 1994; 23:S41–S46.
22. Larregue M, Trincal D, Bressieux JM, Fusade T, Tanzer J, Menguy C. Early acroparesthesia in females: a sign disclosing heterozygote Fabry's disease. Ann Dermatol Venereol 1991; 118(3): 191–197.
23. Ledvinova J, Elleder M. Filipin test for diagnosis of Niemann-Pick disease type C. Sb Lek 1993; 94(2):137–143.
24. Lejoyeux M, Dubois G, Turpin JC, Baumann N, Lemperiere T. Assays of arylsulfatase activity in psychotic patients. Review of the literature and results of a study of 22 patients. Encephale 1991; 17(2):87–92.
25. Lieberman PH, Jones CR, Steinman RM, et al. Langerhans cell (eosinophilic) granulomatosis—a clinicopathologic study encompassing 50 years. Am J Surg Pathol 1996; 20(5):519–552.
26. Montgomery EA, Meis JM, Frizzera G. Rosai-Dorfman disease of soft tissue. Am J Surg Pathol 1992; 16(2):122–129.
27. Risdall RJ, McKenna RW, Nesbit ME, et al. Virus-associated hemophagocytic syndrome. Cancer 1979; 44:993–1002.
28. Roff CF, Goldin E, Comly ME, et al. Niemann-Pick type C disease: deficient intracellular transport of exogenously derived cholesterol. Am J Med Genet 1992; 42(4):593–598.
29. Rousselet M-C, Francois S, Croue A, Maigre M, Saint-Andre J-P, Ifrah N. A lymph node interdigitating reticulum cell sarcoma. Arch Pathol Lab Med 1994; 118:183–8.
30. Sidransky E, Dietrich KM, Ginns EI. False-positive pregnancy tests in Gaucher disease. Lancet 1994; 344:1156.
31. Suzuki K, Saul R. Korey lecture. Molecular genetics of Tay-Sachs and related disorders: a personal account. J Neuropathol Exp Neurol 1994; 53(4):344–350.
32. Tanaka A. Tay-Sachs disease. Nippon Rinsho 1993; 51(9):2281–2285.
33. Vanier MT, Rodriguez-Lafrasse C, Rousson R, et al. Prenatal diagnosis of Niemann-Pick type C

disease: current strategy from an experience of 37 pregnancies at risk. Am J Hum Genet 1992; 51(1):111–122.
34. Whittington R, Goa KL. Alglucerase. A review of its therapeutic use in Gaucher's disease. Drugs 1992; 44(1):72–93.
35. Monocyte and macrophage disorders. In: Williams WJ, Beutler E, Erslev AJ, Lichtman MA, eds. Hematology. 4th ed. New York: McGraw-Hill, 1990:886–892.
36. Willman CL, Busque L, Griffith BB, et al. Langerhans cell histiocytosis (histiocytosis X)—a clonal proliferative disease. N Engl J Med 1994; 331(3):154–160.
37. Yu RC, Chu C, Bulewala L, Chu AC. Clonal proliferation of Langerhans cells in Langerhans cell histiocytosis. Lancet 1994; 343(8900):767–768.
38. Weisz B, Spirer Z, Reif S. Neimann-Pick disease. New classification based on genetic mutations of the disease. Adv Pediatr 1994; 41:415–426.
39. Niemann A. Ein unbekanntes Krakheitbild, Jarb Kinderheilkd. 1914; 79:11–17.
40. Crocker AC. The cerebral defects in Tay-Sachs and Neimann-Pick disease. J Neurochem 1961; 7: 69–78.

7

Benign Disorders of Leukocytes

Gene L. Gulati and Zoran Gatalica
Jefferson Medical College, Thomas Jefferson University, Philadelphia, Pennsylvania

Bong H. Hyun
Ajou University School of Medicine, Suwon City, Korea, and Jefferson Medical College, Thomas Jefferson University, Philadelphia, Pennsylvania

I. INTRODUCTION

Disorders of leukocytes can be classified into two groups, a malignant or neoplastic and a benign or reactive type. Malignant disorders result from autonomous proliferation of a clone of abnormal leukocytes, whereas benign disorders represent a reaction to underlying nonmalignant condition(s). Benign disorders can be further subclassified into two groups, quantitative disorders and qualitative disorders. The conditions associated with either an increase above normal or a decrease below normal in the number of one or more types of white blood cells comprise the group of quantitative leukocyte disorders. The qualitative leukocyte disorders include conditions associated with morphologic changes and/or functional defects in one or more types of white blood cells. Although many of the conditions included in the group of nonmalignant or benign disorders of leukocytes are clinically benign, some, such as Chediak-Higashi syndrome and chronic granulomatous disease, as discussed later, are associated with major clinical problems. Salient features of the common as well as some of the not-so-common reactive disorders of leukocytes, both quantitative and qualitative, and inherited and acquired, are presented in this chapter.

II. QUANTITATIVE DISORDERS OF LEUKOCYTES

A. Leukocytosis

Leukocytosis refers to an increase in the white blood cell (WBC) count to over the upper limit of normal for the age and ethnic origin, usually over 11.0×10^9/L for white adults and over 10.0×10^9/L for black adults. It may be physiologic or pathologic. The former is produced by factors that do not involve tissue damage, such as stress, exercise, and injection of epinephrine.

The latter, on the other hand, is brought about by a disease and usually involves tissue damage. Although an increase in the number of any one or more of the white cell types (neutrophils, eosinophils, basophils, lymphocytes, and monocytes) may be responsible for leukocytosis, it is most often due to an increase in the number of circulating neutrophils.

B. Neutrophilia (Fig. 1)

Neutrophilic leukocytosis or neutrophilia may be defined as an increase in circulating neutrophils to over the upper limit of normal, usually over 7.5×10^9/L in adults. An increase in only the percentage of neutrophils (including bands) to over 80 is referred to as *relative neutrophilia* and carries little, if any, clinical significance. Additional features that generally accompany a nonleukemic neutrophilic leukocytosis or reactive neutrophilia include (a) "shift to the left," toward more immature neutrophilic cells, primarily bands, but a few metamyelocytes and myelocytes may be present—blasts and promyelocytes are generally absent; and (b) toxic changes including toxic granulation (primary azurophilic granules), vacuolization, and Döhle bodies (remnants of RNA) in the cytoplasm of neutrophils and bands (Fig. 1). Neutrophilia may result from (a) a shift of neutrophils from the marginal pool to the circulating pool, (b) reduced exit rate of cells from the circulation, (c) increased release of cells from the bone marrow stores, (d) increased production in the bone marrow, or (e) any combination of these. The conditions associated with neutrophilia are summarized in Table 1.

C. Leukemoid Reaction (Fig. 2)

A leukemoid reaction is characterized by either (a) leukocytosis of 50.0×10^9/L or higher with a shift to the left, or (b) the presence of a considerable number of immature cells (metamyelo-

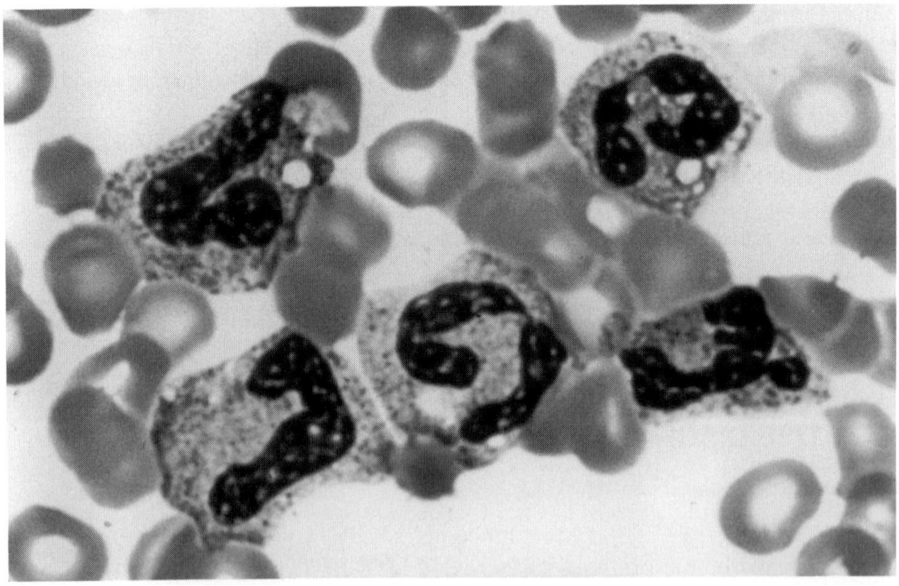

Figure 1 Neutrophilia with left shift: a blood smear from a patient with pneumonia, showing two neutrophils, three bands, and the toxic granulation, vacuolization, and Döhle bodies. (×1000)

Table 1 Conditions Associated with Neutrophilia

1. *Hereditary neutrophilia*: cyclic, familial, etc.
2. *Physiologic neutrophilia*: neonatal state (1–2 days), pregnancy (third trimester), labor, purperium, postprandial, nausea, vomiting, convulsions, exercise, emotional stress, etc.
3. *Infections*: primarily bacterial, but also rickettsial, fungal, parasitic, and viral (at least initially)
4. *Metabolic disorders*: diabetic acidosis, uremia, gout, eclampsia, etc.
5. *Neoplastic disorders*: myeloproliferative disorders (chronic myelogenous leukemia, polycythemia vera, etc.), lymphomas, melanoma, carcinoma of lung, thyroid, gallbladder, etc.
6. *Tissue necrosis*: myocardial infarction, burns, extreme cold, trauma, etc.
7. *Drugs*: epinephrine, serotonin, chlorpropamide, digitalis, lithium, steroids, vaccines, etc.
8. *Chemicals*: benzene, ethylene glycol, turpentine, lead, mercury, etc.
9. Myeloid growth factor therpy: granulocyte-colony stimulating factor (G-CSF), granulocyte/monocyte-colony stimulating factor (GM-CSF), etc.
10. *Others*: acute hemorrhage, hemolysis, electric shock, smoking, postsplenectomy state, idiopathic, etc.

cytes, myelocytes, promyelocytes, and even an occasional blast cell) in the peripheral blood, mimicking leukemia (Fig. 2). In the latter case, the WBC count may be above normal, normal, or rarely below normal. Depending on the predominant cell type, the leukemoid reaction may be neutrophilic, eosinophilic, or lymphocytic. Monocytic and basophilic leukemoid reactions, if they occur, are rare. Among the various types of leukemoid reactions, neutrophilic is the one most frequently encountered in clinical practice. In fact, it is so common that the term *leukemoid reaction* is presumed to refer to neutrophilic reaction unless specified otherwise. Neutrophilic leukemoid reaction may occur in many of the conditions associated with neutro-

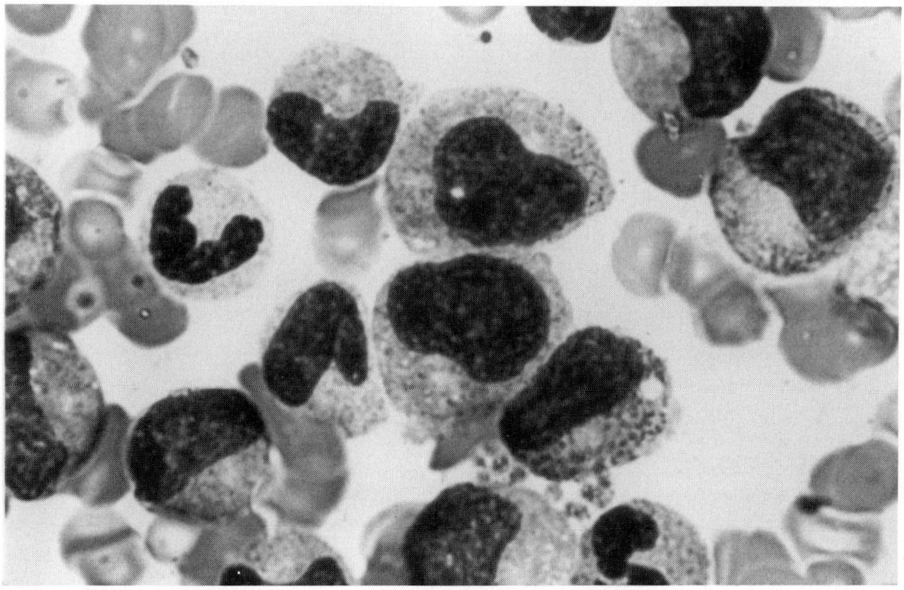

Figure 2 Leukemoid reaction: a blood smear from a patient with metastatic carcinoma, showing immature granulocytes (myelocytes, metamyelocytes, and bands). (×1000.)

Table 2 Conditions Associated with Leukemoid Reaction

1.	Severe or chronic infections.
2.	Severe hemolysis, severe hemorrhage
3.	*Toxic conditions*: severe burns, eclampsia, etc.
4.	*Malignant disorders*: myelofibrosis, Hodgkin's disease, metastatic carcinoma, etc.
5.	*Myeloid growth factor therapy*: G-CSF, GM-CSF, etc.

philia (Table 2). Cytoplasmic changes, such as toxic granulation, vacuolization, and Döhle bodies, along with a high neutrophil alkaline phosphatase (NAP) score, help to differentiate the leukemoid reaction from chronic myelogenous leukemia (CML), which is generally characterized by a large proportion of myelocytes, eosinophilia, basophilia, and a low NAP score. The diagnosis of CML is confirmed by the presence of Philadelphia chromosome or BCR-ABL gene rearrangement, both of which are absent in the leukemoid reaction. The leukemic hiatus, a characteristic of acute leukemia, is also absent in the leukemoid reaction. Eosinophilic leukemoid reactions usually occur in children and are generally caused by parasitic infections. Lymphocytic leukemoid reactions may occur in whooping cough, infectious lymphocytosis, infectious mononucleosis, and tuberculosis.

Based on clinical findings, the laboratory investigation of neutrophilia, neutrophilic or leukemoid reaction, particularly persistent neutrophilia, neutrophilic or leukemoid reaction, may include any of the following studies:

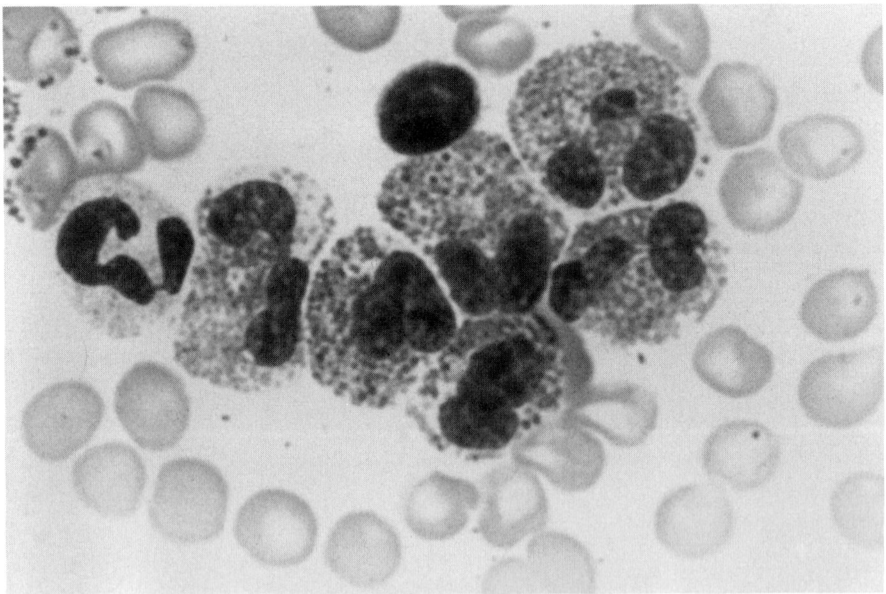

Figure 3 Eosinophilia: a blood smear from a patient with visceral larva migrans due to *Toxocara cati* infection, showing six eosinophils, one neutrophil, and one lymphocyte. (×1000.)

1. Blood smear examination
2. Bone marrow examination, particularly if a malignancy is suspected
3. Neutrophil alkaline phosphatase score
4. Cytogenetic studies, e.g., Philadelphia chromosome
5. Molecular diagnostic studies, e.g., BCR-ABL gene rearrangement
6. Test(s) for underlying condition(s)

D. Eosinophilia (Fig. 3)

An absolute eosinophil count exceeding the upper limit of normal, usually over 0.5×10^9/L of blood, is defined as eosinophilia. The most common causes of eosinophilia are allergic reactions, parasitic infections, skin disorders, and reactions to drugs. A list of conditions known to be associated with eosinophilia is presented in Table 3.

Based on clinical findings, the laboratory evaluation of eosinophilia, particularly persistent eosinophilia, may include any of the following studies:

1. Blood smear examination
2. Test(s) for suspected or identified underlying condition(s), e.g., feces examination for ova and parasite, and serum IgE determination
3. Bone marrow examination, if a malignancy is suspected.

Table 3 Conditions Associated with Eosinophilia

1. Hereditary eosinophilia (rare)
2. *Allergic/hypersensitivity reactions*: hay fever (seasonal rhinitis), bronchial asthma, urticaria, food sensitivity, drug sensitivity, etc.
3. *Parasitic infections*: trichinosis, amoebiasis, ascariasis, tapeworm, hookworm, filariasis, schistosomiasis, visceral larva migrans (*Toxocara cati* and *canis*), liver fluke, etc.
4. *Skin disorders*: psoriasis, pemphigus, dermatitis herpetiformis, etc.
5. *Collagen diseases*: polyarteritis nodosa, rheumatoid arthritis, Wagner's granulomatosis, systemic necrotizing vasculitis, etc.
6. Pulmonary eosinophilic syndromes
7. *Malignancies*: myeloproliferative disorders (chronic myelogenous leukemia, eosinophilic leukemia), Hodgkin's disease, lymphomas, carcinoma of lung, ovary, stomach, etc.
8. *Others*: splenectomy, GM-CSF therapy, rarely bacterial, viral or fungal infections
9. Idiopathic hypereosinophilic syndrome

E. Basophilia

Basophilia refers to an increase in circulating basophils to over the upper limit of normal, usually over 0.1×10^9/L. It is seen most frequently in association with myeloproliferative disorders, particularly chronic myelogenous leukemia and acute basophilic leukemia. Allergic reactions make up the second most common cause of basophilia. A list of conditions associated with basophilia is presented in Table 4.

Based on clinical findings, the laboratory evaluation of basophilia, particularly persistent basophilia, may include any of the following studies:

1. Blood smear examination
2. Test(s) for suspected or identified underlying condition(s)
3. Bone marrow examination, if a malignancy is suspected
4. Cell marker studies, as needed, to establish or confirm the specific cell lineage.

Table 4 Conditions Associated with Basophilia

1. Hypersensitivity reactions
2. *Hematologic malignancies*: chronic myelogenous leukemia, acute basophilic leukemia, systemic mast cell disease, etc.
3. Radiation therapy
4. *Miscellaneous*: myxedema, chronic sinusitis, smallpox, ulcerative colitis, postsplenectomy state, chronic hemolytic anemia, etc.

F. Lymphocytosis (Fig. 4)

Lymphocytosis is defined as an increase in circulating lymphocytes to over the upper limit of normal, usually over 4.0×10^9/L for adults and over 8.0×10^9/L for children. Relative lymphocytosis, an increase in only the percentage of lymphocytes to above the upper limit of normal, usually over 45 for adults and over 70 for children, is commonly associated with conditions causing neutropenia. Absolute lymphocytosis may result from (a) increased production in the bone marrow and/or lymphoid tissues, (b) prolonged survival in the circulation, or (c) a combination of these. The most common cause of absolute lymphocytosis is viral infections, particularly the Epstein-Barr virus (EBV) infection. Viral-induced absolute lymphocytosis is frequently accompanied by a variable number of circulating atypical lymphocytes. The atypical lymphocytes, also known by the names of reactive lymphocytes, stimulated lymphocytes, and variant lymphocytes, are generally characterized by their large size (equal to or larger than a normal neutrophil), often irregular shape, abundant cytoplasm which stains deep blue either throughout the cell or at least at the periphery, and nuclear chromatin of variable density (Fig.

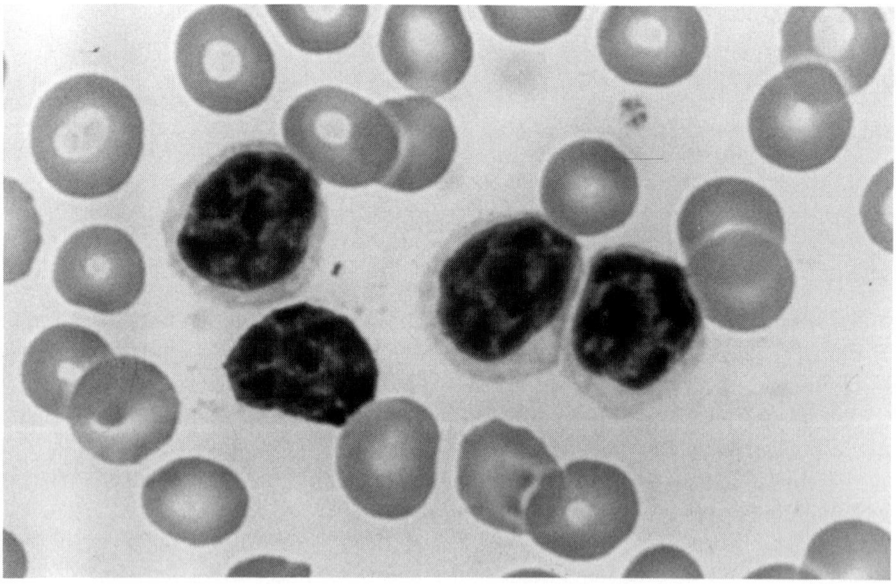

Figure 4 Lymphocytosis: a blood smear from a child with whooping cough, showing four mature lymphocytes. (×1000.)

6). The nucleus of an atypical lymphocyte may be as mature as that of a normal lymphocyte or as immature as that of a blast cell. The cytoplasm of atypical lymphocytes may contain a few azurophilic granules and rarely even a few vacuoles. This pleomorphism of cell size, shape, and nuclear chromatin density characterizing atypical lymphocytes helps differentiate benign lymphoproliferative disorders from malignant lymphoproliferative disorders. The conditions associated with lymphocytosis are summarized in Table 5.

Based on clinical findings, the laboratory evaluation of lymphocytosis, particularly persistent lymphocytosis, may include any of the following studies:

1. Blood smear examination
2. Serologic test(s) for infectious agent(s)
3. Lymph node biopsy, particularly when serologic tests are nondiagnostic
4. Bone marrow examination, if a malignancy is suspected
5. Cell marker studies, as needed, (a) to determine if the lymphocyte population is monoclonal (suggestive of malignancy) or polyclonal (nonmalignant) and (b) subclassify the lymphoid cells as T, B, common, and null. Assessment of maturational stage(s) of the cell-population of interest is also possible with specific cell marker studies. Such studies may be performed on blood, bone marrow, and/or lymph node specimens
6. Test(s) for other suspected or identified underlying condition(s)

Table 5 Conditions Associated with Lymphocytosis

1. *Viral infections*: infectious mononucleosis, cytomegalovirus infection, infectious hepatitis, acute infectious lymphocytosis, herpes simplex or zoster, varicella, influenza, mumps, measles, rubella, human immunodeficiency virus (HIV), mycoplasma pneumonia, etc.
2. *Bacterial infections*: pertussis (whooping cough), tuberculosis, syphilis, brucellosis, listeriosis, etc.
3. *Protozoal infections* (*uncommon*): toxoplasmosis, malaria, etc.
4. *Drug sensitivity* (*uncommon*): Phenytoin, para-aminosalicylic acid (PAS), sulfasolazine, etc.
5. *Malignant conditions*: chronic lymphocytic leukemia, acute lymphoblastic leukemia, leukemic phase of lymphoma, Waldestron's macroglobulinemia, etc.
6. *Others*: trauma, stress related to medical emergencies (such as vaso-occlusive crisis in sickle-cell anemia), smoking, hyposplenism, splenectomy, hyperthyroidism, congenital adrenal hyperplasia, etc.

Infectious mononucleosis, the most common condition associated with lymphocytosis, particularly atypical lymphocytosis, is considered in detail.

G. Infectious Mononucleosis (Fig. 5)

Infectious mononucleosis (IM) is an acute, sporadic, self-limited infection that usually occurs in young adult Caucasians. Males and females are equally affected. It is transmitted through saliva during prolonged kissing, hence the name "kissing disease." The etiologic agent is the Epstein-Barr virus, which infects B lymphocytes. Characteristic clinical findings include fever, frequently with chills and sweating, sore throat due to pharyngitis, and lymphadenopathy (cervical, axillary, and inguinal). Splenomegaly develops in 50% of patients, and hepatomegaly accompanies splenomegaly in about one-fourth of patients. Splenic rupture, although rare, is an important cause of death in this disease. Jaundice may develop in some patients (about 10% of cases). Other, less commonly encountered clinical features are malaise, nausea, anorexia, skin rash, gingivitis, conjunctivitis, photophobia, abdominal pain, and headache.

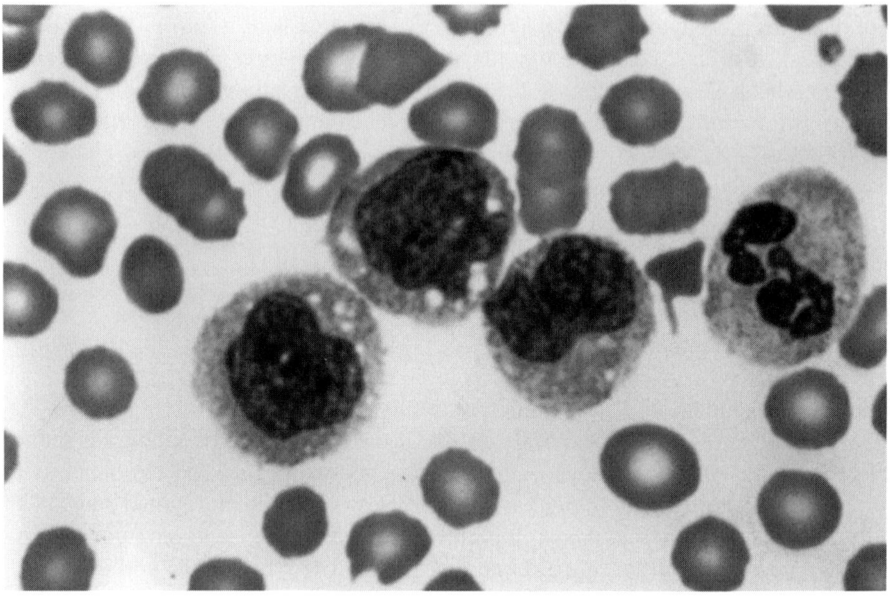

Figure 5 Atypical lymphocyte in a blood smear from a patient with infectious mononucleosis. (×1000.)

Characteristic laboratory finding is the presence of many atypical lymphocytes (over 10% of white cells) in the peripheral blood. The WBC count may be increased, normal, or rarely decreased. Lymphocytes often constitute over 50% of leukocytes, but absolute lymphocytosis may or may not be present in the early phase of the disease. Moreover, a slight to moderate left shift of neutrophils is not an uncommon finding during the initial stage of the disease. Although the total number of both B and T lymphocytes is increased in the peripheral blood, the majority of the atypical lymphocytes are activated T cells capable of killing the EBV-infected B cells. The clinical diagnosis of IM is confirmed by serologic tests. A heterophile antibody test, such as Mono test, is routinely performed on every suspected case of IM. The EBV-antibody tests are used primarily to diagnose heterophile negative IM. Antiviral capsid antigen (anti-VCA) antibodies appear early as IgM antibodies and hence are useful in the diagnosis of acute IM. Later in the course of the disease, the anti-VCA antibodies appear as IgG antibodies, which persist for life. Anti-early antigen (anti-EA) antibodies appear early (during the first week) and peak during the second or third week after onset. The serologic tests help in the differential diagnosis of IM, which can be confused with cytomegalovirus infection, posttransfusion syndrome, infectious hepatitis, PAS hypersensitivity, etc. Liver function test results, including alkaline phosphatase, glutamic oxaloacetic transaminase (GOT), and glutamic pyruvic transaminase (GPT), are also abnormal in many IM patients. Mild to moderate elevation in the serum bilirubin level is seen in about one-third of patients.

H. Monocytosis (Fig. 6)

An absolute monocyte count above the upper limit of normal, usually over 1.0×10^9/L, is defined as monocytosis. Slight monocytosis is normal during the first two weeks of life. Monocytosis is often transient and correlates poorly with specific disorders. Among the conditions

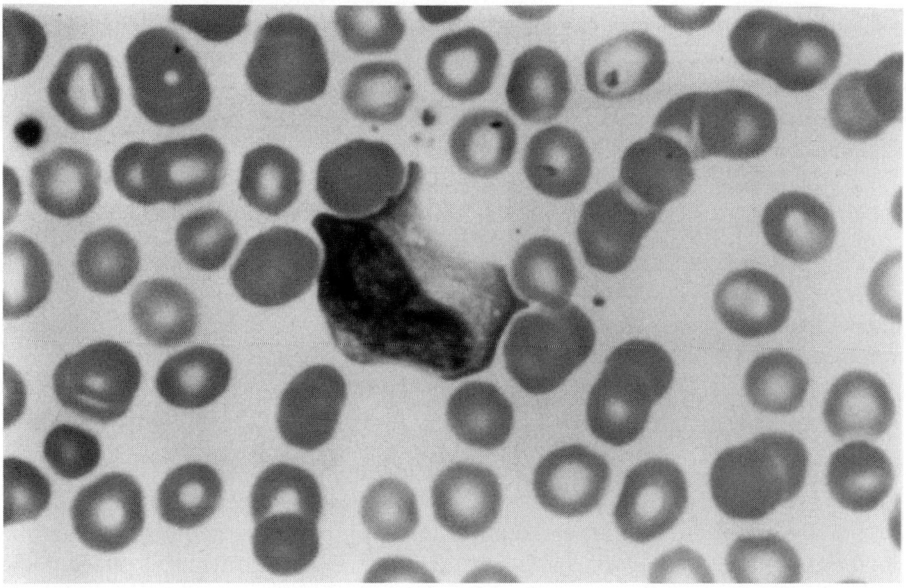

Figure 6 Monocytosis: a blood smear from a patient with tuberculosis showing three monocytes and a neutrophil. (×1000.)

associated with monocytosis (Table 6), neutropenic disorders, indolent infections, convalescence from infection/inflammation, and malignancies, particularly hematologic, stand out as the most common causes.

Based on clinical findings, the laboratory evaluation of monocytosis, particularly persistent monocytosis, may include any of the following studies:

Table 6 Conditions Associated with Monocytosis

1. *Chronic infections*:
   Bacterial: tuberculosis, brucellosis, syphilis, subacute bacterial endocarditis, leprosy, etc.
   Rickettsial: typhus, Rocky Mountain spotted fever, etc.
   Protozoal: malaria, trypanosomiasis, kala-azar, etc.
2. *Hematologic disorders*: acute and chronic monocytic and myelomonocytic leukemias, myelodysplastic syndromes, neutropenic disorders, Hodgkin's disease, lymphomas, myeloma, lipid storage diseases, etc.
3. *Nonhematologic malignancies*
4. *Connective tissue disorders*: rheumatoid arthritis, polyarteritis, myositis, systemic lupus erythematosus, etc.
5. *Granulomatous diseases*: sarcoidosis, regional enteritis, ulcerative colitis, etc.
6. *Postradiotherapy, postchemotherapy*
7. *Myeloid growth factor therapy*: GM-CSF, monocyte/macrophage-colony stimulating factor (M-CSF), etc.
8. *Others*: postsplenectomy state, chronic high-dose steroids administration, tetrachlorethane poisoning, etc.

1. Blood smear examination
2. Test(s) for suspected or identified underlying condition(s)
3. Bone marrow examination, if a malignancy is suspected
4. Cell marker studies, as needed, to establish or confirm the monocytic lineage of the cell population of interest

I. Leukopenia

Leukopenia refers to a decrease in the white blood cell count below the lower limit of normal, usually below 4.0×10^9/L for white adults and below 3.0×10^9/L for black adults. Although a decrease in the number of any one or more of the white cell types may contribute to leukopenia, it is most often due to decreased number of circulating neutrophils and/or lymphocytes.

J. Neutropenia

An absolute neutrophil count below the lower limit of normal, usually below 1.8×10^9/L for white adults and below 1.0×10^9/L for black adults, is defined as neutropenia. The term *agranulocytosis* is generally used to denote severe neutropenia often revealing no neutrophils in the peripheral blood and myeloid hypoplasia and/or maturation arrest at the myelocyte stage in the bone marrow. When the neutrophil count falls below 0.5×10^9/L, the patient is very likely to have recurrent infections, necessitating the inclusion of isolation precautionary measures in the management plan. Neutropenia may result from (a) decreased production in the bone marrow, (b) ineffective production, (c) increased removal from the blood, (d) shift of cells from the circulating pool to the marginal pool, or (e) any combination of these. Neutropenia may be selective or part of a general pancytopenia, which refers to a reduction in all three cell lines, leukocytes, erythrocytes, and thrombocytes in the peripheral blood. Frequently, neutropenia is associated with relative lymphocytosis. The conditions associated with neutropenia are listed in Table 7.

Based on clinical findings, the laboratory evaluation of neutropenia, particularly persistent neutropenia, may include any of the following studies:

1. Blood smear examination
2. Complete blood counts on family members, if hereditary or familial neutropenia is suspected

Table 7 Conditions Associated with Neutropenia

1. Hereditary neutropenia, familial neutropenia, cyclic neutropenia
2. *Nutritional deficiency*: vitamin B_{12} deficiency, folate deficiency
3. *Drugs*: antiinflammatory, antibacterial, antirheumatics, anticonvulsants, antithyroids, hypoglycemics, psychotropics, chemotherapy
4. *Radiation*
5. *Infections*: hepatitis, HIV, influenza, typhoid, tuberculosis, parvovirus, etc.
6. *Immune neutropenias*: autoimmune neutropenoia, systemic lupus erythematosus, hypersensitivity reaction, anaphylaxis
7. *Hematologic disorders*: lymphoproliferative disorders, myelodysplastic syndromes, acute leukemia, myelofibrosis, megaloblastic anemia, etc.
8. *Hypersplenism*
9. *Others*: severe chronic neutropenia, idiopathic neutropenia, etc.

3. Bone marrow examination
4. Antibodies against neutrophils
5. Neutrophil function test(s)
6. Test(s) for suspected or identified underlying condition(s)

K. Lymphocytopenia

Lymphocytopenia is defined as an absolute lymphocyte count below the lower limit of normal, usually below $1.5 \times 10^9/L$ for adults and below $3.0 \times 10^9/L$ for children. Decreased production, increased loss from circulation due to mechanical interference, destruction by viruses, radiation, or drugs, or any combination of these may be responsible for the development of lymphocytopenia. The conditions associated with lymphocytopenia are summarized in Table 8.

Based on clinical findings, the laboratory evaluation of lymphocytopenia, particularly persistent lymphocytopenia, may include any of the following studies:

1. Blood smear examination
2. Cell marker studies, particularly flow cytometry, as needed, to determine the cell lineage (T or B) and maturation stage(s) (subsets of T and B cells) of the lymphoid cell population
3. Bone marrow examination
4. Quantitative immunoglobulin determination
5. Test(s) for suspected or identified underlying condition(s)

L. Monocytopenia, Eosinopenia, and Basopenia

A decrease in circulating monocytes below the lower limit of normal, usually below $0.2 \times 10^9/L$, is defined as monocytopenia. Chronic administration of corticosteroids often results in monocytopenia.

Eosinopenia is defined as a decrease in circulating eosinophils below the lower limit of normal, usually below $0.04 \times 10^9/L$. Eosinophils show diurnal variation; their level is lowest in the morning and highest at night. Acute stress, acute inflammation, Cushing's syndrome, and corticosteroid therapy are some of the conditions associated with eosinopenia.

Table 8 Conditions Associated with Lymphocytopenia

1.	*Immune deficiency disorders*:	
	T-cell defects:	Thymic aplasia, purine nucleoside phosphorylase (PNP) deficiency, AIDS, Hodgkin's disease, non-Hodgkin's lymphoma, drugs (cyclosporine, steroids, etc.), etc.
	B-cell defects:	X-linked agammaglobulinemia, acquired common variable hypogammaglobulinemia, selective IgA or IgG deficiency, myeloma, nephrotic syndrome, etc.
	T- and B-cell defects:	severe combined immunodeficiency, Blooms' syndrome, Wiskott-Aldrich syndrome, chronic lymphocytic leukemia, postradiotherapy, postchemotherapy, post-bone marrow transplantation, etc.
2.	*Corticosteroids and other immunosuppressive therapy*	
3.	*Intestinal lymphocyte loss*: intestinal lymphangiectasia, Whipple's disease, obstruction of thoracic duct or intestinal lymphatics	
4.	*Severe bone marrow failure*: aplastic anemia, etc.	
5.	*Others*: tuberculosis, sarcoid, systemic lupus erythematosus, etc.	

Basopenia exists when the absolute basophil count falls below the lower limit of normal, usually below $0.01 \times 10^9/L$. Basophils, like eosinophils, show diurnal variation; their level is lowest in the morning and highest at night. Acute stress, acute infection, hyperthyroidism, and sustained treatment with adrenal glucocorticoids are some of the conditions known to be associated with basopenia.

Clinical significance of all three of these conditions, monocytopenia, eosinopenia, and basopenia, remains poorly understood.

III. QUALITATIVE DISORDERS OF LEUKOCYTES

Qualitative disorders of leukocytes are characterized by either abnormal leukocyte morphology with or without functional abnormality or are associated with abnormal leukocyte function with or without morphologic abnormality. The abnormalities, morphologic and functional, may involve any one or more types of leukocytes and may be inherited or acquired. Salient features of some of the qualitative disorders of leukocytes, particularly those involving neutrophils, are presented below:

A. Disorders Characterized by Abnormal Leukocyte Morphology

1. Pelger-Huet Anomaly (Fig. 7)

Pelger-Huet anomaly is a benign autosomal dominant anomaly affecting primarily granulocytes, which are characterized by either bilobed nuclei (heterozygous form) or rounded nuclei (homozygous form) with coarsely clumped chromatin. The heterozygous form occurs in 1 in 6000 births, while the homozygous form is rare. The appearance of nuclei in neutrophils is

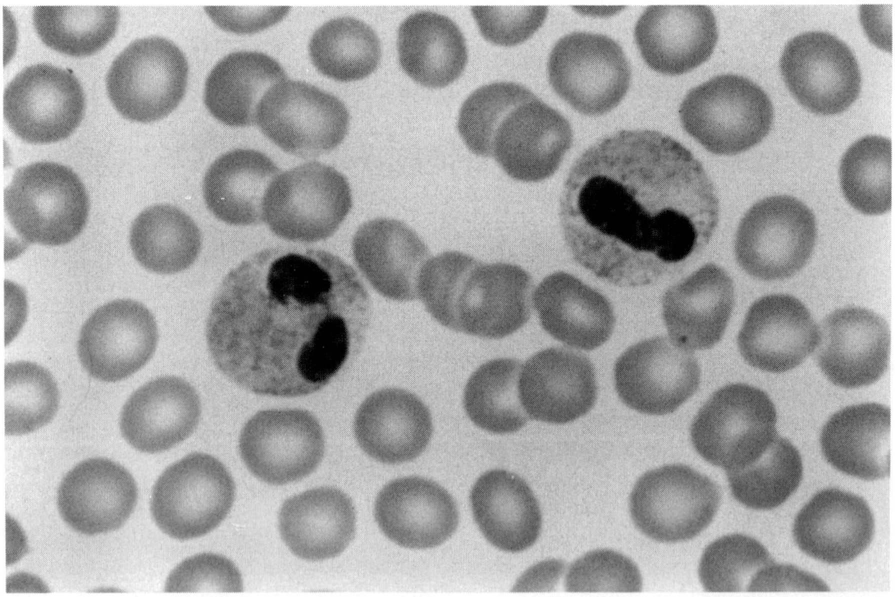

Figure 7 Two neutrophils, one with a bilobed (pince-nez) nucleus and the other with a peanut-shaped nucleus, in a blood smear from a patient with Pelger-Huet anomaly. (×1000.)

classically described as "pince-nez" (a form of spectacles without ear pieces, very popular in Europe in the 1920s and 1930s). The more modern description compares them with the bikini tops (no straps). Nuclear chromatin is clumped in essentially all nucleated cells of the blood and bone marrow. In the heterozygous form, approximately 80% of neutrophils have classical bilobed nuclei, while a minor proportion has oblong, dumbbell, or peanut-shaped nuclei. A few neutrophils may have three-lobed nuclei, but it is rare, if not almost impossible, to find a four-lobed neutrophil. Pelger-Huet neutrophils are sometimes mistakenly identified as left shift, leading to unnecessary treatment. These cells function and survive normally. Affected individuals have normal resistance to infection. Acquired or pseudo-Pelger-Huet anomaly is more common and is associated with myelodysplastic syndromes, acute and chronic myeloid leukemias, HIV infection, and with the use of sulfonamides, colchicine, taxoid, etc. This acquired nuclear aberration is usually seen in minority of granulocytes and is a transient finding.

2. *Alder-Reilly Anomaly (Figs. 8 and 9)*

Alder-Reilly anomaly is a rare autosomal recessive disorder characterized by the presence of larger than normal azurophilic granules in the cytoplasm of leukocytes and macrophages of the blood and bone marrow. These granules, also known as "Alder-Reilly bodies," stain dark lilac by Wright-Giemsa. Lymphocytes and macrophages containing Alder-Reilly bodies have been named Gasser's cells and Berhot's cells, respectively. Affected cells reportedly do not show impairment of their function. Similar morphologic abnormality is also seen in patients with various types of mucospolysaccharidoses (MPS), including Hurler syndrome, Hunter syndrome, Sanfilipo's syndrome, and Morquio's syndrome. The MPS results from deficiency of any one of the several enzymes involved in sequential degradation of glycosaminoglycans (GAGs). The undegraded GAGs accumulate in connective tissue cells, macrophages, endothelial cells, neurons, and hepatocytes.

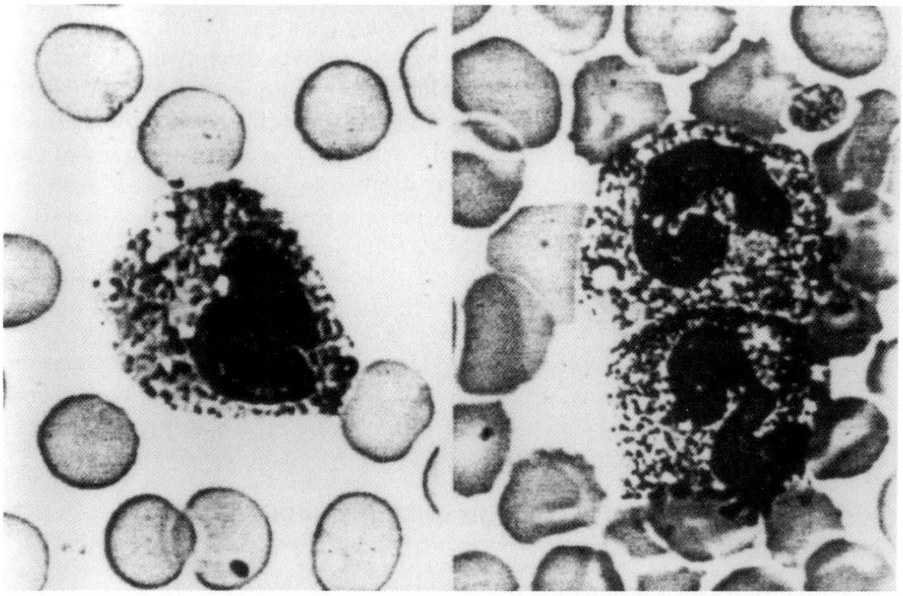

Figure 8 Alder-Reilly inclusions in granulocytes in a blood smear from a patient with mucopolysaccharidosis. (×1000.) (Reproduced with permission.)

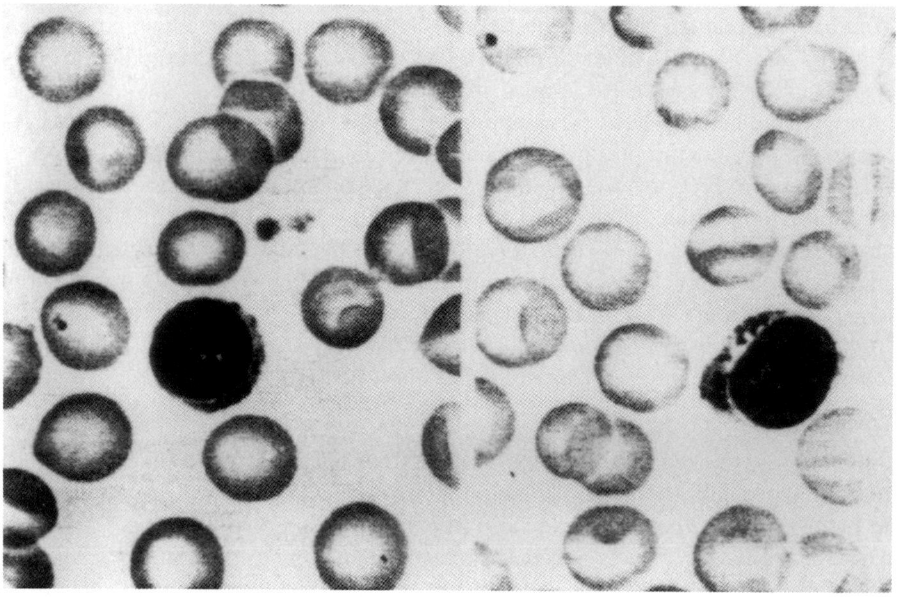

Figure 9 Alder-Reilly inclusions in lymphocytes (also known as Gasser cells) in a blood smear from a patient with mucopolysaccharidosis. (×1000.) (Reproduced with permission.)

3. *May-Hegglin Anomaly (Fig. 10)*

May-Hegglin anomaly is a rare autosomal dominant disorder characterized by (a) Döhle bodies-like inclusions in granulocytes and monocytes, (b) poorly granulated giant platelets, and in some cases (c) mild to moderate thrombocytopenia, sometimes with hemorrhagic manifestations. The leukocyte inclusions are larger and more prominent than the Döhle bodies associated with infections, toxic states, pregnancy, and myeloproliferative disorders. Electron microscopic studies reveal that these inclusions consist of spherical particles and randomly distributed rods surrounded by cisternae of rough endoplasmic reticulum. They stain blue with Wright-Giemsa and pink with methyl-green-pyronin, both denoting RNA. Giant platelets are believed to be the result of some defect in megakaryocyte maturation. Thrombocytopenia is often found incidently, as many patients are asymptomatic. However, detailed history does reveal excessive bleeding after tooth extraction, easy bruising, menorrhagia, and unexpected bleeding following surgical procedures in about half of the patients. May-Hegglin anomaly has not been associated with increased susceptibility to infection.

4. *Hereditary Hypersegmentation of Neutrophils (Fig. 11)*

Hereditary hypersegmentation of neutrophils is a rare autosomal dominant disorder characterized by many large neutrophils containing more than five nuclear lobes. The hypersegmented neutrophils function normally. The main significance of this disorder is that it is not due to a defect in vitamin B_{12} or folate metabolism.

B. Disorders Associated with Functional Abnormalities of Leukocytes

1. *Chronic Granulomatous Disease*

Chronic granulomatous disease (CGD) is characterized by the inability of granulocytes and other phagocytic cells to kill ingested bacteria, resulting in chronic local granulomatous inflam-

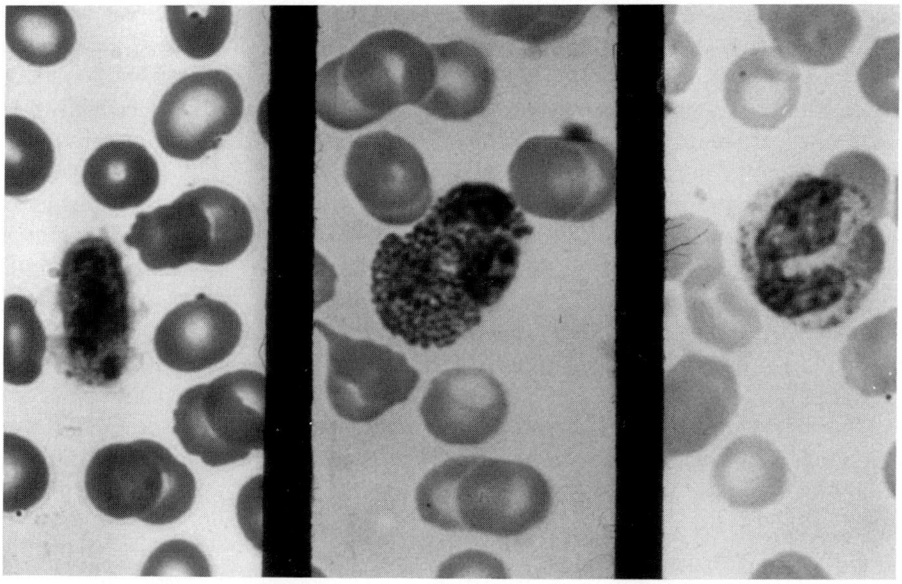

Figure 10 A giant platelet (a), Döhle bodies-like inclusions in an eosinophil (b), and a band (c) along with lack of platelets (thrombocytopenia) in a blood smear from a patient with May-Hegglin anomaly. Left to right: a, b, c. (×1000.)

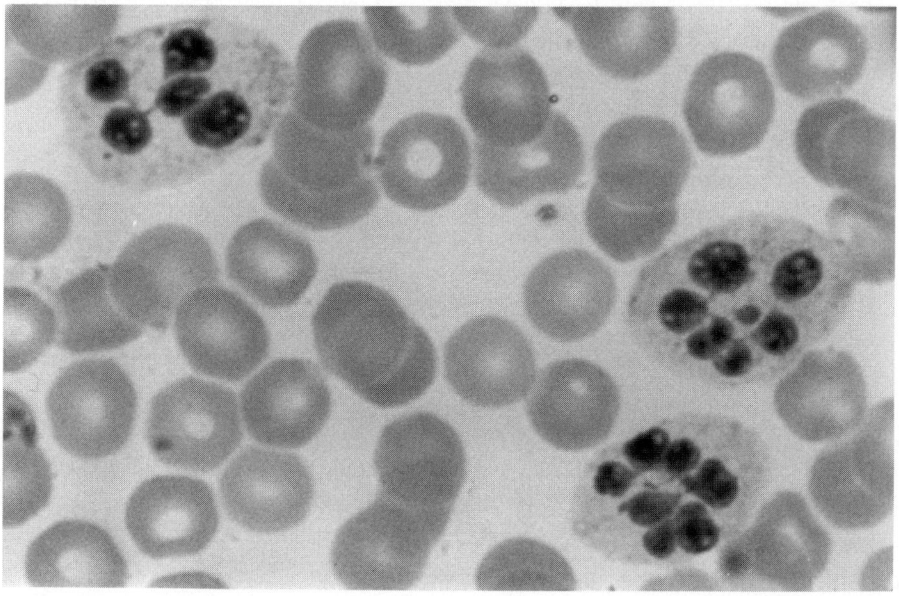

Figure 11 Hypersegmented neutrophils in a blood smear from a patient with hereditary hypersegmentation of neutrophils. (×1000.)

mation. The disease typically presents in the first few weeks of life with recurrent bacterial and fungal infections involving the skin, respiratory tract, gastrointestinal tract, and lymph nodes. Abscesses may form in various organs of the body. The disease is caused by the failure of NADPH oxidase in phagocytic leukocytes to generate superoxide needed for the killing of the microorganisms, particularly catalase positive bacteria, e.g., *Staphylococcus aureus*. NADPH oxidase is a multicomponent enzyme consisting of at least five subunits. Mutations in both integral membrane units (p22-phox and gp91-phox) as well as in two cytoplasmic units (p47-phox and p67-phox) have been found in patients suffering from CGD. The most common mutation (50% of cases) affects gp91-phox. The gene for gp91-phox is located on the X chromosome. Approximately one-third of the cases are inherited in autosomal recessive fashion. Mutations in the fifth unit (GTP-binding protein) have not been described. Morphologically, the neutrophils and monocytes appear normal. The most widely used test for the diagnosis of CGD is the nitroblue tetrazolium (NBT) reduction assay. In this assay, neutrophils are activated and the superoxide generated by the respiratory burst reduces the yellow NBT dye to blue formazan, which precipitates on the activated cells as a deep blue pigment. Since the neutrophils from CGD patients generate little or no superoxide, the NBT test is negative.

2. *Leukocyte Adhesion Protein Deficiency*

Leukocyte adhesion protein deficiency (LAD) is a rare autosomal recessive disorder of leukocyte adhesion and chemotaxis. Leukocytes from patients with LAD adhere poorly to endothelial cells and exhibit defective margination and chemotaxis, leading to recurrent severe infections. Leukocyte adhesion deficiency 1 (LAD1) is caused by defects in CD18 gene, which codes for the common beta-2 subunit of the leukocyte integrins LFA-1 (CD11a/CD18), Mac-1 (CD11b/CD18), and p150,95 (CD11c/CD18). Patients with LAD2 exhibit normal expression of CD18 but lack sialyl Lewis X antigen (selectin ligand) and similarly do not adhere to endothelial cells. Neutrophil adherence and aggregation deficits in general population are most commonly drug induced (glucocorticoids, alcohol, etc.), or acquired (hemodialysis, myelodysplastic syndromes, etc.). Patients with LAD have persistent leukocytosis ($15–20 \times 10^9$/fL), but the leukocytes appear morphologically normal. The laboratory diagnosis of LAD is generally made by flow cytometric analysis of blood neutrophils using antibodies specific for CD11 or CD18 antigens.

3. *Myeloperoxidase Deficiency*

Complete or partial deficiency of myeloperoxidase (MPO), a benign autosomal recessive disorder, occurs in 1 of 2000 people, making it the most common among the inherited disorders of phagocytes. The genetic defect results in abnormal posttranslational processing of proMPO, and lack of mature MPO. The lack of MPO reduces microbicidal activity of phagocytic cells, but the host defense system in general is not significantly impaired unless there is additional compromising disease, e.g., diabetes mellitus. Partial MPO deficiency has been reported also in patients with myelodysplastic syndrome, acute myeloid leukemia, and chronic myeloid leukemia. Morphologically, all leukocytes appear normal and only the neutrophils and monocytes, not eosinophils, reveal absence of peroxidase when examined cytochemically. Most of the cases are found incidentally due to aberrant leukocyte counts obtained with automated analyzers that utilize cytochemical demonstration of myeloperoxidase.

C. Disorders Associated with Functional and Morphologic Abnormalities of Leukocytes

1. *Chediak-Higashi Syndrome (Fig. 12)*

Chediak-Higashi Syndrome (CHS) is an autosomal recessive disease characterized by recurrent pyogenic infections, partial oculocutaneous albinism, photosensitivity, and a mild bleeding

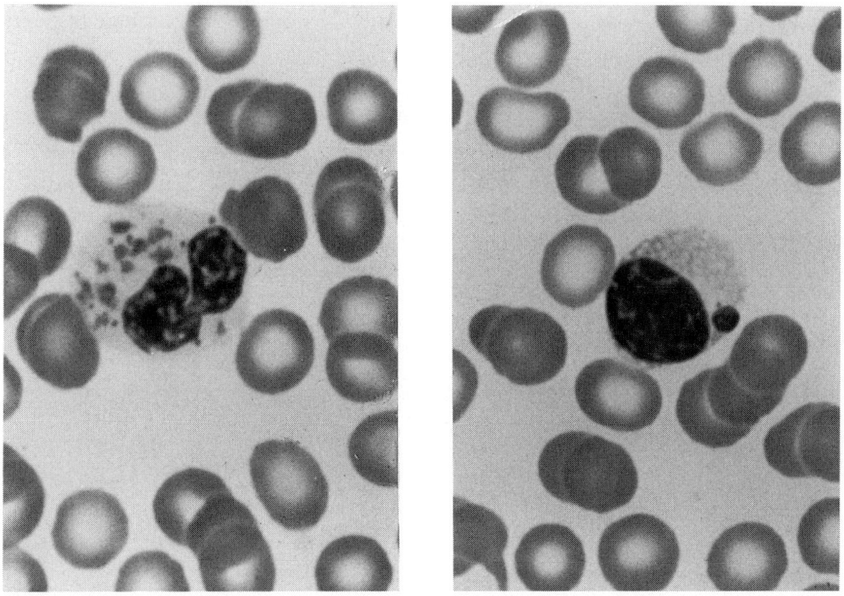

Figure 12 Giant lysosomal granules in a neutrophil and a lymphocyte in a blood smear from a patient with Chediak-Higashi syndrome. (×1000.)

diathesis. An accelerated lymphoma-like phase characterized by pancytopenia, diffuse lymphoid and histiocytic proliferation in the liver, spleen, and bone marrow, and neurologic abnormalities, is experienced by over 80% of patients, usually before the age of 10 years. Intercurrent infection and hemorrhage are the main causes of death. The main laboratory findings include neutropenia and the presence of large intracellular inclusions of lysosomal origin (byproducts of fusion among primary granules or primary and secondary granules) in granule-containing cells, most notably the leukocytes (including granular lymphocytes and monocytes) in the blood and/or bone marrow. These granules stain positive for myeloperoxidase (denoting primary granules) and often also for acid phosphatase (denoting secondary granules). Other cells affected by the disease include platelets, melanocytes, Schwaan cells, macrophages of the reticuloendothelial system, and granular cells of gastric mucosa, pancreas, renal tubular epithelium, and thyroid. The giant granule formation is thought to be due to an abnormal protein involved in membrane fusion. The cells containing the giant granules are functionally defective; impaired chemotaxis and phagocytic activity have been noted.

D. Laboratory Evaluation of Qualitative Leukocyte Disorders

Based on clinical findings, the laboratory evaluation of qualitative leukocytic disorders may include any of the following studies:

1. Complete blood count (CBC)
2. Differential leukocyte count
3. Blood smear examination (morphology evaluation)
4. Immunoglobulin quantitation
5. Complement quantitation
6. Serum IgE determination

7. T and B lymphocyte function
8. Leukocyte adhesion protein(s)
9. Motility and chemotaxis
10. Superoxide generation (NBT test)
11. HIV antibody screen
12. Others

CASE STUDY

Patient

Twenty-six-year-old female.

Chief Complaint

Fever (101°F), fatigue, malaise, anorexia, sore throat with dysphagia, and headache for approximately a week.

Medical History

Unremarkable.

Medications

Tylenol for headache and fever.

Physical Examination

Pharyngitis, jaundice, cervical lymphadenopathy, and enlarged spleen (one fingerbreadth below the costal margin).

Laboratory Results

	Patient	Normal
CBC:		
WBC ($\times 10^9$/L)	12.0	4.0–11.0
RBC ($\times 10^{12}$/L)	1.8	3.7–5.2
HGB (g/dL)	6.1	12.5–15.0
HCT (%)	17.0	36–46
MCV (fL)	95	81–99
MCH (pg)	33.9	27–32
MCHC (g/dL)	35.9	32–36
RDW (%)	18.5	11.5–14.5
PLT ($\times 10^9$/L)	350	140–400
Differential:		
Neutrophil (%)	22	40–73
Lymphocytes (%)	30	20–44
Atypical lymphocytes (%)	20	0–5
Monocytes (%)	6	3–13
Eosinophils (%)	3	0–6
Basophils (%)	1	0–3
Bands (%)	18	0–9
Blood Smear examination:		
Red cell agglutination 4+		
Polychromosia 3+		

Questions

1. What is the most likely diagnosis?
2. What is the cause of severe anemia in this patient?
3. What additional test(s), if any, would help make or confirm the diagnosis?

Additional Laboratory Results

	Patient	Normal
Mono test	Reactive	Nonreactive
Reticulocyte count (%)	14.0	0.5–1.5
Bilirubin (mg/dL)	3.0	0.2–1.2
Coomb's test	Positive	Negative
Antibody screen	Anti-i	Negative
Cold agglutinin titer	1:1280	—

Diagnosis

Infectious mononucleosis with autoimmune hemolytic anemia.

Discussion

Clinical findings are suggestive of infectious mononucleosis. Initial laboratory findings of slight leukocytosis, absolute lymphocytosis, many atypical lymphocytes, and left shift of neutrophils are also consistent with the suspected clinical diagnosis of infectious mononucleosis. The diagnosis of infectious mononucleosis was confirmed by the positive Mono test (a serologic test for heterophile antibody). The hemoglobin level of 6.1 g/dL, however, is not consistent with the sole diagnosis of infectious mononucleosis. Peripheral blood smear examination revealed marked agglutination of red cells and polychromasia, in addition to the presence of many atypical lymphocytes. In fact, the CBC results given above were obtained after incubating the blood specimen at 37°C for 15 min. These findings are indicative of cold-antibody-mediated hemolytic process, which was confirmed by a positive Coomb's test, a reticulocyte count of 14%, bilirubin of 3 mg/dL, and the cold agglutinin titer of 1:1280. The antibody screen revealed anti-i antibody. Thus, the clinical and laboratory findings together led to the definitive diagnosis of infectious mononucleosis with autoimmune hemolytic anemia. Autoimmune hemolytic anemia develops as a complication of infectious mononucleosis in 5–10% of cases.

Bibliography

1. Hoeprich PD, Flynn NM. Infectious mononucleosis and related disorders. In RL Bick, ed. Hematology: Clinical and Laboratory Practice. Philadelphia: Mosby, 1993:659–662.
2. Nakamura RM, Smith RS. Laboratory evaluation of mononucleosis syndrome. In RL Bick, ed. Hematology: Clinical and Laboratory Practice. Philadelphia: Mosby, 1993: 663–672.
3. Chetham MM, Roberts KB. Infectious mononucleosis in adolescents. Pediatr Ann 1991; 20(4):206–213.

SELECTED READINGS

1. Abramson JS, Wheeler JG, eds. The Neutrophil. New York: Oxford University Press, 1993.
2. Agamanolis DP. The pathology of lysosomal storage diseases. Pathol Ann 1995; 30:247–285.
3. Baetz K, Isaaz S, Griffiths GM. Loss of cytotoxic function in Chediak-Higashi syndrome arises from a secretory defect that prevents lytic granule exocytosis. J Immunol 1995; 154:6122–6131.
4. Becker R, Pfluger KH. Myeloperoxidase deficiency: an epidemiologic study and flow-cytometric detection of other granular enzymes in myeloperoxidase-deficient subjects. Ann Hematol 1994; 69: 199–203.
5. Bogomolski-Yahalom V, Matzner Y. Disorders of neutrophil function. Blood Rev 1995; 9:183–190.
6. Brunning RD. Morphologic alterations in nucleated blood and marrow cells in genetic disorders. Hum Pathol 1970; 1:99–124.
7. Chanarin I, Harrisingh D, Tidmarsh E, et al. Significance of lymphocytosis in adults. Lancet 1984; 2:897–899.
8. Dale DC, Hammond WP. Cyclic neutropenia: a clinical review. Blood Rev 1988; 2:178–185.
9. Davey FR, Huntington S. Age-related variation in lymphocyte sub-populations. Gerontology 1977; 23:381–389.
10. Etzioni A, Phillips LM, Paulson JC, Harlan JM. Leukocyte adhesion deficiency (LAD)II. Ciba Found Symp 1995; 189:51–58.
11. Fauci AS, Harley JB, Roberts WC, et al. The idiopathic hypereosinophilic syndrome. Clinical, pathophysiological, and therapeutic considerations. Ann Intern Med 1982; 97:78–92.
12. Foucar K, Duncan MH, Smith KJ. Practical approach to the investigation of neutropenia. Clin Lab Med 1993; 13(4):879–894.
13. Friedenberg WR. Disorders of granulocytes: quantitative and qualitative. In Mazza JJ, ed. Manual of Clinical Hematology. Boston: Little, Brown, 1995:163–189.
14. Gieselmann V. Lysosomal storage disease. Biochem Biophys Acta 1995; 1270:103–136.
15. Greinacher A, Mueller-Eckhardt. Hereditary types of thrombocytopenia with giant platelets and inclusion bodies in leukocytes. Blut 1990; 60:53–60.
16. Gulati GL, Ashton JK, Hyun BH. Benign lymphocytosis, monocytosis, and plasmacytosis. In RL Bick, ed. Hematology, Clinical and Laboratory Practice. St. Louis: Mosby, 1993:651–658.
17. Jandl JH. Leukocyte anomalies. Blood: Textbook of Hematology, Chapter 19. Boston: Little, Brown, 1987:571–588.
18. Juneja S, Januszewicz E, Wolf M, Cooper F. Post-spleenectomy lymphocytosis. Clin Lab Haematol 1995; 17(4):335–337.
19. Juneja SK, Matthews JP, Fan Y, et al. Association of Pelger-Huet anomaly with taxoid therapy. Br J Haematol 1996; 93:139–141.
20. Kay NE. Benign lymphocyte disorders. In: Mazza JJ, ed. Manual of Clinical Hematology. Boston: Little, Brown, 1995:227–293.
21. Kettle AJ, Winterbourn CC. Superoxide-dependent hydroxylation by myeloperoxidase. J Biol Chem 1994; 269:17146–17151.
22. Maladonado JE, Hanlon DG. Monocytosis: a current appraisal. Mayo Clin Proc 1968; 40:246–251.
23. Mazzone A, Ricevuti G. Leukocyte CD11/CD18 integrins: biological and clinical relevance. Haematologica 1995; 80:161–175.
24. Naiman JL, Oski FA, Allen FH, et al. Hereditary eosinophilia: report of a family and review of the literature. Am J Hum Genet 1964; 16:195–203.
25. Nauseef WM, Olsson I, Arnljots K. Biosynthesis and processing of myeloperoxidase: a marker for myeloid differentiation. Eur J Haematol 1988; 40:97–110.
26. Peterson L, Hrisinko MA. Benign lymphocytosis and reactive neutrophilia. Laboratory features provide diagnostic clues. Clin Lab Med 1993; 13(4):863–877.
27. Reed WW, Diehl LF. Leukopenia, neutropenia, and reduced hemoglobin levels in healthy american blacks. Arch Intern Med 1991; 151:501–505.
28. Roos D. The genetic basis of chronic granulomatous disease. Immunol Rev 1994; 138:121–157.

29. Salama A, Mueller-Eckhardt C. Immune-mediated blood cell dyscrasias related to drugs. Semin Hematol 1992; 29:54–63.
30. Schmitz LL, Litz CE, Brunning RD. Morphologic and quantitative alterations in hematopoietic cells associated with growth factor therapy: review of the literature. Hematol Pathol 1994; 8(3):55–73.
31. Schmitz LL, McClure JS, Litz CE, et al. Morphologic and quantitative changes in blood and marrow cells following growth factor therapy. Am J Clin Pathol 1994; 101:67–75.
32. Schoentay RA, Cangiarella J. The nuances of lymphocytopenia. Clin Lab Med 1993; 13(4):923–936.
33. Sievers EL, Dale DC. Non-malignant neutropenia. Blood Rev 1996; 10:95–100.
34. Strand Cl, Goldstein D, Cantella A. Value of cytoplasmic vacuolization of neutrophils in the diagnosis of blood-stream infection. Lab Med 1991; 22:263–266.
35. Stroncek DF. Drug-induced immune neutropenia. Transf Med Rev 1993; 7(4):268–274.
36. Wilkinson PC. Defects of leukocyte locomotion and chemotaxis: prospects assays and lessons from Chediak-Higashi neutrophils. Eur J Clin Invest 1993; 23:690–692.
37. Zacharski LR, Linman JW. Lymphocytopenia: its causes and significance. Mayo Clin Proc 1971; 46:168–173.

8

Acute Leukemia and Myelodysplastic Syndromes

Mark D. Brissette
Madigan Army Medical Center, Tacoma, Washington

James D. Cotelingam
Louisiana State University Medical Center, Shreveport, Louisiana

I. GENERAL

A. Definition

Acute myeloid leukemia (AML) and acute lymphoblastic leukemia (ALL) are malignant bone marrow disorders of hematopoietic precursor cells. The hallmark of these diseases is the presence of increased blast cells in the bone marrow and often the presence of blasts in the peripheral blood.

B. Etiology

The cause of human leukemia is unknown. There are known risk factors—some are established causes and others are presumed causes of leukemia. These include radiation, chemicals, chromosomal abnormalities, and viruses.

1. Radiation

Exposure to moderate to high doses of ionizing radiation increases the incidence of leukemia. Fetuses and young children exposed to smaller doses of ionizing radiation also have an increased incidence of acute leukemia. Leukemia that develops after radiation exposure differs from de-novo AML in that a preleukemic phase is often present, chromosomal aberrations are frequent, treatment is less successful, and survival time is short.

2. Chemicals

Several chemicals and drugs are leukemogenic. Exposure to high doses of benzene causes AML. The incidence of leukemia is increased in patients treated with alkylating agents (e.g.,

---

The opinions and assertions contained herein are the private views of the authors and are not to be considered as official or as representing the views of the Departments of the Army or Defense.

melphalan, chlorambucil), epipodophyllotoxins (e.g., etoposide), anthracyclines, and actinomycin D. Most patients developing leukemia after exposure to these agents develop AML. Similar to radiation-induced leukemia, chemical-induced leukemia usually has a preleukemic phase, chromosomal abnormalities, poor response to treatment, and short survival.

3. *Chromosomal and Genetic Factors*

A small number of childhood leukemias are associated with chromosomal disorders, such as Down syndrome and Klinefelter's syndrome. Several inherited disorders also predispose to leukemia, including Bloom's syndrome, Fanconi's anemia, and Li-Fraumeni syndrome. Patients with structural abnormalities of the retinoblastoma gene on chromosome 13 are also at increased risk of developing leukemia.

4. *Viruses*

Viruses have been found to cause leukemia in animals. Viruses are also implicated in human leukemogenesis, especially in the chronic leukemias and lymphomas.

C. Epidemiology

The current overall age-adjusted annual incidence of leukemia in the United States is 10–11 per 100,000. The incidence of AML increases exponentially after age 40. There are two peak ages for ALL—one at age 3 and the other in later life, after age 60.

D. Ancillary Studies in the Diagnosis of Acute Leukemia

1. *Cytochemistry*

The cytochemical stains most widely used in the diagnosis of leukemia include:

Myeloperoxidase (MPO)
Sudan black-B (SBB)
Chloroacetate esterase (CAE)
α-Naphthyl-acetate esterase (A-EST) and α-naphthyl-butyrate esterase (B-EST) (the nonspecific esterases)
Periodic acid Schiff (PAS)

Myeloperoxidase activity is found in the primary granules of the granulocytic series and in the lysosomes of monocytes (lymphocytes are uniformly negative). Thus myeloperoxidase can be considered specific for the myelomonocytic series. SBB stains various lipids and nonlipid material. It is positive in the granulocytic series and monocytes. Thus, a positive reaction for SBB supports the diagnosis of AML. This is not absolute, however, as cases of ALL with blasts positive for SBB have been reported.

Chloroacetate esterase, also known as "specific esterase," is found only in the granulocytic series. Monocytes and lymphocytes show no or low activity. AML with granulocytic differentiation will show positivity.

The nonspecific esterases (A-EST and B-EST) are strongly positive in normal and leukemic monocytes, and the reaction is inhibited by fluoride pretreatment. Normal and leukemic granulocytes are negative for both nonspecific esterases. A-EST positivity can also be seen in T cells, T-ALL, megakaryocytes, and megakaryoblastic leukemia. B-EST is more specific for monocytes, but can be positive in megakaryocytes and megakaryoblasts.

The PAS reaction is used to identify glycogen, glycoproteins, glycolipids, and other carbohydrate-containing substances. It has been used to differentiate ALL from AML. In many cases of ALL, blasts show granules or blocks of PAS-positive material, often encircling the nucleus in a "rosary bead" fashion. However, similar findings can be seen in acute myeloblastic and acute monoblastic leukemias, as will be discussed later. Also, in erythroleukemia, immature normoblasts may show PAS-positive blocks and more mature normoblasts may show a diffuse red "blush" cytoplasmic staining.

2. *Immunophenotyping*

Cell surface marker immunophenotyping is an important adjunct to the diagnosis of acute leukemia, especially ALL and some types of AML. Many monoclonal antibodies are available, but only a few are necessary for assessing cell lineage. A list of the most commonly used antibodies is given in Table 1. Surface marker immunophenotyping requires fresh blood, bone marrow, or other tissue. These studies are most commonly performed by flow cytometry.

Immunoperoxidase stains can be done on air-dried or fixed smears, touch preps, paraffin-embedded fixed tissue, and frozen tissue. The most common antigens for which antibodies are available include myeloperoxidase (myeloid cells), CD15 (granulocytic cells), CD20 and CD45RA (B cells), and CD3 (T cells).

3. *Electron Microscopy*

Electron microscopy (EM) is used much less frequently since the introduction of immunohistochemistry and immunophenotyping, but it can still be a useful aid in the diagnosis of some types of AML.

II. ACUTE LYMPHOBLASTIC LEUKEMIA

A. Incidence

ALL is the most frequent malignancy of childhood, with the peak incidence at age 3. However, ALL can occur at any age.

Table 1 Selected Hematopoietic Antigens for which Antibodies are Available for Immunophenotyping

Myelomonocytic	*B cell*	*Megakaryocytic*
CD13	CD19	CD 41
CD33	CD20	CD 42
	CD22	CD 61
	CD10 (CALLA)[a]	
Granulocytic	*T-Cell*	*Erythroid*
CD15[a]	CD2	CD71[a]
Myeloperoxidase	CD3	Glycophorin
	CD4[a]	
Monocytic	CD5	*Multiple lineages*
CD14	CD7[a]	HLA-DR
Progenitor cells		
CD34[a]		
TdT[a]		

[a]Antigens that are not lineage specific.

B. Clinical Findings

The most common signs and symptoms in children include fatigue, weight loss, fever, and bone pain. Hepatosplenomegaly and lymphadenopathy may also be present. With T-ALL, a mediastinal mass may be present.

C. Laboratory Findings

1. Peripheral Blood

The white blood cell count can be elevated, but is frequently normal or low. Blasts are usually present in the peripheral smear. A normocytic, normochromic anemia is commonly present and may be severe. Thrombocytopenia is also usually present and is generally severe. Blast cells in the peripheral blood, associated with anemia and thrombocytopenia, is strongly suggestive of acute leukemia.

2. Bone Marrow

Bone marrow examination almost always reveals replacement of normal marrow elements by lymphoblasts. The marrow is hypercellular as a rule, but on occasion may be hypocellular or necrotic.

D. Classification

1. Morphology

The French-American-British (FAB) classification is used to separate ALL into three groups by morphology. This classification is shown in Table 2. Amount of cytoplasm and the presence or absence of nucleoli are the most important criteria in distinguishing between L1 and L2. A scoring system has been devised to help classify L1 and L2 (Table 3). The leukemia is classified as L1 if the score is 0 to +2, and as L2 if the score is −1 or less. Blasts should exceed 30% of all nucleated cells in the bone marrow and are commonly more than 50%. Examples of L1, L2, and L3 ALL are shown in Figs. 1–3. L1 accounts for over 80% of ALL cases in

Table 2 FAB Classification of Acute Lymphoblastic Leukemia

Morphology	L1	L2	L3
Cell size	Predominantly small	Large, heterogeneous	Large, uniform
Nuclear features			
Shape	Smooth contour, occasional clefting or indentation	Irregular, clefting and indentation common	Smooth contour, oval to round
Chromatin	Homogeneous in any one case	Variable, heterogeneous in any one case	Finely stippled and homogeneous
Nucleoli	Small and inconspicuous or not visible	One or more present, often large	Prominent, one or more
Cytoplasm	Scanty; slight or moderate basophilia	Moderate to abundant; variable basophilia	Moderately abundant; deeply basophilic
Cytoplasmic vacuoles	Variable	Variable	Often prominent

Source: Modified from Bennett JM, Catovsky D, Daniel MT, et al. Proposals for the classification of the acute leukemias: French-American-British (FAB) Cooperative Group. Br J Haematol 1976; 33:451–458.

Table 3 Scoring System for FAB L1 and L2 Subclasses

Criteria	Score[a]
Nuclear/cytoplasmic ratio:	
High ≥75% of cells	+
Low ≥25% of cells	−
Nucleoli:	
0 to 1 (small) ≥75% of cells	+
1 or more (prominent) ≥25% of cells	−
Irregular nuclear membrane ≥25% of cells	−
Large cells ≥50% of cells	−

[a]Positive (+); negative (−). If total score is 0 to +2 = L1; −4 to −1 = L2.

Source: Modified from Bennett JM, Catovsky D, Daniel MT, et al. The morphological classification of acute lymphoblastic leukemia: concordance among observers and clinical correlations. Br J Haematol 1981; 41:553–561.

childhood and 30% in adults. The majority of ALL cases in adults are L2. L3 makes up 3–5% of ALL cases in children and adults.

2. *Cytochemistry*

ALL cells are characteristically negative for MPO, SBB, CAE, and the nonspecific esterases. PAS stain often demonstrates coarse red granules or blocks of positive material in some or many of the lymphoid cells. The granules and blocks are found in a clear background, in

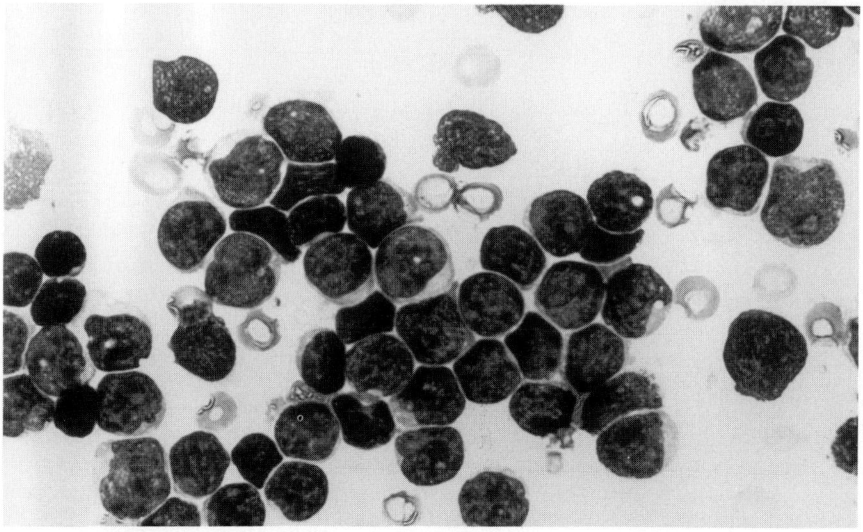

Figure 1 Acute lymphoblastic leukemia, L1. Small cells with high nuclear:cytoplasm ratio predominate. (Original magnification ×1000.)

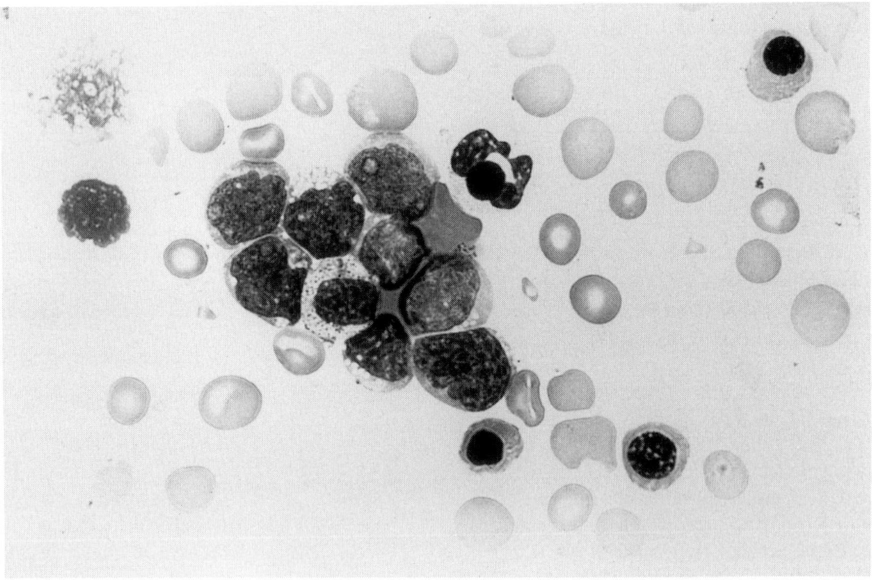

Figure 2 Acute lymphoblastic leukemia, L2. Larger cells with irregular nuclei and nucleoli predominate. (Original magnification ×1000.)

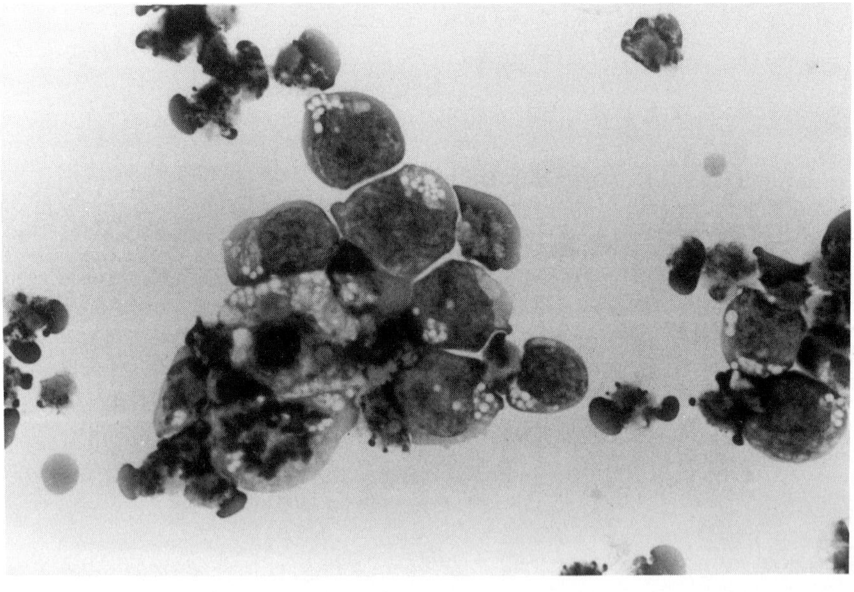

Figure 3 Acute lymphoblastic leukemia, L3. Uniform large cells with vacuolated basophilic cytoplasm predominate. (Original magnification ×1000.)

contrast to AML (especially M1, M4, M5, and M6), where there is a finely granular or diffusely positive background. Acid phosphatase will stain the lymphoblasts of T-ALL. The blasts will show strong, focal, paranuclear acid phosphatase activity which appears as a red dot-like structure located in the Golgi zone next to the nucleus. ALL L3 blasts often stain with oil red 0 due to the presence of neutral lipids within the cytoplasmic vacuoles.

Terminal-deoxynucleotidyl transferase (TdT) is a deoxynucleotide polymerizing enzyme. It can be detected using an immunoperoxidase or immunofluorescent procedure, or by flow cytometry. The majority of blasts in ALL are TdT positive. Blasts in lymphoblastic crisis of chronic myeloid leukemia (CML) are also usually positive. Occasionally, myeloblasts in AML will express TdT, but usually <50% of the blasts will be positive. ALL L3 blasts are characteristically negative.

3. Immunophenotyping

ALL can also be classified by immunophenotyping (see Table 4). Over 50% of ALL cases have common ALL phenotype. About 20% are pre-B-ALL, up to 5% are B-ALL, and 1–2% are early B-precursor-ALL. Twenty percent have a T phenotype. Early B-precursor-ALL and common ALL can have FAB L1 or L2 morphology. Pre-B-ALL usually has L1 morphology; and B-ALL has L3 morphology. T-ALL usually has L2 morphology.

CD34 may be positive in any of the subtypes. It is considered a good prognostic indicator, in contrast to AML, where CD34 expression is considered a poor prognostic indicator.

4. Cytogenetics

More than 70% of ALL cases have one or more chromosomal abnormalities. These can be numerical or structural. In childhood ALL, hyperdiploidy of the leukemic blasts with a DNA index of ≥1.15 or a chromosome count of >50 is associated with longer survival than a normal karyotype. Likewise, patients with a normal karyotype have a better prognosis than those with a chromosome count less than 46 or with structural aberrations.

The most common structural chromosomal abnormality is the Philadelphia chromosome, t(9;22) (q34;q11). This translocation is seen in 15–25% of adult patients and in 3–5% of pediatric patients. On the cytogenetic level, the t(9;22) appears to be the same as the translocation in CML, but on the molecular level, the break in the *BCR* gene is at the minor-bcr region. This translocation is associated with L1 and L2 morphology and the phenotypes of early B-precursor, common, and pre-B-ALL.

Table 4 Immunologic Classification of Acute Lymphoblastic Leukemia

	Cell Markers								
Category	TdT	HLA-DR	CD19	CD20	(CALLA) CD10	cμ[a]	sIg[b]	CD7	CD2
Early B-precursor ALL	+	+	+	−	−	−	−	−	−
Common ALL	+	+	+	−	+	−	−	−	−
Pre-B-ALL	+	+	+	+	+	+	−	−	−
B-ALL	−	+	+	+	+/−	−/+	+	−	−
Early T-precursor ALL	+	−	−	−		−	−	+	−
T-ALL	+	−	−	−	−/+	−	−	+	+

[a]Cytoplasmic mu heavy chain.
[b]Surface immunoglobulin (with kappa or lambda light-chain restriction).

The chromosomal aberration t(4;11) (q21;q23) is seen in about 5% of all ALL cases, being equal in frequency among adults and infants younger than 1 year. This translocation is associated with L1 and L2 morphology and the early B-precursor phenotype. The blasts often express the myeloid antigen CD15. These patients tend to have a high white blood cell count and splenomegaly at diagnosis. The prognosis is poor.

The t(1;19) (q23;p13) is associated with L1 morphology and pre-B-ALL phenotype. Patients with this abnormality have a poor prognosis.

The t(8;14) (q24;q32) is seen in the majority of cases with L3 morphology and B-ALL phenotype, as well as Burkitt's lymphoma. The *c-myc* proto-oncogene on chromosome 8 is translocated adjacent to the immunoglobulin heavy-chain gene on chromosome 14. This results in activation of the *c-myc* gene, leading to production of multiple copies of the protein. Patients with this abnormality have a high rate of central nervous system involvement and a poor prognosis.

E. Differential Diagnosis

Diagnosis of ALL is usually not difficult. However, the following are conditions which may be confused with ALL: AML M1 (in the adult), neuroblastoma, infectious mononucleosis, prolymphocytic leukemia, Sezary syndrome (especially the blastic type), and hairy cell leukemia. These can be distinguished on the basis of clinical setting, morphology, or immunophenotyping and/or immunohistochemistry.

F. Course and Treatment

Most children and 80% of adults with ALL achieve complete remission with treatment. Over one-third of adults and over one-half of children have long-term survival. Prognostic factors in childhood ALL are listed in Table 5.

Poor prognostic factors in adult ALL include older age, male gender, presence of CNS involvement, high white blood cell (WBC) count, B-ALL phenotype, CD10 absence, and presence of the t(9;22).

Remission induction therapy usually consists of combination chemotherapy. Postremission treatment includes consolidation and maintenance chemotherapy. Central nervous system involvement is common at relapse, thus CNS prophylaxis is an integral part of postremission treatment. Relapse can also occur in the testes.

Table 5 Prognostic Factors in Childhood Acute Lymphoblastic Leukemia

Poor	Good
Male	Age 2–10
<2 years old; >10 years old	Lower WBC count
High WBC count (>30 × 10^9/L)	No mediastinal mass or lymph node involvement
Platelet count (<50 × 10^9/L)	Hyperdiploid (DNA index >1.15; chromosome number >50)
Mediastinal mass or marked lymphadenopathy	CD10 expression
Structural cytogenetic abnormalities	
CD10-negative	
sIg positive	
pre-B phenotype[a]	

[a]Especially with t(1;19) (q23;p13).

Allogeneic bone marrow transplantation is usually reserved for patients in second remission (remission after relapse) and possibly for those with refractory leukemia, especially if they are young (<30 years). Autologous bone marrow reinfusion (marrow removed from the patient during remission) may be a consideration for selected patients.

The principal cause of death in ALL patients is infection due to neutropenia. Other causes of death include hemorrhage and leukemic infiltration of the CNS or of vital organs.

G. Hand-Mirror Cell Variant

Hand-mirror cells (HMCs) are lymphocytes and blasts with a uropod. The shape of these cells resembles the shape of a hand mirror (Figs. 4a and 4b). Hand-mirror cells can be seen in unusual variants of leukemia, and their significance is not known.

III. ACUTE MYELOID LEUKEMIA

A. Incidence

AML occurs at any age, but the incidence increases progressively into middle age, with a median age of about 60 years. There is a slight male predominance.

B. Clinical Findings

The most common signs and symptoms in AML include fatigue, fever, bleeding, joint pain, and hepatomegaly. Disseminated intravascular coagulation is common in promyelocytic leukemia (AML M3). Skin infiltration (diffuse, plaquelike violaceous lesions) and gum hypertrophy suggest acute myelomonocytic or monocytic leukemia (AML M4, M5).

C. Laboratory Findings

1. Peripheral Blood

The white blood cell count is usually elevated, but it may be normal or low. Blast cells are usually seen in the peripheral smear, and neutrophils are decreased. Rarely, blasts are absent (aleukemic leukemia). These aleukemic patients are commonly leukopenic and frequently have hypoplastic marrows, but the majority of marrow cells are blasts (hypocellular leukemia).

Anemia is a common finding and is usually normocytic, normochromic. Nucleated red cells are occasionally seen in the peripheral blood. Thrombocytopenia is extremely common.

2. Bone Marrow

Bone marrow examination reveals >30% blast cells. Myeloblasts can be of three types. Type I blasts have open chromatin, one or more distinct nucleoli, and slightly basophilic cytoplasm with no granules. Type II blasts are similar to type I, except they contain a few azurophilic granules (up to 15 granules according to some authors). Type III blasts are similar to type II, but they have more granules and are usually seen in AML M2 with the t(8;21). Type III blasts do not have a Golgi zone; if present, the cell would be considered a promyelocyte. Also, the chromatin of a promyelocyte shows slight clumping and the nucleus may be eccentric. A distinctive feature of AML is the Auer rod, which is a rod-shaped structure formed by fusion of azurophilic granules. Auer rods are usually found in blasts, but may be seen in maturing granulocytic cells. The number seen varies but, if present, indicates myeloid lineage.

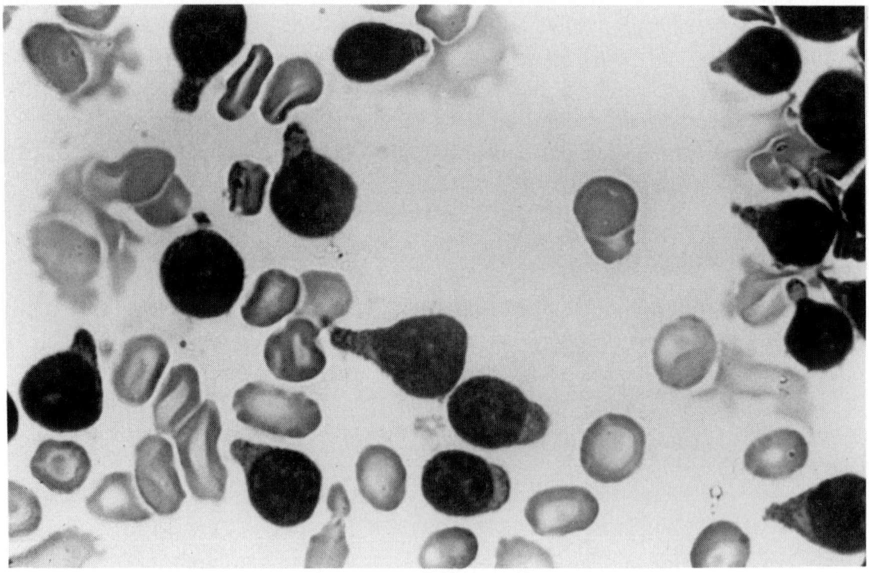

(a)

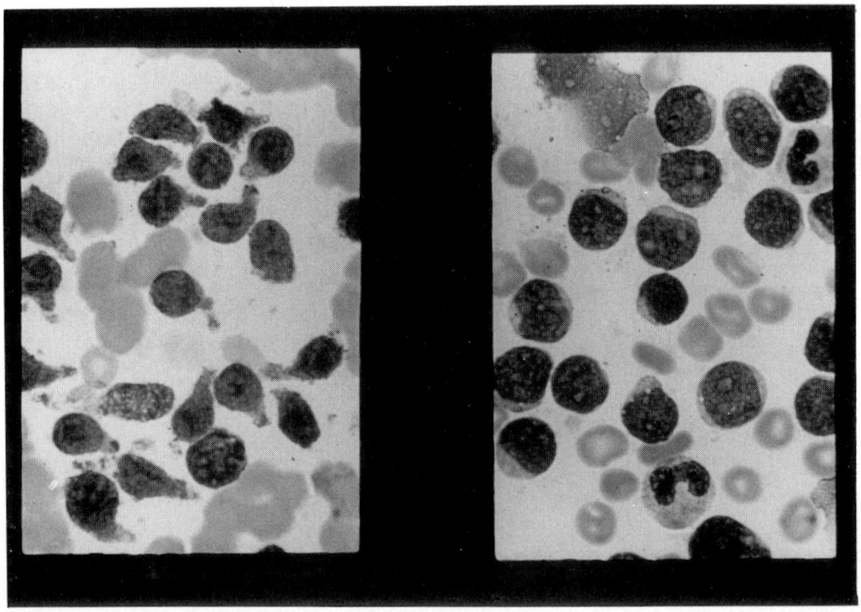

(b)

Figure 4 (a) Acute lymphoblastic leukemia, Hand-mirror cell variant. Several hand-mirror cells are present. (Original magnification ×1000.) (b) Acute lymphoblastic leukemia, Hand-mirror cell variant. Both panels are from the same marrow. The smear shown on the left panel is a direct smear, while the smear on the right was made after collection in EDTA. EDTA removes calcium, which is necessary for microtubule (tubulin) development and cytoskeletal formation. Calcium is necessary for the formation of hand-mirror cells and they will not be seen in bone marrow collected in EDTA. (Original magnification ×1000.)

D. Classification

The French-American-British (FAB) classification is the most widely used classification for AML. There are now eight main types of AML according to the FAB (M0–M7). Each type is classified by cellular morphology of bone marrow using Romanowsky-stained smears and cytochemical reactions. The addition of immunophenotyping, electron microscopy, and cytogenetics help to definitively diagnose some types of AML or to give additional information regarding prognosis or therapy. Diagnostic criteria for each type are given in Table 6. Immunophenotypic and cytogenetic findings are given in Table 7. Additional information is given below.

Table 6 Classification of Acute Myeloid Leukemia by Bone Marrow Findings

M0	>30% blasts Cytochemical stains negative or <3% blasts positive Evidence of myeloid lineage by immunophenotyping, immunohistochemistry, or EM
M1	>30% blasts >3% blasts MPO and/or SBB positive ≤10% maturing granulocytes (from promyelocyte onward) plus monocytes
M2	>30% blasts >10% maturing granulocytes <20% monocytic cells
M3	>30% blasts and promyelocytes Promyelocytes have abnormal morphology (reniform or bilobed nuclei) Auer rods often prominent Hypogranular variant
M4	>30% blasts. >20% granulocytic lineage[a] >20% monocytic lineage[b]
M4E	as for M4 except ≥5% eosinophils
M5a	>80% monoblasts <20% granulocytic lineage
M5b	>80% monoblasts/promonocytes/monocytes At least 30% monoblasts plus myeloblasts
M6	>50% of ANC[c] are nucleated erythroid cells If ≥30% of ANC are myeloblasts then AML M6 If <30% of ANC are myeloblasts, recalculate blast count as a percentage of the NEC[d] If ≥30% of NEC are myeloblasts, then AML M6 If <30% of NEC are myeloblasts, then myelodysplastic syndrome
M7	>30% megakaryoblasts Blasts identified as megakaryoblasts by immunophenotyping (expression of CD41, CD42, CD61) or by EM (platelet peroxidase)

Percentages are of all nucleated cells except for M6.
[a]Myeloblasts, promyelocytes, myelocytes, metamyelocytes, neutrophils.
[b]Monoblasts, promonocytes, monocytes. The peripheral blood monocyte count is usually 5×10^9/L or more. If less than this, either serum/urine lysosome must be elevated three times above the lab reference range, and/or cytochemistry using A-EST or B-EST must confirm marrow monocytic lineage >20% of NEC.
[c]All nucleated cells.
[d]Nonerythroid cells.

Table 7 Immunophenotype and Cytogenetics of Acute Myeloid Leukemia

FAB Type	Immunophenotye	Cytogenetics
M1	CD13 and/or CD33, HLA-DR + CD15, CD34, CD7 +/–	No specific abnormality
M2	Same as M1	t(8;21)(q22;q22)
M3	CD13, CD33 + CD15, CD2 +/– HLA-DR –	t(15;17)(q22-24;q11-21)
M4	CD13, CD33, CD15, HLA-DR + CD14, CD4, CD34 +/–	No specific abnormality
M4Eo	Same as M4	Structural abnormalities of chromosome 16 inv(16)(p13;q22) and t(16;16)(p13;q22)
M5	CD13, CD33, HLA-DR + CD15, CD14, CD4, CD34, CD7 +/–	t(9;11)(q22;q23) Other structural abnormalities of long arm of chromosome 11
M6	Erythroid: Glycophorin A + CD 71, CD45 +/– Myeloblasts: Same as M1	No specific abnormality
M7	CD41, CD42, and/or CD61 + CD13, CD33 +/–	t(1;22)(p13;q13) Abnormalities of long arm of chromosome 3
M0	CD13 and/or CD33, CD34, MPO, HLA-DR + TdT, CD7 +/– B and T cell markers –	No specific abnormality

+ = positive; – = negative; +/– = variable positive.

1. M1

M1 is myeloblastic leukemia without maturation and comprises 20% of AML (Fig. 5, Tables 6 and 7). Most of the time, 90% or more of the nonerythroid cells (NECs) are blasts. Auer rods may be identified. CAE may also be positive. A-EST and B-EST are negative.

2. M2

M2 is myeloblastic leukemia with maturation, which makes up 25–30% of AML (Fig. 6, Tables 6 and 7). More than 10% of cells are maturing granulocytes (promyelocytes to segmented neutrophils), while less than 20% of cells are of monocytic origin. Auer rods may be seen. The t(8;21) (q22;q22) is commonly seen in AML M2.

3. M3

M3 is promyelocytic leukemia, and comprises 5–10% of AML (Fig. 7, Tables 6 and 7). The abnormal promyelocytes are usually heavily granulated and have a bilobed or kidney bean-shaped nucleus with a nucleolus. Auer rods are often prominent, and some cells contain multiple Auer rods. There is also a microgranular variant. This variant has nuclear features identical to hypergranular AML M3, but granules are not apparent by light microscopy. However, granules can be visualized using electron microscopy.

Both types of M3 show positivity for MPO, SBB, and CAE. Nonspecific esterases are negative. As opposed to all other types of AML (except possibly M7), HLA-DR is usually negative.

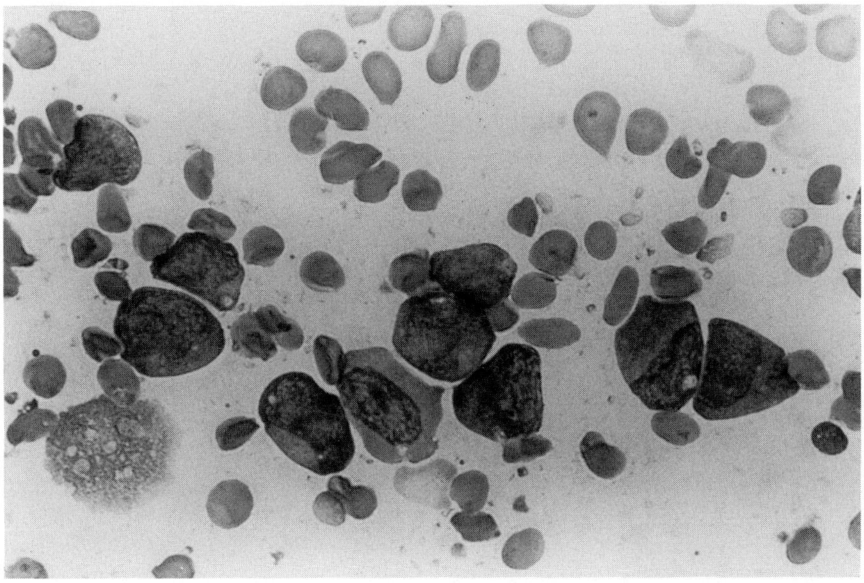

Figure 5 Acute myeloblastic leukemia without maturation, M1. Blasts have round to oval nuclei and one or more nucleoli. (Original magnification ×1000.)

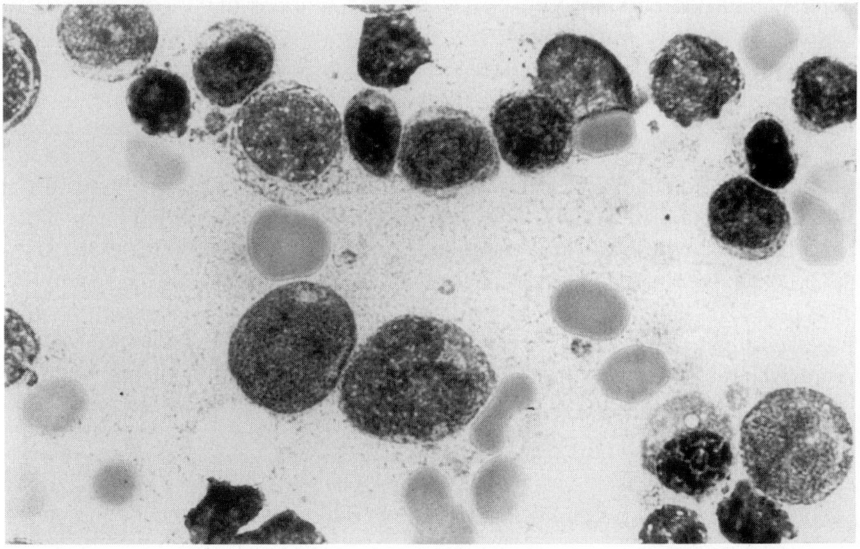

Figure 6 Acute myeloblastic leukemia with maturation, M2. Blasts and more mature, granulated forms are present. (Original magnification ×1000.)

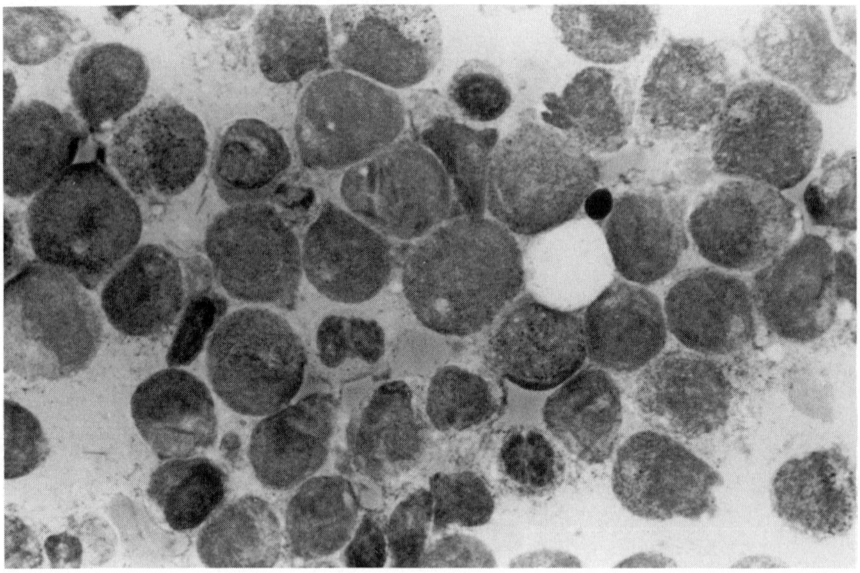

Figure 7 Acute promyelocytic leukemia, M3. Predominantly large cells with granules and Auer rods. (Original magnification ×1000.)

The t(15;17) (q22-24; q11-21) is seen in virtually all cases of M3. The genes involved in this translocation are *PML* (promyelocytic leukemia) on chromosome 15 q22-24 and *RARα* (retinoic acid receptor alpha) on chromosome 17 q11-21. A few cases of M3 are cytogenetically normal, but can be found to have the *PML-RARα* rearrangement by Southern blot or PCR. If this rearrangement is not found by either cytogenetics or molecular techniques, the diagnosis of M3 is unlikely.

4. M4

M4 is myelomonocytic leukemia and makes up 20–25% of AML (Fig. 8, Tables 6 and 7). As the name implies, there is both granulocytic and monocytic differentiation. Peripheral blood promonocyte/monocyte count will usually be greater than 5×10^9/L, or serum or urine lysozyme will be three times above the laboratory reference range for serum or urine, respectively.

There is a subtype of M4 called M4Eo, which is myelomonocytic leukemia with eosinophilia. The marrow findings are the same as for M4, except there are increased eosinophils (usually 5% or more). These eosinophils are abnormal, as they may contain eosinophilic and large basophilic granules and may have a single unsegmented nucleus (Fig. 9). As opposed to normal eosinophils, those in M4Eo stain positively with CAE and PAS.

5. M5

M5 is monocytic leukemia and comprises 10% of AML. Monoblasts, promonocytes, and monocytes constitute 80% or more of ANC in bone marrow. There are two subtypes determined by the percentage of monoblasts: M5a and M5b (Figs. 10 and 11, Tables 6 and 7). Monocyte differentiation is shown by positivity for A-EST and/or B-EST.

6. M6

M6 is erythroleukemia, and makes up 5% of AML (Fig. 12, Tables 6 and 7). More than 50% of all nucleated bone marrow cells are nucleated erythroid cells. These erythroid cells usually

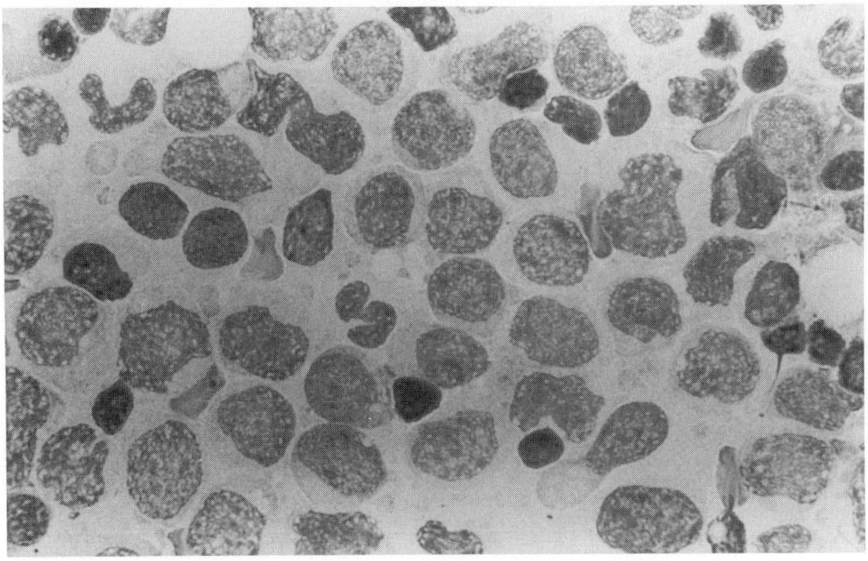

Figure 8 Acute myelomonocytic leukemia, M4. Both immature monocytic and granulocytic cells are present. (Original magnification ×1000.)

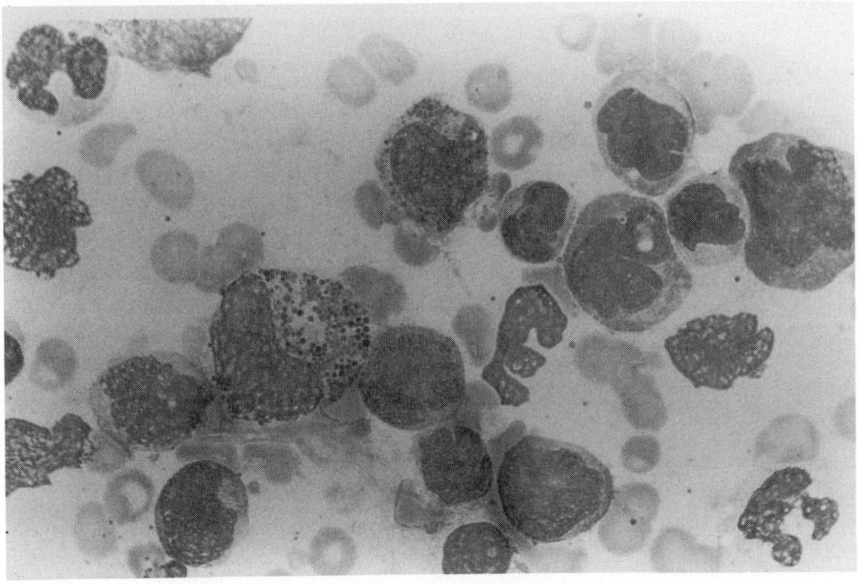

Figure 9 Acute myelomonocytic leukemia with eosinophilia, M4E. Immature myeloid and monocytic cells and an abnormal eosinophil with many basophilic granules. (Original magnification ×1000.)

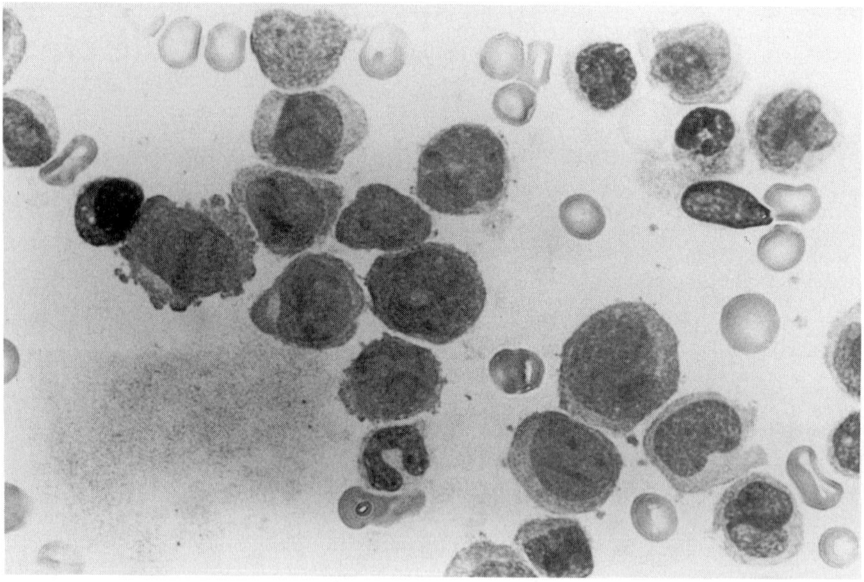

Figure 10 Acute monocytic leukemia, M5a. Predominantly monoblasts with abundant cytoplasm, irregular nuclei, and nucleoli. (Original magnification ×1000.)

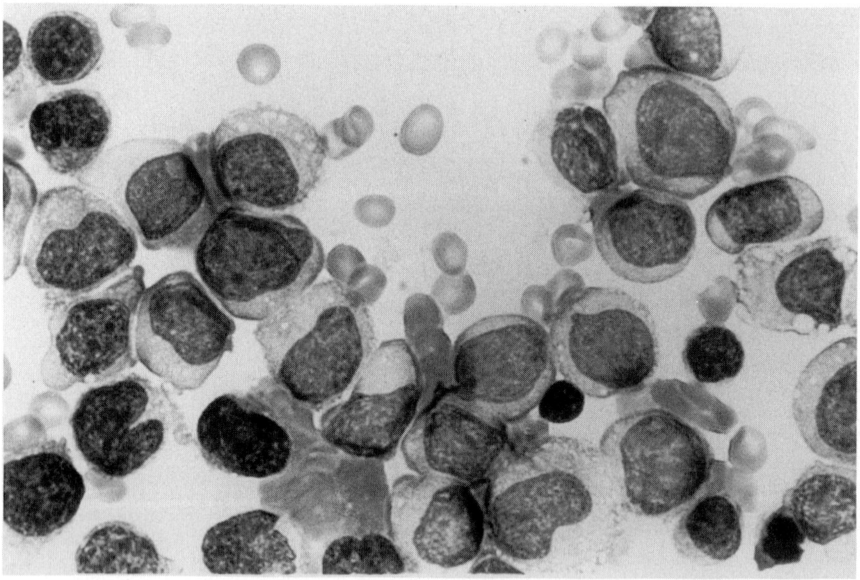

Figure 11 Acute monocytic leukemia, M5b. Note predominance of monocytes and promonocytes. (Original magnification ×1000.)

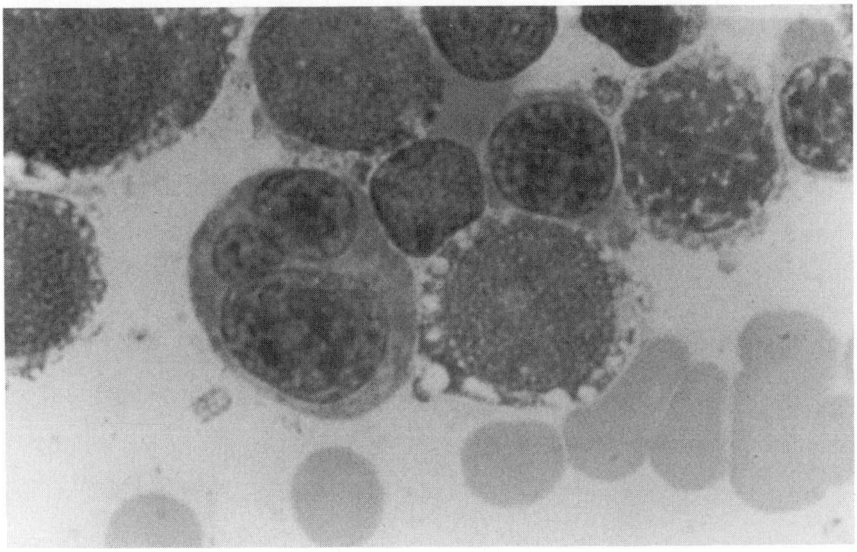

Figure 12 Erythroleukemia, M6. Note several large proerythroblasts with deeply basophilic cytoplasm, a multinucleated normoblast, and nuclear:cytoplasmic dyssynchrony. (Original magnification ×2500.)

show dysplastic features and often have bizarre morphology. Myeloblast counts are determined by one of two methods, as shown in Table 6. Cytochemistry and immunophenotyping of the myeloblasts is not well characterized. The erythroid precursors are PAS-positive, showing block positivity in the most immature and blush positivity in the more mature cells.

7. M7

M7 is megakaryoblastic leukemia and makes up 5–7% of AML (Fig. 13, Table 6). The megakaryoblasts vary in size and have a high nuclear:cytoplasmic ratio. The cytoplasm is pale blue and agranular. Cytoplasmic blebs resembling budding platelets may be seen. Cytochemical stains are usually negative except for nonspecific esterases and PAS.

Definitive identification of megakaryoblasts requires EM or immunophenotyping (Table 7). Platelet peroxidase activity is detected by EM and is probably the most sensitive and specific test for megakaryoblastic differentiation. In megakaryoblasts, peroxidase is localized to the nuclear membrane and endoplasmic reticulum as opposed to myeloblasts, where peroxidase activity occurs in cytoplasmic granules and the Golgi area.

8. M0

This is minimally differentiated acute myeloid leukemia and comprises 2–3% of AML (Fig. 14, Table 6). Blasts tend to be large with agranular cytoplasm and have nuclei with open chromatin and prominent nucleoli (can be single). The blasts occasionally resemble FAB L2-type lymphoblasts. Cytochemical reactions are uniformly negative. Immunophenotype is shown in Table 7. MPO can also be detected using anti-MPO antibody by flow cytometry or by immunohistochemistry. MPO can be detected in small granules by EM. Thus the diagnosis of M0 requires the use of immunologic and/or ultrastructural methods.

9. Acute Basophilic Leukemia

Acute basophilic leukemia is AML with basophil precursors. This is a newly described entity, and the incidence is not known with certainty. These cases resemble M2, but some blasts

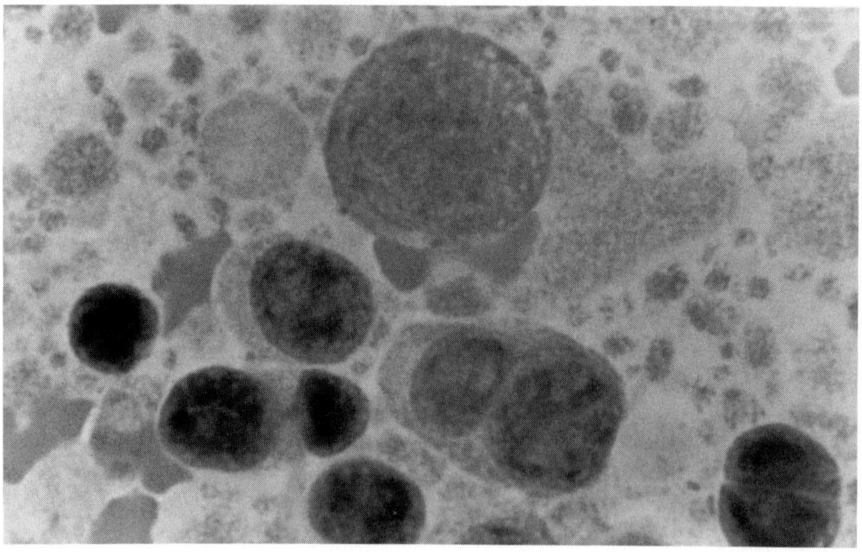

Figure 13 Acute megakaryoblastic leukemia, M7. Large blast with abundant cytoplasm and nucleolus. (Original magnification ×2500.)

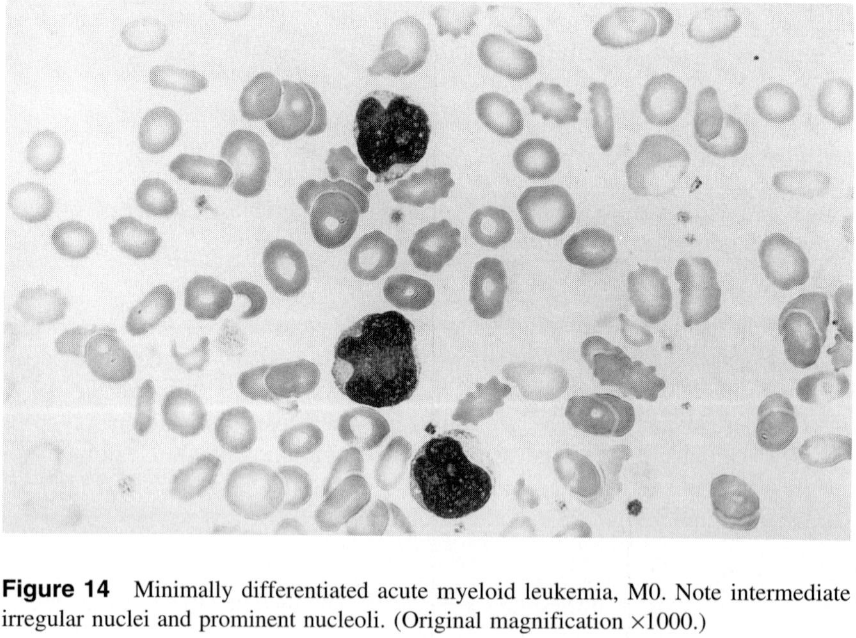

Figure 14 Minimally differentiated acute myeloid leukemia, M0. Note intermediate sized blasts with irregular nuclei and prominent nucleoli. (Original magnification ×1000.)

contain basophilic granules in their cytoplasm. By EM, the granules are immature basophil granules, theta granules, and/or immature mast cell granules. They can be seen in blasts that do not have granules by light microscopy. Cytogenetic associations are ill defined.

10. Myelodysplasia and AML

In 10–15% of AML cases, trilineage dysplasia is present. It can be seen in all types of AML except M3. It is most common in M6 and M7, and least common in M1. These cases may represent myelodysplastic syndrome that has not been detected until leukemia develops. Similar findings can be seen in secondary leukemia—leukemia occurring after treatment for other malignancies, especially after use of alkylating agents or exposure to other toxic agents. Cytogenetic abnormalities include monosomy 7 (−7), deletion of part of the long arm of chromosome 7 (7q−), and deletion of part of the long arm of chromosome 5 (5q−).

11. Hypocellular AML

Hypocellular AML is defined as more than 30% blasts in a marrow that is less than 30% cellular. Fibrotic areas are excluded when determining cellularity. Determining the blast count is often difficult, as the smears may be hypocellular.

12. Peripheral Acute Leukemia

There are reports of patients with more than 30% peripheral blood blasts, but less than 30% marrow blasts, who progressed to AML within 1–2 months. Several of these patients have had cytogenetic abnormalities typical of AML [e.g., t(8;21)]. These reports suggest that patients who have more than 30% peripheral blood blasts should be considered as having acute leukemia, even if the marrow blasts are less than 30%.

E. Differential Diagnosis

Some types of AML can be confused with ALL L-2 and peripheralized large cell lymphoma in adults. Myelodysplastic syndromes may also be difficult to separate from AML. A leukoerythroblastic reaction with a high blast count in peripheral blood may also mimic AML.

Transient myeloproliferative disorder (TMD) is seen in newborns and can mimic AML. TMD is associated with trisomy 21 and can be seen in patients with Down syndrome or phenotypically normal infants with trisomy 21 in marrow cells. These patients require no treatment, and the TMD resolves spontaneously. However, the incidence of subsequent AML is increased, especially in patients with Down syndrome.

F. Treatment and Course

The mainstay of treatment is chemotherapy. Complete remission rates range from 60% to 90% in patients younger than 60 years. After remission is achieved, intensive consolidation treatment is used to further reduce the number of leukemic cells. The relapse rate for conventional chemotherapy is 50–60%.

Allogeneic bone marrow transplant (BMT) is also used as a postremission treatment strategy. The disease-free survival for patients undergoing allogeneic BMT in first remission is 40–60%. BMT is usually limited to patients under age 60 because of treatment-related toxicity. Autologous bone marrow reinfusion has also been used, especially in patients lacking an HLA-identical donor.

In adults, previous myelodysplastic syndrome or chemotherapy, high white blood cell count, and older age are poor prognostic indicators. In children, high white blood cell count and younger age are poor prognostic indicators. AML M4Eo with inv(16) and AML M2 with the t(8;21) appear to have a better prognosis, while M5 with abnormalities of 11q and any AML with the t(9;22) [Philadelphia chromosome] have a poorer prognosis.

IV. MIXED-PHENOTYPE ACUTE LEUKEMIA

Widespread use of immunophenotyping and immunohistochemistry has shown that leukemias often express antigens of different lineages. Likewise, some antigens are not lineage specific, as previously thought. An example is the finding of CD7 or CD2, once thought to be specific for lymphocytes, on myeloblasts.

There is no agreed-upon definition for mixed-phenotype (hybrid or biphenotypic) acute leukemia (AMLL). Most authorities feel that at least two antigens from another lineage must be expressed by leukemic blasts in order to be classified as mixed lineage (e.g., AML expressing myeloid antigens as well as CD19 and CD20). This "lineage infidelity" would include MPO demonstrated by immunologic or ultrastructural means in ALL. One author has devised a scoring system based on currently known antigen specificity for a particular lineage (Catovsky et al., 1991; see Selected Readings).

Chromosomal abnormalities such as the t(9;22) and the t(4;11) have been associated with AMLL. The treatment for these leukemias is ill-defined at this time.

V. ACUTE UNDIFFERENTIATED LEUKEMIA

In acute undifferentiated leukemia, blasts have a morphology that is not typical of AML or ALL, and show no or minimal (<3%) reactivity with cytochemical stains. In addition, immunophenotyping is negative except for CD34, CD7, TdT, and/or HLA-DR. MPO is not detected by immunologic or ultrastructural methods.

VI. MYELODYSPLASTIC SYNDROMES

A. General

Myelodysplastic syndromes (MDS) are a group of clonal bone marrow disorders characterized by dysplastic changes in one or more of the marrow cell lines (myeloid, erythroid, or megakaryocytic). There may also be an increase in the number of myeloblasts or monocytes. MDS can be primary or secondary to previous chemotherapy or radiotherapy. Primary MDS usually occurs in patients older than 50 years, while therapy-related MDS (t-MDS) can occur at any age.

Dyserythropoiesis is characterized in the marrow by nuclear/cytoplasmic dyssynchrony; nuclear budding, blebbing, or indentations; multinuclearity; nuclear fragmentation (karyorrhexis), and formation of Howell-Jolly bodies.

Dysgranulopoiesis is characterized by hyposegmentation and decreased primary and/or secondary granules leading to hypogranularity. There may be an increase in myeloblasts.

Dysmegakaryopoiesis is indicated by finding large megakaryocytes with mature cytoplasm but nonlobated or hypolobated nuclei, micromegakaryocytes, and megakaryocytes with multiple separate nuclei (pawn-ball forms).

Dysplastic changes are best appreciated in aspirate smears. The biopsy often shows architectural distortion, with clusters of myeloid blasts found in the central marrow region rather than in their normal position near the trabecular surface. This is called abnormal localization of immature precursors (ALIP).

Most cases of MDS show cytogenetic abnormalities with complex multiple chromosomal defects as the most frequent finding. Common single defects include monosomy 5, 5q–, monosomy 7, 7q–, and trisomy 8.

B. Classification

The FAB recognizes five types of MDS. Two others have been added by some authors for cases that do not fit into one of the FAB groups. The criteria for diagnosing each subtype are listed in Table 8. Additional information is given below.

1. *Refractory anemia* (RA): The bone marrow is normocellular to hypercellular with erythroid hyperplasia and/or dyserythropoiesis. Ringed sideroblasts may be present but are <15%. Granulocytes and megakaryocytes show slight to no dysplasia.
2. *Refractory anemia with ringed sideroblasts* (RARS): The patients sometimes have dimorphic red cell populations—hypochromic and normochromic or normocytic and macrocytic populations.
3. *Refractory anemia with excess blasts* (RAEB): The marrow is usually hypercellular with variable panmyelosis (hyperplasia of all three cell lines).
4. *Refractory anemia with excess blasts in transformation* (RAEB-T): The presence of Auer rods in blasts or maturing myeloid cells when the marrow or blood blast count

Table 8 Myelodysplastic Syndromes

Subtype	Criteria
Refractory anemia (RA)	PB[a]: anemia, reticulocytopenia, <1% blasts BM[b]: dyserythropoiesis, <5% blasts
Refractory anemia with ringed sideroblasts (RARS)	PB: anemia, reticulocytopenia, <1% blasts BM: dyserythropoiesis, <5% blasts, >15% ringed sideroblasts
Refractory anemia with excess blasts (RAEB)	PB: cytopenia in 2 or 3 cell lines; <5% blasts BM: Trilineage dysplasia; 5–20% blasts
Refractory anemia with excess blasts in transformation (RAEB-T)	PB and BM: same as RAEB plus: (1) >5% circulating blasts and/or (2) 21–29% blasts in marrow and/or (3) Auer rods
Chronic myelomonocytic leukemia (CMML)	PB: monocytosis $>1.0 \times 10^9$/L BM: similar to RAEB except usually increased monocytes and promonocytes
Chronic myelomonocytic leukemia in transformation (CMML-T)	PB and BM: same as CMML plus: (1) >5% circulating blasts and/or (2) 21–29% blasts in marrow and/or (3) Auer rods
Refractory cytopenia with multilineage dysplasia (RCMD)	All cases of MDS that do not fulfill the criteria of the other subtypes

[a]Peripheral blood.
[b]Bone marrow.

is <20% or ≤5%, respectively, allows a diagnosis of RAEB-T. Other criteria are listed in Table 8.

5. *Chronic myelomonocytic leukemia* (CMML): Circulating blasts are <5%.
6. *Chronic myelomonocytic leukemia in transformation* (CMML-T): The peripheral blood and bone marrow findings resemble CMML, but have one or more of the findings associated with RAEB-T.
7. *Refractory cytopenia with multilineage dysplasia* (RCMD): The majority of these cases resemble RA, with <5% blasts in the marrow and <5% ringed sideroblasts. However, there is moderate to severe dysplasia in the granulocytic and megakaryocytic lines which precludes a diagnosis of RA. Most cases of t-MDS fall into this group. Other cases of MDS that do not fulfill the criteria for the other subtypes should be put into this category.

C. Course and Treatment

Patients with MDS may develop progressive bone marrow failure with cytopenias or may progress to acute leukemia. RAEB-T and CMML-T have the highest risk of progressing to acute leukemia, usually within months.

Treatment is usually supportive, with use of blood products as needed. Chemotherapy is also used in selected patients. Allogeneic bone marrow transplantation has been used to treat younger patients (<50 years) with MDS.

STUDY CASE 1

Patient

Newborn female.

Chief Complaint

Multiple petechial and purpuric lesions on skin over most of the body.

Medical History

A 3985-g, 41-week-gestational-age female was delivered vaginally. Meconium was present in the amniotic fluid at birth, and APGAR at 1 min was 4 and at 5 min was 6.

Physical Examination

Multiple indurated, purpuric lesions and petechiae over most of the skin surface ("blueberry muffin" appearance) and hepatosplenomegaly were present.

Laboratory Results

Screening procedures showed WBC, 298×10^9/L with 67% blasts; HCT, 0.37; platelets, 42×10^9/L; PT, 25.4 sec; PTT, 57 sec; fibrinogen, 55 mg/dL; FSP >20 μg/mL; and D-dimer 1–2 μg/mL. The blasts were predominantly large, with a high nucleus:cytoplasm ratio, prominent single or multiple nucleoli, and occasional convoluted nuclear membranes (Fig. 15).

Hospital Course

Peripheral blood findings were considered consistent with acute leukemia. Complete remission was achieved after chemotherapy, but the child relapsed at age 6 months. She had several more short-lived remissions and relapses and died before 1 year of age.

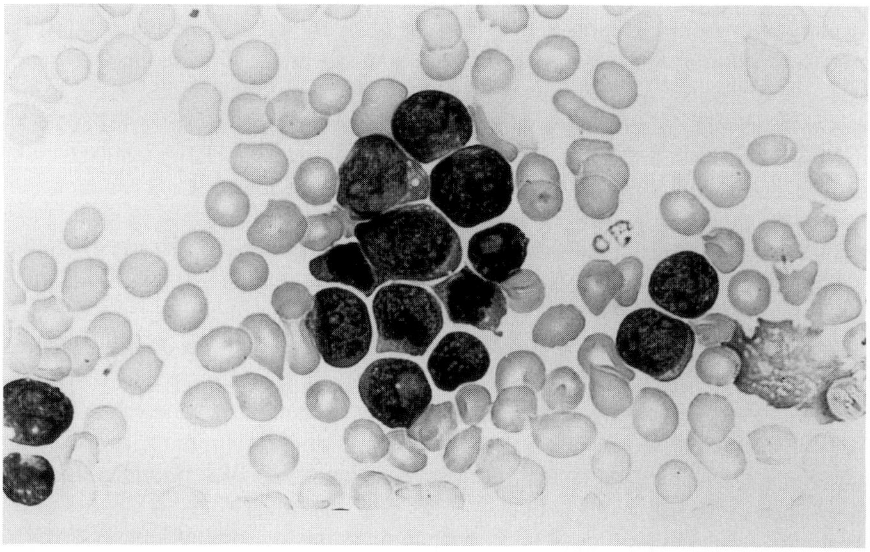

Figure 15 Large blasts with a high nuclear:cytoplasm ratio, round to irregular nuclei, and prominent nucleoli. (Original magnification ×2500.)

Questions

1. What conditions are in the differential diagnosis?
2. What are the features of acute leukemia with abnormalities of 11q23?

Confirmatory Laboratory Results

Cytochemistry: Blasts were negative for myeloperoxidase, Sudan black B, chloroacetate esterase, and PAS, and positive for α-naphthyl butyrate esterase (B-EST).

Immunophenotyping: Blasts expressed CD45, CD19, CD22, CD15, HLA-DR, CD34 (dim), and TdT. Blasts did not express CD3, CD5, CD7, CD4, CD8, CD20, CD10, CD13, CD33, or CD14.

Cytogenetics: Performed on leukemic cells from peripheral blood. 46XX with t(4;11) (q21; q23).

Diagnosis

Early B-precursor acute lymphoblastic leukemia (congenital ALL).

Discussion

t(4;11) (q21;q23) is the most common cytogenetic abnormality identified in congenital ALL, and is seen in about one-half of patients. At presentation, patients frequently have hyperleukocytosis, often greater than 200×10^9/L. Hepatosplenomegaly is very common, and lymphadenopathy can be seen. Anemia and thrombocytopenia are usual findings. CNS involvement is common.

Blasts are usually lymphoid in appearance, but occasionally granulated blasts may be identified. In rare cases, a dimorphic population of lymphoid and myeloid blasts may be seen. Cytochemical stains are uniformly negative except for PAS and occasionally nonspecific esterase. In most cases with t(4;11), there is an unique immunophenotype: CD19+, HLA-DR+, TdT+, CD24–/+, CD10–, and often CD15+. This is an early B-precursor ALL phenotype with aberrant expression of the myeloid antigen CD15 and often aberrant loss of CD24, which is a B-cell antigen present on the vast majority of B-lineage ALLs.

Most cases of t(4;11) ALL do not show hyperdiploidy (>50 chromosomes or DNA index >1.15). Most are diploid, with rare cases classified as near-tetraploid.

The differential diagnosis of congenital leukemia is large, thus the diagnosis is often one of exclusion. Congenital infections, including toxoplasmosis, rubella, cytomegalovirus, Herpes simplex, adenovirus, and syphilis can all mimic the blood findings of congenital leukemia. Serologic tests, as well as bone marrow aspiration/biopsy, will usually be necessary to rule these out. Bacterial infections, hypoxia, hemolytic anemia (usually alloimmune), and infiltrative marrow processes, such as histiocytosis X and neuroblastoma, may also mimic congenital leukemia. These were all excluded in our patient.

Transient myeloproliferative disorder (TMD) closely simulates congenital leukemia (CL). It is found in Down syndrome infants and phenotypically normal infants who are mosaic for trisomy 21 or who have the trisomic karyotype restricted to hematopoietic cells. TMD is morphologically identical to acute leukemia. However, the blasts always show trisomy 21 and often express megakaryocytic antigens. These patients essentially always have spontaneous remission. These features are rarely seen in congenital acute leukemia. Also, patients with CL usually appear more ill and often have leukemia cutis, which is not seen in TMD.

Treatment for CL varies, but all include combination chemotherapy. Many patients die within days of diagnosis due to respiratory failure or cerebral hemorrhage as a consequence of leukostasis and hyperviscosity. Even with the institution of chemotherapy, many fail induction, and progressive organ involvement and hemorrhage occur. The median survival ranges from 2 to 7 months, depending on the study.

Bibliography

1. Borowitz MJ. Acute lymphoblastic leukemia. In: Knowles DM, ed. Neoplastic Hematopathology. Baltimore: Williams & Wilkins, 1992:1295–1314.
2. Brissette MD, Duval-Arnould BJ, Gordon BG, et al. Acute megakaryoblastic leukemia following transient myeloproliferative disorder in a patient without Down syndrome. Am J Hematol 1994; 47:316–319.
3. Childs CC, Hirsh-Ginsberg C, Culbert SJ, et al. Lineage heterogeneity in acute leukemia with the t(4;11) abnormality: implications for acute mixed lineage leukemia. Hematol Pathol 1988; 2:145–157.
4. McCoy JP, Overton WR. Immunophenotyping of congenital leukemia. Cytometry 1995; 22:85–88.
5. Parkin JL, Arthur DC, Abramson CS, et al. Acute leukemia associated with the t(4; 11) chromosome rearrangement: ultrastructural and immunologic characteristics. Blood 1982; 60:1321–1331.
6. Pui CH, Frankel LS, Carroll AJ, et al. Clinical characteristics and treatment outcome of childhood acute lymphoblastic leukemia with the t(4;11) (q21;q23): A collaborative study of 40 cases. Blood 1991; 77:440–447.

STUDY CASE 2

Patient

Sixty-two-year-old man.

Chief Complaint

Weakness and nights sweats for several weeks.

Medical History

The patient had served in the Navy and was exposed to rocket fuel and solvents.

Physical Examination

Afebrile. Hepatosplenomegaly and lymphadenopathy were absent.

Laboratory Results

Screening procedures showed WBC, 1.7×10^9/L with a normal differential count; Hb, 6.0 g/dL; HCT, 0.18; MCV, 97.8 fL; platelets, 85×10^9/L.

Clinical Course

The diagnosis of a myelodysplastic syndrome was made after bone marrow aspiration and biopsy. Over the next 7 months, the patient had decreasing peripheral blood counts and the appearance of blasts in the peripheral blood. He elected to receive supportive care only and died 1 month thereafter.

Questions

1. According to the FAB classification, how many marrow blasts are required to diagnose refractory anemia with excess blasts, refractory anemia with excess blasts in transformation, and AML?
2. What are the most common cytogenetic abnormalities seen in MDS?

Confirmatory Laboratory Results

Peripheral blood: Seven months after diagnosis, the WBC count had normalized, but there were now 33% circulating blasts.

Bone marrow analysis: Marrow at presentation was hypercellular with erythroid predominance. There were dysplastic changes in all three cell lines. The blast count was 14%. The second bone marrow aspirate showed 25% blasts and the final aspirate showed >30% blasts (Fig. 16).

Cytochemistry: Not performed.

Immunophenotyping studies: Blasts expressed CD45, CD33, CD4, CD34, and HLA-DR.

Cytogenetics: Performed on second bone marrow aspirate-45XY, t(13q;15q).

Diagnosis

Myelodysplastic syndrome (refractory anemia with excess blasts evolving into refractory anemia with excess blasts in transformation), transforming to acute myeloid leukemia.

Discussion

MDS usually affects older individuals, especially those over 50 years of age. It can be seen in younger adults and children, especially those previously treated for other malignancies. Twenty

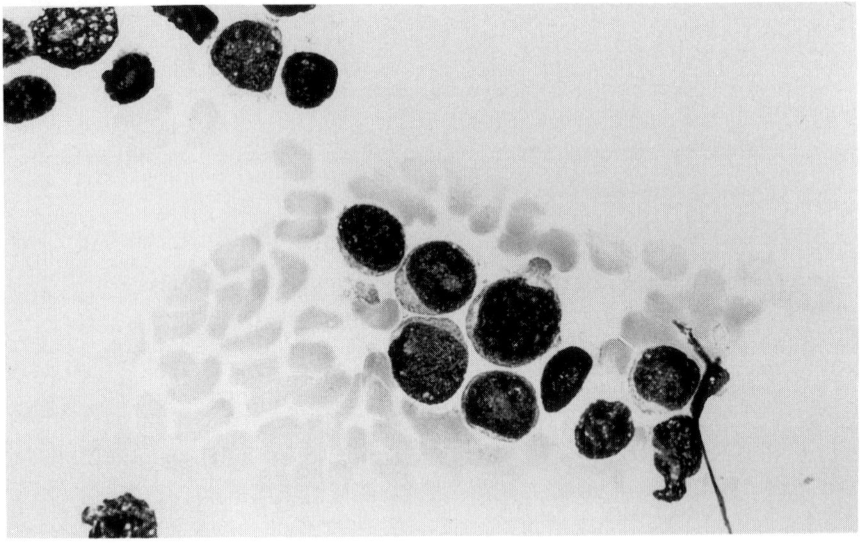

Figure 16 Intermediate-sized to large blasts with high nuclear:cytoplasm ratio and nucleoli. (Original magnification ×2500.)

to thirty percent of patients progress to AML; 60–80% die from complications of pancytopenia, hemorrhage, or infection; while 10–20% have stable disease and die of other causes.

The typical bone marrow and peripheral smear findings in MDS as well as the FAB classification of MDS were previously discussed in this chapter. Frequency, survival and leukemic progression data are shown in Table 9. The frequencies of the two new proposed categories, chronic myelomonocytic leukemia in transformation and RCMD, have not been determined. Our patient was diagnosed with RAEB (blasts 5–20%), but then progressed to RAEB-T (blasts 21–29%), and lastly, AML (blasts ≥30%).

At least 39–79% of patients with de-novo MDS have cytogenetic abnormalities at diagnosis. Frequencies by FAB subtype are RA (56%), RARS (25%), RAEB (76%), RAEB-T (100%), and CMML (42%). The most common cytogenetic finding is a complex karyotype with two or more abnormalities. This often includes monosomy 7 or 7q–, monosomy 5 or 5q–, and monosomy 17 or 17p–. Single isolated abnormalities included monosomy 7 or 7q– (most

Table 9 Frequency, Median Survival, and Leukemic Progression of Patients with Primary MDS

Subtype	Frequency (%)	Median survival (mo)	Leukemic progression (%)
RA	28	50	12
RARS	24	51	8
RAEB	23	11	44
RAEB-T	9	5	60
CMML	16	11	14

Source: Modified from Third MIC Cooperative Study Group (1988).

common), 5q−, trisomy 8, and 20q−. The cytogenetic abnormality found in our patient is unusual and is not well characterized.

Many negative prognostic factors of MDS have been identified. These include: ≥5% blasts in bone marrow; circulating blasts; karyotypic abnormalities, especially if complex; granulocytopenia; thrombocytopenia; monocytopenia; anemia; ineffective erythropoiesis (adequate iron incorporation); and exposure to radiation or past chemotherapy.

Another negative prognostic factor is CD34+ blasts. Circulating CD34+ cells are associated with progression to AML and poor survival. It has also been shown that the finding of aggregates of CD34+ cells in a bone marrow biopsy is also associated with shorter survival. This correlation is best seen in patients with RAEB or RAEB-T.

In adults, treatment is usually supportive, especially in lower-grade MDS (RA, RARS). This may consist of blood transfusions and use of cytokines, such as granulocyte-colony stimulating factor. For the more aggressive types (RAEB, RAEB-T, CMML, and CMML-T), intensive chemotherapy followed by allogeneic bone marrow transplantation may be the treatment of choice. However, this treatment is currently given only to patients under 50 years of age.

Bibliography

1. Bennett JM, Catovsky D, Daniel MT, et al. Proposals for the classification of the myelodysplastic syndromes. Br J Haematol 1982; 51:189–199.
2. Bick RL, Laughlin WR. Myelodysplastic syndromes. Lab Med 1993; 24:712–716.
3. Brunning RD. Myelodysplastic syndromes. In: Knowles DM, ed. Neoplastic Hematopathology. Baltimore: Williams & Wilkins, 1992:1367–1404.
4. Soligo DA, Oriani A, Annaloro C, et al. CD34 immunohistochemistry of bone marrow biopsies: prognostic significance in primary myelodysplastic syndromes. Am J Hematol 1994; 46:9–17.
5. Sullivan SA, Marsden KA, Lowenthal RM, et al. Circulating CD34+ cells: an adverse prognostic factor in the myelodysplastic syndromes. Am J Hematol 1992; 39:96–101.
6. Third MIC Cooperative Study Group. Recommendations for a morphologic, immunologic, and cytogenetic (MIC) working classification of the primary and therapy-related myelodysplastic disorders. Cancer Genet Cytogenet 1988; 32:1–10.
7. Yunis JJ, Brunning RD. Prognostic significance of chromosomal abnormalities in acute leukemias and myelodysplastic syndromes. Clin Haematol 1986; 15:597–620.

ADDENUM 1: PROPOSED WORLD HEALTH ORGANIZATION (WHO) CLASSIFICATION OF ACUTE MYELOID LEUKEMIA*

Acute Myeloid Leukemia (de novo)
- Acute Myeloblastic Leukemia, minimally differentiated (AML-M0)
- Acute Myeloblastic Leukemia without maturation (AML-M1)
- Acute Myeloblastic Leukemia with maturation (AML-M2)
  - Acute myeloblastic leukemia with maturation with associated t(8;21) (q22;q22)
  - Acute myeloblastic leukemia with maturation and increased marrow basophils with associated t(6;9) (p23;q34)
- Acute Promyelocytic Leukemia

*The threshold blast percentage for a diagnosis of acute leukemia is 20%, down from the previous requirement of 30%.

Hypergranular (AML-M3)
Microgranular (AML-M3V)
Acute Myelomonocytic Leukemia (AML-M4)
Acute myelomonocytic leukemia with increased marrow eosinophils (AML-M4 EO) with inv or del 16(q22)
Acute Monocytic Leukemia
Acute monoblastic leukemia (AML-M5A)
Acute monocytic leukemia with maturation (AML-M5B)
**Acute Erythroid Leukemia
Acute pure erythroid leukemia (AML-M6A)
Acute erythroleukemia (AML-M6B)
Acute Megakaryoblastic Leukemia
Acute myeloblastic leukemia/transient myeloproliferative disorder associated with Down syndrome
Acute Panmyelosis with Myelofibrosis (Acute Myelofibrosis)
Hypocellular (Hypoplastic) Acute Myeloid Leukemia
Acute Basophilic Leukemia
Myeloid Sarcoma
Acute Myeloid Leukemia, Therapy-Related
Alkylating agent-related type
Topoisomerase II-related type
Acute Myeloid Leukemia Evolving from a Myelodysplastic Syndrome

ADDENDUM 2: PROPOSED WORLD HEALTH ORGANIZATION (WHO) CLASSIFICATION OF MYELODYSPLASTIC SYNDROMES

De novo Myelodysplastic Syndromes
Refractory Anemia (RA)
Refractory Anemia with Ringed Sideroblasts (RARS)
RARS with unilineage dysplasia
RARS with multilineage dyplasia
Refractory Cytopenia with Multilineage Dysplasia (RCMD)
Refractory Anemia with Excess Blasts (RAEB)
Refractory Anemia with Excess Blasts in Transformation (RAEB-T)
Myelodysplastic syndrome, unclassified
Therapy Related Myelodysplastic Syndromes
Classify as de novo, but add the qualifying term, "therapy-related"
If the case cannot be classified, diagnose as "therapy-related MDS, unclassified"

SELECTED READINGS

1. Bennett JM, Catovsky D, Daniel MT, et al. Proposals for the classification of the acute leukemias: French-American-British (FAB) Cooperative Group. Br J Haematol 1976; 33:451–458.
2. Bennett JM, Catovsky D, Daniel MT, et al. The morphological classification of acute lymphoblastic

**Work by author and literature indicate classification as: Acute erythroleukemia AML-M6A
Acute pure erythroleukemia AML-M6B

Source: Vardiman JW, Head D, et al. Society for Hematopathology: The myelodysplastic syndromes (MDS) and related disorders. Mod Path 1999, 12:101–106.

leukemia: concordance among observers and clinical correlations. Br J Haematol 1981; 41:553–561.

3. Bennett JM, Catovsky D, Daniel MT, et al. Proposals for the classification of the myelodysplastic syndromes. Br J Haematol 1982; 51:189–199.
4. Bennett JM, Catovsky D, Daniel MT, et al. Criteria for the diagnosis of acute leukemia of megakaryocyte lineage (M7): a report of the French-American-British Cooperative Group. Ann Intern Med 1985; 103:460–462.
5. Bennett JM, Catovsky D, Daniel MT, et al. Proposed revised criteria for the classification of acute myeloid leukemia: a report of the French-American-British Cooperative Group. Ann Intern Med 1985; 103:626–629.
6. Bennett JM, Catovsky D, Daniel MT, et al. Proposal for the recognition of minimally differentiated acute myeloid leukemia (AML-MO). Br J Haematol 1991; 78:325–329.
7. Brissette MD, Duval-Arnould BJ, Gordon BG, et al. Acute megakaryoblastic leukemia following transient myeloproliferative disorder in a patient without Down syndrome. Am J Hematol 1994; 47: 316–319.
8. Brunning RD. Myelodysplastic syndromes. In: Knowles DM, ed. Neoplastic Hematopathology. Baltimore: Williams & Wilkins, 1992:1367–1404.
9. Catovsky D, Matutes E, Buccheri V, et al. A classification of acute leukemia for the 1990s. Ann Hematol 1991; 62:16–21.
10. Cheson BD, Cassileth PA, Head DR, et al. Report of the National Cancer Institute-sponsored workshop on definitions of diagnosis and response in acute myeloid leukemia. J Clin Oncol 1990; 8: 813–819.
11. Clare N, Hansen K. Cytogenetics in the diagnosis of hematologic malignancies. Hematol Oncol Clin N Am 1994; 8:785–807.
12. Devine SM, Larson RA. Acute leukemia in adults: recent developments in diagnosis and treatment. CA Cancer J Clin 1994; 44:326–352.
13. First MIC Cooperative Study Group. Morphologic, immunologic, and cytogenetic (MIC) working classification of acute lymphoblastic leukemias. Cancer Genet Cytogenet 1986; 23:189–197.
14. Hirsch-Ginsberg C, Huh YO, Kagan J, et al. Advances in the diagnosis of acute leukemia. Hematol Oncol Clin N Am 1993; 7:1–46.
15. Klobušická M. Possibilities and limitations of cytochemical methods in diagnosis of acute leukemia. Micron 1994; 25:317–329.
16. Kowal-Vern A, Cotelingam J, Schumacher HR. The prognostic significance of proerythroblasts in acute erythroleukemia. Am J Clin Pathol 1992; 98:34–40.
17. Maeda K, Alessio RC, Hawley RC. Recent advances in diagnosis of leukemia. Jpn J Clin Oncol 1993; 23:79–84.
18. Peterson LC, Parkin JL, Arthur DC, et al. Acute basophilic leukemia: a clinical, morphologic and cytogenetic study of eight cases. Am J Clin Pathol 1991; 96:160–170.
19. Sandler DP. Epidemiology and etiology of acute leukemia: an update. Leukemia 1992; 6:3–5.
20. Second MIC Cooperative Study Group. Morphologic, immunologic, and cytogenetic (MIC) working classification of the acute myeloid leukemias. Cancer Genet Cytogenet 1988; 30:1–15.
21. Traweek ST. Immunophenotypic analysis of acute leukemia. Am J Clin Pathol 1993; 99:504–512.
22. Vogel VG, Fisher RE. Epidemiology and etiology of leukemia. Curr Opin Oncol 1993; 5:26–34.
23. Wilbowo A, Pankowsky D, Mikhael A, et al. Adult acute leukemia: hand mirror cell variant. Hematopathol Mol Hematol 1996; 10:85–98.

9

Chronic Leukemias

Scott J. Graham
Naval Medical Center, Portsmouth, Virginia

James D. Cotelingam
Louisiana State University Medical Center, Shreveport, Louisiana

I. INTRODUCTION

Chronic leukemias are clonal proliferations of myeloid or lymphoid cells which, in contrast to acute leukemias, are characterized by the accumulation of relatively more mature cells within the blood, bone marrow, and parenchymal organs.

Chronic leukemias are divided into lymphoid (T- and B-cell) and myeloid (granulocytic and/or monocytic) lineages. Table 1 illustrates a general classification scheme for the chronic leukemias.

Accurate diagnosis depends on a multidisciplined approach which takes into account complete blood count (CBC) data, peripheral blood and bone marrow examination, specific cytochemical reactions, immunophenotype analysis, cytogenetic studies, and molecular genetic studies. The relative value of individual studies varies among the different disease processes. Cytogenetic and molecular genetic studies play a much more important role in the diagnosis of chronic myeloproliferative disorders than in chronic lymphoid leukemias, where flow cytometric immunophenotyping often provides more compelling supportive information.

II. SPECIAL STUDIES USED IN EVALUATING CHRONIC LEUKEMIAS

A. Cytochemical Reactions

1. Leukocyte Alkaline Phosphatase

Leukocyte alkaline phosphatase (LAP) activity helps differentiate cases of chronic myelogenous leukemia (CML) from other chronic myeloproliferative disorders and leukemoid reactions. LAP activity is limited principally to granulocytes, and is expressed objectively as an "LAP score." Normal scores range from approximately 20 to 200, varying slightly between laboratories.

Low LAP scores are characteristic of typical CML, and may be observed in infectious mononucleosis, sickle cell anemia, and paroxysmal nocturnal hemoglobinuria. Chronic neutro-

Table 1 Classification of Chronic Leukemias

I. Lymphoid leukemias
A. B-cell leukemias
Chronic lymphocytic leukemia (CLL)
B-cell prolymphocytic leukemia (B-PLL)
Hairy cell leukemia (HCL)
Lymphosarcoma cell leukemia, B-cell (LSCL)
Plasma cell leukemia
B. T-cell leukemias
T-gamma lymphoproliferative diseases (TGLD)
Adult T-cell leukemia/lymphoma (ATLL)
T-cell prolymphocytic leukemia (T-PLL)
Mycosis fungoides/Sezary syndrome (MF/SS)
II. Myeloid leukemias
Chronic myelogenous leukemia (CML)
Juvenile chronic myelogenous leukemia (JCML)
Chronic neutrophilic leukemia (CNL)
Chronic myelomonocytic leukemia (CMML)
Chronic monocytic leukemia (CMoL)
Hypereosinophilic syndromes/chronic eosinophilic leukemia (EL)
Mast cell leukemia (MCL)

philic leukemia, polycythemia rubra vera, pyogenic infections, pregnancy, and steroid therapy are characterized by elevated LAP scores. LAP scores tend to normalize in blast crisis of CML.

2. Acid Phosphatase

Acid phosphatase (AP) has seven isoenzymes. All but isoenzyme 5, which is present in the lymphoid cells of hairy cell leukemia (HCL), are sensitive to tartrate inhibition, and are the basis of the tartrate resistant-acid phosphatase (TRAP) reaction in HCL. TRAP-positive hairy cells demonstrate a multifocal cytoplasmic granular positivity. A Golgi zone-restricted TRAP positivity can often be demonstrated in T-cell lymphoproliferative disorders.

3. Nonspecific Esterases

Alpha-naphthyl acetate esterase (A-EST) and alpha-naphthyl butyrate esterase (B-EST) stains are used in both acute and chronic leukemias to demonstrate monocytic or histiocytic differentiation.

4. Terminal Deoxynucleotidyl Transferase

Terminal deoxynucleotidyl transferase (Tdt) is a nuclear enzyme which is evaluated by immunologic methods, and is demonstrable principally in lymphoid blasts. Tdt is valuable in differentiating lymphoblastic disorders from chronic lymphoproliferative processes, and as an adjunct for identifying lymphoblastic crisis of CML.

5. Toluidine Blue O

Toluidine blue O (TBO) is a basic dye which stains acid mucopolysaccharides, and is valuable in identifying mast cells and basophils, producing metachromatic granular cytoplasmic positivity.

B. Immunophenotype

Immunophenotyping is the process of identifying lineage and differentiation specific cell surface molecules by immunologic methods. Each molecule, or marker, has been cataloged by the

Nomenclature Committee of the International Workshop on Human Leukocyte Differentiation Antigens, and given a cluster designation (CD) number.

The use of immunophenotyping in the specific diagnosis of chronic myeloproliferative processes is limited by lack of narrow specificity. In CML, however, immunophenotyping easily distinguishes between lymphoblastic and myeloblastic crises.

In contrast, phenotypic data are quite useful in supporting or confirming the diagnosis of chronic lymphoid proliferations. Many chronic lymphoid leukemias possess a fairly unique pattern of immunoreactivity which, together with morphologic, histologic, cytochemical, and clinical findings, leads to accurate diagnosis. Table 2 contains the typical immunophenotypic profiles of the chronic lymphoid leukemias.

C. Cytogenetics and Molecular Genetics

Many hematopoietic malignancies demonstrate nonrandom chromosomal abnormalities. Table 3 outlines the most common cytogenetic findings reported for the chronic leukemias.

Table 2 Typical Immunophenotypes for Chronic Lymphoid Leukemias

	B-CLL	B-PLL	T-PLL	LSCL	HCL	ATLL	MF/SS	TGLD	MM/PCL
CD2			+			+	+	+	
CD3			+			+	+	+	
CD5	+	+/– dim	+			+	+	+/–	
CD7			+			+/–		+	
CD4			+			+	+		
CD8			+/–′					+	
CD19	+	+		+	+				–
CD20	+ dim	+		+	+				–
CD11c					+				
CD10		+/– dim		+/–					
CD25	+/– dim	+/–	+/–		+	+	+/–		–
CD38			+/–			+			+
CD45	+	+	+	+	+	+	+	+	–
Ig	sIg dim	sIg		sIg	sIg				cIg
HLA-DR	+	+		+		+	–	+/–	–

(+) = >70% of cases are positive
(–) = Relevant negative reactions
sIg = Surface immunoglobulin
(′) = About 10% of T-PLL will be CD4–, CD8+
+/– = <50% of cases are positive
dim = Low intensity
cIg = Cytoplasmic Immunoglobulin

B-CLL = B-cell chroinc lymphocytic leukemia
B-PLL = B-cell prolymphocytic leukemia
T-PLL = T-cell prolymphocytic leukemia
LSCL = lymphosarcoma cell leukemia (B-cell)
HCL = hairy cell leukemia
ATLL = adult T-cell leukemia/lymphoma
MF/SS = mycosis fungoides/Sezary syndrome
TGLD = T-gamma lymphoproliferative diseases
MM/PCL = multiple myeloma/plasma cell leukemia

Note: TGLD are often positive for CD11b, CD16, CD56, and CD57 in addition to the immunophenotypic findings listed above.

Table 3 Most Frequently Observed Cytogenetic Abnormalities

Chronic myelogenous leukemia	t(9;22)(q34;q11)/Ph
Chronic neutrophilic leukemia	No consistent abnormality
Chronic myelomonocytic leukemia	Trisomy 8
	del(11)(q23)
	Absence of chromosome 5
	Absence of chromosome 7
	del(5q)
	del(7q)
Chronic monocytic leukemia	No consistent abnormality
Eosinophilic leukemia	No consistent abnormality
Mast cell leukemia	No consistent abnormality
Chronic lymphocytic leukemia	Trisomy 12
	Abnormal 13(13q14)
	t(14;19)
	t(11;14)
B-cell prolymphocytic leukemia	Abnormal 14(14q32)
	t(11;14)
	t(6;12)
	Trisomy 12
T-cell prolymphocytic leukemia	Abnormal 2 and 8
	inv14(q11;q32)
Hairy cell leukemia	14q+
Lymphosarcoma cell leukemia (B-cell)	t(14;18)
Mycosis fungoides/Sezary syndrome	Abnormal 6 and 1
	Trisomy 7q
	inv(17q)
Adult T-cell leukemia/lymphoma	Trisomy 3, 7, and 21
	del(6)(q21)
	del(10)(p13)
	Translocations of 14q11
	Absence of X chromosome
Multiple myeloma/plasma cell leukemia	14q+(14q32)
	t(11;14)

Cytogenetic abnormalities represent detectable microscopic events with molecular consequences, and may involve one of many cellular oncogenes present in eukaryotic cells which involve proliferation and differentiation. Table 4 lists the most common reported oncogenes expressed in chronic leukemic processes.

Southern blot DNA analysis is useful in identifying clonal gene rearrangements, which are demonstrable in many chronic lymphoid neoplasms.

III. LYMPHOPROLIFERATIVE DISORDERS

A. Chronic Lymphocytic Leukemia

Chronic lymphocytic leukemia (CLL) is the most common adulthood leukemia, accounting for about 30% of all leukemias diagnosed in the Western hemisphere. The incidence is much lower in Asia. Males outnumber females by 2.5 : 1. The median age at diagnosis is 55 years, and

Table 4 Oncogene Expression

Chronic myelogenous leukemia	*abl*
Chronic myelomonocytic leukemia	*K-ras*
Chronic lymphocytic leukemia	*N-ras*
	K-ras
B-cell prolymphocytic leukemia	*bcl-1*
Lymphosarcoma cell leukemia (B-cell)	*bcl-2*
	bcl-1
Adult T-cell leukemia/lymphoma	Viral (HTLV-1)
Multiple myeloma/plasma cell leukemia	*ras*
	bcl-2

there appears to be a genetic predisposition. CLL is an indolent disorder resulting in the accumulation of small round lymphocytes in the blood, bone marrow, and parenchymal organs, and has a variety of late-stage complications.

Minimal diagnostic criteria for CLL according to the National Cancer Institute-sponsored Working Group include:

1. At least 5×10^9/L small, mature-appearing lymphocytes occur in the peripheral blood.
2. At least 30% of all nucleated cells in the bone marrow are lymphocytes.
3. Most peripheral blood lymphocytes should be CD19-, CD20-, or CD24-positive B cells with coexpression of CD5, and low-intensity surface immunoglobulin, with kappa or lambda restriction.

The total white blood cell (WBC) count ranges from the minimal numeric criteria for diagnosis up to 600×10^9/L or more. Many patients are discovered incidentally.

In typical cases, most WBCs are small lymphocytes with round nuclei, condensed, blocky chromatin, absent to inconspicuous nucleoli, and scant cytoplasm (Fig. 1). Peripheral blood smears often contain numerous "smudge" or "basket" cells, which are a technical artifact. In a small percentage of cases, the nuclei have slight irregularities or plasmacytoid features. Up to 10% of circulating lymphocytes may be classified as prolymphocytes, which have more abundant cytoplasm, nuclei with more open chromatin, and a single prominent nucleolus. When prolymphocytes account for 11–55% of lymphoid cells, the designation prolymphocytic transformation of CLL (CLL/PLL) is appropriate. If >55% of lymphoid cells are prolymphocytes, the diagnosis of de-novo prolymphocytic leukemia (PLL) is likely.

Table 5 outlines the common hematologic and clinical manifestations of CLL.

Bone marrow infiltration is best evaluated on biopsy sections, and is described as nodular, interstitial, mixed nodular and interstitial, or diffuse. Infiltrates are composed of small round lymphocytes, occasionally with scattered larger nucleolated forms. Prognostically, the diffuse pattern portends a more aggressive clinical course.

Almost all CLL patients develop lymphadenopathy and splenomegaly. Affected lymph nodes reveal a diffuse infiltrate of small lymphocytes with scattered "proliferation centers" (also known as "pseudofollicles" or "growth centers"), which are composed of slightly larger cells with more open chromatin, visible nucleoli, more abundant cytoplasm, and conspicuous mitotic activity. Splenic involvement consists of white pulp infiltrates which may extend modestly into the red pulp.

Immunophenotypic data readily support the diagnosis of CLL. The characteristic pheno-

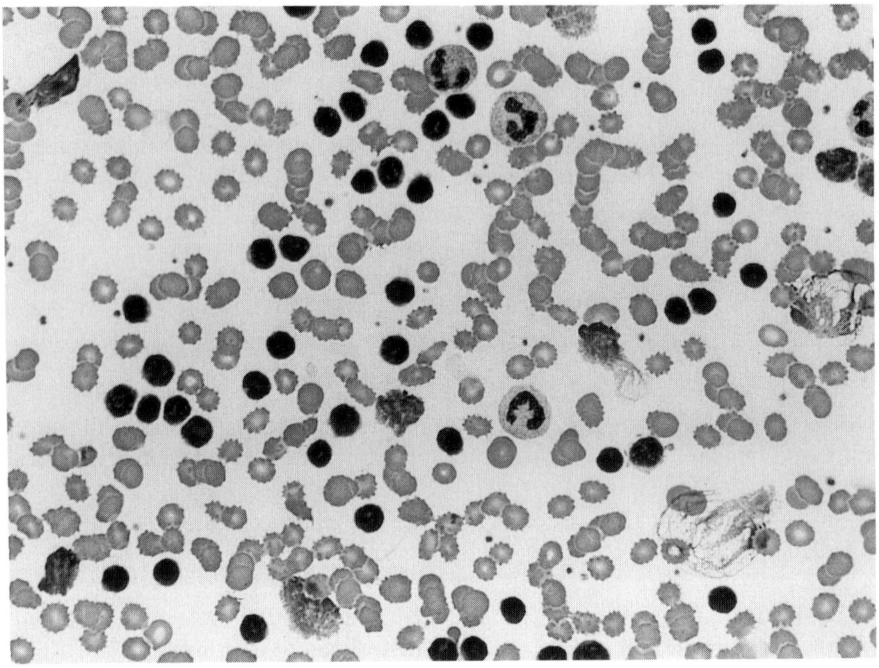

Figure 1 Peripheral blood smear, CLL. Numerous small lymphocytes with round nuclei, coarsely clumped chromatin, and scant cytoplasm. Scattered smudge and basket cells are present. (×200.)

Table 5 Clinical and Hematologic Features of Chronic Lymphocytic Leukemia

Anemia	(50%)
Pure red cell aplasia may occur	
Anemia and thrombocytopenia	(25%)
Autoimmune hemolytic anemia	(10–20%)
Immune thrombocytopenia	(5–10%)
Hypogammaglobulinemia	(50%)
Monoclonal gammopathy	(50%)
Neutropenia	
Only with extensive CLL bone marrow infiltrates	
Secondary malignancies	
Possibly increased incidence of melanoma, sarcomas, GI and lung carcinoma	

Percentages are approximate frequency of occurrence.

Table 6 Chronic Lymphocytic Leukemia Staging

Rai	Binet
Stage 0: Lymphocytosis	Stage A: No anemia No thrombocytopenia Involvement of <3 lymphoid areas
Stage I: Lymphocytosis, lymphadenopathy Stage II: Lymphocytosis, hepatomegaly/splenomegaly	Stage B: No anemia No thrombocytopenia Involvement of ≥3 lymphoid areas
Stage III: Lymphocytosis, anemia (Hgb < 11 g/dL) Stage IV: Lymphocytosis, thrombocytopenia	Stage C: Anemia (Hgb <10 g/dL) or thrombocytopenia
Low-risk disease = stage 0; intermediate risk = stages I, II; high risk = stages III, IV	Lymphoid areas defined as cervical, axillary, inguinal lymph nodes, liver, and spleen

Thrombocytopenia = platelets $<100 \times 10^9/L$.

typic profile is illustrated in Table 2. Presence of the T-cell marker CD5 is particularly noteworthy.

Cytogenetic studies demonstrate abnormalities in almost 50% of cases. Table 3 contains the most frequent cytogenetic findings.

Staging in CLL has been shown to be of prognostic significance. The Rai and Binet systems are the most frequently utilized, and are outlined in Table 6.

About 40% of CLL patients develop cytologic transformation to a more aggressive morphology at some time during their course. Prolymphocytic transformation occurs in about 30% of CLL patients, and is considered when 11–55% of circulating leukemia cells have prolymphocytic features. Richter's syndrome is a parenchymal transformation with the appearance of a pleomorphic large cell lymphoma.

B. Prolymphocytic Leukemia

Prolymphocytic leukemia (PLL) is clinically aggressive. Both B-cell and T-cell phenotypes are recognized, and share many common clinical and pathologic features. The incidence of PLL is about 10% that of CLL. The ratio of B-cell to T-cell phenotypes is about 2–3 : 1.

1. B-Cell Prolymphocytic Leukemia

B-Cell prolymphocytic leukemia (B-PLL) is a disease of elderly adults, with a slight male predominance. Table 7 outlines common clinical and hematologic parameters.

Prolymphocytes are larger than small lymphocytes. The nuclei are round to oval, central

Table 7 Clinical and Hematologic Features of B-Cell Prolymphocytic Leukemia at Presentation

Leukocytosis $>100 \times 10^9/L$	(75%)
Anemia	
Thrombocytopenia	
Neutropenia	
Hepatosplenomegaly	
No significant lymphadenopathy	

or eccentric, have mature chromatin, and a single prominent central nucleolus. The cytoplasm is light blue and moderately abundant (Fig. 2). The presence of >55% prolymphocytes in peripheral blood helps distinguish de-novo PLL from CLL and CLL/PLL.

Flow cytometric immunophenotyping provides supportive data in suspected cases. The typical B-PLL phenotype is illustrated in Table 2.

Significant bone marrow involvement is characteristic, with the leukemic infiltrate demonstrating interstitial, diffuse, or mixed patterns. The purely nodular pattern as seen in some cases of CLL has not been observed.

Involved lymph nodes demonstrate diffuse effacement with scattered pseudofollicles or "growth centers." The usually massive spleen shows white pulp infiltration producing a nodular pattern. Leukemic involvement of the red pulp is also evident in most cases.

Typical cytogenetic findings are listed in Table 3.

2. *T-Cell Prolymphocytic Leukemia*

T-cell prolymphocytic leukemia (T-PLL) accounts for about one-third of cases morphologically consistent with PLL. Most patients are elderly adults presenting with fatigue, weight loss, and skin lesions. Table 8 contains the most common clinical and hematologic manifestations.

The leukemic cells may be indistinguishable from their B-cell counterparts, or have irregular nuclear contours and somewhat less cytoplasm.

Bone marrow biopsies show an interstitial, diffuse, or mixed leukemic infiltrates. Increased reticulum fibrosis is frequently observed. Spleens demonstrate predominantly red pulp infiltra-

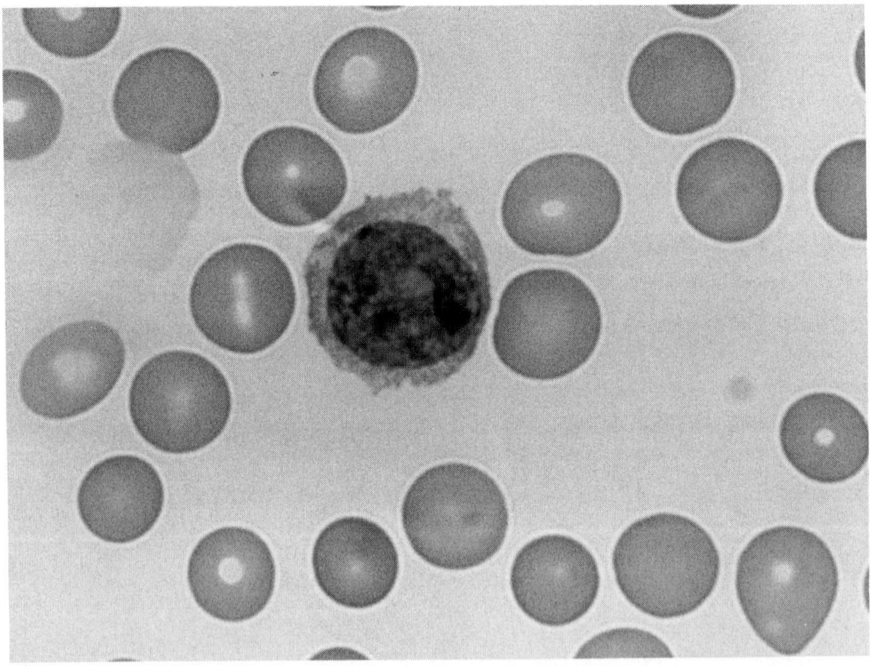

Figure 2 Peripheral blood smear, prolymphocyte morphology. The cell is larger than a small lymphocyte with a round to oval nucleus, prominent central nucleolus, and moderately abundant cytoplasm. (×1000.)

Table 8 Clinical and Hematologic Features of T-Cell Prolymphocytic Leukemia at Presentation

Anemia	(35%)
Thrombocytopenia	(50%)
Leukocytosis $>200 \times 10^9$/L	(60%)
Lymphadenopathy	(50%)
Hepatosplenomegaly	(55%)
Skin lesions	(25%)

Percentages are approximate frequency of occurrence.

tion, but concurrent involvement of the white pulp is often present. Skin lesions have a dense perivascular and periadnexal leukemic infiltrate without epidermotropism.

Typical immunophenotypic data and cytogenetic findings are presented in Tables 2 and 3. Molecular genetic analysis often demonstrates clonal rearrangement of the beta T-cell receptor gene.

The most frequently encountered differential diagnosis of B-PLL and T-PLL is prolymphocytic transformation of CLL. Examination of the peripheral blood smear with adherence to numerical criteria make it possible to distinguish between these two entities. Differences in immunophenotypic profiles provide further support.

C. Hairy Cell Leukemia

Hairy cell leukemia (HCL) is a relatively rare disorder of middle-aged adults, with males outnumbering females. Common hematologic and clinical manifestations are outlined in Table 9.

Because hairy cells are usually observed in only small numbers, buffy coat smears of peripheral blood are often made for easier morphologic evaluation and to demonstrate tartrate-resistant acid phosphatase (TRAP) activity, which is present in >95% of cases at presentation. True leukemic presentation with $>5 \times 10^9$ hairy cells/L is uncommon, but may be seen after splenectomy.

Hairy cell morphology is unique but not specific. The cells are slightly larger than small lymphocytes, have round to oval central or slightly eccentric nuclei, evenly distributed lacy chromatin, and one or two inconspicuous nucleoli. The abundant cytoplasm is pale gray-blue

Table 9 Clinical and Hematologic Features of Hairy Cell Leukemia at Presentation

Normochromic normocytic anemia	(70%)
Thrombocytopenia	(85%)
Neutropenia	(70%)
Monocytopenia	(85%)
Splenomegaly	(80%)
Hepatomegaly	(50%)
Lymphadenopathy	
May develop centrally, rare peripherally	(5–10%)

Percentages are approximate frequency of occurrence.

with "hairy" borders (Fig. 3). In most cases, bone marrow aspirates result in a "dry tap" due to reticulum fibrosis. Bone marrow biopsies reveal the characteristic diffuse, monomorphic infiltrate of hairy cells with typical round to oval nuclei surrounded by abundant clear cytoplasm (Fig. 4). A reticulum stain accentuates well-defined cell borders. Similar histology is characteristic of the splenic red pulp. Extravasated red blood cells (RBCs) are often observed within the neoplastic infiltrate, and are referred to as "pseudosinuses" and "blood lakes."

Typical immunoreactivity and cytogenetic findings are presented in Tables 2 and 3.

T cells morphologically similar to hairy cells have been described in association with HTLV-II seropositivity.

The differential diagnosis of HCL includes CLL, lymphosarcoma cell leukemia, PLL, and splenic lymphoma with villous lymphocytes. The combination of TRAP reactivity, bone marrow biopsy morphology, and immunophenotype clarifies most cases.

D. Lymphosarcoma Cell Leukemia

Lymphosarcoma cell leukemia (LSCL) is the term used to describe the leukemic phase of non-Hodgkin's lymphomas (NHL), not including entities which have previously named leukemic manifestations [such as lymphoblastic lymphoma (ALL-L1 and L2), Burkitt's lymphoma (ALL-L3), mycosis fungoides (Sezary syndrome), and adult T-cell leukemia/lymphoma]. The term LSCL should be reserved to describe cases in which the number of circulating lymphoma cells results in an absolute lymphocytosis; fewer cells should be considered tumor peripherali-

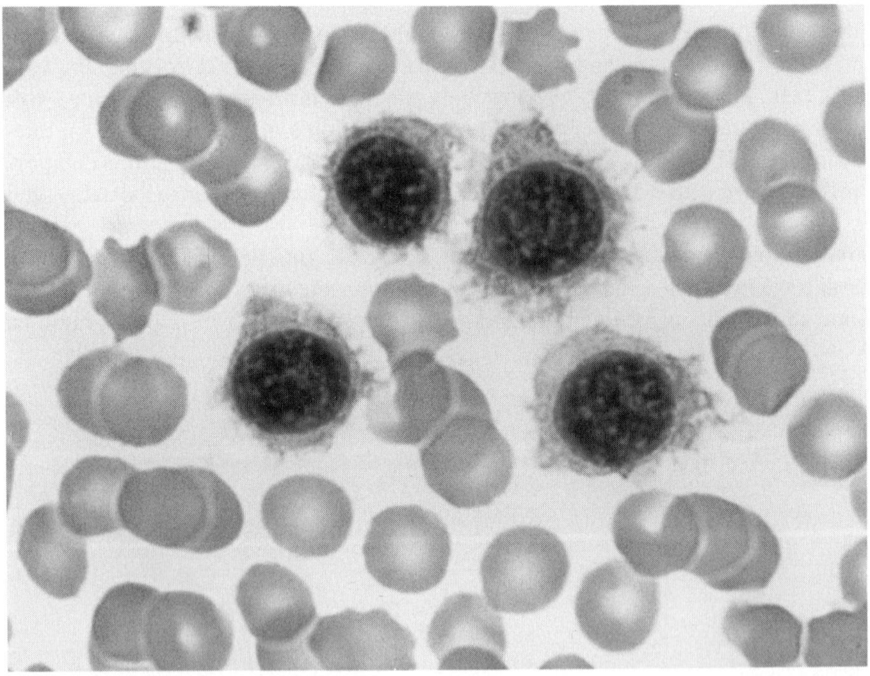

Figure 3 Buffy coat smear, HCL. Several hairy cells slightly larger than small lymphocytes, round to oval nuclei, evenly distributed chromatin, inconspicuous nucleoli, and moderately abundant ruffled cytoplasm. (×1000.)

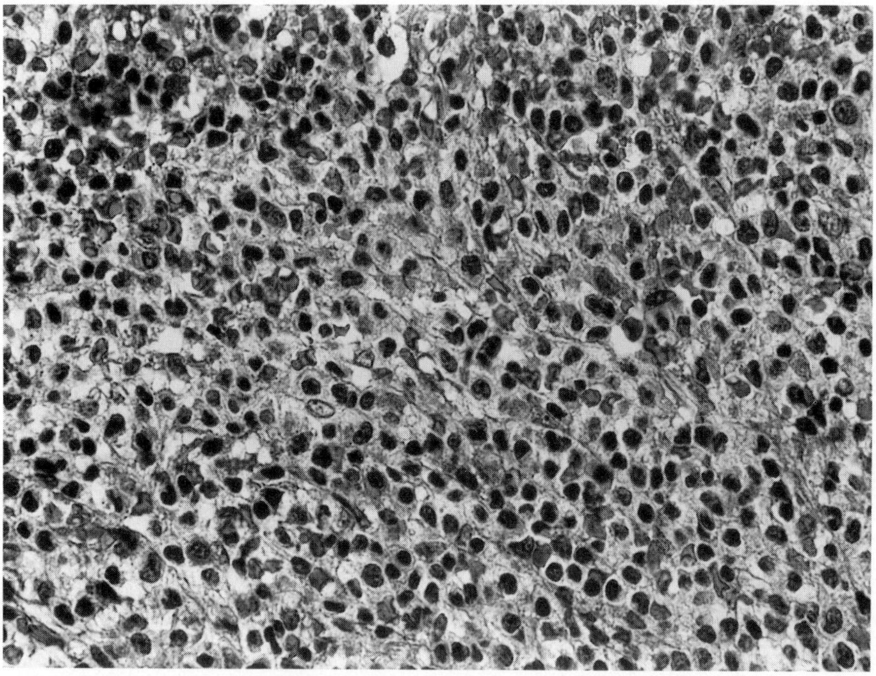

Figure 4 Bone marrow biopsy, HCL. Diffuse monomorphic infiltrate of small lymphoid cells with round to oval nuclei, abundant clear cytoplasm, and distinct cell borders. (×200.)

zation, not LSCL. LSCL does not appear to have independent prognostic significance, as most patients with LSCL have more advanced disease than their nonleukemic counterparts.

Like lymphomas in general, most LSCLs are of B-cell phenotype. While the most frequently encountered lymphocyte morphology in LSCL is the small cleaved cell of small cleaved follicular center cell lymphomas (Fig. 5), circulating lymphoma cells have been documented in most other types of lymphomas, including both B-cell and T-cell phenotypes.

The morphology of the circulating lymphosarcoma cell is often but not necessarily related to the parenchymal lymphoma morphology. Small cleaved cells tend to have small nuclei, condensed chromatin, and a prominent nuclear cleft, while large cells have nuclei with open chromatin, prominent nucleoli, variable nuclear contours, and basophilic cytoplasm.

Most patients present with parenchymal disease, and develop LSCL late in their course. Occasionally, the presentation of lymphoma and leukemic manifestations occur simultaneously, and the designation lymphoma-leukemia is appropriate.

E. Plasma Cell Leukemia

Plasma cell leukemia (PCL) is a rare disorder in which circulating plasma cells account for >20% of the differential WBC count, or the absolute plasma cell count is $>2 \times 10^9$/L. When PCL follows the diagnosis of multiple myeloma (MM), *secondary* PCL is the appropriate designation. Secondary PCL occurs in about 2% of late-stage MM patients. The term *leukemic myelomatosis* is used when PCL precedes or is diagnosed concurrently with multiple myeloma, and is extremely rare.

Circulating plasma cells have been reported in up to 17% of MM patients, but most have

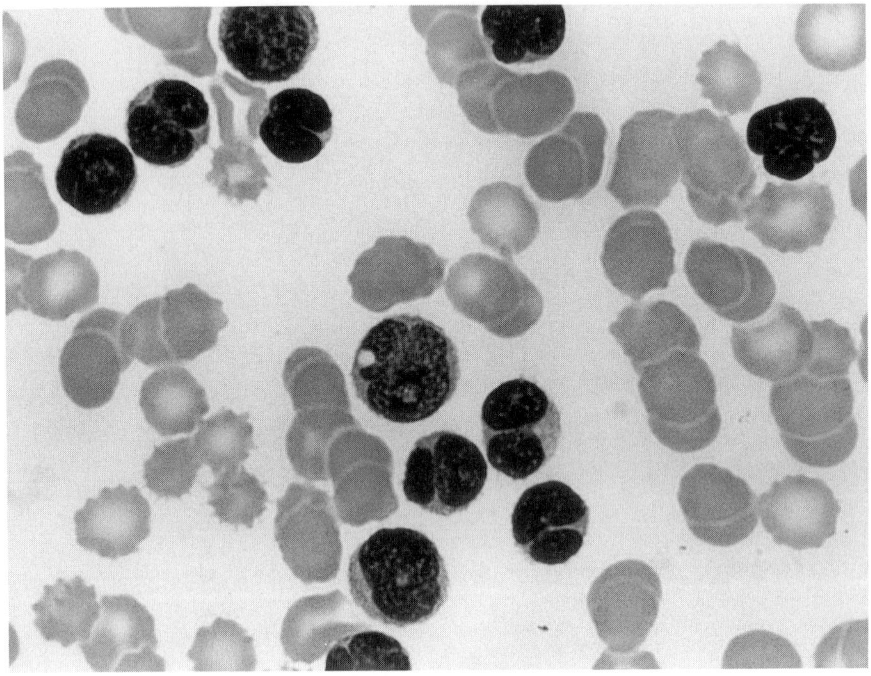

Figure 5 Peripheral smear, LSCL. Lymphoid cells of varying size, coarsely clumped chromatin, and prominant nuclear clefts. (×1000.)

fewer than required for the diagnosis of PCL, and therefore have tumor peripheralization, not leukemia.

All immunoglobulin classes are represented as monoclonal manifestations of PCL, and parallel the incidence of paraproteins in nonleukemic MM. One exception, IgE myeloma, while extremely unusual, manifests a leukemic phase in over 25% of cases.

Examination of peripheral blood reveals total WBC counts from 20 to 100×10^9/L. The morphology of the leukemic cells varies from easily recognizable plasma cells (Fig. 6), to large cells with open chromatin, prominent nucleoli, and higher nuclear to cytoplasm ratios. These latter cases require immunophenotypic analysis for accurate classification.

Bone marrow aspirate material generally demonstrates numerous plasmacytoid cells, many with binucleate and trinucleate morphology. Prominent nucleoli usually indicate an aggressive process. The bone marrow biopsy invariably reveals a diffuse plasma cell infiltrate. Immunoperoxidase studies for kappa and lambda light chains performed on paraffin-imbedded tissue reveal a clonal excess, and should correlate with serum or urine protein electrophoresis with immunofixation.

Flow cytometric evaluation of PCL has demonstrated positivity for specific plasma cell markers, including PC-1, PCA-1, PCA-2, as well as CD38. LCA, CD19, and CD20 are usually negative.

Commonly reported cytogenetic abnormalities are presented in Table 3. Molecular genetic studies demonstrate clonal rearrangement of the light- and heavy-chain immunoglobulin genes.

The differential diagnosis of PCL includes Waldenstrom's macroglobulinemia, CLL, and B-PLL, all of which may have circulating lymphoplasmacytoid cells and paraproteinemia.

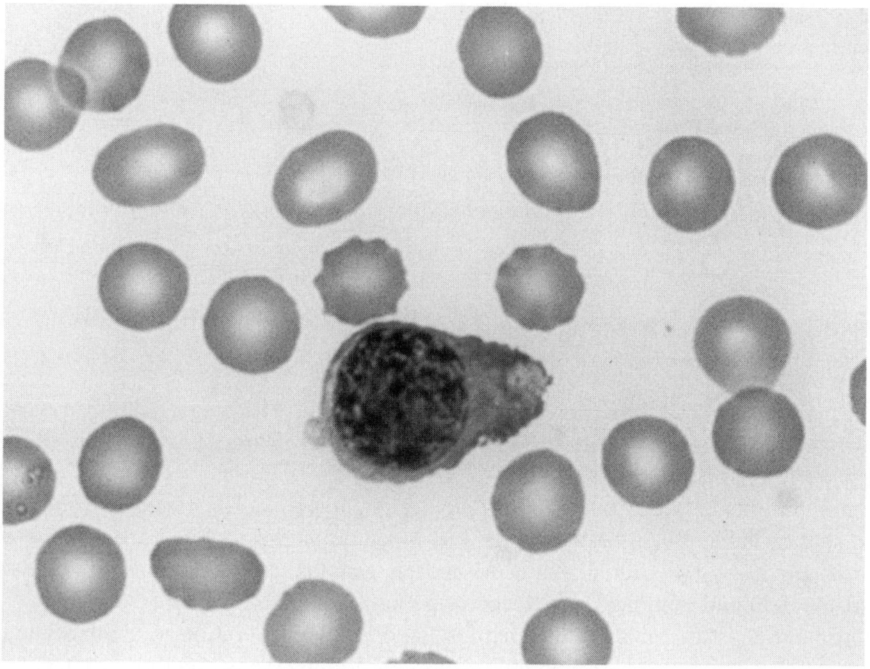

Figure 6 Peripheral smear, PCL. This circulating plasma cell has the usual round eccentrically placed nucleus, coarse chromatin, abundant cytoplasm, and a perinuclear golgi zone. (×1000.)

Immunophenotypic analysis, together with clinical and radiographic data, usually leads to accurate diagnosis.

F. Adult T-Cell Leukemia/Lymphoma

HTLV-1-associated adult T-cell leukemia/lymphoma (ATLL) was first described in southwest Japan in 1977, and is the only chronic leukemia with a well-established viral etiology. Endemic areas, where seropositivity is reported as high as 37%, now include the Caribbean islands, the southeastern United States, parts of southern Italy, South America, and Africa.

ATLL affects adults of all ages, with a median age of about 55 years. Males outnumber females by 1.5 : 1.

Characteristic clinical manifestations are outlined in Table 10. Sixty to 70% of patients present with peripheral blood involvement. Total WBC counts range from normal up to >500 × 10^9/L. The leukemic cells are larger than small lymphocytes, with nuclei demonstrating coarse chromatin, inconspicuous nucleoli, and marked irregularities, including the so-called flower or propeller morphology (Fig. 7). Others demonstrate two or more deep nuclear folds. Cytoplasm is variably abundant and basophilic, occasionally vacuolated.

Involved lymph nodes have varied histologic appearances. The neoplastic infiltrate may be composed of exclusively small lymphocytes, a mixture of small and large cells, or mostly large cells, occasionally with immunoblastic morphology.

Skin infiltrates may be perivascular, periadnexal, or diffuse. Epidermotropism with Pautrier's microabscesses are observed in some cases.

Bone marrow involvement occurs in over 50% of cases. On aspirate smears, the leukemic

Table 10 Clinical Features of Adult T-Cell Leukemia/Lymphoma at Presentation

Skin rash	(50%)
Perivascular, periadnexal, or diffuse infiltrates	
May have epidermotropism	
Lymphadenopathy	(70%)
Hepatomegaly	(75%)
Splenomegaly	(55%)
Hypercalcemia	(35%)

Percentages are approximate frequency of occurrence.

cells have features similar to those observed in the peripheral blood. Histologic sections reveal a focal interstitial nonparatrabecular infiltrate. Patients with hypercalcemia have increased osteoclastic activity.

Immunophenotyping usually demonstrates a T-helper phenotype as illustrated in Table 2.

Cytogenetic studies have shown trisomy 3 or 7 in Japanese studies, while chromosome 6 abnormalities predominate in the United States. Molecular genetic studies demonstrate clonal rearrangement of the beta and gamma T-cell receptor genes.

Sezary syndrome (SS) is the principal differential diagnostic consideration. As both SS and ATLL may have similar cutaneous and immunophenotypic findings, the distinction depends on a combination of cytologic, serologic, and clinical parameters. Nuclei of Sezary cells demon-

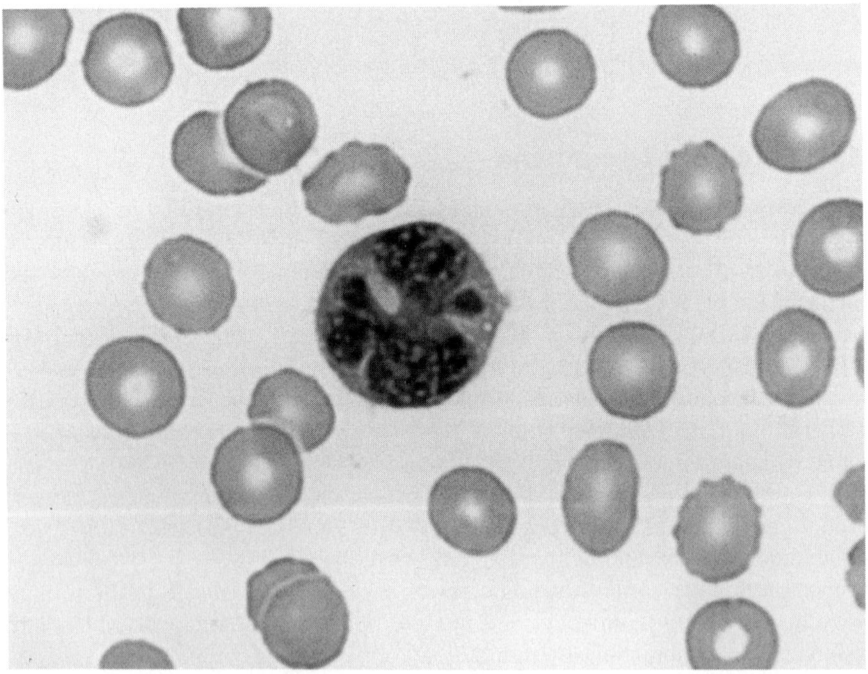

Figure 7 Peripheral smear, ATLL. Lymphoid cell with prominent nuclear irregularities, characteristic of ATLL. (×1000.)

strate more internal convolutions, whereas those of ATLL are more externally irregular. Additionally, HTLV-1-associated antibodies and hypercalcemia are infrequent in Sezary syndrome.

G. T-gamma Lymphoproliferative Disease

T-gamma lymphoproliferative disease (TGLD) is a heterogeneous group of chronic T-cell disorders which have in common the presence of large granular lymphocytes (LGLs) in the peripheral blood. Most cases of TGLD are indolent, although a small percentage develop a rapidly progressive course with lymphocytosis, tissue infiltration, and fatal infections.

TGLD occurs in adults over 50 years of age, with a slight male predominance. About 25% of patients are discovered incidentally.

Recent studies have divided the TGLDs into two major groups based on immunophenotype. The larger group, containing about 80% of cases, are known as T-cell lymphoproliferative disorders of granular lymphocytes (T-cell LDGL), commonly express CD2, CD3, CD8, often CD16 and CD57, demonstrate antibody-dependent cellular cytotoxicity in vitro, have weak or absent natural killer (NK) activity, and often have detectable clonal rearrangements of the TCR beta or gamma genes. These patients manifest the characteristic clinical findings of neutropenia, hepatosplenomegaly, evidence of autoimmune phenomena such as rheumatoid arthritis, and recurrent infections. The smaller group, accounting for about 20% of cases, are known as NK cell LDGL, express CD2, CD16, CD56, variable CD8 and CD57, demonstrate natural killer cytotoxicity in vitro, and have no detectable TCR gene rearrangement. Patients with this form often have hepatosplenomegaly, but rarely manifest neutropenia or autoimmunity.

Immunophenotypic profiling may provide prognostic information, as weak or absent CD57 expression has been associated with a more aggressive clinical course.

Examination of the peripheral blood reveals varying numbers of large lymphocytes with irregular nuclei and abundant pale cytoplasm containing azurophilic granules of variable size and number (Fig. 8). Absolute LGL counts range from 2.0 to 7.0×10^9/L. The accompanying neutropenia, if present, may be cyclical. Slight anemia and thrombocytopenia is often observed. Pure red cell aplasia has occasionally been reported.

Bone marrow involvement is seen in most patients, and consists of small, loosely formed lymphoid aggregates or more extensive nodular, interstitial, or diffuse patterns. Infiltrates are composed predominantly of small lymphocytes with condensed chromatin, slightly irregular nuclear contours, inconspicuous nucleoli, and scant cytoplasm. Scattered larger transformed lymphocytes and plasma cells are occasionally observed.

No consistent cytogenetic abnormalities have been observed, although trisomy 8 and trisomy 14 have been reported.

The differential diagnosis of TGLD includes CLL, HCL, T-PLL, LSCL, and reactive lymphocytosis. In most cases, careful attention to the clinical, morphologic, and immunophenotypic profile permits distinction among these entities.

Distinction between TGLD and Felty's syndrome (LGLs, neutropenia, splenomegaly, and rheumatoid arthritis) is made on temporal grounds, as most Felty's patients have a long history of arthritis prior to onset of hematologic disease. In TGLD, the clinical and hematologic manifestations present simultaneously.

H. Mycosis Fungoides and Sezary Syndrome

Mycosis fungoides (MF) is a relatively rare cutaneous T-cell lymphoproliferative disorder characterized by skin infiltration resulting in scaly pruritic and erythematous patches, plaques, and

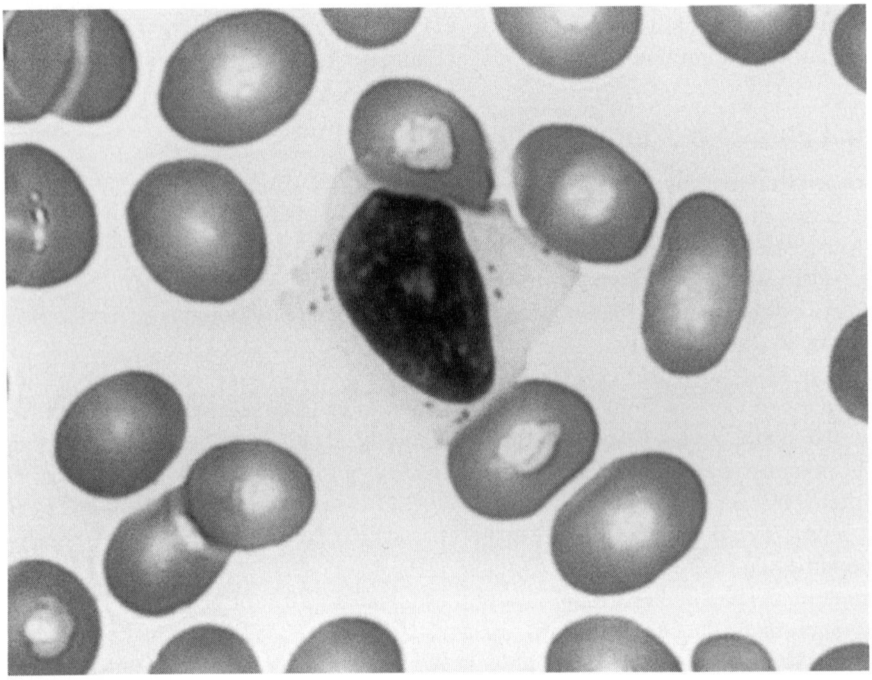

Figure 8 Peripheral smear, TGLD. Large lymphoid cell with an irregular nucleus, abundant clear cytoplasm, and scattered cytoplasmic granules. (×1000.)

tumor nodules. Most patients are initially evaluated by a dermatologist, and diagnosis is established after one or more skin biopsies.

Sezary syndrome (SS) is considered a systemic or leukemic manifestation of MF. Patients present with diffuse erythroderma and numerous peripheral blood atypical convoluted lymphocytes.

The diagnosis of MF is made upon examination of skin biopsy material. Characteristic is a bandlike superficial dermal infiltrate of small, atypical, convoluted lymphocytes, often with variable numbers of eosinophils and plasma cells. The term *epidermotropism* is used to describe single and small groups of atypical convoluted lymphocytes surrounded by clear halos present within the nonspongiotic epidermis. The small collections of atypical convoluted lymphocytes are known as *Pautrier's abscesses*, and together with the single cell pattern, constitute the primary diagnostic criteria (Fig. 9).

Sezary cells rarely number $>20 \times 10^9$/L in peripheral blood. Two types of circulating MF (Sezary) cells have been characterized. The small cell variant is similar in size to normal small lymphocytes, except for its internally convoluted ("cerebriform") nucleus and coarsely clumped chromatin (Fig. 10). The large (or transformed) variant has a nuclear diameter two to three times larger than a small lymphocyte, more open chromatin, occasional small nucleoli, and more abundant cytoplasm. The nuclei tend to be clefted or folded rather than convoluted.

Histopathologic staging in MF/SS has prognostic value, and includes evaluation of skin lesions, peripheral blood, lymph nodes, and bone marrow. Twenty percent or more of periph-

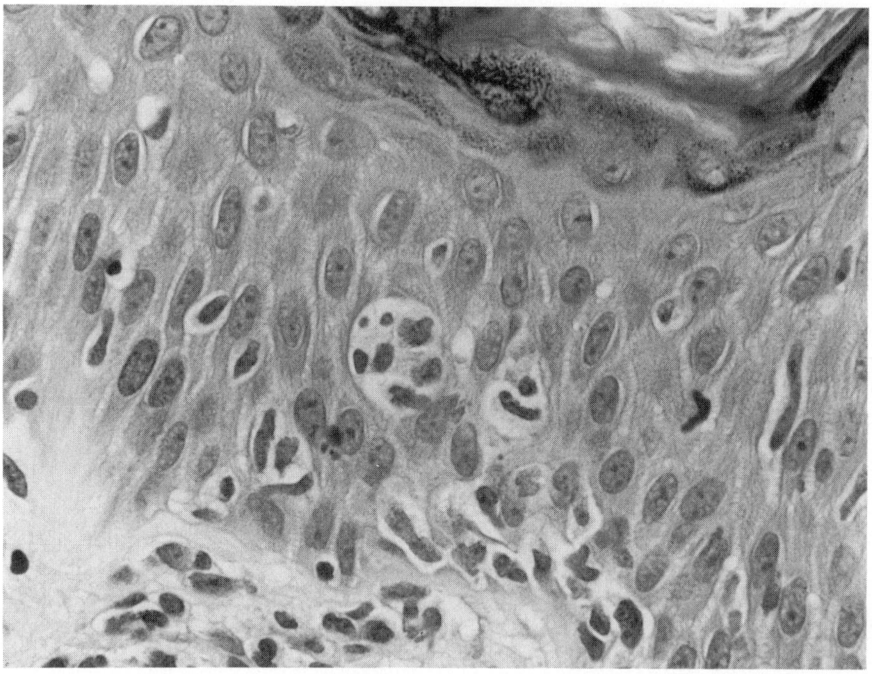

Figure 9 Skin biopsy, MF. Atypical convoluted lymphocytes within the epidermis, occurring singly and in clusters (Pautrier's microabscess), surrounded by clear halos are characteristic. (×400.)

eral blood lymphocytes, morphologically consistent with either large or small Sezary cells, are adequate to consider the peripheral blood positive for involvement. Lymph node biopsies have traditionally been graded according to the guidelines established by Matthews and Gazdar, as illustrated in Table 11. LN-3 or LN-4 histology are considered positive. Bone marrow lesions are seen in up to 20% of cases at diagnosis, and consist of paratrabecular or intertrabecular aggregates of atypical convoluted lymphocytes, occasionally with accompanying small round lymphocytes and scattered large transformed cells. Advanced cases may demonstrate a diffuse infiltrating pattern.

The immunoprofile of MF/SS is illustrated in Table 2. Proof of clonality is best demonstrated using Southern blot analysis, identifying a clonal T-cell receptor gene rearrangement.

Cytogenetic studies have revealed no consistent abnormalities in either MF or SS, but random abnormalities are frequently observed.

For many years it has been suspected that MF/SS was caused by HTLV-I or II, although there was no supportive serologic evidence. Recent studies utilizing combined polymerase chain reaction (PCR) and Southern blot technology have reported finding HTLV pol and/or tax or tax/rev proviral sequences in a high percentage of cases.

The principal differential diagnostic consideration is HTLV-I-associated ATLL. Immunophenotypic analysis and cutaneous manifestations can be similar in both disorders. Morphologically, MF/SS cells are more often characterized by internal nuclear convolutions, whereas ATLL demonstrates more external nuclear irregularities. Positive routine viral serologies for HTLV-I and hypercalcemia support the diagnosis of ATLL, as both are unusual in MF/SS.

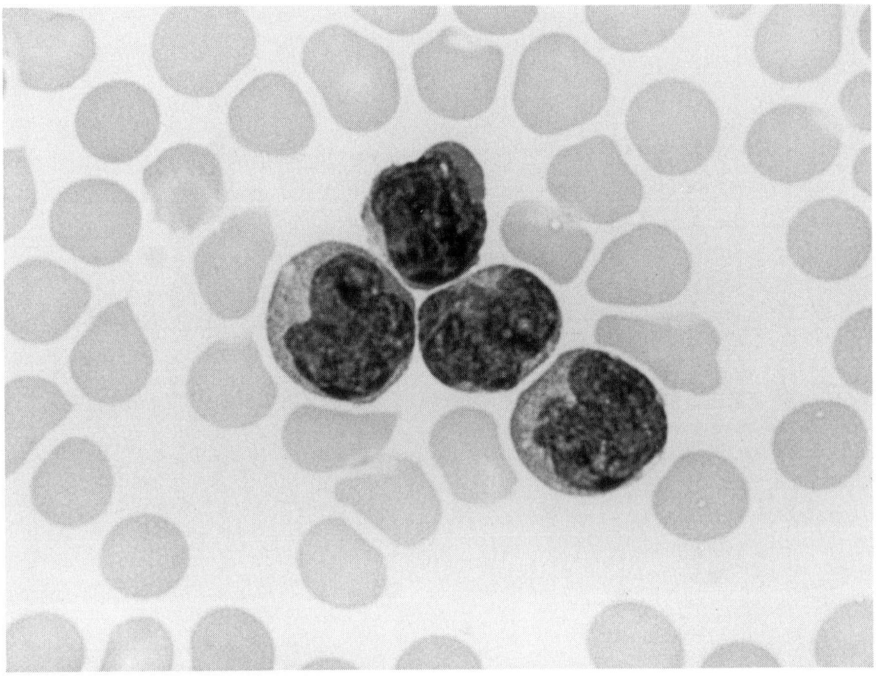

Figure 10 Peripheral blood, SS. Sezary cells demonstrating irregular clumped chromatin, inconspicuous nucleoli, and marked nuclear convolutions. (×1000.)

IV. MYELOPROLIFERATIVE PROCESSES

A. Chronic Myelogenous Leukemia

Chronic myelogenous leukemia (CML) is a clonal neoplasm of pleuripotential hematopoietic stem cells in which granulocytic differentiation dominates the process. Table 12 outlines key features distinguishing CML from the other common chronic myeloproliferative disorders.

CML is a disease primarily affecting adults, with a median age of about 50 years, although

Table 11 Lymph Node Staging in Mycosis Fungoides/Sezary Syndrome (Mathews and Gazdar, NCI-NAVY)

LN0:	Dermatopathic lymphadenitis, no atypical lymphocytes
LN1:	Dermatopathic lymphadenitis, scattered single lymphocytes in paracortex
LN2:	Dermatopathic lymphadenitis, small clusters (<6 cells) of atypical lymphocytes
LN3:	Dermatopathic lymphadenitis, large clusters (>6 cells) of atypical lymphocytes
LN4:	Partial or complete lymph node effacement by atypical lymphocytes

Table 12 Characteristics of the Chronic Myeloproliferative Disorders

	Chronic myelogenous leukemia	Myelofibrosis with myeloid metaplasia	Polycythemia vera	Essential thrombocythemia
Hemoglobin	Usually decreased	Usually decreased	Increased	Normal or decreased
Granulocytic leukocytosis	Usually >50,000	Usually <30,000	Usually <25,000	Usually <25,000
Differential	Immature myeloid, all stages neutrophils and myelocytes predominate	Immature myeloid, all stages	Usually mild left shift	Usually mild left shift
Basophilia and/or eosinophilia	Present	Usually present	May be present	May be present
Erythrocyte morphology	Usually normal	Numerous teardrop poikilocytes, anisocytosis	Normal to hypochromic and microcytic	Hypochromic and microcytic to normal
nRBCs in peripheral blood	Occasional	Common	Rare	Rare
Platelet count	Normal or increased	Normal, increased, or decreased	Normal to increased	Markedly increased
LAP	Markedly decreased	Usually increased	Usually increased	Normal
Bone marrow	Marked myeloid proliferation, panmyelosis	Hypercellular, panmyelosis, "dry tap," and fibrosis	Hypercellular, panmyelosis, and decreased iron stores	Hypercellular, panmyelosis, marked megakaryocytic proliferation with abutment
Splenomegaly	Moderate to marked	Marked	Mild or absent	Absent or mild
Special studies	Philadelphia chromosome in all hematopoietic cells	Marrow imaging, normal urine hydroxyproline, occasional 13 q–	Increased RBC mass, normal arterial O_2 saturation, decreased to normal erythropoietin, increased histamine	Abnormal in-vitro platelet aggregation studies

about 10% of cases are reported in children and adolescents. Males slightly outnumber females.

Clinical symptoms are usually nonspecific, and include fatigue, weight loss, anorexia, and headache. Significant splenomegaly develops in 80–90% of patients, and may cause abdominal discomfort. Lymphadenopathy is unusual at presentation. Up to 50% of patients may be asymptomatic.

Peripheral blood findings are highly suggestive of the diagnosis. Total WBC counts are typically $>25 \times 10^9$/L, and in at least half of cases number $>100 \times 10^9$/L. All stages of granulocytic maturation are present, with myelocytes and neutrophils predominating (Fig. 11). Up to 3% myeloblasts are acceptable. Eosinophilia and basophilia are usually present; monocytosis is occasionally observed. Thrombocytosis occurs in >50% of patients, with counts up to $1{,}000{,}000 \times 10^9$/L in some. Thrombocytopenia is observed in <10% of cases. Giant and hypogranular platelets may be identified. Most patients have a mild to moderate normocytic, normochromic anemia, although occasional cases have normal or elevated hemoglobin concentrations. Small numbers of nucleated RBCs are often present.

Bone marrow aspirate smears closely resemble the peripheral blood, with granulocytic maturation predominant. Neutrophils and myelocytes are most numerous, and myeloblasts represent <5% of nucleated elements. The myeloid-to-erythroid ratio is usually >10 : 1. Megakaryocytes are usually small but mature. Erythropoiesis is adequate or relatively decreased and normoblastic. Scattered mast cells and pseudo-Gaucher cells are often present.

Bone marrow biopsy material demonstrates hypercellularity with granulocytic predominance and occasional early reticulum fibrosis. Megakaryocytic abutment and exaggerated nuclear lobation is generally not observed.

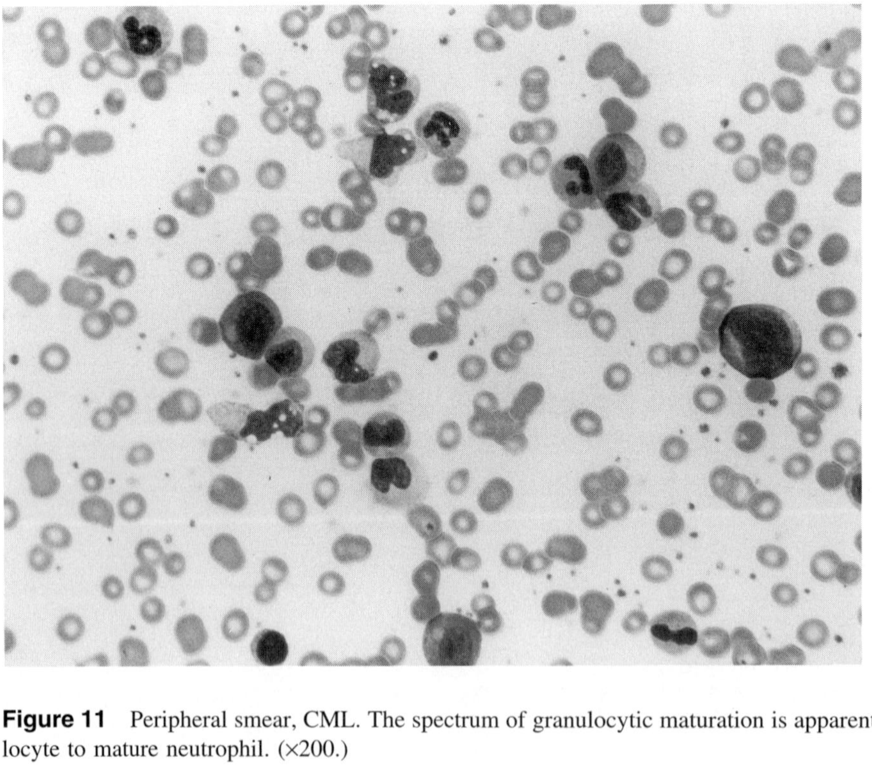

Figure 11 Peripheral smear, CML. The spectrum of granulocytic maturation is apparent, from promyelocyte to mature neutrophil. (×200.)

A low or absent LAP score provides initial supportive diagnostic evidence. Elevated serum B_{12} and B_{12}-binding proteins are also present.

Cytogenetic analysis demonstrates the Philadelphia chromosome (Ph) [t(9;22) (q34;q11)] in about 90% of cases resembling CML. Of the remaining 10%, about 5% will have a demonstrable *bcr-abl* molecular genetic equivalent. The remaining cases often have atypical clinical and pathologic features and may represent difficult-to-classify chronic myeloproliferative diseases.

After the initial chronic phase, which lasts an average of 3–4 years, most patients develop "accelerated phase" or "blast crisis," which resembles evolving and acute leukemia, respectively. Diagnostic criteria for accelerated phase is imprecise, but usually includes a peripheral blood or bone marrow blast count of 15–29%. Blast crisis is recognized when peripheral blood or marrow blasts meet or exceed 30%. These changes are usually accompanied by increased reticulum fibrosis, dyserythropoiesis, and dysmegakaryopoiesis. The LAP score may normalize, and cytogenetic studies usually demonstrate additional abnormalities, often including a second Ph. Cytochemical and immunophenotypic analysis of the blasts demonstrate myeloid differentiation in about 70% of cases. Monoblastic, megakaryoblastic, erythroblastic, and mixed-lineage leukemias have all been reported. In the remaining 30%, blast crisis is lymphoblastic, with French-American-British cooperative group (FAB) L1 or L2 morphology, and a Tdt-positive, CALLA+, precursor B-cell phenotype. The median survival after metamorphosis to blast crisis is 2–6 months.

The differential diagnosis of chronic-phase CML includes reactive granulocytosis, leukemoid reaction, CNL, CMML, and other chronic myeloproliferative disorders. The LAP score, presence or absence of basophilia, eosinophilia, and peripheral blood myeloblasts are features helpful in distinguishing reactive processes from CML.

Juvenile CML (JCML) is an uncommon Ph-negative, bcr-abl-negative myeloproliferative disorder which usually affects male children under the age of 4 years. There is an increased incidence of JCML in patients with neurofibromatosis. Recently, the term *juvenile chronic myelomonocytic leukemia* (CMML) has been introduced for this disorder.

Clinical presentation includes fatigue, fever, bleeding, or rash. Hepatosplenomegaly is commonly observed; lymphadenopathy is less frequent.

Peripheral blood findings include leukocytosis, absolute monocytosis, all stages of granulocyte maturation, including small numbers of blasts. Nucleated RBCs, thrombocytopenia, elevated hemoglobin F levels, and polyclonal hypergammaglobulinemia are additional findings.

Bone marrow examination demonstrates increased monocytes and trilineage dyspoiesis. Some cases terminate in acute leukemia.

Cytogenetic and molecular genetic studies show no Ph or *bcr-abl* abnormalities. Monosomy 7 has been observed, but is not specific. Mutations involving the *N-ras* gene have been identified in some cases using PCR technology.

B. Chronic Neutrophilic Leukemia

Chronic neutrophilic leukemia (CNL) is an unusual disorder of adults over 50 years of age, with a slight male predominance. Clinical features and associated conditions are outlined in Table 13.

Mature neutrophils account for 90–95% of circulating WBCs (Fig. 12). Rare patients have more immature granulocytes or nucleated RBCs.

Bone marrow studies reveal granulocytic hyperplasia with normal blast count, slightly diminished normoblastic erythropoiesis, and numerically normal or minimally increased mega-

Table 13 Clinical and Hematologic Features of Chronic Neutrophilic Leukemia

Neutrophilia (>25–50 × 10^9/L)	
No toxic granulation/no Dohle bodies	
Anemia	
Splenomegaly	(85%)
Hepatomegaly	
Lymphadenopathy	Rare
Other associations	
Gouty arthritis, monoclonal gammopathy, multiple myeloma, and polycythemia rubra vera	

karyocytes without abutment or prominent endoreduplication. Myelofibrosis is generally not observed.

The LAP score is elevated in CNL. Cytogenetic studies are usually normal, although random chromosomal abnormalities are occasionally detected. The Ph is not observed.

The differential diagnosis includes CML and leukemoid reaction. The former is most easily distinguished from CNL by LAP score and cytogenetic or molecular genetic analysis.

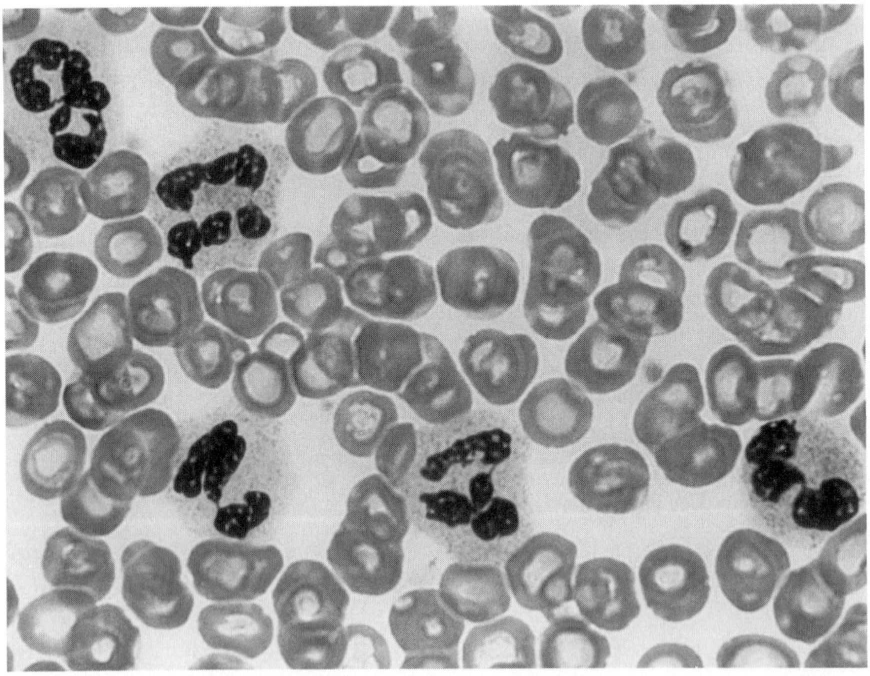

Figure 12 Peripheral smear, CNL. Mature neutrophils with normal nuclear segmentation and cytoplasmic granularity. (×1000.)

C. Chronic Myelomonocytic Leukemia

Chronic myelomonocytic leukemia (CMML) is most often classified as a myelodysplastic disorder and shares with other myelodysplastic syndromes (MDS) findings of peripheral cytopenias and trilineage dyspoiesis in the bone marrow.

CMML usually occurs in patients over 60 years of age; men outnumber women 3 : 1. Presenting symptoms are related to cytopenias, including fatigue, bleeding, or infection. Hepatosplenomegaly is observed in about 40% of cases. Increased serum and urine lysozyme levels are often present.

The common hematologic manifestations of CMML are illustrated in Table 14. A minimum absolute monocyte count of 1×10^9/L is required for diagnosis. As with other MDS, cases of CMML usually demonstrate dyspoietic neutrophils, including Pelgeroid nuclei and cytoplasmic hypogranularity (Fig. 13). Immaturity is often present, with less than 5% blast forms.

Bone marrow aspirates demonstrate granulocytic and monocytic predominance. Up to 19% of nucleated cells may be blasts. Both type I and type II blasts are included in the count (type I with no granules, type II with <15 azurophilic granules). When 20–29% of nucleated cells are blasts, the process is designated CMML in transformation (CMML-T).

Myelomonocytic differentiation can be demonstrated utilizing cytochemical reactions, including Sudan black B, myeloperoxidase, nonspecific esterases (A-EST, B-EST), and chloroacetate esterase. Occasional cells with dual granulocytic/monocytic differentiation may be demonstrated by combined chloroacetate and nonspecific esterase methods.

Dysmegakaryopoiesis is manifest by decreased nuclear segmentation ("pawn ball" forms) and "micromegakaryocytes." Dyserythropoietic changes include megaloblastoid nuclei, dyskinetic nuclear divisions, basophilic stippling, and variable numbers of ringed sideroblasts.

Bone marrow biopsies are usually hypercellular, often with abnormal localization of myeloid precursors away from the bony trabeculae. Myelofibrosis usually does not develop.

Cytogenetic abnormalities are commonly observed in CMML, but are nonspecific. The most common karyotypic aberrations are listed in Table 3. Overexpression of the *K-ras* oncogene has been associated with a t(5;12) abnormality. Neither the Ph or *bcr-abl* molecular equivalent have been observed.

The differential diagnosis of CMML includes Ph-negative, *bcr-abl*-negative CML, and the other myelodysplastic syndromes. Cases of Ph-negative CML which lack basophilia and have

Table 14 Hematologic Features of Chronic Myelomonocytic Leukemia

Leukocytosis	(65%)
Monocytosis ($>1 \times 10^9$/L)	
Required for diagnosis	
Neutropenia	(50%)
Pelgeroid forms, hypogranularity present	
Neutrophilia	(50%)
Thrombocytopenia	(25%)
Abnormal forms present	
Macrocytic anemia	
Coarse basophilic stippling, polychromasia, and occasional nucleated RBCs	

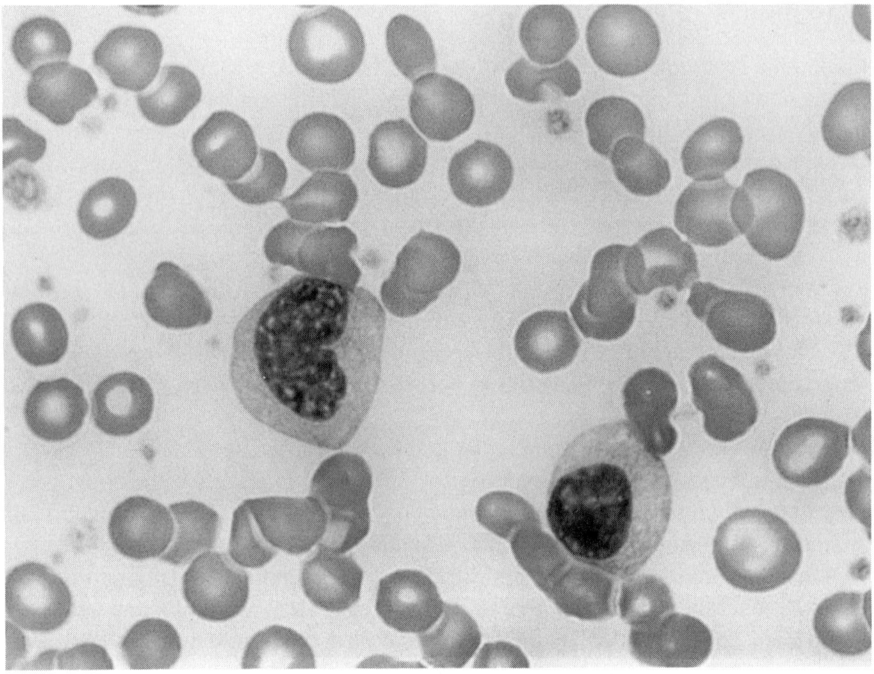

Figure 13 Peripheral blood smear, CMML. Monocyte and adjacent neutrophil demonstrating nuclear hyposegmentation characteristic of the myelodysplastic syndromes. (×1000.)

pronounced monocytosis can be difficult to distinguish from CMML with more proliferative than dysplastic features, and may require reevaluation at appropriate intervals to discover the true nature of the disease.

D. Chronic Monocytic Leukemia

Chronic monocytic leukemia (CMoL) is a rare disorder which lacks complete diagnostic criteria. The best-documented cases are in adults; males predominate. Presenting symptoms include fatigue, fever, and abdominal discomfort secondary to splenomegaly. Hepatomegaly is frequently observed.

Peripheral blood evaluation reveals a mild normocytic, normochromic anemia. The total WBC count varies from low to increased, up to about 25×10^9/L. Thrombocytopenia is present in about half of patients. Absolute monocytosis develops immediately, or up to 2 years after splenectomy. Circulating monocytes have normal morphology (Fig. 14). Occasionally, promonocytes are identified. No monoblasts, Auer rods, or myelodysplastic changes are observed. Infiltration of parenchymal organs frequently occurs.

Bone marrow biopsies before splenectomy are hypocellular or normocellular, and may lack significant monocytic infiltrates. After splenectomy, the monocytic infiltrate develops progressively, at the expense of normal hematopoietic elements. Erythrophagocytosis and platelet phagocytosis are observed in some cases. Myelofibrosis is usually absent.

No consistent cytogenetic or molecular genetic anomalies have been reported in CMoL. Absence of the Ph is important to document.

The differential diagnosis of CMoL includes CMML, other chronic monocytic/histiocytic

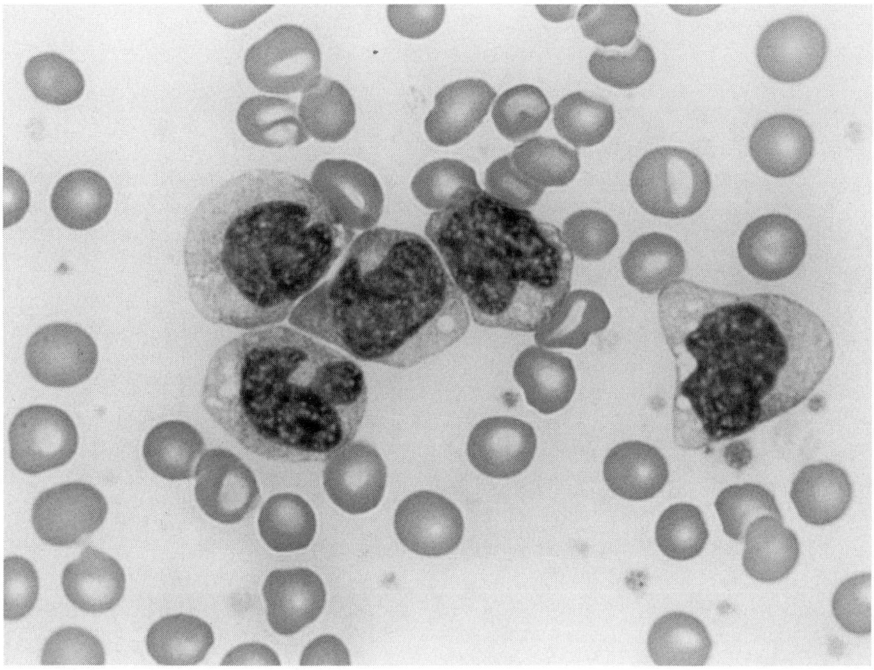

Figure 14 Peripheral smear, CMoL. Several mature monocytes with folded or lobed nuclei, abundant occasionally vacuolated cytoplasm. (×1000.)

neoplasms, HCL, and AML-M4 and M5. The presence or absence of TRAP-positivity, myelodysplasia, and bone marrow blast counts helps differentiate CMoL from the most common entities. Clinical and cytologic features are important in distinguishing CMoL from the malignant histiocytoses.

E. Hypereosinophilic Syndromes

Eosinophilia occurs during the course of a variety of disorders, and may be considered reactive (associated with a recognized nonneoplastic stimulus), idiopathic (sustained eosinophilia of 1.5 $\times 10^9$/L for at least 6 months without recognized stimulus), or associated with neoplasia.

Reactive eosinophilia ($>600 \times 10^9$/L) is associated with numerous conditions, including allergies, drug reactions, parasitic infections, and connective tissue disorders. The eosinophilia is usually transient, and resolves following appropriate therapy for the underlying disorder.

Patients which fulfill the diagnostic criteria for idiopathic hypereosinophilia may encompass both neoplastic and nonneoplastic proliferations, and may result in widespread tissue damage. Some cases represent eosinophilic leukemoid reactions, while others may be classified as myeloproliferative disorders. In this latter category, the eosinophils often demonstrate dysmorphic cytologic features such as nuclear hypersegmentation or hyposegmentation and cytoplasmic vacuolization (Fig. 15).

Eosinophilia associated with lymphoproliferative disorders is generally considered reactive. Most are T-cell processes, and include mycosis fungoides, T-cell lymphomas, and acute lymphoblastic leukemia. Eosinophilia accompanying Hodgkin's disease and solid parenchymal neoplasms is also considered reactive.

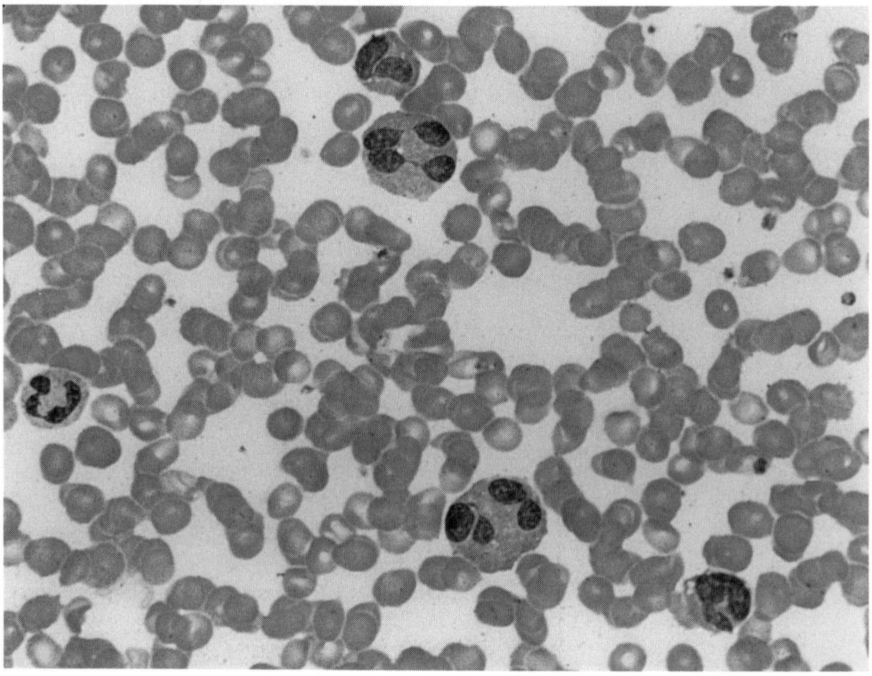

Figure 15 Peripheral smear, hypereosinophilic syndrome. Several eosinophils, including two large forms with nuclear hypersegmentation. (×400.)

In contrast, there is morphologic and cytogenetic evidence that the eosinophils in acute and chronic myeloproliferative processes, including AML (FAB-M4Eo) and CML, are part of the neoplastic proliferation.

True eosinophilic leukemia has been documented in over 100 cases, but lacks well-defined diagnostic criteria because the peripheral eosinophil counts have varied considerably and consistent blast counts have not been observed.

F. Mast Cell Leukemia

Mast cell proliferations have been divided into indolent, aggressive, and leukemic forms. Indolent mast cell proliferations tend to be diagnosed in infancy and childhood, are dominated by cutaneous manifestations, and usually resolve at puberty. Mast cell proliferations arising in adulthood may be indolent, or may behave more aggressively; the latter form manifesting with urticaria pigmentosa, hepatosplenomegaly, and constitutional symptoms.

Cases of indolent mastocytosis do not have circulating peripheral blood mast cells. Small numbers of circulating mast cells may be observed in aggressive mastocytosis, but do not imply leukemic transformation.

The least common manifestation of systemic mast cell disease is mast cell leukemia (MCL), which is a rare disorder. Patients frequently present with constitutional symptoms and peptic ulcer disease. Total WBC counts are variable (ranging from 8.5 to 66.0×10^9/L), with absolute mast cell counts ranging from 0.65 to 47.0×10^9/L. Mast cells should constitute a minimum of 10% of the WBC differential to establish the diagnosis of MCL. The number of circulating mast cells does not seem to correlate with either tumor burden or survival.

Bone marrow involvement is reported in up to 75% of cases, including indolent forms. Bone marrow aspirates reveal numerous atypical mast cells in all forms of the disease. Bone marrow biopsy material usually demonstrates focal lesions in indolent mastocytoses, while the more aggressive systemic forms reveal diffuse and extensive infiltrates. The neoplastic mast cells usually acquire a spindle shape with round to oval nuclei, inconspicuous nucleoli, and fairly abundant pink granular cytoplasm. Mitotic figures are sparse, and varying degrees of accompanying fibrosis are observed.

The pattern of bone marrow involvement is reported to have prognostic significance. Favorable histology consists of focal paratrabecular and perivascular infiltrates with an admixed fibroinflammatory component, reticulum fibrosis, and normal intervening bone marrow. Intermediate prognosis histology includes sheets of mast cells in a perivascular or paratrabecular location, myelofibrosis, osteosclerosis, and granulocytic hyperplasia in the intervening marrow. Diffuse lesions are predictive of a poor prognosis and MCL.

Toluidine blue stain demonstrates a metachromatic granular cytoplasmic pattern in mast cells, supporting the diagnosis. Immunophenotyping studies have demonstrated variable positivity with CD2, CD4, CD11b, CD33, and CD45. No consistent cytogenetic abnormalities have been recognized.

The differential diagnosis includes HCL, idiopathic myelofibrosis, Hodgkin's disease, eosinophilic fibrohistiocytic lesion, AML-M3, angioimmunoblastic lymphadenopathy with dysproteinemia, and blast crisis of CML with basophilic and mast cell precursors.

CASE STUDY 1

Patient

Thirty-year-old male.

Chief Complaint

Four- to 6-month history of increasing fatigue, weight loss, and easy bruising. Two-week history of increasing abdominal girth.

Medical History

G6PD deficiency.

Physical Examination

Splenomegaly palpable to the level of the umbilicus; no hepatomegaly or significant adenopathy.

Laboratory Results

Screening procedures showed WBC 340×10^9/L with the following differential count: segmented neutrophils 46%, band forms 9%, metamyelocytes 7%, myelocytes 9%, blasts 8%, lymphocytes 5%, eosinophils 10%, basophils 5%, 4 nRBC/100WBC. HCT was 0.22, and platelets 226×10^9/L. PT was 11.7 sec, and aPTT was 36.3 sec.

Questions

1. What diagnosis should be considered?
2. What additional laboratory studies should be performed to confirm the diagnosis?
3. How do the results of molecular genetic studies influence the diagnosis and clinical course?

Additional Laboratory Results

1. Bone marrow examination (Fig. 16) revealed panmyelosis with myeloid : erythroid > 10 : 1. Myeloblasts accounted for 9% of all nucleated cells. No significant reticulum fibrosis was observed.
2. Leukocyte alkaline phosphatase: markedly decreased.
3. Cytogenetic studies: 46XY.
4. Molecular genetic studies: positive for *bcr/abl* gene fusion by Southern blot and specific DNA probe analysis.

Diagnosis

Chronic myelogenous leukemia, chronic phase, Philadelphia chromosome (Ph) negative, *bcr/abl* positive.

Discussion

This case demonstrates the need to pursue molecular genetic studies in cases clinically and morphologically consistent with CML, but lacking a Ph chromosome on routine cytogenetic analysis. The diagnostic criteria for Ph-negative CML are the same as for Ph-positive CML, except for the absence of the Ph on cytogenetic studies.

CML can be subdivided according to cytogenetic and molecular genetic features. Approximately 90% of cases demonstrate the t(9;22)(q34;q11) Ph chromosome. As CML is a stem cell disorder, the Ph chromosome can be demonstrated in all hematopoietic bone marrow cells, as well as many B lymphocytes. Since occasional cases of T-cell lymphoblastic crises of CML have been described, it is likely that some T lymphocytes also contain the Ph chromosome.

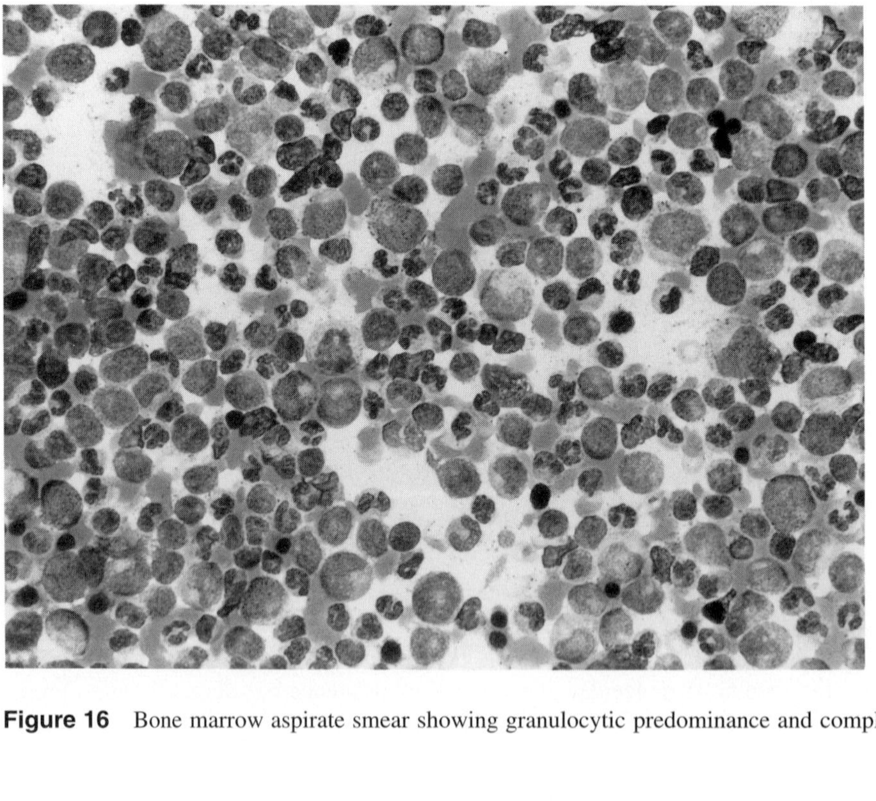

Figure 16 Bone marrow aspirate smear showing granulocytic predominance and complete maturation.

Variations of the Ph chromosome which can be identified by cytogenetic studies account for about 5% of CML cases. The remaining 5% of cases morphologically consistent with CML have normal karyotypes or have cytogenetic aberrations which involve neither chromosome 9 nor 22. These cases are classified as Ph-negative CML. Almost half of these Ph-negative patients have demonstrable *bcr/abl* fusion genes by molecular methods, and resemble their Ph-positive counterparts both clinically and hematologically.

The Ph chromosome and the *bcr/abl* fusion gene are not unique to chronic-phase CML, but are also identified in blast crisis of CML (both lymphoid and myeloid phenotypes) and in de-novo acute leukemias. Rearrangements of *bcr/abl* are present in approximately 20% of adult ALLs, 10% of childhood ALLs, and in a small percent of adult AMLs.

Subtle molecular differences in the *bcr/abl* fusions result in an 8.5-kb mRNA and a 210-kD fusion protein product in CML, and a 7.3-kb mRNA, 190-kD protein product in many de-novo acute leukemias.

Clinical and pathologic differences have been observed between *bcr/abl*-positive and *bcr/abl*-negative CML. In general, *bcr/abl*-negative patients tend to be older (median age 65 years) than *bcr/abl*-positive patients, are more likely to complain of weight loss and fatigue, and have hepatosplenomegaly, lymphadenopathy, and peripheral cytopenias. LAP scores may be diminished, elevated, or normal. Fewer *bcr/abl*-negative patients terminate in blast crisis, but are more likely to succumb to bleeding or infection.

As CML may be accompanied by monocytosis and mild to moderate dysplastic changes, CMML is often considered in the differential diagnosis. CMML has more clinical and laboratory similarities to *bcr/abl*-negative CML than *bcr/abl*-positive disease. The *bcr/abl* gene rearrangement has not been described in CMML. Up to 50% of CMML cases have cytogenetic abnormalities, but rarely involve chromosomes 9 and 22.

Summary

Morphology: typical CML
Cytogenetics: 46XY
Molecular genetics: positive for *bcr/abl* chimeric gene
Diagnosis: Ph-negative, *bcr/abl*-positive CML

Bibliography

1. Bartram CR. Rearrangement of the c-abl and bcr genes in Ph-negative CML and Ph-positive acute leukemias. Leukemia 1988; 2:63–64.
2. Croce CM, Huebner K, Isobe M, et al. Mapping four distinct BCR-related loci to chromosome 22q11: order of BCR loci relative to CML and ALL breakpoints. Proc Natl Acad Sci USA 1987; 84:7174–7178.
3. Hirsch-Ginsberg C, Childs C, Chang K-S, et al. Phenotypic and heterogeneity in Philadelphia chromosome-positive acute leukemia. Blood 1988; 71:186–195.
4. Kantarjian HM, Shtalrid M, Kurzrock R, et al. Significance and correlations of molecular analysis results in patients with Philadelphia chromosome-negative chronic myelogenous leukemia and chronic myelomonocytic leukemia. Am J Med 1988; 85: 639–644.
5. Kantarjian HM, Kurzrock R, Talpaz M. Philadelphia chromosome negative chronic myelogenous leukemia and chronic myelomonocytic leukemia. Hematol Oncol Clin N Am 1990; 4:389–404.
6. Kawasaki E, Clark SS, Coyne MY, et al. Diagnosis of CML and ALL by detection

of leukemia-specific mRNA sequences amplified in vitro. Proc Natl Acad Sci USA 1988; 85:5698–5702.
7. Kurzrock R, Gutterman J, Talpaz M. The molecular genetics of Philadelphia chromosome positive leukemias. N Engl J Med 1988; 319:990–998.
8. Shtalrid M, Talpaz M, Blick M, et al. Philadelphia-negative chronic myelogenous leukemia with bcr rearrangement: molecular analysis and clinical characteristics. J Clin Oncol 1988; 6:1569–1575.

CASE STUDY 2

Patient

Sixty-nine-year-old male.

Chief Complaint

Malaise, fatigue, fevers for 2 weeks.

Medical History

Chronic lymphocytic leukemia for 3 years, controlled with prednisone and chlorambucil.

Physical Examination

Moderate hepatosplenomegaly, mild peripheral lymphadenopathy.

Laboratory Results

Screening procedures showed WBC 1.2×10^9/L with the following differential count: segmented neutrophils 56%, lymphocytes 44%. HCT was 0.26, Hgb was 8.6 g/dL, platelets were 17×10^9/L. Serum chemistries revealed a significant metabolic acidosis and elevated liver function studies.

Hospital Course

Ischemic bowel was suspected, and the patient was taken to surgery for exploratory laparotomy. At operation, the liver was dusky gray and nodular, consistent with hepatic necrosis. A needle biopsy of the liver was performed (Fig. 17), and an abdominal lymph node was sampled (Fig. 18).

Questions

1. How does one prove clonality in cases of cytologically transformed CLL?
2. What are the different types of cytologic transformation described in CLL?

Additional Laboratory Results

Immunoperoxidase studies on paraffin-imbedded material: Leukocyte common antigen +, L-26 +, UCHL-1 −, S-100 protein −, cytokeratin −

Flow cytometric immunophenotyping on lymph node material: LCA +, CD19 +, CD20 +, CD22 +, CD5+, IgM +, lambda +

Diagnosis

Richter's syndrome.

Discussion

Richter's syndrome (or Richter's transformation), first described in 1928, is defined as the development of a large cell lymphoma during the course of chronic lymphocytic leukemia

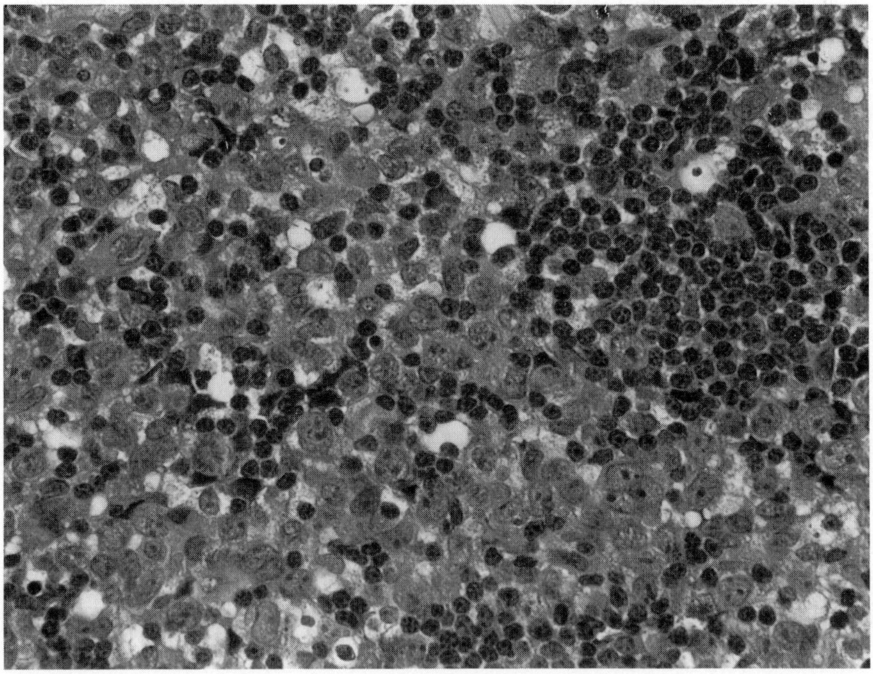

Figure 17 Liver biopsy demonstrating a mixture of large nucleolated cells and a background of small round lymphocytes. (×400.)

(CLL). Richter's transformation occurs in about 8% of CLL patients, and can be suspected when a CLL patient suddenly develops unexplained weight loss, fever, organomegaly, and rapidly increasing lymphadenopathy.

It is thought that cytologic transformation begins in nodal tissue, then rapidly involves extranodal sites, including spleen, liver, bone marrow, and other parenchymal organs, especially the gastrointestinal tract. Peripheral blood involvement by the transformed cells is unusual.

Examination of lymph node biopsy material demonstrates transformed lymphoid cells infiltrating in a diffuse pattern, often leaving foci of small, round, CLL lymphocytes in the background. The large cells have irregular nuclei with marginated chromatin and one or two prominent nucleoli. Cytoplasm is variably abundant and often basophilic. Reed-Sternberg-like cells are frequently observed.

Prolymphocytic transformation of CLL (CLL/PLL) is the most frequent type, occurring in about 25% of cases, and is defined as 11–55% of peripheral blood lymphocytes having prolymphocytic features. Prolymphocytic transformation is accompanied by increasing leukocytosis, anemia, thrombocytopenia, lymphadenopathy, and splenomegaly.

Transformation of CLL to acute leukemia is rare. Cases of transformation to AML are usually associated with prior exposure to alkylating chemotherapeutic agents or radiotherapy. Transformation to ALL has been supported by immunologic and cytogenetic studies.

Plasmacytoid transformation of CLL occurs even less frequently than acute leukemic transformation, and is defined as the development of multiple myeloma during the course of CLL. Morphologic features of the plasma cell proliferation are similar to de-novo multiple myeloma.

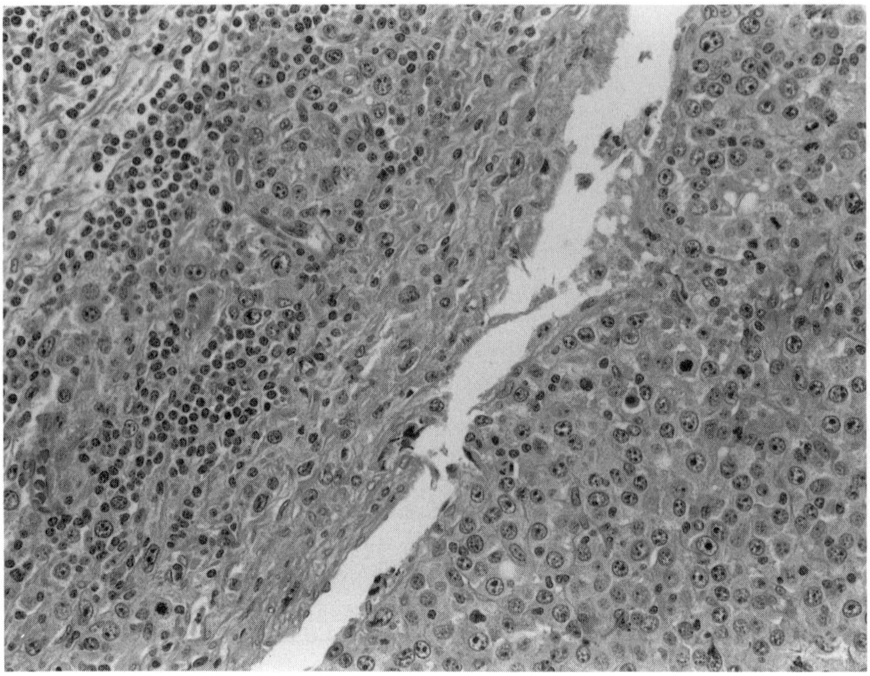

Figure 18 Lymph node biopsy showing large pleomorphic cells with prominent nucleoli replacing the normal architecture. Collections of small round lymphocytes are seen within the thickened capsule. (×200.)

Paraimmunoblastic transformation is the most recently described variant of transformed CLL. Small numbers of paraimmunoblasts are normally seen within the proliferation centers of lymph nodes involved by CLL, and are of intermediate size, have open nuclear chromatin, a conspicuous central nucleolus, and a moderate amount of pale-staining cytoplasm. When paraimmunoblasts are seen in a diffuse pattern, the designation *paraimmunoblastic transformation* is appropriate (Fig. 19). Occasional patients present initially with diffuse paraimmunoblastic proliferations. In such cases, the diagnosis of paraimmunoblastic variant of small lymphocytic lymphoma/leukemia can be rendered.

Proof of a clonal relationship between the small lymphoid population of CLL and the transformed cells can be supported by consistent light-chain restriction, cytogenetic findings, and identical immunoglobulin gene rearrangements by Southern blot analysis. Consistent CD5 positivity is demonstrable in many cases.

It has been recently emphasized that demonstration of clonality by molecular means requires analysis of both the heavy- and light-chain immunoglobulin genes, as postrearrangement mutations in the heavy-chain genes are fairly common, but are less likely to affect the light-chain genes.

The clinical course of CLL after cytologic transformation is variable, but generally accelerated. Richter's and prolymphocytic transformations are associated with a median survival of 12 months or less from the time of onset. Paraimmunoblastic transformation has a reported median survival of slightly more than 2 years.

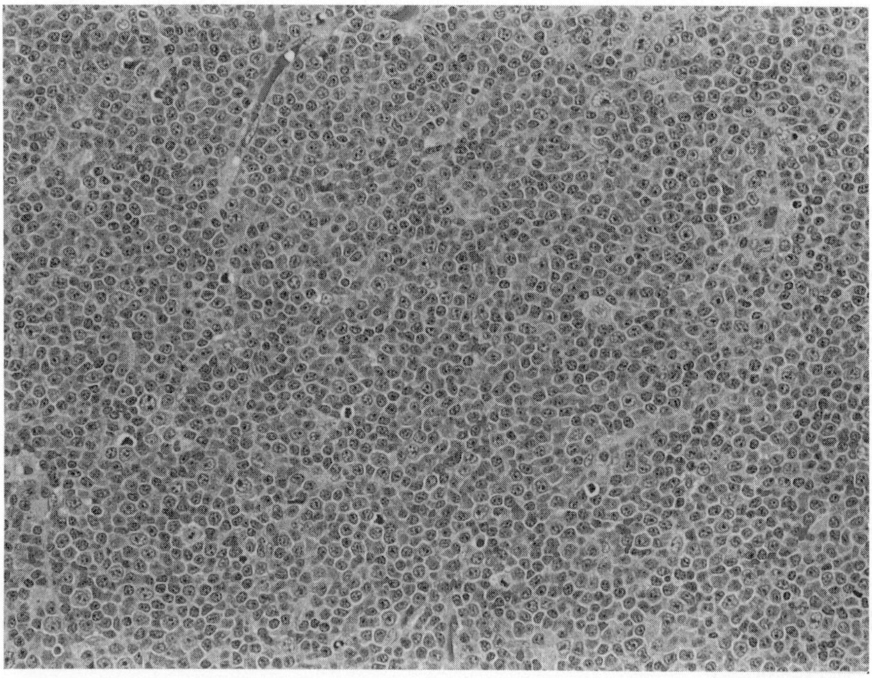

Figure 19 Lymph node biopsy demonstrating the diffuse pattern characteristic of paraimmunoblastic transformation. The cells are intermediate in size, have open chromatin, conspicuous nucleoli, and a moderate amount of cytoplasm. (×100.)

Summary

Morphology: malignant large cell infiltrate in the setting of CLL
Paraffin imbedded immunoperoxidase: LCA +, L26 +, UCHL-1 –, S-100 protein –, cytokeratin –
Flow cytometry immunophenotyping: LCA+, CD19+, CD20+, CD22+, CD5+
Cytogenetics: not performed, but usually shows trisomy 12 or 14q+
Molecular genetics: not performed, but usually shows clonal immunoglobulin gene rearrangement
Diagnosis: Richter's syndrome

Bibliography

1. Foucar K, Rydell RE. Richter's syndrome in chronic lymphocytic leukemia. Cancer 1980; 46:118–134.
2. Kjeldsberg CR, Marty J. Prolymphocytic transformation of chronic lymphocytic leukemia. Cancer 1981; 48:2447–2457.
3. Lane PK, Townsend RM, Beckstead JH, Corash L. Central nervous system involvement in a patient with chronic lymphocytic leukemia and non-Hodgkin's lymphoma (Richter's syndrome), with concordant cell surface immunoglobulin isotypic and immunophenotypic markers. Am J Clin Pathol 1988; 89:254–259.
4. Miyamura K, Osada H, Yamauchi T, et al. Single clonal origin of neoplastic B-cells

with different immunoglobulin light chains in a patient with Richter's syndrome. Cancer 1990; 66:140–144.
5. Pines A, Ben-Bassat I, Selzer G, Ramot B. Transformation of chronic lymphocytic leukemia to plasmacytoma. Cancer 1984; 54:1904–1907.
6. Pugh WC, Manning JT, Butler JJ. Paraimmunoblastic variant of small lymphocytic lymphoma/leukemia. Am J Surg Pathol 1988; 12:907–917.
7. Richter MN. Generalized reticular cell sarcoma of lymph nodes associated with lymphatic leukemia. Am J Pathol 1928; 4:285–292.
8. Saltman DL, Ross JA, Banks RE, et al. Molecular evidence for a single clonal origin in biphenotypic concomitant chronic lymphocytic leukemia and multiple myeloma. Blood 1989; 74:2062–2065.
9. Scully RE, Mark EJ, McNeely WF, McNeely BU (editors). Richter's syndrome. Case Records of the Massachusetts General Hospital (Case 18-1991). N Engl J Med 1991; 324:1267–1277.
10. Sun T, Susin M, Desner M, et al. The clonal origin of two cell populations in Richter's syndrome. Hum Pathol 1990; 21:722–728.
11. Tohda S, Morio T, Suzuki T, et al. Richter's syndrome with two B cell clones possessing different surface immunoglobulin gene rearrangements. Am J Hematol 1990; 35:32–36.

SELECTED READINGS

1. Brunning RD, McKenna RW. Tumors of the Bone Marrow, in Atlas of Tumor Pathology, Third Series, Fascicle 9. Washington, DC: Armed Forces Institute of Pathology, 1994.
2. Canellos GP, ed. Chronic leukemias. Hematol/Oncol Clin N Am 1990; 4:319–506.
3. Fenoglio-Preiser CM, Willman CL. Molecular Diagnostics in Pathology. Baltimore: Williams & Wilkins, 1991.
4. Foucar K. Bone Marrow Pathology. Chicago: American Society of Clinical Pathologists Press, 1995.
5. Keren DF, Hanson CA, Hurtubise PE. Flow Cytometry. 2d ed. Chicago: American Society of Clinical Pathologists Press, 1994.
6. Schumacher HR, Cotelingam JD. Chronic Leukemia. New York: Igaku-Shoin, 1993.
7. Sun T, Li CY, Yam LT. Atlas of Cytochemistry and Immunochemistry of Hematologic Neoplasms. Chicago: American Society of Clinical Pathologists Press, 1985.

10

Myeloproliferative Disorders

Powers Peterson
Sentara Norfolk General Hospital, Norfolk, Virginia

DEFINITION

The chronic myeloproliferative disorders (MPDs) include a group of clonal stem cell disorders characterized by self-perpetuating and differentiating proliferation of seemingly only one of the myeloid lines in bone marrow. The term was originally coined by Dameshek (1951) and includes a group of closely related diseases shown in Table 1. The acute myeloproliferative disorders originally in this classification are discussed elsewhere in this volume. With the exception of chronic myelogenous leukemia, the chronic MPDs are discussed below.

POLYCYTHEMIA VERA (PRIMARY POLYCYTHEMIA) AND OTHER ERYTHROCYTOSES

Definition

Polycythemia in the broad sense denotes an overabundance of circulating red blood cells (RBCs). However, the term is not synonymous with erythrocytosis. The diagnosis of polycythemia vera (PV) depends on an absolute increase in the red cell mass. If the hemoglobin (Hb) level or hematocrit (Hct) is only slightly increased, it may be that a reduced plasma volume has produced only a relative polycythemia. Under these circumstances, determination of the red cell mass (RCM) may be warranted (Fig. 1).

The RCM is determined directly by labeling erythrocytes with ^{51}Cr. The RCM is directly proportional to the dilution of the ^{51}Cr -labeled cells; i.e., the greater the dilution, the larger the RCM.

Classification

The polycythemias are classified in four broad groups:

1. Polycythemia vera (primary polycythemia): a clonal stem-cell disorder, in which all marrow cellular production is variant
2. Secondary polycythemias: a group of unrelated disorders in which increased amounts of erythropoietin (Epo) are produced. The underlying pathophysiology may be physiologic (tissue hypoxia) or nonphysiologic.

Table 1 Myeloproliferative Disorders

Acute
Erythroleukemia
DiGuglielmo's syndrome—M6a—myeloblastic predominant
DiGuglielmo's disorder—M6b—proerythroblastic predominant
M6c—combined M6a and M6b
Acute myelogenous leukemia (AML)
Acute megakaryocytic leukemia (FAB AML, M7)
Chronic
Polycythemia vera
Chronic myelogenous leukemia
Essential thrombocythemia
Myelofibrosis with myeloid metaplasia

3. Familial polycythemias: rare primary erythrocytoses occurring in two or more family members.
4. Stress polycythemia (Gaisböck's syndrome): an erythrocytosis secondary to decreased plasma volume with only a small increase in RCM.

Polycythemia Vera (Primary Polycythemia)

Clinical Findings

Polycythemia vera (PV) is a clonal disease primarily of middle-aged and older adults. Males are affected slightly more than females. The disease appears to be as common among Jews as among other Caucasians, although it is probably less common in blacks.

Patients are often asymptomatic, especially in the very early stages of the disease; the

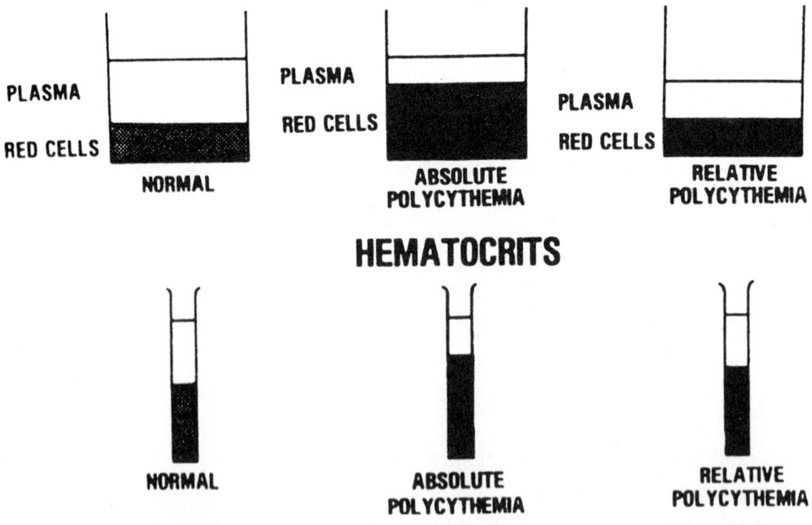

Figure 1 Hematocrit in relation to red cell mass and plasma volume in normal person and in patients with absolute and relative polycythemia.

disorder may be discovered accidently. Complaints of headaches, dizziness, weakness, malaise, fatigue, or visual disturbances are common. Symptoms of vascular disease may manifest as angina, intermittent claudication, and cerebral insufficiency. Thrombotic episodes—myocardial infarcts, erythromelalgia, hepatic vein thrombosis (Budd-Chiari syndrome)—are well documented. Paradoxically, patients with PV tend to bleed, especially from the upper gastrointestinal tract. Intense pruritis may occur following bathing (especially after a hot shower). Almost half of patients have asymptomatic hyperuricemia.

Important physical findings in polycythemia vera include splenomegaly without lymphadenopathy; plethora of the face, hands, feet, ears, and mucous membranes; and engorgement of the retinal and conjunctival veins. Hepatomegaly is detected in 40% of patients at presentation.

Laboratory Findings and Diagnosis

Peripheral Blood Findings. The RBC count is elevated, as is the Hb level and the Hct. The RBCs appear crowded on peripheral smear, even in the thin area of the slide. There are no histological changes in the RBCs that might suggest a diagnosis of PV. In addition to increased numbers of RBCs, a leukocytosis is also common. The cells are predominantly neutrophils and other granulocytes, and the white blood cell (WBC) counts are moderately elevated (12,000 to 25,000/μL). As in the other chronic MPDs, an absolute increase in numbers of basophils and eosinophils may occur.

The platelet count is usually increased, often remarkably so. Some patients present with platelet counts of >1,000,000/μL. Morphologically the platelets may be abnormally large and bizarre.

Hemorrhagic complications occur for the following reasons:

1. Defects in platelet aggregation
2. Increased blood viscosity
3. Defects in platelet metabolism, granules, surface membrane

Bone Marrow. The marrow aspiration and biopsy is a standard part of the evaluation of a patient suspected of having a chronic MPD. Bone marrow examination shows:

1. Increased marrow cellularity (85% to 90% of patients)
2. Absence of marrow iron stores in >95% of patients
3. Increased numbers and size of megakaryocytes
4. Increased volume of the venous sinuses
5. Increased reticulin fiber content (variable finding at diagnosis)

A marrow sample should also be obtained for cytogenetic studies. Although cytogenetic studies in PV have not shown a consistent chromosomal abnormality, it is necessary to exclude the Philadelphia chromosome (Ph^1) or a *bcr* rearrangement.

Erythrocyte Mass. The measurement of absolute RCM is an important procedure in the diagnosis of PV. Increased RCM is defined as ≥36 mL/kg in males and ≥32 mL/kg in females.

Leukocyte Alkaline Phosphatase. The leukocyte alkaline phosphatase (LAP) level is usually increased in patients with PV. The test has limited positive predictive value, but evaluated levels are one of the accepted secondary diagnostic criteria.

Arterial Oxygen Saturation. Adequate oxygenation of tissues results from a concert of synchronous events. In PV and in erythrocytoses due to nonphysiologic increases in Epo, arterial sO_2 is normal. Physiologic increases in Epo secretion resulting from altered oxygen affinity of abnormal Hb are not accompanied by a reduced sO_2. Similarly, arterial sO_2 is normal in polycythemia (PV) due to excessive endogenous or exogenous androgens. On the other hand, erythrocytoses due to a physiologic increase in Epo secretion are characterized by decreased arterial sO_2. These include erythrocytoses resulting from:

1. Cardiopulmonary dysfunction
2. Vascular malformations with arterial-venous shunting
3. Methemoglobinemia and carboxyhemoglobinemia
4. Decreased barometric pressure (high altitudes)

Therefore, the arterial sO_2 is a key test in evaluating an erythrocytosis.

Oxygen Dissociation Curve. Proper tissue oxygenation depends on amount of environmental or available oxygen, Hb concentration, and affinity of oxygen for Hb [pO_2 (0.5)]. The point of reference for affinity of oxygen for Hb has been designated as that partial pressure of oxygen at which the Hb is one-half saturated, i.e., the P_{50}. Under standard conditions of temperature (37°C) and pH (7.4), the P_{50} of normal Hb A is 26.6 mm Hg (Fig. 2). If the value is lower, the P_{50} has shifted to the left; this indicates an increased affinity of Hb for oxygen. Conversely, if the P_{50} value is >26.6 mm Hg, the oxygen affinity of Hb has decreased and the P_{50} has shifted to the right. Those abnormal Hbs with amino acid substitutions resulting in increased oxygen affinity retain oxygen. This retention results in tissue hypoxia, increased Epo formation, and an erythrocytosis. Some examples are Hemoglobins Chesapeake, Vanderbilt, Little Rock, Syracuse.

Erythropoietin. In many erythrocytoses, the aforementioned tests will distinguish between primary and secondary disorders. If not, assays for serum levels of Epo are available, but they lack strong predictive values.

Serum B_{12} and Unsaturated B_{12} Binding Capacity ($UB_{12}BC$). Serum levels of B_{12} and $UB_{12}BC$ are increased in the chronic MPDs, including CML. Both levels are usually increased in PV but are not increased in the other erythrocytoses.

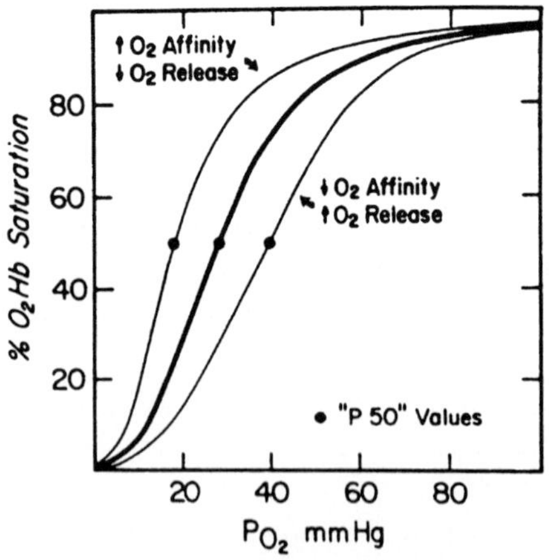

Figure 2 Oxygen dissociation curve of hemoglobin. Affinity of hemoglobin for oxygen is increased when curve shifts to left and decreased when curve shifts to right. (From Oski et al. [1970].)

Other Findings

The serum uric acid in PV may be normal or increased, and patients may have secondary gout. Because of the high blood viscosity, the erythrocyte sedimentation rate may be reduced or even zero mm/h.

Differential Diagnosis

The key diagnostic studies in the evaluation of a patient with elevated Hb are shown in Table 2. These include:

1. Clinical history and physical examination to exclude causes of secondary erythrocytoses and to evaluate for splenomegaly
2. Arterial oxygen saturation
3. Evaluation of Hb (Hb electrophoresis, $P_{50}O_2$, RBC enzymes)
4. Serum Epo levels (to assess familial polycythemias)

Evaluation of RCM with ^{51}Cr may be necessary, but this study is increasingly difficult to obtain.

Diagnosis

In sum, the diagnosis of PV requires obtaining a clinical history, physical exam, and appropriate studies. The Polycythemia Vera Study Group criteria for the diagnosis of PV (Table 3) are widely accepted.

Complications and Course

In addition to increased risks of thrombosis and hemorrhage, there are two other major complications in PV. The first is acute leukemia (AL), or blastic transformation. AL does occur in patients not treated with chemotherapy or radiation, but the incidence is many times higher in treated patients. The AL is most often myelogenous, and survival after the diagnosis of AL is uniformly brief.

Table 2 Differential Diagnosis of Polycythemia

Diagnosis	Key diagnostic test
Polycythemia vera	See Table 3
Secondary polycythemia	
Physiologic	Arterial oxygen saturation
1. Cardiovascular shunts	
2. Pulmonary disease	Arterial oxygen saturation
3. High altitude	Arterial oxygen saturation
4. Obesity (Pickwickian)	Arterial oxygen saturation
5. Smoking	Carboxyhemoglobin level
6. Hemoglobin abnormalities	$P_{50}O_2$, hemoglobin analysis, red cell enzyme analysis
Nonphysiologic	
1. Tumor (kidney, liver, uterus)	Pertinent clinical history and physical examination
2. Renal disease (cysts, hydronephrosis, posttransplant)	Radiological studies
Stress polycythemia (Gaisböck's syndrome)	Carboxyhemoglobin level
Familial erythrocytosis	Erythropoietin level

Table 3 Diagnostic Criteria for Polycythemia Vera

Polycythemia vera is diagnosed if A, B, and C are present:
  A. Red cell mass ≥ 36 mL/kg in males or ≥ 32 mL/kg in females
  B. Arterial oxygen saturation ≥ 92%
  C. Splenomegaly
If splenomegaly is absent, then any two of the following can substitute for C:
  1. Thrombocytosis (platelet count ≥ 400,000/μL)
  2. Leukocytosis without fever or infection (WBC ≥ 12,000/μL)
  3. Leukocyte alkaline phosphatase score ≥ 100
  4. Serum vitamin B_{12} level ≥ 900 pg/mL or $UB_{12}BC$ ≥ 2,200 pg/mL

Source: Polycythemia Vera Study Group.
$UB_{12}BC$: unsaturated B_{12} binding capacity.

The second complication is postpolycythemic myelofibrosis (PPMM), or "spent" PV. PPMM occurs in 15% to 20% of patients with PV regardless of the mode of treatment. Characterized by progressive splenomegaly with anemia and extramedullary hematopoiesis (EMH), the bone marrow exhibits reticulin fibrosis. This change usually occurs later in the disease, from 8 to 12 years after diagnosis. Median survival after the diagnosis of PPMM is variable, but there is a further increased risk of progression to AL.

Treatment

The primary goals of PV treatment are to alleviate symptoms, to reduce the risk of vascular (thrombotic/hemorrhagic) events by suppressing marrow cellular production, and to minimize potential consequences of long-term therapy. Treatment modalities include:

1. Phlebotomy of 250–500mL of blood two to three times a week until Hct is between 40% and 45%.
2. Treatment with radioactive phosphorus (^{32}P). Because of the increased risk of AL after 7 to 10 years of ^{32}P therapy, this drug is usually restricted to patients over 60 years.
3. Administration of appropriate myelosuppressive drugs. These include hydroxyurea, interferons, and alkylating agents. The alkylating agents (such as chlorambucil) are prescribed infrequently now because of the unacceptably high risk of transformation to AL after 5 to 7 years of treatment.

Secondary Polycythemia

The secondary polycythemias can be divided into two large groups: those that are hypoxic (physiologic or compensatory), and those that are nonhypoxic (not physiologic or compensatory) (Table 2). The hypoxic group is characterized by chronic tissue anoxia which stimulates Epo production (e.g., cardiovascular shunts, pulmonary disease, smoking). Patients with nonhypoxic polycythemias have tumors (e.g., renal or hepatocellular carcinomas, cerebellar hemangioma, uterine leiomyomas, etc.) or renal disorders (e.g., cysts, hydronephrosis, posttransplantation complications).

Patients with secondary polycythemia usually exhibit physical and laboratory findings different from patients with PV. These include:

1. Absence of splenomegaly
2. Absence of leukocytosis and/or thrombocytosis
3. Normal LAP value

4. In patients with chronic anoxia, arterial sO_2 is ≥92%
5. Patients with abnormal Hb may show abnormalities in oxygen dissociation curve (P_{50}), Hb electrophoresis, or RBC enzymes
6. Bone marrow examination does not show the marked hypercellularity and megakaryocytic hyperplasia typical of PV

Hemoglobin Electrophoresis

Detection of a high oxygen affinity Hb is often possible by standard electrophoretic methods; i.e., cellulose acetate at pH 8.4 to 9.0, citrate agar gel at pH 6.0 to 6.2, isoelectric focusing. But it may still be necessary to determine the P_{50}.

Methemoglobin and Carboxyhemoglobin

Methemoglobinemia is a disorder characterized by the presence of heme iron in the oxidized or trivalent state so that the Hb molecule is incapable of combining with oxygen. It can be an acquired or an inherited disorder.

Carboxyhemoglobin (COHb) is formed when carbon monoxide binds reversibly to the ferrous iron of the Hb molecule. Carboxyhemoglobinemia is a major cause of polycythemia in smokers. Patients with "smoker's" polycythemia usually have elevated levels of COHb (≥4%).

Red Cell Enzymes

RBC enzyme abnormalities may occasionally underlie a polycythemia. Intracellular organic phosphates such as 2,3-diphosphoglycerate (2,3-DPG) can alter Hb oxygen affinity. Decreased levels of this enzyme in the glycolytic (Embden-Meyerhof) pathway result in a shift of the oxygen dissociation curve to the left and reduced oxygen release to the tissues. Hemoglobin Hiroshima has reduced levels of 2,3-DPG, resulting in mild tissue hypoxia and secondary polycythemia.

Stress Polycythemia (Spurious Polycythemia, Gaisböck's Syndrome)

Stress polycythemia is a disorder of hypertensive, obese, middle-aged males who smoke heavily. These patients may demonstrate a slight plethora but they lack splenomegaly. The laboratory studies usually show:

1. Hb level is slightly elevated
2. WBC and platelet counts are normal
3. LAP score is within normal limits
4. Arterial oxygen saturation is normal, but COHb levels are elevated

Familial Erythrocytosis

This group of erythrocytoses has been found in members of the same family and apparently is not a single entity. The underlying pathophysiologic mechanisms are not entirely clear, but two theories are:

1. Increased Epo production uninfluenced by alterations in the oxygen carrying capacity of the blood.
2. An expanded erythropoietic precursor pool responsive to Epo.

MYELOFIBROSIS WITH MYELOID METAPLASIA

Definition

Myeloid metaplasia (agnogenic myeloid metaplasia [AMM]) with myelofibrosis (MF) is characterized by fibrosis in the bone marrow and extramedullary hematopoiesis (EMH), proliferation of the myelogenous elements in the spleen, liver, and lymph nodes. AMM may occur without MF. This occurrence is characterized by progressive anemia and increasing splenomegaly. Marrow studies show absence of Ph^1 chromosome and histologically demonstrable fibrosis.

Clinical Findings

Early in AMM, many patients are asymptomatic. As the disease progresses, patients complain of malaise, weight loss, bleeding, splenic pain, gout, renal colic, and fevers. Patients with AMM may have:

1. Splenomegaly (very common)
2. Hepatomegaly
3. Petechiae and bleeding (secondary to thrombocytopenia)
4. Lymphadenopathy (rare)
5. Ascites and jaundice
6. Portal hypertension and cirrhosis (Budd-Chiari syndrome)

Laboratory Findings

Peripheral Blood

Slight anemia with nucleated red blood cells (NRBC) in the peripheral blood is present at diagnosis and becomes progressively severe. The RBCs may show only slight poikilocytosis and polychromasia at onset. As the disease progresses, the RBCs show marked shape changes with teardrop cells (dacrocytes), striking anisocytosis, and NRBCs. Splenomegaly contributes to this anemia in the following ways:

1. Increase in plasma volume secondary to massive splenomegaly
2. Splenic sequestration of RBCs
3. Intrasplenic destruction of RBCs with a shortened RBC survival

The leukocyte count may vary considerably. However, it is unusual to see an AMM patient with a leukocyte count in excess of 10,000/μL unless the patient has had a splenectomy. Myelocytes and metamyelocytes are observed in films of most patients, and a few promyelocytes and myeloblasts may also be present.

Platelet count is variable at the onset of AMM, but as the disease progresses, thrombocytopenia is the norm. The platelets are bizarre forms which may be agranular, clear blue, or giant granular forms. In addition, small megakaryocyte nuclei and megakaryocytic fragments are occasionally observed.

The above findings of NRBCs, immature WBCs but <10% blasts, and abnormal platelets on the peripheral smear are collectively referred to as the leukoerythroblastic blood picture. Acute leukemic transformation can be diagnosed with certainty when the blast count meets standard criteria. This group of patients, however, may be clinically leukemic even with a blast count <20%. Other disorders may give a similar peripheral blood picture—e.g., metastatic carcinoma in the marrow.

Bone Marrow

Attempts to aspirate the marrow of a patient with MF yield only scanty material ("dry tap"). Therefore, a bone marrow biopsy is needed and usually shows:

1. Increased, histologically aberrant bony trabeculae with evidence of bone remodeling
2. Marrow spaces largely devoid of hematopoietic elements but showing increase in reticulin fiber content
3. Scattered residual islands of distorted marrow elements

Other Findings

Associated findings in AMM are:

1. Hyperuricemia and uricosuria resulting in gouty arthritis and urate nephropathy.
2. Variable LAP scores
3. No consistent pattern of chromosomal abnormalities
4. Increased levels of lactate dehydrogenase (LDH) and normal to increased levels of serum B_{12} and $UB_{12}BC$
5. Abnormalities of humoral immune mechanisms

Radiological studies frequently reveal osteosclerosis. The osteosclerosis tends to be symmetric in distribution and commonly involves the vertebral bodies, pelvis, ribs, clavicles, and metaphyseal portion of the femur.

Differential Diagnosis

The anemic individual with striking RBC changes (anisopoikilocytosis, teardrop RBCs, NRBC) in the peripheral blood, documented marrow fibrosis, and significant splenomegaly is readily classified as having AMM. Less obvious cases of AMM can be difficult to differentiate from other chronic MPDs.

The key distinguishing features for chronic MPDs are shown in Table 4. Myelodysplastic syndromes (MDS) can often be to distinguished from AMM by the hypercellular, iron-overloaded marrow biopsy without fibrosis and the absence of splenomegaly. Lysosomal storage diseases and portal hypertension can usually be excluded by the absence of marrow fibrosis.

Diagnosis

Since EMH is a defining characteristic of AMM, its demonstration would seem essential. But one can be reasonably certain of the diagnosis on other grounds. Key features to the diagnosis include:

1. The characteristic leukoerythroblastic peripheral blood findings of immature granulocytes, NRBCs, and teardrop RBCs
2. Massive splenomegaly often associated with hepatomegaly
3. Characteristic "dry tap" marrow aspiration with biopsy findings of prominent and malformed trabeculae and fibrosis of the marrow spaces

Table 4 Chronic Myeloproliferative Syndromes, Distinguishing Features

	Essential thrombocythemia	Polycythemia vera	Agnogenic myeloid metaplasia	Chronic myelogeous leukemia	Erythroleukemia (AML, M7)
Erythrocytes					
Number	Normal	Increased	Decreased	Usually decreased	Decreased
Morphology	Normal	Normal	Marked anisocytosis with teadrps and NRBC	Normal	Dysplasia with NRBC
Granulocytes					
Number	Normal	Normal or increased (<30,000/uL)	Usually increased (<50,000/uL)	Increased (>35,000/uL)	Normal or low
Morphology	Normal	Normal			Variable
Platelets					
Number	Increased	Normal or increased	Variable	Increased or normal	Normal or decreased
Morphology	Abnormal	Normal or abnormal	Usually abnormal	Normal or abnormal	Normal or abnormal
Bone marrow					
Cellularity	Megakaryocytic hyperplasia	Erythroid hyperplasia	Variable	Granulocytic hyperplasia	Erythroid hyperplasia with dyspoiesis
Fibrosis	Usually absent	Frequent	Present	Variable	Absent
Spleen	Normal or slightly enlarged	Enlarged	Very enlarged	Enlarged	Slightly enlarged or normal
Leukocyte alkaline phosphatase	Normal or high	Normal or high	Normal or high	0–10	Variable
Ph^1 or *bcr* rearrangement	Absent	Absent	Absent	Present in >95%	Absent

Course, Complications, Treatment

The usual course of AMM is one of progressive deterioration associated with increasing splenomegaly and marrow fibrosis. The mean life span from diagnosis is variable. Clinical complications include:

1. Weight loss and inanition
2. Anemia requiring repeated transfusions
3. Infections secondary to granulocytopenia
4. Hemorrhages secondary to thrombocytopenia
5. Portal hypertension with esophageal varices and ascites (Budd-Chiari syndrome)
6. Acute myelogenous leukemia (AML), the terminal event in >10% of patients

Treatment is usually directed toward specific complications since to date no therapy has any beneficial effect on the pathologic process. Therapies include:

1. Allopurinol to control the serum uric acid level
2. Androgens and growth factor therapy to stimulate hematopoiesis, e.g., fluoxymesterone, Epo, GM-CSF, G-CSF, thrombopoietin, etc.
3. Chemotherapy in some cases to control thrombocytosis, leukocytosis, and splenomegaly; agents used include hydroxyurea, interferons alpha and gamma, and busulfan
4. Splenectomy to alleviate symptoms of hypersplenism

ESSENTIAL THROMBOCYTHEMIA (HEMORRHAGIC OR PRIMARY THROMBOCYTHEMIA)

Definition

The term "thrombocythemia" should be confined to instances where the platelet count is persistently elevated to >600,000/μL on at least three separate occasions. Such values are common in patients with chronic MPD. The term "thrombocytosis," a general designation for elevated platelet count, denotes patients with platelet count elevations generally associated with benign disorders.

Essential thrombocythemia (ET) is a chronic MPD characterized by platelet counts >600,000/μL, marked megakaryopoiesis, and recurrent hemorrhage and thrombosis. A slight splenomegaly is detected in only 25% to 40% of patients. Since the patients bleed frequently, a slight anemia may be present. As with other chronic MPDs, ET is a clonal disorder of the pluripotent stem cell.

Clinical Findings

ET occurs equally in male and female patients and affects all adult age groups. It may be the most common chronic MPD. Important clinical manifestations include:

1. Weakness, headache, paresthesias, dizziness
2. Bleeding, often from the gastrointestinal tract or skin
3. Thrombosis, both venous and arterial
4. No splenomegaly (>75% of patients)

Laboratory Findings

Peripheral Blood

The platelet count often exceeds $1.0 \times 10^6/\mu L$. The peripheral blood film shows increased numbers of platelets clumped in large masses. The platelets show striking changes in size, shape, and granularity. Both giant and small platelets and fragments of megakaryocytes may be present.

The RBCs in ET are usually normocytic but may be microcytic and hypochromic if chronic blood loss results in iron deficiency.

The WBC count is usually normal or slightly elevated.

Bone Marrow

The bone marrow in ET shows megakaryocytic hyperplasia. The large groups of clustered megakaryocytes produce large masses of visually striking platelets.

Other Findings

The LAP score is usually normal. Serum B_{12} and uric acid levels are frequently high. The thrombocytosis may cause:

1. Spurious results in serum potassium levels
2. Abnormalities in serum levels of acid phosphatase, uric acid, LDH
3. A hypercoagulable state

Cytogenetic studies are usually normal.

Differential Diagnosis

ET can be distinguished from other thrombocytoses but not without difficulty. "Benign" thrombocytosis is associated with iron-deficiency anemia, infections, and inflammations. ET can be distinguished from other thrombocytoses by the following:

1. Both bleeding and thrombosis occur in ET.
2. Splenomegaly occurs in ET but is absent in benign thrombocytoses.
3. Increased platelet counts (>600,000/μL) persist in ET but are temporary in other thrombocytoses.
4. Platelet morphology is abnormal in ET.

Distinguishing between ET and other chronic MPDs may be extremely difficult.

Diagnosis

ET is a distinctive primary clonal condition which hematologically and pathologically is one of the chronic MPDs. The diagnosis should be considered when:

1. Hemorrhagic and thrombotic episodes occur in association with a sustained increase in the platelet count to >600,000/μL.
2. Iron stores are replete.
3. The marrow shows marked megakaryocytic hyperplasia with clustering.

4. Ph^1 chromosome and *bcr* rearrangement are absent.
5. Uric acid and serum B_{12} levels and LAP score are elevated.

Course, Complications, and Treatment

The course of undiagnosed ET is generally characterized by hemorrhagic and thrombotic episodes. Many patients live with their disease for years without treatment. However, a thromboembolic event such as a cerebral or myocardial infarct or severe gastrointestinal bleeding may be fatal. Occasionally the patient develops AML as a terminal event; the frequency of this transformation is increased in patients given myelosuppressive therapy.

Early in the course of the disease, especially in patients under 40, therapy may not be indicated. If the platelet counts are $>1 \times 10^6/\mu L$ and thrombotic/bleeding complications ensue, definitive treatment should be initiated. Treatment consists of:

1. Myelosuppression with hydroxyurea, anagrelide, or interferon-α to lower the platelet count. Alkylating agents (busulfan, melphalan) and ^{32}P are not considered appropriate therapy. In some patients over 60 years, however, ^{32}P is used and may be the therapy of choice.
2. Antiplatelet agents, e.g., aspirin, dipyridamole, ticlopidine. Antiplatelet agents used in conjunction with myelosuppressive agents may significantly increase the risk of hemorrhage.
3. Thrombocytopheresis for patients with life-threatening hemostatic problems.

NOTE ADDED IN PROOF

Since the manuscript was completed there have been changes proposed for classification, for diagnostic criteria, and for therapies of this group of disorders. The most notable is the World Health Organization classification scheme (the WHO Proposed Classification of Neoplastic Diseases of the Hematopoietic and Lymphoid Tissues), to which the reader is referred.

BIBLIOGRAPHY

1. Berglund S, Zettervall O. Incidence of polycythemia vera in a defined population. Eur J Haematol 1992; 67:285–291.
2. Berk PD, Goldberg JD, Silverstein MN, et al. Increased incidence of acute leukemia in polycythemia vera associated with chlorambucil therapy. N Engl J Med 1981; 304:441–447.
3. Berlin NI. Diagnosis and classification of the polycythemias. Semin Hematol 1975; 12:339–351.
4. Berlin NI (Ed). Polycythemia vera. Semin Hematol 1997; 34:1–80 (entire issue).
5. Buss DH, O'Conner ML, Woodruff RD, et al. Occurrence, etiology, and clinical significance of extreme thrombocytosis: a study of 280 cases. Am J Med 1994; 96:247–253.
6. Dameshek W. Some speculations on the myeloproliferative syndromes. Blood 1951; 6:372–375.
7. Ellis JT, Peterson P, Geller SA, Rappaport H. Studies of the bone marrow in polycythemia vera and the evolution of myelofibrosis and second hematologic malignancies. Semin Hematol 1986; 23: 144–155.
8. Hasselbalch H. Idiopathic myelofibrosis: a clinical study of 80 patients. Am J Hematol 1990; 34: 291–300.
9. Iland HJ, Laszlo J, Peterson P, et al. Essential thrombocythemia: clinical and laboratory characteristics at presentation. Trans Assoc Am Physicians 1983; 96:165–174.
10. Iland HJ, Laszlo J, Case DC, et al. Differentiation between essential thrombocythemia and polycythemia vera with marked thrombocytosis. Am J Hematol 1987; 25:191–201.
11. McIntyre KJ, Hoagland HC, Silverstein MN, Petitt RM. Essential thrombocythemia in young adults. Mayo Clin Proc 1991; 66:149–154.
12. Peterson P, Ellis JT. The bone marrow in polycythemia vera. In: Wasserman LR, Berk PD, Berlin

NI, eds. Polycythemia Vera and the Myeloproliferative Disorders. Philadelphia: W.B. Saunders, 1995:31–53.
13. Wanless IR, Peterson P, Das A, et al. Portal hypertension in agnogenic myeloid metaplasia (AMM) and polycythemia vera (PV): a clinicopathological study. Hepatology 1990; 12:1166–1174.
14. Ward HP, Block MH. The natural history of agnogenic myeloid metaplasia (AMM) and a critical evaluation of its relationship with the myeloproliferative syndrome. Medicine 1971; 50:357–420.
15. Wolf BC, Banks PM, Mann RB, Neiman RS. Splenic hematopoiesis in polycythemia vera. A morphologic and immunohistologic study. Am J Clin Pathol 1988; 89:69–75.
16. Berlin NI, Berk PD, Wasserman LR, eds. Polycythemia and the myeloproliferative disorders. Philadelphia: W.B. Saunders Co, 1995.
17. Fruchtman SM, Mack K, Kaplan ME, et al. A PVSG report on hydroxyurea in patients with polycythemia vera. Semin Hematol 1997; 34:17–23.
18. Gruppo Italiano Studio Policitemia. Polycythemia vera: the natural history of 1213 patients followed for 20 years. Ann Intern Med 1995; 123:656–664.
19. Randi ML, Fabria F, Cella G, et al. Cerebral vascular accidents in young patients with essential thrombocythemia: relation to other known cardiovascular risk factors. Angiology 1998; 49:477–481.
20. Schwartz RS. Polycythemia vera—chance, death, and mutability. N Engl J Med 1998; 338:613–615.
21. Van Gendered PJJ, Mulder PGH, Waleboer M, et al. Prevention and treatment of thrombotic complications in essential thrombocythemia: efficacy and safety of aspirin. Br J Haematol 1997; 97: 179–184.
22. Vardiman J. The overlap between MDS and chronic myeloproliferative disorders, including CMML. Mod Pathol 1999; 12:104–106.
23. Visani G, Finelli C, Castelli U, et al. Myelofibrosis with myeloid metaplasia: clinical and haematological parameters predicting survival in a series of 133 patients. Br J Haematol 1990; 75:4–9.

CASE 1

Patient: 57-year-old male

Chief Complaint: The patient complained to his internist of recurring headaches and intermittent visual disturbances (blurred vision, “floaters”).

Medical History: The patient had experienced a myocardial infarct 3 years earlier. He recovered uneventfully. He also has a 10-year history of hypertension.

Drug History: Calcium-channel blocking agent.

Physical Examination: The patient’s spleen was palpable 6 cm below the LCM. There was no hepatomegaly or lymphadenopathy.

Laboratory Results

A. Screening Procedures

	Patient	Ref. range
Hb	12 g/dL	13.1–16.5 g/dL
Hct	37%	39–50%
RBC count	$4.6 \times 10^6/\mu L$	$4.2–5.6 \times 10^6/\mu L$
MCV	80 fL	81–98 fL
RDW	16.7	11.6–14.8
WBC count	$9.7 \times 10^3 \mu L$	$4.5–11.2 \times 10^3/\mu L$
Platelet count	$655 \times 10^3/\mu L$	$150–450 \times 10^3/\mu L$

Blood Film Examination: Unremarkable red and white cell morphology and differential. Platelets increased in number with large forms.

Questions

1. What is the likely etiology of this patient's anemia and thrombocytosis?
2. Explain the etiology of the patient's headaches and visual disturbances (chief complaint).
3. Of what significance is the patient's splenomegaly in terms of a differential diagnosis?

Laboratory Results

B. Additional Studies

	Patient	Ref. range
Serum iron	12 μg/dL	60–160 μg/dL
Serum ferritin	18 ng/mL	20–250 ng/mL
Leukocyte alkaline phosphatase	136	30–130
Arterial blood gas pO_2	95%	≥92%
Bone marrow aspiration and biopsy	Erythroid and megakaryocytic hyperplasia; absent iron stores	
Cytogenetic and molecular studies	46, XY; no Ph^1 or *bcr* rearrangement detected	
Stool guaiac	Positive	Negative

Diagnosis: Polycythemia vera with iron deficiency.

Discussion

This case is an example of polycythemia vera (PV). The low normal hemoglobin level, the increased RDW, and the increased platelet count all suggest iron deficiency. But this degree of splenomegaly indicates the likelihood of a concomitant myeloproliferative disorder. Although heart attacks are common in this age group, this thrombotic event may be due to platelet abnormalities characteristic of PV.

The results of serum iron and ferritin levels and the absence of iron stores in the marrow confirm an iron deficiency. The normal arterial sO_2, the bilineage hyperplasia on marrow studies, and the normal karyotype strongly suggest iron-deficient PV. This diagnosis should be made only after the patient is iron-replete. In this case, the patient was placed on oral iron for 1 month. The Hb level rose to 17 g/dL, the Hct to 51%, the MCV to 93 fL, and the RBC count to $5.5 \times 10^6/\mu L$. A rise in the Hb of more than 1 g/dL after an adequate iron trial strongly favors PV as the diagnosis. The RCM study performed after the patient was iron-replete was 39.4 mL/kg.

PV has protean clinical manifestations, but hemorrhagic and/or thrombotic events are very common. This patient's gastrointestinal bleeding is an example of hemorrhage. His neurological complaints of headache and visual disturbances are the result of intermittent circulatory interruptions secondary to increased blood viscosity (increased numbers of circulating RBCs and platelets).

Because of the potentially long clinical course of PV, the choice of therapy is based on age and hematological data as well as on severity of symptoms. Currently accepted treatment modalities include phlebotomy, hydroxyurea, the interferons, radioactive phosphorus (^{32}P), and some alkylating agents and mustards. One long-term complication of radiation/myelosuppression is acute leukemia, or blastic transformation. A myelodysplasia may precede overt transformation. Independent of mode of treatment, approximately 10% of patients will experience the spent phase, or postpolycythemic myeloid metaplasia (PPMM).

Bibliography

1. Berlin NI, ed. Polycythemia vera. Semin Hematol 1997; 34:1–80 (entire issue).
2. Buss DH, O'Conner ML, Woodruff RD, et al. Occurrence, etiology, and clinical significance of extreme thrombocytosis: a study of 280 cases. Am J Med 1994; 96:247–253.
3. Peterson P, Ellis JT. The bone marrow in polycythemia vera. In: Wasserman LR, Berk PD, Berlin NI, eds. Polycythemia Vera and the Myeloproliferative Disorders. Philadelphia: W.B. Saunders, 1995:31–53.

CASE 2

Patient: 37-year old female

Chief Complaint: The patient's physician noted a platelet count of $725 \times 10^3/\mu L$ at the time of her annual gynecological exam.

Medical History: The healthy woman had delivered her two children, now ages 8 and 5, uneventfully.

Drug History: No medications.

Physical Examination: Unremarkable. There were no cutaneous, mucosal, or ocular signs of bleeding or thrombosis.

Laboratory Results

A. Screening Procedures

	Patient	Ref. range
Hb	11.6 g/dL	11.7–15.5 g/dL
Hct	36%	35–45%
MCV	82 fL	82–98 fL
RBC count	$4.4 \times 10^6/\mu L$	$3.8–5.1 \times 10^6/\mu L$
WBC count	$8.7 \times 10^3/\mu L$	$4.5–11.2 \times 10^3/\mu L$
Platelet count	$725 \times 10^3/\mu L$	$150–450 \times 10^3/\mu L$

Blood Film Examination: Unremarkable red and white cell morphology and differential. Platelets increased in number with large and giant forms and clumping.

Questions

1. What is the most likely diagnosis in this patient?

2. What other entities should be considered in the differential diagnosis?
3. Should this patient be treated? Why or why not?

Laboratory Results

B. Confirmatory Procedures

	Patient	Ref. range
Repeat platelet count	$678 \times 10^3/\mu L$	$150–450 \times 10^3/\mu L$
Serum iron	48 μg/dL	50–150 μg/dL
Serum ferritin	15 ng/mL	10–120 ng/mL
LAP score	97	30–130
Bone marrow aspiration and biopsy	Megakaryocytic hyperplasia with decreased iron stores	
Cytogenetic and molecular studies	46, XX; no Ph^1 chromosome or *bcr* rearrangement detected	

Diagnosis: Essential (primary) thrombocythemia.

Discussion

This case is an example of essential (or primary) thrombocythemia (ET). The differential diagnosis in this patient includes iron deficiency; undiagnosed inflammatory states; subclinical chronic infection, e.g., subacute bacterial endocarditis; undiagnosed carcinoma; and the other chronic myeloproliferative disorders such as PV. The low normal serum iron and ferritin levels indicate that iron deficiency alone cannot explain the asymptomatic thrombocytosis. This is confirmed by the presence of iron stores, albeit decreased, in the bone marrow aspirate and biopsy.

This patient's asymptomatic presentation is typical of many ET patients, especially those under 45 years. Symptomatic presentations include hemorrhagic ones, e.g., recurrent epistaxis and nose bleeds, gastrointestinal bleeding, menorrhagia, and abnormal bleeding in surgical/obstetrical conditions. Other symptomatic presentations reflect thromboses, e.g., strokes and heart attacks, erythromelalgia, headaches and transient ischemic attacks, mesenteric thrombosis, and Budd-Chiari syndrome.

The natural history of untreated ET is not really known. Asymptomatic patients may have the disease for years. Symptomatic patients may die secondary to a massive thrombotic event without the disease having been suspected or diagnosed. Since the disease occurs in adults of all ages, treatment options are based on age and hematological data as well as on severity of symptoms. Younger adults, especially those in their childbearing years, may not be treated unless they are symptomatic. Older adults, especially those in whom concomitant diabetes mellitus and/or atherosclerosis is present, almost always require some form of myelosuppressive therapy. Agents currently used included hydroxyurea, anagralide, interferons, ^{32}P, and some of the alkylating agents. Antiplatelet agents such as aspirin may be employed as solitary therapy in young patients.

Bibliography

1. Buss DH, O'Conner ML, Woodruff RD, et al. Occurrence, etiology, and clinical significance of extreme thrombocytosis: a study of 280 cases. Am J Med 1994; 96:247–253.

2. Iland HJ, Laszlo J, Peterson P, et al. Essential thrombocythemia: clinical and laboratory characteristics at presentation. Trans Assoc Am Physicians 1983; 96:165–174.
3. Iland HJ, Laszlo J, Case DC, et al. Differentiation between essential thrombocythemia and polycythemia vera with marked thrombocytosis. Am J Hematol 1987; 25:191–201.
4. McIntyre KJ, Hoagland HC, Silverstein MN, Petitt RM. Essential thrombocythemia in young adults. Mayo Clin Proc 1991; 66:149–154.

11

Anemia: Approach to Diagnosis

William F. Baker, Jr.
U.C.L.A. Center for Health Sciences, Los Angeles, California

I. DEFINITION

The definition of anemia is primarily quantitative and is based on a reduction of hemoglobin, in grams per 100 mL, to at least two standard deviations below the mean, adjusted for age, sex, and altitude of residence. For women of child-bearing age, normal values are 10% lower than in men. Normal values increase in proportion to elevation above sea level (Table 1). The normal value for hemoglobin is adjusted upward in smokers. The hematocrit for adult men residing at sea level is 47 with a range of 42–52, and for women it is 42 with the range of 37–47. Normal hemoglobin is 16 g/100 mL for men with a range of 14–18 g/100 mL, and for women the mean is 14 g/100 mL with a range of 12–16 g/100 mL (Tables 2–4). As Htoo et al. (1) and Yip et al. (2) have noted, although an increase in ineffective erythropoiesis and iron stores occurs in the elderly, hemoglobin concentration does not change sufficiently to warrant the establishment of new geriatric norms. Since anemia is frequently both underdiagnosed and

Table 1 Adjustments in Hemoglobin for Altitude of Residence

Altitude (ft)	Change in hemoglobin (g/100 mL)
<3,000	0.0
3,000–3,999	+0.2
4,000–4,999	+0.3
5,000–5,999	+0.5
6,000–6,999	+0.7
7,000–7,999	+1.0
8,000–8,999	+1.3
9,000–9,999	+1.6
>10,000	+2.0

Source: Bessman JD, Gilmer PR Jr, Gardner F. Improved classification of anemias by MCV and RDW. Am Soc Clin Pathol 1983; 80:322–326.

Table 2 Lower Limit of Normal Hemoglobin for White, Middle-Class Children, Nonpregnant Women, and Men[a]

Age	Hemoglobin
Children—both sexes	
1–1.9	11.0
2–4.9	11.2
5–7.9	11.4
8–11.9	11.6
Males	
12–14.9	12.3
15–17.9	12.6
≥18	13.6
Females	
12–14.9	11.8
15–17.9	12.0
≥18	12.0
Elderly	12.0

[a]1 g/dL or less decrease in normal values in blacks; not adjusted for smoking history or elevation above sea level.
Source: Yip R, Johnson C, Dallman PR. Age-related changes in laboratory values used in the diagnosis of anemia and iron deficiency. Am J Clin Nutr 1984; 39:427–436.

overtreated, it is critical to avoid assuming that age per se is a cause of anemia. Anemia may be found more commonly in the elderly because the underlying pathologic conditions resulting in anemia are more common. Although the age-related incidence of various etiologies of anemia may differ, the primary pathophysiology does not.

In infants and children, blood analysis is frequently done by obtaining capillary samples after a prick with a lancet. Hemoglobin values from these samples are always 3–4 g/100 mL higher during the first few hours after birth than in samples obtained by venepuncture. Screening of 1-year-old infants reveals that 37% of blacks and 22% of whites have a hemoglobin below 11.5 g/100 mL.

Since anemia is defined in terms of concentration rather than total red cell mass, it is important to note that a spurious anemia may be diagnosed during rapid plasma volume expansion. Anemia, a hemoglobin below the 95% reference range for age and gender, is determined to exist when the hemoglobin is below 13.0 g/100 mL in men and below 12.0 g/100 mL in women. Black women may have a 1.0 g/100 mL reduction in the normal hemoglobin compared to white women of the same age and socioeconomic status.

II. CLINICAL FEATURES

A. History

Although anemia is defined by quantitative laboratory analysis, a detailed history and physical examination are essential to correct diagnosis. Basic historic data are of critical importance. Sex, age, racial and ethnic background, occupation, gravida and para state of women, and numerous other historical clues provide an index of suspicion which may guide the search for

Table 3 Elderly Adults: Normal Hemoglobin[a]

Age	Median hemoglobin, control
Males	
65–72	14.50 + 2.53
73–80	13.66 + 3.85
81–88	13.83 + 3.89
89–96	14.42 + 3.63
All >65	14.09 + 3.43
Females	
65–72	13.74 + 3.02
73–80	13.51 + 280
81–88	12.74 + 2.65
89–96	12.96 + 4.47
All >65	13.37 + 3.08

[a]Establishment of new geriatric norms not generally recommended.
Source: Htoo SH, Kogkoff RL, Freedman ML. Erythrocyte parameters in the elderly: an argument against new geriatric normal values. J Am Ger Soc 1979; 27:547–551.

symptoms and signs of a specific etiology of anemia. Anemias commonly seen in specific populations are listed in Table 5.

1. History of Present Illness

The development of symptoms associated with anemia is related primarily to the rate at which the anemia develops, the severity of the anemia, and the presence of underlying disease. Compensatory mechanisms such as expansion of the plasma volume, changes in 2–3-DPG and

Table 4 Normal Hemoglobin Values in Pregnancy: Pregnant Women, 5th Percentile Values

Gestation in weeks	Hemoglobin
12	11.0
16	10.6
20	10.5
24	10.5
28	10.7
32	11.0
36	11.4
40	11.9

Source: Goodman RA, ed. Current trends—CDC criteria for anemia in children and child bearing-aged women. MMWR 1989; 38:400–404.

Table 5 Common Types of Anemia in Specific Populations

Age/sex	Type of anemia	Presentation	Diagnosis
Infants and young children	Microcytic	Asymptomatic unless severe	Iron deficiency
Infants and young children	Microcytic Normocytic	Failure to thrive, growth impairment, symptomatic crises	Thalassemia or other red cell abnormality
Teens and young adults			
Male	Microcytic	Asymptomatic unless severe	Iron deficiency
Female	Microcytic	History of heavy menstrual blood loss or pregnancy, fatigue, lightheadedness, pica, etc.	Iron deficiency
Male or female	Normocytic	Fever, chills, inanition, myalgia, arthralgia	Anemia of chronic disease or hemolysis
Male or female	Macrocytic	Neurologic or gastrointestinal symptoms; fever, chills, inanition	Vitamin B_{12} or folate deficiency, anemia of chronic disease
Adults			
Male or female	Microcytic Normocytic	Asymptomatic (unless acute or severe) or gastrointestinal symptoms	Iron deficiency or acute blood loss
Female	Microcytic Normocytic	History of heavy menstrual blood loss or multiple pregnancies, fatigue, lightheadedness, heat intolerance, etc.	Iron deficiency or acute blood loss
Male or female	Normocytic	Asymptomatic or symptoms of chronic disease, fevers, chills, inanition, myalgia, arthralgia	Anemia of chronic disease or hemolysis
Male or female	Macrocytic	Neurologic or gastrointestinal symptoms	Vitamin B_{12} deficiency
Geriatric	Microcytic Normocytic	Acute blood loss, gastrointestinal symptoms	Acute blood loss or iron defiency
	Microcytic Normocytic	Asymptomatic or fatigue, lightheadedness, weight loss, and positive occult blood tests of stool (cancer screening); weight loss, fever, chills, arthralgia myalgia, changes in mental status or other focal organ system symptoms; also acute infection (sepsis)	Anemia of chronic disease; myelophthistic anemia; aplastic anemia; myelo fibrosis
Geriatric	Macrocytic	Dementia, changes in mental status, focal neurologic symptoms, gastrointestinal symptoms	Vitamin B_{12} deficiency

associated shift in the oxyhemoglobin dissociation curve, increase in cardiac output, and other physiologic adjustments are related directly to the presence of symptoms. Since plasma volume expansion after acute blood loss requires approximately 2 days to reach hemodynamic equilibrium, acute blood loss will be accompanied by significant symptoms. The insidious development of chronic anemia is more commonly asymptomatic until the hemoglobin levels drop below 8. Mild anemia, with hemoglobin greater than 10 g/dL, is generally asymptomatic except during heavy physical exertion or serious cardiovascular compromise. Some patients may tolerate hemoglobin levels of 6 g/dL or lower, especially if they are otherwise healthy and sedentary. Dawson et al. (3) have determined that pallor is the only symptom usually associated with the severity of anemia. It was also found that dizziness (orthostatic hypotension due to acute blood loss), anorexia, and painful tongue (with vitamin B_{12} deficiency) are among the few symptoms that are helpful in identifying the type of anemia. Table 6 presents a summary of symptoms which occur with any anemia, as well as those which suggest a specific type.

It is important in obtaining the history to determine whether the anemia has developed gradually or acutely. The present hemoglobin and hematocrit values should be compared with results from a prior evaluation. Women of child-bearing age are at a significant risk for iron deficiency. During pregnancy, 20–60 % of women have hemoglobin levels below 11 g/100 mL.

2. Dietary History

Dietary history should include details of the usual daily diet, especially the presence or absence of red meat. Ernst and Phillip (4) report specific elimination of sources of iron in the diet as an example of covert child abuse. Key aspects of the dietary history which may explain an anemia include the following.

Table 6 Symptoms of Anemia

Symptoms common to all anemia.
Weakness, fatigue, lightheadedness, lassitude, shortness of breath (if severe).
Acute blood loss
Syncope or near-syncope, headache. Symptoms also referable to site of bleeding including hematemesis, melena, abdominal pain, back pain, crush injury, major lacerations, pain from fractures of long bones.
Iron deficiency
Diminished work capacity, behavioral and learning disorders, palpitations, sicca. Craving for clay (geophagia), cornstarch (amylophagia), ice (pagophagia), etc. Dysphagia (thin membranous webs in the postcricoid area—Patterson-Kelly/Plummer-Vinson syndrome).
Vitamin B_{12} deficiency
Vertigo, tinnitus, palpitations, chest pain, paroxysmal nocturnal dyspnea, orthopnea, dependent edema, sore tongue anorexia, weight loss, diarrhea, hypesthesia, parasthesia, ataxia, poor fine-motor coordination, diminished sphincter control, diminished proprioception, variable changes in mental status from irritability and forgetfulness to dementia or psychosis.
Folic acid deficiency
Vertigo, tinnitus, palpitations, chest pain, paroxysmal nocturnal dyspnea, orthopnea, dependent edema, anorexia, weight loss, diarrhea, psychosis, dementia, neurosis.
Sickle cell anemia
Impairment of growth and development, high risk for serious infections (especially pneumococcal), skin ulcers, visual difficulties, painful crises with abdominal pain, chest pain, polyarthralgia, fever, dyspnea, acute arthritis, stroke, seizure, coma, death.

1. Strict vegetarians (such as Hindu Indian families), who abstain from vitamin and mineral supplements may develop iron deficiency anemia and lose weight. This may be corrected by the administration of ascorbic acid. After many years of strict avoidance of animal products, cobalamin deficiency may develop.
2. Food fads, with elimination of certain foods, may underlie a hypoproliferative, nutritional anemia.
3. Tannin-containing beverages such as tea, in association with a vegetarian diet, impair iron absorption and cause iron deficiency.
4. A diet that is deficient in vitamin C may lead to reduced absorption of iron as well as mucosal degeneration, with bleeding, intravascular hemolysis, and altered folate metabolism, all contributing to the 75% incidence of anemia seen in scurvy.
5. Supplementation with excessive amounts of vitamin C may cause erythrocyte damage and hemolysis in premature infants.
6. Folate deficiency, with macrocytic anemia, may occur within 3 weeks of inadequate dietary intake, as in the elderly, chronic alcoholics, and hospitalized patients.

3. Childhood History

In addition to obtaining information regarding the usual childhood diseases and any lasting complications from these, a number of special clinical situations may relate to the development of anemia. These include the following.

1. A history of prematurity or low birth weight, which constitutes a special risk for iron deficiency.
2. Unsupplemented milk feeding in infants who are exclusively breast or bottle fed for 9 months or longer may predispose to iron deficiency.
3. Children, as well as adults, from developing countries may be particularly prone to anemia of various causes. Table 7 correlates type of parasitic infection, anemia, and geographic location.
4. A history of congenital malformations with anemia suggests Fanconi's anemia or Diamond-Blackfan syndrome.

4. Past Medical History

The details of prior medical and surgical problems must be included in the medical history. Chronic conditions such as heart disease; kidney disease; rheumatic fever; diabetes mellitus; chronic infections (such as tuberculosis, coccidioidomycosis, histoplasmosis, or infestation with parasites); a history of pregnancy; malignancy (with TNM staging and details of therapy); history of gallbladder disease, peptic ulcer disease, colitis and neurologic disease may all be directly relevant to the etiology of anemia. The most recent laboratory studies (especially complete blood count), gastrointestinal endoscopic procedures, and radiographic studies should be detailed.

5. Surgical History

The surgical history may be key to the diagnosis. Gastrointestinal surgery is especially important. Procedure notes and pathology reports should be obtained. Blood transfusions given in resuscitation from trauma or surgery must be detailed as to date, number of units, and diagnosis. Once transfused red cells with their shortened half-life begin to disappear from the circula-

Table 7 Worldwide Distribution of Parastic Diseases Associated with Anemia

Parasite	Anemia	Distribution
Malaria sp.	Hemolytic	Worldwide in tropical and some temperate zones
Plasmodium malariae	Tropical splenomegaly syndrome	Worldwide, patchy distribution in tropical and some temperature zones
Schistosoma mansoni	Hypersplenism	Africa and Latin America
Schistosoma japonicum	Hypersplenism	Southeast Asia and Western Pacific
Leishmania donovani (visceral leishmaniasis or Kala-azar)	Hemolysis, gastrointestinal blood loss, splenomegaly	Ethiopia, India, Kenya, Sudan, Latin America
Ancyclostoma duodenale	Microcytic, iron deficiency	Mediterranean Basin, Middle East, Northern India, China, Japan
Necator americanus	Microcytic, iron deficiency	Tropical Africa, Asia, America
Diphylloboytrium latum	Macrocytic, vitamin B_{12} deficiency	Baltic countries, Scandinavia, Japan, Russia, Switzerland, Italy, Chile, Central Africa, North-central United States, Florida, Pacific coast

ion, inadequate iron replacement or nutritional complications of the primary illness may result in the development of a late postoperative anemia.

Specific surgical procedures which are well recognized to be associated with anemia are as follows:

1. Gastric surgery: Vitamin B_{12} deficiency, folate deficiency, iron deficiency (gastritis, anastomotic ulcers)
2. Resection of the terminal ileum: Vitamin B_{12} malabsorption
3. Short bowel syndrome: Multifactorial, hypoproliferative anemia
4. Resection of the colon: Anemia of chronic disease and iron deficiency
5. Resection of the duodenum: Anemia due to copper deficiency
6. Cholecystectomy: Cholelithiasis due to hereditary spherocytosis, red cell enzymopathy and hemoglobinopathy, and other chronic hemolytic anemias
7. Splenectomy: The treatment of choice for chronic hemolytic anemias such as hereditary spherocytosis, red cell enzymopathy, and hemoglobinopathy
8. Cardiac valve replacement or any cardiovascular surgery: Mechanical hemolysis or anemia of chronic disease

6. Family History

Knowledge of the family history is essential to determine whether an anemia is congenital or acquired. Sickle cell anemia, sickle cell trait, and double-heterozygous variants, other hemoglobinopathies, and glucose-6-phosphate dehydrogenase deficiency are more commonly seen in blacks and Asians. Thalassemia is more common in blacks, Asians, and those of Mediterranean extraction. Regional origin is a much less reliable clue to the etiology of anemia due to gene dispersion, changing endemicity of malaria, and the concurrence of abnormal hemoglobins, thalassemia, and glucose-6-phosphate dehydrogenase deficiency.

7. Social History

Chronic alcohol consumption may cause anemia of several etiologies. Cigarette smoking is a major cause of cancer, cardiovascular disease, and peptic ulcer disease. Recreational injectable drug use predisposes to anemia as a result of bacterial endocarditis, vasculitis, infectious hepatitis, and acquired immunodeficiency syndrome. Nasal mucosal injury with epistaxis may result in iron deficiency as the result of cocaine use.

A travel history may indicate exposure to parasites that may potentially be responsible for anemia (Table 7).

Occupational or leisure-time exposure to toxic chemical agents may include lead exposure in welders or carbon tetrachloride in gun enthusiasts. Distance running, karate, forced marching, and conga drumming may cause hemolytic anemia. Astronaut anemia associated with space flight results from both hemolysis due to oxidative injury to red cells from a hypobaric, hyperoxic environment and from suppression of erythropoiesis due to weightlessness. The consequences of acquired immunodeficiency syndrome with its multiple complications, including anemia, and the worldwide epidemic of other venereal diseases, makes the sexual history highly significant.

8. Medications

The medication history must include both prescription and nonprescription drugs. Vitamins and minerals, especially iron, may be used to compensate for a symptom of anemia, without medical supervision.

An increasingly large number of drugs are recognized as potential sources of any of several types of anemia. Aspirin is a common cause of gastrointestinal hemorrhage and iron deficiency anemia. Antineoplastic drugs or exposure to therapeutic doses of radiation for neoplasia may explain several types of anemia. The specific diagnosis for which therapy was provided and the frequency and duration of treatment is important. Folic acid may correct the megaloblastic changes of vitamin B_{12} deficiency while neurologic dysfunction worsens. Therapeutic trials of folate and vitamin B_{12} are not indicated. Sulfa drugs and quinine derivatives may cause intermittent hemolysis in patients with glucose-6-phosphate dehydrogenase deficiency. Alpha-methyl-DOPA may cause hemolytic anemia resulting from the formation of anti-Rh antibodies. Chloramphenicol may cause aplastic anemia even months after exposure.

9. Review of Systems

Symptoms may be general or related to a specific etiology of anemia. Frequently, few or no symptoms may be present, and those noted may be nonspecific and of insidious onset. Fatigue, intolerance of exertion, weakness, and lassitude may be associated with several types of anemia. Impaired thermogenesis, diminished work capacity, and behavioral and intellectual changes may result from iron deficiency. Lightheadedness, fatigue, anorexia, weight loss, or cold intolerance may be due to endocrine failure or occult neoplasia associated with anemia of chronic disease. Fevers, chills, and night sweats may be associated with acute or chronic infection. Sexual dysfunction may be the only symptom of an adverse drug reaction, diabetes mellitus, tabes dorsalis, peripheral vascular disease, neuropathy, or another serious chronic disorder. Both impotence and priapism may occur with chronic granulocytic leukemia or sickle cell disease. The only symptom which correlates with the severity of anemia is pallor.

Table 8 Physical Signs of Anemia

Common to all types of anemia	
	Pallor, systolic flow murmur, tachycardia
Acute blood loss	
	Hypotension (with orthostatic changes), focal signs referable to site of blood loss
Iron deficiency	
	Koilonychia (nails dry, brittle, ridged with concave surface), angular stomatitis, glossitis, esopheal webs (if severe)
Vitamin B_{12} deficiency	
	Icterus, cardiomegaly, hepatosplenomegaly, low-grade fever, smooth beefy red tongue, hypesthesia, impaired proprioception, weakness, ataxia, abnormal Rhomberg test, poor fine-motor coordination, diminished sphincter tone, hyper- or hyporeflexia, Babinski sign abnormal, decreased memory, disorientation, confusion, psychosis
Folic acid deficiency	
	Icterus, cardiomegaly, hepatosplenomegaly, glossitis, cheilosis, wasting, cachexia
Sickle cell anemia	
	Black, physically immature for chronologic age; cachexia; conjunctival icterus, conjunctival sickling sign; cardiomegaly, hyperdynamic precordium, S3 and S4 gallop rhythms, pulmonary rales; abdominal tenderness with bowel sounds and rebound tenderness; erythematous, warm, immobile, tender, effusive joints; retinal infarctions, arteriovenous anomalies of retina, vitreous hemmorrhage, retinitis proliferans, retinal detachment; chronic skin ulcers; priapism; hemiplegia, seizures, coma, visual field defect

B. Physical Examination

The patient's body stature and general appearance may suggest the presence of chronic disease. A cachectic appearance implies nutritional deficiency or a serious chronic illness. The obese patient has a statistically higher incidence of numerous chronic and malignant diseases. Table 8 summarizes presenting signs associated with classic causes of anemia. Pallor is the most common cutaneous and mucosal finding in patients with anemia.

Cardiovascular manifestations of anemia occur only in severe chronic anemia, with hemoglobin less than 7–8 g/100 mL. An upward shift in the cardiac index reflects the severity and type of anemia. The significant physical finding of splenomegaly is associated with a number of illnesses that cause anemia, as summarized in Table 9.

III. LABORATORY EVALUATION

By the time a clinical problem is identified, laboratory evaluation has already begun. *Anemia is not, however, a diagnosis.* An index of suspicion, combined with basic laboratory studies, will guide further investigation. As all anemias have an underlying etiology, it is essential that the workup proceed to a specific diagnosis before the institution of therapy.

The first step in laboratory evaluation is to repeat the hemoglobin within 24–72 hr. While the hemoglobin concentration is highly accurate and reproducible, laboratory error or other factors may be present which could lead erroneously to the initiation of an extensive laboratory evaluation doomed to be unrevealing. The hematocrit is affected by volume changes and is not a reliable index of the presence or absence of either blood loss or anemia. With electronic counters, the hematocrit value is calculated from other data and thus is subject to variability if red cell anisocytosis is present, as in sickle cell disease, hemolysis, or iron deficiency. A variation in hematocrit of as much as 2% may be present in 95% of determinations, and a

Table 9 Splenomegaly Associated with Anemia

Disease	Anemia
Infection	
Subacute bacterial endocarditis, brucellosis, tuberculosis, syphilis, histoplasmosis, malaria, Kala-azar, schistosomiasis, Epstein-Barr virus (acute mononucleosis), cytomegalovirus mononucleosis, infectious hepatitis (type A, B, C,), splenic abcesses	Chronic disease, iron deficiency (coagulopathy due to severe hepatitis with associated blood loss, genitourinary blood loss due to schistosomiasis)
Collagen vascular	
Rheumatoid arthritis, systemic lupus erythematosus, Felty's syndrome	Chronic disease, iron deficiency (gastrointestinal bleeding due to ulcerogenic medications) Hemolytic (Coomb's positive—rare)
Hematologic malignancy	
Lymphoma, histocytoses, myeloproliferative syndromes, chronic lymphocytic leukemia, acute leukemia	Chronic disease, myelophthistic, iron deficiency (coagulopathy with associated blood loss, hemolytic (chronic lymphocytic leukemia)
Congestive splenomegaly—portal hypertension	
Hepatic cirrhosis, acute fulminant hepatitis, splenic vein obstruction, myeloid metaplasia, toxin-induced hepatic necrosis	Chronic disease, iron deficiency (coagulopathy with associated blood loss, hemolytic (alcoholic cirrhosis), megaloblastic anemia (folate deficiency)
Hemolytic anemia	
Hemoglobinopathies, autoimmune, hereditary spherocytosis, etc.	Hemolytic

hemoglobin range of 1.5% is within acceptable limits of accuracy. A 5–10% variation in hemoglobin and hematocrit values may result from postural changes. Combining the variation in laboratory values due to acceptable laboratory error and the changes which occur with posture, a hematocrit of 45 might fall to 39.5 and a hemoglobin of 15 to 13.2, in the absence of any demonstrable pathology.

After establishing an appropriate index of suspicion and considering the accuracy of laboratory values, anemia is established as a definite clinical problem and secondary laboratory studies are ordered. Laboratory studies are guided by a knowledge of test reliability and sensitivity.

The electronically determined complete blood count provides essential information. Further evaluation is guided primarily by red cell numbers, indices, and morphology. Modern hematology autoanalyzers perform electronic counting of red cell number (RBC count), impedance measurement of the red cell volume (MCV), and calculation of the red blood cell size distribution width (RDW) with presentation of the associated histogram. The mean corpuscular hemoglobin concentration (MCHC) and hematocrit (Hct) are calculated based on this data. The white blood cell number and differential count and platelet number and morphology are key to the diagnosis of disorders such as leukemia, preleukemic states, disseminated intravascular coagulation, anemia of acute or chronic infection, and megaloblastic anemia. A moderate neutrophilic leukocytosis with a left shift may occur early after acute blood loss, but is generally not associated with chronic anemia. In both acute and chronic blood loss, thrombocytosis is common. Most problems with the laboratory workup of anemia occur as a result of failure to utilize the information in the red cell indices and simple oversight.

Although review of the peripheral blood smear may be useful in directing further analysis, Jen et al. (5) have demonstrated that personal review of the smear by the physician is poorly reproducible and not superior to combined analysis by the hematologic autoanalyzer and review by a well-trained laboratory technician. Review of the peripheral smear by the primary physician remains an important teaching tool, but is otherwise reserved for the difficult and unusual cases as seen by the internal medicine or hematology specialist or clinical pathologist.

The basic laboratory studies include: (a) complete blood count: including hemoglobin, hematocrit, red blood cell count, red cell indices, and size-distribution width; (b) a Wright-stained peripheral blood smear; and (c) a reticulocyte count. The reticulocyte index is then calculated in order to correct for the degree of anemia and the longer life span of reticulocytes in severe anemia. Alternatively, the absolute reticulocyte count may be measured with flow cytometry. The formula for calculating reticulocyte index is shown below. The normal value for both the reticulocyte index and the reticulocyte count is 1.0, with a range of 0.5 to 2.0.

$$\begin{array}{c}\text{Reticulocyte Index}\\ (\text{normal} = 1.0)\end{array} = \frac{\text{reticulocyte count}}{\text{maturation index}}$$

$$\begin{array}{c}\text{Maturation index}\\ (\text{normal} = 1.0)\end{array} = \frac{\text{measured hematocrit}}{\text{normal hematocrit}}$$

Maturation index	Measured hematocrit
1	45
1.5	35
2	25
2.5	15

As the result of the basic laboratory studies, the anemia is first classified into one of three morphologic categories: (a) normocytic, (b) microcytic, or (c) macrocytic. Further diagnostic studies to determine a specific etiologic classification are guided by the initial classification.

IV. CLASSIFICATION AND ETIOLOGIES

A. Normocytic Anemia

The etiologies of normocytic anemia include acute blood loss, hemolytic anemia, anemia of chronic disease, anemia of chronic renal disease, hematologic malignancy, myelophthisic anemia, aplastic anemia, and the anemia associated with endocrinopathies. The most common cause of normocytic anemia is acute hemorrhagic anemia, the second most common cause of anemia in the United States (22–25% of cases).

Normocytic anemia not resulting from acute blood loss is divided into one of two categories that can be separated by the reticulocyte index. The reticulocyte index rises as the result of either acute blood loss or destruction of red cells. The clinical presentation, history, and physical examination will often suggest a source of blood loss. In the absence of a clear diagnosis, then, the clinician must obtain a reticulocyte index, review serial hemoglobin and hematocrit values, and follow the patient clinically until hemorrhage is excluded.

The patient with normocytic anemia who has no evidence of acute blood loss but has an elevated reticulocyte index is probably hemolyzing. Etiologies of hemolytic anemia include hereditary membrane defects, red cell enzyme defects, hemoglobinopathies, acquired membrane abnormalities, splenomegaly, immune-mediated hemolysis, mechanical red cell trauma, toxic effects, drug effects, and infectious agents. Infants and children with hemolysis will usually be found to have an inherited hemoglobinopathy, enzymopathy, or immune-mediated hemolysis. Laboratory and clinical features similar to those found in adults lead to accurate diagnosis. An initial step in the laboratory evaluation is review of the peripheral smear in search of schistocytes, helmet cells, or fragmented red cells, which are highly specific for intravascular hemolysis.

Sickle cell and other hemoglobinopathies result in extravascular hemolysis and accompanying elevations of serum lactate dehydrogenase and total and unconjugated bilirubin. Hemoglobin crystals and target cells in hemoglobin C disease and the sickle cells of sickle cell SS disease are typical abnormalities of anisocytosis. Heterozygous sickle cell disease may be identified by a sickle cell prep, and hemoglobin electrophoresis will help to identify other abnormal hemoglobins. Anemias combining the disorders of sickle cell disease, iron deficiency, thalassemia, hemoglobin C disease, and red cell enzymophathies present challenging diagnostic problems requiring additional laboratory testing including free erythrocyte protoporphyrin, transferrin saturation, hemoglobin electrophoresis, enzymatic, and genetic studies. When other causes of hemolysis are excluded and there is no evidence of abnormal hemoglobin, a red cell enzymopathy should be considered. Congenital or acquired defects may be found, as in patients with pyruvate-kinase deficiency, which may be associated with the development of preleukemia.

Anemia of chronic disease is associated with a normal or low reticulocyte index in the patient with normocytic indices. The diverse etiologies of anemia of chronic disease include chronic inflammation and infection, collagen vascular diseases, malignancy, renal failure, endocrinopathy, and liver disease. The growth factor erythropoietin, responsible for regulating proliferation and maturation of the erythroid cell line, is depressed or rendered ineffective in a number of chronic illnesses.

The primary goal of laboratory evaluation is to exclude other causes of anemia and to determine the nature of the underlying disorder. A depressed reticulocyte count or pancytopenia suggests a myelophthisic process, or aplastic anemia. A depressed serum iron and total iron-binding capacity distinguish iron deficiency from anemia of chronic disease. In the absence of a primary hematologic disorder, the serum chemistry analysis may reveal abnormalities suggestive of uremia, hepatic dysfunction, or even Addison's disease. An elevated sedimentation rate may indicate an autoimmune disorder, acute or chronic infection, or an occult malignancy. Disease-specific laboratory, radiographic, and invasive studies should be guided by the composite clinical presentation. A bone marrow aspiration and biopsy is frequently required to characterize the anemia fully.

If anemia of chronic disease is felt to arise from occult malignancy, a thorough evaluation to identify the primary is essential. Myelophthisic anemia, in which neoplastic cells invade the bone marrow directly, is most often the result of carcinoma, malignant melanoma, and hematologic malignancies. While iron deficiency, myelophthisic anemia and anemia of chronic disease are the usual correlates of a variety of malignancies; hemolysis, megaloblastic anemia, aplastic anemia, and several other varieties of anemia also occur.

B. Microcytic Anemia

The microcytic anemias (MCV less than 80 mm^3) include iron deficiency, thalassemia, hemoglobinopathies, sideroblastic anemia, lead toxicity, and occasionally anemia of chronic disease or copper deficiency. A correct diagnosis is the result of a history, physical, and appropriate laboratory evaluation. The principal etiologies of microcytic anemia may be separated using the RBC count, MCV, reticulocyte count, serum iron, total iron-binding capacity, and serum ferritin.

C. Macrocytic Anemia

Macrocytic anemias (MCV greater than 100 mm^3) may be megaloblastic or nonmegaloblastic. Typical etiologies include vitamin B_{12} deficiency, folic acid deficiency, hemolytic anemia, acute blood loss, chronic liver disease, postsplenectomy, hypothyroidism, myelophthisic anemia, aplastic anemia, and sideroblastic anemia. Megaloblastic, macrocytic anemias are due to acquired or inherited abnormalities of deoxyribonucleic acid synthesis, usually related to folate or vitamin B_{12} deficiency.

Nonmegaloblastic, macrocytic anemias are multifactorial and include compensatory reticulocytosis following acute hemolysis or blood loss, increased red cell membrane surface area in chronic liver disease or after splenectomy, myxedema, myelophthisic, hypoplastic or aplastic anemias. Hemolytic anemia may present with erythrocyte macrocytosis, distinguished from other causes of macrocytic indices by obtaining a reticulocyte index or absolute reticulocyte count by flow cytometry.

V. DIFFERENTIAL DIAGNOSIS

The differential diagnosis is the product of the history and physical examination, basic and then confirmatory laboratory studies. Laboratory error is a potentially costly pitfall, so poor laboratory-to-clinical correlation requires a repeat of the basic hematologic evaluation before additional studies are obtained.

After the history and physical examination and complete blood count, including red cell indices, the clinician should obtain a reticulocyte count. Laboratory chemistries or other studies should be ordered based on the clinical suspicion of nonhematologic illness. The red cell indices and reticulocyte count guide further evaluation.

Upon classification of the anemia as a normocytic, microcytic, or macrocytic, a differential diagnosis will be proposed, followed by the ordering of specific studies which result in a diagnosis specific as to type of anemia and etiology. Algorithms summarizing the evaluation of normocytic (Fig. 1), microcytic (Fig. 2), and macrocytic anemia (Fig. 3) illustrate the sequential diagnostic evaluation. A complete evaluation to a certain conclusion is essential, since failure to identify the underlying cause of the anemia will frequently have serious consequences.

CASE STUDY

Patient

Fifty-one-year-old female.

Chief Complaint

Fatigue.

Medical History

The patient presented to the hospital emergency room complaining of fatigue and lightheadedness. Although she had had fatigue for over a year, her symptoms had been worsening rapidly over the previous 3 weeks. She had experienced dyspnea with climbing stairs for about 6 months, and a sore, red, and discolored tongue for 1 year. She had low abdominal pain,

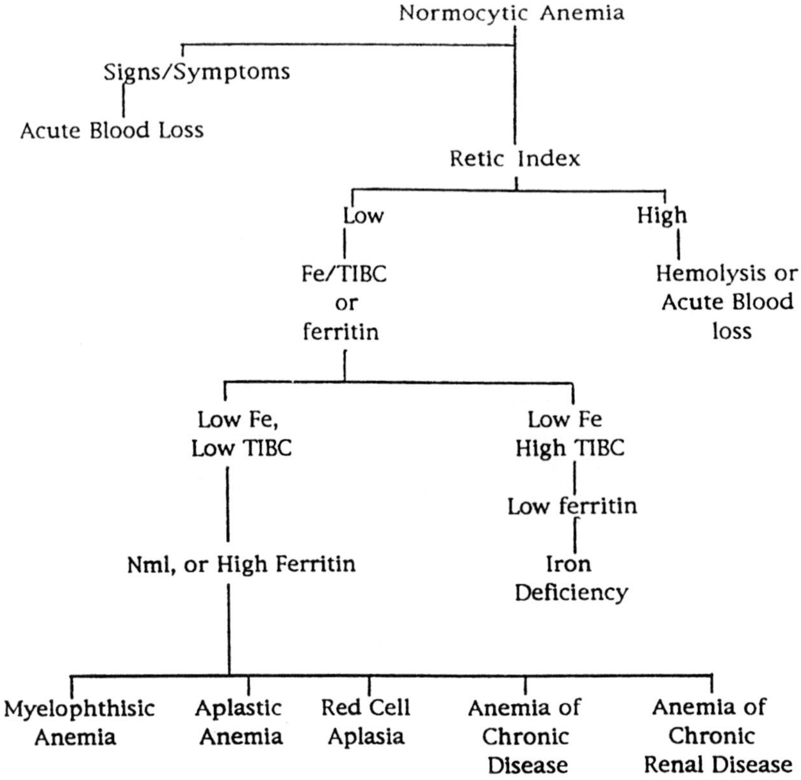

Figure 1 Differential diagnosis of normocytic anemia.

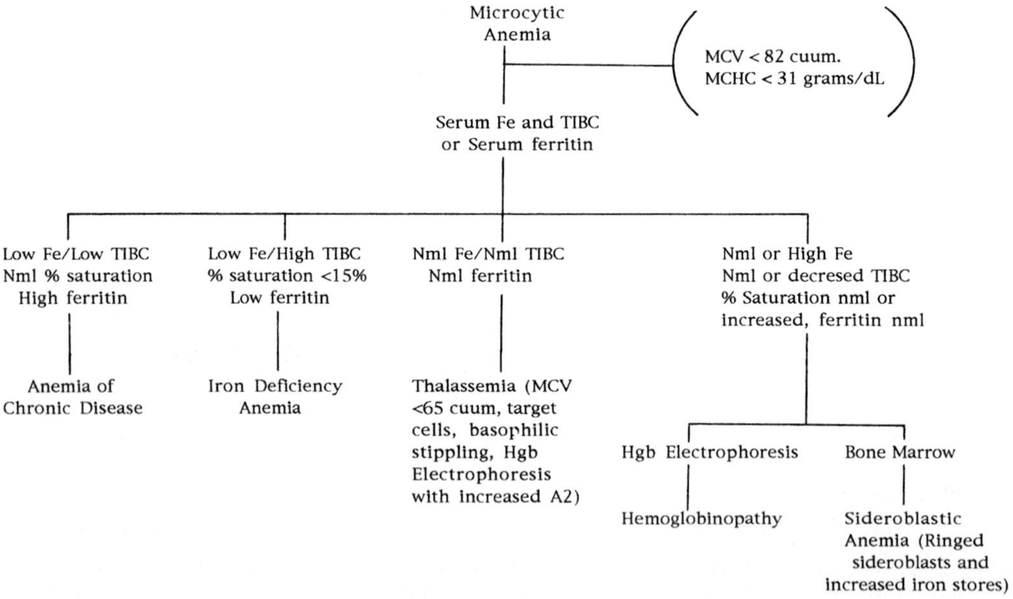

Figure 2 Differential diagnosis of microcytic anemia.

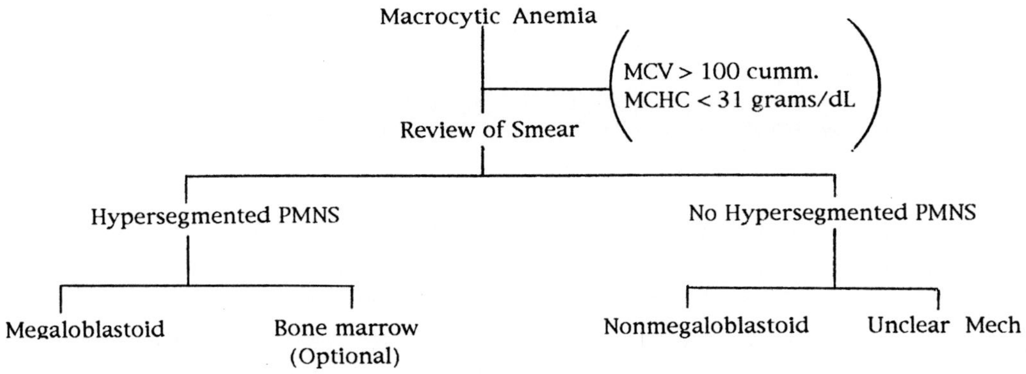

Figure 3 Differential diagnosis of macrocytic anemia.

bilateral hand parasthesia, a 10-lb weight loss over a 2-month period of time, a decreased appetite, and cardiac tachycardia with any brisk movement. Anemia had been diagnosed 8 months prior, and an extensive gastrointestinal evaluation was performed which revealed a normal esophagogastroduodenoscopy and colonoscopy. She has a history of hypothyroidism. She had nausea for 1 year and an episode of melena 6 months prior.

She was referred for consultation regarding the etiology of anemia. The referring physician and the patient were concerned about the possibility of a hematologic malignancy.

Family History

Mother and father with heart disease but no history of anemia or malignancy.

Medications

Loestrin, 1/20 oral contraceptive; thyroid, USP 90 mg/day; omeprazole 5 mg qid.

Physical Examination

Marked pallor of the skin, palmar crease, and mucous membranes was readily apparent. The tongue was denuded and shiny. Lymph nodes were not enlarged, and the skin was normal. The abdomen was mildly tender in the lower quadrants and moderately tender in the left upper quadrant, but there was not palpable splenomegaly.

Laboratory Results

	Patient	Normal
Hemoglobin	8.2 g/dL	12–16 g/dL
RBC count	2.08 M/mm^3	4.7–6.1 M/mm^3
MCV	119.4 fL	79–100 fL
RDW	21.2	11.5–14.8
Reticulocyte index	1.0%	1.0%
White blood count	2.0 Th/mm^3	4.8–11.0 Th/mm^3
Platelet count	120 Th/mm^3	150–400 Th/mm^3
LDH	485 IU/L	90–200 IU/L
Total bilirubin	1.8 mg/dL	0–1.5 mg/dL
Peripheral smear	3+ anisocytosis, 1+ polychromasia, teardrops, and schistocytes	3+ macrocytosis

Questions

1. Based on the clinical presentation and the findings on the initial laboratory studies, what is the differential diagnosis?
2. Which clinical features may be explained by a severe anemia of any type or etiology and which provide clues to the specific etiology in this patient?
3. What additional studies are necessary to determine a clear diagnosis and to guide therapy?
4. Is a trial of therapy indicated prior to additional evaluation?

Additional Laboratory Results

	Patient	Normal
Serum B_{12} level	27 pg/mL	171–953 pg/mL
RBC folate level	255 ng/mL	110–700 ng/mL
Schillings test	0.2%	>5%

Bone marrow aspiration and biopsy findings were consistent with megaloblastic anemia with a nucleocytoplasmic dyssynchrony consistent with mild vitamin B_{12} or folate deficiency. A preleukemic state could not be excluded due to the ill-defined nature of the changes.

An upper gastrointestinal tract with small bowel radiographic study was normal except for a focal area of gastritis in the gastric cardia, with normal terminal ileum.

Diagnosis

Pernicious anemia, autoimmune.

Discussion

This patient presented with symptoms typical of any severe anemia, such as fatigue, lightheadedness, intolerance of exertion, and cardiac tachycardia with exertion. In addition, she had characteristic symptoms of pernicious anemia, including weight loss, anorexia, sore tongue, and parasthesia. Remarkably, all of these symptoms resolved completely with administration of vitamin B_{12}. The finding of leukopenia and thrombocytopenia resulted from the severe deficiency of cyanocobalamin and, as is not uncommon, the mild hyperbilirubinemia, elevation of the serum LDH, and schistocytes reflected the mild degree of hemolysis frequently observed with severe vitamin B_{12} deficiency. This patient also had hypothyroidism (as is recognized with increased frequency in patients with pernicious anemia), and somewhat later in her course developed a mild normocytic anemia as the result of inadequate thyroxine replacement. The normocytic anemia corrected with the normalization of the thyroid-stimulating hormone level corresponding to therapy with levothyroxine.

REFERENCES

1. Htoo SH, Kogkoff RL, Freedman ML. Erythrocyte parameters in the elderly: an argument against new geriatric normal values. J Am Ger Soc 1979; 27:547–551.
2. Yip R, Johnson C, Dallman PR. Age-related changes in laboratory values used in the diagnosis of anemia and iron deficiency. Am J Clin Nutr 1984; 39:427–436.

3. Dawson AA, Ogston D, Fullerton HW. Evaluation of diagnostic significance of certain symptoms and physical signs in anemic patients. Br Med J 1969; 3:436–439.
4. Ernst TN, Phillip M. Severe iron deficiency anemia. West J Med 1986; 144:358–359.
5. Jen P, Woo B, Rosenthal P, Bunn F, Loscalzo A, Goldman L. The value of the peripheral blood smear in anemic inpatients: the laboratory's reading vs a physician's reading. Arch Intern Med 1983; 143:1120–1125.

SELECTED READINGS

1. Baker WF. Clinical evaluation of the patient with anemia. In: Bick RL. Hematology: Clinical and Laboratory Practice. St. Louis: Mosby, 1993:203–229.
2. Beaver PC, Jung RC, Cupp EW. Clinical Parasitology. 9th ed. Philadelphia: Lea & Febiger, 1984.
3. Bergin JJ. Evaluation of anemia. Postgrad Med 1985; 77:253–254, 256, 261–269.
4. Bessman JD, Gilmer PR Jr, Gardner F. Improved classification of anemias by MCV and RDW. Am Soc Clin Pathol 1983; 80:322–326.
5. Carpentieri U, Smith LR, Daeschner CW, Haggard ME. Why is my child so pale? Evaluation of anemia in children. Tex Med 1983; 79:71–73.
6. Casadevall N, Dupuy E, Molho-Sabatier P, Tobelem G, Varet B, Mayenx P. Autoantibodies against erythropoietin in a patient with pure red-cell-aplasia. N Engl J Med 1996; 334:630–633.
7. Cazzola M, Messinger O, Battisel V, et al. Recombinant human erythroeitin in the anemia associated with multiple myeloma or non-Hodgkin's lymphoma: dose finding and identification of predictors of response. Blood 1995; 86:4446–4453.
8. Centers for Disease Control. Reference criteria for anemia screening. MMWR 1989; 38:400–404.
9. Clark R, Topley E, Flear CTG. Assessment of blood-loss in civilian trauma. Lancet 1955; 268:629.
10. Dallman PR. Manifestations of iron deficiency. Semin Hematol 1982; 19:19.
11. Dallman PR, Yip R, Johnson C. Prevalence and causes of anemia in the United States, 1976–1980. Am J Clin Nutr 1984; 39:437–445.
12. Dawson AA, Ogston D, Fullerton HW. Evaluation of diagnostic significance of certain symptoms and physical signs in anaemic patients. Br Med J 1969; 3:436–439.
13. Delaunay J, Alloisio N, Morlie L, Pothier B. The red cell skeleton and its genetic disorders. Mol Aspects Med 1990; 11:161–241.
14. Ernst TN, Phillip M. Severe iron deficiency anemia. West J Med 1986; 144:358–359.
15. Freedman ML. Anemias in the elderly: physiologic or pathologic? Hosp Pract 1982; 17:121.
16. Goodman RA, ed. Current trends—CDC criteria for anemia in children and child bearing-aged women. MMWR 1989; 38:400–404.
17. Gottfried E. Erythrocyte indexes with the electronic counter. N Engl J Med 1979; 300:1277.
18. Herbert V, Tisman G. Hematologic effects of alcohol. Ann NY Acad Sci 1975; 252:307.
19. Htoo SH, Kogkoff RL, Freedman ML. Erythrocyte parameters in the elderly: an argument against new geriatric normal values. J Am Ger Soc 1979; 27:547–551.
20. Jen P, Woo B, Rosenthal P, Bunn F, Loscalzo A, Goldman L. The value of the peripheral blood smear in anemic inpatients: the laboratory's reading vs a physician's reading. Arch Intern Med 1983; 143:1120–1125.
21. Lacombe C. Resistance to erythropoietin. N Engl J Med 1996; 334:660–662.
22. McPhee SJ. The evaluation of anemia. West J Med 1982; 137:253–257.
23. Nonnally RM. Hemoglobin and hematocrit levels: effects of posture and test variability. J La State Med Soc 1977; 129:97–98.
24. Savage D, Lindenbaum J. Anemia in alcoholics. Medicine 1986; 65:322–338.
25. Smith MA, Knight SM, Maddison PJ, Smith JG. Anemia of chronic disease in rheumatoid arthritis: effect of the blunted response to erythropoietin and of interleukin production by marrow macrophage. Ann Rheum Dis 1992; 51:753–757.

26. Varat M, Adolph R, Fowler N. Cardiovascular effects of anemia. Am Heart J 1972; 83:415–426.
27. Wallerstein R. Role of the laboratory in the diagnosis of anemia. JAMA 1976; 236:490–493.
28. Wallerstein R Jr. Laboratory evaluation of anemia. West J Med 1987; 146:443–451.
29. Wheeler L, Brecher G, Sheiner L. Clinical laboratory use in the evaluation of anemia. JAMA 1977; 238:2709–2714.
30. Yip R, Johnson C, Dallman PR. Age-related changes in laboratory values used in the diagnosis of anemia and iron deficiency. Am J Clin Nutr 1984; 39:427–436.
31. Recommendations to prevent and control iron deficiency in the United States. Centers for Disease Control and Prevention. MMWR Morb Mortal Wkly Rep 1998; 47:1–29.
32. Bain BJ. Pathogenesis and pathophysiology of anemia in HIV infection. Curr Opin Hematol 1999; 6:89–93.
33. Bothwell TH. Overview and mechanisms of iron regulation. Nutrition Review 1995; 53:237–245.
34. Carmel R. A focused approach to anemia. Hosp Pract (Off Ed) 1999; 34:71–78, 81–85, 89–90; discussion 90–91.
35. Fonseca R, Tefferi A. Practical aspects in the diagnosis and management of aplastic anemia. Am J Med Sci 1997; 313:159–-169.
36. Lindsay JO, Robinson, SD, Jackson JE, Walters JR. The investigation of iron deficiency anemia—a hospital based audit. Hepatogastroenterology 1999;46:2887–2890.
37. Little DR. Ambulatory management of common forms of anemia. Am Fam Physician 1999; 59: 1598–1604.
38. Ludwig H, Fritz E. Anemia in cancer patients. Semin Oncol 1998; 25:2–6.
39. Means RT, Jr. Advances in the anemia of chronic disease. Int J Hematol 1999; 70:7–12.
40. Moore RD. Human immunodeficiency virus infection, anemia, and survival. Clin Infect Dis 1999; 29:44–49.
41. Osaki T, Ueta E, Arisawa K, Kitamura Y, Matsugi N. The pathophysiology of glossal pain in patients with iron deficiency and anemia. Am J Med Sci 1999; 318:324–329.
42. Rangan AM, Blight GD, Binns CW. Iron status and non-specific symptoms of female students. J Am Coll Nutr 1998; 17:351–355.
43. Sadahiro S, Suzuki T, Tokunaga N, Mukai M, Tajima T, Makuuchi H, Saito T. Anemia in patients with colorectal cancer. J Gastroenterol 1998; 33:488–494.
44. Sayetta RB. Pica: an overview. Am J Fam Physician 1986; 33:181–187.
45. Shiga S, Furukawa T, Koyanagi I, Yamagishi M, Yoshida Y, Takahashi T, Kannagi R, Mori T. Laboratory diagnosis of anemia and related diseases using multivariate analysis. Am J Hematol 1997; 54:108–117.
46. Thomas ML. Impact of anemia and fatigue on quality of life in cancer patients: a brief review. Med Oncol 15 Suppl 1998; 1:S3–S7.
47. van den Broek NR, Letsky EA, White SA, Shenkin A. Iron status in pregnant women: which measurements are valid? Br J Haematol 1998; 103:817–824.
48. Weiss G. Iron and anemia of chronic disease. Kidney Int Suppl 1999; 69:S12–S17.

12

Iron Deficiency Anemia

Donald P. Skoog and James R. Newland
University of Nebraska College of Medicine, Omaha, Nebraska

I. DEFINITION

Iron deficiency anemia (IDA) has variably decreased hemoglobin caused by insufficient iron. In advanced cases the anemia is severe and markedly microcytic and hypochromic, but early on, hemoglobin and mean corpuscular volume (MCV) are only minimally decreased.

II. INCIDENCE

Worldwide, iron deficiency is the most common nutritional deficiency, and IDA, likewise, is the most common anemia. Its underlying cause tends to vary according to age, sex, and socioeconomic group (1).

III. CLINICAL FEATURES

A. Secondary to the Anemia Itself

Because the anemia is insidious in onset, compensatory mechanisms usually prevent symptoms until the hemoglobin falls to the range of 8 g/dL. Coexisting disease of the cardiopulmonary system may act jointly with less advanced anemia to produce symptoms typical of more severe anemia. When anemia is sufficiently advanced to be solely responsible for symptoms, the physical examination usually reveals pallor, and, occasionally, koilonychia, angular stomatitis, and glossitis, as well as splenomegaly.

B. Secondary to the Underlying Condition

Iron deficiency anemia results from three abnormalities affecting iron: loss from abnormal bleeding, deficient diet, and malabsorption.

1. Blood Loss

Blood loss is the most common cause of IDA in adults living in developed countries. Gastrointestinal blood loss is the most frequent cause in males and postmenopausal females. Heavy menstrual bleeding is a frequent cause of IDA in women of child-bearing age. Pregnancy, which requires approximately 1000 mg of iron, is also a common cause (2).

Intestinal parasites, such as hookworms and schistosomes, often cause IDA in underdeveloped regions, but are rarely found in developed countries.

2. Deficient Diet

In a broad sense, iron deficiency develops when intake does not keep pace with utilization and loss of iron. Worldwide, the most common cause is a low content of dietary iron, especially in readily absorbable forms such as in meat. In developed countries, dietary inadequacy is uncommon except when it is relative to increased need, as in the premature infant. Term infants may also develop iron deficiency, especially when bottle fed. Female adolescents, with increased need for iron because of both rapid growth and onset of menses, have a relatively high incidence of iron deficiency.

3. Malabsorption

Malabsorption is an uncommon cause of IDA. Some patients with the short bowel syndrome, nontropical sprue, or a history of gastrectomy cannot absorb iron normally. Increased blood loss contributes to their anemia, and the majority have symptoms or a history of gastrointestinal disease.

IV. LABORATORY FINDINGS

Laboratory tests are essential for detecting or confirming anemia and for determining that it is caused by iron deficiency, but they are of limited value in ascertaining the deficiency's cause. The latter is determined by the history and physical examination, supplemented by endoscopic and radiographic evaluation of the gastrointestinal tract. Following is a discussion of laboratory tests commonly used for evaluating IDA.

A. Hemoglobin Level

In severe, chronic iron deficiency, the hemoglobin may be as low as 3–4 g/dL. The degree of anemia is related directly to the severity and duration of deficiency, and the spectrum of hemoglobin values ranges downward from normal. Hemoglobin is the key test for detecting the presence of anemia and for following its response to treatment.

B. Red Cell Indices, Including RDW

The MCV is of great importance in determining that iron deficiency is causing anemia. As with hemoglobin, the MCV varies downward from normal, depending on the severity of anemia. When hemoglobin is in the 3 to 4-g/dL range, the MCV will be 50–60 fl. A discordance between the two values, for example, a hemoglobin of 6 g/dL associated with an MCV that is only mildly decreased, is indicative of IDA complicated by another process, such as significant acute blood loss, or of an entirely different type of anemia.

The MCH and MCHC are less important, especially the latter. Most laboratories use automated cell counters that do not detect decreased MCHC until there is marked hypochromia and microcytosis.

The RDW appears not to be a valuable discriminator between IDA and other causes of microcytic anemia (3). A normal value tends to exclude IDA, but an elevated value lacks specificity.

C. Reticulocyte Count

The reticulocyte count is not an important test in the evaluation of IDA. It is usually essentially normal, as it is in the disorders from which iron deficiency must be differentiated.

D. White Cell and Platelet Counts

There are no characteristic or diagnostically important changes in white cells or platelets. Elevated white cell and platelet counts occasionally occur, and, rarely, the latter exceed 1 million. There may also be thrombocytopenia, which in rare cases may be severe.

E. Red Cell Morphology

Microcytosis, anisocytosis, poikilocytosis, and hypochromia are readily seen in the peripheral blood smear of individuals with moderate to marked IDA. However, because of inconsistent and inaccurate interpretation of the blood smear, as well as the superior sensitivity and accuracy of automated determination of red cell indices, morphologic findings do not contribute significantly to the accurate diagnosis of IDA (4,5).

F. Serum Ferritin

In a recent meta-analysis, Guyatt and associates (6) found serum ferritin to be much more powerful than all other blood tests for diagnosing iron deficiency. In the absence of disorders that produce an acute-phase reaction, there is excellent correlation between the serum ferritin level and iron stores. Unfortunately, conditions such as malignancy, infection, and noninfectious inflammatory disorders cause serum ferritin to act as an acute-phase reactant, producing "false" elevations that make interpretation difficult. With very rare exceptions, a subnormal ferritin level indicates absent iron stores, even if the acute phase reaction is present. When the latter is occurring, values in iron deficiency may range upward to 100 ng/mL, with decreasing likelihood of iron deficiency as the value approaches 100.

G. Serum Iron, Transferrin, and Transferrin Saturation

Before the serum ferritin test was available, these were the preferred blood tests for assessing iron stores. However, the acute-phase reaction decreases serum iron to less than normal and also frequently decreases transferrin. These tests have less diagnostic power than the serum ferritin and should no longer be used to test for iron deficiency, especially in sick, hospitalized patients (7).

H. Serum Transferrin Receptor

Elevated concentrations of serum transferrin receptor are found in both iron deficiency and erythroid hyperplasia (8). There is indication that this test, which is currently used only in research settings, may help evaluate iron stores when the acute-phase reaction is present (9; see Ref. 10 for a negative opinion).

I. Red Cell Protoporphyrin

Iron deficiency, like lead poisoning, increases red cell protoporphyrin. The availability of accurate and easily operated hematoflourometers has increased the use of this test in screening for these two conditions. However, red cell protoporphyrin levels lack the sensitivity and specificity of serum ferritin for iron deficiency (6).

J. Fecal Occult Blood

Because gastrointestinal bleeding frequently leads to anemia, testing the stool for blood has a time-honored place in the investigation of IDA. However, many foods, such as meat, broccoli, and bananas, as well as liquid stool samples and oral iron therapy, may cause false positive reactions. Administration of ascorbic acid, as well as degradation of hemoglobin when there is upper gastrointestinal bleeding, may cause false negative reactions (11). In addition, many lesions probably bleed only intermittently, producing negative reactions on stools from non-bleeding intervals. For these reasons, the sensitivity and specificity of tests for occult blood are relatively low. Negative tests should not be a deterrent from endoscopic or radiographic evaluation of the gastrointestinal tract in patients with unexplained microcytic anemia or other indications for such examination.

K. Bone Marrow Examination

Erythrocytic hyperplasia and deficient hemoglobinization of red cell precursors are usually found in the marrow, particularly in more advanced cases. However, these changes have only modest diagnostic significance, and the pivotal finding is the absence of marrow iron stores. This is the "gold standard" for determining iron deficiency. Marrow examination is not required for most patients but should be carried out when the diagnosis is in doubt, especially when the serum ferritin has an equivocal value, or when a trial of iron therapy fails. Normal infants and children have little or no stainable iron stores, and evaluation of marrow iron does not distinguish depleted from normal stores.

V. PATHOPHYSIOLOGY

A. Iron Metabolism

The major portion of body iron is in hemoglobin, myoglobin, and various enzymes. Nearly all of the remainder is in storage in the reticuloendothelial system, primarily in the bone marrow, liver, and spleen.

1. Absorption

Normally, dietary absorption is limited to the amount of iron necessary to produce hemoglobin, myoglobin, and enzymes, to compensate for losses, and to build stores. When losses increase or there are other causes of increased need, absorption may not keep pace because it can increase only modestly.

2. Loss

Adults daily lose approximately 1 mg of iron, mainly in desquamated epidermal, urinary, and gastrointestinal cells. Menstrual bleeding adds, on average, slightly more than 1 mg to the daily loss, as does lactation.

3. Transport

Transferrin is the primary vehicle for transporting iron entering the plasma. Essentially all proliferating cells have on their surfaces transferrin receptors whose affinity increases with the latter's iron content and whose synthesis and release into the blood increases with decreasing availability of iron. Erythroid precursors and hepatic and placental cells have more receptors than other cells.

4. Storage

Ferritin is the primary storage protein for iron, and its production and cellular content, as well as the amount circulating in plasma, are increased by increasing amounts of cellular iron. Ferritin, present in essentially all cells, readily gives up iron and serves as the storage compartment for cellular utilization. Hemosiderin, a more stable storage form, holds most of the iron in the reticuloendothelial system's macrophages.

B. Progression of Iron Deficiency

When absorption does not keep pace with utilization and loss, iron stores are used. As stores become depleted, the individual passes through three stages of iron deficiency.

1. Latent Stage

Iron stores are depleted, and marrow contains no stainable iron. However, hemoglobin production has not yet decreased, and there is no anemia or microcytosis. Serum ferritin, reflecting body iron stores, is decreased. Serum transferrin receptors, serum iron, transferrin, transferrin saturation, and red cell protoporphyrin are normal.

2. Early Stage

As the imbalance between absorption and need continues, insufficient iron is available for hemoglobin synthesis, and the various markers of deficiency begin to be established. The hemoglobin decreases through the normal range into the subnormal. Red cells being produced are smaller and have decreased content of hemoglobin and increased zinc protoporphyrin. However, early in this stage, because the abnormal cells are mixed in the peripheral blood with a much larger number of normal cells, routine studies of red cell parameters continue to be normal. Therefore, especially if the patient's baseline MCV is in the upper portion of the normal range, early IDA can be normocytic. Serum ferritin, already below normal during latent deficiency, can undergo no further measurable decrease, and thus is not helpful in determining the degree of deficiency. Serum transferrin receptors, however, become increased in the early stage of iron lack and progressively increase as the deficiency worsens.

3. Established Stage

As the deficiency progresses, under the stimulation of increasing amounts of erythropoietin, erythroid precursors are more numerous in the marrow, and the lack of iron causes the more mature forms to have visibly less cytoplasm that has deficient hemoglobinization. Anemia worsens, and progressively smaller red cells with lesser amounts of hemoglobin become more numerous in the peripheral blood. As the duration and severity of deficiency increase, and as more of the previously produced normal cells become senescent and are removed, the RDW increases and red cell histogram widens. The MCV and MCH decrease and become progressively more abnormal, in proportion with the decrease in hemoglobin. Likewise, there is a proportionate increase in serum transferrin receptors.

C. Relative Iron Deficiency

Under maximal stimulation from erythropoietin, whether endogenous or experimentally or therapeutically administered, the expanded erythroid population's need for iron may outstrip the capacity of the delivery system, even when storage iron is plentiful (12,13). Examples include hemolytic anemia and treatment with erythropoietin.

D. Nonhematologic Consequences of Iron Deficiency

Although the effects of iron deficiency itself may be difficult to distinguish from those of the anemia it causes, there is increasing awareness that iron deficiency itself is harmful (14). For example, compared with other anemias, IDA causes increased risk of preterm delivery (15). IDA produces significantly decreased work performance, but in addition, nonanemic iron-deficient subjects gain increased work capacity from iron therapy before there is a significant increase in hemoglobin. Infants with IDA have impaired mental function which may not be completely reversible with iron therapy. The increased absorption of iron that results from iron deficiency is accompanied by increased absorption of additional metals, including lead, making iron-deficient children more susceptible to lead poisoning.

VI. DIAGNOSIS

When the anemia is severe, the routine blood count provides the information needed for diagnosis, and additional studies are needed only to establish the etiology of the deficiency. The medical history and physical findings relative to the gastrointestinal tract and, in women, to the genital tract will most often reveal the reason for anemia. Endoscopic and/or radiographic evaluation of the gastrointestinal tract is frequently required to reveal the source of blood loss. When the anemia is mild to moderate, more extensive evaluation is necessary to establish that iron deficiency is its cause. Serum ferritin is the key test for making this determination, but the acute-phase reaction may interfere with its interpretation, necessitating a bone marrow examination or a trial of iron therapy to establish the presence of iron deficiency. Table 1 shows the characteristic laboratory findings in iron deficiency and the common disorders from which it must be distinguished.

VII. DIFFERENTIAL DIAGNOSIS

A. Anemia of Chronic Disease

IDA and anemia of chronic disease (ACD) are both very common, and they frequently coexist. Also, microcytosis is frequent in ACD. Therefore, it is often necessary to determine whether a patient has IDA, ACD, or both. Differentiation hinges on the serum ferritin level. In a patient who may have both IDA and ACD, a value below the usually quoted normal, 10–12 ng/mL, confirms iron deficiency. If, as is more likely, the level is in the normal range, the closer it is to the lower limit of normal, the more likely is iron deficiency. Some authors state that a normal RDW argues against iron deficiency, because the test has a high sensitivity for IDA (16). However, the preponderance of evidence suggests that the test lacks sufficient sensitivity (3) to supplement the diagnostic power of serum ferritin (6). In some cases a clear-cut distinction can not be made on the basis of clinical and laboratory findings, and a trial of iron therapy or a bone marrow examination may be required.

B. Thalassemia

Heterozygous alpha and beta thalassemia are common microcytic anemias. The combination of low normal to slightly decreased hemoglobin, high normal to slightly increased red cell count, moderately decreased MCV, and target cells is characteristic of thalassemia minor. In iron deficiency when the hemoglobin is comparable to that typical of thalassemia minor, the MCV is usually less abnormal. Serum ferritin and hemoglobin A2 levels usually suffice to make the distinction.

Table 1 Summary of Laboratory Findings in the Differential Diagnosis of Iron Deficiency Anemia

Condition	Definition	Hemoglobin concentration	MCV	Serum ferritin	Serum transferrin receptors
Latent iron deficiency	Absent iron stores but iron adequate for hemoglobin production	Normal	Normal	Decreased	Normal
Early iron deficiency anemia	Insufficient iron for hemoglobin production	Low normal to slightly decreased	Low normal to slightly decreased	Decreased	Slightly increased
Established iron deficiency anemia	Chronic iron deficiency with significant anemia	Moderately to markedly decreased	Moderately to markedly decreased	Decreased	Moderately to markedly increased
Anemia of chronic disease	Normocytic or microcytic anemia caused by a variety of chronic diseases	Slightly to moderately decreased	Normal to mildly decreased	Normal or increased	Normal or slightly increased
Anemia of chronic disease with superimposed iron deficiency	Same as above but with iron deficiency, usually from blood loss	Slightly to moderately decreased	Normal to mildly decreased	Variable. Below 45 makes iron deficiency likely; above 100, unlikely	Increased
Thalassemia minor	Genetically determined deficiency of globin chain production	Low normal to slightly decreased	Mildly to moderately decreased	Normal to increased	

C. Hemoglobinopathy

Hemoglobin E, common in Southeast Asians, causes microcytosis that is mild in heterozygotes and marked in homozygotes (17). Heterozygotes are usually not anemic and homozygotes only mildly so. Hemoglobin electrophoresis is diagnostic.

D. Lead Poisoning

In the past, lead poisoning was considered in the differential diagnosis of microcytic anemia, but it is now thought that both anemia and microcytsis are secondary to coexisting iron deficiency, which is common in underprivileged children, a group in which plumbism is often found (18).

VIII. TREATMENT

The first goal of therapy is to eliminate the cause of the deficiency. Until this has been accomplished, a full response to replacement of iron is unlikely. In addition, further harm may accrue to a patient with a serious underlying disorder if it is unrecognized and allowed to progress while the anemia is being treated. After managing the underlying problem, most patients' iron deficiency can be successfully treated with oral iron. The few patients who cannot tolerate or are unable to absorb oral iron can be given intravenous iron, which, however, is considerably more expensive and has the potential for causing life-threatening anaphylactic reactions. Red cell transfusions are only rarely indicated: for example, when the patient has angina or severe heart failure associated with moderate or severe anemia, or when a seriously anemic patient must undergo a major surgical procedure.

Noncompliance with oral therapy, use of an iron preparation that delivers suboptimal amounts of iron, continued blood loss, and presence of a disorder causing ACD are the usual causes of incomplete response. Failure to achieve normalization of the hemoglobin after treatment deserves an aggressive evaluation (19). After causes have been carefully excluded, consideration should be given to more unusual causes such as malabsorption, iron loss secondary to intestinal parasites or paroxysmal nocturnal hemoglobinuria, and sequestration, as in idiopathic pulmonary hemosiderosis.

CASE STUDY 1

Patient

Fifty-six-year-old man.

Chief Complaint

Intermittently tarry stools.

Medical History

The patient had been well until approximately 4 months ago, when he began to notice that his stools were intermittently darker than usual. The most recent episode led to his seeking medical advice. Hypertension was being successfully treated with an ACE inhibitor. He denied the use of other drugs, including aspirin. There was no personal or family history of easy bleeding.

Laboratory Results

	Patient	Normal
Hemoglobin	8.9 g/dL	13–17 g/dL
MCV	70 fL	82–98 fL
MCHC	31.1%	32–36
Platelets	540,000/μL	150,000–450,000/μL

Additional Laboratory Results

	Patient	Normal
Ferritin	10 ng/mL	35–250 ng/mL
Serum Iron	32 μg/dL	50–190 μg/dL
Transferrin	450 mg/dL	200–400 mg/dL
Transferrin saturation	7.1%	20–55%

A peripheral blood smear from this patient is shown in Fig. 1.

Upper and lower gastrointestinal tract radiographic studies were normal. A biopsy of duodenal mucosal friability was interpreted as a leiomyoma.

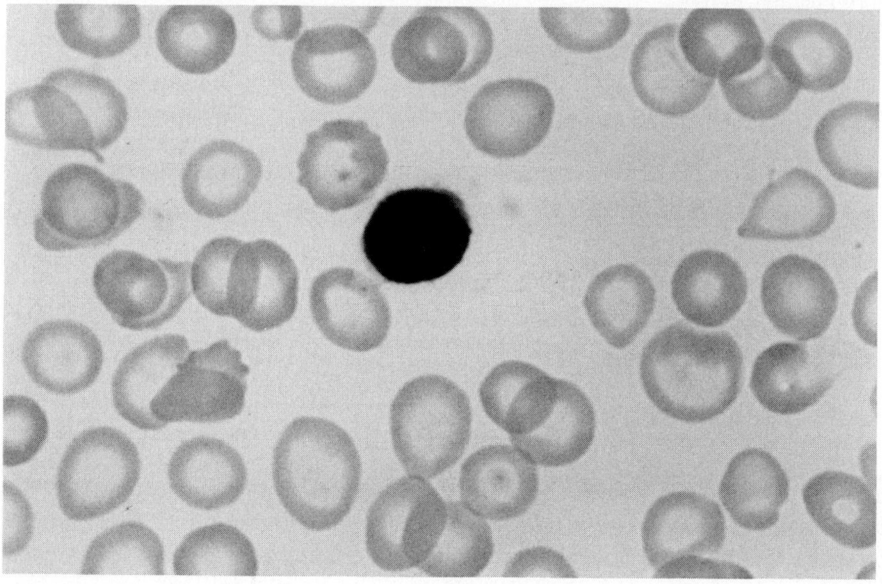

Figure 1 Peripheral blood smear in iron deficiency anemia. These microcytic, hypochromic red blood cells have a diameter less than that of the nucleus of the small lymphocyte and a central pallor greater than one-third the diameter of the red cell. (×1000.)

Questions

1. Using the morphologic approach, classify this man's anemia.
2. List the differential diagnosis in this case.
3. Compare the use of serum ferritin versus serum iron and transferrin in the study of patients with possible iron deficiency anemia.

Discussion

This is a microcytic hypochromic anemia related to iron deficiency due to chronic blood loss from a duodenal leiomyoma. Other causes of microcytic anemia include alpha and beta thalassemia, anemia of chronic disease, and sideroblastic anemia. In adults, chronic blood loss is almost always the cause of IDA, the gastrointestinal tract being the most common source. Young children may develop IDA, so-called milk-and-crackers anemia, while pregnant women may become iron deficient due to fetal demands for iron. There are two general etiologies for microcytic anemia: (a) abnormal iron metabolism, as in this patient; and (b) abnormal globin metabolism, as in the thalassemias and hemoglobin E.

Although the literature documents the superiority of serum ferritin, serum iron and transferrin, regrettably, are still widely used. Ferritin levels in the serum reflect total body iron stores; however, the level rises as an acute-phase reactant in conditions such as febrile illnesses, chronic infections, noninfectious inflammatory disorders, and malignancies. Nevertheless, under these circumstances it is still possible to interpret ferritin values, as shown below. Interpretation of ferritin values can be improved using sex-based reference values, also indicated below.

Typical Laboratory Findings in IDA

A. Initial studies		B. Additional studies	
Hemoglobin	Decreased	Ferritin	Decreased
MCV	Decreased	Serum iron	Decreased
MCHC	Normal or decreased	Transferrin	Increased
Platelets	Normal or increased	Transferrin saturation	Decreased
Reticulocytes	Normal or increased		
C. Normal serum ferritin values		D. Serum ferritin values in acute phase reaction	
Premenopausal women	10–100 ng/mL	Probably iron deficient	10–50 ng/mL
Postmenopausal women	25–150 ng/mL	Possibly iron deficient	50–75 ng/mL
Men	35–250 ng/mL	Indeterminate	75–100 ng/mL
		Unlikely to be iron deficient	>100 ng/mL

It is usually not necessary to obtain a bone marrow specimen to evaluate for IDA, but when it is necessary, marrow smears have a lack of stainable iron. Metarubricytes retain blue-staining cytoplasm caused by lack of hemoglobin. The cell borders have a ragged appearance, as shown in Fig. 2.

Treatment

Treatment for iron deficiency requires finding and treating the underlying disease, followed by oral iron therapy.

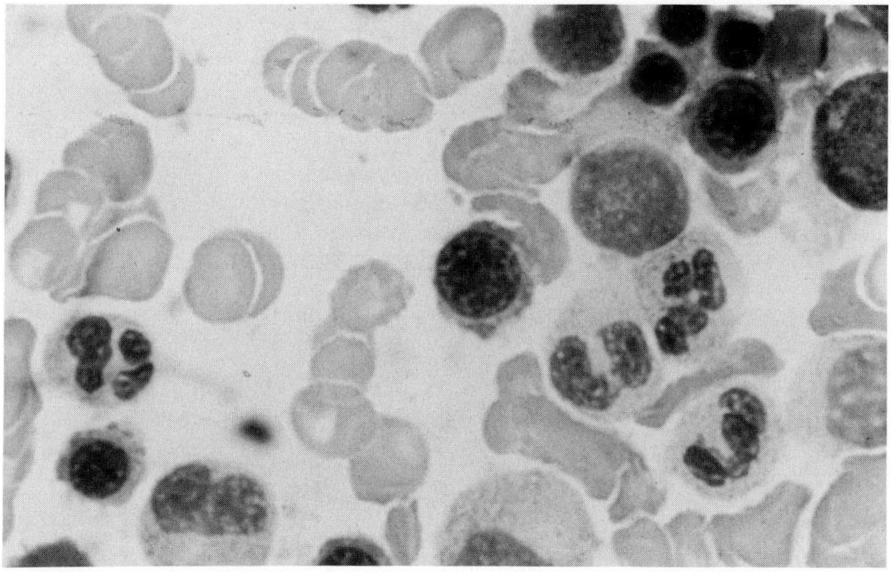

Figure 2 Bone marrow aspirate in iron deficiency anemia. The metarubricyte in the center has a darker cytoplasm than normal due to deficient hemoglobinization, and the cytoplasm also has a ragged appearance.

CASE STUDY 2

Patient

Sixty-year-old woman.

Chief Complaint

The patients has a long history of rheumatoid arthritis. She reports increasing joint pain over the past month.

Medical History

In the past 2 weeks, there has been increasing fatigue. There is a recent history of a small amount of blood on her stool. She has had no black stools. Salicylate treatment for the rheumatoid arthritis has been successful in limiting her symptoms.

Physical Examination

There are moderate deformities of her hands, consistent with rheumatoid arthritis.

Laboratory Results

	Patient	Normal
Hemoglobin	7.9 g/dL	11.5–15.5 g/dL
MCV	78 fL	82–98 fL
MCHC	34%	32–36%
Platelets	350,000/μL	150,000–450,000/μL
Reticulocytes	115,000/μL	25,000–125,000/μL

Additional Laboratory Results

	Patient	Normal
Ferritin	125 ng/mL	25–150 ng/mL
Serum Iron	35 μg/dL	50–190 μg/dL
Transferrin	220 mg/dL	200–400 mg/dL
Transferrin Saturation	16%	20–55%

The appearance of the peripheral smear of this patient is shown in Fig. 3.

Stools were negative for occult blood. Endoscopy revealed anal fissures. There were no lesions in the colon.

Questions

1. Using the morphologic approach, classify this patient's anemia.
2. Given the laboratory data and clinical information, suggest the most likely reason for this patient's anemia.
3. How does one differentiate IDA and a microcytic ACD?
4. What therapy could be used for this patient?

Discussion

The patient has a microcytic normochromic anemia due to ACD. Approximately 20% cases of ACD are microcytic rather than normocytic. Although the serum iron is decreased, the transferrin does not have the increase characteristic of IDA, and the pattern here is quite typical of

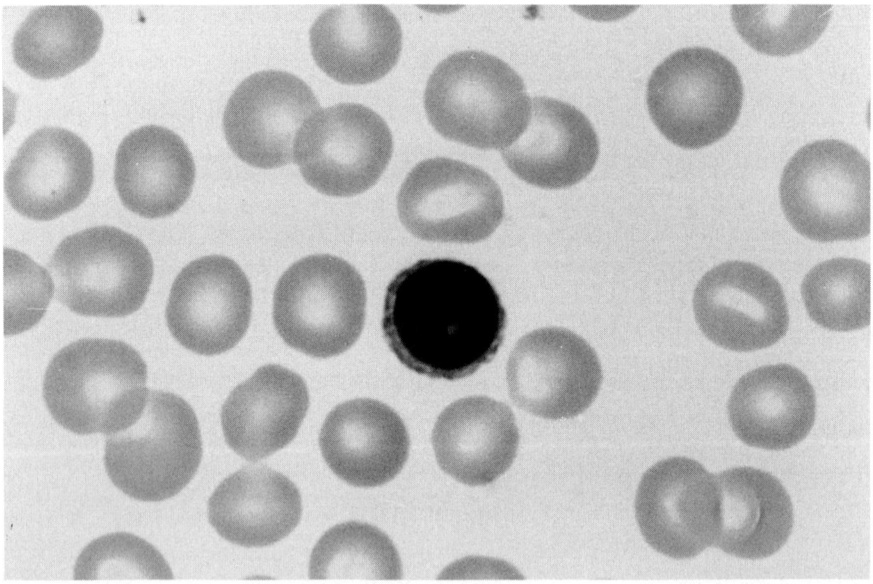

Figure 3 Peripheral blood smear in anemia of chronic disorders. About 20% of cases of anemia of chronic disorders are microcytic like this one. Note that the diameters of the red cells are generally less than that of the nucleus of the central small lymphocyte.

ACD. Also, the ferritin value in this patient is too much into the normal range to be indicative of an underlying IDA.

Clinical Picture and Laboratory Findings

Patients with ACD usually have an obvious chronic disorder such as rheumatoid arthritis or cancer. Anemia is mild to moderate and, unless complicated by another mechanism, is never severe. Platelets and reticulocytes are usually normal. In ACD, serum ferritin is normal or increased, while serum iron is decreased, and transferrin is either normal or decreased. As indicated in Case Study 1, a serum ferritin less than 50 ng/mL in a patient with a condition associated with ACD is likely to indicate superimposed iron deficiency.

Treatment

The treatment for ACD is aimed primarily at the underlying chronic disorder. Recombinant human erythropoietin has resulted in improvement of the anemia.

Bibliography

1. Brown RG. Determining the cause of anemia: general approach, with emphasis on microcytic, hypochromic anemias. Postgrad Med 1991; 89(6):161–170.
2. Hardin RI, Lux SE, Stossel TP. Blood: Principles and Practice of Hematology. Philadelphia: Lippincott, 1995.
3. Massey AC. Microcytic anemia: differential diagnosis and management of iron deficiency anemia. Med Clin N Am 1992; 76:549–565.
4. Mohler E. Iron deficiency and anemia of chronic disease: clues to differentiating these conditions. Postgrad Med 1992; 92(4):123–128.

REFERENCES

1. Looker AC, Dallman PR, Carroll MD, Gunter EW, Johnson CL. Prevalence of iron deficiency in the United States. JAMA 1997; 277:973–976.
2. Schwartz WJ, Thurnau GR. Iron deficiency anemia in pregnancy. Clin Obstet Gynecol 1995; 38: 443–454.
3. Savage RA. The red cell indices: yesterday, today and tomorrow. Clin Lab Med 1993; 13:773–785.
4. Fairbanks VF. Is the peripheral blood smear reliable for the diagnosis of iron deficiency anemia? Am J Clin Pathol 1971; 55:447–451.
5. Simmons JO, Noel GL, Diehl LF. Does review of peripheral blood smears help in the initial workup of common anemias? J Gen Intern Med 1989; 4:473–481.
6. Guyatt GH, Oxman AD, Ali M, Willan A, McIlroy W. Laboratory diagnosis of iron-deficiency anemia: an overview. J Gen Intern Med 1992; 7:145–153.
7. Burns ER, Goldberg SN, Lawrence C, Wenz B. Clinical utility of serum tests for iron deficiency in hospitalized patients. Am J Clin Pathol 1990; 93:240–245.
8. Cook JD, Baynes RD, Skikne BS. The physiologic significance of circulating transferrin receptors. Adv Exp Biol Med 1994; 352:119–126.
9. Ferguson BJ, Skikne BS, Simpson KM, Baynes RD, Cook JD. Serum transferrin receptor distinguishes the anemia of chronic disease from iron deficiency anemia. J Lab Clin Med 1992; 19: 385–390.
10. Kurer SB, Seifert B, Michel B, Ruegg R, Fehr J. Prediction of iron deficiency in chronic inflammatory rheumatic disease anaemia. Br J Haematol 1995; 91:820–826.
11. Van Dam J, Bond JH, Sivak MV. Fecal occult blood screening for colorectal cancer. Arch Intern Med 1995; 155:2389–2402.
12. Finch CA, Huebers H. Perspectives in iron metabolism. New Engl J Med 1982; 306:1520–1528.

13. Brugnara C, Coella GM, Cremins J, et al. Effects of subcutaneous recombinant human erythropoietin in normal subjects: development of decreased reticulocyte hemoglobin content and iron deficient erythropoiesis. J Lab Clin Med 1994; 123:660–667.
14. Yip R. Iron deficiency: contemporary scientific issues and international programmatic approaches. J Nutr 1994; 124:1479S–1490S.
15. Scholl TO, Hediger ML, Fischer RL, Shearer JW. Anemia vs iron deficiency: increased risk of preterm delivery in a prospective study. Am J Clin Nutr 1992; 55:985–988.
16. van Zeben D, Bieger R, van Wermeskerken RKA, Castel A, Hermans J. Evaluation of microcytosis using serum ferritin and red blood cell distribution width. Eur J Haematol 1990; 44:105–108.
17. Monzon CM, Fairbanks VF, Burgert EO Jr, Sutherland JE, Elliot SC. Hematologic genetic disorders among Southeast Asian refugees. Am J Hematol 1985; 19:27–36.
18. Clark M, Royal J, Seeler R. Interaction of iron deficiency and lead and the hematologic findings in children with severe lead poisoning. Pediatrics 1988; 81:247–254.
19. Ascari E. Iron-deficiency anemia resistant to iron therapy. Haematologica 1993; 78:178–182.

SELECTED READINGS

1. Ascari E. Iron-deficiency anemia resistant to iron therapy. Haematologica 1993; 78:178–182.
2. Berger M, Brass LF. Severe thrombocytopenia in iron deficiency anemia. Am J Hematol 1987; 24: 425–428.
3. Brugnara C, Coella GM, Cremins J, et al. Effects of subcutaneous recombinant human erythropoietin in normal subjects: development of decreased reticulocyte hemoglobin content and iron deficient erythropoiesis. J Lab Clin Med 1994; 123: 660—667.
4. Burns ER, Goldberg SN, Lawrence C, Wenz B. Clinical utility of serum tests for iron deficiency in hospitalized patients. Am J Clin Pathol 1990; 93:240–245.
5. Clark M, Royal J, Seeler R. Interaction of iron deficiency and lead and the hematologic findings in children with severe lead poisoning. Pediatrics 1988; 81:247–254.
6. Cook JD, Baynes RD, Skikne BS. The physiologic significance of circulating transferrin receptors. Adv Exp Biol Med 1994; 352:119–126.
7. Cook JD, Skikne BS. Iron deficiency: definition and diagnosis. J Intern Med 1989; 226:349–355.
8. Fairbanks VF. Is the peripheral blood smear reliable for the diagnosis of iron deficiency anemia? Am J Clin Pathol 1971; 55:447–451.
9. Ferguson BJ, Skikne BS, Simpson KM, Baynes RD, Cook JD. Serum transferrin receptor distinguishes the anemia of chronic disease from iron deficiency anemia. J Lab Clin Med 1992; 19: 385–390.
10. Finch CA, Huebers H. Perspectives in iron metabolism. New Engl J Med 1982; 306:1520–1528.
11. Guyatt GH, Oxman AD, Ali M, Willan A, McIlroy W. Laboratory diagnosis of iron-deficiency anemia: an overview. J Gen Intern Med 1992; 7:145–153.
12. Hercberg S, Galan P. Nutritional anemias. Baillieres Clin Haematol 1992; 5:143–168.
13. Kurer SB, Seifert B, Michel B, Ruegg R, Fehr J. Prediction of iron deficiency in chronic inflammatory rheumatic disease anaemia. Br J Haematol 1995; 91:820–826.
14. Looker AC, Dallman PR, Carroll MD, Gunter EW, Johnson CL. Prevalence of iron deficiency in the United States. JAMA 1997; 277:973–976.
15. McIntyre AS, Long RG. Prospective survey of investigations in outpatients referred with iron deficiency anaemia. Gut 1993; 34:1102–1107.
16. Monzon CM, Fairbanks VF, Burgert EO Jr, Sutherland JE, Elliot SC. Hematologic genetic disorders among Southeast Asian refugees. Am J Hematol 1985; 19:27–36.
17. Oski FA. Iron deficiency in infancy and childhood. New Engl J Med 1993; 329:190–193.
18. Patterson C, Guyatt GH, Singer J, Ali M, Turpie MB. Iron deficiency in the elderly: the diagnostic process. Can Med Assoc J 1991; 144:435–440.
19. Rockey DC, Cello JP. Evaluation of the gastrointestinal tract in patients with iron-deficiency anemia. N Engl J Med 1993; 329:1691–1695.

20. Savage RA. The red cell indices: yesterday, today and tomorrow. Clin Lab Med 1993; 13:773–785.
21. Scholl TO, Hediger ML, Fischer RL, Shearer JW. Anemia vs iron deficiency: increased risk of preterm delivery in a prospective study. Am J Clin Nutr 1992; 55:985–988.
22. Schwartz WJ, Thurnau GR. Iron deficiency anemia in pregnancy. Clin Obstet Gynecol 1995; 38: 443–454.
23. Siegel RM, LaGroin DH. The use of zinc protoporphyrin in screening young children for iron deficiency. Clin Pediatr 1994; 33:473–479.
24. Simmons JO, Noel GL, Diehl LF. Does review of peripheral blood smears help in the initial workup of common anemias? J Gen Intern Med 1989; 4:473–481.
25. Van Dam J, Bond JH, Sivak MV. Fecal occult blood screening for colorectal cancer. Arch Intern Med 1995; 155:2389–2402.
26. van Zeben D, Bieger R, van Wermeskerken RKA, Castel A, Hermans J. Evaluation of microcytosis using serum ferritin and red blood cell distribution width. Eur J Haematol 1990; 44:105–108.
27. Yip R. Iron deficiency: contemporary scientific issues and international programmatic approaches. J Nutr 1994; 124:1479S–1490S.

13

Megaloblastic Anemias

LoAnn C. Peterson
Northwestern University Medical Center, Chicago, Illinois

I. DEFINITION

The megaloblastic anemias comprise a group of disorders that share a characteristic morphologic appearance in the blood and bone marrow. The common biochemical feature causing the morphologic change is defective deoxyribonucleic acid (DNA) synthesis with relatively unimpaired ribonucleic acid (RNA) synthesis. This unbalanced growth is characterized by nuclear/cytoplasmic asynchrony. Nuclear maturation is arrested or immature, while cytoplasmic maturation proceeds normally. The microscopic appearance of this dissociation is morphologically described as megaloblastic. Megaloblastic cells tend to be large, with cell nuclei that appear less mature than the cytoplasm. Most megaloblastic anemias are due to the deficiency of vitamin B_{12} (cobalamin) or folate or both.

II. PATHOPHYSIOLOGY

A. Vitamin B_{12}

Vitamin B_{12} is a large, complex organometallic compound known as cobalamin. It is composed of a corrin ring (similar to porphyrin) and a nucleotide. The trace element cobalt is located centrally within the corrin ring. Cobalamins cannot be synthesized by the human body and most be supplied in the diet. The only dietary sources of cobalamin are animal products such as meat and dairy foods.

Vitamin B_{12} is released from its tight polypeptide linkages in food during gastric digestion by the action of hydrochloric acid and pepsin. The free vitamin B_{12} attaches to salivary and gastric R-binding proteins (R because of their rapid electrophoretic mobility). On entering the duodenum, the R–B_{12} complexes are digested by pancreatic proteases. The released vitamin B_{12} then attaches to intrinsic factor, a glycoprotein produced by normal gastric parietal cells that is essential for absorption of vitamin B_{12}. The vitamin B_{12}–intrinsic factor complexes pass into the small intestine, where they adhere to specific receptors on the mucosal brush border of the distal ileum. The vitamin B_{12}–intrinsic factor complex is taken into the mucosal cell, where the intrinsic factor is destroyed and the vitamin is transferred to another transport protein, transcobalamin II (TC-II). The B_{12}–TC-II complex is then secreted into the plasma and rapidly taken up by bone marrow, liver, and other proliferating cells.

The recommended minimal daily requirement for vitamin B_{12} is 1–3 μg for adults, and 0.3–1.0 μg for infants and children. The total body content of vitamin B_{12} is approximately 2000–5000 μg in an adult male, with the liver being the main site of storage. Reserves in the body are usually sufficient for 3–6 years if intake or absorption is stopped abruptly.

B. Folate

Folic acid or pteroylmonoglutamic acid is synthesized by many plants and microorganisms. Leafy vegetables and fruits are rich sources of folate. Some forms of dietary folate are very heat labile and are readily destroyed by cooking.

Folates in foods are largely conjugated to polyglutamic acid. In order for folate to be absorbed, conjugases in the bile and small intestine convert the polyglutamates to mono- and diglutamates. These are readily absorbed in the proximal jejunum. Most of the plasma folate is in the form of N^5-methyltetrahydrofolate. The majority is loosely bound to albumin and is readily taken up by folate receptors present on cells throughout the body. Once in the cell, the folate is reconverted to the polyglutamate form.

The recommended minimum daily requirement for folate is about 50 μg but may be increased severalfold during periods of increased demand such as pregnancy. The normal total stores of folate are about 5,000–20,000 μg, primarily in the liver. Deficiency will occur within months if intake or absorption is curtailed.

C. Functions and Interrelationships of Vitamin B_{12} and Folate

The primary function of folate is to act as an intermediate in the transfer of one-carbon unit such as methyl ($—CH_3$), methylene ($—CH_2—$), or formal (HCO) in a variety of reactions related to the synthesis of DNA. The most important metabolic processes dependent on these one-carbon transfers are (a) synthesis of purines; (b) synthesis of methionine from homocysteine, a reaction that also requires vitamin B_{12}; and (c) synthesis of deoxythymidylate monophosphate (dTMP).

Two reactions in humans are known to require vitamin B_{12}. Vitamin B_{12} provides coenzymatic activity in (a) the conversion of homocysteine to methionine and (b) the isomerization of methylmalonyl coenzyme A to succinyl coenzyme A.

The formation of methionine is central to DNA synthesis and requires both vitamin B_{12} and folate. Methylcobalamin, a form of vitamin B_{12} is an essential cofactor for methyltransferase in the conversion of homocysteine to methionine (Fig. 1). N^5-methyltetrahydrofolate acts as the original methyl donor in this reaction. The methyl group is first transferred from N^5-methyltetrahydrofolate to the enzyme-bound cobalamin to form methylcobalamin; methylcobalamin then transfers the methyl group to homocysteine to generate methionine. The importance of this reaction is that it generates tetrahydrofolate. Tetrahydrofolate is required (through its derivative N^5, 10-methyltetrahydrofolate) for the conversion of deoxyuridine monophosphate (dUMP) to deoxythymidine monophosphate (dUMP), an immediate precursor of DNA.

It has been postulated that the cause of impaired DNA synthesis in vitamin B_{12} deficiency is the decreased availability of tetrahydrofolate. In the absence of vitamin B_{12}, N^5-methyltetrahydrofolate cannot be demethylated and therefore cannot be converted to other forms of tetrahydrofolate. This is the so-called methylfolate trap hypothesis. Since N^5-methyltetrahydrofolate is a poor substrate for conjugating enzyme, it largely remains in the unconjugated stage and slowly leaks from the cell. Tissue folate depletion develops even though serum levels of

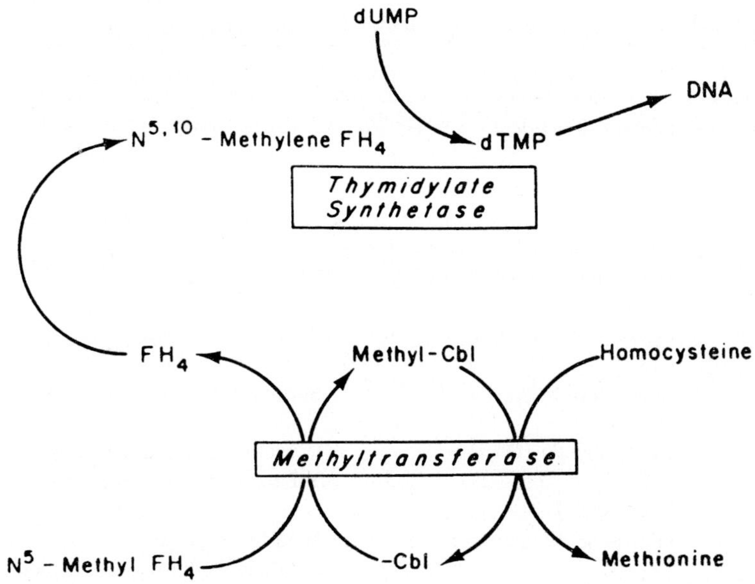

Figure 1 Reaction that requires methylcobalamin (methyl-Cbl) and transfers the methyl group of N^5-methyltetrahydrofolate (N^5-methyl FH_4) to homocysteine to form methionine and tetrahydrofolate. Tetrahydrofolate is required for the conversion of deoxyuridine monophosphate (dUMP) to deoxythymidinne monophosphate (dTMP), an immediate precursor of DNA. (From Beck WS. Metabolic aspects of vitamin B12 and folic acid. In: Williams WJ, et al., eds. Hematology. New York: McGraw-Hill, 1983: 311.)

folate may be normal or elevated. The hypothesis that deficiency of folate is the fundamental cause of anemia in vitamin B_{12} deficiency is supported by the fact that large doses of folate can produce a partial hematologic remission in patients with vitamin B_{12} deficiency.

III. CLASSIFICATION OF THE MEGALOBLASTIC ANEMIAS

The most common causes of megaloblastic anemia are deficiencies of vitamin B_{12}, folate, or both. The classification of the megaloblastic anemias secondary to vitamin B_{12} and folate deficiency is shown in Tables 1 and 2.

A. Vitamin B_{12} Deficiency

1. Inadequate Intake

The dietary intake of vitamin B_{12} is more than adequate for daily requirements, except for individuals on a purely vegetable diet and breast-fed infants of such individuals. Therefore, deficiency of vitamin B_{12} due to inadequate intake is rare.

2. Defective Absorption

Pernicious anemia is the most common cause of decreased absorption of vitamin B_{12}. Several other potential causes of defective absorption exist (Table 1), but are encountered in clinical practice only rarely. In fact, pernicious anemia is the most common cause of vitamin B_{12} deficiency in the United States. The fundamental defect in pernicious anemia is severe gastric

Table 1 Classification of Megaloblastic Anemias Due to Vitamin B_{12} Deficiency

Causes	Mechanisms	Clinical conditions
Inadequate intake	Dietary deficiency	Strict vegetarian, breast-fed infants of deficient mothers
Defective absorption	Decreased intrinsic factor	Pernicious anemia, juvenile pernicious anemia, gastrectomy
	Inadequate pancreatic proteases	Pancreatic insufficiency
	Inactivation of pancreatic proteases	Zollinger-Ellison syndrome
	Parasitic or bacterial overgrowth	Fish tapeworm, blind loop syndrome
	Mucosal defects	Sprue, surgical resection, amyloidosis
	Drug-induced effect	Colchicine, para-aminosalicylate, neomycin, colestyramine
	Decreased TC-II	Congenital TC-II deficiency
Increased requirements	Increased utilization or loss	Hemolysis, pregnancy, lactation, infancy, adolescence, hemodialysis
Disorders of metabolism	Inhibition of suppression of enzymes	Inborn enzyme error, nitrous oxide inhalation

Table 2 Classification of Megaloblastic Anemias Due to Folate Deficiency

Causes	Mechanisms	Clinical conditions
Inadequate intake	Dietary deficiency	Alcoholism, drug addiction, indigent and elderly individuals
Increased requirements	Growth, proliferative states, or loss exceeds intake	Pregnancy, growth spurts in infancy and adolescence, increased hematopoiesis, malignant diseases, hemodialysis, exfoliative skin disorders
Defective absorption	Gastrointestinal abnormalities	Sprue and other small bowel disorders, surgical resection, amyloidosis, congenital malabsorption
	Interference of absorption by drugs	Phenytoin, primidone, phenobarbitol
Disorders of metabolism	Inhibition of folate metabolism	Inhibitors of dihydrofolate reductase: methotrexate, pentamidine, pyrimethamine; alcohol
	Inherited disorders	Congenital enzyme deficiencies (dihydrofolate reductase), others (rare)

atrophy, with loss of all gastric secretions including intrinsic factor, the presence of which is necessary for absorption of vitamin B_{12}. Pernicious anemia is a disease of insidious onset that usually begins in middle age or later. It is rare under age 30, although children can be affected (juvenile pernicious anemia). It is found in all ethnic groups. Pernicious anemia is currently believed to result from immunologically mediated destruction of gastric mucosa. There is a significant association of pernicious anemia with other autoimmune disorders such as Grave's disease, Hashimoto thyroditis, and vitiligo.

About 90% of patients with pernicious anemia have antiparietal cell IgG antibodies in the serum, while 60% have serum anti-intrinsic factor antibodies. These antibodies are not specific for pernicious anemia, since antiparietal cell antibodies are found in 50% of patients with gastric atrophy without pernicious anemia. Unaffected relatives of patients with pernicious anemia may have anti-intrinsic factor antibodies in their serum.

3. Increased Requirement

Vitamin B_{12} stores are usually abundant. Deficiency states due to increased use or loss occur (Table 1) but are rare.

4. Metabolic Disorders

Inborn errors of metabolism resulting in megaloblastic anemia are rare; in these disorders megaloblastic anemia is present, but serum folate and vitamin B_{12} levels are normal. Nitrous oxide therapy inactivates coenzyme forms of vitamin B_{12} resulting in functional intracellular vitamin B_{12}deficiency.

B. Folic Acid Deficiency

1. Inadequate Intake

Folate malnutrition is common in alcoholics, whose main source of calories is alcoholic beverages that are virtually devoid of folic acid. Individuals addicted to drugs may be folate deficient due to malnutrition. Many indigent or elderly persons with diets lacking in fresh foods are folate deficient.

2. Increased Demand

Tissues with a relatively brisk mitotic rate such as the bone marrow have a high requirement for folate. Therefore, patients with hemolytic anemia or other very active hematopoiesis may become folate deficient. Increased folate is also required during periods of rapid growth and development, such as in pregnancy, infancy, and adolescence. Folic acid is lost during hemodialysis, and these patients may become deficient if not supplemented.

3. Deficient Absorption

Folic acid deficiency is common in sprue and may also be present in patients with other small bowel disorders. Congenital malabsorption of folate has also been documented. Several drugs may inhibit absorption of folate although the megaloblastic anemia caused by these agents is mild.

4. Disorders of Metabolism

Chemotherapeutic drugs that inhibit folate metabolism (Table 2) cause megaloblastic changes. Alcohol may also inhibit folate metabolism. Rare hereditary disorders of folate metabolism secondary to enzyme deficiencies have been reported.

IV. CLINICAL MANIFESTATIONS OF MEGALOBLASTIC ANEMIA

A. Vitamin B_{12} Deficiency

A patient with vitamin B_{12} deficiency may have a wide range of symptoms affecting various organ systems or may be completely asymptomatic and identified because of a macrocytosis detected on a screening blood count. In symptomatic patients, the symptoms may be related to the anemia or to other manifestations of vitamin B_{12} deficiency. The anemia may be severe, with hemoglobin values as low as 3 g/dL; the anemia is often surprisingly well tolerated because it develops so slowly. Weakness, easy fatiguability, dyspnea, palpitations, or angina may be present, depending on the severity and rapidity of onset of the anemia. Rarely, purpura is present due to thrombocytopenia. The patient may be pale or slightly jaundiced, depending on the degree of ineffective erythropoiesis.

Gastrointestinal manifestations related to the defective DNA synthesis of rapidly proliferating epithelium may also be present. The patient s tongue may be sore and appear smooth and beefy red secondary to villous atrophy. Loss of appetite related to the painful tongue or other problems mentioned above may also be present. The patient may complain of episodic diarrhea, which may be due to megaloblastic changes in the epithelium of the gastrointestinal tract and associated with malabsorption.

Neurologic manifestations beginning with demyelonization, followed by axonal degeneration, and lastly neuronal death occurs with vitamin B_{12} deficiency and may not fully remit with therapy. Neurologic damage involves peripheral nerves first and gradually progresses to involve the posterior and lateral columns of the spinal cord. Signs and symptoms include numbness and parathesias in the extremities, weakness, ataxia, loss of deep tendon reflexes, decreased position sense, and decreased vibration sense. Mental disturbances range from mild irritability and memory deficits to frank psychosis ("megaloblastic madness"). The biochemical basis for neuropathy in vitamin B_{12} deficiency is not clear. Earlier studies focused on the defect in succinyl coenzyme A synthesis as the possible mechanism. However, more recent studies suggest that defective methionine synthesis may be responsible.

B. Folic Acid Deficiency

Since the body stores of folate are relatively low, megaloblastic anemia secondary to dietary deficiency or increased metabolic demand can occur rather quickly. The clinical manifestations of patients with folate deficiency are similar to those of vitamin B_{12} deficiency, although patients with folate deficiency are more likely to appear malnourished. In addition, in contrast to vitamin B_{12} deficiency, neurologic abnormalities do not occur.

V. HEMATOLOGIC MANIFESTATIONS OF MEGALOBLASTIC ANEMIA

A. Blood Counts and Indices

The hemoglobin values in megaloblastic anemia vary from normal to markedly decreased levels as low as 3 g/dL. Most patients have a macrocytosis with mean corpuscular volumes (MCV) ranging from 100 to as high as 160 fL. Macrocytosis may be present in a variety of disorders (see Table 3), but megaloblastic anemia should be strongly suspected if the MCV is greater than 110–120 fL. The MCV may be normal in megaloblastic anemia if concurrent iron deficiency, thalassemia, or anemia of chronic disease is present; it is occasionally normal in

Table 3 Causes of Macrocytosis

Megaloblastic anemia
Liver disease
Alcoholism
Reticulocytosis
Hypothyroidism
Arsenic or chlordane intoxication
Congenital dyserythropoietic anemia
Aplastic anemia
Myelodysplastic syndromes
Myeloproliferative disorders
Myeloid leukemias
Chemotherapy

the absence of other disorders. The mean cell hemoglobin concentration (MCHC) in megaloblastic anemia is normal; the red cell distribution with (RDW) is increased. The reticulocyte count is low. Occasional patients exhibit neutropenia and/or thrombocytopenia.

B. Blood Smear Morphology

The peripheral blood smears are characterized by the presence of numerous oval macrocytes (Fig. 2) as well as occasional microcytes, fragmented red blood cells, and teardrop forms. Howell-Jolly bodies and basophilic stippling are frequently identified. Circulating nucleated red blood cells are often present.

Hypersegmentation of neutrophils, designated as six or more lobes in one or more neutrophils, is present in most cases (Fig. 3). Hypersegmented neutrophils appear early in the devel-

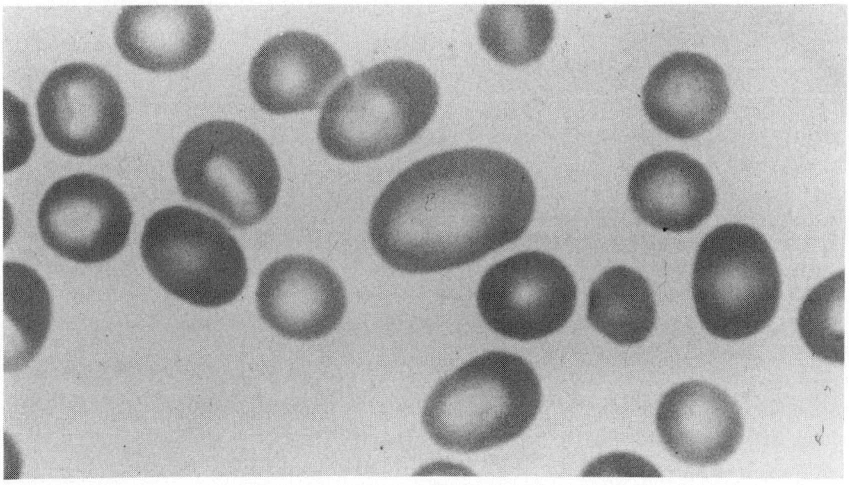

Figure 2 Blood smear from patient with pernicious anemia showing marked anisocytosis and oval macrocytes.

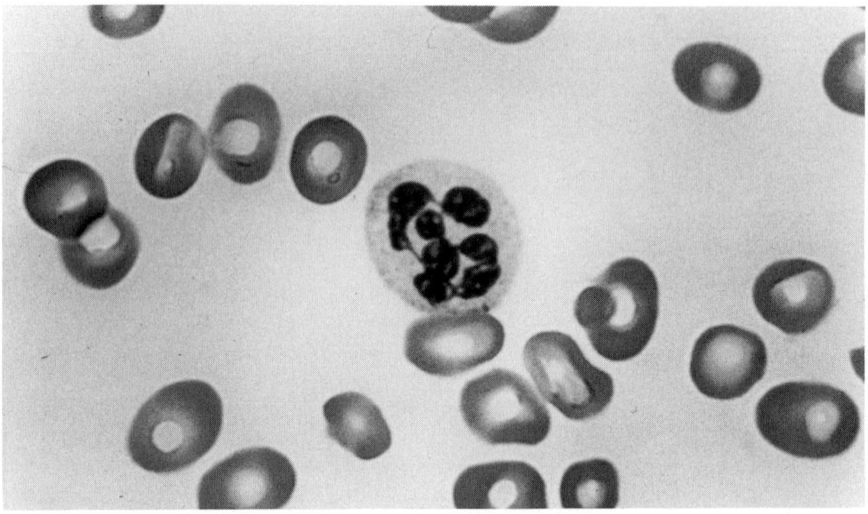

Figure 3 Hypersegmented neutrophil in blood from patient with megaloblastic anemia.

opment of megaloblastic anemia and typically precede the macrocytosis and anemia. However, they persist longer after therapy.

C. Bone Marrow Morphology

The bone marrow in megaloblastic anemia is hypercellular, with erythroid precursors predominating. A shift to immaturity is characteristically present, and mitotic figures may be numerous. The hypercellular bone marrow with peripheral cytopenias is a reflection of intramedullary death (inefffective erythropoiesis) secondary to the defect in DNA synthesis (nuclear maturation defect). The erythroid precursors are large, with a finely dispersed chromatin pattern (Fig. 4). The cytoplasm is more mature than the nucleus. The granulocyte precursors also display nuclear/cytoplasmic asynchrony (Fig. 5). The most striking changes occur in the band and metamyelocyte stages (giant bands and metamyelocytes). The cells are large, with nuclei that exhibit "immature chromatin" as compared with the stage of maturation of the cytoplasm. The nuclei may have bizarre shapes, and segmentation of the nuclei may begin while the chromatin pattern is still "immature". Megakaryocytes may also be large and hypersegmented.

VI. IDENTIFICATION OF SPECIFIC VITAMIN DEFICIENCIES

A. Serum Vitamin B_{12}, Serum Folate, and Red Cell Folate Determinations

Measurements of serum vitamin B_{12}, serum folate, and red cell folate are the primary tests used to determine whether there is a specific vitamin deficiency. The serum vitamin B_{12} level is a useful measure of the patient s vitamin B_{12} stores and is decreased in pernicious anemia and other anemias secondary to vitamin B_{12} deficiency. Decreased serum folate levels are typically found in patients with megaloblastic anemia secondary to folate deficiency. However, red cell folate quantitation is more reliable in determining whether folate deficiency is responsible for the megaloblastic anemia, since serum folate levels fluctuate considerably with recent diet. A

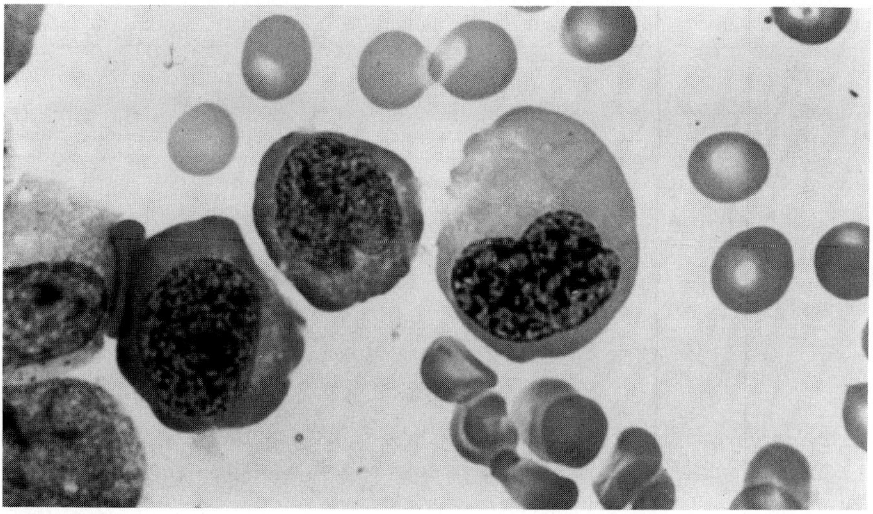

Figure 4 Megaloblastic erythroid precursors (megaloblasts) in bone marrow from patient with megaloblastic anemia.

deceased serum folate level indicates a negative folate balance, whereas a decreased red cell folate concentration more accurately reflects tissue stores. In the evaluation of megaloblastic anemia it is desirable to obtain all three measurements (Table 4). In vitamin B_{12} deficiency, the serum vitamin B_{12} level is low; the serum folate level is normal or high and the red cell folate level is normal or low. This has been attributed to the "methylfolate trap" hypothesis. A decrease in all three levels indicate deficiency of both vitamin B_{12} and folate, but also occurs in some patients with folate deficiency alone. Spuriously low vitamin B_{12} levels may be seen

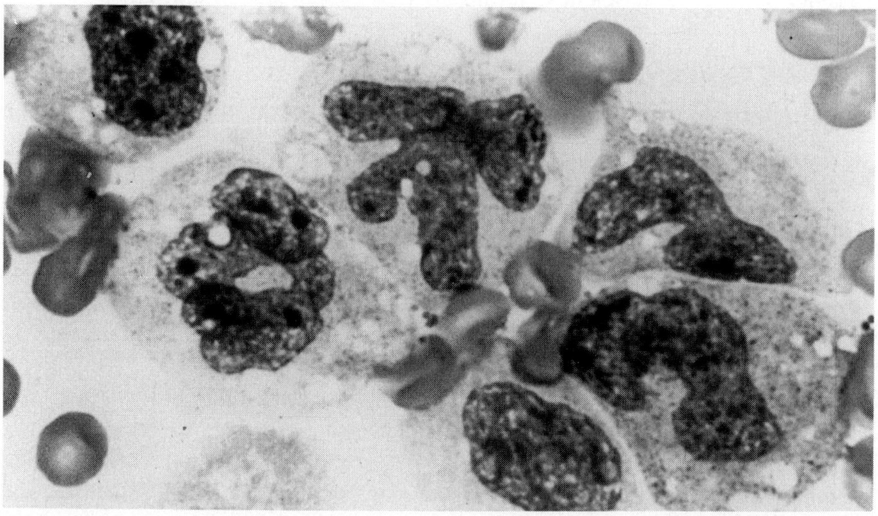

Figure 5 Giant metamyelocytes in bone marrow from patient with megaloblastic anemia.

Table 4 Characteristic Serum Values in Vitamin B_{12} and Folate Deficiency

	Serum vitamin B_{12}	Serum folate	RBC folate	Serum Methylmalonic acid	Serum homocysteine
Vitamin B_{12} deficiency	Low	Normal	Normal/low	High	High
Folate deficiency	Normal	Low	Low	High	Normal
Negative folate balance	Normal	Low	Normal	High	High
Combined vitamin B_{12} and folate deficiency	Low	Low	Low	High	High

with pregnancy, oral contraceptive use, multiple myeloma and acquired immunodeficiency syndrome, and transcobalamin-I deficiency. Importantly, a low level may represent a deficiency state even in the absence of anemia. Normal or elevated vitamin B_{12} levels may occur in vitamin B_{12}-deficient patients with liver disease or myeloproliferative disorders because of increased levels of vitamin B_{12} binders in the blood.

B. Serum Methylmalonic Acid and Homocysteine

Data suggest that measurement of serum methylmalonic acid and homoocysteine are highly sensitive for detecting intracellular vitamin B_{12} deficiency. Serum methylmalonic acid and homocysteine are elevated in more than 95% of patients with vitamin B_{12}deficiency (Table 4). Normal levels rule out a deficiency with near certainty. Furthermore, elevated levels are more specific for detecting vitamin B_{12} deficiency states that low serum B_{12} levels, which can be decreased without evidence of deficiency. One limitation, however, is that elevations in serum methylmalonic acid can also be seen in patients with renal dysfunction. Measurement of these metabolites is available through reference laboratories and can be done to confirm vitamin B_{12} deficiency when serum vitamin B_{12} levels are in the low normal range. Serum homocysteine is elevated in patients with folate deficiency; serum methylmalonic acid is normal.

VII. TESTS TO DETERMINE PATHOGENESIS OF VITAMIN B_{12} DEFICIENCY

A. Schilling Test

The most common method for evaluating vitamin B_{12} adsorption is the Schilling test. In the first stage (stage I) of this test, the patient ingests radiolabled vitamin B_{12}. This is followed by a parenteral dose of unlabeled vitamin B_{12} to displace the radiolabled B_{12} from receptors in plasma and tissues. Urine is collected over 24 hr, and the amount of radioactivity in this sample is measured. In pernicious anemia, the oral radioactive dose does not appear in the urine. In this situation, the test is repeated with intrinsic factor added to the oral dose (stage II). Patients with pernicious anemia will then have normal excretion of radiolabled vitamin B_{12}. An abnormal stage II result indicates that the patient may have malabsorption of vitamin B_{12} for reasons other than pernicious anemia.

The most common problems with the Schilling test are incomplete urine collection and renal insufficiency. In addition, the test may also be abnormal in pernicious anemia, due to the effect of vitamin B_{12} deficiency on the terminal ileum. In this situation, the second stage of the

Schilling test with intrinsic factor should be performed after the patient has received vitamin B_{12} therapy.

B. Serum Intrinsic Factor and Parietal Cell Antibodies

Serum intrinsic factor antibodies are present in 50–60% of patients with pernicious anemia. False positives are rare, so the presence of these antibodies in a patient with megaloblastic anemia secondary to vitamin B_{12} deficiency is essentially diagnostic of pernicious anemia. Serum parietal cell antibodies are present in 90% of patients with pernicious anemia, but false positives are common (10% of people over age 30), making this test less specific in the diagnosis of pernicious anemia.

VIII. OTHER TESTS

Megaloblastic anemia is associated with both ineffective erythropoiesis (intramedullary death) and hemolysis of circulating erythrocytes. Laboratory abnormalities that result from these processes are elevated serum lactic dehydrogenase (LDH) level, increased plasma unconjugated bilirubin, and decreased plasma haptoglobin levels. Serum iron and serum ferritin are usually elevated in untreated megaloblastic anemia.

IX. THERAPY FOR MEGALOBLASTIC ANEMIA

Since the defect in anemia secondary to vitamin B_{12} deficiency is usually one of absorption, the mainstay of treatment is parenteral administration of vitamin B_{12}. This therapy should be lifelong. Folate deficiency is also treated by replacement therapy, usually oral folate. The duration of therapy depends on the cause of the deficiency state. Therapy for several weeks is usually adequate in an alcoholic who begins to eat a normal diet. Patients with chronic conditions such as hemolytic anemia, malabsorption, or exfoliative skin diseases should continue oral folate supplementation indefinitely.

Specific therapy results in a prompt improvement in the hematologic parameters. The bone marrow begins to convert from megaloblastic to normoblastic erythropoiesis within 12–24 hr, with complete resolution in 48–96 hr. A reticulocytosis begins 2–3 days after therapy and peaks at 5–8 days. A full normalization of hematocrit occurs at 4–8 weeks. Neutrophils reach normal values within 5–7 days, while giant metamyelocytes and hypersegmented neutrophils may persist for 12–14days. The platelet count is corrected within 7–10 days.

The neurologic manifestations of patients with pernicious anemia improve and do not progress further with vitamin B_{12} therapy. However, they may not resolve completely. Large doses of folate will improve the hematologic abnormalities of vitamin B_{12}, but the neurologic disease will progress.

CASE STUDY

Patient

Fifty-eight year-old female.

Chief Complaint

The patient presented to her physician because of tiredness and fatigue of several months duration, which was increasing in severity. She also complained of tingling and numbness in her feet and legs for the past 3–4 weeks.

Medical History

The patient had been previously healthy, except for an appendectomy at age 18.

Drug History

No medications.

Physical examination

The patient was pale, and her skin had a sallow appearance. Neurologic exam revealed diminished vibratory sense and decreased sensation in the lower extremities.

Laboratory Results

	Patient	Normal
Hgb	8.2 g/dL	14.0–18.0 g/dL
Hct	25.0%	40–54%
MCV	116 fL	80–99 fL
RDW	20.7%	11–15%
Leukocyte count	7.2×10^9/L	$4.0–11 \times 10^9$/L
Platelet count	165×10^9/L	$150–350 \times 10^9$/L

Blood Film Examination

Decreased red cells with marked anisopoikilocytosis and numerous oval macrocytes. Frequent hypersegmented neutrophils.

Questions

1. What is the most likely diagnosis in this patient?
2. How do the presenting clinical features relate to the diagnosis?
3. How should this patient be treated?

Additional Laboratory Results

	Patient	Normal
Vitamin B_{12}, serum	<50 pg/mL	200–1000 pg/mL
Folate, serum	15 ng/mL	2.5–17 ng/mL
Folate, red cell	121 ng/mL	120–600 ng/mL
Schilling test		Abnormal stage I test. Normal absorption when cobalamin is given with intrinsic factor

Diagnosis

Pernicious anemia.

Discussion

This case is an example of pernicious anemia. The decreased hemoglobin/hematocrit with the markedly elevated MCV suggest the possibility of a megaloblastic anemia. The morphologic findings in the blood smear including the presence of oval macrocytes and hypersegmented neutrophils support this diagnosis. Results of the testing for serum vitamin B_{12} and serum and red cell folate levels indicate that the patient has a megaloblastic anemia due to vitamin B_{12} deficiency. The most common cause of megaloblastic anemia in the United States is pernicious anemia. A Schilling test was performed, and the results were characteristic of pernicious anemia.

The two principal manifestations of classical vitamin B_{12} deficiency are anemia and neurologic symptoms. In this patient, the anemia was manifested clinically by tiredness, weakness. This patient also had some signs and symptoms of neurologic abnormalities associated with cobalamin deficiency. Neurologic abnormalities are very common in vitamin B_{12} deficiency and typically consist of sensory neuropathy that begins in the feet and lower legs, as in this patient. They may be present in the absence of anemia or macrocytosis. Neurologic damage from cobalamin deficiency is progressive and, if untreated, may be permanent.

The mainstay of treatment for pernicious anemia is vitamin B_{12} replacement therapy. Since the defect is one of absorption, replacement therapy should be administered parentrally, specifically intramuscular cyanocobalamin. Treatment should be lifelong. Improvement in the hematologic status will begin quickly, with reticulocytosis appearing in a few days. Most improvement in the neurologic status occurs within the first 6 months of therapy. However, neurologic abnormalities may not resolve completely.

Bibliography

1. Green R, Kinsella LJ. Current concepts in the diagnosis of cobalamin deficiency. Neurology 1995; 1435–1440.
2. Pruthi RK, Tefferi A. Pernicious anemia revisited. Mayo Clin Proc 1994; 69:144–150.
3. Schilling RF, Williams WJ. Vitamin B_{12} deficiency: underdiagnosed, overtreated? Hosp Practice 1995; 30:47–54.

CASE STUDY 2

Patient

Sixty-one-year-old man.

Chief Complaint

The patient was brought in by his family for evaluation. The patient lived alone and had been "going downhill" over the past few months. He had become so weak recently that he was unable to care for himself. He was able to walk into the clinic, but needed assistance from family members.

Medical History

The patient has a long history of alcoholism. He had been treated 5 years earlier for a gastrointestinal hemorrhage.

Drug History

No medications.

Physical Examination

The patient appeared lethargic and was in mild distress. The skin was pale and slightly jaundiced. Spider nevi were apparent. The heart rate was 105 per minute. Scattered bruises were noted on trunk and extremities.

Laboratory Results

	Patient	Normal
Hgb	3.2 g/dL	14.0–18.0 g/dL
Hct	9.6%	40–54%
MCV	120 fL	80–99 fL
RDW	25.0%	11–15%
Reticulocyte count	0%	0.5–1.5%
Leukocyte count	3.0×10^9/L	4.0–11 × ^{9}/L
Platelet count	30×10^9/L	150–350 × 10^9/L

Blood film examination

Markedly decreased red cells with marked anisopoikilocytosis and oval macrocytes. Hypersegmented neutrophils. Thrombocytopenia.

Questions

1. Which is the most likely diagnosis in this patient?
2. What is the cause of the thrombocytopenia in this patient?
3. What is the treatment for folate deficiency?

Additional Laboratory Results

	Patient	Normal
Vitamin B_{12}, serum	300 pg/mL	200–1000 pg/mL
Folate, serum	<0.5 ng/mL	2.5–17 ng/mL
Folate, red cell	<50 ng/mL	120–600 ng/mL

Diagnosis

Megaloblastic anemia secondary to folate deficiency.

Discussion

This case is an example of megaloblastic anemia secondary to folate deficiency. One of the most common settings for dietary folate deficiency in adults is alcohol abuse accompanied by poor diet. Daily requirements of folate constitute about 1% of the body folate stores. This is considerably higher than in the case for vitamin B_{12} and accounts for the much greater frequency of dietary folate deficiency. Alcohol also has multiple effects on folate. Alcohol interferes with folate absorption and also appears to interfere with the enterohepatic circulation of folate.

Pancytopenia with a markedly elevated MCV is characteristic of a megaloblastic anemia. The MCV can be elevated in alcohol abuse and liver disease, but in those situations the MCV is usually less than 110 fL. The results of the blood film examination support the diagnosis of a megaloblastic anemia with the findings of marked anisopoi-kilocytosis with oval macrocytes and hypersegmented neutrophils. This patient also has a thrombocytopenia. Thrombocytopenia occurs less commonly than anemia, but occasional thrombocytopenia including severe thrombocytopenia with a platelet count less than $50 \times 10^9/\mu L$ is seen. A neutropenia is also occasionally present. All of the cytopenias result from megaloblastic changes occurring secondary to the vitamin deficiency. In this patient, alcohol suppression of the bone may have also contributed to the cytopenias. The jaundice in this patient was secondary both to liver disease and the ineffective erythropoiesis present in megaloblastic anemia associated with an increase in bilirubin.

Oral folic acid therapy is the treatment for folate deficiency. Therapy limited to several weeks is usually adequate in an alcoholic patient who begins to eat a normal diet. In patients with chronic conditions, oral folate is continued indefinitely. Red cell transfusions are rarely required because of the well-compensated state of even severely anemic patients. This patient, however, was given red cell transfusions because of cardiac symptoms associated with severe anemia. The hematologic abnormalities due to folate deficiency respond rapidly to therapy. Reticulocytosis begins in a few days. Neutrophil and platelet counts usually return to normal within a week to 10 days.

Bibliography

1. Carmel R. Clinical aspects of megaloblastic anemia. In: Bick RL, ed. Hematology, Clinical and Laboratory Practice. Vol. 1. St. Louis: Mosby, 1993:459–469.
2. Antony AC. Megaloblastic anemias. In: Hoffman R, Benz EJ, Shattil SJ, Furie B, Cohen HJ, Silberstein LE, eds., Hematology—Basic Principles and Practice. 2d ed. New York: Churchill-Livingston, 1995:1523–1529.

SUGGESTED READINGS

1. Allen RH. Megaloblastic anemias. In: Wyngaarden JB, Smith LH, Bennett JC, eds. Cecil Textbook of Medicine. 19th ed. Philadelphia: Saunders, 1992:846–854.
2. Antony AC. Megaloblastic anemias. In: Hoffman R, Benz EJ, Shattil SJ, Furie B, Cohen HJ, Silberstein LE, eds. Hematology—Basic Principles and Practice. 2nd ed. New York: Churchill-Livingston, 1995:552–586.
3. Babior BM. The megaloblastic anemias. In: Beutler E, Lichtman MA, Coller BS, Kipps TJ, eds. Williams Hematology. New York: McGraw-Hill, 1995:471–489.
4. Babior BM. Metabolic aspects of folic acid and cobalmin. In: Beutler E, Lichtman MA, Coller BS, Kipps TJ, eds. Williams Hematology. New York: McGraw-Hill, 1995:380–394.
5. Beck WS. Diagnosis of megaloblastic anemia. Annu Rev Med 1991; 43:311–322.
6 Carmel R. Clinical aspects of megaloblastic anemia. In: Bick RL, ed. Hematology Clinical and Laboratory Practice. Vol. 1. St. Louis: Mosby, 1993:459–469.
7. Chanarin I, Deacon R, Lumb M, Perry J. Cobalamin and folate: recent developments. J Clin Pathol 1992; 45:277–283.
8. Green R, Kinsella LJ. Current concepts in the diagnosis of cobalamin deficiency. Neurology 1995; 1435–1440.
9. Lindenbaum J, Heaton EB, Savage DG, et al. Neuropsychiatric disorders caused by cobalamin deficiency in the absence of anemia or macrocytosis. N Engl J Med 1988; 318:1720–1728.
10. Peterson L, McKenna RW. Laboratory evaluation of megaloblastic anemia. In: Bick RL, ed. Hematology. Clinical and Laboratory Practice. Vol 1. St. Louis: Mosby, 1993:459–469.
11. Pruthi RK, Tefferi A. Pernicious anemia revisited. Mayo Clin Proc 1994; 69:144–150.
12. Savage DG, Lindenbaum J, Stabler SP, Allen RH. Sensitivity of serum methylmalonic acid and total homocysteine determinations for diagnosing cobalamin and folate deficiencies. Am J Med 1994; 96:239–246.
13. Schilling RF, Williams WJ. Vitamin B_{12} deficiency: underdiagnosed, overtreated? Hosp Practice 1995; 30:47–54.
14. Stabler SP, Allen RH, Savage DG, Lindenbaum J. Clinical spectrum and diagnosis of cobalamin deficiency. Blood 1990; 76:871–881.
15. Tefferi A, Pruthi RK. The biochemical basis of cobalamin deficiency. Mayo Clin Proc 1994; 69: 181–186.

14

Anemias of Chronic Disorders and Nonhemolytic Normochromic, Normocytic Anemias

Robert T. Means, Jr.
Medical University of South Carolina and R. H. Johnson VA Medical Center, Charleston, South Carolina

I. DEFINITION

The term *anemia of chronic disorders* is generally used to refer to the anemia frequently observed in patients with chronic infectious, inflammatory, or neoplastic diseases, and which does not arise from blood loss or replacement of bone marrow by tumor or fibrosis (1–3). However, this syndrome is sometimes observed in association with a number of diseases that are not chronic. The disorders which produce this syndrome are characterized by increased production of the cytokines which mediate the immune or inflammatory response, such as tumor necrosis factor (TNF), interleukin-1, and the interferons (IFNs). For this reason, the anemia observed in severe acute infections results from the same mechanisms as the anemia of chronic disorders. The diagnostic hallmark of the anemia of chronic disorders is hypoferremia in the presence of normal or increased reticuloendothelial (RE) iron stores.

II. INCIDENCE

It is generally conceded that the anemia of chronic disorders is the most common etiology of anemia other than blood loss with consequent iron deficiency. Cash and Sears (1) reviewed all anemic patients admitted to the medical service of a busy county hospital over 4 months in 1985–1986. After patients with bleeding, hemolysis, and known hematologic malignancies were excluded, 52% of the remaining patients met laboratory criteria for the anemia of chronic disorders. This syndrome is observed in 58% of newly diagnosed patients admitted to inpatient rheumatology units and as many as 27% of outpatients followed in rheumatology practices (4).

III. ASSOCIATED SYNDROMES

As mentioned above, the anemia observed with acute infections has the same pathophysiology, and not all anemic patients with a chronic disease have the "anemia of chronic disorders." The association between the following syndromes and the anemia of chronic disorders is well established.

Acute infections: acute bacterial infections; acute fungal infections; acute viral infections
Chronic infections: tuberculosis and other mycobacterial infections; infective endocarditis; osteomyelitis; human immunodeficiency virus infection; chronic urinary tract infections; chronic fungal diseases such as histoplasmosis
Chronic noninfectious inflammatory disorders: rheumatoid arthritis (4); collagen vascular diseases; polymyalgia rheumatica; other inflammatory arthropathies; decubitus ulcers; sarcoidosis
Malignancy: disseminated nonhematologic malignancies; lymphoproliferative malignancies (the anemia of malignancy is discussed later in greater detail).

IV. CLINICAL FEATURES

The anemia of chronic disorders is typically a mild anemia, with hemoglobin ≥9 g/dL, and so its clinical features are essentially those of the associated syndrome. The degree of anemia parallels the activity of the associated disease, and typically requires 2–3 months to develop.

V. LABORATORY FINDINGS

1. Seventy-five percent of patients with the anemia of chronic disorders have hemoglobin levels ≥9 g/dL; however, a significant minority may be sufficiently anemic to require red cell transfusion.
2. Approximately 80% of patients will have a normocytic, normochromic anemia; the remainder will be microcytic.
3. The reticulocyte count is typically slightly low for the degree of anemia; extreme reticulocytopenia (<0.2%) is very uncommon.
4. The serum or plasma iron is decreased; this test cannot be used to distinguish iron deficiency from the anemia of chronic disorders.
5. Serum transferrin and transferrin saturation are decreased. The serum transferrin saturation is typically ≥16%; however, when the serum transferrin level is <150 μg/dL, a very low transferrin saturation (<10%) can be observed in this syndrome.
6. Serum ferritin levels are normal or (more typically) elevated; it must be remembered that serum ferritin levels may be elevated out of proportion to iron stores in inflammatory states, and so a normal serum ferritin may not reflect the presence of reticuloendothelial iron (RE).
7. Serum transferrin receptor levels are elevated in iron deficiency, but not in the anemia of chronic disorders.
8. Free erythrocyte protoporphrin elevations will not distinguish the anemia of chronic disorders from iron deficiency.
9. RE iron stores, as assessed by a Prussian blue-stained marrow specimen, are normal or increased (Fig. 1).
10. Leukocyte and platelet counts are not altered in the anemia of chronic disorders per se, and reflect the associated syndrome.
11. Although there are bone marrow abnormalities characteristic of the anemia of chronic disorders, such as increased plasma cells and decreased siderocytes, these features

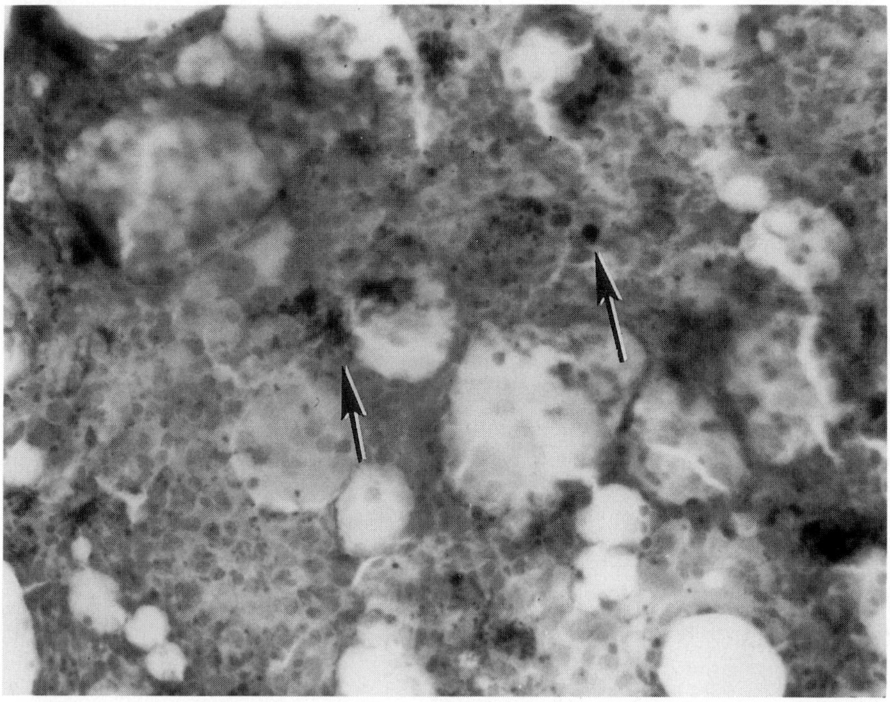

Figure 1 Bone marrow aspirate stained with Prussian blue reaction in a patient with anemia of chronic disorders. Note large block iron granules (blue in color). (Original magnification ×400.)

are not diagnostic. The primary indication for marrow examination in the anemia of chronic disorders is definitive identification of RE iron stores.

VI. PATHOPHYSIOLOGY

The development of the anemia of chronic disorders requires three processes:

1. Shortened red cell survival, creating an increased demand for red cell production by the marrow

The marrow is unable to respond to this increased demand because of:

2. Impaired erythropoietic response and
3. Impaired mobilization and utilization of iron for erythropoiesis

Although the decrease in red cell survival is very modest and would usually be easily compensated for by the marrow, the impaired erythropoiesis prevents this. The impaired erythropoietic response reflects both a blunted erythropoietin response to anemia (less erythropoietin is produced than would be seen in an equally anemic iron-deficient patient) and a reduced ability of erythroid progenitors to respond to the erythropoietin which is available. Iron metabolism is impaired both at the level of iron mobilization by the RE system and at the level of iron uptake by the erythroid precursor. In-vivo and in-vitro studies have demonstrated that all of these processes can be attributed to cytokine effects (5,6).

VII. DIAGNOSIS

The diagnosis is established by demonstrating hypoferremia with adequate marrow iron stores in an anemic patient with an appropriate clinical history. Adequate iron stores can be demonstrated by a serum ferritin >200 ng/mL, or marrow examination (7–9).

VIII. DIFFERENTIAL DIAGNOSIS

The major disorder from which the anemia of chronic disorders must be distinguished is iron-deficiency anemia. Demonstration of adequate iron stores will permit this distinction.

Confusion in the differential diagnosis may be observed in the following situations:

1. Underlying renal failure.
2. Concomitant iron deficiency or chronic blood loss. Up to 25% of patients with rheumatoid arthritis and the anemia of chronic disorders are also iron deficient.
3. Bone marrow replacement by tumor or fibrosis.

IX. THERAPY

Iron therapy is of no use in the anemia of chronic disorders. Patients with complicating iron deficiency will correct their anemia on iron therapy only to the degree that iron deficiency is involved. Recombinant human erythropoietin (rhEPO) can correct the anemia of chronic disorders, but should be reserved for that minority of patients with symptomatic anemia or who require transfusion. Patients who wish to donate blood for autologous transfusion at elective surgery may also benefit from rhEPO administration (10,11).

X. ANEMIA OF MALIGNANCY

The anemia of malignancy represents a special case. Transfusion-requiring anemia is observed in 18% of patients with malignancies other than leukemia undergoing their first cycle of chemotherapy. In addition to the mechanisms associated with the anemia of chronic disorders, anemia in cancer patients may result from marrow replacement by tumor or tumor-induced fibrosis, or from the effects of therapy, which include marrow toxicity, renal toxicity (impairing erythropoietin production), and poor nutrition. The anemia associated malignancy responds well to rhEPO therapy (Figs. 2–4).

XI. NONHEMOLYTIC NORMOCHROMIC, NORMOCYTIC ANEMIA

In addition to the anemia of chronic disorders, a variety of other syndromes result in nonhemolytic anemia that is typically normochromic and normocytic. All of these syndromes except acute blood loss are associated with an inappropriately low reticulocyte response for the degree of anemia.

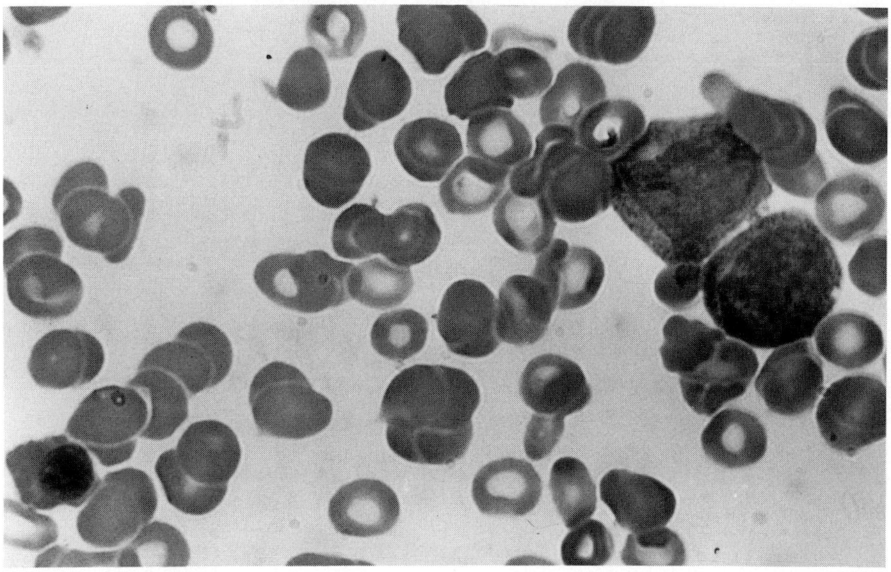

Figure 2 Peripheral blood showing leukoerythroblastic picture from patient with metastatic carcinoma. Note promyelocytes (right) and nucleated red blood cell in left lower corner. (Original magnification ×1000.)

XII. ACUTE BLOOD LOSS ANEMIA

Chronic blood loss eventually results in iron deficiency and a microcytic, hypochromic anemia associated with a decreased reticulocyte response. Acute blood loss, in contrast results in a normocytic anemia associated with reticulocytosis (12).

The symptoms of acute blood loss depend on the quantity of blood lost, and the rapidity of the loss. A 500-mL blood loss (roughly the equivalent of a blood donation) over an hour may either be asymptomatic or minimally symptomatic (diaporesis, dizziness while upright which is relieved by reclining); if lost over a 4-day period, this quantity of blood would probably not result in symptoms at all. When more than 30% of the blood volume is lost acutely, organ perfusion is compromised.

1. The hemoglobin concentration is normal for approximately 24 hr following an acute blood loss; the process of transcapillary refill leads to replacement of the lost blood volume from the extracellular volume, and the decline in hemoglobin concentration begins. Red cell and plasma volume require 2–3 days to equilibrate.
2. Reticulocytosis begins approximately 72 hr after blood loss. Statistically significant elevations of endogenous EPO are not observed until the hematocrit falls below 38%.
3. A large-volume blood loss associated with a brisk reticulocytosis may also result in leukoerythroblastosis, with nucleated erythrocytes and myelocytes detectable on blood smears.
4. A moderate elevation of platelet count usually accompanies significant acute blood loss.

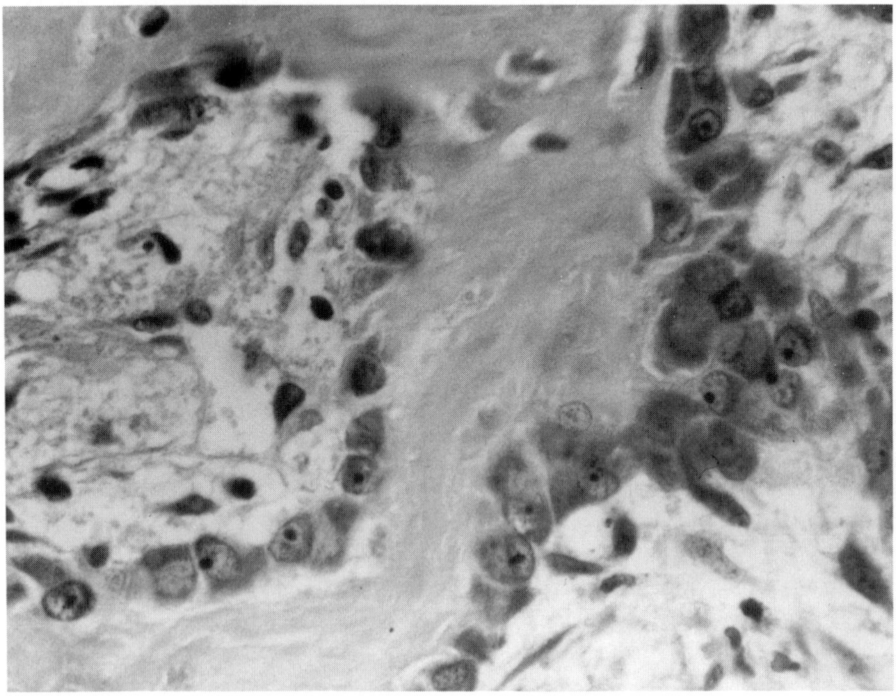

Figure 3 Bone marrow biopsy showing osteoblastic activity in a patient with metastatic prostatic carcinoma. (Original magnification ×400.)

The diagnosis of acute blood loss is generally straightforward. The goal of therapy is restoration of blood volume to preserve tissue perfusion, and, if necessary, red cell transfusion to restore oxygen delivery. Blood losses less than 750 mL can generally be treated with crystalloid alone, unless the clinical picture suggests impaired oxygen delivery. Whole blood is often recommended for resuscitation of acute blood loss; crystalloid and packed red blood cells work as well, particularly if 6 units of platelets and 4 units of fresh frozen plasma are administered after every 6–8 units of packed red cells, to prevent "washout" of platelets and coagulation factors.

XIII. ANEMIA OF RENAL FAILURE

In the era prior to the use of rhEPO, 98% of patients maintained on hemodialysis were anemic. Although the primary cause of anemia in renal failure is EPO deficiency, other factors contribute. Factors that contribute to anemia of renal failure include the following.

1. *EPO deficiency*. This is the major factor in the development of anemia in renal failure.
2. *Decreased red cell survival*. This is due both to extracorpuscular defects related to the severity of anemia, and to increased red cell susceptibility to oxidative injury from depleted cellular glutathione.
3. *Iron deficiency*. Patients on hemodialysis lose 1–2 g iron/year, mostly due to blood loss during dialysis.

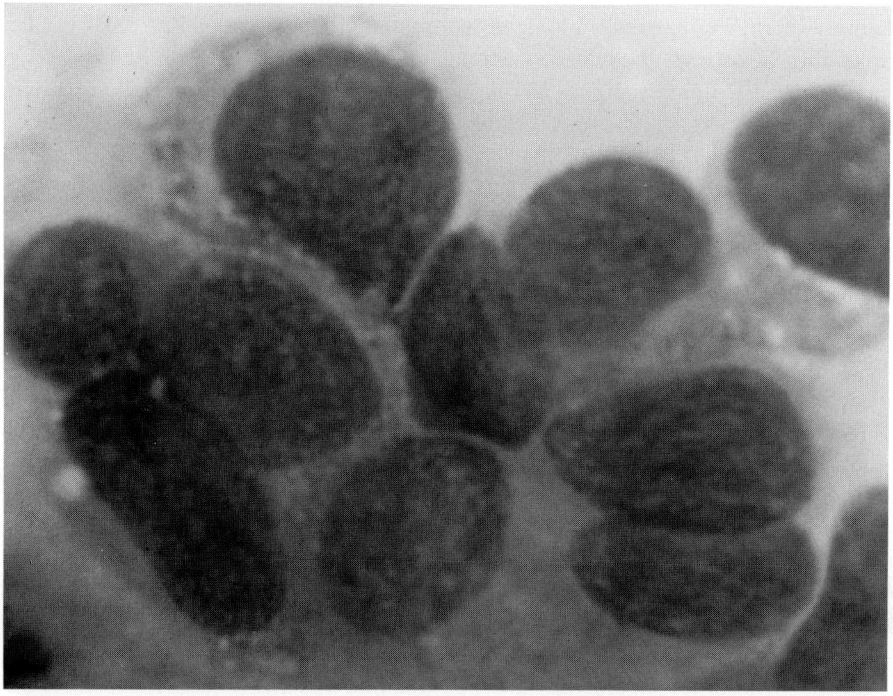

Figure 4 Bone marrow aspirate from a patient with metastatic breast carcinoma. Note cluster of large cells showing nuclear molding. (Original magnification ×1000.)

4. *Folate deficiency*. Folate deficiency is common in patients on hemodialysis, since folate is dialyzable.
5. *Aluminum toxicity*. Aluminum toxicity may produce a microcytic anemia in patients with adequate iron stores.
6. *Hyperparathyroidism*. Elevated parathormone levels may produce marrow fibrosis.
7. *Circulating inhibitors*. A number of substances which inhibit erythropoiesis in vitro are detectable in the serum of uremic patients. However, the effects of these substances are generally not specific for erythropoiesis, and the clinical relevance of this phenomenon is not clearly established.

Features of the anemia of renal failure include the following.

1. More than 80% of patients have normocytic red cells (4% microcytic, 15% macrocytic).
2. Reticulocytopenia is present, with uncorrected reticulocyte count typically <2%.
3. Patients on peritoneal dialysis tend to be less severely anemic than patients on hemodialysis.
4. Iron and/or folate deficiency may also be present.
5. Echinocytes (burr cells; Fig. 1) are present in significantly uremic patients.
6. The bone marrow is typically normocellular or slightly hypercellular; the myeloid: erythroid ratio may be slightly increased

The availability of rhEPO has revolutionized the treatment of the anemia of renal failure. Administration of rhEPO corrects the anemia of the vast majority of patients on hemodialysis. Failure to respond to rhEPO therapy suggests complicating iron or folate deficiency, aluminum toxicity, or inflammation.

XIV. ANEMIA OF LIVER DISEASE

A. Chronic Liver Disease

Anemia is observed in 40–65% of patients with chronic liver disease (12). Mechanisms responsible for anemia include the following.

1. *Dilution.* A majority of cirrhotic patients exhibit a significantly increased plasma volume. In contrast to the situation in pregnancy, this is usually accompanied by an absolute reduction in red cell mass.
2. *Folate deficiency.* This may result from poor dietary intake or from impaired ability to retrieve folate from tissue stores.
3. *Hypersplenism* from cirrhosis, resulting in red cell sequestration.
4. *Hemolysis.* Several hemolytic syndromes have been observed in chronic liver disease patients:
   (a) Acute spur cell anemia (12,13).
   (b) Zieve's syndrome—hemolysis in hyperlipidemic patients with cirrhosis. It is unclear if this is a distinct syndrome or a stage in the natural history of cirrhosis (12,13).
   (c) Autoimmune hemolytic anemia in primary biliary cirrhosis.
   (d) Nonimmune hemolysis not described above (i.e., Wilson's disease).
5. *Iron deficiency.* Patients with cirrhosis may have gastrointestinal blood loss (as from esophageal varices) contributing to anemia.

Clinical and laboratory features are as follows.

1. The majority of patients exhibit a moderate macrocytosis.
2. Morphologically abnormal red cells, such as acanthocytes (spur cells) and target cells (Figures 5 and 6), are common.
3. Bone marrow cellularity is usually normal or increased, but there is considerable variation.

B. Acute Viral Hepatitis

Nonimmune hemolysis and aplastic anemia may complicate the course of acute viral hepatitis.

C. Alcohol Abuse

Any of the disorders described for chronic liver disease (particularly Zieve's syndrome and spur cell anemia) may arise in patients with chronic liver disease due to alcohol abuse (6). Aside from its contributions to the development of chronic liver disease, alcohol exhibits its own effects on erythropoiesis. Anemia following heavy acute alcohol ingestion is not uncommon, and is typically normocytic or slightly macrocytic. The erythropoietin response of these patients appears to be intact. The marrow of chronic alcoholic patients or individuals taking

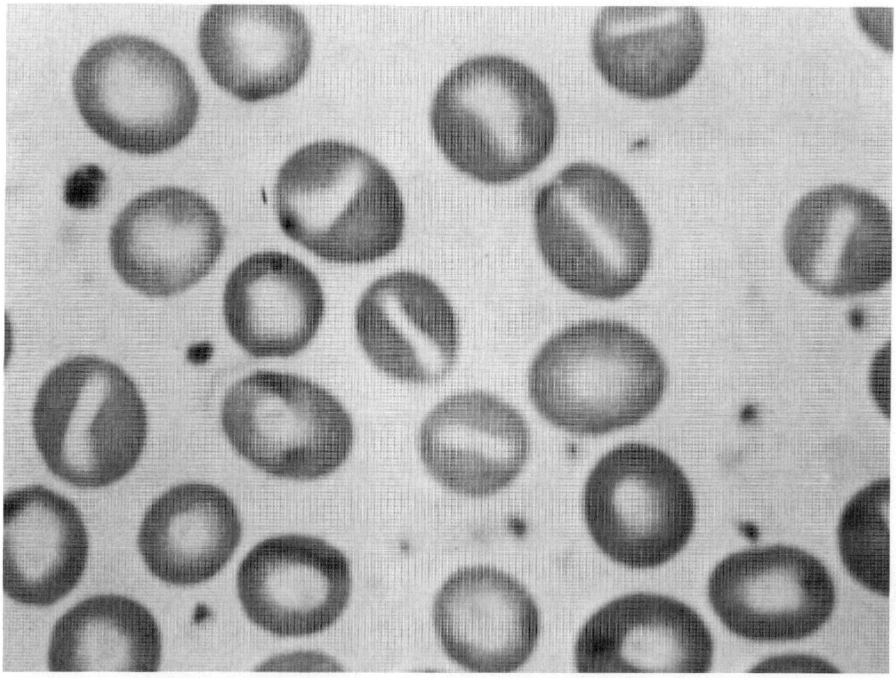

Figure 5 Peripheral blood smear showing stomatocytes in an acute alcoholic. (Original magnification ×1000.)

large quantities of ethanol over short periods of time exhibits a variety of abnormalities, including megaloblastic changes, vacuolization of erythroid precursors, and/or ringed sideroblasts. Folate-deficient alcoholics taking ethanol fail to respond to therapeutic doses of folate, indicating that ethanol impairs utilization of folate by erythroid precursors. Ringed sideroblasts are seen in almost half of marrows from alcohol abusers and appear to result from impaired marrow conversion of pyridoxine to pyridoxal phosphate in the presence of ethanol; ringed sideroblasts may resolve with pyridoxal phosphate therapy, but not with pyridoxine. These marrow changes are transient and resolve after alcohol cessation (Fig. 5).

D. Treatment

The treatment of anemia in liver disease is primarily supportive: alcohol cessation, adequate nutrition, and folate therapy. Patients with autoimmune hemolytic anemia or aplastic anemia should receive specific therapy for those syndromes.

XV. ANEMIA OF ENDOCRINE DISORDERS

A mild anemia is occasionally observed in patients with various endocrine disorders (Table 1). This anemia typically results from a reduction in basal metabolism, with consequent reduction in erythropoietic demand. Exceptions include the anemia observed in hyperthyroidism, which appears to result from impaired red cell survival, and the anemia of hyperparathyroidism, which results from parathormone-induced marrow fibrosis. Most anemias associated with endo-

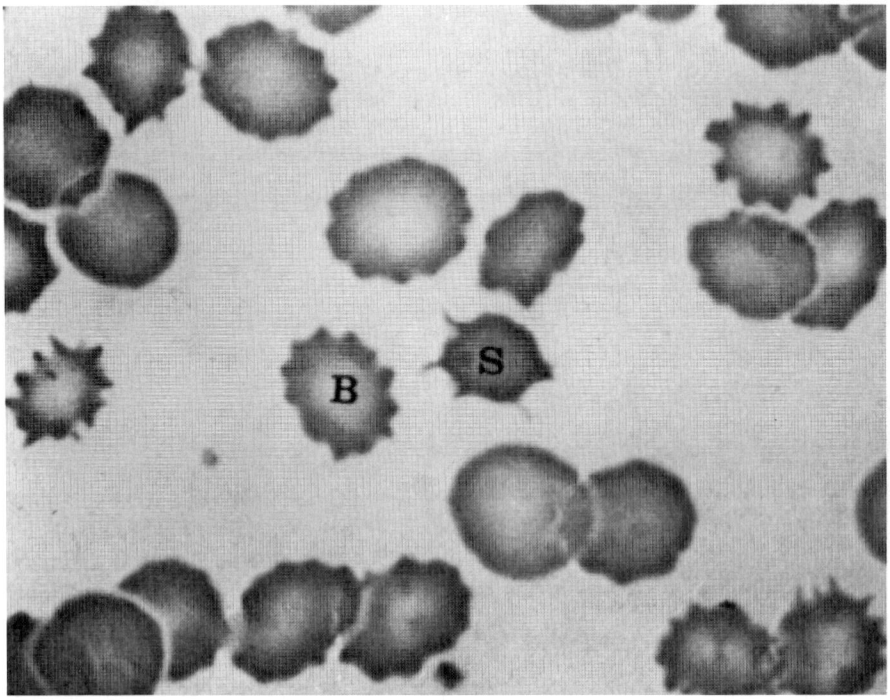

Figure 6 Peripheral blood smear from a patient with terminal Laennec's cirrhosis showing burr cell (B) and spur cell (S) for comparison. Note other burr and spur cells. (Original magnification ×1000.)

crinopathies exhibit normochromic and normocytic red cells, although the anemia of hypothyroidism characteristically involves a mild macrocytosis (MCV typically less than 110 fL). The anemias associated with endocrinopathies exhibit an impaired reticulocyte response, and correct with specific treatment of the underlying disorder.

XVI. CONGENITAL DYSERYTHROPOIETIC ANEMIAS

Congenital dyserythropoietic anemias (CDA) are associated with peripheral blood anisocytosis and basophilic stippling. Chronic ineffective erythropoiesis often leads to systemic iron over-

Table 1 Endocrine Disorders Associated with Anemia

Hypothyroidism
Hyperthyroidism[a]
Hypopituitarism
Hypogonadism (male)
Adrenal insufficiency
Hyperparathyroidism
Anorexia nervosa

[a]Anemia is uncommon in this disorder.

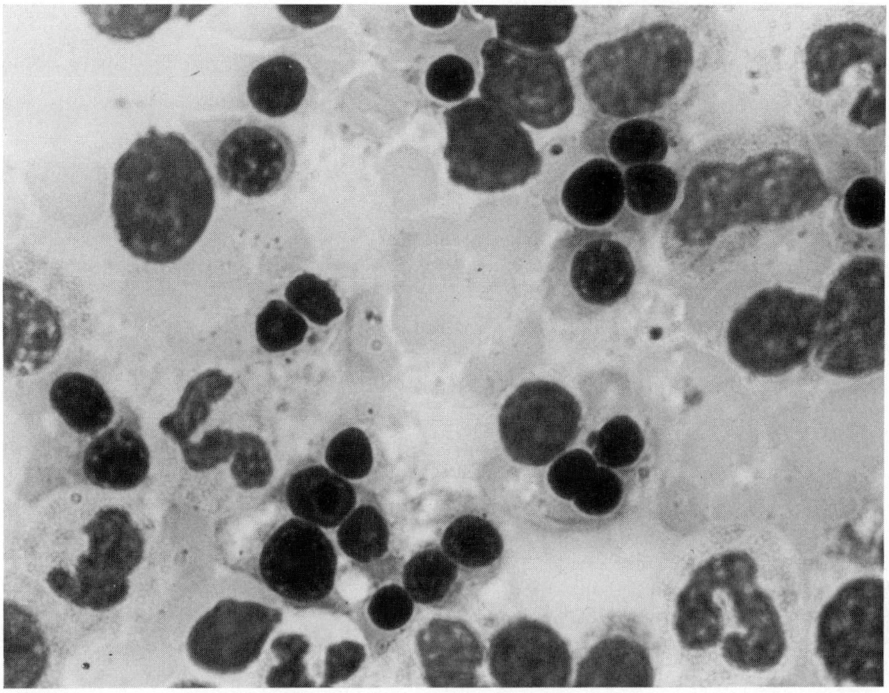

Figure 7 Bone marrow aspirate of patient with HEMPAS. Note multinucleated normoblasts. (Original magnification ×1000.)

load, and adults have been diagnosed with CDA whose initial presentation was hemochromatosis (14). These uncommon familial disorders are classified into three groups.

Type I CDA is characterized by marrow erythroid hyperplasia, with multinucleated erythroblasts exhibiting internuclear bridging. Type II CDA is also referred to as HEMPAS (hereditary erythroblast multinuclearity with positive acidified serum test) and is the most common of these syndromes. The abnormal marrow erythroblasts are typically binucleate and uncommonly exhibit internuclear bridging (Fig. 7). The diagnosis requires a positive acid hemolysis test. Type III CDA is characterized by gigantic pronormoblasts ("gigantoblasts"), and erythroblasts containing large number of nuclei. All three syndromes exhibit a chronic clinical course.

CASE STUDY 1

Patient

Seventy-three-year old male.

Chief Complaint

The patient was referred for evaluation of a chronic anemia. He maintained a hematocrit of approximately 30.0%, with hemoglobin 10.7 g/dL and MCV 86 fL. Leukocyte and platelet count were normal. The patient had been treated empirically with iron and vitamin B_{12} prior to referral, without benefit.

Medical History

The patient had undergone hemicolectomy for polyps 2 years prior to referral. The history was otherwise unremarkable.

Medications

Cimetidine.

Review of Systems

The patient reported feeling lethargic and having decreased interest in activities. He also noted that he did not need to shave every day.

Physical Examination

Physical examination was unremarkable. Stool examination did not reveal occult blood.

Laboratory Results

	Patient	Normal
Serum iron	66 μg/dL	35–140 μg/dL
Serum transferrin	188 μg/dL	200–400 μg/dL
Serum ferritin	171 ng/dL	25–250 ng/dL

Questions

1. Are the data presented sufficient to make a diagnosis?
2. If not, how could the diagnosis be further narrowed?

Additional Laboratory Studies

Bone marrow examination was unremarkable. Normal stainable iron was present.

Questions

1. What are the diagnostic possibilities now?
2. Does the patient's clinical picture suggest any possibilities to be evaluated?

Diagnostic Laboratory Studies

	Patient	Normal
Thyroid–stimulating hormone	3.8 μU/mL	<6 μU/mL
Serum testosterone	0.3 ng/mL	3–10 ng/mL
Serum cortisol	17 μg/dL	5–20 μg/dL

Diagnosis

Anemia due to hypogonadism.

Discussion

The patient had an interesting and complex problem. The initial consideration in any anemic older male, particularly one with a history of gastrointestinal pathology, must always be iron deficiency. Iron studies do not support this diagnosis, but a serum ferritin <200 ng/dL makes it difficult to rule out. The low transferrin suggests the anemia of chronic disorders, but the mid-range serum iron level is not consistent with the diagnosis. Iron deficiency was definitively ruled out by marrow examination.

At this point, the most likely diagnosis remains the anemia of chronic disorders, although the laboratory picture is not entirely typical. Of greater significance is the lack of a clinical syndrome compatible with the anemia of chronic disorders. The patient's history suggests an endocrine disorder, although the history cannot distinguish thyroid, adrenal, gonadal, or pituitary insufficiency. Further studies following the identification of the patient's hypogonadism demonstrated that this was a result of pituitary dysfunction; his anemia resolved with testosterone replacement.

CASE STUDY 2

Patient

Sixty-four-year-old male.

Chief Complaint

The patient was referred for consideration of parenteral iron replacement. The patient had a microcytic anemia (hematocrit 28.4%, hemoglobin 9.4 g/dL, mean corpuscular volume 75.4 fL) with low serum iron (33 μg/dL), leading to a diagnosis of iron deficiency anemia, but had failed to respond to oral iron therapy. Endoscopic examination of the upper and lower abdominal tract demonstrated gastritic and gastroesophageal reflux, and sigmoid diverticulosis.

Medical History

The patient's history was notable for severe inflammatory arthritis which had developed over the preceding 3 months. This had been associated with acute joint and synovial swelling, fever and weight loss, and extreme elevations of the erythrocyte sedimentation rate (>120 mm/sec). The patient had responded remarkably well to steroids, with improvement in systemic symptoms.

Medications

Acetaminophen, oxycodone, omeprazole, cimetidine, ferrous sulfate.

Review of Systems

Joint pain and stiffness, especially in the morning.

Physical Examination

Physical examination was notable for synovial thickening. Stool heme was negative.

Laboratory Results

	Patient	Normal
Serum iron	15 μg/dL	35–140 μg/dL
Serum transferrin	118 μg/dL	200–400 μg/dL
Serum ferritin	230 ng/dL	25–250 ng/dL
Serum B_{12}	347 pg/mL	200–800 pg/mL
Serum folate	3.9 ng/mL	1.9–4.0 ng/mL

Questions

1. Was the patient's original diagnosis correct?
2. At this point, can a diagnosis be made?
3. Which diagnostic tests ordered above were unnecessary?
4. What study would absolutely secure the diagnosis?

Additional Laboratory Studies

Bone marrow examination was remarkable for a modest increase in reactive plasma cells. Ample iron stores were present.

Diagnosis

Anemia of chronic disorders.

Discussion

This patient has a classic presentation for his hematologic disorder; the torturous course by which he came to the diagnosis is also classic. The major diagnosis with which the anemia of chronic disorders is confused is iron deficiency, because both are common, both are associated with hypoferremia, and a significant minority (20–25%) of patients with the anemia of chronic disorders have microcytic erythrocytes. The serum ferritin and the examination of a Prussian blue-stained marrow specimen are the most reliable methods for assessing iron stores: Neither had been evaluated in the early part of this patient's history.

The failure to respond to iron therapy was another important clue: The most common reason for failure to respond to iron is noncompliance, and the second most common reason is that the patient is not iron deficient. The tests obtained at that point (hypoferremia, hypotransferrinemia, and serum ferritin >200 ng/mL), with the clinical history, are diagnostic of the anemia of chronic disorders. With significant hypotransferrinemia, the transferrin saturation (12.7% in this case) is not helpful in identifying iron deficiency. Vitamin B_{12} and folate deficiency are rarely associated with microcytosis, and then only in the setting of concommitant iron deficiency, so those tests were not indicated in the absence of a clear-cut diagnosis of iron deficiency. The bone marrow examination for demonstration of iron stores, to rule out iron deficiency absolutely, is useful in cases less clear than this one.

Bibliography

1. Baer AN, Dessypris EN, Krantz SB. The pathogenesis of anemia in rheumatoid arthritis. A clinical and laboratory analysis. Semin Arthritis Rheum 1990; 14:209–223.
2. Cartwright GE. The anemia of chronic disease. Semin Hematol 1966; 3:351–375.
3. Mazza J, Barr RM, McDonald JWD, Valberg LS. Usefulness of the serum ferritin concentration in the detection of iron deficiency in a general hospital. Can Med Assoc J 1978; 119:884–886.

NOTE ADDED IN PROOF

Since the completion of this chapter, new contributions to the therapy and pathogenesis of the anemia of renal failure have appeared. Besarab and colleagues have emphasized the benefits and possible risks of aggressive iron replacement in anemic dialysis patients (15). Rice et al. have clarified the contribution of hemolysis to anemia in dialysis patients by demonstrating the occurrence of selective hemolysis of young erythrocytes ("neocytolysis") in renal failure patients, and observing that this condition is associated with withdrawal of rhEPO (16). Finally, Allen and colleagues have reported that serum from uremic patients with inflammatory disorders inhibits erythroid colony formation in vitro, and that this inhibitory effect is substantially reversed by neutralizing antibodies to either tumor necrosis factor (TNF) or interferon (IFN)-γ. This particular finding is perhaps no great surprise, but it is coupled with a demonstration that the inhibitory effect of serum from uremic patients *without* concurrent inflammatory disorders is also corrected by a combination of neutralizing antibodies to TNF and IFN-γ (17). The findings of this study, if confirmed, suggest the need to re-examine the current paradigms dealing with the pathogenesis of the anemia of renal failure, and imply that the pathogenetic mechanisms of the anemia of chronic disorders are shared by the anemia of renal failure (18).

REFERENCES

1. Cash JM, Sears DA. The spectrum of diseases associated with the anemia of chronic disease. A study of 90 cases. Am J Med 1990; 87:638–644.
2. Lee GR. The anemia of chronic disease. Semin Hematol 1983; 20:61–80.
3. Means RT, Dessypris EN. The anemia of chronic disease, renal failure, and endocrine disease. In: Bick RL, Bennett JM, Byrnes RK, et al., eds. Hematology: Clinical and Laboratory Practice. St. Louis: Mosby-Yearbook, 1993:419–429.
4. Baer AN, Dessypris EN, Krantz SB. The pathogenesis of anemia in rheumatoid arthritis. A clinical and laboratory analysis. Semin Arthritis Rheum 1990; 14:209–223.
5. Means RT. Pathogenesis of the anemia of chronic disease: a cytokine-mediated anemia. Stem Cells 1995; 13:32–37.
6. Means RT, Krantz SB. Progress in understanding the pathogenesis of the anemia of chronic disease. Blood 1992; 80:1639–1647.
7. Lee MH, Means RT. Extremely elevated serum ferritin levels in a university hospital: associated diseases and clinical significance. Am J Med 1995; 98:566–571.
8. Mazza J, Barr RM, McDonald JWD, et al. Usefulness of the serum ferritin concentration in the detection of iron deficiency in a general hospital. Can Med Assoc J 1990; 119:884–886.
9. Witte DL. Can serum ferritin be effectively interpreted in the presence of the acute phase response? Clin Chem 1991; 37:484–485.
10. Means RT. Clinical application of recombinant human erythropoietin in the anemia of chronic disease. Hematol/Oncol Clin N Am 1994; 8:933–944.
11. Means RT. Erythrocyte-stimulating factors. In: DeVita LVT, Hellmann S, Rosenberg SA, eds. Biologic Therapy of Cancer. 2d ed. Philadelphia: Lippincott, 1995:190–201.
12. Means RT, Dessypris EN. The anemias of pregnancy, liver disease, and acute blood loss. In: Bick RL, Bennett JM, Byrnes RK, et al., eds. Hematology: Clinical and Laboratory Practice. St. Louis: Mosby-Yearbook, 1993:431–435.
13. Eichner ER, Hillman RS. The evolution of anemia in alcoholic patients. Am J Med 1971; 50: 218–232.
14. Halpern Z, Rahmani R, Levo Y. Severe hemochromatosis: the predominant clinical manifestation of congenital dyserythropoietic anemia type 2. Acta Haematol 1985; 74:178–180.
15. Besarab A, Bolton WK, Browne JK, et al. The effects of normal as compared to low hematocrit values in patients with cardiac disease who are receiving hemodialysis and epoetin. N Engl J Med 1998; 339:347–354.
16. Rice L, Alfrey CP, Driscoll T, et al. Neocytoloysis contributes to the anemia of renal disease. Am J Kidney Dis 1999; 33:59–62.
17. Allen DA, Breen C, Yaqoob MM, et al. Inhibition of CFU-E colony formation in uremic patients with inflammatory disease: role of IFN-γ and TNF-α. J Invest Med 1999; 47:204–211.
18. Means RT. Commentary: An anemia of chronic disease, after all? J Invest Med 1999; 47:203.

15

Sideroblastic Anemia and Porphyrias

Lawrence Kass
Case Western Reserve University School of Medicine and
Metro Health Medicine Center, Cleveland, Ohio

I. SIDEROBLASTIC ANEMIA

Sideroblastic anemia comprises a heterogeneous group of disorders characterized by ring sideroblasts in the bone marrow, intramedullary cell death of erythroblasts leading to ineffective erythropoiesis, and anemia. Sideroblastic anemia can be hereditary, in which case the disorder is inherited as an autosomal dominant trait. More often, sideroblastic anemia is acquired. In this form, it may occur after exposure to a variety of drugs such as chloramphenicol or isoniazid, to heavy metals such as arsenic or lead, or to ethyl alcohol (Table 1).

Sideroblastic anemia can also result from a defect(s) at the stem cell level in the marrow, in which the disorder has been called idiopathic sideroblastic anemia (ISA) or refractory anemia with ring sideroblasts (RARS). Currently, RARS is regarded as a part of the myelodysplastic group of panmyelotic marrow disturbances. In a small percentage of cases, RARS may evolve into acute nonlymphoblastic leukemia.

A. Formation of Ring Sideroblasts

By mechanisms not fully understood, iron in the form of ferritin accumulates in the lamellae and cristae of mitochondria in developing erythroblasts (Fig. 1). Accumulation of substantial amounts of ferritin leads to decreased activity of mitochondrial enzymes required for hemoglobin synthesis. These enzymes include ferrochetalase (heme synthetase) and delta ALAase. With decline in activities of enzymes required for hemoglobin synthesis, anemia develops. Ferritin also acts as a mitochondrial poison, leading to premature death of erythroblasts in the bone marrow and worsening anemia.

Sideroblasts can be identified using acidified potassium nitroferricyanide. Potassium nitroferricyanide is also known as Prussian blue stain. It demonstrates iron in the 3+ or ferric hydroxide form as found in ferritin. As seen under the light microscope, siderotic granules actually represent ferric iron contained in mitochondria.

Proerythroblasts are the earliest recognizable erythroid precursors. In these cells siderotic granules are not identified. Instead, siderotic granules are detectable in erythroblasts which display hemoglobinization as manifested by cytoplasmic polychromasia. Morphologically, these erythroblasts are identified as early and late intermediate normoblasts, or orthochromic normoblasts. Siderotic granules may be numerous, up to 20 or more, and surround the nucleus

Table 1 Sideroblastic Anemias

	Hereditary	Acquired
Age at presentation	20–40	50–80
CBC findings	Usually normochromic normocytic	Often macrocytic
Peripheral smear	Anisocytosis, rare macrocytes	Macrocytosis, anisocytosis, poikilocytosis; there may also be leukopenia and monocytosis
Bone marrow	Marked erythroid normoblastic hyperplasia	Marked megaloblastoid erythroid hyperplasia; granulocytic precursors and megakarocytes may also be abnormal
Ring sideroblasts	Yes	Yes
Ferritin	High	High
Cause	Genetic	Primary acquired, or secondary to ethanol, isoniazid, chloramphine, heavy metals
Treatment	Pyridoxine may lead to improvement; anemia usually recurs when pyridoxine is stopped	Pyridoxine, folic acid, desferrioxamine; usually refractory to most agents used alone or in combination); may be reversible if offending agent (e.g., isoniazid) is stopped
Leukemic evolution	Rare	7–10% in primary acquired variety

simulating a "ring". In normal erythroblasts, several small punctate siderotic granules are seen rarely.

B. Hereditary Sideroblastic Anemia

Hereditary sideroblastic anemia is inherited as an autosomal dominant trait. In afflicted individuals, anemia becomes manifest in young adulthood, and may be severe enough to require blood transfusions. Peripheral blood smears from affected individuals may show hypochromia and microcytosis, and bone marrow displays erythroid hyperplasia and ring sideroblasts. Serum ferritin levels are markedly elevated. Administration of pyridoxine (vitamin B_6) in pharmacologic amounts of 200 mg/day may lead to amelioration of the anemia. If pyridoxine is stopped, anemia usually recurs.

C. Acquired Sideroblastic Anemia

Exposure to chloramphenicol, isoniazid or heavy metals can lead to sideroblastic anemia. Likewise, alcoholism may result in sideroblastic anemia. Usually, withdrawal of the offending substance(s) leads to improvement of the anemia.

In most cases of idiopathic acquired sideroblastic anemia, individuals are 40–80 years old (Case Study 1). Anemia may be asymptomatic, or symptomatic requiring blood transfusions

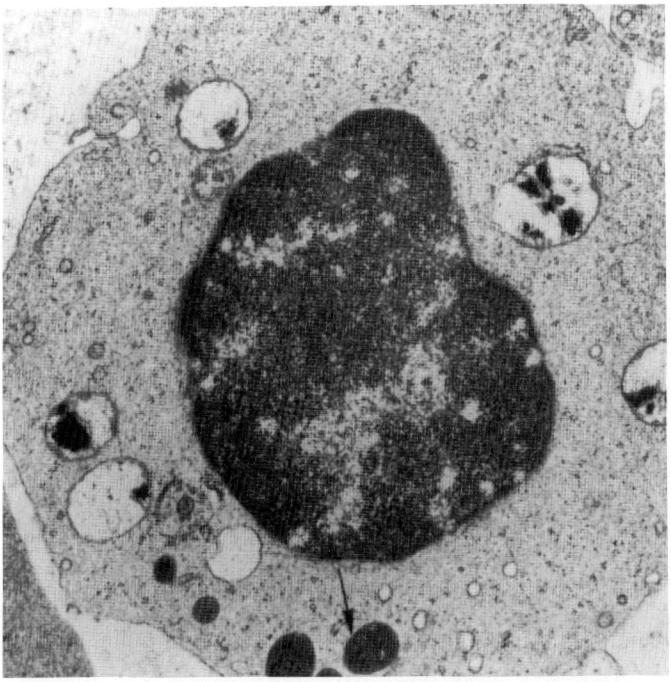

Figure 1 Electron micrograph of intermediate normoblast in refractory anemia with ring sideroblasts (RARS). Ferritin (black) distends and disrupts lamellae and cristae of mitochondria. Arrow denotes a cytoplasmic dense body.

to maintain the hemoglobin at or greater than 8 g/dL. Serum ferritin values are markedly elevated, and may exceed 2000 ng/ml.

Hematologically, the anemia is usually normochromic and normocytic, but is often macrocytic with mean corpuscular volume exceeding 110 fL. Sometimes, leukopenia and thrombocytopenia occur, signifying a generalized disturbance of the bone marrow. Peripheral blood smears from afflicted individuals demonstrate anisocytosis and poikilocytosis of erythrocytes, giant macrocytes, occasional teardrop poikilocytes, basophilic stippling, and rarely Pappenheimer bodies (Fig. 2, top). Platelets are small or large, and demonstrate multiple vacuoles and either hypergranularity or hypogranularity (Fig. 2, bottom). Neutrophils may be decreased in number. Some display the pseudo-Pelger Huet anomaly of nuclear hyposegmentation (Fig. 3, top). Monocytes can be increased in number (Fig. 3, bottom).

Bone marrow aspirates from patients with idiopathic sideroblastic anemia show intense megaloblastoid erythroid hyperplasia (Fig. 4, top and bottom). Proerythroblasts are often increased in number, and sometimes occur in clusters of two to six cells. Megakaryocytes are often small and atypical (Fig. 5). Macrophages are numerous, and contain hemosiderin as well as erythrocytes and degenerating erythroblasts. Erythrophagocytosis by macrophages constitutes evidence for intramedullary cell death (Fig. 6, top). Often, mast cells are increased.

Using the Prussian blue stain, many ring sideroblasts can be identified on smear preparation, but only rarely on a formalin-fixed paraffin-embedded section (Fig. 6, middle). The PAS

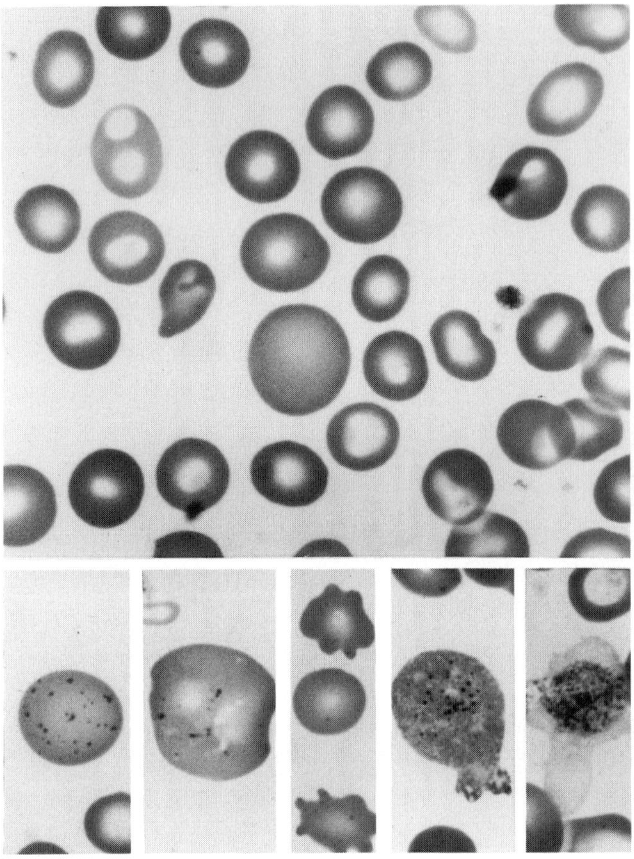

Figure 2 Peripheral blood smear, refractory sideroblastic anemia. Top: Variation in size (anisocytosis) and shape (poikilocytosis) of erythrocytes, including giant macrocytes. Bottom, left to right: Basophilic stippling, Pappenheimer bodies, schistocytes, giant platelet, giant hypergranular platelet with prominent pseudopodia.

stain for glycogen may be positive in a blocklike pattern in proerythroblasts and normoblasts (Fig. 6, bottom). More often, the staining reaction is negative in erythroblasts.

Patients with idiopathic sideroblastic anemia may be asymptomatic and not require blood transfusions. Other symptomatic patients require blood transfusions at regular intervals. In these individuals, repeated transfusions can lead to hemosiderosis. Some require an iron chelating agent, such as desferrioxamine, for removal of excessive amounts of iron. Certain individuals respond rapidly and dramatically to desferrioxamine, with a fall in ferritin levels to the normal range. In these patients, there may be a diminution or even a temporary cessation of blood transfusions. Various hematinics such as folic acid and pyridoxine have been tried alone or in combination. For the most part these agents are ineffective, and many patients are transfusion dependent (Table 2).

In approximately 7–10% of patients with idiopathic sideroblastic anemia, evolution into acute nonlymphoblastic leukemia occurs. Leukemia of this type that has evolved from a prior hematologic disorder may be particularly resistant to treatment with chemotherapy.

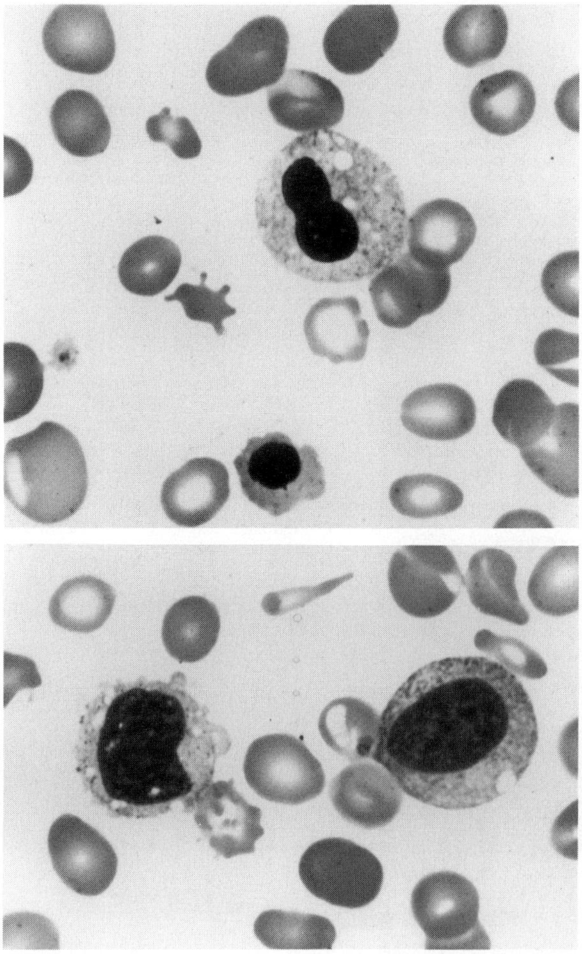

Figure 3 Peripheral blood smear, refractory sideroblastic anemia. Top: Granulocyte showing pseudo-Pelger-Huet anomaly. A normoblast is also seen. Bottom: Monocytes.

II. PORPHYRIAS

Porphyrias are inherited disorders of enzymes involved in the biosynthesis of heme. As a result of the enzyme disorder, excessive amounts of porphyrins or their precursors accumulate, leading to characteristic clinical manifestations and findings (Table 3).

A. Heme Synthesis

As shown in Fig. 7, the synthesis of hemoglobin begins in mitochondria with the condensation of glycerin and succinylcoenzyme A to form delta aminolevulinic acid (δ ALA), a reaction catalyzed by ALA synthase. Following this mitochondrial reaction, subsequent steps in heme synthesis occur in the cytoplasm of erythroblasts. In the cytoplasm, two molecules of ALA condense to form porphobilinogen (PBG). Next, four molecules of PBG condense to form hydroxymethylbilane. This intermediate cycles into either urophophyrinogen I or uroporphyrinogen III.

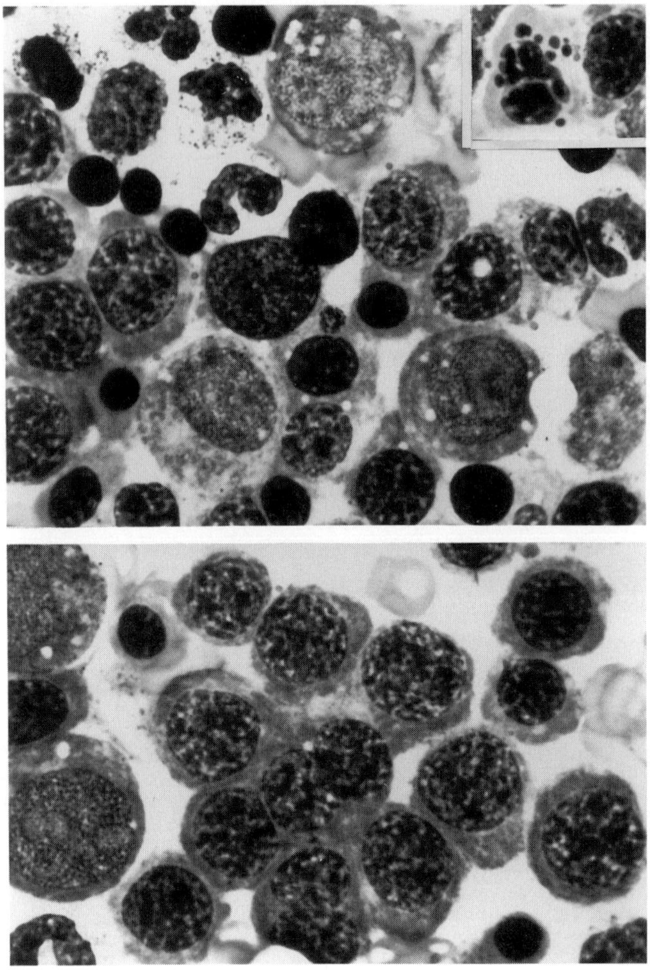

Figure 4 Bone marrow refractory sideroblastic anemia. Top and bottom display marked erythroid hyperplasia. Megaloblastoid nuclear chromatin patterns are shown. Inset, upper right: Normoblast with multiple Howell-Jolly bodies.

Uroporphyrinogen III is converted to coproporphyrinogen III by an enzymatic reaction catalyzed by uroporphyrinogen decarboxylase. From its site of synthesis in the cytoplasm, coproporphyrinogen III reenters the mitochrondria and, in an enzyme reaction catalyzed by coproporphyrinogen oxidase, is converted to protoporphyrinogen IX. In a reaction catalyzed by protoporphyrinogen oxidase, protoporphyrinogen IX is oxidized to protoporphyrin IX. Finally, heme is produced by a reaction catalyzed by ferrochetalase or heme synthetase, in which a ferrous iron atom is inserted in the center of the protoporphyrin IX ring.

B. Porphyrias

As a result of an inherited enzyme defect in any of the steps leading to the biosynthesis of hemoglobin, intermediates accumulate and lead to clinical manifestations. For example, in

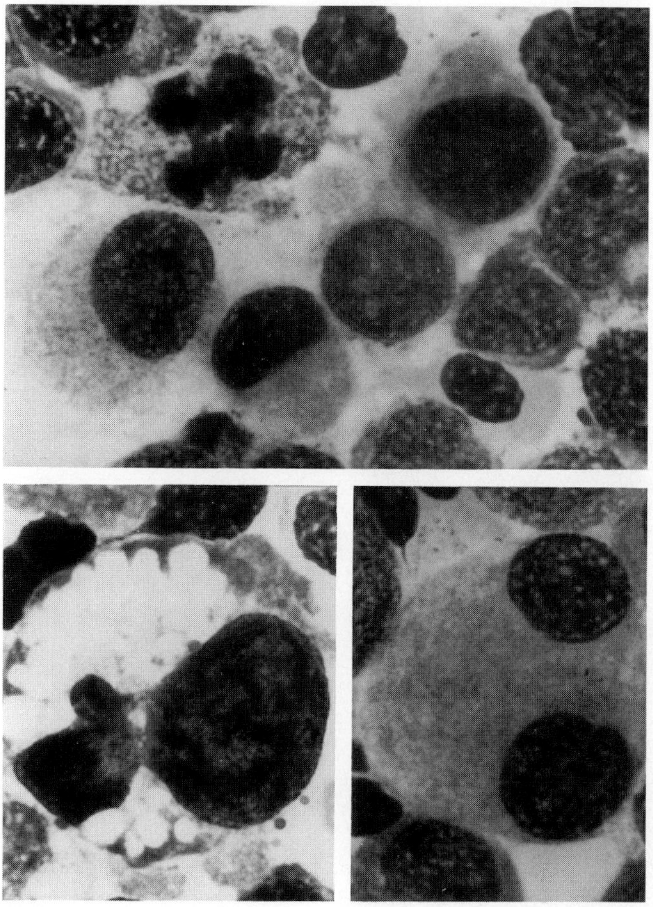

Figure 5 Bone marrow, refractory sideroblastic anemia. Top: Micromegakaryocytes. Bottom, left and right: Small atypical megakaryocytes.

acute intermittent porphyria, ALA and PGB accumulate, and patients display neurologic signs and symptoms. In contrast, if uroporphyrins, coproporphyrins, or protoporphyrins accumulate, the primary manifestations are dermatologic.

C. Laboratory Diagnosis of the Porphyrias

In acute intermittent porphyria, PBG and/or ALA accumulate, and can be detected in the urine. Drugs, hormones, or alcohol may lead to increased amounts of PBG and ALA in the urine, and precipitate an acute attack. In variegate porphyria due to a defect in protoporphyrinogen oxidase, protoporphyrinogen and protoporphyrin can accumulate. In hereditary coproporphyria due to a defect in coproporphyrinogen oxidase, coproporphyrinogen and coproporphyrin accumulate in the urine. In variegate porphyria and hereditary coproporphyria, substrates produced in excessive amounts due to the enzyme defects also inhibit PBG deaminase. This in turn causes an increase in ALA and PBG, leading to both neurologic and cutaneous manifestations in these patients.

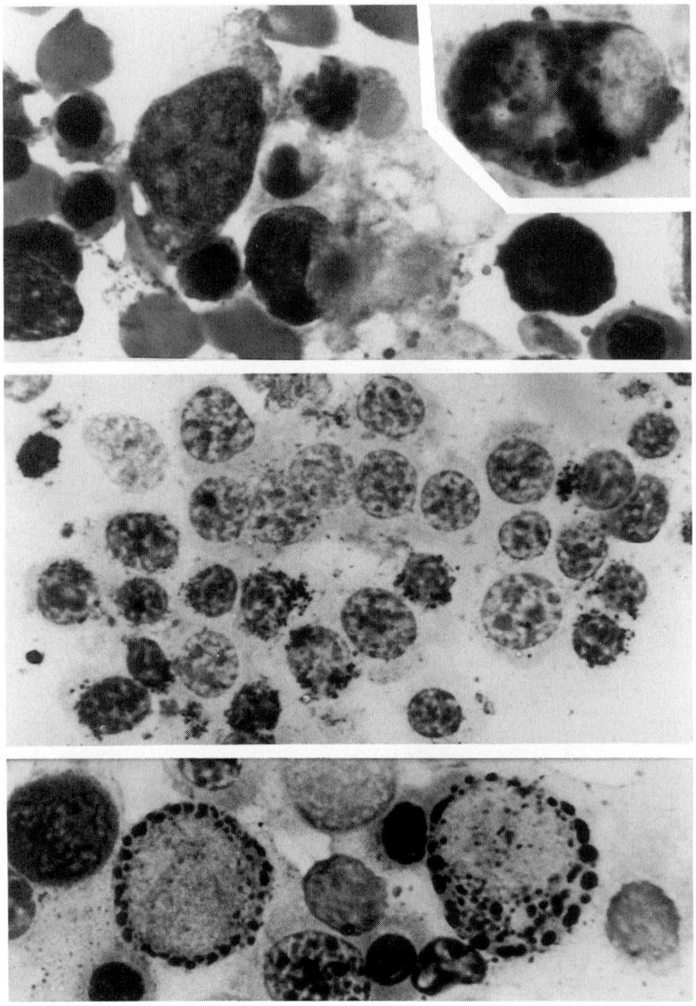

Figure 6 Bone marrow, refractory sideroblastic anemia. Top and inset: Macrophages. The cell in the center shows erythrophagocytosis, signifying ineffective erythropoiesis. Middle: Ring sideroblasts, Prussian blue stain. Bottom: PAS stain, demonstrating blocklike pattern in erythroblasts.

Table 2 Treatment of Refractory Anemia with Ring Sideroblasts

1. Pyridoxine (200 mg/day)
2. Folic acid
3. Iron chelating agents (desferrioxamine)
4. Blood transfusions in symptomatic individuals and/or if hemoglobin 8 gm/dL or less

Table 3 Enzymatic Defects in Porphyrias

Type of porphyria	Enzymatic defect	Elevated porphyrin precursors
Acute intermittent porphyria	Uroporphyrinogen I synthetase	PBG, ALA
Variegate porphyria	Protoporphyringen oxidase	ALA, PBG, protoporphyrin, coproporphyin
Hereditary coproporphyria	Coproporphyringen oxidase	Coproporphyin III, PBG, ALA
Porphyria cutanea tarda	Uroporphyrinogen decarboxylase	Uroporphyrin
Congenital erythropoietic porphyria	Uroporphyrinogen cosynthetase	Uroporphyrin I and coproporphyrin I
Protoporphyrin	Ferrochetalase	Protoporphyrin

In porphyria cutanea tarda, approximately 50% of patients demonstrate decreased activity of erythrocyte uroporphyrinogen decarboxylase. In acute intermittent porphyria, urinary levels of ALA or PBG or both are increased during and between attacks. In the neurocutaneous porphyrias, fecal porphyrins are increased during and between acute attacks. For example, in acute intermittent porphyria, normal or only slightly increased amounts of stool porphyrin are found. In variegate porphyria, protoporphyrin predominates in the stool, and there may also be increased amounts of coproporphyrin. In hereditary coproporphyria, coproporphyrins predominate in the stool, and excretion of protoporphyrin is normal. In porphyria cutanea tarda, excessive amount of uroporphyrin occur in the urine.

In nonporphyric diseases, urinary porphyrin excretion can be increased. For example, in lead poisoning, coproporphyrins and ALA are increased in the urine. In alcoholism and liver disease, coproporphyrins are increased. In hereditary tyrosinemia, ALA may be increased; and in chronic renal failure during dialysis, uroporphyrin may be increased.

D. Clinical Manifestations

Acute intermittent porphyria is inherited as an autosomal dominate trait, leading to deficiency of PBG deaminase. The disorder is characterized by abdominal pain, paresthesias and pain in the extremities, constipation, nausea and vomiting, and chest pain (Case Study 2). Tachycardia, dark urine, peripheral motor deficits and confusion occur frequently. Drugs reported to exacerbate acute intermittent porphyria include glutethemide, carbamazepine, valproic acid, ergots, danazol, barbiturates, ethanol, griseofulvin, hydantoins, meprobamate, oral contraceptives, and sulfonamides. Acute attacks are treated with glucose, chlorpromazine, and intravenous heme given in the dose of 3–5 mg/kg of body weight every 12 hr. Used appropriately, heme almost always decreases hepatic overproduction of ALA and PBG, leading to improvement in symptomatology in cases of recent onset. Rarely, intravenous heme has been associated with a coagulopathy.

Hereditary coproporphyria, a disorder caused by an enzyme defect in coproporphyrinogen oxidase, is inherited as an autosomal dominant trait. It is characterized by neurologic manifestations as in acute intermittent porphyria, or cutaneous manifestations in the form of a vesiculobullous eruption similar to that in porphyria cutanea tarda. Treatment of the acute episode involves the use of sunscreens and avoidance of sunlight.

Variegate porphyria is caused by a deficiency of activity of protoporphyrinogen oxidase, and is common in South Africa. Clinically, patients with the disease demonstrate acute neuro-

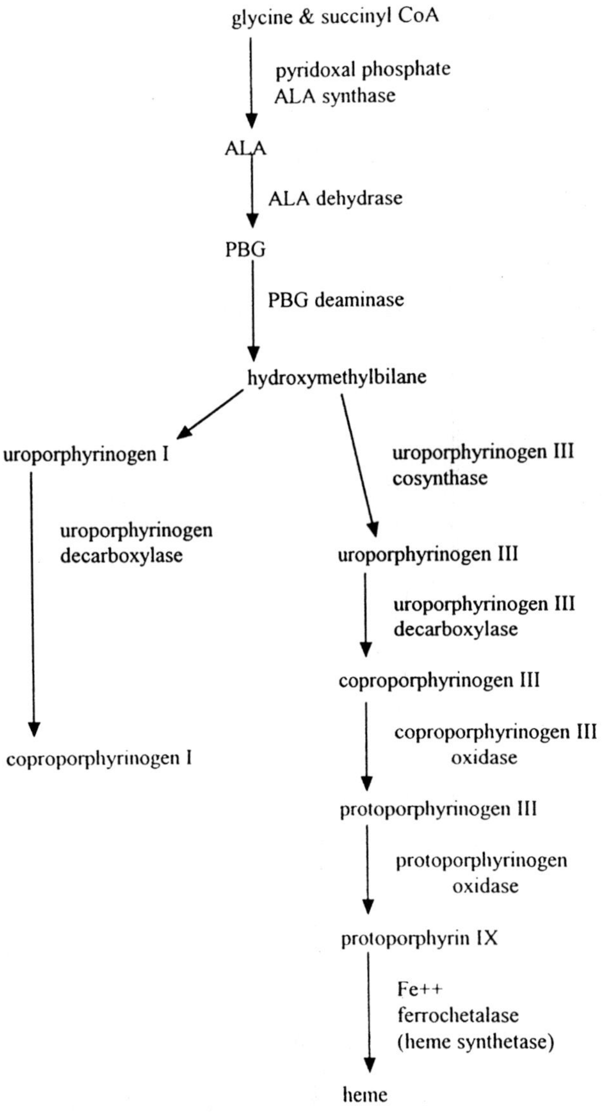

Figure 7 Diagrammatic representation of the biosynthetic pathway of heme.

logic symptoms and photodermatitis. In variegate porphyria, increased amount of protoporphyrin occur in the stool. For acute attacks, glucose, chlorpromazine, and intravenous heme are used.

Porphyria cutanea tarda can be acquired or inherited, and is the most common form of porphyria in the United States. It is characterized by a marked increase in urinary uroporphyrins and heptacarboxyl porphyrins. It presents as a dermatologic disorder, with blisters, sores, and vesicles that develop at sites of mild trauma. Porphyria cutanea tarda occurs in alcoholism, in women using oral contraceptives, in patients on chronic hemodiaylis, and in cases of iron overload. Treatment involves stopping alcohol, contraceptives, and removal of iron. In patients with unusually high excretion of urinary uroporphyrin, phlebotomy is used along with low doses of chloroquine. Avoidance of sunlight is important, although sunscreens are not effective because they do not screen out light in the Soret band of the spectrum.

Congenital erythropoietic porphyria is a very rare disorder transmitted as an autosomal recessive trait and caused by a defect in activity of uroporphyrinogen III synthase. The first sign of this disorder in infants is red urine that stains the diaper. Clinically, the disorder is characterized by photosensitivity, a cutaneous eruption following exposure to sunlight, and mutilation of nose, cartilage, and digits. There may also be hypertrichosis and erythrodontia, in which the teeth display red fluorescence under ultraviolet light, due to deposits of porphyrins in the dentin. Enlargement of the liver and spleen occurs. Treatment involves avoidance of sunlight and trauma to the skin. Suppression of erythropoiesis by hypertransfusion may also lead to amelioration of symptoms.

E. Secondary Porphyrias

Secondary porphyrias are characterized by a mild to moderate increase in urinary porphyrin excretion, and particularly coproporphyrin. Significantly, there is no increase in urinary ALA and PBG in these disorders, in contrast to acute intermittent porphyria, in which ALA and PBG are markedly elevated. Some of the disorders that produce secondary porphyrinuria include aplastic anemia, hemolytic anemia, pernicious anemia, leukemia, Hodgkin's disease, liver diseases including alcoholic hepatitis and cirrhosis, diabetes mellitus, and heavy metal intoxication.

CASE STUDY 1

Patient

Seventy-four-year-old white female.

Chief Complaint

Weakness and fatigue, shortness of breath.

Medical History

Overall, the patient had been in good health.

Medications

None.

Review of Systems

Exertional dyspnea, fatigue, ankle edema.

Physical Examination

Pallor, tachycardia, and pitting ankle edema, stool negative for occult blood.

Laboratory Results

	Patient	Normal
Hemoglobin	8.0 g/dL	13.5–18 g/dL
Hematocrit	23.2%	42–52%
MCV	112 fL	80–100 fL
Reticulocyte count	1.2%	0.5–1.5%
Platelet count	558×10^3	$150–400 \times 10^3$

A peripheral blood smear displayed anisocytosis, macrocytosis, and an occasional schistocyte. Hypersegmented neutrophils were not observed.

Questions

1. What blood tests should be ordered to evaluate the patient's macrocytic anemia?
2. Why would a bone marrow aspiration and biopsy be useful in determining the diagnosis?
3. How would you counsel the patient regarding her long-term prognosis?

Additional Laboratory Studies

Vitamin B_{12} and folate levels were normal. Ferritin was markedly elevated, at greater than 2000 ng/ml (normal is 10–291 ng/ml). A Coombs' test was negative, and bone marrow showed striking megaloblastoid erythroid hyperplasia. Leukemic blasts were not identified. An iron stain of the bone marrow demonstrated many ring sideroblasts.

Diagnosis

Refractory anemia with ring sideroblasts.

Discussion

This patient came to the doctor complaining of weakness and fatigue. After a blood count was obtained, it was clear that she had significant anemia, and that the anemia was most likely the cause of her weakness. Hematologic indices showed macrocytosis, and the differential diagnosis included deficiency of vitamin B_{12} and/or folate, hypothyroidism, and myelodysplastic disorder such as refractory anemia with or without ring sideroblasts. Laboratory studies for the anemia showed that levels of B_{12}, folate, and free thyroxine were normal, but the ferritin level was markedly elevated at greater than 2000 ng/ml. A bone marrow aspiration and biopsy and iron stain revealed marked megaloblastoid erythroid hyperplasia with ring sideroblasts. The patient was treated with pyridoxine in pharmacologic amounts, but had little if any rise in hemoglobin. Initially and subsequently, she required blood transfusions for amelioration of symptoms referable to the anemia. She was counseled that her anemia would persist, and most likely would require ongoing transfusions. She was also counseled that repeated transfusions could lead to overload of iron, causing transfusional siderosis. The possibility of using a chelating agent such as desferrioxamine was explained to the patient. Finally, she was informed that she had a risk of developing acute leukemia, that the risk was small (approximately 7–10%), and that her blood counts would be closely monitored to note any significant change.

Bibliography

1. Goasguen JE, Bennett JM. Classification and morphologic features of the myelodysplastic syndromes. Semin Oncol 1992; 13:4–13.
2. Cazzola M, Barosi G, Gobbi PG, et al. Natural history of idiopathic refractory sideroblastic anemia. Blood 1988; 71:305–312.

CASE STUDY 2

Patient

Forty-three-year-old black female.

Chief Complaint

Severe colicky abdominal pain for 5 days, anxiety, and depression.

Medical History

The patient related a decade-long history of depression, requiring treatment with a variety of psychiatric medications, including phenothiazines on several occasions.

Medications

None.

Review of Systems

Colicky and diffuse abdominal pain for 5 days, no evidence of darkening of stools, normal biliary sonogram 1 week earlier. Two years earlier she had a seizure.

Physical Examination

Anxiety alternating with periods of depression, diffuse abdominal tenderness, no rebound tenderness.

Laboratory Results

CBC was normal, and the only abnormal blood chemistry was serum sodium, 122 mEq/dL. A 6-h-old urine sample brought to the emergency department by the patient was virtually black. A freshly voided urine specimen was colorless. A CT scan of the abdomen and pelvis was normal, and MRI of the brain was normal.

Questions

1. What is the differential diagnosis of abdominal pain in the patient?
2. What was the clue that the patient might have an abnormality of heme synthesis?
3. What additional tests should be performed to make the correct diagnosis?

Diagnosis

Acute intermittent porphyria.

Discussion

This patient is a typical example of acute intermittent porphyria. Often, patients with this disorder come to medical attention by way of the emergency department. They seek help during periods of colicky abdominal pain which can mimic other disorders such as perforated duodenal ulcer, acute cholecystitis, renal colic and acute diverticulitis, to name only a few. Patients with acute intermittent porphria may also have psychiatric disturbances such as depression and/or anxiety. In some instances they may have seizures. Hyponatremia may occur in acute intermittent porphyria, as was the case with this patient. The diagnosis was suspected by the finding of very dark urine, and was confirmed by the detection of porphobilinogen in the urine. The patient was counseled that her psychiatric and abdominal abnormalities were likely connected, and part of the symptom complex of acute intermittent porphyria. She was treated with intravenous heme and improved significantly, with abatement of symptoms. She was advised to avoid barbiturates, sulfonamides, and hydantoins, since all of these are known to provoke attacks of acute intermittent porphyria.

Bibliography

1. Bloomer JR, Bonkovsky HL. The porphyrias. Disease-a-Month 1989; 35:1–54.
2. Werman HA. The porphyrias. Emerg Med Clin N Amer 1989; 7:927–940.

NOTE ADDED IN PROOF

Since this chapter was written, considerable advances have been made in understanding genetic abnormalities in acquired idiopathic sideroblastic anemia (15). In pyridoxine-responsive x-linked sideroblastic anemia, missense mutations in the erythroid-specific ALA synthase gene ALAS2 may be the primary cause of the disorder (16–18). After treatment with the cytoprotective agent amifostine (19), some patients with primary acquired refractory sideroblastic anemia, a myelodysplastic disorder, demonstrate rises in leukocyte, platelet, and red blood cell counts, and decrease in transfusion requirements.

Advances in the understanding of porphyrias have also occurred. In a family with variegate porphyria, a nonsense mutation in the protoporphyrinogen oxidase gene was identified as the underlying mutation. Other studies further defined the molecular defect of a genetic mutation leading to partial deficiency of protoporphyrinogen oxidase in homozygous variegate porphyria (21). For detection of urinary porphyobilinogen in acute intermittent porphyria, a commercial semi-quantitative bit (Trace) is described as more sensitive and specific than the standard Watson–Schwartz test (22).

SELECTED READINGS

Sideroblastic Anemia

1. Bottomley SS. Pathophysiology of heme synthesis. Semin Hematol 1988; 25:282–302.
2. Cazzola M, Barosi G, Gobbi PG, Invernizzi R, Riccardi A, Ascari E. Natural history of idiopathic refractory sideroblastic anemia. Blood 1988; 71:305–312.
3. Cotter PD, Rucknagel DL, Bishop DF. X-linked sideroblastic anemia: identification of the mutation in the erythroid-specific delta aminolevulinate synthase gene ($ALAS_z$) in the original family described by Cooley. Blood 1994; 84:3915\n]\3924.
4. Cox TC, Bottomley SS, Wiley JS, Bowden MJ, Matthews CS, May BK. X-linked pyridoxine-responsive sideroblastic anemia due to the Thr^{388}-to-Ser substitution in erythroid 5-aminolevulinate synthase. New Engl J Med 1994; 330:675–679.
5. Cox TC, Bowden MJ, Abraham N, et al. Erythroid 5-aminolevulate synthase is located in the X-chromosome. Am J. Hum Genet 1990; 45:107–111.
6. Goasguen JE, Bennett JM. Classification and morphologic features of the myelodysplastic syndromes. Semin Oncol 1992; 19:4–13.
7. Greenberg PL. Treatment of myelodysplastic syndromes with hemopoietic growth factors. Semin Oncol 1992; 19:106–114.
8. Levine EG, Bloomfield CD. Leukemias and myelodysplastic syndromes secondary to drug, radiation, and environmental exposure. Semin Oncol 1992; 19:47–84.
9. Sano T, Ban K, Ichiki T, et al. Molecular and genetic analyses of two patients with Pearson's marrow-pancreas syndrome. Pediatr Res 1993; 34:105–110.

Porphyrias

10. Bloomer JR, Bonkovsky HL. The porphyrias. Disease-a-Month 1989; 31:1–54.
11. Meola T, Lim HW. The porphyrias. Dermatol Clin 1993; 11:583–596.
12. Poh-Fitzpatrick MB. The porphyrias. Dermatol Clin 1987; 5:55–61.
13. Tefferi A, Golberg LA, Ellefson RD. Porphyrias: clinical evaluation and interpretation of laboratory tests. Mayo Clin Proc 1994; 69:289–290.
14. Tefferi A, Golberg LA, Ellefson RD. The porphyrias: diagnosis and management. Mayo Clin Proc 1994; 69:991–995.
15. Gatterman N, Retzlaff S, Wang YL, Hofhaus G, Heinisch J, Aul C, Schneider W. Heteroplasmic point mutrations of mitochondrial DNA affecting subunit I of cytochrome c oxidase in two patients with acquired idiopathic sideroblastic anemia. Blood 1997; 90:4961–4972.
16. May A, Bishop DF. The molecular biology and pyridoxine responsiveness of x-linked sideroblastic anemia. Haematologica 1998; 83:56–70.

17. Edgar AJ, Vidyatilake HM, Wickramasinghe SN. X-linked sideroblastic anaemia due to a mutation in the erythroid 5-aminolaevulinic synthase gene leading to an arginine 170 to leucine substitution. Europ J Haematol 1998; 61:55–58.
18. Cotter PD, May A, Li L, Al-Sabah AI, Fitzsimons EJ, Cazzola M, Bishop DF. Four new mutations in the erythroid-specific 5-aminolevulinate synthase (ALAS2) gene causing x-linked sideroblastic anemia: incresed pyridoxine responsiveness after removal of iron overload by phlebotomy and coinheritance of hereditary hemochromatosis. Blood 1999; 93:1757–1769.
19. List AF. Use of amifostine in hematologic malignancies, myelodysplastic syndrome, and acute leukemia. Seminars in Oncology 1999; 26(2, Suppl 7): 61–65.
20. Frank J, Jugert FK, Kalka K, Goerz G, Merk HF, Christiano AM. Variegate porphyria; identification of a nonsense mutation in the protoporphyrinogen oxidase gene. J Investigative Dermatology 1998; 110:449–451.
21. Roberts AG, Puy H, Dailey TA, Morgan RR, Whatley SD, Dailey HA, Martasek P, Nordmann Y, Deyback JC, Elder GH. Molecular characterization of homozygous variegate porphyria. Human Molecular Genetics 1998; 7:1921–1925.
22. Deacon AC, Peters TJ. Identification of acute porphyria: evaluation of a commercial screening test for urinary porphobilinogen. Ann Clin Biochem 1998; 35:726–732.

16

Anemias of Bone Marrow Failure

Robert T. Means, Jr.
Medical University of South Carolina and R. H. Johnson VA Medical Center, Charleston, South Carolina

I. DEFINITION AND INCIDENCE

Aplastic anemia is a disorder characterized by pancytopenia in the presence of significant marrow hypoplasia or aplasia. The term usually refers to persistent aplasia (as distinguished from the transient aplasia, which routinely follows cancer chemotherapy) which is not due to an underlying hematologic disease, such as paroxysmal nocturnal hemoglobinuria or hypocellular myelodysplastic syndromes. Aplastic anemia is said to be severe when the marrow shows cellularity less than 25% of that expected for age, and at least two of the following: peripheral blood granulocytes $<500/\mu L$, reticulocytes $<20{,}000/\mu L$, or platelets $<20{,}000/\mu L$. The age-adjusted annual incidence rate for aplastic anemia is 4.7–7.1 cases per million population.

II. ETIOLOGY

The etiologies of aplastic anemia are shown in Table 1.

A. Congenital Aplastic Anemia

Congenital aplastic anemias are typically associated with dysmorphic physical features, such as growth retardation, limb hypoplasia, and cardiac or renal abnormalities. Shwachman-Diamond syndrome is associated with pancreatic insufficiency. Fanconi's anemia is characterized by an impaired ability to repair damaged DNA crosslinks.

B. Secondary Aplastic Anemia

1. Drugs

Table 2 lists a variety of drugs that have been clearly established to be associated with aplastic anemia. The list is by no means exhaustive. It should be recalled that aplastic anemia is not a frequent occurrence in patients treated with any of these agents.

Among *antibiotics*, chloramphenicol has the best-known association with aplastic anemia. A reversible hypoproliferative anemia occurs in approximately 50% of patients receiving chloramphenicol. Aplastic anemia is much more rare, occurring in 1 of 10,000 administrations. It is more frequent following oral administration of the drug. This has suggested that chloram-

Table 1 Etiologies of Aplastic Anemia

Congenital
Fanconi's anemia
Shwachman-Diamond syndrome
Secondary
Drug-induced (see Table 2)
Radiation
Industrial toxins—benzene, other aromatic hydrocarbons, pesticides
Arsenic
Viral—hepatitis B, parvovirus B19, Epstein-Barr virus
Pregnancy
Idiopathic

phenicol metabolites produced by intestinal bacteria are predominantly responsible for marrow aplasia. Aplastic anemia is observed with a variety of other classes of antibiotics as well (Table 2).

Anticonvulsants are the drugs most commonly implicated in blood dyscrasias. Aplastic anemia has been described in association with most of the commonly used anticonvulsants, including the hydantoin compounds, valproic acid, and carbamazepine.

Analgesics, particularly nonsteroidal anti-inflammatory agents, have a strong association with aplastic anemia. Although acetylsalicylic acid (aspirin) has been clearly implicated in some cases of marrow aplasia, the widespread, generally unregulated use of this product suggests that it is extremely rare.

Gold salts, used in the management of advanced rheumatoid arthritis, were associated with 1.6 aplastic anemia-related deaths per 10,000 prescriptions in 1984. The mechanism of aplasia is unclear.

Ticlopidine is an antiplatelet agent used following cerebrovascular accidents and myocardial ischemia. Reversible agranulocytosis is observed in 2.4% of patients; aplastic anemia is much less frequent. These events are characteristically observed in the first 12 weeks of therapy.

A variety of *other drugs*, including oral hypoglycemic drugs, neuroleptics (particularly phenothiazines), antithyroid agents, and diuretics, have been associated with aplastic anemia (Table 2).

2. *Radiation*

Individuals exposed to acute high-dose whole-body irradiation typically develop marrow aplasia (often fatal) at 3–6 weeks. However, aplastic anemia is not a long-term complication observed in atomic bomb survivors. Chronic exposure to low-dose radiation may result in aplastic anemia, presumably as a result of hematopoietic stem cell injury.

3. *Industrial Hydrocarbons and Pesticides*

The association between industrial hydrocarbons such as benzene and pancytopenia or aplastic anemia is well established. The toxic effects of benzene are associated with its concentration in marrow fat and are attributed to metabolites, particularly hydroxyquinone phenols. Toluene, xylene, and *n*-alkylbenzenes lack hematopoietic toxicity. Organochloride and organophosphate pesticides are associated with aplastic anemia based on epidemiologic data. No mechanism has been proposed.

4. *Arsenic*

Arsenic poisoning is associated with deposition of crystalline arsenic in marrow and presumed direct toxicity toward hematopoietic progenitors/precursors resulting in aplasia. Arsenic-associated marrow aplasia has been reported to progress to acute leukemia.

5. *Viral Infections*

Aplastic anemia has been associated with a variety of viral infections, including hepatitis B, parvovirus B19, and Epstein-Barr virus. Hepatitis-associated aplasia carries a particularly poor prognosis. Some investigators have suggested that antiviral therapy should be considered early in the treatment of aplastic anemia.

6. *Pregnancy*

The onset of aplastic anemia occasionally is observed during pregnancy; whether this is coincidental or related to immunologic alterations in pregnancy is a controversial point. Interruption of the pregnancy may result in correction of the aplasia.

C. Idiopathic Aplastic Anemia

Despite efforts to identify an etiology, approximately 50% of cases of aplastic anemia appear to be of idiopathic origin. The success of immunosuppressive therapy in managing these patients (discussed below) suggest that immunologic mechanisms may be involved in a majority of these cases.

Table 2 Drugs Reported to Cause Aplastic Anemia

Analgesics	Tranquilizers/psychoactive drugs
Phenylbutazone[a]	Meprobamate
Acetylsalicylic acid	Phenothiazines
Oxyphenbutazone	Chlorodiazepoxide
Diclofenac[a]	Lithium
Indomethacin	Anticonvulsants
Anti-infectives	Phenytoins (diphenylhydantoin)[a]
Chloramphenicol, thiamphenicol[a]	Carbamazepine[a]
Sulfonamides[a]	Valproic acid
Isoniazid[a]	Felbamate
β-Lactam antibiotics[a]	Others
Pyrimethamine[a]	Allopurinol[a]
Flucytosine	Penicillamine[a]
	Sulfonylureas[a]
	Propylthiouracil
	Methimazole, carbimazole
	Antineoplastic drugs[a]
	Ticlopidine
	Gold[a]
	Furosemide

[a]Also associated with pure red cell aplasia (PRCA).

III. CLINICAL AND LABORATORY FEATURES

A. Clinical Features

Patients typically exhibit clinical manifestations of anemia. In addition, petechiae/purpura or frank bleeding may be observed in severely thrombocytopenic patients, and severely neutropenic patients may be febrile or exhibit the manifestation of the sepsis syndrome (hypotension, multiorgan system failure, etc.). Splenomegaly is distinctly uncommon. Patients with secondary aplastic anemia may exhibit manifestations of the associated state (hepatitis, neuropathy in arsenic poisoning, etc.).

B. Laboratory Findings

1. Hematologic Findings

As noted above, patients typically exhibit varying degrees of neutropenia, thrombocytopenia, and reticulocytopenic anemia. Red cells are often slightly macrocytic (mean corpuscular volume $<$105 fL). This finding may precede the onset of pancytopenia and, in treated patients, may herald its recurrence. Erythrocytes containing fetal hemoglobin are increased in patients with familial aplastic anemia.

2. Bone Marrow Findings

As discussed above, the diagnosis of aplastic anemia requires pancytopenia, reticulocytopenia, and a hypocellular marrow. This determination is made most accurately on a biopsy (Fig. 1).

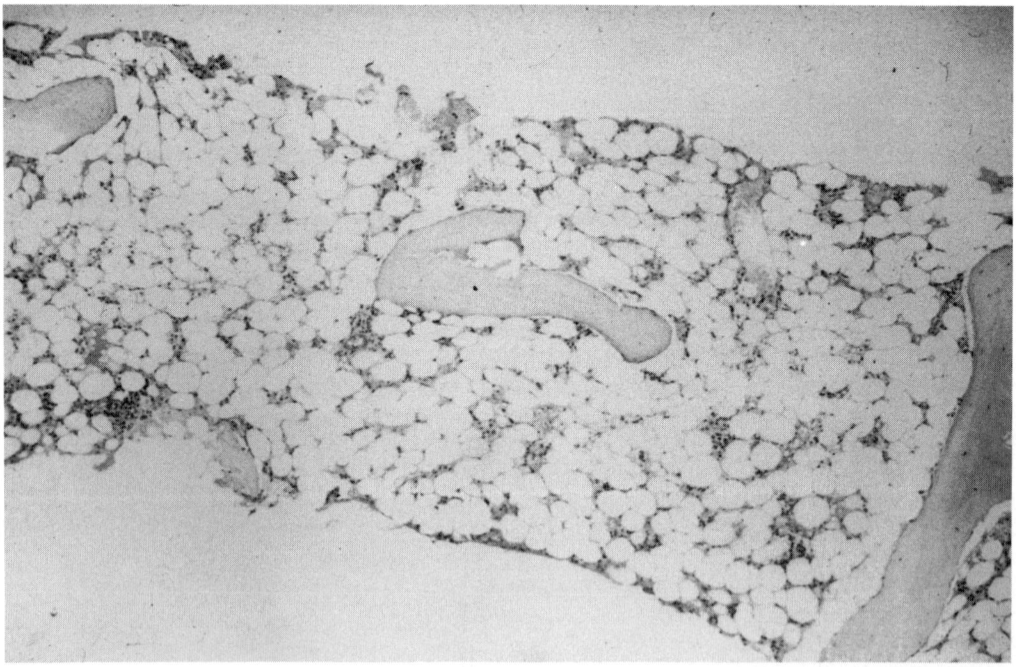

Figure 1 Bone marrow biopsy from a patient with severe aplastic anemia. (Original magnification ×400.)

Marrow cellularity is not distributed uniformly, so aspirates may be misleading; a hypocellular aspirate may reflect a hypocellular marrow, but may also reflect sampling error or technical problems (i.e., excessive blood dilution or a fibrotic marrow). Efforts should be made to obtain a large biopsy specimen to rule out sampling errors; residual hematopoiesis may result in hypercellular areas surrounded by aplasia. Special studies which should be obtained on bone marrow specimens include cytogenetics and flow cytometry; both are to evaluate the possibility of pancytopenia due to other clonal marrow syndromes.

In children, diepoxybutane studies should be obtained to demonstrate chromosomal fragility for the diagnosis of Fanconi's anemia.

3. *Other Laboratory Features*

In the absence of liver disease or disseminated intravascular coagulation, coagulation factor levels are normal. Serum or plasma erythropoietin levels are typically extremely elevated, with concentrations >10,000 mU/mL not uncommon.

IV. DIFFERENTIAL DIAGNOSIS

The differential diagnosis includes all etiologies of pancytopenia, including megaloblastic anemias, acute leukemia, and myelodysplastic syndromes. Most of these disorders will be identified on marrow examination, or by clinical features. The following disorders, which are associated with pancytopenia and a hypocellular marrow, require special attention.

A. Paroxysmal Nocturnal Hemoglobinuria

Paroxysmal nocturnal hemoglobinuria (PNH) should be considered in the differential diagnosis of pancytopenia with a hypocellular marrow. Typically the PNH patient will exhibit evidence of intravascular hemolysis (elevated serum bilirubin, elevated serum lactate dehydrogenase, hemosiderinuria, decreased serum haptoglobin), and may have a history of recurrent thrombosis. A sugar water or sucrose lysis test will be positive in PNH.

B. Hypocellular Myelodysplastic Syndromes

Hypocellular myelodysplastic syndromes (MDS) may be extremely difficult to distinguish from aplastic anemia. Characteristics of hypocellular MDS may include abnormal cytogenetics, micromegakaryocytes, abnormal megakaryocyte distribution, and marrow fibrosis. Hypocellular acute leukemias are also occasionally observed.

V. TREATMENT

A. Initial Evaluation

A careful history of medication use and toxic exposures should be taken on all patients with aplastic anemia. Many drug-induced aplasias, particularly those associated with phenothiazines, antithyroid drugs, and antineoplastic agents, will resolve, and only support is required in most cases.

B. Supportive Care

All patients with aplastic anemia will require supportive care. Transfusion of red cells and/or platelets, and empiric administration of broad-spectrum antibiotics for fever while neutropenic, may be necessary depending on the circumstances of individual cases. Administration of myeloid colony-stimulating factors may provide transient correction of neutropenia during episodes of fever or infection.

C. Bone Marrow Transplantation/Antithymocyte Globulin

Eighty percent of untreated aplastic anemia patients die within 1 year. Patients whose aplastic anemia fails to resolve in 4–6 weeks require aggressive therapy. Bone marrow transplantation should be considered for eligible patients, particularly those under 40 years of age. For all other patients, antithymocyte globulin should be administered. Patients who fail to respond to an initial course of antithymocyte globulin may respond to a second course using a product prepared in a different species of animal. The addition of cyclosporine appears to improve the response rate to antithymocyte globulins. Patients who respond to either antithymocyte globulin or bone marrow transplantation have prolonged survival.

D. Other Drugs

High-dose corticosteroids, high-dose cyclophosphamide, acyclovir, and intravenous immunoglobulin have also been reported to produce responses in aplastic anemia. Androgens, long a mainstay of therapy, are no longer felt to have a role the treatment of aplastic anemia.

VI. PURE RED CELL APLASIA (PRCA)

Pure red cell aplasia (PRCA) is a syndrome of reticulocytopenic anemia associated with selective erythroid hypoplasia in an otherwise normocellular marrow. A classification of PRCA is given in Table 3.

A. Congenital PRCA

Diamond-Blackfan anemia is a congenital anemia characterized by selective erythroid hypoplasia. Unlike the majority of cases of adult PRCA or transient erythroblastopenia of childhood,

Table 3 Classification of Pure Red Cell Aplasia

Congenital pure red cell aplasia
Diamond-Blackfan anemia
Acquired pure red cell aplasia
Primary pure red cell aplasia
Transient erythroblastopenia of childhood
Immune/idiopathic
Myelodysplastic
Secondary pure red cell aplasia
Thymoma
Malignancy
Lymphoproliferative disorders
Parvovirus
Other infectious agents
Collagen vascular disease
Pregnancy
Drugs and chemicals
Megaloblastic anemia

it appears to result from an intrinsic erythroid progenitor defect which alters responsiveness to erythropoietin. Diamond-Blackfan anemia is often associated with other congenital anomalies.

B. Primary PRCA

1. Transient Erythroblastopenia of Childhood

Transient erythroblastopenia of childhood is a transient PRCA typically follows a viral illness, and is produced by IgG antibodies directed against erythroid progenitors.

2. Immune/Idiopathic PRCA

PRCA most commonly presents as an autoimmune or presumably autoimmune disorder. In many cases, antibodies directed against erythroid precursors or progenitors can be demonstrated; in other cases, T-cell-mediated suppression of erythroid differentiation/proliferation can be demonstrated in vitro.

3. Myelodysplastic PRCA

MDS may present with a clinical picture resembling PRCA. These patients typically fail respond to immunosuppression.

C. Secondary PRCA

PRCA is frequently a consequence of other disorders or of exposure to drugs or toxins. In most cases, these are drug- or disease-associated autoimmune reactions, and may respond to immunosuppression.

1. Thymoma

The association between PRCA and thymoma is well known. PRCA is observed in 1–15% of patients with thymoma; thymoma is observed in 10–50% of cases of PRCA. Although most PRCA-associated thymomas are benign, association with thymic carcinoma has also been reported. Thymomas with PRCA are observed almost exclusively in adults, and in women more than men. Thymoma may precede the development of PRCA by many years; cases of PRCA following thymoma resection have also been described.

2. Malignancy

Infrequent cases of thymoma associated with nonthymic malignancies have been reported. Associated malignancies include carcinomas of the stomach, breast, hepatobiliary system, and lung, as well as chronic myelogenous leukemia, agnogenic myeloid metaplasia, and Kaposi's sarcoma.

3. Lymphoproliferative Disorders

The incidence of PRCA in chronic lymphocytic leukemia has been reported to be as high as 6%. It has also been reported in association with non-Hodgkins lymphomas, although less frequently.

4. Parvovirus Infection

Parvovirus B19, the agent responsible for the childhood exanthem, Fifth disease, has assumed great importance in the pathogenesis of PRCA. Initially, it was reported to produce transient aplastic crises in patients with chronic hemolytic anemias; more recently, it has been shown to be responsible for a significant number of cases of PRCA observed in individuals infected with the human immunodeficiency virus (HIV). Parvovirus exerts its effects by infection of erythroid precursors.

5. Other Infectious Agents

PRCA has been reported in association with meningococcal or staphylococcal infections, as well as with hepatitis, mononucleosis, mumps, and cytomegalovirus infection.

6. Collagen Vascular Diseases

PRCA in association with rheumatoid arthritis and with systemic lupus erythematosus.

7. Pregnancy

Like aplastic anemia, PRCA has been described in association with pregnancy. In some cases, anemia may resolve following pregnancy.

8. Drugs and Chemicals

PRCA has been described in association with many drugs and chemicals. A number of these drugs are indicated in Table 2.

9. Megaloblastic Anemia

Severe B_{12} or folate deficiency, particularly in the presence of underlying protein-calorie malnutrition, may present a picture resembling PRCA. Megaloblastic myeloid changes will typically identify these patients and distinguish them from individuals with other etiologies of PRCA.

D. Diagnosis

1. Hematologic Features

Patients with PRCA exhibit anemia with severe reticulocytopenia. Uncorrected reticulocyte percentages less than 0.3% are typical. White cell and platelet counts are typically normal. Abnormalities of these other counts call the diagnosis of PRCA into question.

2. Bone Marrow Features

The bone marrow in PRCA is normocellular and remarkable primarily for the absence or extreme reduction of erythroid precursors (Fig. 2). Plasma cells and lymphocytes are often slightly increased in a nonspecific pattern. In PRCA secondary to chronic myelogenous or lymphocytic leukemia, agnogenic myeloid metaplasia, or lymphoma involving the marrow, evidence of the primary disease is also present. Parvovirus-induced PRCA may be associated with giant pronormoblasts (Fig. 3), often with cytoplasmic blebbing; however, this finding is not specific. Chromosome studies should be obtained to identify myelodysplastic syndromes presenting as PRCA.

3. Parvovirus Studies

Studies to identify the presence of parvovirus should be performed on all patients with PRCA. These studies can be performed on either blood or bone marrow. Parvovirus genome should be identified by dot blot hybridization or polymerase chain reaction; demonstration of antibody to parvovirus is not adequate for diagnosis.

4. Other Tests

Other laboratory tests are typically normal in PRCA or exhibit evidence of associated diseases. Serum or plasma erythropoietin levels, as in aplastic anemia, are greatly elevated.

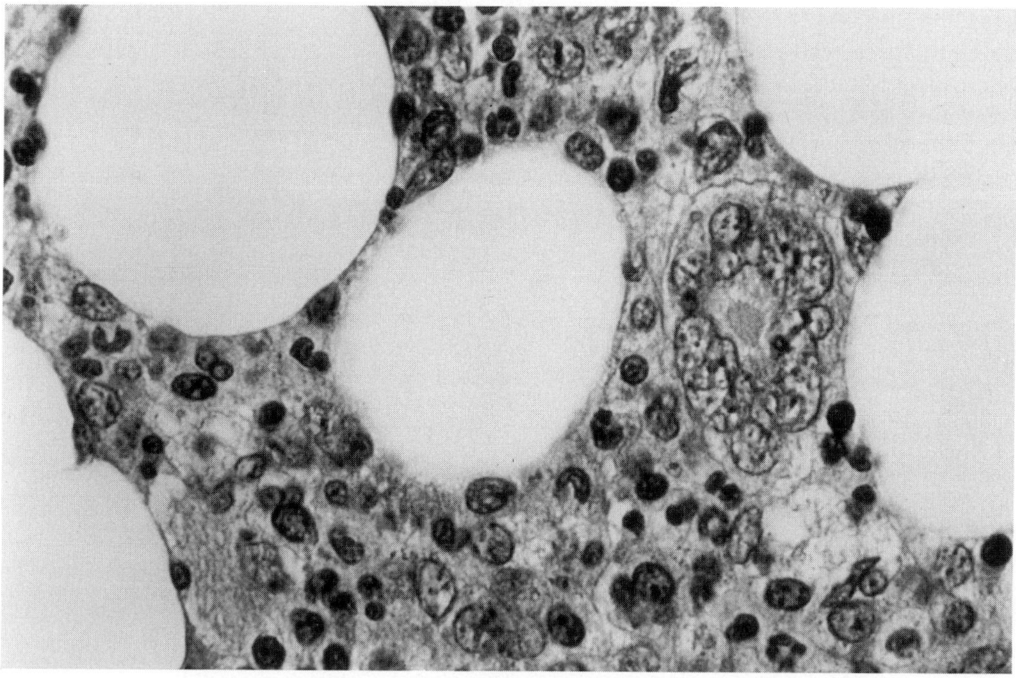

Figure 2 Bone marrow biopsy from a patient with idiopathic pure red cell aplasia. (Original magnification ×1000.)

E. Management

1. *Initial Evaluation*

The initial evaluation should focus on medication history, toxic exposures, and evidence of associated diseases. Drug cessation or treatment of associated diseases will often correct secondary PRCA. Thymomas should be sought radiographically.

2. *Thymectomy*

Patients with PRCA and a thymoma should undergo thymectomy. This will produce a remission in 25% of cases. Nonresponding or relapsing patients should receive immunosuppression. Mediastinal exploration in the absence of a demonstrated thymoma is not useful.

3. *Management of Parvovirus Infection*

Patients with documented parvovirus infection should receive intravenous immunoglobulin. This will typically lead to a prompt reticulocytosis.

4. *Immunosuppression*

Patients with primary PRCA or secondary PRCA who do not respond to treatment of the underlying illness or drug cessation should receive immunosuppression. Initially, corticosteroids should be used, at doses of 1 mg/kg/day. If the patient fails to respond within 6 weeks, oral cyclophosphamide or azathioprine can be added. Treatment should be slowly tapered in responding patients, beginning after correction of the anemia. This approach will produce responses in approximately two-thirds of patients. Cyclosporine A has been used in refractory

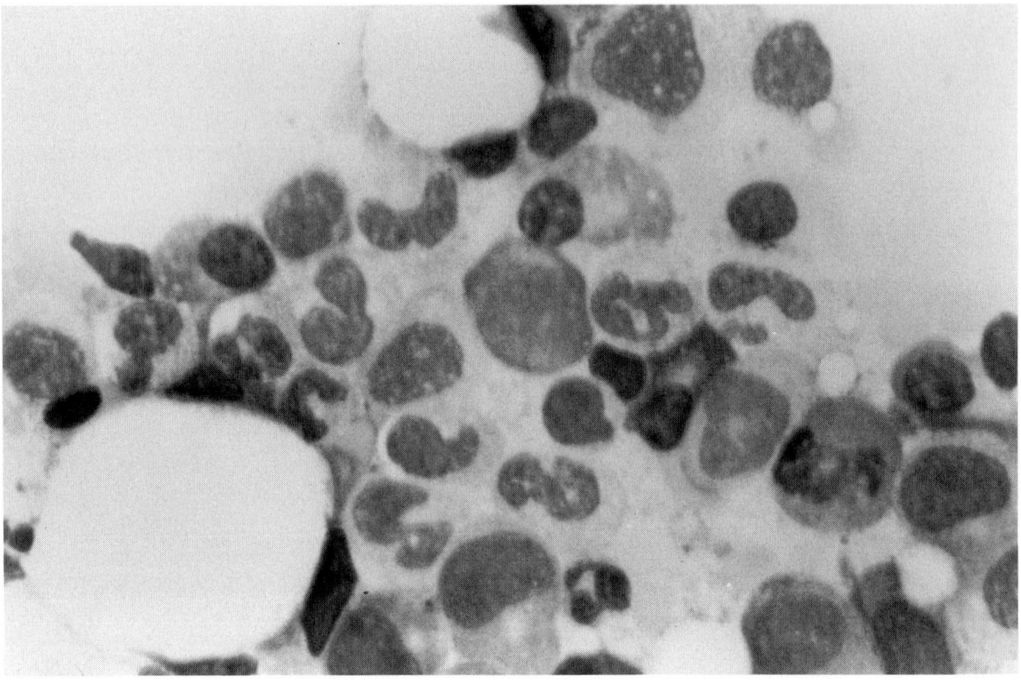

Figure 3 Bone marrow aspirate from a patient with parvovirus-induced pure red cell aplasia. Giant pronormoblast in center. (Original magnification ×1000.)

patients with good success; late occurrence of lymphoproliferative malignancies is a concern which limits its first-line use. Other second- and third-line agents include antithymocyte globulin, intravenous immunoglobulin, and plasmapheresis. Unfortunately, a significant percentage of responding patients will relapse later, and require further immunosuppression.

5. Childhood PRCA

Patients with Diamond-Blackfan anemia typically respond to corticosteroid therapy. Transient erythroblastopenia of childhood is self-limited and usually does not require specific therapy. A therapeutic dilemma may be presented by cases of primary PRCA presenting in childhood, which typically become confused with Diamond-Blackfan anemia, and which require more vigorous immunosuppression. In-vitro studies of erythroid progenitors may be required to distinguish the two syndromes.

CASE STUDY

Patient

Thirty-six-year-old male.

Chief Complaint

Pallor, dyspnea, tiredness for 2 months.

Medical History

Chronic vitiligo, celiac sprue.

Medications

None.

Physical Examination

Remarkable for patchy vitiligo on arms, trunk.

Laboratory Results

Hemoglobin	7.9 g/dL
Hematocrit	24.1%
MCV	87 fL
Reticulocytes	0.1%

White blood count, differential, platelet count, serum ferritin, B_{12}, and folate were normal.

Question

1. What test is indicated in the evaluation at this point?

Additional Laboratory Results

Bone marrow examination revealed a normocellular marrow with absent erythroid precursors. Myeloid maturation was normal. Plasma cells were slightly increased. Iron stores were increased. Cytogenetics were normal.

Question

1. What further studies are indicated at this point?

Further Studies

Parvovirus genome was not detected on a blood specimen amplified by polymerase chain reaction.

Diagnosis

Pure red cell aplasia (PRCA).

Discussion

Patients with PRCA not infrequently show evidence of other autoimmune disorders. B_{12} measurement was indicated despite a normal MCV because of the history of sprue and potential malabsorption. In reticulocytopenic anemias, marrow examination is indicated when serum iron, B_{12}, and/or folate studies fail to provide a diagnosis. Parvovirus infection, for which effective and specific (but expensive) therapy is available, should be ruled out in all cases of PRCA.

Bibliography

1. Dessypris EN. Pure Red Cell Aplasia. Baltimore: Johns Hopkins University Press, 1988.

SUGGESTED READINGS

1. Aggio MC, Zuuni C. Reversible pure red cell aplasia in pregnancy. N Engl J Med 1977; 297:221.
2. Champlin R, Ho W, Gale RP. Antithymocyte globulin treatment in patients with aplastic anemia. A prospective randomized trial. N Engl J Med 1983; 308:113–118.

3. Chikkappa G, Zarrabi MH, Tsuan M-F. Pure red cell aplasia in patients with chronic lymphocytic leukemia. Medicine 1986; 65:339–351.
4. Clark DA, Dessypris EN, Krantz SB. Studies on pure red cell aplasia. XI. Results of immunosuppressive therapy of 37 patients. Blood 1984; 63:277–286.
5. Dessypris EN. Pure Red Cell Aplasia. Baltimore: Johns Hopkins University Press, 1988.
6. Dessypris EN, Krantz SB, Roloff JS, et al. Mode of action of the IgG inhibitor of erythropoiesis in transient erythroblastopenia of childhood. Blood 1982; 59:114–123.
7. Doney K, Leisenring W, Storb R, et al. Primary treatment of acquired aplastic anemia: outcomes with bone marrow transplantation and immunosuppressive therapy. Ann Intern Med 1997; 126: 107–115.
8. Feder HM. Chloramphenicol: what have we learned in the last decade? South Med J 1986; 79: 1129–1134.
9. Fohlmeister I, Fischer R, Modder B, et al. Aplastic anaemia and the hypocellular myelodysplastic syndrome: histomorphological, diagnostic, and prognostic features. J Clin Pathol 1985; 38:1218–1224.
10. Gibson J, McGirr EE, York J, et al. Aplastic anemia in association with gold therapy for rheumatoid arthritis. Austral NZ J Med 1983; 13:130–134.
11. Girdwood RG. Death after taking medications. Br Med J 1984; 1:1266–1268.
12. Gomez-Almaguer D, Marfil-Rivera J, Kudish-Wersh A. Acyclovir in the treatment of aplastic anemia. Am J Hematol 1988; 29:172–173.
13. Harris JW. Parvovirus B19 for the hematologist. Am J Hematol 1992; 39:119–130.
14. Ikehara O. Drug-induced blood dyscrasias in Okinawa. Rinsho Ketsueki 1991; 32:709–711.
15. International Agranulocytosis and Aplastic Anemia Study. Risks of agranulocytosis and aplastic anemia: a first report of their relation to drug use with special references to analgesics. JAMA 1986; 256:1749–1757.
16. Lesesve JF, Callat M-P, Lenormand B, et al. Hematologic toxicity of Ticlopidine. Am J Hematol 1994; 47:149–150.
17. McSweeney PA, Carter JM, Green GJ, et al. Fatal aplastic anemia associated with hepatitis B viral infection. Am J Med 1988; 85:255–256.
18. Means RT. Toxic effects on erythrogenesis. In: Bloom JC, ed. Toxicology of the Hematopoietic System. Vol. 4 (Comprehensive Toxicology). New York: Elsevier/Pergamon, 1997:87–106.
19. Means RT, Dessypris EN, Krantz SB. Treatment of refractory pure red cell aplasia with cyclosporine A: in vitro correlation of clinical response. Br J Haematol 1991; 78:114–119.
20. Means RT, Krantz SB, Dessypris EN, et al. Retreatment of aplastic anemia with antithymocyte globulin or antilymphocyte serum. Am J Med 1988; 84:678–682.
21. Najean Y, Arrago JP, Delsol G, et al. Diagnostic and prognostic value of bone marrow biopsy in aplastic anemia. Nouv Rev Fr Hematol 1986; 28:281–285.
22. Rozman C, Nomadieu B, Marin P, et al. Criteria for severe aplastic anaemia. Lancet 1987; 2: 955–957.
23. Szklo M, Sensenbrenner L, Markowitz J, et al. Incidence of aplastic anemia in metropolitan Baltimore: a population-based study. Blood 1985; 66:115–119.
24. Tichelli A, Gratwohl A, Nissen C, et al. Morphology in patients with severe aplastic anemia treated with antilymphocyte globulin. Blood 1992; 80:337–345.
25. Weinsheimer W, Szepesi T, Fliedner TM. Early indicators of response to accidental radiation exposure and the relevance for clinical management strategies. Prog Clin Biol Res 1991; 372:155–165.

17

Hemoglobinopathies and Thalassemias

Donald L. Rucknagel
University of Cincinnati College of Medicine, and Cincinnati Comprehensive Sickle Cell Center, Children's Hospital Medical Center, Cincinnati, Ohio

I. INTRODUCTION

Over 700 different inherited variants of hemoglobin have been described in humans. Most are of no clinical consequence. Some, however, significantly alter molecular stability or function, resulting in anemia or other disease manifestations. Most of the clinical abnormalities are explainable in terms of the structural abnormality.

II. HEMOGLOBIN STRUCTURE

Hemoglobin is a tetramer of two pairs of different globin chains with a molecular weight of 64,000 daltons. The sequence of the 141 amino acid residues of the α-globin of normal adult hemoglobin and 146 of the β-globin chains (the primary structure) are similar and are arranged in seven or eight helical regions (the secondary structure), designated A through H from the amino terminus (Fig. 1). The α-chains have no D helix, however. Short linear sequences are interspersed between the helices and at the ends of the chain. They are designated by the termini and the two helical regions before and after—e.g., the NA and AB regions on either side of the A helix. Each chain is folded into a compact tertiary structure such that hydrophobic amino acids are oriented toward the interior of the molecule and charged or hydrophilic amino acids tend to be oriented toward the surface.

The heme group, a protoporphyrin IX, is interposed between two histidine imidazole groups in the E and F helices at (E7) and (F8), respectively. The 60 atomic contacts between the various amino acids and the heme groups that stabilize the molecule have been precisely determined by X-ray diffraction. The interior of the molecule is devoid of water.

Oxygen molecules enter the heme pockets between the iron atom of the heme group and the histidine molecule in the E helix at residue 57 of the α- and 63 of the β-globin chain. These are called the distal histidines. The oxygen atom in each pocket tugs on the iron molecule of the heme, pulling it into the plane of the heme group (Fig. 2), in turn pulling the histidine on the opposite side of the heme iron at F8 (residue 87 of the α- and 92 of the β-globin chains), closer to the E helix; this initiates complex conformational changes in the tertiary structure that accompany oxygenation. The changes in the relationship among the four chains of the

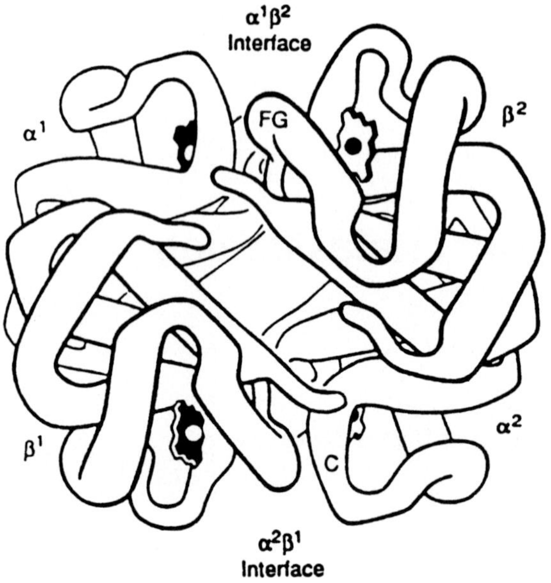

Figure 1 Diagrammatic representation of the tertiary structure of a β-globin chain, showing the heme group and the location of variant hemoglobins that impart physical instability to the molecule. (From Embury et al., 1994.)

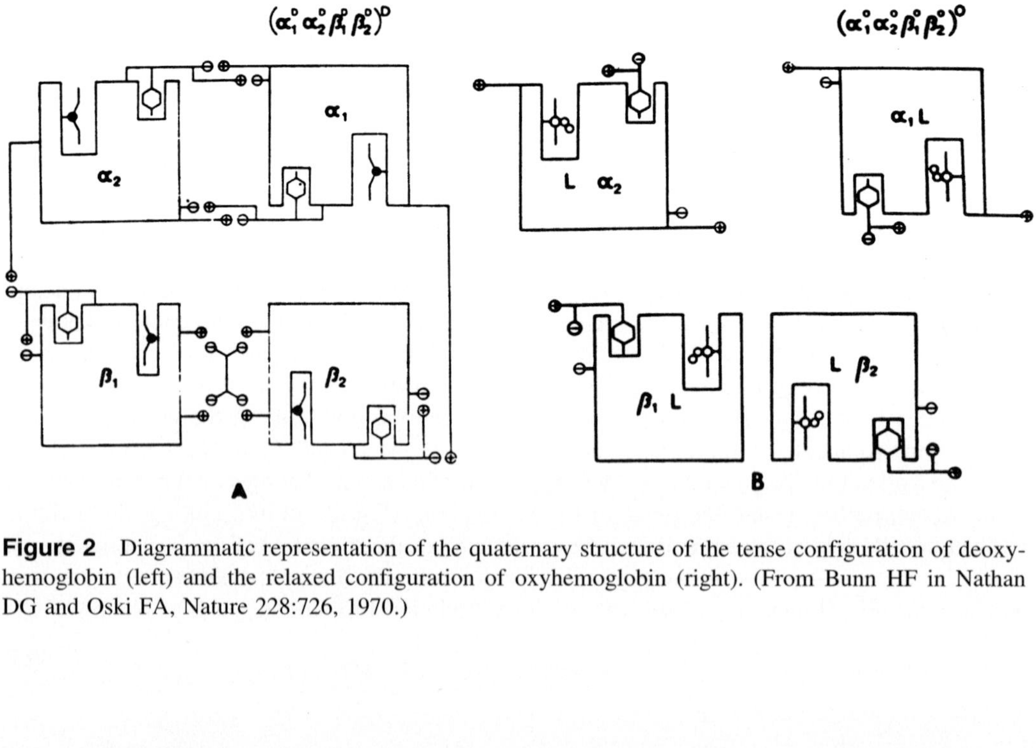

Figure 2 Diagrammatic representation of the quaternary structure of the tense configuration of deoxy-hemoglobin (left) and the relaxed configuration of oxyhemoglobin (right). (From Bunn HF in Nathan DG and Oski FA, Nature 228:726, 1970.)

hemoglobin molecule, the quaternary structure, as oxygen enters and leaves the hemoglobin tetramer produce, explain in part the changes in oxygen binding responsible for the oxyhemoglobin dissociation curve.

The hemoglobin molecules, when fully oxygenated, are in a less compact tertiary structure called the relaxed form; a small percentage are dissociated into $\alpha\beta$ dimers (Fig. 2). The number of atomic contacts between α- and β-chains in a dimer, called the $\alpha_1\beta_1$ interface, is larger than the number between the α-chain of one $\alpha\beta$ dimer and the β-chain of the opposite dimer (called the $\alpha_1\beta_2$ interface). As oxygen is removed from the hemoglobin tetramer, each chain from which it is removed assumes a more compact conformation (called the tense form), and the equilibrium of the quaternary structure shifts toward the tetrameric form. Involved in these changes is translation or sliding of dimers along the $\alpha_1\beta_2$ interface. These changes will be discussed further below in the context of mutants that alter hemoglobin function.

III. NOMENCLATURE

Six different globin chains produced in humans combine to form the various tetramers present in red cells (Fig. 3). Hb Gower 1 (z2E2) is produced in yolk sac cells early in embryogenesis followed by Hb Gower 2 (α_2E_2) later in the embryonic period when α-chain synthesis commences. Subsequently Γ-chain synthesis and then β-chain synthesis are reciprocally switched on to combine with α-chains to form Hbs F then A. A few months after birth δ-chain synthesis begins; these chains combine with α-chains to form Hb A_2. Thus, α-globin chains are produced nearly throughout development. The adult level of Hb A_2 of 2% to 3.5% of the total hemoglobin is not attained until approximately 2 years of age. Several glycosylated hemoglobins accumulate in red cells at a rate proportionate to the concentration of glucose in the blood; measure-

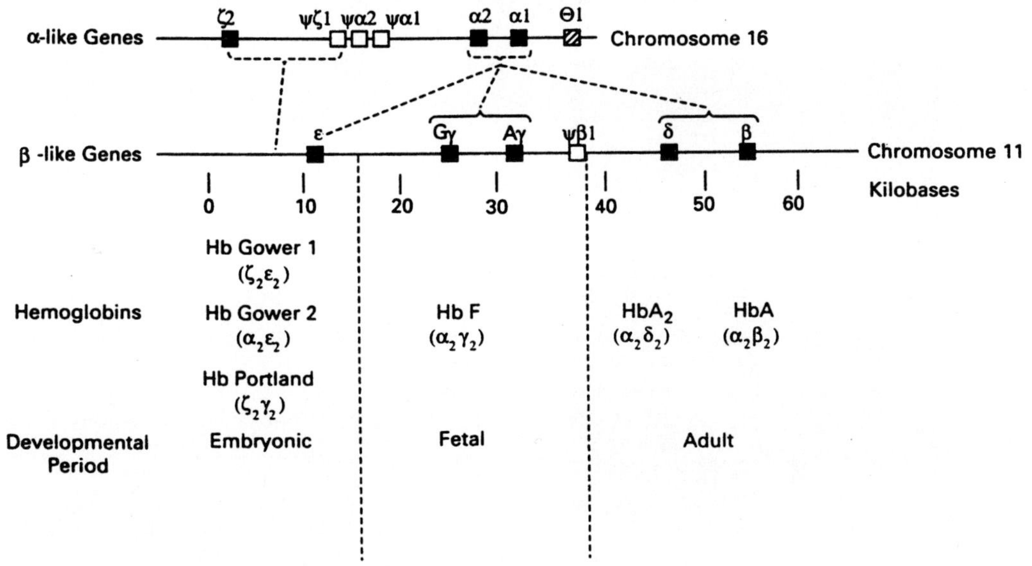

Figure 3 Chromosomal organization of the globin genes and their expression during ontogeny. The switch from embryonic to fetal hemoglobin production begins at approximately 6 weeks of gestation and from fetal to adult beginning at approximately 10 weeks. (From Embury et al., 1994.)

ment of glycosylated hemoglobin provides an estimate of the average blood glucose level over the life span of the red cells, aiding in the regulation of diabetes.

Most abnormal hemoglobins are due to amino acid substitutions that change net ionic charge, thereby altering electrophoretic mobilities (Fig. 4). Variants were initially designated alphabetically—Hb A for normal adult, F for fetal and S for sickle; variants were named in order of discovery—hemoglobins C, D, E, and G were the next variants detected. Over 50 variants with the mobility of Hb S (+2 net charges per tetramer) have been described. These are referred to generically as hemoglobins D if the substitution is in the β-globin chain and Hb G if in the α-chain. (The first such variant, described also under various other names, was Hb G_{α}-Philadelphia.) When it became clear that the number of variants would exceed the alphabet, geographic names were employed to designate new hemoglobins. To this a chemical designation describing the location of the amino acid substitution in sequence in the chain, and the corresponding helix has been added. Thus, the symbol for sickle cell hemoglobin is Hb Sβ6(A3)Glu → Val, indicating that a glutamic acid has been replaced by valine at the sixth position of the β-globin chain or the third position of the A helix. Hemoglobin G-Philadelphia, α68(E17)Asn → Lys, is the most common alpha-chain variant. Relative mobilities of selected variants by cellulose acetate electrophoresis at alkaline pH (CAE) and citrate agar gel electrophoresis (CAGE) at acid pH are compared in Figure 5. The amino acid substitutions of frequently encountered variants are summarized in Table 1.

IV. LABORATORY METHODS FOR DIAGNOSING HEMOGLOBINOPATHIES

A. Standard Hematologic Methods

Most hemoglobin structural variants do not affect erythrocyte morphology, including some with significant functional abnormalities. Some do, however. Since most states include electro-

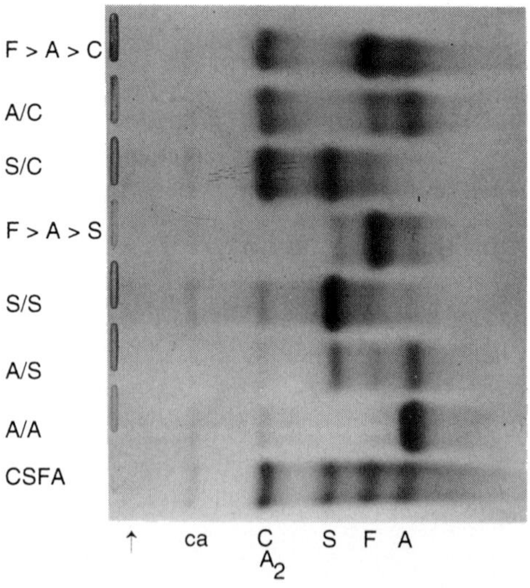

Figure 4 Cellulose acetate electrophoresis of hemoglobin from various sickle cell diseases; Tris buffer, pH 8.4; migrating to the right (anode); Ponceau S stain. Arrow: point of application; ca, carbonic anhydrase enzyme.

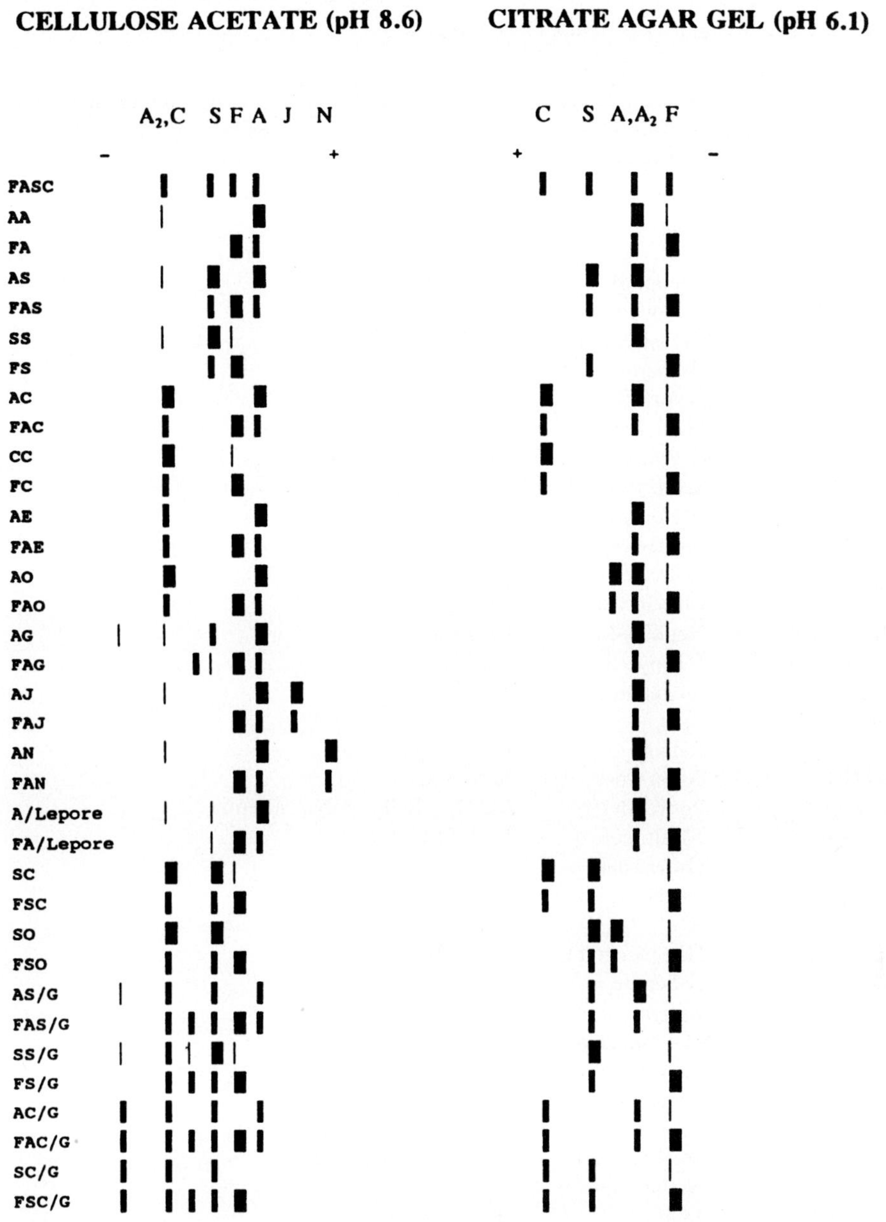

Figure 5 Comparative mobilities in standard electrophoretic methods (CAE and CAGE; see text) of hemoglobin of the most common variant hemoglobins. The fetal phenotypes are designated with the letters in descending order of concentration in the blood; e.g., FAS = F > A > S. Other hemoglobins migrating with the mobility of Hb S on CAE are Hbs S, D, G-Philadelphia, and Lepore. Those migrating with the mobility of Hb C or A_2 are Hbs E, O-Arab, and the G/S hybrid molecule of compound heterozygotes of Hb S and G_α ($\alpha_2^G\beta_2^S$). The hemoglobin migrating between the positions Hbs S and C is the Hb G derivative of Hb F ($\alpha_2^G\Gamma_2$) (From Adams in Embury et al., 1994.)

Table 1 Selected Clinically Significant Hemoglobin Variants

Substitution	Name	Property
Alpha chain variants		
5 (A3) Ala → Asp	J-Toronto	
11 (A9) Lys → Glu	Anantharaj	SE Asia
12 (A10) Ala → Asp	J-Paris	
16 (A14) lys → Glu	I	Af-Am
23 (B4) Glu → Gln	Memphis	Af-Am with Hb S
30 (B11) Glu → Gln	G-Honolulu	
47 (CE5) Asp → Gly	Umi, Beilinson	Unstable
Asp → His	Hasharon	
57 (E6) Gly → Asp	J-Norfolk	
58 (E7) His → Tyr	M-Boston	Methemoglobinemia
68 (E17) Asn → Lys	G-Philadelphia	Often cis to α-thal
78 (EF7) Asn → Lys	Stanleyville-II	With Hb S
85 (F6) Asp → Asn	G-Norfolk	Inc O_2 Affinity
Asp → Val	Inkster	With β-thal
87 (F8) His → Tyr	M-Iwate	Methemoglobinemia
92 (FG4) Arg → Leu	Chesapeake	Inc O_2 affinity
112 (G19) His → Asp	Hopkins-II	Unstable
115 (GH3) Ala → Asp	J-Tongariki	cis to α-thal
141 (HC3) Arg → Pro	Singapore	
β-Globin variants		
1 (NA1) Val → AcAla	Raleigh	Decr O_2 affinity
7 (A4) Glu → Gly	G-San Jose	Slt unstable
9 (A6) Ser → Cys	Porto Alegre	Inc O_2 affinity, polymerization
16 (A13) Gly → Asp	J-Baltimore	With S, C, β-thal
22 (B4) Glu → Ala	G-Coushata	
Glu → Gln	D-Iran	
26 (B8) Glu → Lys	E	Thal phenotype
42 (CD1) Phe → Ser	Hammersmith	Unstable
61 (E5) Lys → Glu	N-Seattle	With S
63 (E7) His → Arg	Zurich	Unstable
His → Tyr	M-Saskatoon	Methemoglobinemia
67 (E11) Val → Glu	M-Milwaukee-I	Methemoglobinemia
73 (E17) Asp → Asn	Korle-Bu	With S
89 (F5) Ser → Asn	Creteil	Inc O_2 affinity
92 (F8) His → Tyr	M-Hyde Park	Methemoglobinemia
95 (FG2) Lys → Glu	N-Baltimore	
97 (FG4) His → Gln	Malmo	Inc O_2 affinity
98 (FG5) Val → Met	Koln	Unstable
99 (G1) Asp → Asn	Kempsey	Inc O_2 affinity
Asp → His	Yakima	Inc O_2 affinity
Asp → Ala	Radcliffe	Inc O_2 affinity
Asp → Tyr	Ypsilanti	Inc O_2 affinity, asymmetric hybrids
Asp → Gly	Hotel-Dieu	Inc O_2 affinity
Asp → Val	Chemilly	Inc O_2 affinity
102 (G4) Asn → Lys	Richmond	Asymmetric hybrids
112 (G14) Cys → Arg	Indianapolis	Very unstable
121 (GH4) Glu → Gln	D-Los Angeles	With S, Inc O_2 affinity

Table 1 Continued

Substitution	Name	Property
Glu → Lys	O-Arab	With S, β-thal
136 (H14) Gly → Asp	Hope	Unstable, decr O_2 affinity
145 (HC2) Tyr → His	Bethesda	Inc O_2 affinity
Tyr → Cys	Ranier	Inc O_2 affinity
Tyr → Asp	Fort Gordon	Inc O_2 affinity
Tyr → Term	McKees Rocks	Inc O_2 affinity
146 (HC3) His → Asp	Hiroshima	Inc O_2 affinity
His → Pro	York	Inc O_2 affinity
His → Arg	Cochin-Port Royal	
His → Leu	Cowtown	Inc O_2 affinity
Variants having two amino acid substitutions in one chain		
β6 (A3) Glu → Val 73 (E17) Asp → Asn	C-Harlem	
β6 (A3) Glu → Val 142 (H20) Ala → Val	S-Travis	Inc O_2 affinity
Variants having extended chains		
α141Term → Gly	Constant Spring	31 amino acids appended to C-terminus
α139-140 -1 frame-shift	Wayne	Two terminal amino acids replaced by unique sequence of 10
Fusion genes		
δβ hybrid chain	Lepore	Formed by unequal crossover
Γβ hybrid chain	Kenya	Unequal crossover between Γ and β

phoresis of hemoglobin in newborn screening programs, most abnormal hemoglobins in the United States are detected at birth.

B. Hemoglobin Diagnostic Techniques

With a given electrophoretic technique some abnormal hemoglobins comigrate with other variants or Hb A. Therefore, several techniques are necessary to assure detection of most hemoglobin variants.

1. The standard zone electrophoretic methods employing buffers at pH 8.4 to 8.6 separate the various hemoglobins on the basis of net charge. Cellulose acetate (CAE) is the simplest matrix (Fig. 4).

2. Comparison of mobilities of variants by cellulose acetate (CAE) with citrate agar gel electrophoresis (CAGE) at pH 6.1 (Fig. 5). CAGE separates Hb S from Hbs D or G; the latter migrate as Hb A. Use of this technique with CAE allows accurate identification in most cases. By CAGE of cord blood the large amount of Hb F present migrates faster than Hb A, allowing more accurate assessment of the relative amounts of Hb A and Hb S.

3. Isoelectric focusing (IEF) is a newer method and has exceptionally high resolution (Fig. 6).

4. High-pressure liquid chromatography (HPLC) has good resolution (Fig. 7) and can be automated with the use of automatic injection. A short cationic column (Poly LC Co.) measures

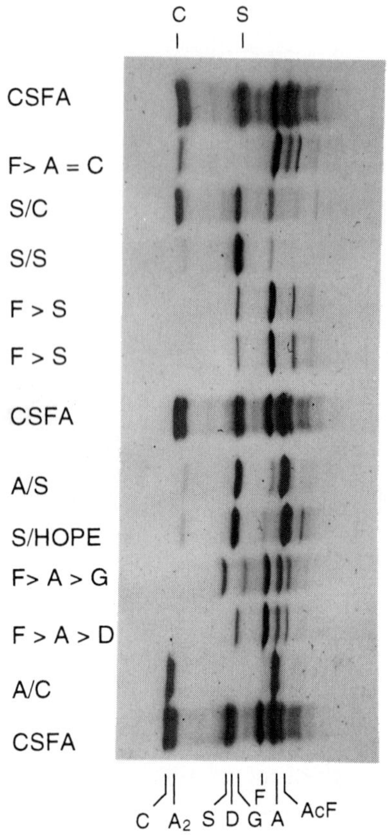

Figure 6 Isoelectric focusing pattern of common hemoglobin genotypes in newborns and adults. **CSFA**, controls; **F > A = C**, cord blood with Hb C trait; **S/C**, sickle cell Hb C disease with increased Hb F; **S/S** with small amounts of Hb A_2 and Hb F; **F > S** twice, cord blood with sickle cell anemia having small amount of Hb S and large amount of Hb F and faster-migrating N-acetyl Hb F; **CSFA**, control; **A/S**, adult sickle cell trait; **S/HOPE**, compound heterozygote with Hb HOPE migrating faster than Hb A; **F > A > G**, cord blood Hb G-Philadelphia trait (Note that the leftmost band is the F/G hybrid); **F > A > D**, cord with Hb D-Los Angeles trait; **A/C**, adult Hb C trait; **CSFA**, control. The band to the right of Hb A AcF is N-acetylated Hb F.

a specimen every 10 to 12 min and allows quantification of all of the major and minor components in a sample, including glycosylated hemoglobin for regulation of diabetes.

5. Micro–column chromatography with small commercially available disposable plastic columns measure Hbs A_2 and F.

6. Determination of the amino acid substitution by reverse-phase HPLC coupled with amino acid analysis or sequencing of tryptic peptides.

7. In many cases direct sequencing of the mutant gene is easier than globin structure determination.

8. Sickle cell solubility test detects only the presence of Hb S. It does not differentiate the various sickle genotypes. It is not recommended for most hemoglobin screening; CAE or IEF is preferable. Lipidemia may give a false-positive, anemia a false-negative test.

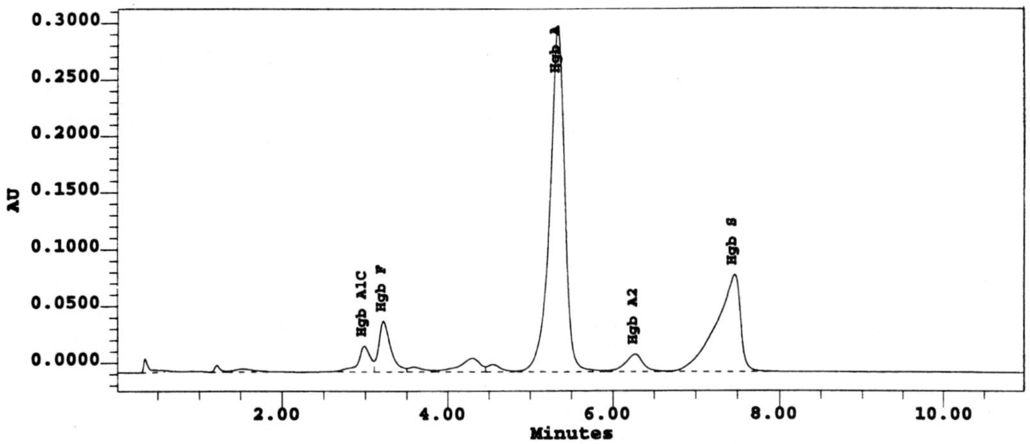

Figure 7 Cationic HPLC of the hemoglobin of a patient with sickle cell anemia who has received blood transfusions. The chromatographic resin, bonded to silica particles, is packed into steel tubes (Poly LC Co.), and the chromatographic solvent (the mobile phase) is pumped through under pressure between 1000 and 2000 lb/in^2. A wide variety of resins (stationary phases) for both anionic and cationic chromatography are commercially available. Mobility and resolution are controlled by buffer composition and slope of the gradient. Reverse-phase columns allow separation of the various globin chains present.

9. Heat stability test for Coomb's-negative hemolytic anemia. Heating a hemolysate of washed red cells in neutral phosphate buffer at 55°C or in isopropanol solution at 37°C will cause unstable hemoglobin variants to denature (precipitate). It may detect variants even in the absence of abnormal electrophoretic mobility.

V. SICKLE CELL HEMOGLOBIN

A. Definition

Hb S, $\alpha_2\beta^{6(A3)Glu\rightarrow Val}{}_2$, is due to the substitution in the β-globin gene of GTG for GAG in that codon. One in 12 African-Americans is a heterozygote. In 1 in 144 matings between two African-Americans, both partners have this trait. If both have it, the odds are 1 in 4 that each child will have homozygous sickle cell anemia. Thus, 1 in 600 newborns (or 0.0016) in this population have sickle cell anemia. Other compound heterozygous states are shown in Table 2.

Table 2 Classification of Sickle Cell Diseases in Order of Decreasing Severity Among African-Americans

Disease	Symbol	Severity	Frequency
Sickle cell anemia	S/S	++++	1 in 600
Sickle cell-β^0-thalassemia	S/β^0-thal	+++	1 in 25,000
Sickle cell-Hb D LA disease	S/D Los Angeles	+++	1 in 10^{-6}
Sickle cell-hemoglobin C ds	S/C	++	1 in 1250
Sickle cell- β^+-thalassemia	S/β^+ thal	+	1 in 3000

Physiology of Sickling

Deoxygenation of Hb S causes a number of changes in cell structure and physiology:

1. The deoxygenated conformation allows Hb S molecules to aggregate into long chains.
2. Fourteen parallel chains aggregate to form a microfibril.
3. Myriad microfibrils, packed into parallel arrays visible by electron microscopy, form a gel and stretch the sickle cell into its characteristic shape.
4. The internal viscosity of cells and bulk blood viscosity increase and deformability of the sickled cells decreases.
5. Water and potassium leak from the cell through the damaged membrane. Although sickling is reversible in young cells, the lost water and solute are not replaced when reoxygenation occurs.
6. As the cells age they become increasingly hyperchromic and dense, exceeding the density of the densest normal cells, and sickling becomes irreversible.
7. Young sickled cells adhere to postcapillary venular endothelium, perhaps mediated by adhesion molecules stimulated by infection or inflammation, thereby narrowing the lumen of venules.
8. Reversibly sickled cells and older, dense, irreversibly sickled cells adhere to each other, completing the process of occluding the narrowed venular lumena.

Many more details of this chain of events remain to be elucidated.

Studies of the physiology of sickling have been confounded by cellular heterogeneity. The increased amount of Hb F present in SCA is restricted to a subset of cells, called F-cells, each of which contains ⅓ Hb F and ⅔ Hb S. The remainder of the cells contain mostly Hb S. S-cells have survival times of 2 weeks and F-cells of 2 months.

B. Sickle Cell Trait

One in 12 (8.3%) of African-Americans is heterozygous for the gene for Hb S or has sickle cell trait. It should not be considered a disease. Inability to concentrate urine does not predispose to end-stage renal disease. An uncertain but small proportion of patients have hematuria that may be intermittent and self-limiting; it may frequently be chronic. Persons with sustained, significant hypoxia, say, from flight above 12,000 feet in planes with unpressurized cabins, may have splenic infarction. Since the advent of jet flight there have been no reports confirming this complication in the trait. Life expectancy is normal.

In a large study of military veterans the trait was found not to be associated with any of the common diseases or to shorten life expectancy. Approximately 30 military recruits per million with sickle cell trait have been shown to die during basic training in the United States Armed Forces versus 1 per million recruits without sickle trait. It has since been shown that these deaths can be prevented by closer attention to hydration during strenuous exercise. Isolated cases of infarction of bone in persons with sickle cell trait must be scrutinized carefully to assure that sickle cell-β^{+}-thalassemia has not been misdiagnosed as sickle cell trait.

VI. SICKLE CELL ANEMIA

A. Definition

SCA is the most severe of a group of clinically significant sickle cell diseases characterized by chronic hemolytic anemia punctuated by episodes of pain. In addition, acute and chronic organ damage contribute to morbidity and short life span. Although morbidity varies for each genotype, any of the complications can be equally severe for any genotype.

A collaborative prospective natural history study sponsored by the National Institutes of Health has documented a death rate for SCA of approximately 8% in the first two decades. A projected median life span for males is 42 years and for females 48 years. The projected life span for sickle cell-Hb C disease is normal.

B. Clinical Findings

The large amount of Hb F present in cord blood protects newborns with SCA. A pathognomonic sign of the disease is acute dactylitis in which fingers and toes and the dorsa of hands and feet become swollen, erythematous, hot, and exquisitely tender. The corresponding bones develop myriad osteolytic lesions and elevated periostea within a week. Infection in infancy is frequently the earliest manifestation of the disease. Administration of prophylactic penicillin twice each day from 4 months to 5 years of age has nearly eliminated fulminating, often fatal pneumococcemia.

1. Pain

Vaso-occlusion of bones is the principal cause of the pain in SCA. No bone is exempt. Whereas the average patient has two or three episodes per year requiring medical intervention, in the Natural History Study, one-third of children had no pain in 5 years. Pain may be mild or severe, transient or persistent for many days. (Although these are often referred to as sickle cell crises, many clinicians avoid this term in favor of the less emotionally charged vaso-occlusion.) If the vaso-occlusion is severe enough, frank bone infarction may occur; the hemoglobin concentration often falls to as low as 4 g/dL in a day or so; reticulocytosis and an increase in the number of nucleated RBCs suggest increased hemolysis. The platelet count may fall, perhaps being sequestered in areas of vaso-occlusion. Two life-threatening complications are stroke and acute chest syndrome.

2. Strokes

Cerebral vascular accidents may present either as transient ischemic attacks or as acute events and are most prevalent in SCA. Approximately 11% of patients experience strokes, primarily infarctive, by age 20. The cause in these is bilateral stenosis of lumina of the main branches of the internal carotid arteries due to deposition of fibrin, predictable by demonstration of increased blood flow using transcranial Doppler. Another 4% have hemorrhagic strokes between ages 20 and 29. Magnetic resonance imagery of asymptomatic children also show small infarcts and perfusion abnormalities in the watershed area. Their etiology and relationship to hemorrhagic stroke or to the stenosis of large vessels is unknown.

3. Acute Chest Syndrome

Children and adults with sickle cell diseases are prone to pulmonary complications referred to as the acute chest syndrome (ACS). An epidemiologic study has shown that new infiltrates occur in 12.8 per 100 patient-years. In young children the ACS was more apt to be due to infection and is seldom associated with pain. In older children and adults concomitant rib infarction, demonstrable by radionuclide bone scintigraphy in 50% of cases, is the primary event. Presumably the inflammation surrounding infarcts in ribs creates pleuritis, splinting, atelectasis, hypoxemia, and increased sickling. The clinical picture may rapidly proceed to adult respiratory distress syndrome or multiorgan failure. (See below for therapy.) The number of episodes of ACS determines life expectancy. Severe episodes of bone infarction may result in embolism of necrotic marrow into the lungs, brain, kidney, and other organs. It is difficult to recognize and is usually fatal.

Many other acute and chronic complications contribute to the morbidity of SCA. A partial list appears in Table 3.

C. Laboratory Findings and Diagnosis

The electrophoretic pattern contains primarily Hb S migrating midway between Hb A and Hb A_2. Increased amounts of Hb F are present, depending on the patient's age and sex. The Hb F present is heterogeneously distributed by the Kleihauer-Betke or cytoimmunofluorescent stains. F-cells containing ⅓ Hb F and ⅔ Hb S survive 2 months; the remaining S-cells contain predominantly Hb S and survive 2 weeks.

Additional hematologic and biochemical abnormalities are:

1. Anemia with hemoglobin concentrations between 7 and 9 g/dL
2. Reticulocyte counts vary between 5% and 30% but are not clinically useful unless the total hemoglobin falls much below baseline in which case they help to differentiate hyperhemolysis from aplasia
3. Sickle forms visible in peripheral blood films
4. Polychromatophilia
5. Hyperbilirubinemia, predominantly indirect acting
6. Elevated AST (SGOT) due to hemolysis; ALT (SGPT) is normal in the steady state
7. Elevated alkaline phosphatase concentrations to 150% of normal are common even in the steady state

The severity of SCA is inversely related to the concentration of Hb F present. The gene for Hb S has been found on five different haplotypes (Fig. 8), named for the regions of Africa or the Middle East and Asia where they are believed to have originated. Each haplotype has a different combination of 14 cleavage sites for 10 restriction endonucleases in the vicinity of the β-globin locus. Each haplotype, plus genetic modifiers on the X-chromosome, contributes additively to the proportion of Hb F with the Senegal and Indian contributing more than Benin, Bantu, and Cameroon. The restriction cleavage sites merely mark each chromosome. The genetic difference responsible for the variation in Hb F are unknown. Genes linked to the X-chromosome are responsible for higher Hb F levels in females than in males.

Table 3 Complications of Sickle Cell Diseases

Retinal hemorrhages
Hepatic sequestration
Acute cholecystitis or cholelithiasis
Splenic sequestration of red cells initiated by acute viral infection
Acute aplasia, associated with infection with parvovirus B-19 may be one of the few indications for bone marrow aspiration; it is also a life-threatening complication
Salmonella osteomyelitis
Hematuria with or without papillary necrosis
Avascular necrosis of the femoral or humeral heads
Chronic leg ulcers in adolescents and young adults

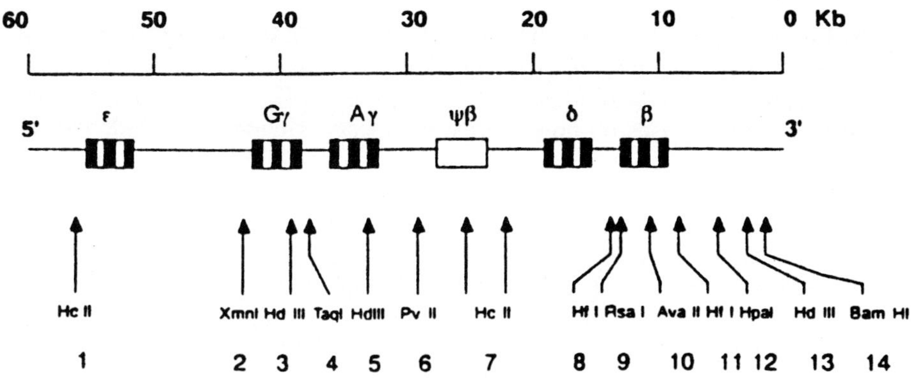

	1	2	3	4	5	6	7	8	9	10	11	12	13	14
Senegal	-	+	+	+	-	+	+ +	+	-	+	+	+	+	+
Benin	-	-	-	-	-	+	- +	-	-	+	+	-	-	+
Bantu	-	-	+	+	-	+	- -	-	+	+	+	+	+	+
Cameroon	-	-	+	+	+	+	- +	+	-	+	-	+	+	-
Indian	+	+	+	+	-	+	+ +	-	+	+	-	+	+	-

Figure 8 Restriction endonuclease polymorphisms in the β-globin cluster. Top, arrows point to the cleavage sites for each of the enzymes. Bottom, haplotypes defined by the patterns of cleavages typical of the regions where each haplotype is most prevalent. (From Nagel in Embury et al., 1994.)

Persons with predominant Hb S in the electrophoretic pattern plus an increased amount of Hb F without anemia or red cell morphologic abnormalities are most likely have sickle cell hereditary persistence of Hb F, defined further in the section on thalassemia.

D. Approaches to Therapy

The acute pneumococcal sepsis formerly common among infants and children to age 5 is preventable with administration of oral penicillin twice daily from 3 months to 5 years of age.

Pain management is essential to therapy. The frequency of emergency department usage and hospitalization are inversely proportionate to effectiveness of outpatient analgesia.

Stroke is treated with emergency red cell pheresis to 25% Hb S or below. The percentage of Hb S is then maintained between 25% and 40% with monthly transfusions of packed red cells. Iron overload is prevented by chelation five nights a week with desferioxamine administered by subcutaneous clysis via a portable battery-powered pump. In asymptomatic children stenosis of cerebral arteries is demonstrable by transcranial Doppler; prophylactic transfusion prevents 90% of clinical strokes.

Chest pain must be treated with aggressive analgesia combined with use of the incentive spirometer to prevent development of pulmonary infiltrates. Adult respiratory distress syndrome may develop if arterial oxygenation cannot be maintained with nasal oxygen; red cell pheresis and intubation may be necessary. Acute, unexpected circulatory collapse may indicate fat embolism syndrome. Emergency red cell pheresis, intubation, intravenous corticosteroids, and systemic support are indicated.

Hydroxyurea prophylaxis diminishes the severity of the disease 50% by increasing the concentration of Hb F; it may also interfere with sickle cell adhesion. The dose must be slowly titrated to optimal effect or to toxicity.

There is no consensus on how to treat leg ulcers. Treatments include topical antibiotics, Una's boots, transfusions until healed or until it is clear that they will not respond, and skin grafts.

Aplasia and sequestration are treated with transfusions. Sequestration tends to recur, so splenectomy may be required.

Hematuria is usually self-limiting. Therapy consists first of vigorous hydration and bed rest, administration of epsilon amino caproic acid, or retrograde instillation of silver nitrate into the renal pelvis.

VII. HEMOGLOBIN C GENOTYPES

A. Definition

Hemoglobin C Trait

Two percent of African-Americans are heterozygotes for the gene for Hb C—β6(A3)Glu → Lys. Hb C has +4 net charge and comigrates with Hb A_2. This genotype is totally asymptomatic. Peripheral blood is microcytic with large numbers of target cells. The electrophoretic pattern is composed of 60% Hb A and approximately 40% Hb C (minus the normal concentrations of Hb F and Hb A_2, of course). No therapy is indicated.

Sickle Cell Hemoglobin C Disease

Clinical Findings. The next most frequent of the clinically significant sickle cell syndromes affects 1 in 1250 African-Americans (Table 2). The average patient probably has a significant episode of pain every 3 or 4 years. Despite having lower morbidity, these patients may nevertheless have severe vaso-occlusive episodes. A majority of case reports of fatal fat embolism syndrome have been pregnant women with Hb SC. Retinopathy and avascular necrosis of the femoral head are more frequent in sickle cell hemoglobin C than in SCA. Although their red cells sickle at lower oxygen tensions than do those of SCA, presumably the higher ambient hematocrit elevates baseline arterial viscosity such that less sickling is required to increase blood viscosity above a threshold sufficient to embarrass perfusion. Splenomegaly may persist into adulthood, and splenic sequestration and aplasia occur although less frequently than in SCA. The Natural History Study projects a normal life expectancy.

B. Laboratory Findings and Diagnosis

The electrophoretic and HPLC patterns contain approximately 55% Hb S and 45% Hb C (Figs. 4–7); included in these percentages are a slightly increased proportion of Hb F and a normal concentration of Hb A_2. Additional hematologic and biochemical abnormalities are:

Total hemoglobin concentration among patients may vary from 10 to 14 g/dL.
Reticulocytosis: Red cell survival time is 60 days.
Few sickled forms in peripheral blood.
Large numbers of target cells.
Distinct intraerythrocytic crystals are present, especially if the cells are placed in hypertonic saline.
Nucleated red cells are present but fewer in numbers than in SCA.

Normal to slightly increased indirect bilirubin concentration.
Remaining liver function studies are normal.

1. Homozygous Hemoglobin C

Affecting one in 10,000 African-Americans, compensated hemolysis and splenomegaly in adulthood are common. Affected individuals are asymptomatic. Large numbers of target cells are present in peripheral blood. The red blood cells contain a normal amount of Hb A_2 and perhaps slightly increased Hb F; the remainder is Hb C. By the standard alkaline electrophoresis the Hb C comigrates with Hb A_2; the two are separable by HPLC, however. The hemoglobin phenotype for Hb C-β^o-thalassemia is identical with C/C except for a twice-normal concentration of Hb A_2 and higher percent Hb F in the former. HPLC will allow differentiation.

2. Sickle Cell Hemoglobins D

Any amino acid substitution in the β-globin chain in which an acidic amino acid is substituted by a neutral residue or a neutral by a basic will comigrate with Hb S at alkaline pH. Over 50 of these have been reported. Because of its clinically significant interaction with Hb S, the most important is Hb D Los Angeles β121(GH4)Glu → Gln, originally reported as Hb D Punjab.

C. Clinical Findings

Sickle cell hemoglobin D Los Angeles is approximately equivalent to sickle cell hemoglobin C disease in incidence of vaso-occlusion and other complications. Acute chest syndrome and chronic leg ulcers occur. Sickle cell hemoglobin D Iran is clinically very mild to asymptomatic.

D. Laboratory Findings and Diagnosis

The hemoglobin phenotype by alkaline electrophoresis (CAE) is identical to that of SCA (Fig. 5). By CAGE the hemoglobin D comigrates with Hb A (Fig. 5). Therefore, Hb D trait has the phenotype of A/A and sickle cell hemoglobin D appears like sickle cell trait. Every ostensibly S/S blood by CAE should have one CAGE to ascertain those that have Hb S/D. By HPLC the Hb D usually elutes differently from Hb S. Sickle cell Hb D Los Angeles is accompanied by somewhat lower hemoglobin concentrations than SCA, with values that can be as low as 6 g/dL.

1. Homozygous Hb D

Hemoglobin D Los Angeles, β121(GH4)Glu → Gln, being the fourth most common variant in the world (behind Hbs S, C, and E), has been found in the homozygous state, which is asymptomatic.

VIII. FUNCTIONALLY ABNORMAL HEMOGLOBINS

A. Unstable Hemoglobins

1. Definition

As noted above, the hemoglobin molecule is densely packed with an oily interior from which water is excluded. There are variants (Table 1) in which the substitution stearically stresses the molecule, allowing water into the interior causing the molecule to denature. A similar result is obtained when a substitution decreases the number of atomic bonds across the $\alpha_1\beta_1$ interface. The unstable molecules may precipitate in vivo in the red cell, resulting in a hemolytic anemia.

Clinical Findings

Anemia and associated symptoms that may be exacerbated by infections or oxidative stress, jaundice, and splenomegaly may be present.

Laboratory Findings and Diagnosis

Test	Result
Complete blood count	Variable hemoglobin level; peripheral
Morphology	Normochromia; polychromatophilia
Reticulocytes	Increased
Coombs test	Negative
Incubation with oxidative dye	Erythrocyte inclusions
Electrophoresis, HPLC	Variant with abnormal mobility may or may not be present
Heat denaturation test	Turbidity
Bilirubin	Increased indirect acting

A few variants are so unstable that little hemoglobin remains in the red cell. The prototype was Hb Indianapolis. The abnormal chains were identified by incubating reticulocytes with isotopically labeled amino acids and conducting the globin peptide mapping on the labeled globin chains and peptides isolated.

B. Hemoglobins M

1. *Definition*

Methemoglobinemia may be acquired or inherited. The latter may be due to defects in the methemoglobinemia reductase enzyme, more recently recognized to be cytochrome B-5 reductase. These defects are recessively inherited. Methemoglobinemia may also be due to a variant hemoglobin, in which case it may be inherited as an autosomal-dominant trait. One-third of variants are new mutations, however, so lack of affected parents does not prove recessive inheritance.

2. *Clinical Findings*

Cyanosis not associated with dyspnea or cardiovascular abnormalities is present from an early age. Blood gas analyses are normal with the exception of 10% to 30% methemoglobin.

3. *Laboratory Findings and Diagnosis*

Methemoglobin reacts with cyanide to form cyanmethemoglobin that migrates with Hb A by electrophoresis or HPLC. Therefore, to detect hemoglobins M (they migrate in proximity to Hb S) by these techniques, the buffers should not contain cyanide. Absorption spectra should be examined with a recording spectrophotometer with and without cyanide added; the met and cyanmet forms may have absorption spectra that differ from met and cyanmet Hb A.

Four different Hbs M are due to substitution of one of the four histidine residues in proximity to the heme iron by tyrosine (Table 1). Hb M-Milwaukee-1 β67(E11)Val $\rightarrow$ Glu also alters heme stability.

C. Variants with High Oxygen Affinity

1. *Definition*

Many variants that have increased oxygen affinity are due to amino acid substitutions on the $\alpha_1\beta_2$ interface that destabilize the hemoglobin tense tetramer configuration which forces the molecule into the high oxygen affinity state. The left shift of the oxyhemoglobin dissociation curve tends to decrease tissue oxygen concentration, thereby increasing erythropoietin production and erythropoiesis, resulting in hemoglobin concentrations as high as 20 g/dL. The first such variant reported was Hb Chesapeake α92(FG4)Arg → Leu. The interaction across the $\alpha_1\beta_2$ interface of Hbs Ypsilanti β99(G1)Asp → Tyr also results in the presence in the electrophoretic pattern of asymmetric heteropolymers—e.g., $\alpha_2\beta^{Ypsilanti}\beta^{A}$.

2. *Clinical Findings*

In polycythemia vera the number of red cells, concentration of hemoglobin, and platelet count are increased and the spleen may be enlarged. Variant hemoglobins with increased oxygen affinity cause only erythrocytosis. Symptoms leading to diagnosis are headache, plethora, or unusual thromboses.

3. *Laboratory Findings*

Test	Result
Complete blood count	Hemoglobin concentration in excess of 18 g/dL, normal WBC and platelet counts
Hemoglobin fractionation	Presence of variant hemoglobin makes the diagnosis
Arterial blood gas analysis	Normal pO_2; Low pO_2 implies secondary erythrocytosis
Oxygen dissociation curve	Measure this even if electrophoretic pattern is normal; P_{50} is <26 mm Hg.

Amino acid substitutions, such as Hb Kansasβ102(G4)Asn → Thr, may also decrease oxygen affinity resulting in normocytic anemia by the converse mechanism.

D. Alpha Chain Variants

1. *Definition*

Because there are two loci for α-globin chains on chromosome 16, variant chains produced by one of these loci are diluted out by a greater number of normal α-globin chains produced under the control of the three remaining α-globin alleles. Thus, in contrast to heterozygotes for β-chain variants that have 40% to 60% of abnormal hemoglobins, α-chain variants have only 15% to 30% abnormal hemoglobin. Also, because α-chains are shared by Hb F and Hb A_2, in heterozygotes for α-globin variants these components are duplicated, too. Since the α- and β-globin genes segregate independently, heterozygotes at both loci have hybrid tetramers. Thus, a heterozygote for the genes for Hb Gα Philadelphia and HbS will have a hybrid molecule, $\alpha^{G}{}_2\beta^{S}{}_2$, with a net charge of +4.

IX. THE THALASSEMIAS

In an older terminology the term *thalassemia major* referred to a severe disease with hemoglobin concentrations <6 g/dL; this is now known to be due to homozygosity for one of many different thalassemia genes. Thalassemia minor denotes the heterozygous state characterized by a mild microcytosis. In thalassemia intermedia, as the name implies, hemoglobin concentration ranges between 7 and 10 g/dL; it is most often the compound heterozygous state for either a structural variant and a thalassemia allele or for two different thalassemia genes. Rare cases with only subtle erythrocyte morphologic abnormalities but who are parents of a child with thalassemia major have been referred to as thalassemia minima, or silent carriers. Understanding the organization of the genes governing the synthesis of hemoglobin allows a genetic classification that connotes depression in the amount of specific globin chains present in cells.

The β-globin locus is in a complex operon (Figs. 3, 8) occupying approximately 100 kb of the short arm of chromosome 11; it consists of five structural loci encoding the epsilon, $^{G}\Gamma$, $^{A}\Gamma$ (differing only in glycine or alanine residues present at position 136), δ- and β-globin genes. As outlined above, these are expressed during ontogeny approximately in that order. The epsilon chains are synthesized in yolk sac cells. interspersed through the complex are 14 polymorphic restriction endonuclease cleavage sites (Fig. 8), where variation among individuals in cleavage sites is great. A given chromosome can be characterized by the combination of cleavage sites present—the haplotype.

On chromosome 16 another smaller complex (Fig. 3) contains the two alpha globin loci. At the 5′ end it also has a primitive zeta locus, also expressed only in embryonic yolk sac cells. Zeta chains combine with epsilon to form a primitive hemoglobin, Gower-1. Later in yolk sac cells and when erythropoiesis shifts to the other sites of hematopoiesis—the liver and then to the spleen and bone marrow—the α-globin genes are activated and remain so throughout life. Then, the α-chains combine with gamma chains, followed by the β- and lastly the δ-globin chains to form in sequence during development hemoglobins F, A, and A_2. The last has no known physiologic function. Hb A_2 does provide a useful marker for β-thalassemia, however.

An LCR at the 5′ end of the α- and β-complexes indicates tandem arrays of four sequences, each approximately 3 kb in size, each including a site hypersensitive to digestion with DNA-ase. Through a mechanism not yet understood, the LCR seems responsible for the progression during ontogeny of transcriptional activation from 5′ to 3′ of the β-complex. All of the globin structural genes possess two introns of comparable size. The first intron is 100 bases long and the second 900 bases in all of the loci; their locations differ slightly. A pseudo α-gene is not expressed.

A. β-Thalassemias

The molecular abnormality of over 100 thalassemic alleles of the β-locus have been defined. Most are the result of single-base-pair substitutions, analogous to those responsible for the structural variants. They cause virtually all of the genetic lesions known to exist (Fig. 9). They are subsumed in two generic categories: β^{o}- and β^{+}-thalassemia. The lesions of β^{o}-thalassemias are more severe, resulting in either no β-globin MRNA transcription or β-globin chains with such abnormal amino acid sequences that all chains produced by that allele are degraded immediately. The β^{+}-thalassemia mutations partially decrease the amount of β-chains present, but some remain. For instance, intron editing at the normal splice sites may be retarded by base-pair substitutions in canonical splice junction sequences; some splicing occurs normally, but is also forced into aberrant splice sites either in introns or in coding sequences, thereby producing β-globin chains with large insertions or deletions. These grossly deranged chains are very unstable and are rapidly degraded.

1. *Clinical Features.*

β-Thalassemia Trait: No clinical or hematological abnormalities differentiate heterozygous β^{+}- from β^{o}-thalassemia. Splenomegaly may be present, but seldom proceeds to hypersplenism. Marked depression of synthesis of one globin chain results in denaturation and pre-

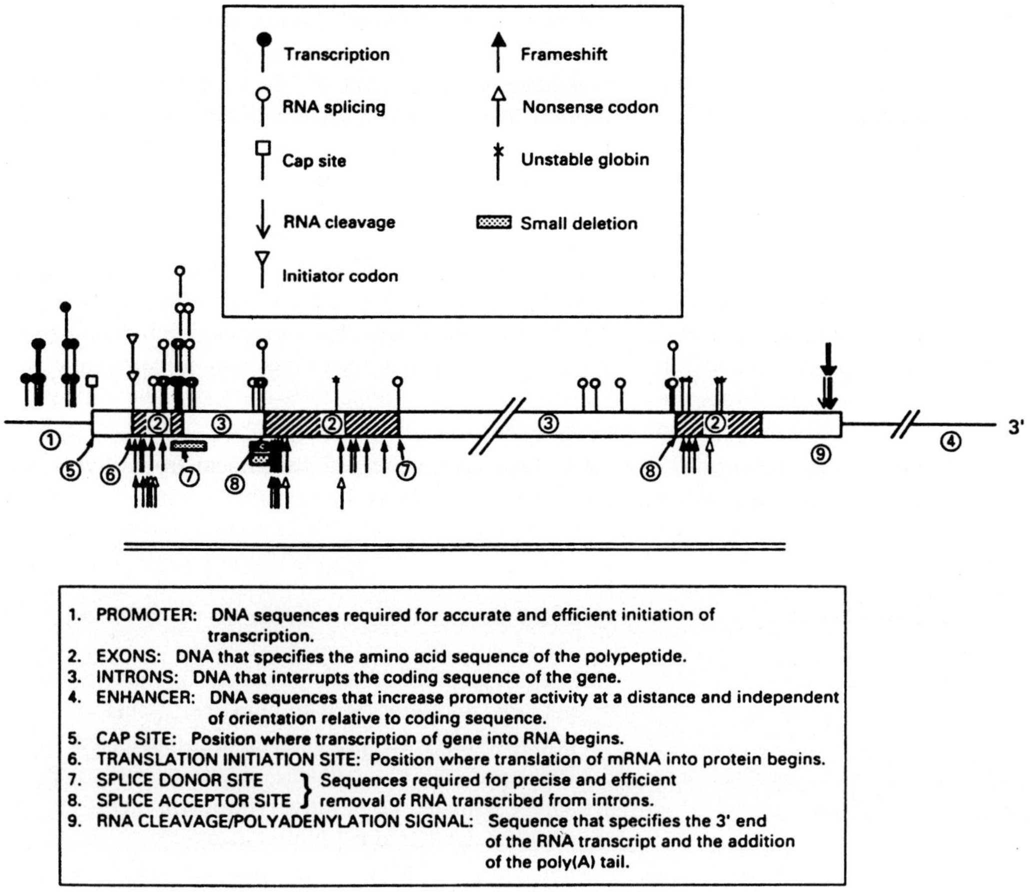

Figure 9 DNA base substitutions in and around the β-globin structural locus responsible for β-thalassemia, categorized according to the genetic mechanism causing the phenotype. (From McDonagh and Nienhuis, 1993.)

cipitation of the complementary chains, contributing to the morphologic abnormality and hemolysis.

Laboratory Features. Most often β-thalassemia trait must be differentiated from iron deficiency. If presumed iron deficiency does not respond to iron, thalassemia should be considered.

Test	Result
Complete blood count	Total hemoglobin concentration 2.5 g/dL below normal; MCV between 70 and 80 fL/cell
Peripheral morphology	Microcytosis, slight hypochromia, polychromatophilia
Reticulocytes	2–5%

Hemoglobin fractionation	Hb A_2 is twice the normal proportion: 4–6% vs. 2–3%; this is pathognomonic if falciparum malaria is not present
Fetal hemoglobin	May or may not be elevated to 5–6%
Globin synthesis	Largely replaced by DNA studies, but if done for special reasons, α/β ratio is 2:3

2. Homozygous β^o-Thalassemia

Newborns are not recognized as having homozygous β^o-thalassemia at birth because hemoglobin production is still under control of fetal programming. In the absence of transfusion, total hemoglobin concentration falls to <6 g/dL. Marked hepatosplenomegaly is evident. Intense erythroid hyperplasia expands the marrow cavity, causing bone deformity or pathologic fractures. Growth of facial bones may be disturbed, causing hypertelorism and malar fullness. In the absence of transfusions growth may be retarded.

Laboratory Findings and Diagnosis. The diagnosis is usually evident from physical examination and peripheral blood morphology.

Test	Result
Complete blood count	Marked anemia, MCV as low as 45 if not transfused
Peripheral morphology	Marked hypochromia and microcytosis, many target cells and large "potato chip" cells, anisopoikilocytosis, Howell Jolly bodies, nucleated RBCs
Inclusion body stain	If splenectomized large intraerythrocytic inclusions of denatured α-globin chains
Hemoglobin fractionation	If not transfused no Hb A, normal amount of Hb A_2, the remainder, Hb F

Homozygous β^+-Thalassemia

Clinical Findings. This is manifest as thalassemia intermedia.

Laboratory Finding and Diagnosis

Test	Result
Complete blood count	7–10 g/dL, MCV 50–70 fL/cell
Peripheral morphology	Marked hypochromia, microcytosis, anisopoikilocytosis but not as severe as in β^o-thalassemia
Hemoglobin fractionation	30–50% Hb F, 4–6% Hb A_2, the remainder Hb A

3. $\delta\beta$-Thalassemia

Clinical and Laboratory Findings. This is a milder form than β-thalassemia, in which globin chain synthesis is less unbalanced. The molecular basis is a deletion of DNA extending from the 5′ end of the δ-globin gene to 80 to 100 kb 3′ of the β-globin gene. Presumably the deletion leaves intact suppressors of Γ-globin expression between the Γ- and δ-globin genes that prevent total compensation of Hb F for the loss of β-globin genes. Heterozygotes have lower than normal percentages of Hb A_2 and 8% to 10% Hb F. Homozygotes have thalassemia intermedia and 100% Hb F.

4. *Hereditary Persistence of Fetal Hemoglobin (HPFH)*

In nonthalassemic HPFH the proportion of Hb F does not fall to normal levels after birth but, rather, levels off at an elevated level that is characteristic for that gene—between 25% and 35% Hb F in the classical HPFH. Globin synthesis is balanced; that is, $\alpha/\beta + \Gamma = 1$. The red cell morphology is normal or nearly so.

Whereas the increased amount of Hb F present in most of the hemoglobinopathies is concentrated in a small subset of red cells (heterocellularly distributed), in classical HPFH each red cell contains the same proportion of Hb F (pancellular distribution). The molecular basis for this impairment of the Hb F switch are deletions, each approximately 100 kb in size but with different breakpoints. The red cell survival time of compound heterozygotes for one of these and the sickle cell gene—sickle cell HPFH—is normal because the dilution of the Hb S in every cell with Hb F diminishes sicklability. In heterocellular HPFH the proportion of Hb F is smaller, the distribution is heterocellular, and the molecular basis is base pair substitutions 5′ to either of the Γ-loci. These inhibit suppressors of Γ-globin gene transcription.

5. *Therapy of the Thalassemias*

Stem cell transfusion is the only definitive cure for thalassemia. In the absence of a matched sibling donor one is left with lifelong transfusions or, more recently, hydroxyurea therapy. The hemoglobin concentration determines whether a regular transfusion program is needed. Maintaining the hemoglobin concentration around 10 g/dL assures normal growth and development. Monthly transfusions equivalent to 2 units of packed red cells in adults causes transfusion hemochromatosis and death in early adulthood. Chelation with desferioxamine for five to seven nights per week, as described above for sickle cell stroke, maintains normal iron balance. Hydroxyurea therapy increases Hb F, as described above for sickle cell anemia, offering an alternative to transfusion.

B. α-Thalassemias

1. *Clinical Findings*

In contrast to the β-thalassemias, most of the family of α-thalassemias are due to deletions of varying numbers of the four α-globin genes (two loci) on chromosome 16 (Fig. 10). The RBC morphology of the heterozygotes is less pronounced than for the β-thalassemias. Hb H is a tetramer of four β-globin chains (β_4), with normal structure. Diagnosis can be made more

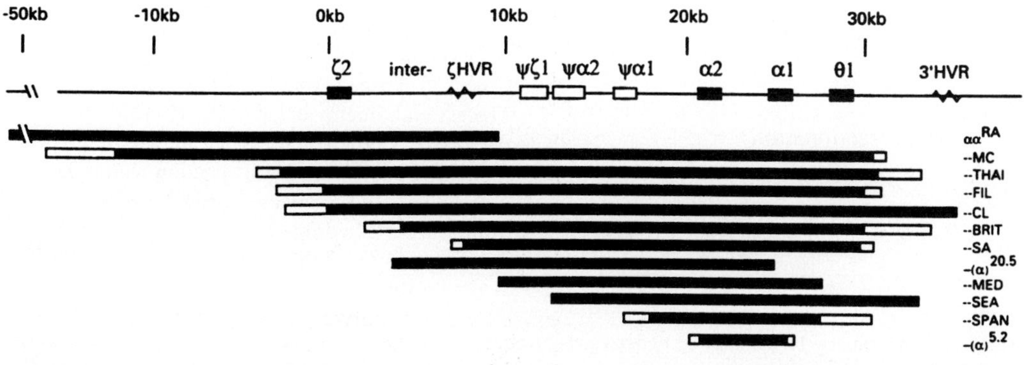

Figure 10 Deletions causing α-thalassemia. The cross-hatched bars denote regions where the precise endpoints of the deletions have not been determined. (From McDonagh and Nienhuis, 1993.)

easily at birth on the basis of the proportion of Hb Bart's (Γ_4) in cord blood. African-Americans have only the α-thalassemia-2 haplotype. Approximately 25% are heterozygotes (–α/αα) and 1.5% are homozygotes (–α/–α). See Table 4.

2. *Laboratory Findings and Diagnosis*

Two different deletions account for the α-thalassemia-2 haplotype or "gene"; the deletion for one 3.7 kb in length is located more 5′ (leftward deletion) to the other 4.2 kb (right). Several different deletions, each approximately 100 kb in size, are responsible for the α-thalassemia-1 haplotype.

3. *Irregular α-Thalassemias*

Children with Hb H disease have been described, one of whose parents has the α-thalassemia-1 deletion; the other parent lacks a deletion. The latter are examples of α^+-thalassemia in which the lesion is a base-pair substitution.

Hb H disease with severe mental retardation has been described. Two forms exist—deletion and nondeletion. The former have large deletions of chromosome 16p13.3 that presumably includes linked loci responsible for the retardation. Another form with intact α-globin genes and genital abnormalities is due to sex-linked mutations. The mutant gene presumably has an epistatic effect on α-globin regulation. An α-thalassemia, including presence of Hb H, has been reported in association with leukemia or preleukemic myelodysplastic syndromes.

Hemoglobin Constant Spring, first detected in a Jamaican family of Chinese origin, is widely distributed in Southeast Asia. It is due to a base-pair substitution in an α-globin gene, changing the chain terminator codon to that for glycine. Another 30 amino acid residues are translated at the carboxyl terminus of the α-chain until another in-frame chain terminator interrupts it. A similar variant is Hb Knosis.

Table 4 Laboratory Findings and Diagnosis

Name	Genotype	% Hb Bart's at birth	Adult phenotype
α-Thalassemia-1[a]	— —/α α[b]	4–10%	Low normal total hemoglobin, MCV 65–75 fL/cell, low Hb A_2. This genotype is uncommon in African-Americans.
α-Thalassemia-2	— α/α α	0–3.5	Normal Hb concentration, nearly normal RBC morphology, normal Hb A_2. Twenty-five percent of African-Americans have this genotype.
Hb H disease	— α/— —	30	Thalassemia intermedia, 5–15% Hb H, 0–10% Hb Bart's, low Hb A_2. Small intraerythrocytic inclusions visible after incubation with oxidative dyes tend to adhere to RBC membranes.
Bart's-Hydrops	— —/— —	100	Stillborn, with hydrops fetalis, severe erythroblastic anemia, marked hepatosplenomegaly, 100% Hb Bart's.

[a]This phenotype can also be obtained by homozygosity for the α-thalassemia-2 haplotype (—α/—α); 1.5% of African-Americans are affected.
[b]—Denotes deletion of one of the α-globin gene alleles. The symbols on either side of the slash denote the haplotype of homologous chromosomes.

X. PRENATAL DIAGNOSIS

The development of the polymerase chain reaction has revolutionized prenatal diagnosis. Most of the clinically significant hemoglobinopathies are prenatally diagnosable in this manner, such as Hbs S, C, E, and D Los Angeles.

A second approach is to employ oligonucleotide hybridization whereby relevant regions of globin DNA are amplified and DNA dots applied to paper are hybridized with 20-mer oligonucleotides containing either the normal or the mutant base in the sequence and end-labeled with ^{32}P or a chemical detector. Hybridization conditions are such that the amplification product with the normal sequence will hybridize with the normal but not the abnormal nucleotide, or, conversely, the abnormal amplification product will hybridize with the abnormal but not the normal oligonucleotide. This approach requires that the precise base substitution of the variant in question be known.

The structural variants of hemoglobin and the thalassemias are amenable to this approach. However, the base substitutions of over 100 different β-thalassemias have been determined. One must have a set of oligonucleotides for each mutant allele for which the patient is at risk. The process can be simplified inasmuch as each population in which thalassemia is prevalent has only approximately six different thalassemia mutants. Reverse dot blotting allows testing all of the variants known to be present in a population or race by only one amplification and hybridization. This is done by fixing oligonucleotide dots for all of the variants and the normal complementary sequence to one membrane. The DNA of the patient is then nick-translated, end-labeled, and hybridized with all of the oligonucleotide simultaneously.

Thalassemias due to deletions, such as α-thalassemia, are diagnosed by either Southern blots or amplifications in which amplification spans the deletion and variants are detected by size fractionation.

XI. SELECTED READINGS

Bellet PS, Kalinyak KA, Shukla R, Gelfand MJ, Rucknagel DL (1995). Incentive spirometry to prevent acute pulmonary complications in sickle cell diseases. N Engl J Med 333:799–703.

Blau CA, Stamatoyannoppulous G (1994). Regulation of fetal hemoglobin. In: Embury SH, Hebbel RP, Mohandas N, Steinberg MH, eds. Sickle Cell Disease. Basic Principles and Clinical Practice. New York: Raven Press, pp. 247–277.

Bunn HF, Forget BG (1986). Hemoglobin: Molecular, Genetic and Clinical Aspects. Philadelphia: W.B. Saunders Co.

Bunn HF (1993). Human hemoglobins: normal and abnormal; methemoglobinemia. In: Nathan DG, Oski FA, eds. Hematology of Infancy and Childhood. Philadelphia: W.B. Saunders Co., pp. 698–731.

Bunn HF (1997). Pathogenesis and treatment of sickle cell disease. N Engl J Med 337:762–769.

Castro O (1996). Systemic fat embolism and pulmonary hypertension in sickle cell disease. Hematol Oncol Clin North Am 10:1289–1303.

Castro O, Brambilla DJ, Thorington B, et al. (1994). The acute chest syndrome in sickle cell disease: incidence and risk factors. Blood 84:643–649.

Chui DHK, Hardison R, Riemer C, et al. (1998). An electronic database of human hemoglobin variants in the World Wide Web. Blood 91:2643–2644.

Dean J, Schechter AN (1978). Sickle cell anemia: molecular and cellular basis of therapeutic approaches. N Engl J Med 299:752–763; 804–811; 863–870.

Embury SH, Hebbel RP, Mohandas N, Steinberg MH (1994). Sickle Cell Disease. Basic Principles and Clinical Practice. New York: Raven Press.

Huisman THJ, Carver MFH, Efremov GD (1996). A Syllabus of Human Hemoglobin Variants. Augusta, GA: Sickle Cell Foundation.

Kark JA, Posey DM, Schumacher HR, Ruehle CJ (1987). Sickle-cell trait as a risk factor for sudden death in physical training. N Engl J Med 317:781–787.
Lucarelli G, Galimberti M, et al. (1990). Bone marrow transplantation in patients with thalassemia. N Engl J Med 322:419–421.
Mc Donagh KT, Nienhuis AW (1993). The thalassemias. In: Nathan DG, Oski FA, eds. Hematology of Infancy and Childhood. Philadelphia: W.B. Saunders Co., pp. 783–879.
Nagel RL (1994). Origin and dispersion of the sickle cell gene. In: Embury SH, Hebbel RP, Mohandas N, Steinberg MH, eds. Sickle Cell Disease. Basic Principles and Clinical Practice. New York: Raven Press, pp. 353–380.
Platt OS, Dover GJ (1993). Sickle cell disease. In: Nathan DG, Oski FA, eds. Hematology of Infancy and Childhood. Philadelphia: W.B. Saunders Co., pp. 732–782.
Ou C-N, Rognerud CL (1993). Rapid analysis of hemoglobin variants by cation-exchange HPLC. Clin Chem 39:820–824.
Platt OS, Brambilla DJ, et al. (1994). Mortality in sickle cell disease. Life expectancy and risk factors for early death. N Engl J Med 330:1639–1644.
Platt OS, Thorington BD, et al. (1991). Pain in sickle cell disease. Rates and risk factors. N Engl J Med 325:11–16.
Powars D, Weidman JA, Odom-Maryon T, Niland JC, Johnson C (1988). Sickle cell chronic lung disease: prior morbidity and the risk of pulmonary failure. Medicine 67:66–76.
Righetti PG, Gianazza E, Bianchi-Bosisio A, Cossu G (1986). Conventional isoelectric focusing and immobilized pH gradients for hemoglobin separation and identification. In: Huisman THJ, ed. The Hemoglobinopathies. Edinburgh: Churchill Livinigstone, pp. 47–71.
Sutcharitchan P, Embury SH (1996). Advances in molecular diagnosis of inherited hemoglobin disorders. Curr Opin Hematol 3:131–138.
Vichinski EP, Styles LA, Colangelo LH, et al. (1997). Acute chest syndrome in sickle cell disease: clinical presentation and course. Blood 89:1787–1792.
Walters MC, Patience P, et al. (1996). Bone marrow transplantation for sickle cell disease. N Engl J Med 335:369–376.
Weatherall DJ (1997). The thalassaemias. BMJ 314:1675–1678.

CASE 1

Patient: 54-year-old African-American male.

Chief Complaint: Left hip pain of 10 years' duration, worse in the past 6 months.

Past Medical History: The patient has been in good health generally with no hospitalizations for vaso-occlusive pain. He had a cataract in the left eye that he attributed to a fall on the job 15 years ago. He overturned a fork lift 10 years ago, following which he had low back and left hip pain necessitating retirement on disability. The pain has been worse for the past 6 months. His primary care physician told him that it was due to his sickle cell trait.

Medications: Ibuprofen, generally once or twice a day.

Review of Systems: Noncontributory.

Physical Examination: African-American male using a cane: his appearance was compatible with his age. The fundus O.S. was not well visualized because of a lenticular opacity. An area of chorioretinitis was evident in the temporal quadrant O.D. The spleen was not palpable but Traub's sign was positive. Full range of motion was present upon flexion and extension of both hips. Internal rotation of the left femur was limited and painful. Rectal examination was negative.

Laboratory Results

	Patient	Normal
Hemoglobin	12.0 g/dL	13.5–17 g/dL
Hematocrit	37.3%	41–47%
Mean cell volume	83.8 fL/cell	82–94 fL/cell
Mean cell hemoglobin	26.9 pg/cell	28–32
RDW	18.7	11–12
Peripheral morphology	Anisopoikilocytosis, increased target cells	
Reticulocytes	5.9%	<1%

Questions

1. Does he have a hemoglobinopathy?
2. Does he have avascular necrosis of the femoral head?
3. Does he have treatable sea fan lesions of the fundi? Is the lenticular opacity due to sickling?

Further Laboratory Tests: Hemoglobin fractionation by HPLC: hemoglobin S, 48.4%; Hb C, 44.5%; Hb F, 3.8%; Hb A_2, 3.3%.

X-Rays: The lumbar spine and pelvis were normal: early avascular necrosis of the left femoral head was present.

Diagnosis: (1) Sickle cell hemoglobin C disease; (2) avascular necrosis of the left femoral head; (3) sickle cell retinopathy.

Discussion: Persons alleged to have sickle cell trait who also have bone and joint pain should be assumed to have sickle cell Hb C disease or sickle cell β^+-thalassemia until proven otherwise. The increased number of target cells in peripheral blood and the retina lesion strongly suggested the former. It is unlikely that the trauma caused the avascular necrosis; it is more likely that the avascular process may have caused the fall. The same may be true of the retinal lesion.

CASE 2

Patient: A 3-month-old infant, both of whose parents were Vietnamese.

Chief Complaint: Patient was referred for evaluation because an abnormal hemoglobin of unknown type was detected by the State/s newborn screening program.

Past Medical History: Irrelevant.

Review of Systems and Family History: No one in the family was known to be anemic.

Physical Examination: Birth weight after normal gestation was 2.7 kg. Subsequent growth has been normal. Liver and spleen were not palpable.

Laboratory Results

	Patient	Normal (child)	Father	Mother
Hemoglobin (g/dL)	8.8	9.5–13.5	14.2	11.8
Hematocrit (%)	26.6%	29–41	42.6	37.9
MCV (fL/cell)	51.8	74–108	82.8	71.1
MCH (pg/cell)	17	25–35	27.5	22.2
Reticulocytes (%)	3.7%	0.5–1.5	1.0	0.5
RDW	19.6	11–14.5	13.6	13.9
Peripheral morphology				
Hypochromia	3+	—	—	2+
Microcytosis	3+	—	—	2+
Polychrom.	2+	—	—	—
Target cells	1+	—	—	—
Schistocytes	1+	—	—	—
Ovalocytes	Occ.	—	—	Occ.
Teardrops	Occ.	—	—	—
Inclusions	1+	—	—	Occ.
Hemoglobin fractionation				
Hb Bart's (%)	10.1	—	—	—
Hb F (%)	10.6		1.1	1.0
Hb A_2 (%)	0.9		2.7	2.4
Hb A (%)	78.4		96.2	96.6

Discussion: A newborn with 10% Hb Bart's would be presumed to have α-thalassemia-1. At birth this child probably had 20% to 30% Hb Bart's, however, and 50% Hb F. The child's hemoglobin phenotype plus the degree of red cell morphologic abnormality and anemia allows a diagnosis of Hb H disease. This is compatible with the parent's phenotype. The mother has unequivocal microcytosis and a low-normal Hb A_2, consistent with α-thalassemia-1. The father's blood was borderline microcytosis, compatible with α-thalassemia-2.

This interpretation should be confirmed by polymerase chain reaction if the parents desire prenatal diagnosis for subsequent pregnancies.

18

Hemolytic Anemias: General Considerations

Robert T. Means, Jr.
Medical University of South Carolina and R. H. Johnson VA Medical Center, Charleston, South Carolina

I. DEFINITION

Hemolytic anemias are defined as those anemias which develop as a result of increased red cell destruction. Bone marrow production of red cells is typically preserved (or actually increased) in these disorders: Anemia develops as a consequence of postproduction events undergone by the erythrocyte. For this reason, hemolysis is typically identified by the combination of (a) evidence of red cell destruction and (b) evidence of adequate or increased red cell production.

II. CLASSIFICATION

A variety of classification schema have been proposed for the hemolytic anemias, based on whether the syndrome is inherited or acquired (Table 1), on the site of hemolysis (Table 2), or on the site of the defect resulting in hemolysis (Table 3). All of the schema described have particular advantages and their advocates; this author favors the system outlined in Table 3 because of the ease with which it is remembered by trainees, and because it provides a more physiologic approach to the diagnosis. However, classification as inherited or acquired (Table 1) is often more easy to perform clinically; and classification by site of hemolysis has significant implications for diagnostic test results (Table 2) (1).

III. CLINICAL FEATURES

The clinical features observed in patients with hemolytic anemia vary according to the defect producing the anemia and the individual circumstances of the patient at a particular point in time (2,3). For example, a patient with typical glucose-6-phosphate dehydrogenase (G-6-PD) deficiency will not be anemic at baseline, but will rapidly develop anemia after exposure to an oxidant drug (4,5). In contrast, a patient with hereditary spherocytosis will frequently exhibit a modest anemia with compensatory reticulocytosis at all times. Following an illness, however, this mild chronic anemia may undergo an acute exacerbation.

General clinical features common to a variety of the hemolytic anemias include the following:

Table 1 Classification of Hemolytic Anemias as Hereditary or Acquired

Hereditary hemolytic anemias
Hemoglobinopathies
Thalassemias
Enzyme deficiencies (such as glucose-6-phosphate dehydrogenase or pyruvate kinase deficiency)
Membrane defects (such as hereditary spherocytosis, hereditary elliptocytosis, etc.)
Acquired hemolytic anemias
Immune hemolytic anemias (autoimmune, alloimmune, drug-induced autoimmune)
Microangiopathic hemolytic anemia (thrombotic thrombocytopenic purpura, disseminated intravascular coagulation, tumor- or chemotherapy-related)
Other mechanical hemolysis (prosthetic heart valve, renovascular hypertension, thermal injury)
Direct toxic effects (clostridial sepsis, malaria, envenomation)
Acquired membrane defects (spur cell anemia, Zieve's syndromem)
Paroxysmal nocturnal hemoglobinuria

1. *Anemia*. As discussed above, this may be chronic, acute, or chronic with acute exacerbations. The degree of anemia may vary from minimal to severe.
2. *Jaundice*. The breakdown of hemoglobin released from hemolyzed red cells results in increased bilirubin production. The degree of jaundice will vary much like the degree of anemia. Mild chronic hemolysis will rarely result in jaundice perceptible on physical examination, while acute hemolysis or acute exacerbations of chronic hemolysis will often result in clinically apparent jaundice.
3. *Splenomegaly*. Some degree of splenomegaly is commonly observed in patients with disorders characterized by hemolysis which is predominantly extravascular (the most common effective meaning of extravascular hemolysis is "in the spleen"; Table 2). The size of the spleen is not predicted by the severity of hemolysis (6), but rather by its chronicity. Splenomegaly is not observed in adult patients with sickle cell syndromes other than sickle hemoglobin C disease or sickle β-thalassemia (7).

Table 2 Classification of Hemolytic Anemias by Site of Hemolysis

Intravascular hemolysis
Microangiopathic hemolytic anemia (thrombotic thrombocytopenic purpura, disseminated intravascular coagulation, tumor or chemotherapy related)
Other mechanical hemolysis (prosthetic heart valve, renovascular hypertension, thermal injury)
Direct toxic effects (clostridial sepsis, malaria, envenomation)
Paraoxysmal nocturnal hemoglobinuria
Hemolytic transfusion reactions
Paroxysmal cold hemoglobinuria
Enzyme deficiencies (such as glucose-6-phosphate dehydrogenase or pyruvate kinase deficiency)
Extravascular hemolysis
Immune hemolytic anemias (other than hemolytic transfusion reaction, paroxysmal cold hemoglobinuria)
Acquired membrane defects (spur cell anemia, Zieve's syndrome)
Hemoglobinopathies
Thalassemias
Hereditary membrane defects (such as hereditary spherocytosis, hereditary elliptocytosis, etc.)

Table 3 Classification of Hemolytic Anemias by Defect Leading to Hemolysis

Defects intrinsic to red cells
Internal/cytoplasmic defects
Hemoglobinopathies
Thalassemias
Enzyme deficiencies (such as glucose-6-phosphate dehydrogenase or pyruvate kinase deficiency)
Membrane defects
Acquired membrane defects (spur cell anemia, Zieve's syndrome)
Hereditary membrane defects (such as hereditary spherocytosis, hereditary elliptocytosis, etc.)
Paroxysmal nocturnal hemoglobinuria
Defects extrinsic to red cells
Immune hemolytic anemias (autoimmune, alloimmune, drug-induced autoimmune)
Microangiopathic hemolytic anemia (thrombotic thrombocytopenic purpura, disseminated intravascular coagulation, tumor or chemotherapy related)
Other mechanical hemolysis (prosthetic heart valve, renovascular hypertension, thermal injury)
Direct toxic effects (clostridial sepsis, malaria, envenomation)

4. *Gallstones.* Bilirubin gallstones are commonly observed in patients with congenital hemolytic anemias.
5. *Bilirubinuria/hemoglobinuria.* Abnormalities of urine pigmentation are frequently observed in hemolytic anemias (discussed in detail below).

Acute episodes of massive intravascular hemolysis (as would be observed following transfusion of ABO-incompatible blood, certain delayed hemolytic transfusion reactions, or clostridial hemolysis) are fortunately uncommon. Clinical findings which could be observed under these circumstances include:

1. Fever, rigors
2. Evidence of systemic hypoperfusion—tachycardia, hypotension, altered sensorium, oliguria
3. Flank or abdominal pain
4. Hemoglobinuria

There are also a number of clinical findings which are characteristic of specific etiologies of hemolysis, such as leg ulcers in sickle cell syndromes, bony abnormalities in the hemoglobinopathies and thalassemias, thrombotic events in paroxysmal nocturnal hemoglobinuria, etc., which are discussed in other chapters.

IV. LABORATORY FEATURES

In this section, the common laboratory features of hemolytic anemias are reviewed. Specific laboratory studies, such as hexose monophosphate shunt enzyme assays, osmotic fragility, sucrose lysis tests, the Coombs test, etc., will be reviewed in the appropriate individual sections.

1. *Anemia.* As noted above, the degree of anemia can range from minimal to severe.
2. *Red cell indices.* Most hemolytic anemias are characterized by a normal or slightly elevated erythrocyte mean corpuscular volume (MCV). The slight elevation usually reflects

reticulocytosis. In contrast, hemoglobinopathies and thalassemias characteristically exhibit microcytosis, but can be distinguished from iron-deficient erythrocytes by a normal or near-normal mean corpuscular hemoglobin concentration (MCHC). Occasionally, patients with chronic intravascular hemolysis develop iron deficiency as a result of urinary hemoglobin loss.

3. *Red cell morphology.* A variety of morphologic abnormalities of red cells—schistocytes, spherocytes, elliptocytes, "blister" cells, etc.—may be helpful in the identification of specific syndromes, and will be reviewed in the appropriate sections.

4. *Reticulocytosis.* There are several ways to utilize the reticulocyte count (typically expressed as the percentage of red cells which are reticulocytes) to evaluate red cell production by the marrow. The reticulocyte count may be expressed as an uncorrected percentage, or as the absolute reticulocyte count (percent reticulocytes multiplied by the red cell count per cubic millimeter), or as the corrected reticulocyte count (percent reticulocytes multiplied by patient's hematocrit/45), or as the reticulocyte production index (corrected reticulocyte count multiplied by a factor which reflects the increased shift of less mature cells to the peripheral blood) (8). All of these modifications are efforts to remind the clinician that a reticulocyte count of 1%, which is perfectly adequate to maintain a hematocrit of 45%, is too low if the patient's hematocrit is 25% (see Table 4 for normal values of reticulocyte evaluations). An elevated reticulocyte count is considered a hallmark of hemolytic anemia. However, as many as 37% of patients with autoimmune hemolytic anemia can present with reticulocytopenia (as defined by a reticulocyte production index <2%), and it is important to remember that absence of reticulocytosis does not rule out a hemolytic anemia (9,10). Individuals with mild chronic hemolysis (particularly patients with hemoglobinopathies or thalassemia) often have a relatively normal hemoglobin concentration and hematocrit but have an elevated reticulocyte count: The shortened red cell survival requires extra marrow production in order to maintain a near-normal hematocrit/hemoglobin. The phenomenon of transient aplastic crises in chronic hemolysis due to B19 parvovirus infection will be discussed elsewhere.

5. *Serum bilirubin.* When hemoglobin is released from the erythrocyte, the porphyrin ring of the heme moiety is metabolized to biliverdin, which in turn is converted to bilirubin in the reticuloendothelial system. This bilirubin circulates bound to albumin, and is described as unconjugated or indirect bilirubin (see Fig. 1). Typically, >85% of serum bilirubin in hemolytic anemia is indirect; however, when the total bilirubin is >5 mg/dL or significant hepatic disease is present, direct-reacting (conjugated) bilirubin becomes a major component (11).

6. *Bilirubinuria/hemoglobinuria.* During intravascular hemolysis, hemoglobin released from lysed erythrocytes becomes bound to haptoglobin and is metabolized in the reticuloendothelial system. The quantity of haptoglobin available for this function is limited, and free hemoglobin that is not bound to haptoglobin is excreted by the kidneys. The jaundice associated with hemolysis is typically "acholuric"; i.e., because the increase in serum bilirubin is

Table 4 Normal Reticulocyte Values

Reticulocyte count (uncorrected)	0.5–2.0%
Absolute reticulocyte count	25,000–75,000/mm^3
Corrected reticulocyte count	0.5–1.5%
Reticulocyte production index	≥3.0
Adequate response to anemia	
Inadequate response to anemia	≤2.0

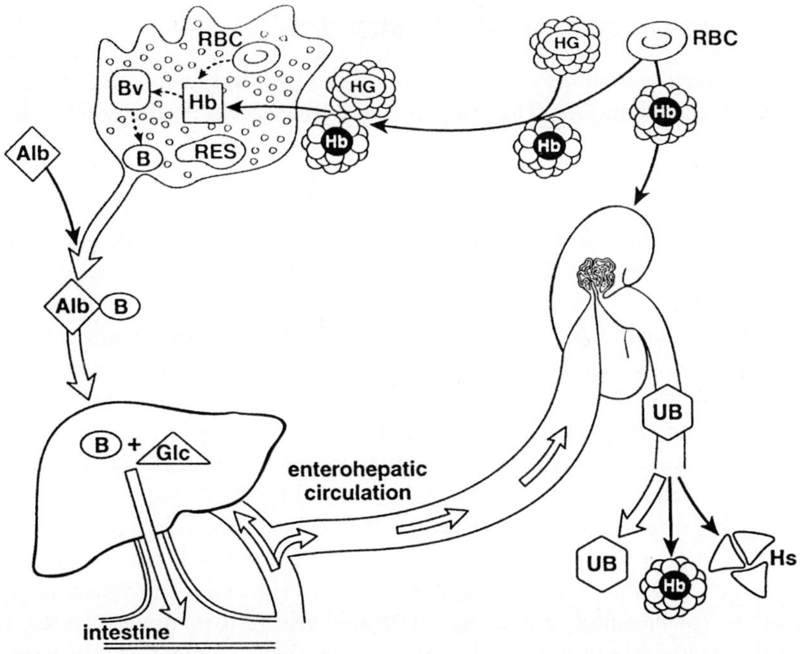

Figure 1 Metabolism of bilirubin released from lysed erythrocytes. The pathway for intravascular hemolysis is represented by a solid line, for extravascular hemolysis by a dashed line, and common metabolite pathways by a double line. Alb, albumen; B, bilirubin; Bv, biliverdin; Glc, glucuronide; Hb, hemoglobin; HG, haptoglobin; Hs, hemosiderin; RBC, red blood cell; RES, reticuloendothelial system; UB, urobilinogen.

primarily in the unconjugated (indirect) fraction, urinary bilirubin products are almost entirely in the form of urobilinogen (see Fig. 1).

7. *Serum lactate dehydrogenase* (LDH). LDH is elevated in hemolysis. The LDH-2 isoenzyme is the major contributor to this elevation. The normal extent of elevation is two to three times the upper limit of normal; microangiopathic hemolysis in thrombotic thrombocytopenic purpura may be associated with LDH levels 10-fold higher than the upper limit of normal.

8. *Serum haptoglobin*. The normal function of haptoglobin is to form a complex with free hemoglobin, and remove it to the reticuloendothelial system for metabolism. The quantity of haptoglobin present in blood is barely adequate to perform this function under normal conditions. During hemolysis, haptoglobin is rapidly consumed, and significantly reduced levels are detected (see Fig. 1). It is often said that haptoglobin is primarily a marker of intravascular hemolysis, but in fact it is a highly sensitive indicator of hemolysis in general. The positive predictive value of a low serum haptoglobin for predicting hemolysis is 87%; the negative predictive value (the likelihood that a patient with normal or elevated haptoglobin is not undergoing hemolysis) is 95% (12).

9. *Plasma hemoglobin/urine hemoglobin*. In intravascular hemolysis, after the collecting capacity of haptoglobin is exceeded, free hemoglobin is present in the plasma, and may also be excreted by the kidney.

V. APPROACH TO THE DIAGNOSIS OF HEMOLYSIS

The diagnosis of hemolytic anemia requires demonstration of red cell destruction and identification of a specific etiology for hemolysis. The latter task is addressed in the individual sections which follow.

Hemolysis is suspected when a decrease in hemoglobin or hematocrit occurs which is too rapid to be explained by marrow suppression only or when anemia occurs with reticulocytosis. In a person beginning with a baseline hemoglobin of ≥13 g/dL and a hematocrit of 40%, this means a decrease in hemoglobin >0.9 g/dL/week or >3 hematocrit percentage points/week. The differential diagnosis is hemolysis, bleeding, or hemodilution. Anemia with jaundice or with gallstones in a young person should also lead to a suspicion of hemolysis. Since some patients with milder variants of the hereditary hemolytic anemias may be able to maintain a normal hemoglobin by a brisk reticulocyte response, hemolysis should be considered part of the differential diagnosis of acholuric jaundice in any patient, anemic or not.

The initial laboratory evaluation should include examination of a peripheral blood smear, determination of the reticulocyte count, serum LDH, and serum bilirubin. Reticulocytosis with elevated bilirubin and LDH is presumptive evidence of hemolysis. The other possibilities which might present this picture are (a) bleeding into a closed space, such as the retroperitoneum or soft tissue, in which breakdown of collected blood will lead to a picture resembling extravascular hemolysis; or (b) bleeding in a patient with preexisting liver disease. Both of these situations should be identifiable by clinical history and physical examination. Examination of the peripheral blood smear may provide supportive evidence of hemolysis by demonstrating characteristic morphologic abnormalities (spherocytes, schistocytes, sickle cells, target cells, etc.) and may guide further workup. The peripheral blood smear also may help support a diagnosis of hemolytic anemia in cases where bilirubin is only minimally elevated or in cases where the degree of reticulocytosis is initially limited.

Haptoglobin levels generally are not helpful in the initial evaluation of hemolysis: Low serum haptoglobin rarely adds anything to the information obtained from the studies described above, and often is not available on an emergency basis. A low haptoglobin level is most valuable in settings where the diagnosis of hemolysis is not clear, i.e., when reticulocytes are low or there is complicating liver disease.

VI. APPROACHES TO THE TREATMENT OF HEMOLYTIC ANEMIA

Detailed discussion of the treatment of particular etiologies of hemolytic anemia will be discussed in the individual chapters dealing with those etiologies. A few general points are outlined below.

1. Many patients with chronic hemolytic anemia live in symbiosis with their shortened red cell survival, maintaining nearly normal hemoglobin concentrations through increased reticulocyte responses. Anemia in these patients often develops rapidly following infections or some systemic stressor, such as surgery. The increased reticulocyte response creates an increased demand for folic acid, and these patients should be supplemented routinely.

2. Chronic hemolysis is associated with increased cholelithiasis, and evaluation for biliary obstruction and cholecystitis needs to be considered rapidly in patients with right upper quadrant symptoms.

3. Although red cell transfusions should be used cautiously in patients with hemolysis, they should be given when tissue oxygen delivery is potentially compromised. Transfusion

does not typically exacerbate hemolysis. Packed red cells should be infused slowly and under careful observation. Patients with cold-reacting autoimmune hemolytic anemia should be transfused using a blood warmer. Autoantibodies often make cross-matching difficult or impossible; the blood bank should provide the least incompatible blood available.

4. Splenectomy is most helpful in patients with extravascular hemolysis, particularly in patients with hereditary membrane defects and warm autoimmune hemolytic anemia.

CASE STUDY 1

Patient

Sixty-eight-year-old male.

Chief Complaint

The patient was referred for evaluation of anemia and jaundice.

Medical History

The patient had been in good health, other than a history of well-controlled hypertension and exertional angina.

Medications

α-Methyldopa, hydrochlorothiazide, isorbide dinitrate.

Review of Systems

The patient reported weakness, dyspnea, and chest pain at rest.

Physical Examination

Remarkable for pallor, jaundice, and tachycardia. The spleen tip was palpable. Rectal examination did not reveal occult blood.

Laboratory Results

	Patient	Normal
Hematocrit	22%	41–47%
Hemoglobin	7.1 g/dL	13.5–17 g/dL
Reticulocyte count	9.2%	0.5–1.5%
Serum bilirubin	4.5 mg/dL	0.2–1.2 mg/dL
Serum LDH	530 IU/L	20–220 IU/L

Peripheral blood smear revealed polychromasia and spherocytes. Other chemical liver function tests were normal.

Questions

1. Are the data presented sufficient to make a diagnosis of hemolysis?
2. Would haptoglobin determination add to the diagnosis?
3. What further studies are needed?

Additional Laboratory Studies

Direct antiglobulin (Coombs) test showed strong IgG sensitization but no complement reaction. The eluted antibody did not agglutinate Rh-null cells.

Diagnosis

Autoimmune hemolytic anemia induced by methyldopa.

Discussion

The patient's diagnosis is readily apparent from the initial studies obtained. The peripheral blood smear supports a hemolytic process. Haptoglobin determination (as is usual) would not have added to the diagnosis. Having established the presence of hemolytic anemia, a specific etiology should be determined. The usual first step is performance of a direct antiglobulin (Coombs) test. The patient's history of methyldopa therapy increased the likelihood that this test would be helpful. Up to 40% of patients treated with methyldopa develop a positive direct antiglobulin test, but only about 1% develop a hemolytic anemia. The responsible antibody is an IgG molecule directed against the Rh locus. This patient responded well to corticosteroids and cessation of methyldopa.

The patient had known coronary artery disease and was having angina at rest, mandating transfusion. Cross-matching could not be performed effectively, so type-specific blood was transfused slowly with frequent monitoring, and fortunately with no adverse effects.

Bibliography

1. Kelton JG. Impaired reticuloendothelial function in patients treated with methyldopa. N Engl J Med 1985; 313:596–600.
2. LoBuglio AF, Jandl JH. The nature of the alpha-methyldopa red-cell antibody. N Engl J Med 1967; 276:658–665.
3. Petz LD, Garratty G. Acquired Immune Hemolytic Anemias. New York: Churchill Livingstone, 1980.

CASE STUDY 2

Patient

Sixty-seven-year-old male.

Chief Complaint

Acute decline in hemoglobin/hematocrit, and red urine.

Medical History

Five days prior to the event described above, the patient was admitted to the hospital with neutropenia, anemia (hemoglobin 5.8 g/dL, hematocrit 17.0%), and moderate thrombocytopenia (platelets 121,000/μL). He was transfused to a hemoglobin of 7.9 g/dL. Bone marrow examination on the second hospital day revealed acute nonlymphocytic leukemia. On the fourth hospital day (while arrangements for induction chemotherapy were being made), the patient had an episode of fever and was treated empirically with Ceftazidime. The following day, the patient became confused, had a second episode of fever, and developed pink urine.

Medications

As indicated above.

Review of Systems

The patient complaint of recent easy fatigability, the symptoms of a chronic demyelinating neuropathy, and of chronic obstructive pulmonary disease.

Physical Examination

The patient was pale, with a slight yellow coloration of his skin. Stool examination did not show occult blood.

Laboratory Results

	Patient	Normal
Hematocrit	13.6%	41–47%
Hemoglobin	4.9 g/dL	13.5–17 g/dL
Reticulocyte count	1.2%	0.5–1.5%
Serum bilirubin	5.7 mg/dL	0.2–1.2 mg/dL
Serum direct bilirubin	0.4 mg/dL	0–0.4 mg/dL
Serum LDH	4138 IU/L	300–550 IU/L

Peripheral blood smear revealed nucleated red blood cells (not noted earlier), but no schistocytes. RPR was nonreactive. PT/PTT, plasma fibrinogen and fibrin split products were normal. Urinalysis revealed pink urine with 4+ blood detected on dipstick. Rare red blood cells were seen on microscopic examination.

Questions

1. What is the differential diagnosis at this point?
2. What further tests are indicated?

Additional Laboratory Results

Direct and indirect antiglobulin (Coombs) tests were negative. Blood cultures from the hospital day 4 grew *Clostridium perfringens.*

Diagnosis

Acute intravascular hemolysis due to *Clostridium perfringens.*

Discussion

The rapid decline in hemoglobin/hematocrit, lack of evidence of bleeding, and indirect hyperbilirubinemia makes the diagnosis of hemolysis apparent, even in the absence of significant reticulocytosis. The limited reticulocyte response undoubtedly reflects functional marrow compromise by acute leukemia. The presence of hemoglobinuria (blood detected on urine dipstick out of proportion to red cells) confirms that this is intravascular hemolysis.

The differential diagnosis is that of intravascular hemolysis (Table 2). Thrombotic thrombocytopenic purpura is the first item on the differential diagnosis of patients with intravascular hemolysis, fever, and altered mental status, but is largely ruled out by the absence of schistocytes on peripheral smear. Other mechanical etiologies of hemolysis are also ruled out by the blood smear and by history and physical examination. Disseminated intravascular coagulation rarely produces significant hemolysis, and is ruled out by normal coagulation studies. The catastrophic presentation of this hemolysis would be uncommon for paroxysmal nocturnal hemoglobinuria or for paroxysmal cold hemoglobinuria; the latter is largely ruled out by the absence of serologic evidence of syphilis. It would be unusual for a hereditary enzyme deficiency, such as G6PD deficiency, to present so late in life, but this does happen occasionally. The differential diagnosis after the initial laboratory evaluation is delayed hemolytic transfusion reaction versus a direct toxic effect; paroxysmal nocturnal hemoglobinuria or G6PD deficiency remain in the differential but are much less likely.

Delayed hemolytic transfusion reaction is ruled out by the absence of a positive indirect antiglobulin (Coombs) test, and the positive blood cultures imply that this syndrome is due to clostridial hemolysis. The M.D. Anderson Cancer Center has reported an experience of 136 episodes of clostridial bacteremia in cancer patients over a 12-year period. Acute hemolysis was observed infrequently, but was uniformly associated with rapid patient death.

Bibliography

1. Bodey GP, Rodriguez S, Fainstein V, et al. Clostridial bacteremia in cancer patients: a 12 year experience. Cancer 1991; 67:1928–1942.
2. Solanki D, McCurdy PR. Delayed hemolytic transfusion reactions: an often-missed entity. JAMA 1978; 239:729–731.

REFERENCES

1. Tabbara IA. Hemolytic anemias: diagnosis and management. Med Clin N Am 1992; 76:649–668.
2. Engelfriet CP, Overbeeke MAM, von dem Borne AEG. Autoimmune hemolytic anemia. Semin Hematol 1992; 29:3–12.
3. Pirofsky B. Clinical aspects of autoimmune hemolytic anemia. Semin Hematol 1976; 13:251–265.
4. Valentine WN. Hemolytic anemias and erythrocyte enzymopathies. Ann Intern Med 1985; 103: 245–257.
5. Hirono A, Forman L, Beutler E. Enzymatic diagnosis in non-spherocytic hemolytic anemia. Medicine 1988; 67:110–117.
6. Ferrant A, Leners N, Michaux JL, et al. The spleen and haemolysis: evaluation of the intrasplenic transit time. Br J Haematol 1987; 65:31–37.
7. Yam LT, Li C-Y. The Spleen. In: Embury Sh, Hebbel RP, Mohandas N, Steinberg MH, eds. Sickle Cell Disease: Basic Principles and Clinical Practice. New York: Raven Press, 1994: 555–566.
8. Rodak BF. Routine laboratory evaluation of erythrocytes. In: Lotspeich-Steininger CA, Steine-Martin EA, Koepke JA, eds. Clinical Hematology: Principles, Procedures, Correlations. Philadelphia: Lippincott, 1992: 107–123.
9. Conley CL, Lippman SM, Ness P. Autoimmune hemolytic anemia with reticulocytopenia: a medical emergency. JAMA 1980; 244:1688–1690.
10. Liesveld JL, Rowe JM, Licthman MA. Variability of the erythropoietic response in autoimmune hemolytic anemia: analysis of 109 cases. Blood 1987; 69:820–826.
11. Tisdale WA, Klatskin G, Kinsella ED. The significance of the direct-reacting fraction of serum bilirubin in hemolytic jaundice. Am J Med 1959; 13:214–227.
12. Marchand A, Galen RS, Van Lente F. The predictive value of serum haptoglobin in hemolytic disease. JAMA 1980; 243:1909–1911.

19

Hemolytic Anemia Associated with Red Cell Membrane Defects

John C. Winkelmann
University of Cincinnati College of Medicine, Cincinnati, Ohio

I. DEFINITION

Hemolytic anemias result from pathogenic mechanisms extrinsic to the erythrocyte or from intrinsic red cell abnormalities. Intrinsic defects include abnormal hemoglobins and erythrocyte enzymes, considered elsewhere. This chapter delineates intrinsic red cell abnormalities that affect the red cell membrane and the membrane skeleton.

A schematic representation of the erythrocyte membrane skeleton is shown in Fig. 1. Spectrin heterodimers, composed of α and β chains, self-associate into filamentous tetramers that are the main constituent of the membrane skeleton. Approximately six spectrin tetramers are attached to each short actin filament to form a two-dimensional network. This network is attached to the inner face of the lipid bilayer via an adapter protein, ankyrin, and the integral membrane protein band 3 (the anion channel). the spectrin network interacts with a second integral membrane protein, glycophorin C, through protein 4.1, a molecule that also stabilizes the spectrin–actin association. Mutations affecting many of the protein constituents have been described that give rise to inherited hemolytic anemias.

II. CLASSIFICATION

It is both convenient and clinically meaningful to divide red cell membranopathies into hereditary and acquired disorders (Table 1). While hereditary hemolytic anemias may present in adults, there is often a long antecedent history of anemia, hyperbilirubinemia, biliary lithiasis, or splenomegaly. The family history may reveal anemia, splenectomy, or jaundice. In contrast, acquired erythrocyte membrane defects occur typically in patients with previously normal hemoglobin values, in patients with normal family histories, and in certain suggestive clinical settings.

III. HEREDITARY SPHEROCYTOSIS

A. Definition

Hereditary spherocytosis (HS) is a chronic, inherited hemolytic anemia of varying clinical severity that is characterized by circulating spherocytic erythrocytes, absence of red cell auto-

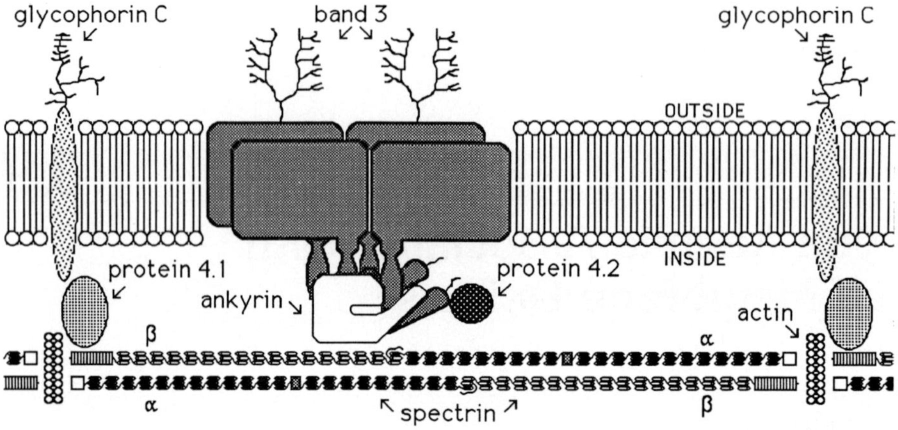

Figure 1 Schematic representation of the erythrocyte membrane skeleton.

Table 1 Hemolytic Anemia Due Primarily to Erythrocyte Membrane Defects

Hereditary
Hereditary spherocytosis
Spherocytic elliptocytosis
Hereditary elliptocytosis
Southeast Asian ovalocytosis
Hereditary pyropoikilocytosis
Hereditary stomatocytosis
Hereditary xerocytosis
Rh antigen deficiency
Hereditary acanthocytosis
Abetalipoproteinemia
McLeod Syndrome (Kell antigen deficiency)
Chorea-acanthocytosis syndrome
In(Lu)
Acquired
Acquired spherocytosis
Clostridia septicemia
Thermal burn
Hypophosphatemia
Zieve's syndrome
Snake, spider, and insect bites
Acquired acanthocytosis
Spur cell anemia
Vitamin E deficiency
Infantile pyknocytosis
Paroxysmal nocturnal hemoglobinuria

antibodies, deficiency of the erythrocyte membrane skeleton protein spectrin (Fig. 1), and a beneficial clinical response to splenectomy.

B. Incidence and Genetics

HS is the most common inherited hemolytic anemia affecting northern Europeans, occurring in approximately 1 in 5000 individuals. HS afflicts all ethnic groups, but its frequency in non-Caucasians is unknown. The most common forms of HS are inherited in an autosomal dominant fashion. In some cases, HS may be secondary to a recessively inherited mutation, a sporadic new mutation, or a congenital cytogenetic anomaly.

C. Etiology

HS is produced by mutations in the genes encoding several different component proteins of the membrane skeleton (Fig. 1). The most frequent mutations that give rise to HS affect the genes for ankyrin and band 3 (anion channel). Mutations also occur in α spectrin, β spectrin, and protein 4.2 (pallidin). The final common pathophysiologic pathway produced by most HS mutations is spectrin deficiency. Spectrin deficiency leads to membrane loss and spherocytosis. It is a consistent characteristic of HS that most hemolysis occurs selectively in the spleen.

D. Clinical Findings

HS ranges in clinical severity from life-threatening neonatal anemia to mild, compensated hemolysis that eludes clinical detection entirely. The "prototypical" HS patient has mild, lifelong anemia, splenomegaly, biliary stones, and mild unconjugated (indirect) hyperbilirubinemia producing chronic or intermittent jaundice. Cases may be brought to light during routine clinical evaluation or when patients experience acute problems such as aplastic crisis precipitated by B19 parvovirus, megaloblastic crisis resulting from folate deficiency, acute cholecystitis, splenic infarction, progressive anemia due to hypersplenism or pregnancy, or worsened jaundice during a systemic illness. The family history is often positive for anemia, splenectomy, jaundice, biliary lithiasis, or even spherocytosis. Patients with HS and their family members may be mislabeled with Gilbert's disease.

E. Laboratory Findings

1. *Peripheral Blood Smear*

In the evaluation of all anemia patients, especially those with suspected hemolytic anemia, examination of the peripheral blood smear is of paramount importance. The morphologic findings in HS are quite characteristic and are therefore a vital aid in diagnosis (Fig. 2). Spherocytic erythrocytes are recognized by their decreased central pallor. Prior to splenectomy, microspherocytes may abound. Polychromasia suggests reticulocytosis. Postsplenectomy, spherocytosis persists but microspherocytes decrease and polychromasia recedes. Howell-Jolly bodies and acanthocytes are typically found postsplenectomy. In mild HS, the morphology may be subtle and easily missed, even by experienced observers.

In recessive HS, increased microcytosis, poikilocytosis, and polychromasia are evident on examination of the peripheral blood. In spherocytic elliptocytosis, elongated spherocytes are visible. Spheroacanthocytes (spherocytes with hornlike projections) and "pincered" red cell are seen in other variant forms of HS.

It is important to note that loss of central pallor mimicking spherocytosis is an artifact of peripheral smear preparation, particularly near the thin end. Therefore, the observer should

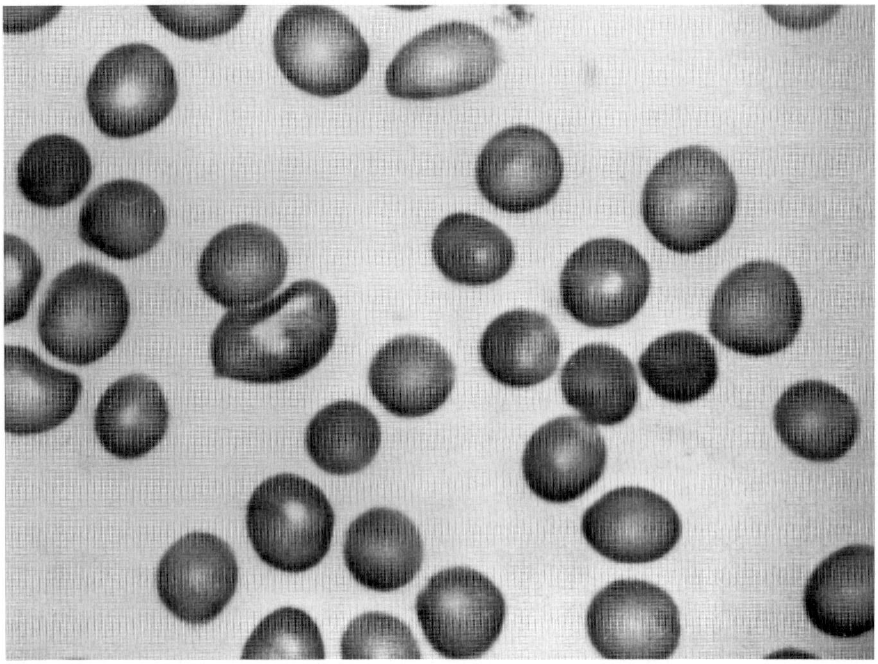

Figure 2 Peripheral blood smear from a patient with hereditary spherocytosis. (Original magnification ×1000.)

evaluate erythrocytes for spherocytosis in an interior part of the smear where some cells have central pallor and yet erythrocytes are well separated.

2. *Routine Laboratory Results*

Patients with HS typically have a mild anemia (Hgb > 10) and reticulocytosis. The MCV is usually normal. The MCHC is often slightly increased. Unconjugated (indirect) hyperbilirubinemia, increased lactate dehydrogenase, and decreased serum haptoglobin suggest hemolysis and often resolve after splenectomy. Bone marrow examination is not usually indicated in the evaluation of HS. Unless other conditions are superimposed, the bone marrow will show erythroid hyperplasia.

3. *Osmotic Fragility (OF)*

One hallmark of spherocytes, regardless of their origin, is increased sensitivity to osmotic lysis. Erythrocytes are suspended for 1 hr in varying hypotonic solutions (usually NaCl and sodium phosphate buffer) that induce swelling by osmotic movement of water into the cells. Normal erythrocytes are able to swell to a significant degree without breaking. Spherocytes, however, have limited capacity to swell. Consequently, red cells from HS patients lyse in solutions less hypotonic than those that lyse normal erythrocytes. Percent hemolysis (calculated by dividing the optical density, read with a visual-spectrum spectrophotometer, of the postcentrifugation supernatant of the sample by that of a completely lysed control) is plotted against the solution tonicity (usually percent NaCl). The resultant sigmoidal curve is shifted in most HS patients toward higher NaCl concentrations (Fig. 3). To help diagnose mild HS, the OF can be made more sensitive by incubating patient blood for 24 hr at 37°C prior to testing. OF measurement is not specific for HS but simply determines the degree of spherocytosis, whatever the cause.

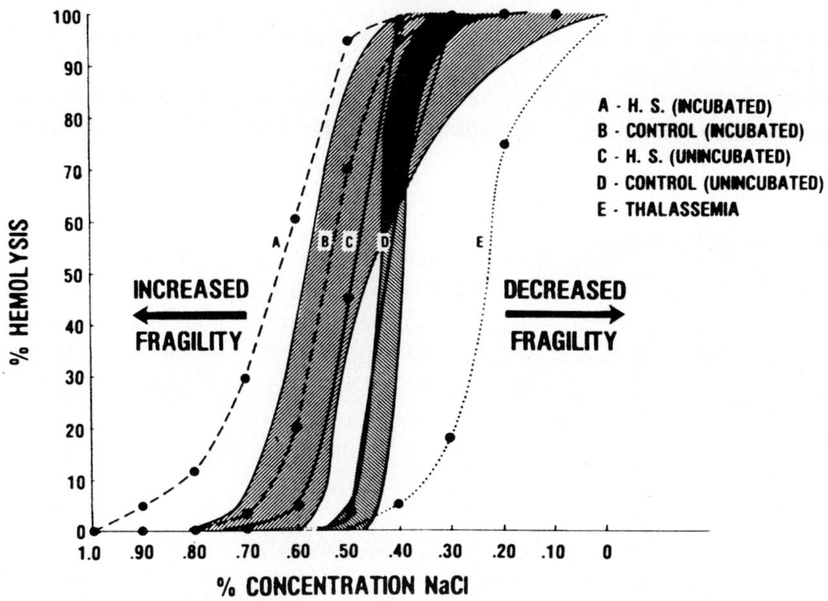

Figure 3 Osmotic fragility (OF) of red cells in hereditary spherocytosis (HS). The OF curve shifts to the left in HS for both unincubated and incubated erythrocytes. The OFs of normal (control) and thalassemic red cells are shown for comparison.

Liver disease or obstructive jaundice that produces target cells in normal individuals may normalize the OF in HS patients. Iron deficiency or coexisting thalassemia may also mask the increased OF in HS.

The autohemolysis test is sometimes used in the diagnosis of HS, but probably does not add significantly to the osmotic fragility test. Various other methods have been devised to diagnose HS, including the glycerol lysis test, the "pink test," and others. None has gained widespread acceptance.

4. Molecular Diagnosis

With the identification of HS mutations in numerous kindreds, it is theoretically possible to apply molecular diagnosis to HS patients. Unfortunately, the great diversity of disease genes and disease-causing mutations precludes routine application of genetic testing to patients. Using biochemical methods (Laemmli and Fairbanks gels), it is sometimes possible to detect spectrin, ankyrin, band 3, and protein 4.2 defects in HS patients. However, to date such studies remain the provenance of research laboratories.

F. Differential Diagnosis

HS must be differentiated from acquired hemolytic anemias that produce circulating spherocytes and abnormal osmotic fragility. Autoimmune hemolytic anemia (AHA) usually produces spherocytes. The direct antiglobulin test (direct Coombs test), readily distinguishes most AHA from HS. On microscopic examination, HS usually produces more uniform spherocytosis than does AHA. An elevated MCHC may also help differentiate HS from AHA. Other causes of acquired spherocytosis such as transfusion reactions, ABO incompatibility, oxidant erythrocyte damage, thermal burns, snake venom, and *Clostridia* sepsis are distinguished from HS by the clinical setting and lack of chronicity.

Unusual inherited conditions occasionally confused with HS include Rh antigen deficiency, hereditary stomatocytosis, unstable hemoglobins, and the oxidant hemolysis of Wilson's disease.

G. Course and Complications

As mentioned above, HS produces a highly variable disease course. Severe, recessive HS patients may have life-threatening anemia, marked jaundice, expanded bone marrow space, growth retardation, delayed puberty, and extramedullary hematopoiesis. In contrast, mild HS may be clinically silent. The large majority of HS patients fall between these extremes. Complications that may afflict HS patients arise from impaired erythropoietic compensation, accelerated hemolysis, splenomegaly, splenectomy, and the consequences of chronic hemolysis.

1. Worsening Anemia

Anything that increases the rate of erythrocyte destruction or impairs bone marrow compensation may lead to progressive anemia in HS patients. Profound, life-threatening anemia can occur in otherwise mild cases. Some HS patients experience progressive hypersplenism or acute sequestration that shortens red cell survival. Immune-mediated hemolysis secondary to, for example, Epstein-Barr virus infection or drugs may be superimposed on HS, leading to exacerbated anemia.

Erythroid hyperplasia increases HS patients' requirements for folate. When pregnancy, malabsorption, or malnutrition produce folate deficiency, a "megaloblastic crisis" can ensue due to impaired compensation. "Aplastic crisis" results from infection by B19 parvovirus. This common viral infection affects bone marrow erythroblasts leading to transient erythroid aplasia and profound anemia in patients with chronic hemolysis. In normal individuals, B19 parvovirus produces a mild viral syndrome that may include a typical exanthem in children, termed "fifth disease."

2. Splenomegaly and Postsplenectomy

HS patients can experience traumatic splenic rupture, splenic infarction, splenic sequestration, or progressive hypersplenism. Postsplenectomy HS patients are vulnerable to overwhelming sepsis caused by encapsulated organisms, including *Streptococcus pneumoniae*. Vaccination to *S. pneumoniae* reduces the likelihood of this complication. Patients who have been immunized to pneumococcus remain susceptible to other encapsulated bacteria such as *Hemphilus influenzae* and *Neisseria meningitidis*.

3. Chronic Hemolysis

Perhaps the most common complication of chronic hemolysis is gallstones composed of radio-opaque calcium bilirubinate. These may remain clinically silent, but can induce biliary colic, acute cholecystitis, or obstructive jaundice due to common bile duct blockage.

Other complications of hemolysis include tumors formed by extramedullary hematopoiesis, chronic skin ulcers of the lower extremity, and iron overload resembling hereditary hemochromatosis. These are ameliorated by splenectomy. Most patients with hemolysis do not get hemochromatosis, so some investigators have postulated that HS patients who load iron have a superimposed defect in iron handling such as heterozygous hemochromatosis.

H. Treatment

Patients with HS may require red cell transfusions for a plastic crisis, chronic folate administration to ward off megaloblastic crisis, or cholecystectomy for biliary lithiasis. The most significant therapeutic decision, however, centers on the issue of splenectomy.

Splenectomy does not eliminate the spherocytic defect but dramatically improves the rate of hemolysis in HS patients. In very mild cases (older age, normal hemoglobin, minimal hemolysis, and no complications), there is no need for splenectomy. In more severely affected individuals (young age, moderate anemia, active hemolysis, and complications), splenectomy is clearly indicated and beneficial. Many HS patients fall between these two groups. There are no solid data on which to base a strong recommendation in borderline cases, so treatment must be individualized. For example, if a patient with mild anemia develops symptomatic gallstones, it is often prudent to recommend splenectomy at the time of cholecystectomy. Newer surgical techniques such as laparoscopic splenectomy and partial splenectomy are beginning to impact on the treatment of HS, but there are insufficient data to ascertain whether the indication for splenectomy has changed. Vaccination against *S. pneumoniae* prior to splenectomy is strongly recommended.

IV. HEREDITARY ELLIPTOCYTOSIS

A. Definition

Hereditary elliptocytosis (HE) is a very heterogeneous group of genetic disorders that share the common characteristic of elongated, elliptical erythrocytes. Only a fraction of patients with HE have clinically significant hemolysis.

B. Incidence and Genetics

In the United States, the prevalence of HE is approximately 3–5 per 10,000. HE appears to be more common in African Americans. Worldwide, HE is more common in regions with endemic malaria. In equatorial Africa, HE is present in ≥0.6% of the population. A particular form of HE, Southeast Asian ovalocytosis (SAO), is found in 30% of the population in some areas. The inheritance mode of HE is almost entirely autosomal dominant.

C. Etiology

A multitude of mutations that cause HE have been identified in several different genes that encode proteins of the erythrocyte membrane skeleton (Fig. 1). The most common mutations causing HE are found in genes for α and β spectrin. These mutations, found mostly in blacks, produce spectrin dimers with defective ability to self-associate into tetramers. Deficient or dysfunctional protein 4.1 is produced by another group of HE mutations. Glycophorin C deficiency, the result of several different mutations, can also give rise to HE. SAO is the consequence of a mutation in band 3.

The pathophysiology common to most HE (with the exception of SAO) is mechanical instability of the erythrocyte membrane skeleton. This can be demonstrated using a technique called ektacytometry, in which red cell membranes are subjected to defined shear stress. In contrast, erythrocyte membranes from patients with HS have normal mechanical properties on ektacytometry. Disruption of the HE membrane skeleton can be visualized on electron microscopy. Presumably, elliptocytic erythrocytes acquire their appearance when, after streaming through the microcirculation, they are unable to resume their normal shape.

The pathophysiology of SAO is unique. In contrast to typical HE, the red cell membrane skeleton in this disorder acquires extra rigidity and hyperstability. There is no significant hemolysis. SAO erythrocytes have been shown to be resistant to malaria invasion in vitro.

C. Clinical Findings

Most HE is subclinical. Cases that are hemolytic may have compensated hemolysis or mild or severe anemia. Like HS, hemolytic HE produces splenomegaly, jaundice, and biliary lithiasis.

E. Laboratory Findings

1. Peripheral Blood Smear

The diagnosis of HE is made by microscopic examination of erythrocyte morphology. Usually >25% of the red cells are elliptical in shape (Fig. 4). Poikilocytosis and microspherocytosis may be evident, depending on the degree of hemolysis. In spherocytic elliptocytosis, rounded ovalocytes with decreased central pallor are characteristic. In SAO, there are predominantly oval erythrocytes, some with transverse ridges or a longitudinal slit.

2. Other Tests

Depending on the degree of hemolysis, HE patients may have laboratory manifestations that reflect chronic hemolytic anemia. Osmotic fragility is normal.

3. Molecular Diagnosis

The plethora of mutations and genes involved in HE precludes the routine application of genetic testing to patients with HE. Biochemical analysis of red cell membrane skeleton protein

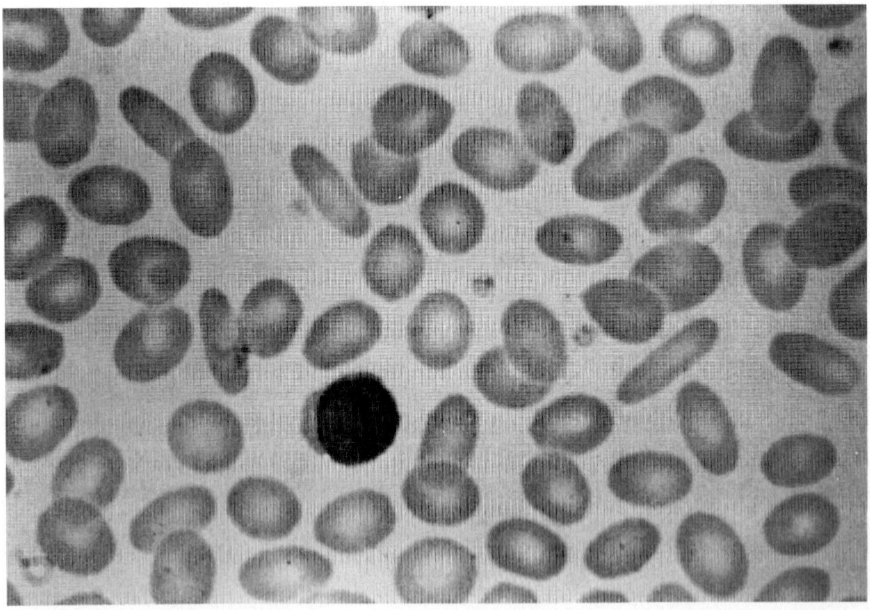

Figure 4 Peripheral blood smear from a patient with hereditary elliptocytosis. (Original magnification ×1000.)

structure and function frequently reveals the defective molecule. These methods, however, are not routinely applicable to clinical practice.

F. Differential Diagnosis

Several other hematologic conditions produce elliptocytes, including iron deficiency, thalassemia, sickle disease, myelophthisic anemias, myelofibrosis, and megaloblastic anemia. It is uncommon for these disorders, however, to result in elliptocytosis as the predominant morphology or elliptocytes in the absence of other poikilocytes. Hereditary pyropoikilocytosis (see below) often demonstrates a significant degree of elliptocytosis. A rare hybrid disorder, hereditary spheroelliptocytosis, has features of both HS and HE. Erythrocytes have both mechanical instability and osmotic fragility. This diagnosis must be considered in cases of hemolytic HE.

G. Course and Complications

Most patients with HE follow a benign clinical course. Patients with hemolytic HE are prone to the same complications as patients with HS (see above).

H. Treatment

Most patients with HE require no treatment. Hemolytic HE, however, responds well to splenectomy. Vaccination to *S. pneumoniae* is recommended prior to splenectomy. All patients with chronic hemolysis should receive folate supplementation.

V. HEREDITARY PYROPOIKILOCYTOSIS

A. Definition

Hereditary pyropoikilocytosis (HPP) is a sever hemolytic anemia presenting in neonates or young children and characterized by marked red cell poikilocytosis, including microspherocytes, budding red cells, fragmented erythrocytes, elliptocytes, teardrop red cells, and numerous bizarre forms (Fig. 5). The disease derives its name from the observation that controlled heating of HPP red cells results in their dissolution at a lower temperature than that affecting normal erythrocytes.

B. Incidence and Genetics

HPP is rare and usually occurs in blacks. It is inherited in an autosomal recessive fashion, although typically one or both parents have mild HE.

C. Etiology

The molecular basis of HPP is spectrin mutation. Invariably, HPP patients have one α spectrin mutation that, alone, causes HE. The opposite α spectrin allele is affected by a mutation that produces a decreased rate of synthesis, analogous to a thalassemia mutation of a globin gene. HPP may also result from homozygous inheritance of two identical HE-causing mutations or compound heterozygous inheritance of two different HE-causing mutations. Some authors classify homozygous and compound heterozygous HE separately from HPP. The clinical and pathophysiologic overlap is sufficient, however, to justify their inclusion under the HPP heading.

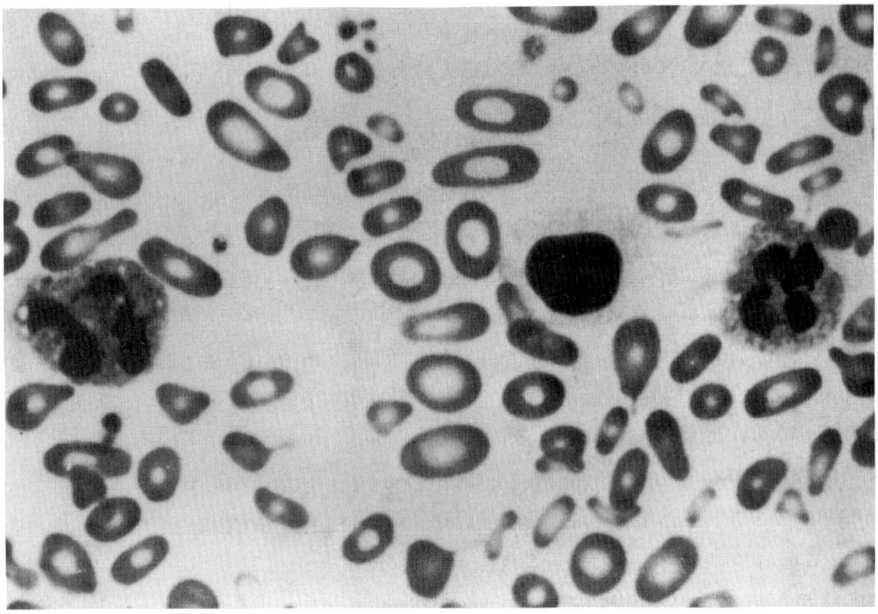

Figure 5 Peripheral blood smear from an infant with hereditary pyropoikilocytosis. Courtesy of Dr. Naomi Luban, Children's Hospital National Medical Center, Washington, DC. (Original magnification ×1000.)

D. Clinical Findings

Patients usually have severe anemia (hemoglobin 4–8 g/dL) with erythroblastosis, jaundice, and splenomegaly.

E. Laboratory Findings

Routine blood evaluation reveals a low MCV due to red cell fragmentation. Abnormal OF and autohemolysis tests are typical, reflecting the presence of microspherocytes. Other laboratory tests demonstrate intense hemolysis.

F. Differential Diagnosis

Some patients with hemolytic HE have a poikilocytic anemia early in life that clinically resembles HPP. These patients appear to "outgrow" their poikilocytosis and manifest typical HE as adults. Clinically, HPP patients resemble severe, recessive HE patients. The predominance of spherocytes among the poikilocytes and the absence of numerous small red cell fragments favors HS.

G. Course and Complications

Skeletal deformities, frontal bossing, growth retardation, and early biliary stone formation are reported complications of HPP. Early therapeutic intervention may help prevent these problems from developing.

H. Treatment

The rate of hemolysis is considerably slowed but not corrected by splenectomy. Chronic folate supplementation is indicated. Vaccination against *S. pneumoniae* prior to splenectomy is recommended.

VI. HEREDITARY STOMATOCYTOSIS AND OTHER HEREDITARY ERYTHROCYTE MEMBRANOPATHIES

A. Hereditary Stomatocytosis

Hereditary stomatocytosis is a rare autosomal dominant disorder typified by circulating erythrocytes that have a central slit or "mouth" on peripheral blood smear. The molecular defect is unknown. Erythrocytes in hereditary stomatocytosis are missing protein 4.9, also called stomatin, and manifest leakiness to sodium. Clinically, patients range from little or no hemolysis to severe anemia. Macrocytosis is typical. Patients with hereditary stomatocytosis must be distinguished from those patients with stomatocytes produced as an artifact of peripheral smear preparation and patients with stomatocytes due to alcohol or medications. Hereditary stomatocytosis patients respond well to splenectomy.

B. Hereditary Xerocytosis

Hereditary xerocytosis (HX) is a rare autosomal dominant disorder in which patients have markedly dehydrated erythrocytes. Erythrocyte morphology may be normal or may demonstrate spiculated and target forms. HX red cells have an increased MCHC and a *decreased* OF. The molecular defect is unknown. The proportion of phosphatidyl choline in the XS red cell membrane is increased. Clinically, most patients have mild to moderate anemia. Splenectomy is *not* beneficial in HX patients.

C. Rh Antigen Deficiency

The rare patients who lack the RH (D) blood group antigen have a moderately severe hemolytic anemia with both spherocytic and stomatocytic features. The OF is only mildly increased in Rh deficiency.

D. Hereditary Acanthocytosis

Acanthocytes are red cells with irregular, hornlike projections. They often coexist with echinocytes, red cells with small, numerous, uniform projections. Both acanthocytes and echinocytes are present in a variety of acquired clinical conditions and may or may not be associated with hemolysis. Several distinct clinical entities have inherited hemolytic anemia with acanthocytosis as the predominant defect.

1. *Abetalipoproteinemia*

Abetalipoproteinemia is a rare, autosomal recessive condition caused by mutations in the microsomal triglyceride transfer protein, resulting in a failure to produce lipoproteins containing apolipoprotein β. Clinically, patients have a progressive neurologic disease, retinitis pigmentosa, and absent β lipoproteins in the blood. From 50% to 90% of the erythrocytes are acanthocytes due to abnormal membrane lipids. Hemolysis is typically mild.

2. McLeod Syndrome

McLeod syndrome is a rare, X-linked recessive disorder resulting from mutation or deletion of the gene encoding Kx, the Kell blood group antigen. Patients have mild compensated hemolysis with acanthocytosis, echinocytosis, and poikilocytosis. Myopathy and/or neuropathy are part of the McLeod syndrome. If transfused, patients may develop antibodies to Kell antigens, whereafter they may only receive blood from Kell-deficient donors.

3. Chorea-Acanthocytosis Syndrome

A diverse group of rare disorders of unknown cause may be considered part of the chorea-acanthocytosis syndrome. Both dominant and recessive inheritance patterns have been reported. A variety of neurodegenerative problems are associated with acanthocytosis. Usually the degree of hemolysis is minor. Serum lipoproteins are normal.

4. In(Lu) Gene

One in 3000 individuals inherits a dominant inhibitor of the Lutheran blood group, called In(Lu). These patients have greatly suppressed expression of Lutheran antigens, CD44, and other red cell surface molecules. Red cell morphology includes acanthocytosis and poikilocytosis. Hemolysis is not significant.

VII. ACQUIRED SPHEROCYTOSIS

A. Clostridial Sepsis

Clostridium perfringens bacteremia is associated, in 10% of cases, with one of the most impressive hemolytic processes seen in any clinical disorder. When hemolysis occurs, the outcome is often fatal. Complete lysis of the red cell mass has been reported. Most likely, the intravascular hemolysis is due to a toxin produced by the organism. Marked microspherocytosis is evident on peripheral blood examination.

B. Thermal Burns

After acute burns affecting 15–20% or more of the skin, patients will develop transient hemolysis with circulating spherocytes. In severe burns, 30% of the red cell mass may undergo hemolysis. The process is self-limited, so no treatment is indicated beyond transfusion and supportive care.

C. Hypophosphatemia

Very low serum phosphate levels are associated with hemolysis. Spherocytes and acanthocytes are present on examination of the blood smear. The pathophysiology is thought to be red cell ATP depletion with resultant metabolic compromise. Treatment with phosphate reverses the hemolysis.

D. Zieve's Syndrome

Zieves syndrome is an unusual and poorly understood condition occurring in patients with alcoholic liver disease. Spherocytes are present on blood smear examination. Hyperlipoproteinemia and jaundice are features of Zieve's. Zieve's must be distinguished from spur cell anemia (see below).

E. Venomous Snake Bites

Pit vipers, including rattlesnakes, copperheads, and cottonmouth snakes, can produce spherocytic hemolysis in victims of bites. The venom includes a potent phospholipase activity that attacks erythrocyte membrane lipids. Administration of antivenin, antitoxin produced from horse serum after immunization with pit viper venom, can reduce the severity of the hemolysis and other systemic effects of venomous snake bites.

F. Spider and Insect Bites

Brown recluse spider bites can produce a delayed spherocytic hemolysis several days after the bite. The venom apparently associates with the red cell membrane and mediates the attachment of IgG and complement to the cell surface, resulting in a positive direct Coombs test. Complement activation causes intravascular hemolysis.

Bees, wasps, and other venomous insects can produce intravascular hemolysis in patients receiving numerous bites through a phospholipase-mediated mechanism. Patients who experience clinically significant hemolysis have circulating spherocytes, falling hemoglobin, and rising potassium. Treatment is supportive.

VIII. ACQUIRED ACANTHOCYTOSIS

Numerous clinical disorders are associated with morphologic acanthocytosis and/or echinocytosis. These include uremia (echinocytosis), malnutrition (acanthocytosis), hypothyroidism (acanthocytosis), postsplenectomy (both), and others. Clinically significant hemolysis, however, is unusual in these disorders. However, acquired hemolytic anemia associated with acanthocytosis is encountered in a few clinical situations.

A. Spur Cell Anemia

The most common acanthocytic hemolytic anemia is associated with severe hepatocellular damage, most commonly alcoholic cirrhosis. Spur cell anemia may produce brisk hemolysis or more chronic, low-grade red cell destruction. Marked indirect hyperbilirubinemia and splenomegaly are typical findings. On peripheral blood smear, acanthocytes are abundant (>20%). Other morphologic alterations due to liver disease, such as target cells, are often also present. Other causes of anemia common in cirrhosis patients may confound the diagnosis (Fig. 6).

The pathophysiology of spur cell anemia involves altered red cell membrane lipids. Erythrocytes acquire increased membrane cholesterol, increasing the cholesterol/phospholipid ratio and surface area. Spur cells are produced by subsequent membrane loss and increased cellular rigidity. Serum from patients with spur cell anemia transforms normal red cells into acanthocytes.

Treatment of spur cell anemia is primarily supportive. Splenectomy may improve red cell survival but is poorly tolerated in most patients with severe liver disease. Consequently, splenectomy should be considered only in the most selected patients in whom surgical risk is minimal and hemolytic anemia is severe.

B. Vitamin E Deficiency

Neonates and patients with malabsorption syndromes may develop vitamin E deficiency. Patients suffer from generalized edema and hemolysis that may be accompanied by acanthocytosis. Thrombocytosis is typically present. The pathophysiology of hemolysis appears to be

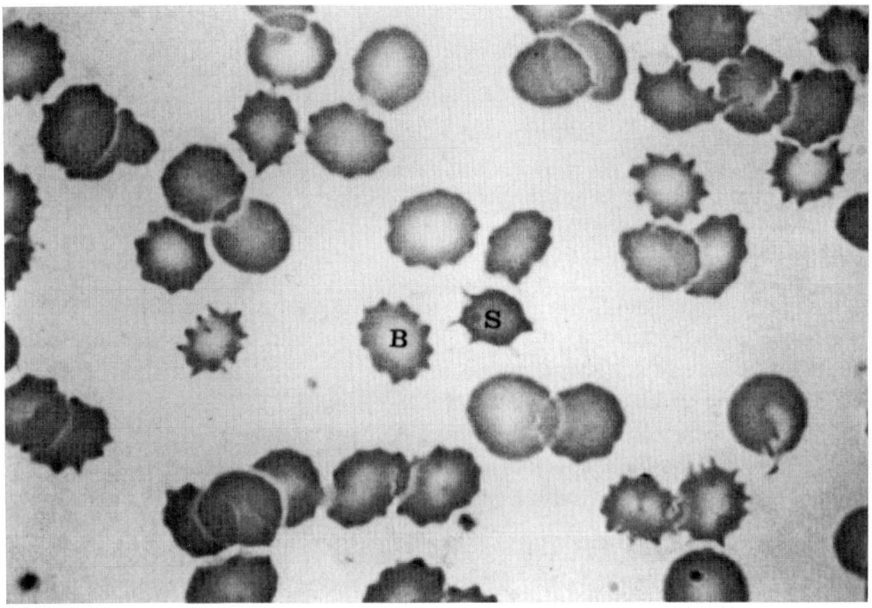

Figure 6 Peripheral blood smear from patient with terminal Laennec's cirrhosis showing a burr cell (B) and an adjacent spur cell (S) for comparison. (Original magnification ×1000.)

decreased red cell resistance to oxidant-mediated damage. Administration of vitamin E can ameliorate this syndrome.

C. Infantile Pyknocytosis

Rarely, newborns develop neonatal jaundice, hepatosplenomegaly, and acanthocytic hemolysis. The erythrocyte morphology was originally described as pyknocytosis, but probably falls within the spectrum of acanthocytosis. Hemolysis persists for several weeks and remits spontaneously. The etiology is unknown. Treatment is supportive.

IX. PAROXYSMAL NOCTURNAL HEMOGLOBINURIA

A. Definition

Paroxysmal nocturnal hemoglobinura (PNH) is an acquired disorder of the hematopoietic stem cell in which abnormal blood cells are produced that lack glycosylphosphatidylinositol (GPI)-linked membrane proteins. This deficiency produces hemolytic anemia, thrombophilia, and defective hematopoiesis that may progress to aplastic anemia, leukemia, or myelodysplasia.

B. Incidence

PNH is rare and may occur in patients of any age.

C. Etiology

The biochemical defect in PNH is the inability of hematopoietic stem cells and their progeny to synthesize GPI linkages. The result is that a host of proteins that normally reside at the cell surface are absent. An essential enzyme in GPI synthesis is called PIG-A. Acquired mutations of this enzyme are responsible for PNH. One consequence is that, over time, the PNH clone overgrows the bone marrow such that a majority of blood cells in symptomatic patients may derive from the defective stem cell. In this sense, PNH resembles clonal stem cell disorders such as myeloproliferative and myelodysplastic syndromes.

Three GPI-linked red cell surface proteins, decay-accelerating factor (DAF), membrane inhibitor of reactive lysis (MIRL), and C8-binding protein, are complement-regulating proteins. Their absence on PNH red cells produces complement sensitivity that is the hallmark of PNH diagnosis and pathophysiology.

D. Clinical Findings

Patients with PNH have chronic or intermittent intravascular hemolysis mediated by complement. The degree of anemia is variable. Hemoglobinuria may be a feature, but uncommonly exhibits the classical nocturnal pattern. Infection may precede an episode of hemolysis, exacerbated anemia, and hemoglobinuria. Acute and chronic renal injury may ensue from intravascular hemolysis. Mild splenomegaly is common in PNH.

PNH patients have a clear prothrombotic tendency. The etiology is not well understood. Venous thrombosis is typically seen, affecting the deep veins of the extremities, the hepatic vein, the portal vein, the splenic vein, the splanchnic veins, the cerebral veins, and others.

Many PNH patients demonstrate evidence of defective hematopoiesis. In its extreme form, aplastic anemia may develop, or may be present at the initial diagnosis of PNH. More commonly, thrombocytopenia or leukopenia may be identified. The erythropoietic response to hemolysis may be blunted, leading to exaggerated anemia.

E. Laboratory Findings

Red cell morphology in PNH patients is typically unremarkable. Reticulocytosis is usually present. PNH patients express biochemical evidence of intravascular hemolysis (urine hemosiderin, plasma free hemoglobin, low serum haptoglobin, etc.) in addition to the more general findings of hemolysis (indirect hyperbilirubinemia, elevated LDH, etc.).

The diagnosis of PNH is established using tests that examine patient red cells for sensitivity to lysis by complement. Maneuvers that activate serum complement produce lysis of PNH red cells. A commonly used screening test is the sucrose hemolysis test, also called the sugar water test. The ionic strength of serum is reduced by dilution with an isoosmotic solution of sucrose. The sucrose hemolysis test is not specific for PNH, but is quite sensitive. In patients with a positive result, a more specific confirmatory test is recommended, the classical Ham test. In this test, the serum is acidified and the Mg^{2+} level is adjusted to achieve maximal sensitivity. The only known false positive Ham test occurs in type II congenital dyserythropoietic anemia. Some research laboratories use the more precise complement lysis sensitivity test that identifies three different populations of PNH red cells based on their differential sensitivity to complement lysis.

Bone marrow biopsy is not routinely indicated in PNH patients. When serious cytopenias are present, bone marrow examination may provide useful information. Usually, erythroid hyperplasia is present in PNH patients. Varying degrees of hypoplasia may also be seen.

There are no useful clinical tests to identify PNH patients who are at high risk of thrombotic complications.

F. Differential Diagnosis

The diagnosis of PNH should be considered in patients with pancytopenia, hemolytic anemia with bland red cell morphology, unexplained thrombosis, unexplained fetal wastage, and unexplained iron deficiency (due to urine hemosiderin loss).

G. Course and Complications

Many of the clinical consequences of PNH have been described above. The mean life span of PNH patients from the time of diagnosis is about 8–10 years. During the course of their disease, PNH patients may manifest any combination of complications arising from hemolysis, thrombosis, bone marrow failure, or clonal evolution. The severity of the clinical course correlates somewhat with the fraction of red cells that are sensitive to complement. Not all PNH patients progress; some patients may improve over time, with waning of the PNH clone.

Hemolysis can lead to profound, life-threatening anemia requiring transfusional support. Acute hemolytic exacerbation may be precipitated by infections, transfusion reactions, or other complement-activating stimuli. Failure to compensate adequately for hemolysis can result from iron deficiency that commonly develops due to loss as urine hemosiderin. Bone marrow failure, parvovirus, or other nutrient deficiencies may impair erythropoietic compensation.

Renal impairment can take the form of acute tubular necrosis after a major hemolytic episode. Chronic renal damage can result in urine concentration defects, renal tubular acidosis, and azotemia.

Most PNH patients develop thrombocytopenia or granulocytopenia during the course of their disease. PNH may progress to aplastic anemia, often a fatal complication. Three to five percent of patients with PNH develop acute leukemia. Leukemic cells derive from the PNH clone.

Finally, thrombotic complications are varied and often severe. PNH patients often die of thrombotic events, particularly hepatic vein thrombosis or pulmonary embolism.

H. Treatment

The only curative approach to a hematopoietic stem cell disorder is to replace the stem cell, correct the defect, or somehow restore the competitive advantage of the residual normal stem cells vis à vis the PNH clone. Bone marrow transplantation (BMT) is the only currently available therapy that achieves any of these goals. Allogeneic BMT is typically reserved for PNH patients who develop aplastic anemia, young PNH patients, or patients with other complications suggesting a poor prognosis. Obviously, not all such patients have a suitable donor. Syngeneic BMT has been used with some success.

Hemolytic episodes may be ameliorated using systemic corticosteroids that, in high doses, interfere with the activation of complement. Transfusion requirements in severely affected patients may be reduced using maintenance prednisone. Iron supplementation is usually necessary to replace iron that is lost in the urine. Transfusion of red cells to PNH patients is often necessary. Occasionally, transfusion may precipitate hemolysis of PNH cells. Transfusion of washed erythrocytes, to eliminate donor complement, prevents this difficulty. Androgenic steroids can increase the hemoglobin and reduce the transfusion requirement. This treatment is poorly tolerated in women. Splenectomy is not helpful in PNH.

Treatment of acute thrombotic complications is similar to other patients with thrombotic diathesis. Thrombolytics may be beneficial. Heparin administration is routine, followed by warfarin. After a thrombotic complication, PNH patients should receive long-term anticoagulation, unless contraindicated.

CASE STUDY 1

Patient

Twenty-two-year-old woman.

Chief Complaint

The patient noticed jaundice during a recent febrile illness. Now she feels extremely weak and tired.

Medical History

The patient's mother says that the patient had jaundice after birth. Except for normal childhood illnesses, she has been healthy. During recent months, several acquaintances at her college have been ill with pharyngitis, fever, and a protracted recovery.

Family History

Her paternal uncle had splenectomy for "anemia." Her father had a cholecystectomy for symptomatic gallstones. Her siblings are healthy.

Physical Examination She has mild scleral icterus and pale conjunctival membranes. Her spleen is palpable 3 cm below her left costal margin.

Laboratory Results

	Patient	Normal
White blood cell count	13×10^9/L	$4–11 \times 10^9$/L
Hemoglobin	6.0 g/dL	13–16 g/dL
MCV	110 fL	80–99 fL
MCHC	37 g/dL	32–36 g/dL
Platelets	210×10^9/L	$150–350 \times 10^9$/L
Corrected reticulocytes	25%	0.5–2.0%
Total serum bilirubin	5.5 mg/dL	0.3–1.0 mg/dL
Direct bilirubin	0.5 mg/dL	0.1–0.3 mg./dL
Indirect bilirubin	5.0 mg/dL	0.2–0.7 mg/dL

Blood smear examination showed numerous atypical lymphocytes. Polychromasia and microspherocytes appeared against background of spherocytes.

Questions

1. Does this patient have any historical or objective findings suggestive of an inherited hemolytic anemia?
2. Is there more than one active problem?

3. Was the patient's hemoglobin always this low?
4. What further workup might be appropriate?

Additional Laboratory Results

	Patient	Normal
EBV acute serology	Positive	Negative
Direct Coomb's	Positive (i antigen specificity)	Negative
Cold agglutinin	Positive	Negative
Osmotic fragility	Positive	Negative

Family Study

The patient's father, uncle, and two siblings were found to have increased osmotic fragility and low-grade hemolysis.

Diagnosis

Clinically silent hereditary spherocytosis (HS) unmasked by an acute exacerbation precipitated by Epstein-Barr virus (EBV) infection with associated cold agglutinin and accelerated red cell destruction.

Discussion

This is a tricky case that underscores general principles pertaining to (HS) and the fact that real patients can present with more than one illness. In general, HS causes compensated hemolysis with mild anemia, splenomegaly, and episodic jaundice. Often, cases are brought to light by supervening conditions. Occasionally, the associated illness confounds the diagnosis, as in this case. In acute exacerbation caused by B19 parvovirus, the low reticulocyte count can mask the presence of hemolysis. In this case, the EBV-induced cold agglutinin worsens red cell destruction and causes a positive direct Coombs test. Usually, a negative Coombs is a hallmark of HS. Autoimmune hemolysis can produce spherocytes that increase the osmotic fragility (OF), although this is less impressive in cold agglutinin-induced hemolysis. Nevertheless, the OF may be nonspecific in this case. The patient's family history, neonatal jaundice, and the background spherocytosis suggest the possibility of HS. Yet, until the family study is done, the diagnosis is not secure. Another alternative, in case the family is unavailable, is to wait for the transient cold agglutinins to resolve and then to retest the patient for HS. This patient is likely to require transfusional support through the acutely worse anemia. Transfused red cells can also confound the evaluation of HS.

The emergence of problematic HS at the age of 22 suggests that this patient might benefit from splenectomy. After the acute illness resolves, the patient is likely to have chronic hemolytic anemia, splenomegaly made worse by EBV, and identifiable gallstones. If so, the patient would be a good candidate for elective splenectomy and cholecystectomy. Vaccination against encapsulated organisms should be done prior to the procedure. Her father and affected siblings should also be evaluated for possible surgery.

Bibliography

1. Hassoun H, Palek J. Hereditary spherocytosis: a review of the clinical and molecular aspects of the disease. Blood Rev 1996; 10(3);129–147.

2. Lux SE, Palek J. Disorders of the red cell membrane. In: Blood: Principles and Practice of Hematology. Philadelphia: Lippencott, 1995:1701–1818.

CASE STUDY 2

Patient

Fifty-eight-year-old man.

Chief Complaint

Increasing jaundice and fatigue.

Medical History

The patient has a long-standing history of alcoholism. He has been in and out of treatment programs for alcohol abuse. He has had numerous medical complications of chronic alcoholism, such as alcoholic hepatitis, pancreatitis, and alcohol withdrawal syndromes. Several months ago he was told he had cirrhosis. Since then, he claims to be abstaining from alcohol. For several weeks he has noticed progressive weakness, fatigue, and jaundice. He has had normal hemoglobin measurements in the past.

Physical Examination

The patient is thin, with numerous stigmata of severe liver dysfunction, such as palmar erythema, gynecomastia, spider angiomata, ascites, hepatomegaly, and mild asterixis. His breath smells of alcohol. He has moderate scleral icterus and splenomegaly.

Laboratory Results

	Patient	Normal
Hemoglobin	6.0 g/dL	14–17 g/dL
MCV	105 fL	80–99 fL
Corrected reticulocytes	8%	0.5–2.0%
Total serum bilirubin	11 mg/dL	0.3–1.0 mg/dL
Direct bilirubin	4 mg/dL	0.1–0.3 mg/dL
Indirect bilirubin	7 mg/dL	0.2–0.7 mg/dL
SGOT	100 U/mL	10–40 U/mL
SGPT	80 U/mL	10–40 U/mL
Alkaline phosphatase	110 IU/L	21–91 IU/L
LDH	300 U/mL	25–100 U/mL
Haptoglobin	10 mg/dL	128 ± 25 mg/dL
Albumin	2.8 g/100 mL	3.5–5.5 g/100 mL

The patient's erythrocytes show prominent acanthocytosis, polychromasia, and target cells. Platelets and leukocytes are unremarkable.

Questions

1. Do any of these findings suggest a hemolytic etiology of the anemia?
2. What are the different causes of anemia in liver disease patients?
3. Why does the patient have both direct and indirect hyperbilirubinemia?
4. How might liver disease confound the laboratory evaluation of hemolysis?

Diagnosis

Spur cell anemia.

Discussion

Spur cell anemia is among the most common hemolytic syndromes. Because, by definition, this disorder arises in patients with liver disease, the diagnosis is often difficult. For example, jaundice, increased LDH, and low haptoglobin are common in cirrhotic patients without hemolysis. Usually the hyperbilirubinemia in liver disease is mostly direct, but the indirect bilirubin is often elevated. In this case, due to hepatocellular damage, there is elevated direct bilirubin more than usual for hemolysis alone. If this direct hyperbilirubinemia is more pronounced, the diagnosis of hemolysis may be obscured.

Diverse pathophysiologies lead to anemia in liver disease patients. These include bleeding varices, blood loss at any site due to coagulopathy, folate deficiency, thiamin deficiency, direct bone marrow toxicity, hypophosphatemia with hemolysis, Zieve's syndrome, spur cell anemia, and others. Blood loss and hemolysis both lead to reticulocytosis. Internal blood loss may give rise to indirect hyperbilirubinemia as well. The peripheral blood morphology provides important diagnostic clues. In spur cell anemia, acanthocytosis is highly suggestive of the diagnosis. Other causes of acquired acanthocytosis must be considered, such as vitamin E deficiency. In this case, congenital hemolytic processes are rendered less likely by the previously normal hemoglobin measurements.

There are no routinely available confirmatory tests for spur cell anemia. Measurement of red cell membrane lipid composition is a research tool. Because there is no single diagnostic test, the physician must use the peripheral smear, laboratory evidence of hemolysis, and the clinical setting to make the diagnosis.

Bibliography

1. Cooper RA. Hemolytic syndromes and red cell membrane abnormalities in liver disease. Semin Hematol 1980; 17(2):103–112.

SELECTED READINGS

1. Allen DW, Manning N. Cholesterol loading of membranes of normal erythrocytes inhibits phospholipid repair and arachidonoyl-CoA:1-palmitoyl-sn-glycero-3-phosphocholine acyl transferase: a model of spur cell anemia. Blood 1996; 87(8):3489–3493.
2. Cooper RA. Hemolytic syndromes and red cell membrane abnormalities in liver disease. Semin Hematol 1980; 17(2):103–112.
3. Gallagher PG, Forget BG. Hematologically important mutations: spectrin variants in hereditary elliptocytosis and hereditary pyropoikilocytosis. Blood Cells Mol Dis 1996; 22(20):254–258.
4. Hassoun H, Palek J. Hereditary spherocytosis: a review of the clinical and molecular aspects of the disease. Blood Rev. 1996; 10(3):129–147.
5. Lux SE, Palek J. Disorders of the red cell membrane. In: Blood: Principles and Practice of Hematology. Philadelphia: Lippencott, 1995:1707–1818.
6. Palek J, Jarolim P. Clinical expression and laboratory detection of red blood cell membranes proteins mutations. Semin Hematol 1993; 30(4):249–283.
7. Parker CJ. Molecular basis of paroxysmal nocturnal hemoglobinuria. Stem Cells 1996; 14(4):396–411.
8. Rosse WF, Ware RE. The molecular basis of paroxysmal nocturnal hemoglobinuria. Blood 1995; 86(9):3277–3286.
9. Winkelmann JC, Forget BG. Erythroid and nonerythroid spectrins. Blood 1993; 81(12):3173–3185.

20

Abnormal Red Cell Metabolism

Abdus Saleem
Baylor College of Medicine, Houston, Texas

I. INTRODUCTION

Energy for red cell function is dependent on the glycolytic pathways (Fig. 1). Several red cell enzymes which play an active role in glycolysis are critical for red cell function and survival. The major pathway is the Embden-Meyerhof pathway (EMF), in which glucose is broken down to lactose and two molecules of ATP are generated, which are sufficient for the energy needs of the red cell. The second pathway, the hexose monophosphate pathway (HMP), which utilizes about 5–10% of the glucose, is the only source of reduced nicotinamide adenine dinucleotide phosphate (NADPH). NADPH is generated from nicotinamide adenine dinucleotide phosphate (NADP) in the HMP pathway by glucose 6-phosphate dehydrogenase (G6PD). NADPH acts as a coenzyme which converts glutathione (GSSH) to reduced glutathione (GSH). GSH protects the red cell from oxidative injury. Many drugs and organisms produce superoxide anion (O^-) and hydrogen peroxide (H_2O_2). These oxidants can destroy red cells. However, GSH rapidly reduces the oxidant anions, and as long as there is adequate supply of NADPH, enough GSH is available to protect the red cells. Although deficiency of any enzyme in the EMF or HMP can cause hemolytic anemia, the most commonly encountered deficiencies are G6PD deficiency and pyruvate kinase deficiency.

II. GLUCOSE 6-PHOSPHATE DEHYDROGENASE DEFICIENCY

G6PD deficiency is an inherited disorder in which the diminished activity of the enzyme results in hemolytic anemia, particularly after the administration of certain drugs (1). As pointed out earlier, G6PD plays an important role in maintaining adequate levels of NADPH and glutathione in reduced form (GSH). GSH preserves the sulfhydryl groups in the red cell membrane and prevents oxidative injury. In G6PD-deficient red cells, the decrease in sulfhydryl groups leads to release of heme from globin, which denatures the globin. Denatured globin attaches itself to the membrane of red cell to form Heinz bodies. The activity of the enzyme G6PD decreases rapidly with the age of the red cell, being highest in the reticulocyte. Thus older red cells are even more susceptible to oxidative injury.

A. Prevalence

G6PD deficiency has been reported from all over the world. A higher frequency is noted in tropical and subtropical areas. More than 350 variants have been reported. There is a great

The Embden-Meyerhof pathway:

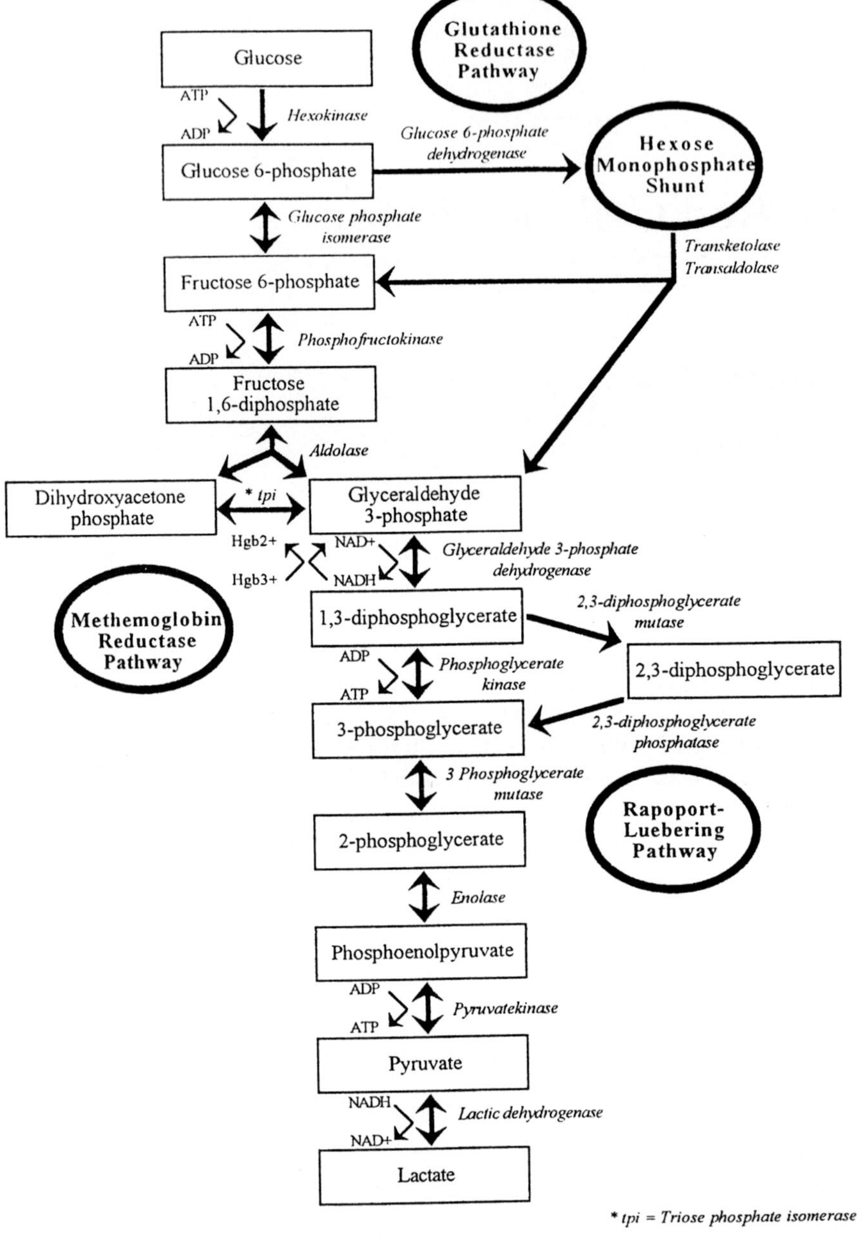

Figure 1 Glucose is broken down anaerobically into lactose in the Embden-Meyerhof pathway, generating ATP, 2′3-DPG in the Rapoport-Luebering pathway, and reducing methemoglobin in the methemoglobin-reductase pathway. An ample supply of reduced glutathione is maintained in the glutathione reductase pathway by aerobic glycolysis in the hexose monophosphate shunt (see text). (Reproduced from Powers LW, ed. Diagnostic Hematology, St. Louis: Mosby Year Book, 1989 with permission.)

variation in the clinical expression of these variant enzymes. The most common type, designated G6PD B, has normal activity. This type is common worldwide. An African variant, G6PD A+, also has normal activity. It is present in 20% of American black males. Another variant, G6PD A–, exhibits only about 5–10% enzymic activity and manifests as moderate to severe hemolysis after exposure to oxidant drugs. G6PD A– is seen in 10% of American blacks. G6PD Mediterranean is common in the white Mediterranean population. G6PD Canton is common in Asians. Both the Mediterranean and Canton types are unstable and exhibit very low G6PD activity (less than 1%); patients may show life-long hemolytic anemia and severe hemolysis after exposure to oxidant drugs (2).

The gene for the expression of G6PD is located on the X chromosome (3). The nucleotide sequence of G6PD has been encoded from cloned cDNA (4). The deficiency is fully expressed in males, and the heterozygous females are apparently normal. G6PD activity in a carrier female is intermediate between that of a normal subject and an affected male.

B. Clinical Features

The clinical features of G6PD deficiency vary greatly. Most patients have no signs or symptoms. Some patients suffer from chronic hemolytic anemia. Episodes of acute hemolysis may occur as a result of (a) administration of oxidant drugs (Table 1), (b) acute infection, (c) a metabolic episode, or (d) spontaneously in infancy. The exact mechanism of red cell destruction by the drugs is still not clear. It is probable that drugs such as methylene blue and phenazine monosulfate act by oxidizing NADPH to NADP, while ascorbic acid, nitrofurantoin, and doxorubicin act by oxidizing GSH (5). Typically, hemolysis occurs 1–3 days after the administration of the offending drug. There is a rapid fall in hematocrit, and the urine turns dark brown to black. Heinz bodies may be seen in erythrocytes. In early stages, hemoglobinemia and hemoglobinuria are present. Later, methemoglobin and methemalbumin are seen in serum. Serum bilirubin is elevated and haptoglobin is absent. Within 4–6 days, hemolysis generally subsides; reticulocytes appear, followed by a rise in hemoglobin and hematocrit. Hemolysis in the G6PD A– type is generally self-limited even if the drug is continued, but in the G6PD Mediterranean type, hemolysis is more severe and continues as long as the drug is being given.

Ingestion of fava beans (*Vicia fava*) in susceptible subjects (favism) may precipitate severe attack of hemolysis (6). Favism is most commonly seen in the Mediterranean countries and in the Middle East, although isolated cases have been reported from all over the world. Favism

Table 1 Oxidant Drugs and Chemicals that May Cause Hemolytic Anemia in G6PD Deficiency

Acetanilide
Chloramphenicol
Dapsone
Methylene blue
Naphthalene
Nitrofurantoin
Phenylhydrazine
Primaquine
Sulfa drugs
Toluidine blue
Trinitrotoluene

occurs most commonly in boys between the ages of 1 and 5 years. Symptoms of acute intravascular hemolysis occur within a few hours after ingestion. Favism is most commonly associated with G6PD Mediterranean. It has not been reported with G6PD A– type.

Infants with G6PD Mediterranean have a higher tendency to develop icterus neonatorum (7). Black Americans with G6PD A– variant appear to be at minimal risk. The cause of neonatal jaundice is not clear. Often there is no history of exposure to drugs by the mother or infant. Phototherapy has been tried successfully in some infants.

Newton and Bass (8) described the first case of hereditary nonspherocytic hemolytic anemia (HNSHA). Variants associated with chronic hemolysis have been reported in black Americans, Caucasians, and Asians. The symptoms appear at birth or in early childhood. These patients are anemic and mildly jaundiced. Administration of oxidant drugs or an acute infection can precipitate acute hemolysis. Splenomegaly is often present; however, splenectomy is not always beneficial.

C. Diagnosis

G6PD deficiency is suspected in patients who develop acute hemolytic anemia after administration of oxidant drugs or after an infectious episode. G6PD deficiency is also suspected in patients with hereditary nonimmune hemolytic anemia. Several commercial kits are available to screen for G6PD deficiency (9). Two commonly used tests are as follows.

Fluorescent spot test: Whole blood is added to a mixture of glucose 6-phosphate, NADP, and saponin. A drop of this mixture is placed on a filter paper and observed for fluorescence in ultraviolet light. In the presence of G6PD, NADP is converted to NADPH, which shows bright fluorescence.

Ascorbate cyanide test: Whole blood is incubated with a mixture of sodium cyanide and sodium ascorbate. Hydrogen peroxide becomes available to oxidize hemoglobin to methemoglobin, showing a brown color. Sodium cyanide is used in the test to inhibit catalase in the red cells. In the absence of G6PD, the reaction takes place more rapidly than in normal cells.

These tests are sensitive for detecting affected male subjects, but are insensitive for detecting female carriers. Also, during a hemolytic episode most of the enzyme deficient cells may be destroyed and younger cells with a high proportion of reticulocytes may have normal levels of enzyme, giving a false negative result. Thus, it may be necessary to repeat the test 2–3 months after an acute attack.

Quantative assays are based on incubation of hemolysate with glucose 6-phosphate and NADP. The rate of reduction of NADP to NADPH is measured spectrophotometrically at 340 nm. The results are expressed in international units per gram of hemoglobin (2).

D. Treatment

No treatment is necessary for patients with few or no symptoms, except for avoidance of oxidant drugs. Acute infection should be treated promptly with appropriate antibiotics.

During a hemolytic episode, the drugs that cause hemolysis should be discontinued immediately. It is important to maintain good flow of urine to avert renal damage caused by hemoglobinuria. Blood transfusion can be life-saving, but the donor should be screened for G6PD deficiency. In newborns with severe neonatal jaundice, exchange transfusion should be considered. Results of splenectomy are generally disappointing.

III. HEXOSE KINASE DEFICIENCY

Hexose kinase (HK) is the first enzyme in the EMF pathway. HK catalyzes the conversion of glucose to glucose 6-phosphate and plays an important role in the regulation of glucose consumption. HK deficiency leads to decreased glucose utilization and decreased adenosine triphosphate (ATP) production. Levels of 2′3-diphosphoglycerate (DPG) are usually low, and the amount of lactose produced is decreased. HK deficiency is a rare disorder that causes hereditary nonspherocytic hemolytic anemia (10). The HK gene has been located on chromosome 10 (11). The disorder is inherited as an autosomal recessive. Heterozygotes are usually normal. In homozygotes a mild to moderate degree of hemolysis is present. The blood picture is normocytic and normochromic. Spherocytes are not seen. Osmotic fragility on a fresh sample is normal. An incubated fragility test, if carefully performed, is sometimes useful. This test measures the amount of spontaneous hemolysis after 48 hr of incubation at 37°C. Normal red cells show little hemolysis (0.2–4.0%) at 48 hr. If hemolysis is measured after addition of glucose or adenosine triphosphate (ATP) prior to incubation, a reduction in hemolysis is seen with normal red cells. Red cells with HK deficiency show mild increase in hemolysis (1.0–6.0%), with some reduction if glucose or ATP is added to the test (type I pattern). In contrast, the pyruvate kinase-deficient red cells show marked hemolysis (8–44%) after 48 hr of incubation. The addition of glucose to the test does not decrease the hemolysis, while addition of ATP significantly corrects the degree of hemolysis (type II pattern).

Generally no treatment is required. Splenectomy improves the red cell life span in some patients.

IV. PYRUVATE KINASE DEFICIENCY

Erythrocytic pyruvate kinase (PK) converts phosphoenolpyruvate (PEP) to pyruvic acid in the EMF pathway. PK is one of the last enzymes in the EMF pathway. However, it participates in generating ATP. In PK deficiency, concentrations of ATP and lactate are decreased, while products prior to the block, including 2′3-DPG, are increased (14). PK deficiency is an uncommon hereditary disorder that sometimes causes nonspherocytic hemolytic anemia (12). PK deficiency is transmitted as an autosomal recessive disorder. Heterozygotes are usually normal, while homozygotes may show highly variable degree of hemolysis ranging from severe neonatal jaundice to a fully compensated hemolytic anemia. The blood smear shows normocytic and normochromic red cells. Splenomegaly is often present in patients with jaundice. Spherocytes are not present. Reticulocytes are increased. Osmotic fragility on fresh blood is normal. Blood incubated at 37°C for 48 hr shows increased hemolysis (8–44%) which is corrected by addition of ATP but not glucose (type II pattern) (13).

PK catalyzes the conversion of PEP to pyruvate, which reduces NADH to NAD. Deficiency of PK leads to loss of fluorescence of NADH which is measured spectrophotometrically at 340 nm. The results are expressed in international units per gram of hemoglobin (2).

No treatment is required for asymptomatic or mild cases. Severe cases may require blood transfusion, especially in infancy or after an episode of acute infection. Splenectomy reduces the need for frequent transfusions and is recommended in severe cases.

V. GLUCOSEPHOSPHATE ISOMERASE DEFICIENCY

Glucosephosphate isomerase (GPI) catalyzes the conversion of glucose 6-phosphate to fructose 6-phosphate. GPI-deficient cells accumulate glucose 6-phosphate and are deficient in ATP and

2′3-DPG. GPI deficiency, although rare, is the third most common red cell enzymopathy after G6PD deficiency and PK deficiency (2). The structural gene is located on chromosome 19. GPI deficiency is inherited as an autosomal recessive. Homozygotes for GPI deficiency show variable degrees of anemia, while heterozygotes are generally asymptomatic. Anemia is nonspherocytic, with marked polychromasia and reticulocytosis. Hemolytic crises may occur during an episode of infection. The spleen is frequently enlarged. Osmotic fragility is normal. Autohemolysis test shows increased hemolysis at 48 hr, and is partially corrected by glucose and ATP (type I pattern). A fluorescent test is available for screening the deficiency, and the diagnosis is established on quantitative assay of the enzyme (2). Patients with a severe form of disease may require repeated transfusions. Splenectomy is not curative, but reduces transfusion requirement (2).

VI. RARE ENZYMOPATHIES

Rare cases of hemolytic anemia as a result of deficiency of phosphofructokinase, triosephosphate isomerase, and 2′3-diphosphoglycerate mutase have been reported. A summary of their clinical features is given in Table 2 (15).

CASE STUDY 1

Patient

Thirty-year-old black male.

Chief Complaint

Weakness, palpitation, shortness of breath, and dark urine.

The patient was admitted to the hospital 2 days after completion of antimalarial therapy with quinine and pamaquine. On admission his urine was black. Physical examination revealed a rapid pulse, icteric sclera, and tenderness over the spleen and liver.

Medical History

The patient is a veteran of the Vietnam War. He recently returned from a visit to Vietnam. Three days before admission he had fever with chills, and his blood smear was positive for falciparum malaria.

Laboratory Tests

Hemoglobin 7.0 g/dL, hematocrit (Hct) 21.1%, white blood cells (WBC) 12.9×10^9/L normal differential. No malarial parasites seen on admission. Serum haptoglobin absent.

Urine: Black, protein +++, blood +++, red blood cells absent, granular casts +++.

G6PD 4.7 IU/G of hemoglobin (normal 7.9–16.2 IU/G of hemoglobin).

Questions

1. What is the most likely diagnosis?
2. Was it necessary to treat the patient with pamaquine?
3. Explain the findings in the urine.
4. Which medications should the patient avoid in future?

Table 2 Erythrocytic Enzymopathies Associated with Hemolytic Anemia

Enzymopathy	Inheritance	Frequency	Clinical severity	Response to splenectomy	Other features	Selected references
Glucose 6-phosphate dehydrogenase	Sex linked	Common	Moderate to severe	—	—	1
Hexose kinase	Autosomal recessive	Rare	Mild to severe	Moderate	Low 2,3-DPG levels, poor tolerance to anemia	11
Glucose phosphate isomerase	Autosomal recessive	Uncommon	Moderate to severe	Good	Propensity for hemolytic crisis during infection	2
Phosphofructokinase	Autosomal recessive	Rare	Mild	None	Myopathy, erythrocytosis, gout	15
Triosephosphate isomerase	Autosomal recessive	Rare	Moderate to severe	Moderate	Neuromuscular disorders, cardiac arrhythmias	15
Phosphoglycerate kinase	Sex linked	Rare	Mild to severe	Moderate	Neurologic and mental defects	2
2,3-Diphosphoglycerate	Autosomal recessive	Rare	None to severe	Not reported	—	2
Pyruvate kinase	Autosomal recessive	Uncommon	Moderate to severe	Moderate	—	12

Source: Modified from Ref. 15.

Diagnosis

G6PD deficiency: hemolysis secondary to oxidant.

Discussion

This case is an example of acute hemolysis in a patient with G6PD deficiency following the administration of an oxidant antimalarial drug, pamaquine, resulting in severe anemia, hemoglobinuria, and renal damage. Pamaquine is useful in *Plasmodium vivax* infections, as it eradicates the exoerythrocytic cycle in the liver. *Plasmodium falciparum* does not colonize in liver, so it is unnecessary to use pamaquine in falciparum infections. After an episode of acute hemolysis, urine may be red due to the presence of hemoglobin. On standing, hemoglobin is oxidized to methemoglobin and urine becomes brown to black. Hemoglobin and methemoglobin give a positive occult blood test. Hemoglobinuria also damages the kidney and it is not uncommon to see albuminuria and granular casts in urine. The patient has moderate deficiency of G6PD, so all oxidant drugs (Table 1) should be avoided.

CASE STUDY 2

Patient

Thirty-seven-year-old male donor.

Presentation

The patient presented to a blood donor center for routine blood donation. He had donated blood six times before. His hemoglobin was over 12.5 g/dL on each occasion. This time his hemoglobin was 11.4 g/dL. He was referred to the medical service for evaluation.

Family History

Mother alive and well. Father suffered from episodes of mild icterus and dark urine.

Drug History

No medication.

Physical Examination

The patient is slightly jaundiced. Liver and spleen are not palpable. Other systems are normal.

Laboratory Results

Hemoglobin 11.4 g/dL, Hct 34.7%, WBC 8.5×10^9/L. Platelets 245×10^9/L.

Blood smear showed normocytic normochromic red cells, moderate polychromasia, moderate anisocytosis, moderate poikilocytosis.

Reticulocytes 10.8%, bilirubin 1.9, haptoglobin absent.

Urine: Bile neg, urobilinogen ++.

Questions

1. What is the most likely diagnosis?
2. Should splenectomy be advised?

Additional Laboratory Results

Osmatic fragility: normal.

Autohemolysis at 48 hr: 20.8% (normal 0–4%). Not corrected by addition of glucose, but corrected by addition of ATP (type II pattern).

Red cell enzyme studies:

G6PD normal
HK normal
PK 5.8 IU/G hemoglobin (normal 11.0–19.0 IU/G hemoglobin)

Discussion

This patient has pyruvate kinase deficiency. Several hereditary red cell enzyme defects can result in nonspherocytic hemolytic anemia. Common among those are G6PD, pyruvate kinase (PK), and hexose kinase (HK) deficiencies. Osmotic fragility is normal in all of the above deficiencies. Autohemolysis test after 48-hr incubation is often abnormal in PK deficiency and HK deficiency. However, the abnormality is corrected with glucose or ATP in HK deficiency, and with ATP only in PK deficiency. The defect should be confirmed by quantitative enzyme levels. Splenectomy should be reserved only for serious cases: It is not curative, but it reduces the transfusion requirement.

REFERENCES

1. Dacie J. Hereditary enzyme-deficiency haemolytic anaemias III: deficiency of glucose-6-phosphate dehydrogenase. In: The Haemolytic Anaemias. Vol. I. Edinburgh: Churchill Livingstone, 1985:364.
2. Beutler E. Hemolytic Anemia in Disorders of Red Cell Metabolism. New York: Plenum, 1978:266.
3. Childs B, et al. A genetic study of a defect in glutathione metabolism of the erythrocyte. Bull Johns Hopkins Hosp 1958; 102:21.
4. Prisco HB, et al. Isolation of human G6PD cDNA clones: primary structure of protein and unusual 5′ non-coding region. Nucleic Acids Res 1986; 14:2511.
5. Beutler E, Dern RJ, Alving AS. The hemolytic effect of primaquine, III. A study of primaquine-sensitive erythrocytes. J Lab Clin Med 1954; 44:177.
6. Vergnes H, et al. Glucose-6-phosphate dehydrogenase Toulouse: a new variant with marked instability and severe deficiency discovered in a family of Mediterranean ancestry. Acta Haematol (Basel) 1974; 51:240.
7. Doxiadis SA, et al. Risk of severe jaundice in glucose-6-phosphate-dehydrogenase deficiency of the newborn: differences in population groups. Lancet 1964; 2:1210.
8. Newton WA Jr, Bass JC. Glutathione-sensitive chronic non-spherocytic hemolytic anemia. J Dis Child 1958; 96:501.
9. Beutler E, Mitchell M. Special modifications of the fluorescent method for glucose-6-phosphate dehydrogenase deficiency. Blood 1968; 32:816.
10. Tanaka KR, Valentine WN, Miwa S. Pyruvate kinase deficiency hereditary nonspherocytic hemolytic anemia. Blood 1962; 19:267.
11. Dallapiccola B, et al. Regional mapping of hexose kinase-I within the short arm of chromosome 10. Hum Hered 1984; 34:156.
12. Mentzer WC Jr. Pyruvate kinase deficiency and disorders of glycolysis. In: Natan DG, Oski FA, ed. Hematology of Infancy and Childhood. Vol. 1. 2nd ed. Philadelphia: Saunders, 1981:584.
13. Dacie J. Hereditary enzyme-deficiency haemolytic anaemia, I: Deficiencies of enzymes of Embden-Meyerhof (EM) pathway. In: Hereditary Haemolytic Anaemia. Vol. I. Edinburgh: Churchill Livingstone, 1985:287.
14. Tanaka KR, Paglia DE. Pyruvate kinase (PK) deficiency. Semin Hematol 1971; 8:367.
15. Saleem A. Hereditary hemolytic anemia associated with erythrocytic enzymopathies. In: Bick RL, ed. Clinical and Laboratory Practice. Vol. I. St. Louis: Mosby, 1993:291.

21

Immune Hemolytic Anemias

Joseph P. Yoe
North General Hospital, New York, New York

Ronald A. Sacher
Georgetown University Medical Center, Washington, D.C.

I. DEFINITION

The immune hemolytic anemias are a heterogeneous group of disorders characterized by in-vivo antibody-mediated destruction of circulating erythrocytes. Immune hemolytic anemias are classified as follows:

1. Alloimmune hemolytic anemias
   a. Hemolytic transfusion reactions
   b. Hemolytic disease of the newborn
2. Autoimmune hemolytic anemias
   a. Warm antibody type
   b. Cold antibody type
   c. Mixed warm/cold type
3. Drug-induced immune hemolytic anemias (Chapter 25)

II. RED BLOOD CELL ANTIBODIES

Destruction of red blood cells (RBCs) by either IgM or IgG antibodies with or without complement causes alloimmune (isoimmune) and autoimmune hemolytic anemias. The antibodies have these general features:

1. IgM antibodies usually cause immediate intravascular destruction of sensitized RBCs, or their sequestration and destruction in the liver.
2. IgG antibodies most often sensitize RBCs that are subsequently sequestered and destroyed in the spleen.

IgM antibodies are referred to as complete antibodies or saline agglutinins, since they are large molecules and can easily bridge the negative repelling charges between RBCs. (This negative charge normally keeps the individual RBCs several hundred angstroms apart.) Since all antibodies have two antigen-combining sites, the IgM molecule that is actually a pentamere can attach to two or more RBCs, causing agglutination. All of the IgM antibodies (including anti-A, -B, and -H antibodies and cold agglutinins) mediate their effects through complement activation. Destruction of RBCs by complement fixation begins in one of two ways:

1. Clq binding by two proximal activated antibody sites. A single IgM molecule can provide such multiple binding sites. This binding results in erythrophagocytosis, usually within the liver.
2. C5–C9 activation causing direct erythrocyte membrane puncture and lysis.

The Clq binding leads to C4 activation, which ultimately produces the major fragment C3b. This fragment adheres firmly to the RBC membrane and is capable of reacting with receptors on phagocytic cells. The C3b may be cleaved by the C3b inactivator (if the cell is not phagocytized), forming fragments C3c and C3d or C3d,g in the case of cold agglutinins. The C3d or C3d,g cannot react with macrophage receptor sites. It appears to prevent further C3b attachment, thereby protecting the cell, and accounts for the positive Coombs test when polyspecific antihuman globulin containing anti-C3 is used.

IgG antibodies are much smaller than IgM antibodies. Clearance of IgG-coated erythrocyte is more complex than that of IgM-sensitized cells and usually not through the complement-mediated intravascular lysis of sensitized erythrocytes. Since the IgG antibodies occupy antigenic sites on the red cell, they may block agglutination of additional RBCs by IgM antibodies, thus the name "blocking" or "incomplete" antibodies. Although the IgG antibody molecule has two binding sites, generally they are unable to react completely with RBCs suspended in saline because of the distance between RBCs imposed by the negative surface charge. Therefore, the IgG antibodies coat the surface of the RBCs but do not cause actual agglutination in saline. Examples of IgG antibodies include:

1. Rh isoantibodies that form after repeated exposure to Rh antigen
2. Warm autoantibodies of idiopathic or secondary acquired autoimmune hemolytic anemia
3. Most drug-related antibodies

There are two mechanisms in the clearance and destruction of IgG-coated red cells: (1) the antibody-mediated adhesion and eventual phagocytosis of sensitized red cells by mononuclear cells, and (2) the augmentation of this process by complement. Adhesion and phagocytosis of IgG-sensitized red cells is mediated by the presence of receptors for the Fc portion of IgG on the phagocytic cells. These receptor sites appear to be specific for IgG1 and IgG3 and do not react with the Fc portions of IgG2, IgG4, or other types of immunoglobulin, including IgM. The concomitant presence of activated complement components (C3b) on the red cell surface greatly augments the clearance of the IgG-sensitized erythrocytes.

In addition to IgM and IgG antibodies causing autoimmune hemolytic anemia, approximately 20–30% of all patients have only C3d on their RBCs. Also, rare patients have been described with only IgA or IgM on the red cell surface. (The IgM was not associated with complement.)

III. ANTI-HUMAN GLOBULIN TEST (COOMBS TEST)

Since the IgG antibodies are too short to bridge the gap between RBCs and cause agglutination, a human antiglobulin serum (Coombs serum) was produced in rabbits or goats, supplying the link necessary for the reaction. Recently, the Coombs serum has been produced by monoclonal antibody techniques. Most of these commercial Coombs sera detect both IgG and C3d on the red cell (polyspecific). However, monospecific antiglobulin sera such as anti-IgG and anti-complement are also available.

There are two kinds of anti-human globulin tests:

1. *The direct anti-human globulin test* detects IgG antibodies and/or C3d coating the circulating RBCs (in vivo). A drop of Coombs serum is added to a saline suspension of the patient's washed RBCs. If either IgG or C3d is attached to the antigenic sites of the RBC membrane, the Coombs serum forms bonds between the RBCs, causing clumping (agglutination) (Fig. 1).
2. *The indirect anti-human globulin test* detects free IgG in the patient's serum (Fig. 2). The patient's serum is incubated with a mixture of group O RBCs that contain most of the known RBC antigens. The RBCs are then washed, suspended in saline, and mixed with anti-human globulin serum. If the patient's serum contains IgG antibodies or C3d that can attach to the group O RBCs during preliminary incubation, the RBCs clump on addition of the anti-human globulin serum. The strength and manner in which they react, including the pattern of reactivity, assist in determining the specificity of the antibody.

The RBCs are often sensitized with IgG and complement, or with either IgG or complement. These proteins are best detected by antiglobulin tests using monospecific antiglobulin sera such as anti-IgG and anticomplement sera. IgA and IgM are sometimes detected, but they are usually found in conjunction with IgG and complement.

The patient's RBCs are checked with dilutions of antiglobulin serum, giving semiquantitative estimates of the amount of protein which is sensitizing the RBCs. This estimate may be particularly useful in following the treatment of a single patient. Although it is acceptable to dilute antiglobulin sera for approximations of RBC-bound IgG, the antiglobulin sera should never be diluted when used for antibody detection or crossmatching.

IV. ALLOIMMUNE HEMOLYTIC ANEMIA

Alloantibodies are antibodies that react with RBCs from the same species but not with RBCs from the individual making the antibody, e.g., antibodies to transfused erythrocyte. Hemolytic

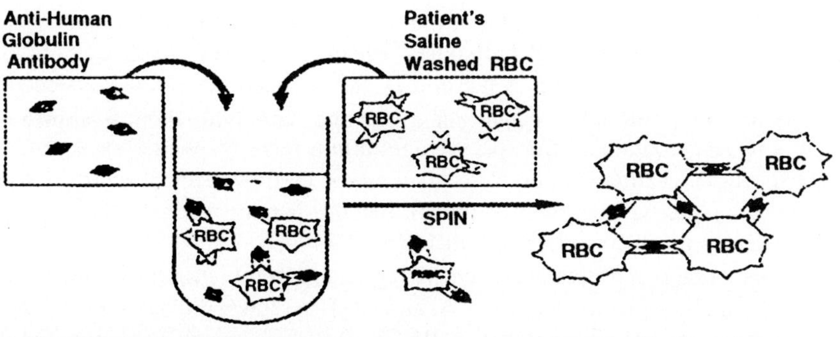

Figure 1 Direct anti-human globulin test.

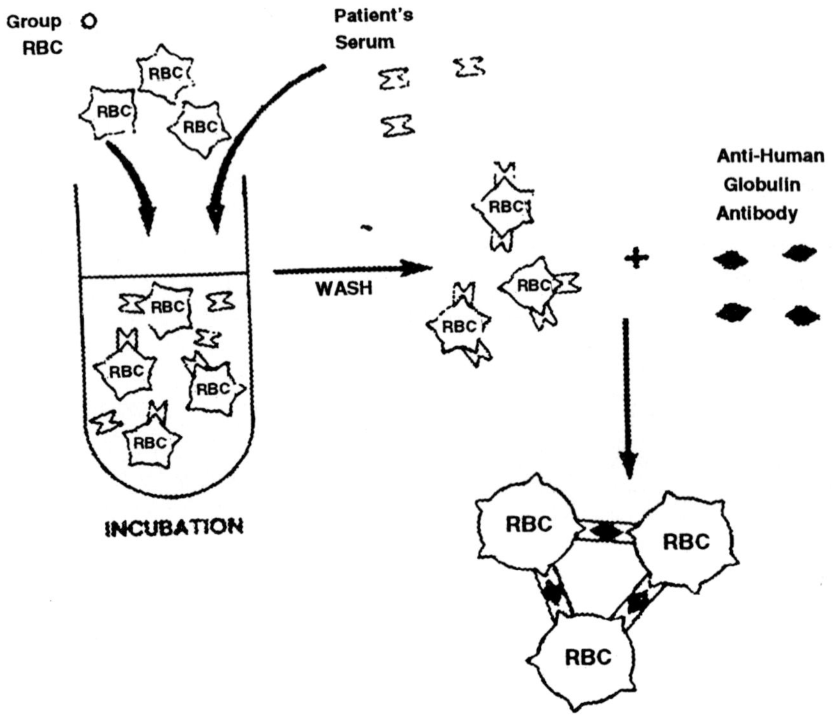

Figure 2 Indirect anti-human globulin test.

anemias caused by these antibodies are divided into two groups: hemolytic transfusion reactions and hemolytic disease of the newborn.

V. HEMOLYTIC TRANSFUSION REACTIONS

A. ABO Incompatibility

Antibodies to the A and B antigens develop naturally in early infancy. Since natural antibodies do not normally develop against one's own cells, persons of blood type B possess anti-A antibodies and persons with blood group A possess anti-B alloantibodies. Individuals with blood type O possess both anti-A and anti-B antibodies, since they possess neither A nor B antigens, and AB persons possess neither anti-A nor anti-B. Severe transfusion reactions occur when a patient is given blood of the mismatched ABO type. In an incompatible transfusion reaction, the recipient's plasma containing the specific agglutinins destroys the donor's RBCs.

Almost all ABO reactions are due to administrative and/or clerical error. Therefore, the greatest emphasis should be placed on properly identifying the patient when collecting the blood sample to be tested and prior to the actual infusion of the blood.

The minor ABO transfusion reaction is observed when plasma from a group O donor with high titers of anti-A and anti-B is given to a group A, B, or AB recipient. In such a situation these antibodies may hemolyze the recipient's own RBCs. However, group O donor blood given as packed red blood cells is usually safe for any recipient, because only a small amount of plasma is present. Even so, the safest transfusion practice is to transfuse only ABO group-specific blood.

B. Rh Reactions

Since the D antigen is the most antigenic of the Rh antigens, hemolysis due to incompatibility occurs in the Rh-negative patient who mistakenly receives Rh-positive blood. However, since anti-D antibodies do not occur naturally, the patient must have been sensitized previously to RBCs containing the D antigen. This situation occurs if:

1. Rh-negative persons of either sex receive Rh-positive RBCs.
2. Rh-negative females are sensitized by Rh-positive fetal cells that gain access to maternal circulation, e.g., during delivery or an abortion.

C. Delayed Hemolytic Reactions

Hemolysis that does not immediately follow transfusion presents a diagnostic problem. Findings may range from a less than expected rise in hemoglobin to an obvious hemolytic transfusion reaction (fever, chills, hemoglobinuria), as with anti-Kidd antibodies. The occurrence of delayed hemolytic transfusion reactions has been observed up to 3 weeks posttransfusion. These findings are the result of an anamnestic immune response in a patient already primarily immunized to a specific blood cell antigen. The delayed transfusion reaction is indicated by:

1. An antecedent transfusion
2. A mixed-field agglutination of the direct antiglobulin test
3. Detection of a new alloantibody

Antibodies responsible for delayed hemolytic transfusions include anti-Jk^a, anti E, c, and e in the Rh system, anti-K, and anti-Fy^a.

D. Management of Hemolytic Transfusion Reactions

The main goal of therapy is to prevent shock, renal, and coagulation complications. Therapy consists of the following:

1. Hydration with either crystalloids or colloid must be initiated immediately to maintain the blood pressure and to increase adequate urine flow rate to 100 mL/hr.
2. Using potent diuretics such as furosemide (80–120 mg i.v., repeated as necessary) to prevent oliguria. Mannitol, an osmotic diuretic, is not of proven value and can add further complications if oliguric renal failure develops.
3. Administering appropriate vasoactive drugs, especially dopamine, may be effective against both hypotension and impaired renal perfusion.
4. Management of coagulopathy: The patient may require support of the defective hemostatic mechanisms with platelets and cryoprecipitate or fresh frozen plasma.
5. Once renal failure is established, further supportive measures including fluid restriction, management of electrolyte balance, and dialysis are required.
6. In the event of massive intravascular hemolytic transfusion reactions, exchange transfusion has been performed, but most reactions may be amenable to conservative therapy.

VI. ALLOIMMUNE HEMOLYTIC DISEASE OF THE NEWBORN (HDN)

A. Etiology

When fetal RBCs cross the placenta into the maternal circulation, they stimulate the production of maternal antibodies against a foreign RBC antigen inherited from the father (i.e., mother Rh negative, father Rh positive, and fetus Rh positive). These antibodies (IgG class) may return to the fetal circulation and lead to the eventual destruction of the fetal RBCs. Although fetal–maternal ABO incompatibility is much more common, most cases of clinically significant HDN are caused by Rh incompatibility. HDN due to Rh incompatibility has been greatly reduced because the widespread use of passive immune therapy with anti-Rh_0 (D)IgG antibodies given to Rh-negative women at risk. Minor or atypical antigens (c, E, K) now account for almost two-thirds of non-ABO isoimmunizations.

B. Clinical Findings

1. Jaundice occurring as a result of RBC destruction is generally absent at birth because bilirubin is transferred readily across the placenta, but it becomes evident within 24 hr. Jaundice occurring within 24 hr of birth almost always indicates a hemolytic anemia.
2. Kernicterus (deposition of indirect bilirubin in the brain tissue) occurs in severe cases if the infant is not given exchange transfusions to lower the circulating bilirubin level. Kernicterus develops when indirect bilirubin is above 200 mg/L, but the critical level is lower in premature infants and those with acidosis.
3. Anemia is usually mild in most erythroblastic infants; little or no pallor is observed. In severe cases, congestive heart failure and even hydrops fetalis occurs.
4. Hepatosplenomegaly varies with the severity of the disease, from absent to massive (as in hydrops fetalis).
5. Intracranial and pulmonary hemorrhage may occur in severe cases. Occasionally, patients have widespread cutaneous "blueberry muffin" lesions caused by islands of dermal erythropoiesis.
6. Others: pulmonary hypoplasia has been described in babies suffering from severe Rh disease. Fetal and neonatal hyperinsulinemia with neonatal hypoglycemia also have been noted.

C. Laboratory Findings

1. Peripheral Blood

1. Marked polychromasia, anisocytosis, and many nucleated RBCs are seen on peripheral smear. Spherocytes are absent in Rh incompatibility, but are seen in ABO incompatibility.
2. Reticulocytes are moderately to markedly elevated.
3. Leukocytosis, as a result of an increase in neutrophils, is frequently present.
4. Thrombocytopenia may be encountered with platelet counts $<50 \times 10^9$/L.
5. Hemoglobin is <140 g/L in cord blood. These values are considered abnormal and occur in about one-half of affected infants. Hemoglobin levels of 30–50 g/L have been observed in hydrops fetalis.

2. Serum Bilirubin

Hyperbilirubinemia is usually related to the unconjugated indirect bilirubin. Values at birth may be only slightly higher than the upper limit of normal (50 μmol/L at birth), because excess bilirubin is handled by the placenta before birth. Cord bilirubin values higher than 90 μmol/L are unusual; when present, they are suggestive of severe disease. In severely affected infants, peak bilirubin levels are reached by the third neonatal day and may reach 550–850 μmol/L. Levels >350 μmol/L greatly increase the risk of kernicterus. Only unbound bilirubin is toxic to the central nervous system, and binding capacity of albumin for bilirubin is therefore of critical importance. Low albumin levels, drugs that displace bilirubin from its albumin-binding sites, and acidosis all decrease the effective binding capacity of albumin. Measurements of the plasma level of free (unbound) bilirubin are considered to provide a reliable index of bilirubin toxicity. Methods that determine the concentration of vacant bilirubin-binding sites on albumin (reserve albumin) also appear to be useful.

3. *Serology*

1. Positive direct antiglobulin test on the infant's cord blood. This finding is presumptive diagnostic evidence of alloimmune hemolytic disease.
2. Mother negative for stimulating antigen and father positive. Cord cells from the infant are positive for the antigen, but typing may be difficult because the mother's antibodies coat the antigen sites on the infant's RBCs.
3. Positive indirect antiglobulin test in the mother, demonstrating the offending serum antibodies. The direct antiglobulin test is negative in the mother, showing lack of antibodies on her RBCs.

4. *Amniotic Fluid Examination*

Generally, women with an irregular antibody titer of 1:16 in albumin (suggesting the presence of IgG antibody) before 34 weeks' gestation and isoimmunized women with a history of previous stillbirths or of babies requiring exchange transfusions, regardless of the titer, should undergo amniotic fluid examination.

The amniotic fluid, which is normally colorless to pale straw, may become bright yellow in severe HDN. This pigment is measured by determining the optical density of the amniotic fluid at 450 nm with a spectrophotometer. The level correlates with the severity of anemia at birth as well as with the infant's prognosis. Important sources of error include: (1) contamination with fetal blood, which may contribute bilirubin; (2) hemolyzed red cells of fetal or maternal origin that yield a false rise in optical density; (3) contamination with meconium or vernix caseosa that causes turbidity and interferes with OD readings; and (4) exposure to light, which reduces pigment concentration by oxidation. The optical density of both normal and abnormal amniotic fluids tends to fall with advancing gestation, an important fact to remember when interpreting optical density data. Amniotic fluid OD 450 measurements correlate well with direct hemoglobin measurements during the third trimester of pregnancy but poorly in the second trimester, when only one-third of measurements reflect the need for transfusion accurately, necessitating other evaluations such as ultrasonography. Direct fetal hemoglobin determination by umbilical blood sampling is the only test capable of distinguishing mild from severe disease in the second trimester, but it is technically impractical before 18–20 weeks.

5. *Fetal Blood Sampling*

During the second trimester and in the presence of severe hemolytic disease, the traditional prognostic indicators tend to be unreliable, and fetal blood sampling for measurement of hematocrit and other parameters represents the most accurate method of assessing hemolysis. This information also permits precise calculation of the volume of blood required. In addition, other causes of fetal hydrops may be excluded and the fetal karyotype may be established.

D. Prevention of Rh Hemolytic Disease of the Newborn

Rh_o(D) hemolytic disease is prevented by eliminating fetal antigens (RBCs) from the maternal circulation using passive antibody therapy. Rh immune globulin is given to Rh-negative mothers within 72 hr of delivery. It is also used in other situations that may lead to immunologic sensitization, such as amniocentesis, or following miscarriages or abortion. The standard prophylactic dose is 300 μg of Rh_o IgG given intramuscularly. In some centers, patients receive smaller amounts of more purified preparations intravenously. Faster elimination of Rh-positive cells from the maternal circulation and a lower incidence of failures have been reported with intravenous doses as compared to intramuscular forms of prophylaxis, but this has not replaced intramuscular therapy because of its higher cost. The intravenous preparation may have applicability in patients who experience a high sensitizing risk, e.g., large fetomaternal hemorrhage or inadvertent administration of Rh-positive cells to an Rh-negative women of child-bearing age. These antibodies destroy or opsonize the fetal RBCs in the mother's circulation and remove the antigenic stimulus to the maternal immune system. All Rh-negative women who have delivered Rh-positive infants or who have had an abortion should receive Rh_o IgG within 72 hr. Even though the risks of immunization with abortion are less than those associated with a normal termination of pregnancy, they nevertheless are considerable, and subsequent fetuses may be severely affected. A dose of 50 μg may be protective in the first trimester. A protective dose of Rh_o IgG after amniocentesis should be given to all Rh-negative women unless the baby's father is known to be Rh negative. The dose should be repeated in 12 weeks if she has not delivered or in 6 weeks if she has had further amniocentesis. Patients with massive transplacental hemorrhage must receive an additional 10 μg of Rh_o IgG/mL of transplacental hemorrhage within 72 hr. Every Rh-negative, nonimmunized woman should receive one prophylactic dose of Rh immune globulin (300 μg) at 28 weeks' gestation, unless the father is known to be Rh negative. The dose should be repeated at 40 weeks if the patient has not delivered.

E. Treatment

Treatment includes proper prenatal care, taking into account history of previous pregnancies, serologic tests (maternal antibody titers and the father's zygosity), and amniotic fluid examinations or direct fetal blood sampling. These results dictate treatment, which ranges from mere observation to early induction or intrauterine fetal transfusion. Postnatal therapy consists of exchange transfusions after considering history or course of action in previous offspring, maternal antibody titer, clinical situation, cord blood hemoglobin, and cord blood bilirubin. If the bilirubin is >85 μmol/L in cord blood at birth or rises rapidly within a few hours after birth and clinical signs suggesting kernicterus at any time or at any bilirubin level are present, exchange transfusion may be necessary.

Phototherapy, which utilizes natural sunlight or fluorescent light, oxidizes bilirubin to biliverdin and ultimately to a nontoxic, water-soluble bilirubin. This therapy reduces toxic indirect bilirubin and decreases the number of exchange transfusions required. However, it is not a substitute for exchange transfusions in severe cases.

VII. HEMOLYTIC DISEASE OF THE NEWBORN DUE TO ABO INCOMPATIBILITY

A. Etiology

ABO-incompatible HDN is about twice as common as Rh-incompatible HDN, but it is rarely so severe and therefore often goes unnoticed with physiologic neonatal jaundice. Statistically, about 20% of all pregnancies involve ABO incompatibilities that may lead to HDN, but the incidence of significant hemolytic disease is only 1 in 150 births and about 1 in 5 of these babies are at risk of developing jaundice. Usually, the mother is group O and the infant is group A or B. This curious phenomenon is attributable to the nature of the anti-A or anti-B antibodies: Only group O mothers produce sufficient quantities of IgG anti-A or anti-B antibodies; the corresponding antibodies of group A or B mothers are confined to the IgM variety that cannot cross the placental barrier. Because group O individuals are naturally presensitized to A and B antigens by exposure to ABO-like substances found in food and other exogenous sources, first-born infants are affected as frequently as those born subsequently. Even when the first infant has suffered from HDN, other incompatible siblings may or may not have the disease. In addition, the severity of the hemolytic process does not increase predictably in succeeding siblings as occurs in association with Rh hemolytic disease. The ability of secretor infants to produce soluble blood group substances does not appear to protect them against ABO hemolytic disease, perhaps because IgG antibodies are more difficult to neutralize by soluble blood group substances than are IgM antibodies. The ratio of secretor to nonsecretor babies is slightly higher than expected, leading to a suggestion that the secreted blood group substances may also play a role in sensitization.

B. Clinical Findings

1. Jaundice in the first 24 hr, rarely causing kernicterus or death
2. Mild pallor secondary to anemia, but this may be absent
3. Hepatosplenomegaly, but much milder than in Rh hemolytic disease

C. Laboratory Findings

1. Anemia is uncommon.
2. Spherocytes are usually present in ABO hemolytic disease, and not observed in Rh hemolytic disease.
3. Polychromasia, increased numbers of nucleated RBCs, and reticulocytosis occur.
4. There is increased osmotic fragility when spherocytes are present. Autohemolysis is not corrected by glucose, as is seen in hereditary spherocytosis.
5. Indirect bilirubin levels are elevated.
6. The direct antiglobulin test is negative to weakly positive. This finding may be related to the fact that A and B antigen sites on the infant's RBCs are farther apart than in adult cells, thereby producing a weaker reaction.
7. Quantitative antibody elution test shows A- or B-specific antibodies which interact strongly with fetal or adult cells.
8. The indirect antiglobulin test is usually positive.

D. Treatment

Phototherapy is used in mild cases and is combined with exchange transfusion in more severe cases. Group O blood of the infant's Rh type should be used, although O cells suspended in AB plasma theoretically are preferable.

VIII. AUTOIMMUNE HEMOLYTIC ANEMIAS (AIHA) DUE TO WARM ANTIBODY TYPES

A. Etiology

Warm antibody AIHA is caused by IgG antibody capable of reacting with the RBC surface at normal body temperature (37°C). The antibody is an autoantibody and thus reacts with the patient's own erythrocyte antigens. Patients with idiopathic AIHA and those anemias associated with lymphomas or collagen disease appear to have IgG antibodies with specificity for a basic structural component of the Rh locus. The antibody does not react with cells that do not contain antigens of the Rh complex (Rh null cells). RBCs sensitized with this IgG antibody are removed in the spleen by macrophages. These macrophages have a membrane receptor for the Fc portion of the IgG immunoglobulin (IgG_1, and IgG_3 subclasses), which allows them to recognize, bind, phagocytize, and ultimately destroy the IgG-coated RBCs. This accelerated destruction results in a reduced red cell survival and subsequent anemia.

B. Classification and Incidence

The classification of warm antibody AIHA appears in Table 1. Idiopathic cases account for 40–50%. Most secondary causes are associated with lymphoid malignancies, collagen vascular disorders, and drug reactions.

The incidence of AIHA is about 1 in 80,000. Females predominate in the idiopathic type. The secondary type occurs with increased frequency after age 45, whereas the idiopathic variety occurs throughout life.

C. Clinical Findings

Patients with idiopathic warm antibody AIHA may demonstrate the following findings:

1. Weakness, perhaps sudden
2. Dizziness
3. Fever
4. Tachycardia, shortness of breath, and other symptoms of cardiac failure
5. Jaundice
6. Hepatosplenomegaly
7. Lymphadenopathy

Patients with secondary AIHA have similar findings with or without the manifestations of their underlying illness (e.g., skin rash in systemic lupus erythematosus, or prominent lymphadenopathy in lymphoma).

Table 1 Classification of Warm Antibody AIHA

Idiopathic
Secondary
Collagen vascular disease, e.g., systemic lupus erythematosus, polyarteritis nodosa
Lymphomas (Hodgkins and non-Hodgkins lymphoma), chronic lymphocytic leukemia
Other benign and malignant neoplasms
Immune deficiency disorders
Drugs, e.g., alpha-methyldopa (Aldomet), stibophen, procainamide
Miscellaneous—cirrhosis, ulcerative colitis, and demyelinating CNS disease

D. Laboratory Findings and Diagnosis

1. Peripheral Blood

1. Spherocytes, anisocytosis, polychromatophilic macrocytes, and frequently, nucleated RBCs
2. Autoagglutination of RBCs (berrylike clusters) may occur but are not as conspicuous as with cold complete antibodies. Autoagglutination must be distinguished from rouleaux formation (poker-chip orientation)
3. Anemia, frequently severe, with hemoglobin values <70 g/L
4. Reticulocytosis markedly elevated and accounting for the macrocytosis observed, since these cells are slightly larger than the older RBCs
5. Lymphocyte counts variable
6. Platelet counts usually normal or elevated, but occasionally decreased (Evans syndrome)

2. Bone Marrow

For typical cases, bone marrow examination is not necessary for diagnosis, but there is a role to exclude a secondary cause. The bone marrow aspirate is hypercellular and shows marked erythroid hyperplasia. Occasionally there are mild megaloblastic changes in the erythroid precursors, owing to the higher folic acid requirements for the increased RBC production.

3. Serology

The direct antiglobulin test is usually positive. Some AIHA occurs with as few as 10 antibody molecules attached to the RBC surface. However, available anti-human globulin sera will only detect RBCs with 100–150 antibodies on their surfaces. Certain techniques can increase the sensitivity of the anti-human globulin test. The majority of these are based on the principle of reducing the RBC-repulsive charge or decreasing the inter-RBC distance. Such manipulations allow the RBCs to attach and agglutinate if they have antibodies on their surfaces. The indirect antiglobulin test may or may not be positive, since it represents autoantibodies in the patient's serum. If excess autoantibody is present after all sites on the RBCs are occupied, the indirect antiglobulin test is positive.

Most cases of AIHA have either IgG or IgM or a combination of these two antibodies. Most IgG antibodies are polyclonal, but specific IgG subclasses predominate. Since IgG_1 and IgG_3 can fix complement, these antibodies have a greater potential for RBC destruction than do IgG_2 and IgG_4, which have little or no complement-fixation ability.

4. Other Tests for Hemolysis

1. Indirect bilirubin moderately elevated
2. Serum haptoglobin low or absent
3. Hemoglobinemia, hemoglobinuria, and hemosiderinuria in severe cases or with complement-fixing antibodies
4. Osmotic fragility increased in direct proportion to the number of spherocytes

E. Treatment

When the diagnosis of AIHA is first made, a search for associated disorders, such as tumors, lymphomas, and collagen vascular diseases is important, because therapy for such disorders will contribute to the permanent resolution of the hemolytic process. The treatment of acute fulminating AIHA requires oxygen corticosteroids and blood transfusion.

1. Blood Transfusion

Blood transfusion may be necessary as an emergency measure. Since the warm antibody AIHA is directed to a basic structure in the Rh locus, it reacts with nearly all potential donors (panagglutinin). Because of "blocking" of antigenic sites by antibody, there is a special problem in typing and matching. Sometimes the offending antibodies can be eluted from the erythrocyte, enabling more accurate phenotyping and identification of the specificity. Other methods of typing include the use of saline instead of albumin-based antisera. Typing can also be accomplished using enzyme-treated red cells. The identification of any clinically significant alloantibodies in the patient's serum is an important part of this workup. Autoabsorption of the autoagglutinin is imperative, since coexisting alloantibodies may be present and may cause an incompatible major transfusion. The panspecific nature of the autoantibody, however, makes finding of totally compatible donor cells unlikely. Thus the physician should administer donor cells most compatible with the patient's major blood group and Rh characteristics. Obviously, if alloantibodies are also identified, red cells appropriately negative for the specificity of the antibody should be used. The risks of a possible transfusion reaction against the benefits of the transfusion in a severely anemic patient must be weighed. Nevertheless, it seems prudent to use only as much blood as is necessary to stabilize the patient. Under all circumstances, imperfectly matched blood should be given slowly and under constant supervision. Most simply, 10–15 mL of donor red cells are infused over 20–30 min and the patient is observed closely for hemoglobinemia and symptoms indicative of hemolytic transfusion reaction. If no hemolysis is observed, the entire unit can be transfused.

2. Corticosteroids

Corticosteroids are the mainstay of medical therapy. Prednisone is given in a dose of 40 mg/m^2 daily initially, but twice this amount or more occasionally may be needed. A median response time is about 7 days. If no response occurs within 3 weeks, further steroid therapy is usually of no benefit. If response occurs, the steroids should be tapered gradually over 3–6 months. As a general strategy, the aim is to reduce steroids rapidly to the equivalent of prednisone 20 mg/m^2 over a 4- to 6-week period, with more gradual reduction and eventual withdrawal over a 3- to 4-month period. The majority of patients (60–70%) achieve either complete remission or control of the disease on low-dose maintenance steroids.

3. Splenectomy

Splenectomy can be considered in those patients who do not respond to steroids during the acute phase of the disease, those with anemia that requires continuous high-dose steroid therapy, or those who have developed serious complications from relatively low doses of steroid. About 50–60% of these patients respond to splenectomy with amelioration of hemolysis or reduction in steroid maintenance. Some authors have found that the results of splenectomy improve greatly by selecting patients who have demonstrated excessive sequestration of ^{51}Cr-labeled red cells within the spleen. Splenic irradiation has been recommended for patients in whom splenectomy is contraindicated.

4. Immunosuppression

Immunosuppression is necessary in about 10% of patients who are resistant to steroids and splenectomy. Azathioprine (Imuran) and cyclophosphamide (Cytoxan) produce a clinical response in about half of these resistant cases.

5. Other Forms of Therapy

Danazol, intravenous immune globulin (IVIG), and other experimental treatments have been tried, and some benefits are noted but not consistently. IVIG, which is highly effective in idiopathic thrombocytopenic purpura, does not seem to have the same success in the management of auto-immune hemolytic anemia. All patients with chronic hemolysis should receive folic acid supplements.

In secondary cases of warm AIHA, treatment of the underlying disorder may eliminate the hemolytic problem, whereas simple removal of the drug may correct the problem in drug-induced AIHA.

IX. AUTOIMMUNE HEMOLYTIC ANEMIAS (AIHA) DUE TO COLD ANTIBODY TYPES

A. Etiology

Cold antibody AIHA is caused by an IgM complement-fixing antibody that binds to the red cell optimally at 4°C and rapidly leaves the RBC surface at warmer temperatures. The antibody attachment at 4°C triggers the complement cascade, which may proceed to C8 and C9 with direct red cell lysis (intravascular hemolysis). More commonly, however, the complement activation is partial (C3b), and as the red cell returns from a cold extremity to body temperature 37°C, the IgM antibody is released from the RBC surface, leaving C3b attached. The C3b continues to accumulate but is ultimately removed in the liver and spleen by macrophages that have a membrane receptor for C3b.

B. Classification

The classification of cold-reactive antibody AIHA is shown in Table 2.

C. Idiopathic Cold Hemagglutinin Disease

1. Clinical Findings

1. Circulatory disturbances occur due to agglutination of RBCs within the capillaries. This agglutination causes mottled blue or red discoloration of the terminal extremities (acrocyanosis). Livedo reticularis may also be seen.
2. Pain and numbness accompanying acrocyanosis.

Table 2 Classification of Cold Antibody Types of AIHA

Idiopathic cold hemagglutinin disease
Secondary
Infections, e.g., infectious mononucleosis, *Mycoplasma pneumoniae*, and other viral infections
Lymphoproliferative disorders, e.g., chronic lymphocytic leukemia, lymphomas
Collagen vascular and immune complex diseases
Paroxysmal cold hemoglobinuria
Idiopathic
Secondary
Syphilis
Viral diseases—upper respiratory infection, measles, mumps, chickenpox

3. Raynaud's phenomenon.
4. Anemia, rarely severe. Hemoglobin levels are usually >70 g/L. Hemolysis is chronic and usually occurs in older patients.
5. Mild jaundice.
6. Mild hepatosplenomegaly.

Cold antibody AIHA of secondary etiology has additional symptoms related to the underlying disease, e.g., infectious mononucleosis (sore throat, fever, lymphadenopathy, splenomegaly) or lymphoma (lymphadenopathy, fever, splenomegaly). In infectious disease the AIHA is usually transient, whereas AIHA with lymphoproliferative disorders usually improves with treatment of the primary disorder.

2. Laboratory Findings

1. Autoagglutination of RBCs on the peripheral blood slide; spherocytosis not striking; nucleated RBCs may be seen.
2. Hemoglobin and hematocrit levels vary with the season in the idiopathic disorder, i.e., lower in the winter months.
3. Reticulocyte count elevated in relation to the level of hemoglobin.
4. Indirect bilirubin mildly elevated, haptoglobin low or absent.
5. Hemoglobinuria and hemosiderinuria present.

3. Serology

1. Cold agglutinin titer elevated. The hemolytic activity correlates more closely with the temperature reaction (thermal amplitude) of the antibody than with the titer.
2. Direct antiglobulin test positive and specific for complement components (C3d); specific anti-gamma-globulin sera typically negative.
3. Complement levels decreased during hemolysis.
4. Cold agglutinins with anti-I/i, P, or Pr specificity.

4. Treatment

Therapy and prevention of hemolytic episodes include the following considerations.

1. Patients should avoid exposure to cold, perhaps even moving to a warmer climate.
2. Patients with chronic hemolysis should have folic acid replacement.
3. Blood transfusions should be avoided if possible. Cross-match should be performed at 37°C, and blood should be warmed to 37°C prior to infusion.
4. Splenectomy and steroid therapy usually are of no benefit, although rare patients respond to steroids and/or alkylating agents.
5. Plasmapheresis can reduce the antibody titer transiently and may be used while other treatments have time to act.
6. Immunosuppressive therapy using cyclophosphamide (Cytoxan) or azathioprine (Imuran) benefits some patients who are not responsive to the usual measures.

D. Paroxysmal Cold Hemoglobinuria (PCH)

PCH is characterized by sudden hemoglobinuria following exposure to cold. The disease has idiopathic and secondary forms (Table 2). A few case reports of underlying neoplastic diseases with PCH are also noted in the literature. The intriguing feature of the disorder is the Donath-

Landsteiner (D-L) antibody, a 7S IgG, remarkably powerful hemolysin even in relatively low concentration. It has a biphasic in-vitro feature in that chilling to 4°C followed by warming to body temperature causes the most severe hemolysis. The requirement for prior cooling depends on the fact that D-L antibodies bind to red cells most avidly at temperatures of less than 15°C. Maximum hemolysis occurs when complement is present in the cold phase. These cold hemolysins have specificity to the P blood group rather than to the I/i group observed in cold agglutinin disease.

These patients pass dark reddish brown or black urine after local or general exposure to cold. They have acute symptoms: chills; fever; pain in the legs, back, or abdomen; general malaise; headache; vomiting; diarrhea. Urticaria and hepatosplenomegaly may be present.

The acute, nonrecurring form of Donath-Landsteiner hemolytic anemia is rare, accounting for only 1.6–5.1% of all cases of AIHA. In children under the age of 5 years, however, more than 40% of all cases of AIHA may be related to the D-L antibody. The course is usually associated with acute viral infections, and recovery is usually rapid, often without therapy.

Laboratory findings reveal evidence of acute intravascular hemolysis. Erythrophagocytosis is a common feature of acute attacks. The serum contains methemalbumin and, later, increased indirect bilirubin. The urine contains hemoglobin and methemoglobin, giving the dark reddish brown to black color. The antiglobulin test is positive if a complement-specific antiserum is used. The Donath-Landsteiner test or one of its refinements indicates a tentative diagnosis. (This test demonstrates hemolysis in a blood sample that is chilled in ice water and then warmed to 37°C.)

1. Treatment

Patients with viral illnesses have PCH of only short duration, and usually recover completely. PCH in patients with syphilis usually improves when the patient is treated. Patients with PCH generally do not respond to corticosteriods or splenectomy. No adequate trials of immunosuppressive agents have been made. The chronic idiopathic PCH patient should avoid cold and should consider moving to a warm climate.

E. Autoimmune Hemolysis with Mixed Warm and Cold Antibodies

In some patients, autoimmune hemolysis appears to be mediated by both warm antibodies and cold antibodies. About 7–8% of all patients with AIHA fall into this category. In most cases (40–50%), no underlying causes can be identified. Collagen vascular diseases, especially lupus erythematosus, constitute the second largest group (20–40%); other associated diseases include non-Hodgkin's disease, and other malignancies in decreasing orders of frequency.

Patients with mixed AIHA often have severe hemolysis, and the disease tends to run a chronic and intermittent course. Dramatic responses to steroid therapy have been reported.

CASE STUDY 1

Patient

Sixty-eight-year-old man.

Chief Complaint

The patient was admitted to the coronary care unit after chest tightness for more than 3 hr that was not relieved completely with sublingual nitroglycerin.

Medical History

The patient had significant past history of aortic stenosis and coronary artery disease. Three months previously, he was diagnosed with chronic lymphocytic leukemia stage III (Rai classification). His CBC revealed total white blood cell count of 60×10^9/L with 80% of mature lymphocytes, hemoglobin of 120 g/L, platelet count of 150×10^9/L. He denied any past blood transfusion. He has been on the same cardiac medication for more than 3 years.

Physical Examination

Pale and slightly jaundiced elderly patient with evidence of chest discomfort and mild shortness of breath. He also had cervical and axillary lymphadenopathy and palpable spleen edge. Cardiac examination revealed ejection systolic murmur without signs of heart failure.

Laboratory Results

CBC: hemoglobin 70 g/L, WBC 65×10^9/L with 85% of mature lymphocyte and platelet count of 140×10^9/L. Peripheral smear revealed mild spherocytosis and polychromasia and a leukocytosis with predominant mature lymphocytes.

Chemistry profile revealed normal electrolytes with LDH of 450 U/L, total bilirubin 60 μmol/L with direct bilirubin of 21 μmol/L with normal transaminases and alkaline phosphatase.

Questions

1. What is the most likely diagnosis of anemia, and how would you confirm the diagnosis?
2. Since the patient has symptomatic anemia, urgent red blood cell transfusion is requested. How would you proceed to obtain the suitable red blood cell?
3. What are the appropriate steps to follow during the transfusion for this type of anemia?
4. What is the appropriate treatment for this type of anemia?

Additional Laboratory Results

1. Additional tests for hemolytic anemia:

Reticulocyte count	10%
haptoglobin	<50 mg/L

2. Confirmatory test for immune hemolytic anemia: direct antiglobulin test

IgG	+3
C3d	neg

3. To exclude unexpected significant alloantibodies: Indirect antiglobulin test with screen cells I, II, and III were positive with panreacting specificity. Following autoabsorption, no alloantibodies were found by a negative repeat indirect antiglobulin test.

   Eluate with untreated and enzyme-treated screen cells were nonreactive.
4. Blood group typing: A with Rh_o (D) positive.

Diagnosis

Autoimmune hemolytic anemia (warm antibody type) secondary to chronic lymphocytic leukemia.

Discussion

This case is an example of autoimmune hemolytic anemia in association with chronic lymphocytic leukemia. Anemia with an elevated LDH and bilirubin suggests a possible hemolytic anemia. An elevated reticulocyte count and low haptoglobin support the diagnosis of hemolytic anemia. Examination of peripheral smear will provide further clues to identify the subtype of hemolytic anemia. Most often, significant spherocytosis will be noted in IgG-mediated immune hemolytic anemia. The most important test to support an immune hemolytic anemia is the direct antiglobulin test (DAT). Most cases of immune hemolytic anemia will have positive DAT. Rare instances of immune hemolytic anemia can be DAT negative. Usually, such cases are suspected in acquired hemolytic anemia with no other apparent underlying causes. A DAT positive must be further evaluated by using monospecific tests to delineate whether it is IgG or C3d related. Most of the IgG-positive DAT are of the warm autoantibody type, and C3d-positive DAT are either IgM cold autoantibody type or mixed types. Once specificity is confirmed, it is important to assess the patient's underlying medical problems, recent medications, and transfusion history. If the patient requires transfusions, it is important to exclude or confirm the presence of unexpected significant alloantibody that may be masked by the autoantibody in the serum.

The patient with IgG autoantibody-mediated hemolytic anemia sometimes can be a great challenge when urgent blood transfusion is warranted. Because of "blocking" of antigenic sites by antibody, there is a special problem in typing and matching. First, proper ABO typing should be done at 37°C with a parallel control test to determine whether autoagglutination is present. If the control test is nonreactive, the results obtained with anti-A and anti-B are valid. When autoagglutination is still present, interpretation of the result can be difficult, but comparing the strength of the observed reaction may be informative. Further Rh characterization and detection of clinically significant allo- or autoantibody must be pursued. The offending antibodies are often removed by elution. Most important is the exclusion or identification of clinically significant alloantibodies in the patient's serum. A large number of donor blood samples must be cross-matched, and the units that give the weakest reaction utilized (NB: concept of least incompatibility).

The risks of a possible transfusion reaction against the benefits of the transfusion in severely anemic and symptomatic patients must be weighed. Nevertheless, it seems prudent to use only as much blood as is necessary to stabilize the patient. Under all circumstances, imperfectly matched blood should be given slowly and under constant supervision.

Since this autoimmune hemolytic anemia is caused by chronic lymphocytic leukemia, the appropriate treatment will be targeted to the underlying leukemia after the hemolytic anemia is controlled by steroids. Combination of alkylating agents and steroids would be the treatment of choice. Recently, nucleoside analogs, especially fludarabine, have been noted to be potent in chronic lymphocytic leukemia; however, their effectiveness over standard alkylating agents plus steroids remains to be seen.

CASE STUDY 2

Patient

Thirty-five-year-old man.

Chief Complaint

The patient was admitted to the hospital during a snowstorm for dizziness and near-syncopal attack.

Medical History

The patient had a recent history of an upper respiratory infection, low-grade fever, and persistent nonproductive cough for 2 weeks. Subsequently he also noted increased malaise and mild shortness of breath. On the day of admission, he felt extremely weak and dizzy and presented to the emergency room for further evaluation. He had no significant past medical history. Recent medications were acetaminophen and Robitussin DM cough syrup.

Physical Examination

A significantly pale and ill-looking young adult with slightly inflamed oropharynx. Lung examination revealed fine rales bilaterally. No lymphadenopathy or hepatosplenomegaly. No other skin abnormality or joint deformity were noted.

Laboratory Results

CBC could not be performed because the blood specimens submitted in the EDTA tubes clotted immediately on two consecutive occasions.

Chemistry profile revealed normal electrolytes with LDH of 688 U/L, total bilirubin 68 μmol/L with direct bilirubin of 10.3 μmol/L, with normal transaminase and alkaline phosphatase.

Chest x-ray showed patchy infiltration, especially at the lower bases.

Questions

1. Why can't a CBC be performed? What can be done to prevent immediate clotting so a CBC can be performed? What are the technical factors, and what can be done to obviate them?
2. Since the patient has symptomatic anemia, urgent red blood cell transfusion is requested. How would you proceed to obtain suitable red blood cells?
3. What are the appropriate investigations to identify the underlying mechanism and cause?
4. What is the appropriate treatment for this type of anemia?

Additional Laboratory Results

Prewarming the EDTA tube prevented clotting (gelling and autoagglutination), allowing the CBC to be performed. CBC revealed hemoglobin of 5 g/dL, WBC of 15,000/μL, and platelet count of 368,000/μL. Peripheral smear revealed rouleaux formation and polychromasia.

1. Confirmatory tests for hemolytic anemia:

Reticulocyte count	8%
Haptoglobin	<50 mg/L

2. Confirmatory tests for immune hemolytic anemia, direct antiglobulin test:

IgG	neg
C3d	+3

3. Cold agglutinin studies:

Anti-I specificity reactive with adult erythrocytes but not with fetal (cord) erythrocytes.
Titer up to 1:640 with thermal amplitude up to 28°C
Polyclonal in nature

4. Exclude unexpected significant alloantibodies: Indirect antiglobulin test with screen cells I, II, and III were positive with panreactivity in room temperature. No alloantibodies were detected with prewarmed autoabsorbed serum.
5. Blood group typing: at 37°C, O with Rh_o (D) positive.

Diagnosis

Autoimmune hemolytic anemia (cold antibody type) secondary to *Mycoplasma pneumoniae.*

Discussion

This case is an example of autoimmune hemolytic anemia (cold antibody type) in association with *Mycoplasma* infection. These patients are not uncommonly identified by a congealed or agglutinated blood in the routine EDTA tube preventing a CBC from being performed. One of the reasons for this is rapid cold agglutination, which an be obviated by using a prewarmed tube and maintaining the sample at 37°C. Anemia with reticulocytosis and elevated LDH and bilirubin suggest hemolytic anemia. Additional tests such as the low haptoglobin support the diagnosis of hemolytic anemia. Examination of peripheral smear will provide further clues to identify the subtype of hemolytic anemia. In this case, significant auto-agglutination was noted in peripheral smear. In severe cold agglutinin disease, sometimes there is evidence of intravascular hemolysis. The most important confirmatory test to support an immune hemolytic anemia is the direct antiglobulin test (DAT). A positive DAT must be further evaluated by using monospecific tests to delineate whether IgG or C3d is involved. In this case, complement C3d was positive, consistent with IgM-mediated or cold-reacting Donath-Landsteiner-type IgG autoantibody. Once cold antibody-type autoimmune hemolytic anemia is suspected, identifying the specificity of the cold agglutinin should be pursued. Identification of the major reactivity (anti-I, -I, or -P/Pr) and its clonal diversity may be clinically informative, since cold agglutinins produced in various diseases show different characteristic patterns of reactivity. In this case it was noted to be anti-I cold agglutinins most often associated with *Mycoplasma* infection. Cold agglutinin titer is the maximal serum dilution at 4°C that retains red cell-agglutinating activity. Clinically significant hemolysis in cold agglutinin diseases is more dependent on thermal amplitude (maximum temperatures beyond which they are unable to combine effectively with their antigen) than titer. Therefore, the closer thermal amplitude is to body temperature, the higher is the chance of clinically significant hemolysis. Once specificity is confirmed, it is important to evaluate the patient's underlying medical problems, recent medications, and transfusion history. If the patient requires transfusions, one must exclude or confirm the presence of unexpected significant alloantibodies in the serum that may be masked by the autoantibody. Since this patient had never received any blood or blood products, no alloantibody problem was anticipated. Nevertheless, alloantibodies must be excluded. Cold agglutinins can also interfere with blood group typing. However, this problem is usually solved by running all the tests at 37°C parallel with the autocontrol. If there is no autoagglutination the results are valid and matched blood may be safely transfused. *Mycoplasma* infection can be confirmed by serologic tests. If the patient is symptomatic, blood transfusion should be considered. At the same time, antibodies such as erythromycin should be started simultaneously. Usually, *Mycoplasma*-related cold agglutination problems are mild and transient.

NOTE ADDED IN PROOFS

Research into the mechanisms of autoimmune hemolytic anemia and the disorders that are associated with it, in particular newer drug associations, continue to be published. A number of more recent articles that discuss these issues in greater detail are also provided as additional bibliography. The reader is referred to these three recent articles (5–7).

SUGGESTED READINGS

1. Hoffman R. Hematology, Basic Principles and Practice. New York: Churchill Livingston, 1995: 710–729.
2. Nydegger UE, Kazatchkine MD, Miescher PA. Immunopathologic and clinical features of hemolytic anemia due to cold agglutinins. Semin Hematol 1991; 28(1):66–77.
3. Rosse WF. Autoimmune hemolytic anemia. Hospital Practice 1985; 15:105–119.
4. Wintrobe MM. Clinical Hematology. Philadelphia: Lea & Febiger, 1994:1146–1196.
5. Garraty G. Auto-Immune Hemolytic Anemia. In: Garraty G, ed. Immunobiology of Transfusion Medicine. New York: Marcel Dekker. 1994:493–521.
6. Dormen RE. An overview of the hemolytic anemia. Cleveland Clin J Med 1998; 65(2), 89–99.
7. Siegel DL. The human immune response to red blood cell antigen as revealed by repertoire cloning. Immunol Res 1998; 17(1–2), 239–252.

22

Carbon Monoxide Poisoning, Methemoglobinemia, and Sulfhemoglobinemia

Ronald L. Nagel
Albert Einstein College of Medicine, Bronx, New York

I. NORMAL HEMOGLOBIN STRUCTURE AND FUNCTION

The adult major hemoglobin (Hb) molecule is a tetramer formed by four polypeptide chains, two α chains and two β chains. Each of these chains is attached to a prosthetic group called a heme, formed by protoporphyrin IX in a complex with an iron molecule (Fig. 1).

The heme is semiburied in the globin heme pocket, because a hydrophobic environment is best for the maintenance of the ferrous state of the iron (Fig. 2). Only the charged propionic side chains are significantly exposed to the solvent at the entrance of the pocket. The pocket is large enough for oxygen to penetrate, but ligands (molecules capable of binding to the iron) that are significantly larger than oxygen, such as CO or the family of isocyanates, have progressive difficulty in reaching the iron in direct proportion to their bulk.

Oxygen transport to the tissues, the ultimate purpose of hemoglobin, is dependent on blood flow, which in turn is affected by cardiac output and by microcirculatory size and distribution, the Hb concentration, and O_2 extraction by the tissues, which in turn is dependent on the shape of the oxygen-binding curve of the red cells and on tissue pO_2. The shape of the oxygen equilibrium curve in Hb is sigmoidal. This shape is determined by the extent of cooperativity: The initial portion of the curve has a very low slope, reflecting a low affinity for oxygen by hemoglobin at the beginning of the loading process. In other words, when Hb is totally deoxygenated, it has a rather poor avidity for oxygen (Fig. 3). As the loading proceeds, and as the molecule binds more oxygen molecules, the slope of the reaction begins to change rapidly and becomes steep. This means that the affinity for oxygen has become much higher in spite of the sluggish beginning. In other words, the initial molecules of oxygen that bind a deoxy-Hb tetramer change this protein avidity for oxygen. This property assures that hemoglobin tetramers, once they begin to accept oxygen, will be fully oxygenated promptly.

At the molecular level, cooperativity is accounted for by the fact that hemoglobin can exist stably in only two fundamentally different conformations, one for the oxygenated molecule (R state), another for the deoxygenated molecule (T state), without intermediate conformations. One molecule of hemoglobin will bind 2 molecules of oxygen in the low-affinity conformation (T state).

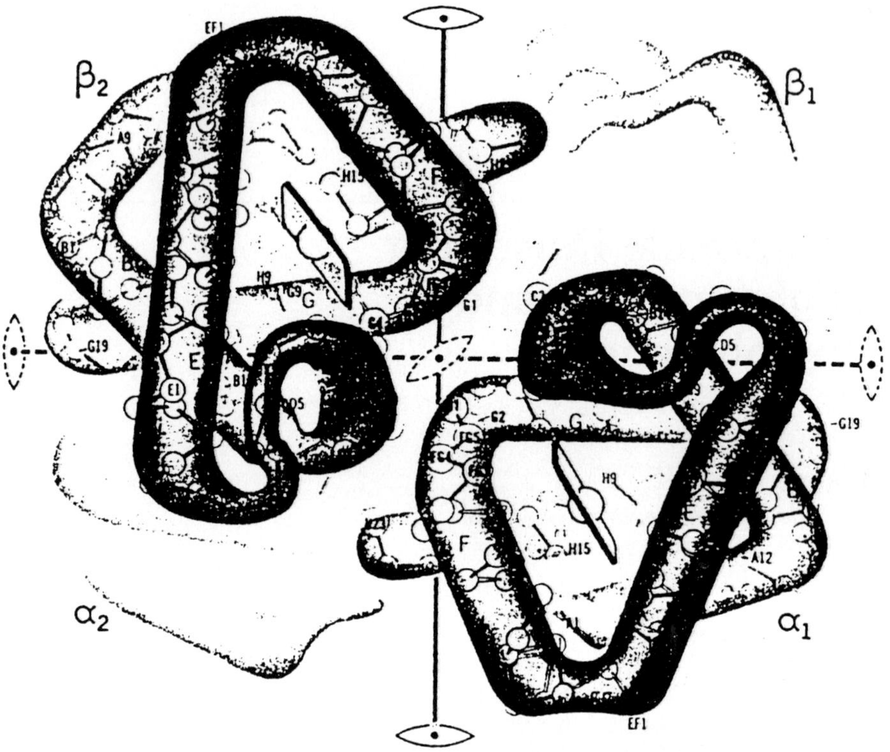

Figure 1 The four chains of hemoglobin. $\alpha_1\beta_2$ contacts (the $\alpha_2\beta_1$ contacts are identical on the back side of the molecule). The two perpendicular pseudo-axes are indicated by dashes. Only the α carbons of the main chains are shown. Those side chains involved in contacts between subunits are given boldface numbers in large circles.

The triggering mechanism at the level of the heme for the conformational change is the following: The iron in deoxy-Hb is slightly out of the plane of the heme (domed configuration) because the pyrrol rings are also slightly pyramidal (Fig. 3). When the ligand binds the sixth coordinating position of the iron, significant stearic stresses are introduced, and to relieve this strain the distal histidine moves 8° to become perpendicular to the heme, significantly decreasing the doming of the iron (the angle between the iron and the heme falls to 4°). There is also the displacement of FG5 in the direction of the histidine F8. The configuration around the heme has now changed to the oxygenated or R state, and a chain of events involving the critical interactions change the conformation of the hemoglobin tetramer.

Hemoglobin binds CO_2 when it is delivering O_2 and releases CO_2 when it is binding oxygen, helping to dissipate the increase in concentration of CO_2 in the tissues and conveniently delivering this metabolic end product to the alveoli of the lungs. It accomplishes this particular task with ease because carbon dioxide is an inhibitor of HbO_2 carrying capacity by decreasing the O_2 affinity of the molecule.

Hb binds hydrogen ions efficiently in a low-pH environment and releases hydrogen ions when it encounters high pH (a phenomena called the Bohr effect). The Bohr effect is the change of O_2 affinity secondary to pH change within a certain range: the lower the pH, the lower is the affinity for O_2. This means that an increased concentration of protons favors low affinity in Hb; deoxy-Hb binds more protons than the oxy-conformer.

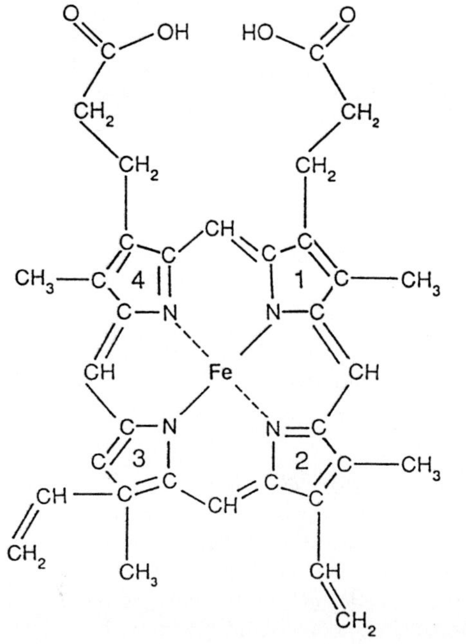

Figure 2 The protoporphyrin IX heme structure consists of four pyrrole rings with the following side-chain replacements: two methyl and two propionic acids in pyrroles 1 and 4; two methyl and two vinyls in pyrroles 2 and 3. Iron is tetracoordinated by the nitrogens of the pyrrole rings.

II. CARBON MONOXIDE POISONING

A. Background

Carbon monoxide is particularly dangerous because it is odorless, colorless, and tasteless. It does have a low solubility in water. Carbon monoxide is a relatively inert gas due to its high bond enthalpy, which is the highest of any molecule. Nevertheless, it combines with high affinity to the heme of hemoglobin (and with lesser affinities, myoglobin and cytochromes) at the same site as O_2. At equilibrium, at physiologic pH and 37°C, its affinity for Hb is about 240 times higher than that of O_2. This very high equilibrium constant is the result of a peculiar kinetic situation as to on and off rates. Actually, contrary to popular belief, CO reacts with the heme of hemoglobin more slowly than oxygen (at 20°C, pH 7.0; k_{on} for CO is 20 versus 470 M^{-1} sec^{-1} for O_2). This is not surprising, since the biatomic carbon monoxide binds perpendicular to the heme and, due to stearic constraints present in the normal heme pocket, has more difficulty reaching the heme. But once CO is bound, its off rate (k_{off} for CO is 0.015 versus 35 sec^{-1} for O_2) is extraordinarily slow, hence, producing a very high affinity constant, and a life-threatening circumstance for living beings.

To complicate matters, and to further endanger those exposed to CO, once two molecules of CO are bound to hemoglobin, the molecule switches to the R state, and hence the two sites left for oxygen binding have a high affinity. This high affinity makes more difficult for the oxygen-binding sites left after exposure to CO to deliver oxygen to the tissues. This is called the *Darling-Roughton effect*. The consequence of this effect is that the oxygen equilibrium curve of blood with a given percentage of CO will be shifted progressively more to the left as the CO level increases.

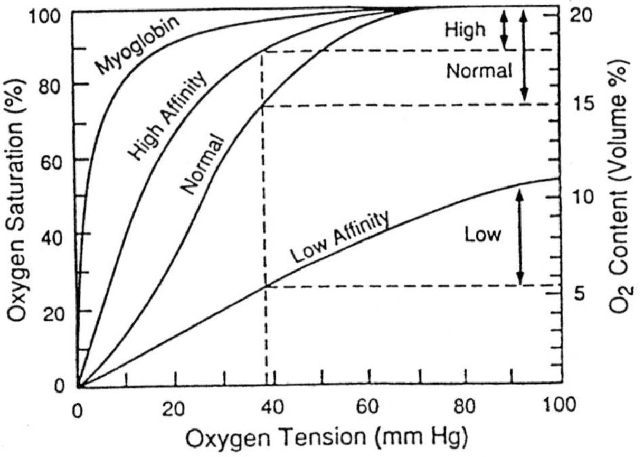

Figure 3 Oxygen equilibrium curves of myoglobin (no cooperativity, hence $n = 1$) and of normal hemoglobin red cells, flanked by curves of high-affinity hemoglobin red cells and low-affinity hemoglobin-containing red cells. Oxygen tension (pO_2) is plotted against percentage of oxygen saturation and oxygen content in volume percentage. Oxygen content takes into account the amount of hemoglobin present. The oxygen extraction is the difference in oxygen content of red cells at a pO_2 of 40 mmHg in the tissues. That subtraction renders about 5 volumes of oxygen for normal Hb. The high-affinity hemoglobin renders 2.5 volumes and causes tissue hypoxia. The very-low-oxygen-affinity hemoglobin results in an extraction of 5 volumes, essentially normal. Nevertheless, any curve between this and the normal will have an *increased* oxygen extraction, and will respond to this increased oxygen delivery with a decrease in the release of erythropoietin and anemia.

In the absence of environmental CO, the blood of adults contains about 1% COHb. This represents about 80% of the total body CO; the rest probably is sequestered in myoglobin and cytochromes. This amount of CO is produced endogenously. The predominant origin is the degradation of heme by the rate-limiting heme oxygenase/cytochrome P-450 complex, which produces CO and biliverdin. Further degradation of biliverdin to bilirubin by biliverdin reductase enables one molecule of hemoglobin to generate one molecule of CO and one molecule of biliverdin.

This *endogenous* production of CO might be important physiologically. Like its analog, NO, which now is known to be vasoactive as well as a member of signal transduction pathways, CO can also bind to the heme of soluble guanydyl cyclase, as well as to the iron/sulfur centers of macrophage enzymes. Since the cyclase regulates the second messenger, cyclic guanosine-3′,5′-monophosphate, controls kinases, transport proteins, and phosphodiasterases, the level of significance of these mechanisms remains to be determined.

Individuals differ as to their level of endogenous CO generation. Gender plays a role, and caloric restriction (increases) and race (Japanese and Amerindians) seem to have higher endogenous levels of CO). Co-presence of hemolytic anemia, hematomas, and infections tend to increase CO production significantly, up to threefold. Age and development also have an effect: fetuses and newborns have double the normal level of COHb, and even higher levels if there is any level of blood group incompatibility.

Not all endogenous production of CO is the product of normal metabolism: Some drugs (such as dephenylidantoin and phenobarbitals), fasting, dehydration, and drugs that produce low-level hemolysis increase endogenous production of CO.

Exogenous sources of CO come from breathing CO present in the atmosphere as a product of incomplete combustion and oxidation of hydrocarbons. Burning of fossil fuels, wood, or other organic matter generates CO.

Another class of risk is presented at high altitude, particularly if the atmospheric CO is increased by an improperly ventilated wood-burning stove. The erythrocytosis and hypoxemia, as well as our imperfect adaptation to high altitude, decreases oxygen intake and prolongs CO excretion, increasing CO blood levels.

In summary, exogenous origins of CO increase circulating COHb levels to 2%, which is among the lowest found in the modern world, to 5% in cases of individuals who are not exposed to a high-risk environment.

B. Carbon Monoxide Chronic Intoxication

1. Clinical Features

In the adult, the normal level of COHb is less than 1%, but this is rarely found in urban centers. Hemolysis can produce a level of 2%. Levels over 3% must have exogenous origins, except for rare conditions such as carriers of the abnormal Hb Zurich.

The U.S. Environmental Protection Agency (EPA) considers 9 ppm over 8 hr and 25 ppm over 1 hr as acceptable. This environmental amount of CO would raise COHb by 1.5%. Any level beyond this might produce symptoms. Pregnant mothers and fetuses are particularly susceptible, since the level of COHb is somewhat elevated already. In addition, HbF is already shifted to the right, due to its lack of susceptibility for right-shifting in the presence of 2,3-DPG, making the Darling-Roughton effect particularly pernicious—this is one of the reasons why cigarette smoking during pregnancy is specially hazardous to the health of the fetus.

In adults, symptoms might include irritability, nausea, lethargy, headaches, and sometimes imitates the flu or a bad cold. Higher COHb levels produce somnolence. Symptoms might include palpitations, cardiomegaly, and hypertension, and might contribute to atherosclerosis. Hematologically, increased levels of COHb might produce erythrocytosis. Chronic CO poisoning can mask the anemia of thalassemia trait or other acquired or genetic chronic hemolysis.

Elimination of CO from the body is achieved by two mechanisms. Pulmonary excretion is by far the principal mechanism. As mentioned above, the removal of CO from Hb is exceedingly slow. At 1 atm pressure, the half-life to COHb is 5 hr and 20 min. Breathing 100% O_2 in a hyperbaric chamber can reduce the half-life to 23 min.

The second mechanism for elimination is the catabolism of CO by cytochrome oxidase. This is a very small component of the CO elimination process.

2. Etiology

The exogenous source of CO must be determined. The most frequent causes are cigarette smoking, which can increase the COHb up to 15%. Pregnant women, fetuses, neonates, and infants are particularly susceptible to CO poisoning by smoking (hence, the warning labels on cigarette packaging), particularly in the latter three groups, in part because of the high levels of the high-affinity HbF. One, two, or three packs a day might generate COHbs from 5% to 15%. Other high-risk occupations for CO intoxication include garage work with improper ventilation, tollbooth attendants, tunnel workers, drivers of vehicles with defective exhaust systems (or opening the rear or tailgate window of a car while driving), firefighters, and inhabitants of houses with defective heating exhaust systems, industrial exposure to paint remover, aerosol propellant, or organic solvents containing dichloromethane.

3. Treatment

Removal of the patient from the source of environment CO is usually sufficient. If the COHb level is high, breathing 100% oxygen will increase the rate of removal. Hyperbaric oxygen, which has complications of its own (bronchial irritation and pulmonary edema), should be reserved for exceptional cases. In most cases, by the time the patient is brought into a hyperbaric chamber, the simple breathing of 100% oxygen has abated COHb sufficient to make the procedure unnecessary.

C. Carbon Monoxide Acute Intoxication

1. *Clinical Features*

Accidental exposure to high environmental levels of CO or suicidal attempts by deliberate exposure to a CO source are the most frequent cause of poisoning deaths in adults in this country. CO is responsible for about 4000 deaths a year.

CO affects rapidly the CNS-PNS and the cardiopulmonary system. Cerebral edema is a common finding, as is alteration of the sensory and peripheral nerve function. By inducing increased permeability in the lung, CO results in acute pulmonary edema. Also, cardiac arrhythmias, generalized hypoxemia, and respiratory failure are common causes of death.

Less severe cases present with the same symptoms as chronic intoxication (although more severe in intensity). In addition to cardiac arrhythmias, myocardial ischemia, lactic acidosis, and convulsions, even coma can occur. An interesting complication observed several days after exposure to CO is the presence of patches of necrotic skin induced by localized hypoxia. Interestingly, significant interpatient variability as to the level of COHb that can elicit any of these symptoms has been observed. In the cases that survive, considerable neurologic deficits can remain.

Acute CO intoxication in children is responsible for about 400 deaths a year. Such intoxication is severe, and occasionally is associated with unique symptomatology (resembling gastroenteritis), and severe sequelae (leukoencephalopathy, white matter destruction, severe myocardial ischemia).

2. *Treatment*

The source of CO should be identified and removed. The patient should be administered 100% O_2 by endotracheal intubation, if necessary. Other support interventions should be related to the symptomatology. As mentioned previously, many of these patients are placed under hyperbaric oxygen, which helps in the removal of CO but can have unwelcome complications. Unless hyperbaric oxygen is essential to the patient, this effort is more dramatic than useful.

3. *Instrumental Diagnosis of COHb*

The most commonly used instrumentation for the detection and quantification of COHb is the CO-oxymeter, which in addition measures levels of oxy-, deoxy-, met-Hb, and total Hb. The instrument is reliable above 5% COHb, but progressively declines as levels decrease from 5%. Bilirubin, methylene blue, and sulf-Hb are sources of interference at low concentrations of COHb. If low levels need to be measured, gas chromatography, a research tool, is the only alternative.

III. METHEMOGLOBINEMIA

A. Definition

Methemoglobinemia (more precisely but more cumbersome, methemoglobincythemia) is the consequence of the oxidation of the iron (from ferrous to ferric) in the center of the protoporphyrin IX ring that forms the prosthetic group (heme) of hemoglobin (Fig. 2). Normally, the level of methemoglobinemia is 0.5%. Production is much higher, but reduction back to ferrous is very efficient in the red cells. Potentially, methemoglobinemia can induce problems since it renders hemoglobin incapable of binding oxygen.

B. Classification

The clinical consequences are generally (but not always) benign, but the change of color of the skin can be quite dramatic. Methemoglobinemia belongs in the differential diagnosis of cyanosis.

Methemoglobinemia can be the consequence of:

1. Hereditary methemoglobinemia: genetic abnormalities of the mechanisms involved in maintaining the hemoglobin in the ferrous state and capable of binding oxygen (hereditary methemoglobinemia)
2. Acquired methemoglobinopathies: exposure to exogenous oxidizing agents capable of penetrating red cells

C. Hereditary Methemoglobinemia

1. Clinical Aspects and Classification

The principal symptom of methemoglobinemia is cyanosis, which can usually be determined by examination of the skin and mucosas. Jaffe (1) calculated that the degree of cyanosis produced by 5 g/dL deoxyHb (in the ferrous state) is equivalent to 1.5 g/dL of met-Hb (ferric state) or 0.5 g/dL of sulfhemoglobin.

Up to now all the mutations associated with methemoglobinemia have been recessive, hence only homozygous individuals express the disease. Nevertheless, the heterozygous individual could be at particular risk for the acquired form of the disease (see below). Hence, other affected members of the pedigree would be sibs—very unlikely—parents or descendants.

A modified clinical classification based on that of Jaffe (1) of hereditary methemoglobinopathies, involves three basic mechanisms: congenital deficiency of the enzyme NADPH-dependent cytochrome, b_5 reductase; congenital deficiency of cytochrome b_5; and mutations of Hb resulting in the stabilization of the ferrous state—the Hb M's.

a. Congenital Deficiency of the Enzyme NADPH-Dependent Cytochrome b_5 Reductase.

i. Red Cell Type (Type I): Classically, these patients are more cyanotic than sick: They show only variable levels of fatigue with strenuous exercise in the worse cases. Survival is normal, and female patients have normal pregnancies. Levels of methemoglobin vary between 20% and 40%. Symptomatic methemoglobinemia can develop on exposure to methemoglobin-inducing drugs or chemicals.

These patients have a decreased activity of the red cell reduced nicotinamide adenine dinucleotide (NADPH)-dependent cytochrome b_5 reductase. NADH-methemoglobin reductase works in conjunction with cytochrome b_5 to reduce methemoglobin. This enzyme has a totally different function in red cell progenitors: It clips the hydrophobic C-terminal portion of microsomal cytochrome b_5.

Treatment is rarely necessary, but methylene blue works in methemoglobin reductase deficiency because it reduces methemoglobin through a different pathway using a NADPH-dependent methemoglobin reductase.

ii. Generalized (Type II): This type of hereditary methemoglobinemia affect about 10–15% of patients. This is a severe and lethal disease, with a strong neurologic component. While the methemoglobinemia can be treated, the neurologic syndrome is refractory. The disease is secondary to a defective NADH-methemoglobin reductase (cytochrome b_5 reductase), in all tissues.

The defect is autosomal recessive, since only the homozygote is affected. There are two NADPH-methemoglobin reductases in the red cell. One is attached to the membrane and another is free in the cytosol, proteolyzed to a state in which it can no longer assemble in the membrane. Since both enzymes were deficient in type II methemoglobinemia patients, the original gene generates both enzyme forms.

Prenatal diagnosis is available for this disease, and is beneficial for future pregnancies. However, such testing is useful only after the propositus is ascertained, since the disease is autosomal recessive.

In early classifications a type III was described, but further studies of the probands demonstrated that they were indeed type I.

b. Congenital Deficiency of Cytochrome b_5. Only one patient has been described, presenting with congenital deficiency of cytochrome b_5 (note, not the enzyme but the cofactor), with a reduction to 23% of the normal level and methemoglobinemia of 12–19%. This disorder has no neurologic symptoms. The cytochrome b_5 reductase level was normal in red blood cells.

c. Mutations of Hb Resulting in the Stabilization of the Ferrous State: The Hb M's. These patients are fundamentally different from other methemoglobinemias because the defect does not involve an enzyme deficiency, but an alteration residing in the hemoglobin molecule itself.

Six types of hemoglobin Ms are known (Table 1). Five correspond to substitutions of the proximal and distal histidines (F8 and E7) by tyrosines in α, β, and γ chains. The sixth involves a residue close to the heme (E11) and the distal histidine.

The substituting residue in all these mutations changes the microenvironment of the heme, producing increased amounts of ferric.

These patients are asymptomatic, except for the presence of a cyanosis, although the color is more brownish or slate, similar to other methemoglobinemias, but not as purple as in cardiopulmonary cyanosis. The abnormal color is present at birth in the α- and γ-chain mutations. Cyanosis appears at about 6 months of age in β-chain mutations. The age difference in expression of the phenotype is in direct accordance with the patter of expression of these globin chains. A mild hemolytic anemia with reticulocytemia has been observed in Hb Hyde Park.

2. Pathophysiology

a. The Ferrous State of Hb. One of the functions of the Hb molecule is to keep the iron molecule inside the heme moiety in the ferrous state so that it can bind O_2 and deliver it to the tissues. The heme niche in Hb is very hydrophobic and, in addition, two residues in each chain are critical: the proximal histidine (His F8) and the distal histidine (His E8) (Fig. 1), highly conserved in most Hbs and myoglobins. The proximal histidine occupies the fifth

Table 1 Hemoglobins Ms

M Hyde Park	β92(F8) His→Tyr
M Saskatoon	β63(E7) His→Tyr
M Iwate	α87(F8) His→Tyr
M Boston	α58(E7) His→Tyr
M Milwaukee	β67(E11)Val→Glu
Fetal M Osaka	γ63(E7) His→Tyr

coordinated position in the iron molecule (the other four are occupied by pyrrol rings). The distal histidine approaches but does not touch the sixth coordinating position, reserved for oxygen and other ligands. Replacement of histidines by tyrosines in ferric heme is limited to the mutated chains, either α or β. These mutated forms of hemoglobin are known as the M Hb variants, M for met-Hb-like.

b. Autooxidation of Hemoglobin. When a hemoglobin solution is left at room temperature (and even faster at 37°C), it turns into a brown material that is predominantly met-Hb. The chemical basis of autoxidation is probably the generation of superoxide anion (O_2^-), catalyzed by H^+, Cl^-, the superoxide anion itself, and probably by partial deoxygenation. Totally deoxygenated Hb, of course, has no oxygen to contribute to the reaction. The α chains of hemoglobin are a preferred site for autoxidation. The autoxidation of Hb is favored by increased temperature, 2,3-DPG, and trace metals.

Oxidation of hemoglobin can occur by exogenous sources. One example is Cu^{2+}, which binds Cys-β93 with high affinity and multiple other sites with low affinity. It converts the iron attached to the heme of the β chains into Met. Drugs can also oxidize hemoglobin (see below). Methemoglobin induces the denaturation of hemoglobin with hemichrome formation. Heinz bodies, made of hemichromes, are common in methemoglobinemia, the product of hemoglobin denaturation. Hemichromes are generated by heme dissociation (favored in met-Hb) from the heme pocket and rebinding elsewhere in globin after the α or β chains. It is understandable, then, that any weakening of the Hb bond with heme will accelerate denaturation.

c. Mechanisms of Reduction of met-Hb in Red Cells. In normal red cell hemolysates, met-Hb is less than 0.5%. Much more is produced but elaborated mechanisms constantly reduce ferric hemes to ferrous (Fig. 4).

The mechanisms capable of reducing met-Hb involve the following.

i. The Cytochrome b_5 Reductase System:

The NADH-dependent enzyme cytochrome b_5 reductase (other names: diaphorase I, NADH-methemoglobin reductase, NADH-dyhyrogenase) (reaction 1, Fig. 4). The membrane-bound cytochrome b_5 cytochrome reductase is found in erythroblasts and has a membrane-binding domain in the N-terminal end. The erythrocyte form results from the membrane-bound form by proteolytic loss of the membrane-binding domain during maturation. The membrane-bond enzyme desaturate and elongate fatty acids in cholesterol biosynthesis and in drug metabolism.

This enzyme has been cloned and consists of 9 exons and 8 introns and covers 30 kb. The cleavage site of the membrane-binding domain was found in the center of the second exon, suggesting an alternative splicing site as mechanism of generation of the soluble form. Some of the mutations that generate NADP-dependent cytochrome b_5 reductase deficiency have been elucidated (Fig. 5).

NADH. This indispensable cofactor for cytochrome b_5 reductase is generated (reaction 1, Fig. 4) by glyceralaldehyde-3-phosphate dehydrogenase, which reduces NADP to NADPH in the process of converting glyceraldehyde-3-phosphate to 1,3-diphosphate in the glycolytic pathway. Conversely, lactic acid dehydrogenase of the glycolytic pathway converts NADPH into NADP in the process of converting pyruvate into lactic acid.

Cytochrome b_5. Cytochrome b_5 is the electron carrier between NADH and met-Hb. Electron transfer between cytochrome b_5 and met-Hb occurs via a complex between these two molecules. The cytochrome binds to four lysines in the heme pocket in both chains.

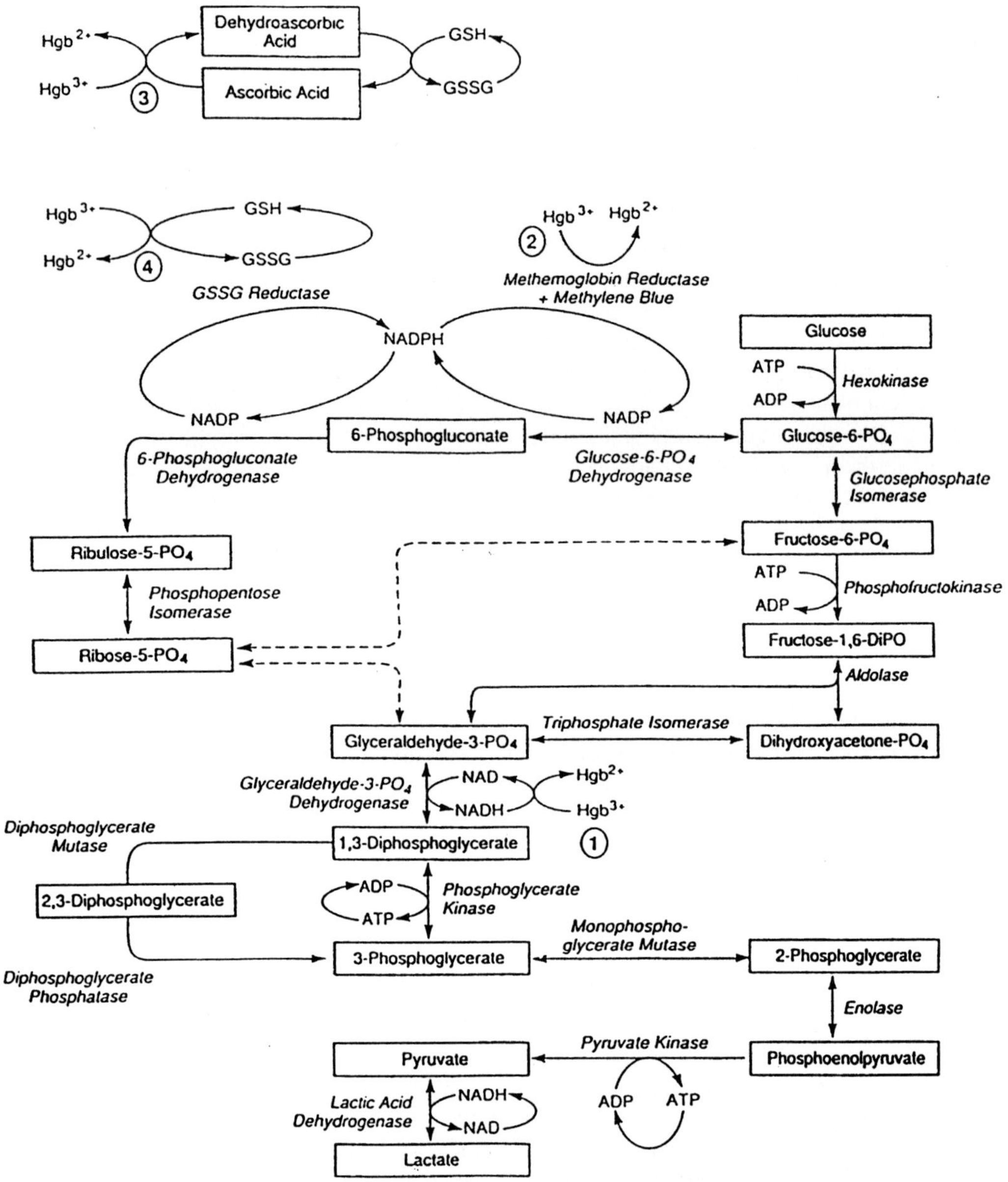

Figure 4 Pathway for the reduction of methemoglobin.

ii. The NADPH-Phosphate Reductase System: This reaction (reaction 2, Fig. 4) is not physiologic, since glucose-6-phosphate dehydrogenase deficiency patients do not have met-Hb. Nevertheless, in the presence of methylene blue, the system is active, and it is the basis for the use of this dye in methemoglobinemia.

iii. Ascorbic Acid: Ascorbic acid can reduce methemoglobin at a low rate in red cells (reaction 3, Fig. 4), in the process of being converted into dehydroascorbic acid, without the help of an enzyme.

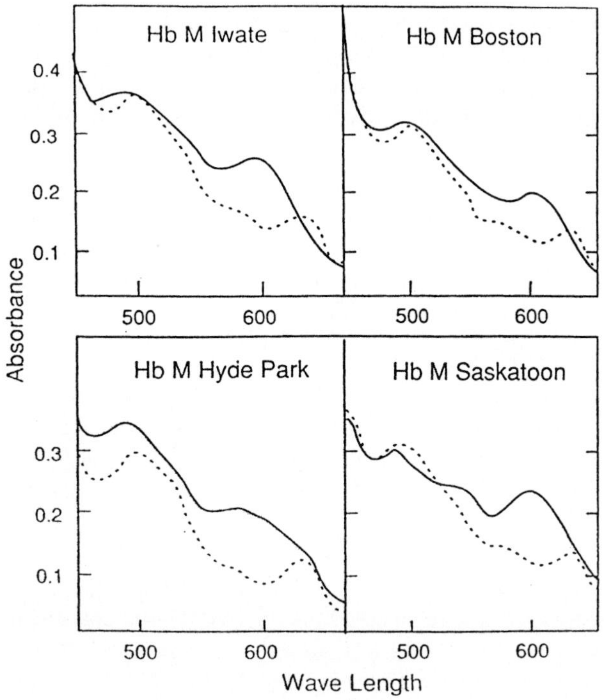

Figure 5 Spectra between 450 and 650 μm of the oxidized form of four M hemoglobins are compared in each case with the normal methemoglobin specrta. In these spectra, the normal chains are met and the abnormal chains have their own particular spectral properties. (After Shibata S, Miyaki T, Iuchi I. Methemoglobin M's of the Japanese. Bull Yamaguchi Med Sch 1967; 14:141.)

iv. Reduced Glutathione System: GSH can reduce met-Hb directly, without enzyme assistance. The resulting oxidized glutathione (GSSG) is reduced by glutathione reductase.

d. Other Protective Mechanisms to Avoid met-Hb Formation. Other protective mechanisms include *superoxide dismutase*, which mops up the toxic superoxide ion, generating H_2O_2, removed by *glutathione peroxidase* and less efficiently by *catalase*. This is why acatalasemia does not show methemoglobinemia, while inherited deficiency for glutathione peroxidase deficiency exhibits some. Low levels of catalase in newborns might explain their susceptibility to acquired met-Hb.

e. Mechanisms by Which the Mutations of the HbMs Favor the Ferric State.

1. *Weak heme attachment.* Deoxy-Hb M Hyde Park loses 20–30% of the heme; the α chains component were normal, but only one of the two β^{HP} chains contained heme.
2. *Binding of the iron to the remaining histidine and to the newly introduced tyrosine.* The proximal histidine (F8) in the β^{M} chains (Hb Hyde Park) moves toward the E helix, allowing the iron to be bound by the distal histidine, accommodating the bulkier side chain of the new tyrosine, and generating a phenolic bond to the sixth coordinating position of the iron, stabilizing the ferric form. *Hb Iwate* is different: The αE helix moves toward the heme, and the distal histidine αE(7)38 of the α chains moves to bind the fifth coordinating position in the α-heme iron.

The interactions of the *distal histidines* (*E7*) substituted by tyrosines in the β^M chain of *HbM Saskatoon* and the α^M chain in *HbM Boston* is also known. In HbM Boston, Tyr-58 (E7) surprisingly fills the fifth coordinating position of the heme iron in spite of the presence of a normal proximal histidine. This bond moves the heme sufficiently to make the interaction between the proximal histidine and the heme iron impossible.

Finally, *Hb Milwaukee* is not a mutation of the proximal or distal histidine, but of a residue nearby (Val-67 E11). The new glutamate occupies the sixth coordination position of the iron, and the proximal histidine retains the fifth coordinating position, stabilizing the abnormal ferric state of Hb Milwaukee. Other mutations of that site, such as HbBristol (Asp) or HbSidney (Ala), are unstable, or have low affinity but do not have met-like heme iron.

3. *Iron Oxidation and Spectral Characteristics*

The M Hbs fundamental characteristic is that their hemes are stabilized in the abnormal ferric state. Hence, they exhibit abnormal visible spectra that can be easily distinguished from regular met-Hb (Fig. 5). This characteristic separates these variants from hemoglobin mutants that have a tendency to form normal met-Hb, such as Hb St. Louis, Hb Bicêtre, I Tolouse, and Hb Seattle, all of which are unstable in addition.

The iron in the abnormal subunits of the M Hb oxidize much more rapidly by molecular oxygen and are resistant, to a variable degree, to reduction by dithionite. Interestingly, HbM Iwate, HbM Hyde Park, and Hb M Boston are not reduced at all by NADH-cytochrome b_5 reductase, but HbM Milwaukee is reduced slowly and M Saskatoon is reduced normally by this enzyme. It is possible that in vivo the latter two MHbs might be less oxidized than expected. Full ferric conversion might occur only in vitro. Older red cells might nevertheless have fully oxidized abnormal chains, in keeping with the presence of clinically apparent cyanosis.

D. Acquired Methemoglobinemia

Several chemical agents and drugs can induce methemoglobinemia. Table 2 (modified from Brown et al. (2)) lists the common offenders. Dyes and anilines reduce molecular oxygen and

Table 2 Agents Implicated in Methemoglobinemia

Local anesthetics
Benzocaine
Lidocaine
Procaine
Aniline dyes
Chlorates
Dapsone
Diarylsulfonylureas (Sulofenur)
Nitrates/nitrites
Sodium nitrites
Nitroglycerine
Amylnitrate
Nitrobenzines
Nitrofurans
Pyridium
Primaquine
Sulfonamides

generate metHb, sometimes in cycles, as the case of phenylhydroxylamine, which, after reducing oxy-Hb, generates nitrobenzene, which is reduced again to phenylhydroxylamine by red cell enzymes and in turn generates more metHb. Nitrites are common offenders, particularly in children, but the mechanism is less well understood. Recreational use of amyl, butyl, or isobutyl nitrites is another cause of acquired methemoglobinemia. In addition, infections might release toxins (including nitrites) that produce methemoglobin. More recently, several life-threatening cases of methemoglobinemia complicating endoscopic premedication have been reported. Interestingly, during the development of sulofenur as an antineoplastic agent, 1 patient in 9 had methemoglobinemia induced by the drug, and was found to be heterozygote for cytochrome b_5 reductase deficiency. In effect, many of the acquired cases might be an interaction between the use of an offending drug and a heterozygous state for a mutation associated, in the homozygous state, with hereditary methemoglobinemia.

E. Diagnosis of Methemoglobinemia

First, distinction is needed between methemoglobinemia resulting from enzyme deficiency or exposure to offending drugs or chemicals, and the HbMs. The best approach is a recorded visible spectrum of the hemolyzate. Enzyme deficiency and acquired methemoglobinemia have a typical met spectra between 450 and 650 μm (Fig. 5). All Hb Ms, in contrast, due to the change of the electronic environment of the heme, have abnormal spectra at 620 μm, clinching the diagnosis. Hb electrophoresis is of limited value, since the oxygenated forms of the M Hbs do not separate in cellulose acetate electrophoresis from normal hemoglobin. Acid agar electrophoresis and isoelectric focusing are better but require experts for correct diagnosis. HPLC separates them more easily but it is not usually available in medical institutions.

Recent or sudden clinically apparent cyanosis, in the absence of cardiopulmonary pathology, suggests *acquired* methemoglobinemia, although sulf-Hb should also be considered. Long standing or presence of the symptom in siblings is compatible with hereditary methemoglobinemia. Since this condition is genetically recessive, it should not be expected in the parents.

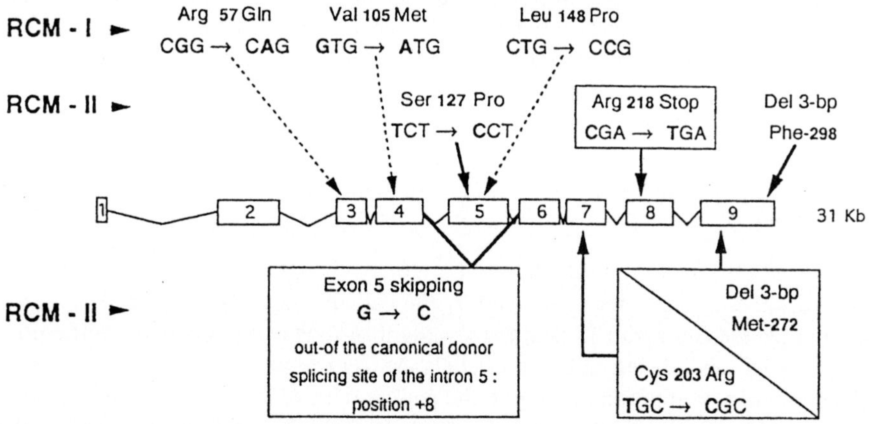

Figure 6 Schematic representation of mutations in types I and II. The structure of 31 kb of the cytb5r gene containing nine exons is shown. The location of mutations within the gene is presented by dashed arrows for type I and solid arrows for type II methemoglobinemia. The mutations described in this report are boxed. (From Ref. 16.)

The differential diagnosis is with hemoglobin Ms and low-affinity Hbs, in which the parents might be affected, since the defect is dominant. Enzymatic assay or spot test are available for the methemoglobin reductases. Prenatal diagnosis is available for type II. The effect of methylene blue is also diagnostic.

There is an unusual high incidence of hereditary methemoglobinemia among Attabaskan Eskimos and Northwest Indians, Navajo Indians, and natives of Yarkusk, Siberia, all of which might be ethnically connected. In addition, it has been observed among Puerto Ricans, African-Americans, and Mediterranean populations.

The incidence of HbM is quite low around the world, except in Shiden village, Iwate Prefecture, Japan, where the disease is known by the popular name of "kuroko" (black child).

F. Treatment of Methemoglobinemia

Acquired methemoglobinemia is treated by stopping the offending agent once it is identified. Methylene blue, 1 or 2 mg/kg, should be administered i.v. in patients with high levels of met-Hb (40–60%), particularly those with symptoms. It does not work in patients with coexisting glucose-6-phosphate dehydrogenase deficiency. In type I this intervention is only cosmetic and can be followed by methylene blue, 100–300 mg p.o., daily, to maintain the hemoglobin reduced. In aniline-induced methemoglobinemia, methylene blue can couple with oxyhemoglobin to generate free radicals, and produce the enhanced hemolysis observed in a few cases. The use of methylene blue should be limited in these cases to two doses. Methemoglobinemia over 70% can be life-threatening, and such patients should be exchange transfused.

Methemoglobinemia associated with HbMs needs no treatment. The diagnosis is important in these patients to avoid costly and sometimes dangerous invasive diagnostic procedures.

IV. SULFHEMOGLOBINEMIA

A. Definition

Sulfhemoglobin is a modification of the hemoglobin molecule that renders it a bright green color due to a sulfur atom incorporated into the porphyrin ring (Fig. 1). It has been associated with certain medications, although mostly when used in higher doses than recommended, in the course of drug abuse, with occupational exposure to sulfur compounds, and with environmental exposure to polluted air. Exposure to molten sulfur does not induce sulfhemoglobinemia. In summary, there is no genetic form of this disease, and all the cases are acquired sulfhemoglobinemia.

B. Clinical Features

Sulfhemoglobinemia is usually asymptomatic except for a change in color of the skin. If chronic and slowly installed, it may not be noticed by the patient or family. Industrial exposure to sulf-Hb-producing agents can result in death. The extent of dyspnea in cases of sulfhemoglobinemia is controversial, and absent unless the levels are very high.

For equivalent amounts of abnormal pigment, the patient with sulfhemoglobinemia appears bluer than the patient with methemoglobinemia, as a result of spectral differences between the pigments, but less symptomatic, as a result of the differences in oxygen affinity.

Sulf-Hb and met-Hb have been reported as coexisting in a number of cases of drug-induced hemoglobinopathy, and the lists of chemicals/drugs reported to produce these syndromes are overlapping.

Acetanilid, usually in the form of Bromo Seltzer, and phenacetin were found to be the main offenders in 62 cases of sulfhemoglobinemia seen at the Mayo Clinic. The aryl hydroxylamine metabolites of these drugs can serve as reducing agents in a cyclic process capable of generating both sulf-Hb and met-Hb. The origin of the sulfur atom in the former case remains unclear, but both H_2S generated by intestinal flora and glutathione have been suggested. It has been noted before that laboratory documentation is often inadequate to distinguish between the entities, and it is likely that sulfhemoglobin is underdiagnosed.

While Acetanilid was removed from Bromo Seltzer a number of years ago and the Food and Drug Administration removed phenacetin from the U.S. market, sulfhemoglobinemia will not disappear. In addition to industrial exposure, sulfonamides, dapsone, and sulfur-containing ointments are reported offenders and are still widely used. Some drugs reported to produce methemoglobin, including acetaminophen, may be found to also produce sulfhemoglobin when more careful analysis is done.

While sulfhemoglobinemia is probably a relatively nontoxic syndrome in individuals with hemoglobin A, it may prove to be a surprisingly toxic syndrome in individuals with Hb S—especially in comparison to methemoglobinemia, which would be expected to ameliorate sickling. The presence of sulfurated subunits will shift the conformation of Hb S tetramers toward the unliganded, polymerizing T form even in the presence of high pO_2. Microvascular occlusion could be exacerbated by the fact that these tetramers remain in the polymerizing conformation in both the arterial and venous circulations.

C. Pathophysiology

The modified hemes, by the addition of sulfur, have a drastically right-shifted oxygenation curve that render the molecule totally ineffective for oxygen transport. The oxygenation curve shows a right shift in the physiologically relevant pO_2 range. Since in most cases only a fraction of the hemes are modified, full saturation of unaltered hemes in the lungs and enhanced oxygen unloading at the tissues would be expected. Since this right shift would ameliorate any decrease in functional hemoglobin mass, by increasing the delivery of oxygen, sulfuration of hemes may have little physiologic significance as long as sufficient unmodified hemoglobin remains. This is fortunate, since there is no known treatment analogous to met-Hb reduction for reconverting sulf-Hb to functional Hb.

Whereas in methemoglobinemia some tetramers have subunits frozen in an oxidized R-like state (Darling-Roughton effect, see above), in sulfhemoglobinemia some tetramers have subunits frozen in a T-like state because they remain unliganded at physiologic pO_2. In the former case, a left-shifted oxygenation curve and impaired oxygen delivery results, while in the latter case a right-shifted curve and enhanced oxygen delivery occurs. The slightly high 2,3-DPG in the blood of patients with sulfhemoglobinemia probably reflects increased binding to the T-like sulfurated tetramers rather than an actual increase in free 2,3-DPG.

D. Diagnosis

Sulf-Hb is a green-pigmented protein that can be accurately identified by spectroscopy (Table 3) and by isoelectric focusing methods proposed by Park and Nagel (3). In the presence of methemoglobinemia, the diagnosis is more difficult and might be missed.

Differential diagnosis between genetic or acquired methemoglobinemia, HbMs and sulfhemoglobinemia in patient presenting with cyanosis (blue person): While the cardiac and pulmonary systems are major targets in the evaluation of a patient with apparent cyanosis, the differential diagnosis of this clinical sign includes two classes of hemoglobinopathies in addi-

Table 3 Laboratory Diagnosis of Cyanosis

Procedure: If a visible spectrum of the hemolysate reveals a peak in the 610–640 nm range, the following sequence of spectra should be taken: (1) the air-equilibrated sample with and without KCN; (2) the sample with dithionite; and (3) the sample with CO.

Interpretation: If only met-Hb is present, the abnormal peak will disappear immediately after the addition of dithionite or cyanide. For Hb M, the peak will disappear slowly and might require hours. For sulfhemoglobin, the peak undergoes a very slow decrease due to instability.

To distinguish sulfhemoglobin from Hb M, compare the spectra of the air- and CO-equilibrated samples. If CO results in an augmentation and downfield shift of the peak, the sample contains sulfhemoglobin.

tion to enzyme-deficient methemoglobinemia: (a) The presence of an abnormal Hb with a normal visible spectrum but a markedly right-shifted p50 results in significant arterial desaturation. (b) In sulf-Hb, met-Hb, and Hb M, the altered visible spectrum of the abnormal pigments is responsible for the gray skin color. The comparative spectral properties of sulf-Hb versus met-Hb are such that less of the former is needed to produce cyanosis, and it is not surprising that patients can be markedly cyanotic with 12% (1.6 gm/dL) sulf-Hb.

The respiratory status of individuals with cyanosis resulting from abnormal hemoglobin varies with the entity. There is general agreement that clinically apparent dyspnea is not associated with the mutant Hbs with right-shifted p50s or with Hbs M, but can be associated with even relatively mild degrees of methemoglobinemia. For sulfhemoglobinemia, there is no agreement. The majority of case reports indicate that dyspnea is not a feature, but others state that the symptoms associated with methemoglobinemia and sulfhemoglobinemia are "identical."

Since the altered hemes in Hb M, sulf-Hb, and met-Hb do not transport oxygen, affected individuals with all three entities may have normal hemoglobin levels but suffer the physiologic affects of an anemia simply because insufficient functional hemes remain. This effect, in isolation, would be clinically significant only in extreme cases of methemoglobinemia and sulfhemoglobinemia or when the overall Hb level is low. Severe cases of these abnormalities have been reported in which the abundance of nonfunctional hemes was the major concern. In contrast, with Hb M, the proportion of normal to abnormal hemes is genetically determined as greater than 75%, so the decrease of oxygen-binding capacity is a problem only when superimposed on underlying anemia.

However, it is important to note that the clinical effects of nonfunctional hemes need not be limited to their inability to transport oxygen. Small amounts of nonfunctional hemes can have clinical significance if their presence in partially modified tetramers produces a physiologically dysfunctional shift in the oxygenation curve. This is the molecular basis of the left-shifted oxygenation curve, the impaired oxygen delivery to the periphery, and the resulting respiratory distress seen in relatively mild degrees of methemoglobinemia. This phenomenon, described above as the Darling-Roughton effect, occurs because the oxidized subunits in partially oxidized tetramers are held in an R-like (or liganded) conformation and this increases the oxygen affinity of the remaining subunits. While mixed venous blood is unusually saturated, the abnormal spectrum of the methemoglobin outweighs this effect and the individual appears cyanotic. An analogous left shift in oxygenation curve occurs, to a more pronounced degree, in CO poisoning, and here too the impaired oxygen delivery is felt to exacerbate dyspnea.

In the Hb Ms, the presence of the abnormal nonfunctional hemes in the affected tetramers results in a marked flattening of the oxygen affinity curve. The curve is also right-shifted, especially in the most physiologically relevant pO_2 range. This leads to normal or even enhanced ability to deliver oxygen to tissues, consistent with the absence of respiratory insufficiency.

The procedure in Table 3 has been suggested by Park and Nagel (3) for evaluating the blood of individuals with pseudocyanosis with exposure to drugs or chemicals associated with methemoglobinemia or sulfhemoglobinemia.

CASE STUDY

Patient

Thirty-eight-year-old male, mine worker.

Chief Complaint

Painful burns over 35% of the skin, due to contact with molten sulfur.

Past Medical History

No diseases, no hospitalizations.

Medication

No history of medications.

Review of Systems and Physical Examination

Besides the skin burns, the rest of the skin had a gray-slate color. No organomegalies.

Laboratory Results

Normal CBC and chemistry. Blood appeared dark brown in color.

Consultation

Surgeon calls our laboratory from Texas, requesting the confirmation of their diagnosis: sulfhemoglobinemia, based on the observation of slate-gray color of the skin and exposure to sulfur.

Questions

1. Is molten sulfur capable of inducing, after contact with the skin and producing third-degree burns, sulfhemoglobin? The answer is no.
2. Then, how is the definitive diagnosis established?

Additional Laboratory Results

A hemolysate spectrophotometric tracing between 650 and 550 μm (see text) excluded the presence of sulfhemoglobin, and detected the presence of an M hemoglobin. Furthermore, examination of the hemolysate 6 months later demonstrated that the abnormal spectra remained identical, while a sulfhemoglobin spectra would have disappeared by then.

Diagnosis

Heterozygous for Hb M Boston-Washington, defined by protein sequence analysis. Also, x-ray crystallography of this hemoglobin was done by Dr. Max Perutz (Nobel Laureate) in Cambridge, England, demonstrating the details of the structure of the heme pocket in this abnormal hemoglobin, and the position of the tyrosine replacing the histidine. This work produced a new understanding of the environment of the iron in the heme, and what is critical to maintain the ferrous state.

Discussion

This patient demonstrates that cases with skin color change (blue men/women) are easy to diagnose if you are somewhat familiar with the subject, and that the largest benefit derived by the patient from the diagnosis is avoiding costly and sometimes dangerous workups for cardiopulmonary disease. The patient described here is indeed a case in point, since further analysis of the pedigree of the proband demonstrated that a son of the patient had undergone a Blalock operation to correct a ductus arteriosus a couple of weeks after birth, due to the detection of a slate-gray coloration to his skin. When we obtained a sample of blood from this patient, he turned out to be a carrier of Hb M Boston-Washington. When performing the Blalock the surgeon did not confirm the presence of the anomaly. Hence, it is very likely that the operation was unnecessary and the abnormal color of the skin, which he retained after the operation, was due to the M hemoglobin.

Unfortunately, when the proband realized this possibility, he terminated his relationships with all physicians. I hope he has changed his mind by now.

REFERENCES

1. Jaffe ER. Methemoglobinemia in the differential diagnosis of cyanosis. Hosp Practice 1985; 20:92.
2. Brown CM, Levy SA, Sussan PW. Methemoglobinemia: life-threatening complication of endoscopy premedication. Am J Gastroenterol 1994; 89:1108.
3. Park CM, Nagel RL. Sulfhemoglobin: clinical and molecular aspects. N Engl J Med 1984; 310:1579.

SUGGESTED READINGS

1. Antionini E, Brunori M. Hemoglobin and myoglobin in their reactions with ligands. In: Neuberger A, Balster RL, Ekelund LG, Grover RF. Evaluation of subpopulations potentially at risk to carbon monoxide exposure. In Air Quality Criteria for Carbon Monoxide. EPA 600/8-90/045F. Research Triangle Park, NC: Environmental Criteria and Assessment Office, Office of Health and Environmental Assessment, Office of Research and Development, U.S. Environmental Protection Agency, 1991:12-1 to 12-23.
2. Basch F. On hydrogen sulfide poisoning from external application of elementary sulfur as an ointment. Arch Exp Pathol Pharmacol 1926; 111:126.
3. Benesch RE, Maeda N, Benesch R. 2,3-Diphosphoglycerate and the relative affinity of adult and fetal hemoglobin for oxygen and carbon dioxide. Biochim Biophys Acta 1972; 257:178–182.
4. Beutler E, Milcus BJ. The effect of methemoglobin formation in sickle cell disease. J Clin Invest 1961; 40:1856.
5. Brown CM, Levy SA, Sussan PW. Methemoglobinemia: life-threatening complication of endoscopy premedication. Am J Gastroenterol 1994; 89:1108.
6. Bunn HF, Forget BG. Hemoglobin: Molecular, Genetic and Clinical Aspects. Philadelphia: Saunders, 1986.
7. Burnett E, King EG, Grace M, Hall WF. Hydrogen sulfide poisoning review of 5 years' experience. Can Med Assoc J 1977; 117:1277.
8. Cumming RLC, Pollock A. Drug-induced sulfhaemoglobinemia and Heinz body anemia in pregnancy with involvement of the foetus. Scott Med J 1967; 12:320.
9. Darling RC, Roughton FJW. The effect of methemoglobin on the equilibrium between oxygen and hemoglobin. Am J Physiol 1942; 137:56.
10. Engel RR, Rodkey FL, O'Neal JD, et al. Relative affinity of human fetal hemoglobin for CO and O_2. Blood 1969; 33:37–45.

11. Environmental Protection Agency. Air Quality Criteria for Carbon Monoxide. EPA 600/8-90/045F. Research Triangle Park, NC: Environmental Criteria and Assessment Office, Office of Health and Environmental Assessment, Office of Research and Development, U.S. Environmental Protection Agency, 1991:1-1 to 12-23.
12. Ford R, Shkov J, Akman WV, et al. Deaths from asphyxia among fishermen. MMWR 1978; 27: 309.
13. Gemelli F, Cattani R. Carbon monoxide poisoning in childhood. Br Med J 1985; 291:1197.
14. Gibson QH. The reduction of methaemoglobin in red blood cells and studies on the cause of idiopathic methaemoglobinaemia. Biochem J 1948; 42:13–23.
15. Jaffe ER. Methemoglobinemia in the differential diagnosis of cyanosis. Hosp Practice 1985; 20:92.
16. Kaplan JC, Leroux A, Beauvais P. Formes cliniques et biologiques de deficit en cytochrome b5 reductase. CR Seances Soc Biol 1979; 173:368.
17. Lambert M, Sonnet J, Mahien P, Hassoun A. Delayed sulfhemoglobinemia after acute dapsone intoxication. Clin Toxicol 1982; 19:45.
18. Mahoney JJ, Vreman HJ, Stevenson DK, et al. Measurement of carboxyhemoglobin and total hemoglobin by five specialized spectrophotometers (CO-oximeters) in comparison with reference methods. Clin Chem 1993; 39:1963–1700.
19. McCutcheon AD. Sulfhaemoglobinaemia and glutathione. Lancet 1980; 2:290.
20. Medeiros MH, Bechara EJ, Naaoum PC, Mourso CA. Oxygen toxicity and hemoglobinemia in subjects from a highly polluted town. Arch Environ Health 1983; 38:11.
21. Nagel RL. Disorders of hemoglobin function and stability. In: Handon RI, Lux SE, Stossel TP, eds. Blood: Principles and Practices of Hematology. Philadelphia: Lippincott, 1995:1591–1613.
22. Nagel RL, Bemski G, Pincus P. Some aspects of the binding of Cu(II) to human hemoglobin and its subunits. Arch Biochem Biophys 1970; 137:428.
23. Nichol AW, Hendry I, Movell DB, Clezy PS. Mechanism of formation of sulfhemoglobin. Biochim Biophys Acta 1958; 156:97.
24. Park CM, Nagel RL. Sulfhemoglobin: clinical and molecular aspects. N Engl J Med 1984; 310: 1579.
25. Passon PG, Hultquist DE. Soluble cytochrome b5 reductase from human erythrocytes. Biochim Biophys Acta 1972; 275:62.
26. Pinkas J, Pjaldetti M, Joshua H, et al. Sulfhemoglobinemia and acute hemolytic anemia with Heinz bodies following contact with a fungicide-zinc ethylanol bisthiocarbamate: in a subject with glucose-6-phosphate dehydrogenase deficiency and hypocatalassemia. Blood 1963; 21:484.
27. Prchal JT, Borgese N, Moore MR, Moreno H, Hegesh E, Hall MK. Cogenital methemoglobinemia due to methemoglobin reductase deficiency in two unrelated American black families. Am J Med 1990; 89:516.
28. Stewart RD, Fisher TN, Hosko MJ, et al. Carboxyhemoglobin elevation after exposure to dichloromethane. Science 1972; 176:295–296.
29. Reynolds TB, Ware AG. Sulfemoglobinemia following habitual use of acetanilid. JAMA 1952; 149:1538.
30. Schwartz JM, Reiss AI, Jaffe ER. Hereditary methemoglobinemia with deficiency of NADH-cytochrome reductase b_5 reductase. In: Stambury JB, Wyngaarden JB, Goldstein IL, Brown ??, eds. The Molecular Basis of Disease. 5th ed. New York: McGraw-Hill, 1983:1654.
31. Vreman HJ, Mahoney JJ, Stevenson DK. Carbon monoxide and carboxyhemoglobin. Adv Pediatr 1995; 42.

23

Practical Approach to Molecular Biology in Hematopathology

Anwar Mikhael and Harold R. Schumacher
University of Cincinnati Medical Center, Cincinnati, Ohio

I. INTRODUCTION

Not too far in the distant past, approaches to the diagnosis of hematologic disorders were based predominantly on clinical criteria, interpretation of cell morphology, cytogenetics, and cytochemistry. It is the interface between hematology and immunology coupled with the recent advancement of molecular tools that has allowed further characterization and classification of lymphoproliferative disorders and acute leukemias. It is the hope that such understanding will allow better prognosis, diagnosis, therapy, and patient management.

For these reasons, a brief background regarding the basic application of molecular biology in diagnostic hematopathology is presented.

II. DETECTION OF CLONAL LYMPHOID POPULATION

A. Organization of the Ig Locus

The immune system has evolved to provide antibody molecules with different combining sites, diverse to a degree to recognize a myriad of antigens.

The process of somatic rearrangement is a prerequisite for the generation and expression of the Ig receptor. In the germline configuration, the single Ig heavy-chain locus consists of a several segments. There are about 100 variable (V) genes located upstream of 10–20 diversity (D) segment region genes and 6 junction (J) segment genes. Over the next 150 kb (kilobases) lies the constant region. It consists, starting from the 5′ end, of the constant region of μ, δ, γ_3, γ_1, α_1, γ_2, γ_4, ε, and α_2. The organization of the gene segments coding for the light chains is similar to that for the heavy chains except for the absence of D segment genes and the presence of only one constant region gene κ (kappa) or λ (lambda). Figure 1 depicts the organization of the Ig heavy- and light-chain loci.

Assembly of both heavy- and light-chain genes involves similar molecular mechanisms. Present at the boundaries of all germline segments are consensus sequences consisting of a conserved palindromic heptamer and nanomer separated by either 12 or 23 bp of non-conserved spacer sequences. Recombination is catalysed by the recombinase (RAG-1 and

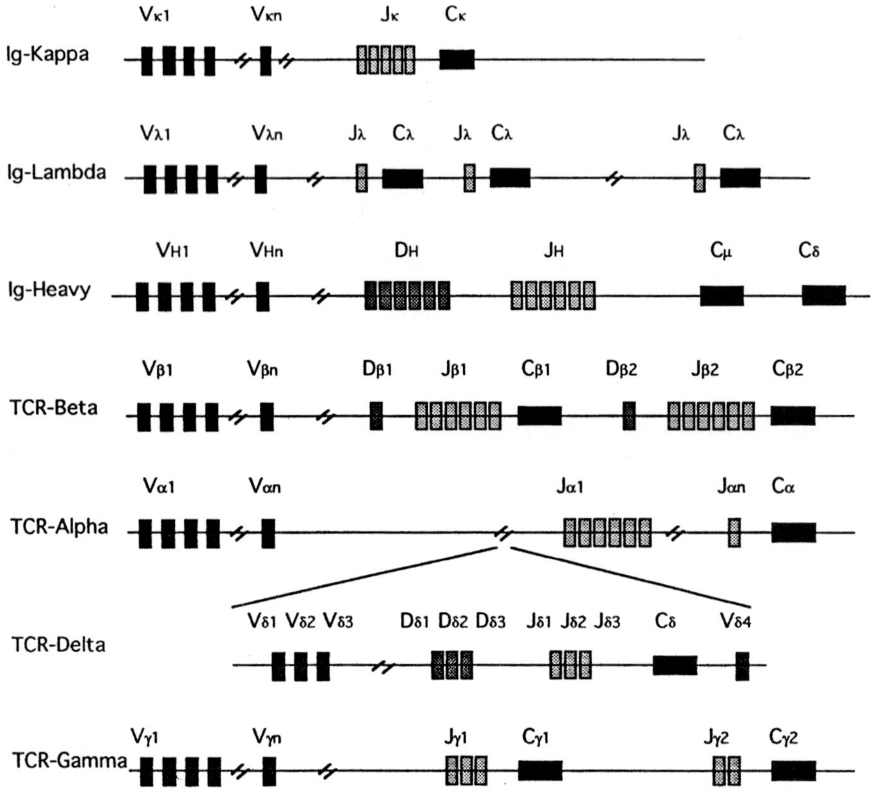

Figure 1 Genomic organization of the immunoglobulin (Ig) and T-cell receptor (TCR) genes. In the germline configuration these genes are composed of multiple segments, the variable (V), the diversity (D), and the joining (J) region gene segments. One segment of each of these genes eventually rearranges.

RAG-2) system. In addition, terminal deoxynucleotidyl transferase (TdT) will add a few nucleotides at the junction, thereby inducing more Ig diversity (1,2).

2. *Ig Rearrangement*

During B-cell ontogeny, B-cell progenitors, present in the bone marrow, undergo Ig heavy-chain gene recombinations. Initially, there is junction of one of the D segments to one of the J segments, with the subsequent recombination of one of the V-gene segment to the newly formed DJ. Rearrangement of the IgH gene segments creates unique DNA sequences at the junction of V, D, and J. These regions are specifically associated with a unique B-cell clone.

A switch site is present upstream of each constant region except the IgD constant region. Upstream of the first switch site (S_{μ}) is the enhancer, which is not deleted during VDJ rearrangements or in the subsequent switching events. Activation of the variable region gene's promotor occurs after VDJ rearrangements, which bring the promotor of the rearranged V-gene segment closer to the enhancer (3) (Fig. 2).

3. *Expression of Ig Chains*

The rearranged gene is transcribed into a primary m-RNA transcript. This nuclear transcript contains noncoding sequences which are spliced out, while the immature transcript is in the

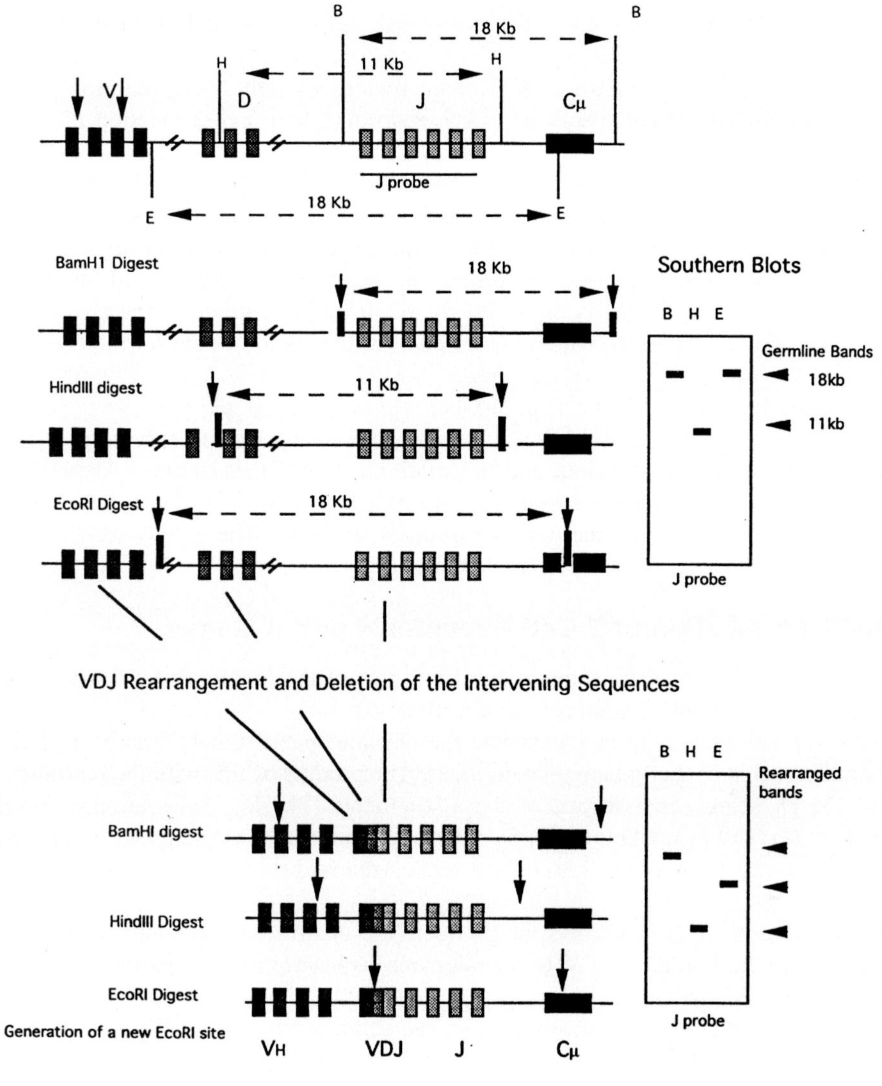

Figure 2 Southern blot analysis of Ig and TCR. DNA extracted from total peripheral blood lymphocytes is digested with three different restriction enzymes. The digested DNA fragments are separated by agarose gel electrophoresis, transfer to nylon filters and hybridized with ^{32}P-labeled probes followed by autoradiography. The upper panel denotes the restriction enzyme map of the germline and the predicted size on a Southern using a J_H probe. Any detectable band different in size from the germline band indicates a rearrangement (lower panel). Vertical lines and arrows indicate the restriction enzyme sites (B, BamHI; H, HindIII, and E, EcoRI).

nucleus. The mature m-RNA is exported to the cytoplasm and is translated into cytoplasmic IgM chain.

The pre-B-cell expressing cytoplasmic IgM chain undergoes light-chain rearrangement. Activation of the kappa-chain locus occurs with V_kJ_k rearrangement and production of cytoplasmic kappa light chain. An IgM-kappa surface-expressing B cell results. In the event of a nonproductive rearrangement of both kappa-chain alleles, the pre-B cells proceed to rearrange the lambda light-chain locus. The productive rearrangement of one of the lambda light chains leads to the expression of cytoplasmic lambda light chain, assembly of heavy and light chains, and expression of cell surface IgM-lambda molecule. The preferential expression of the membrane versus the secreted form of IgM is regulated by the differential usage of the membrane or the secreted exons of the IgM locus, which is located 3′ of the exons coding for the constant domains of the IgM molecule (4).

Association of the heavy- and light-chain variable region generates the variable region of the Ig molecule. Upon exposure to the specific antigen, the mature IgM-expressing B cell undergoes further maturation, cell division, and Ig switching to the other isotypes. Depending on the type of antigen and lymphokines secreted by the T-helper cells, a B cell switches from surface IgM/IgD expression to one of the other Ig isotypes (Roitt I.). These cells secrete high levels of Ig, some of which will eventually differentiate to plasma cells.

B. Genomic Organization of T-Cell Receptor α and β Genes

The genomic organization of the TCR genes is similar to that of the Ig. Figure 1 illustrates the spatial separation of V, D, J, and C segments in T cells (5,6).

The order of β-chain locus rearrangement and the rearrangement signals (haptomer-23nt-nanomer) are similar to that of the Ig heavy-chain locus. The process begins with the rearrangement of one of the D_β segments with one of the J_β segments. The $D_{\beta 1}$ can rearrange to all functional J regions ($J_{\beta 1}$ and $J_{\beta 2}$), whereas the $D_{\beta 2}$ rearrange only to $J_{\beta 2}$ elements with deletion of the intervening sequences. This is followed by a second rearrangement of the newly formed DJ_β to a V_β.

Activation of the α-chain locus follows the productive β-chain rearrangement. Rearrangement consists solely of the joining of a V to a J segment. Transcription and pairing of the α and β chains generate a TCRαβ.

Rearrangement of γ and δ TCR genes occurs by the same mechanisms as Ig and TCR α and β genes. Since the δ gene is entirely located within the α-chain locus, rearrangement of the α locus leads eventually to δ-locus deletion.

C. Detection of Clonal Population by Southern Blot

A nonclonal reactive lymphoid population consists of a mixture of a multitude of B- and T-cell clones. Restriction enzyme digests of the Ig or TCR loci from this polyclonal response results in a multitude of different size DNA fragments. Southern blot analysis will fail to detect a distinct rearranged band. Therefore, a monoclonal proliferative process is the expansion of one clone to a sufficient detectable magnitude that can be characterized by its unique DNA rearrangement pattern. In addition, detection of tumor-associated Ig or TCR DNA rearrangements is achievable provided that an appropriate cloned DNA probe is available. In practice, the probe should detect Ig or TCR rearrangement from a myriad of B- and T-cell tumors.

Typically, extracted DNA is digested with three different restriction enzymes (EcoRI, BamHI, and HindIII), followed by agarose gel electrophoresis, transfer to nylon filter, hybridization with ^{32}P-labeled DNA probe, and subsequent autoradiography. The size of the germ-

Table 1 Guidelines for the Interpretation of Southern Blots

Germline bands only:
Nonlymphoid tissue (normal and neoplastic)
Polyclonal reactive lymphoid response
Nondetectable monoclonal population (<5% neoplastic DNA)
Monoclonal band comigrate with the germline band (rare)
Germline band and rearranged bands:
Homogeneous lymphoid population with one rearranged allele and one germline allele
Monoclonal population mixed with reactive lymphocytes and stromal cells
Rearranged bands only:
Monoclonal population with rearrangement of both alleles

line bands have been determined based on the restriction enzyme map of the Ig and TCR loci (Fig. 2).

Detection of germline band(s) in a DNA sample extracted from a tissue specimen suspected of containing malignant lymphoid cells represents the unrearranged alleles of both the normal cells (stromal and reactive lymphoid) and malignant lymphoid cells. In general, the presence of a rearranged band, usually lower in molecular weight than the germline band, indicates the existence of a monoclonal population. On occasion the rearranged band may comigrate with the germline band. Examination of the other restriction enzyme digestions will reveal the rearranged bands. In general, the ratio of the intensity of the rearranged bands to the germline band should be similar between the different restriction enzymes. Guidelines for the interpretation of Southern blot in the detection of monoclonality are provided in Table 1.

D. Application of Southern Blot Analysis

Analysis of the genomic organization of the Ig and TCR gene loci has become a sensitive tool to assess clonality and to establish cell lineage of lymphoproliferative disorders (Table 2). Gene rearrangement studies are sensitive enough to detect as low as 1–5% tumor-cell associated DNA in a sample Ig and TCR gene rearrangement analysis will determine whether a proliferative process is mono-, poly-, or oligoclonal. This technique has complemented histologic examination in the evaluation of residual and recurrent lymphoproliferative disease. Table 3 provides a guideline for the interpretation of Ig and TCR gene rearrangement results.

1. Acute leukemias

a. Acute Lymphoblastic Leukemias. Virtually all B-lineage acute lymphoblastic leukemias (ALLs) have Ig heavy-chain gene rearrangement; about 40% and only 20% have κ and λ light-chain gene rearrangements, respectively (Table 4). Furthermore, leukemias with imma-

Table 2 Application of Southern Blot Analysis of Ig and TCR to the Diagnosis of Lymphoproliferative Disorders

Distinguish a reactive hyperplasia from non-Hodgkin's lymphoma
Confirm the clonality and lineage of $CD3^-$ surface Ig^- NHL
Demonstrate the clonality of peripheral T-cell lymphoma
Confirm the cell lineage of $CD3^-$ $CD16^+$ proliferative disease
Determine the cell lineage of biphenotypic cases of acute leukemias
Confirm the cell lineage of lymphoid blast crisis of CML
Monitor the response to therapy

Table 3 Interpretation of Gene Rearrangement Studies

IgH	IgL	TCR	
G	G	G	Nonlymphoid neoplasm; immature lymphoid neoplasm
R	G	G	Monoclonal suggestive B cell
R	R	G	B-cell neoplasm
R	G	R	Clonal of undetermined lineage
G	R	G	Probable B lineage, unusual
G	G	R	T-cell neoplasm

ture B-cell precursors (ALL) have greater tendency than mature B-cell lymphoma to rearrange their TCR locus. Nevertheless, in these cases, B-cell lineage assignment is possible. The use of light-chain probes and probes specific for kappa-deleting elements (located in the Jk-Ck intron) will further determine the B-cell lineage (7).

Likewise, the majority of T-ALLs demonstrate T-cell receptor gene rearrangements (δ, β genes). In addition, 14% of immature T-cell precursor ALL demonstrates a nonlineage-specific Ig heavy-chain rearrangement. Although light-chain rearrangement is pathognomonic of B-cell lineage, there are rare cases of κ-gene rearrangements in T-cell ALL (8). Furthermore, early prethymic T cells, with immature T-cell phenotype, may lack any of the TCR genes rearrangements (9). Therefore, in these cases, the final diagnosis should be rendered in the context of more conventional data (Table 4).

b. Acute Myelocytic leukemia. In acute myelocytic leukemias (AML), reports of the frequency of Ig and TCR genes rearrangements vary greatly. These findings stress the nonspecificity of Ig and TCR gene rearrangement studies or, alternatively, may depict a genuine finding present in bilineage leukemias. Approximately 2% of patients with AML have rearrangements of Ig K, supposedly a specific β-cell lineage marker. In any case, the majority of AML that rearrange either their Ig or TCR genes are TdT positive. Although some of these latter may represent bilineage leukemias, it is only recently that this entity has been recognized, and it requires further clinical study and evaluation (Table 4).

Table 4 Frequency of Ig and TCR Rearrangement in Leukemia and Lymphoma

	IgH	Igκ	Igλ	TCRβ	TCRγ	TCRδ
B-cell ALL	98	40	20	33	55	80
T-cell ALL	14	0	0	89	91	96
AML	14	2	0	7	5	9
Childhood ALL	64	18	0	9	0	—
B-NHL	95	95	30	7	0	0
T-NHL	7	0	0	90	95	95
HD	15	10	5	15	—	—
Ki-anaplastic	10	10	0	60	60	—
THL	20	10	0	40	40	—

THL: True histiocytic lymphoma.
Source: Adapted from Refs. 8, 45–48.

2. *Chronic Leukemia*

a. Chronic Lymphocytic Leukemia. The diagnosis of chronic lymphocytic leukemia (CLL) can be easily rendered based on clinical and morphologic criteria. The lymphocytes of CLL are mature B cells, and virtually all CLL lymphocytes rearrange their Ig heavy and Ig light chains. TCR β-chain rearrangement is present in about 10% of cases.

Likewise, in hairy cell leukemia, in addition to immunophenotyping, gene rearrangement studies confirm the B-cell lineage. Virtually all hairy cell leukemias rearrange their Ig heavy-chain gene, and only <5% have a simultaneous TCR-β gene rearrangement.

Southern blot analysis provides genotypic evidence of the existence of subsets of large granular lymphocytosis (LGL). LGL presents with two major phenotypes: T-LGL ($CD3^+$) and NK-LGL ($CD3^-$). Genotypically, T-cell receptor gene rearrangement is present in the former subset and absent in the latter (10).

b. Chronic Myelocytic Leukemia. The hallmark of chronic myelogenous leukemia (CML) is a shortened chromosome 22 (Philadelphia chromosome), which results from a reciprocal translocation involving the long arm of chromosomes 9 and 22. It can be demonstrated in >90% of patients with CML and in 10–25% of adult patients with ALL. The universal association of the Philadelphia chromosome with the earliest detectable stages of CML implies that it has at least an initiating role.

As a consequence of the translocation, sequences of the *ABL* proto-oncogene are moved from chromosome 9 to chromosome 22, where they are located in the 3′ region of the *BCR* gene. The breakpoints on chromosome 9 are widely distributed and range from about 15 to over 40 kb upstream of the most proximal region (first exon) of the *ABL* gene. However, the breakpoint on chromosome 22 occurs over a much shorter region of approximately 5–10 kb. This region is referred as the major breakpoint cluster region (M-bcr) (11).

In CML, this new chimeric gene produces a predicted large transcription product initiated on chromosome 22 and crossing over the translocation breakpoint to the *ABL* sequences. Splicing reduces this structure to a final mRNA of about 8.7 kb which encodes the p210 *BCR-ABL* gene product. The p210 BCR-ABL protein has been reported to occur in both CML and ALL. In Ph-positive acute leukemia, 50–80% of patients have a breakpoint more proximal to the *BCR* region and codes for a 190-kDa protein. This is generally considered to be a lymphoid lineage specific. Southern blot analysis has been used to demonstrate *BCR-ABL* translocation in cases where the karyotypic studies were unconclusive (12). In addition, the lymphoid blast crisis of CML may demonstrate clonal Ig-heavy chain rearrangement as well as *BCR-ABL* translocation (13).

3. *Malignant Lymphoma*

a. Non-Hodgkin's Lymphomas (NHL). Southern blot analysis had the greatest impact on the diagnosis of non-Hodgkin's lymphomas (NHL) (14–16). Table 2 summarizes the different applications of Southern blot in NHL. Virtually all B-cell NHL are mature B cells. Ig heavy and light chains are rearranged in 90% and 100% respectively (17–19). In addition, TCR analysis of mature B-cell lymphoma discloses TCR β rearrangement in only 10% of cases. Likewise, rare cases of T-cell malignancies demonstrate κ or λ light-chain rearrangements (20,21). In these instances the use of probes specific for Ig kappa-deleting element and Ig light chains will help to further determine the cell lineage (7).

T-cell lymphomas are often more challenging than B-cell malignancies. Unlike Ig genes, there is no specific clonal marker for T-cell receptors. Quite often, an accurate diagnosis requires analysis of the genomic organization of the TCR in addition to immunophenotyping (22). Although aberrant expression of T-cell marker(s) may be considered an indication of malignancy, monoclonality should be confirmed by TCR gene analysis (23). In any case, the majority of peripheral T-cell lymphomas (PTCL) display TCR gene(s) rearrangement; only <7% demonstrate a TCR germline configuration (21,22,24), and a similar percentage have rearranged their Ig heavy-chain locus (25).

b. Hodgkin's Lymphoma. Southern blot analysis of DNA of a limited number of cases with large numbers of Reed-Sternberg (RS) cells and their variants (RS/HV) as well as enriched RS/HV populations and the incidence of clonal Ig H rearrangements is high.

More convincing evidence is offered by analysis of individual RS cells which revealed B-cell immunophenotype characterized by rearranged immunoglobulin variable-region heavy-chain genes. Even more interesting, is the findings in a composite lymphoma (follicular lymphoma and Hodgkin's disease) and a B-cell lymphoma followed by Hodgkin's disease three years later (50, 51). In tissue from each patient, the B-cells from the lymphoma had virtually the same rearranged V genes as the Reed-Sternberg cells. Therefore, it is of great importance to uncover the molecular events that drive the precursor in the direction of a RS cell or take it on the road toward a neoplasm of mature B-cells (56, 58).

III. POLYMERASE CHAIN REACTION

A. Introduction

Hybridization of Southern blot with probes specific for leukemic-associated DNA detect rearrangement in samples that contain no less than 1% leukemic cells. Although this technique is highly specific, it lacks the sensitivity required to detect and predict a leukemic relapse. Most patients in remission harbor only a few leukemic cells. Residual malignant cells that resist standard therapy may eventually expand, and a significant percentage of the patients will succumb to their disease. Detection of as few as 1 in 10^6 cells is required to develop treatment strategies.

In theory, polymerase chain reaction (PCR) allows the amplification of DNA from a single cell. This technique can reproducibly detects cells present at a concentration of 1 to 10^4 to 10^5. Because of this sensitivity, PCR has in many instances replaced the use of Southern blot in diagnostic hematopathology (Table 5). More important, it can be applied to small tissue samples (skin biopsies) and to samples with substantial DNA degradation, which are often not suitable for Southern blot technology.

PCR requires knowledge of the DNA sequences of interest. Two sequence-specific primers can be prepared synthetically to hybridize to the DNA sequences of interest. The two sites should not be separated by a large stretch of DNA; rather, it is best utilized with DNA segments less than 1 kb. In the event that the primers are separated by large DNA segments, the use of c-DNA, generated by reverse transcription of m-RNA, as a template, overcomes this problem. Repeated cycles of denaturation, annealing, and extension allow the rapid amplification of the DNA segment of interest. The amplified DNA can be visualized on an electrophoretic DNA gel stained with ethidium bromide (Fig. 3).

Table 5 Application of PCR

Confirm the presence of malignant lymphoma/leukemia
Detect bone marrow involvement
Monitor the response to chemotherapy
Detect minimal residual disease
Diagnosis of relapse before the appearance of clinical symptoms

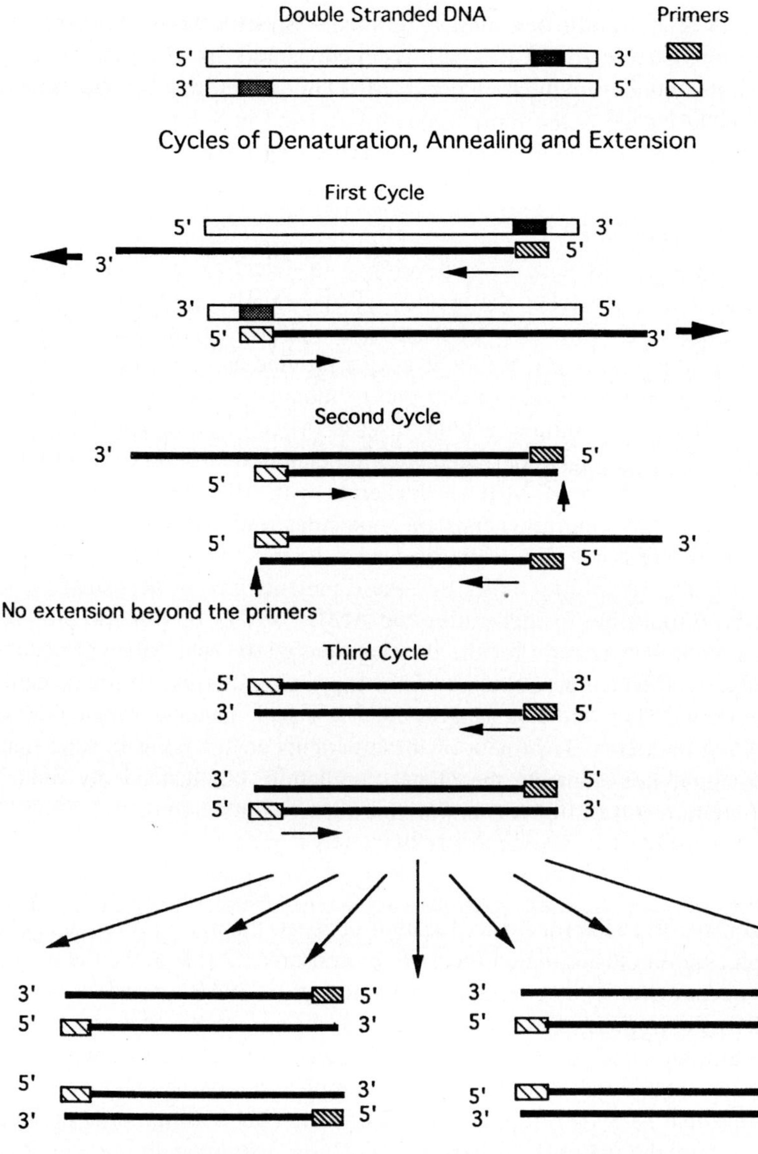

Figure 3 Polymerase chain reaction: amplification of DNA sequences.

B. Application of PCR

1. Acute Lymphoblastic Leukemia

The use of a PCR-based amplification and hybridization strategy (26) allows the detection of the V-gene usage of the leukemic cells in relapse. Such a PCR strategy enables the detection of minimal residual disease, patient surveillance after the induction of a disease-free state, and verification of the effectiveness of purging bone marrow of leukemic cells (Table 5).

In addition to B-ALL, PCR allows the detection of minimal residual disease (MRD) in T-cell ALL. The use of primers specific for TCR-γ and -δ junctions can detect clonal specific PCR products (27). This strategy uncovers the presence of MRD in cases with TCR γ–δ recombinations (27). Since the TAL-1 gene is the most frequently deleted in T-lineage leukemias, detection of TAL-1 gene abnormality strongly indicates the presence of MRD in this subset of T-cell leukemias (28–30).

2. Acute Myelocytic Leukemia (AML)

Reverse transcriptase (RT) PCR assays have been developed to detect the t(15;17)-encoded PML-RARa, the t(8;21)-encoded AMLI-ETO, the inv(16) CBFβ-MYHII, and the most prevalent translocations affecting the MLL gene. Each of these assays allows the rapid and specific detection of the molecular lesions; moreover, RT-PCR assays provide an exceptional level of one leukemic cell among 10^6 normal cells, permitting one to monitor a patient's response to therapy. Detection of the presence of minimal residual disease (MRD) in a patient following documented molecular remission is strongly correlated with impending relapse in cases of t(15; 17)-containing APL. Similarly, evidence of MRD in leukemia with MLL rearrangements id predicative of imminent relapse. By contrast, persistent molecular transcripts have been observed in patients in long-term remission. The significance of the positive result in these patients remains to be defined. The possibility exists that these patients have a persistent clone containing the translocation responsible for generating the AML1 or CBFβ chimeric protein, but lack the cooperating mutations necessary for the development of the full leukemic phenotype. This possibility is supported recent data obtained from expression of these fusion proteins in murine experimental systems. Thus, the data suggest that these patients have a preleukemic clone incapable of producing leukemia. Treatment of these patients at this point in time may be ill advised, in that it might not eradicate the clonal population, but instead my induce secondary mutations that could result in full conversion to a leukemic phenotype (52–55, 57).

3. Chronic Leukemia

In CML, the *BCR/ABL* consist of a reciprocal translocation between the c-abl proto-oncogene present at 9q34 and the breakpoint cluster region (bcr) of chromosome 22q11. Since the breakpoint on chromosome 9 occurs over a long distance, detection of *BCR/ABL* translocation by PCR using genomic DNA as a template may be unsuccessful; the use of RT-PCR may overcome this problem. In addition, PCR can detect *BCR/ABL* translocation in cases where the karyotypic studies have been suboptimal. Many patients in complete remission following bone marrow transplant show residual *BCR/ABL* transcript by RT-PCR. This finding is not predictive of imminent relapse; in fact, the majority of these patients have histologically normal bone marrow. However, the detection of increasing amount of *BCR/ABL* PCR product or conversion to a positive PCR over a period of few months may distinguish those patients who are at greater risk for relapse (35–37).

4. Non-Hodgkin's Lymphomas

About 90% of the follicular B-cell lymphomas and 15–20% of the large diffuse B-cell lymphomas carry the t(14;18)(q32;q21) which involves the Ig heavy-chain locus present on chromosome 14 and the *bcl-2* locus present on chromosome 18. The *bcl-2* breakpoints tend to cluster to two regions: a major and a minor breakpoint cluster region. The Ig heavy-chain region breakpoints occur near the 5′ end of any one of the 5 J_H gene segments. Therefore, a follicular lymphoma B-cell clone has a unique *BCL-2*/JH fusion gene. The use of primers that hybridize to the *BCL-2* gene and to the J_H segments generate a PCR product of a specific size, characteristic of the specific case of follicular lymphoma. This technique allows the detection of residual cells following chemotherapy or bone marrow transplantation, and is useful in monitoring the efficacy of bone marrow purging techniques prior to transplant (38). Detection of residual cells by PCR is associated with a markedly increased risk of relapse.

IV. FLUORESCENCE IN-SITU HYBRIDIZATION

A. Introduction

Since the observation that chromosomal alternations of human neoplasms are nonrandom, conventional karyotyping of banded chromosomes plays an important role in diagnosis, prognosis, and management of patients. This technique suffers from inherent limitations. Conventional karyotyping requires viable dividing cells that can be arrested in metaphase. In addition, cells with low mitotic activity, terminally differentiated cells, and specimens with a large number of normal cells are suboptimal for conventional karyotyping.

During the last decade, in-situ hybridization of nonisotopically labeled probes that can be detected by conventional fluorescence has been used to identify chromosomal alternation of interphase (nonmitotic) cells. This technique can be easily applied to cases that are not suitable for Southern blot analysis and, more important, can detect chromosomal abnormalities in cases where conventional cytogenetic studies are normal and the diagnosis based on cell morphology is debatable.

The technique requires the availability of DNA probes specific for the chromosomal aberrations seen in leukemias. These probes can be:

1. Chromosome-specific, hybridizing to satellite DNA sequences present at the centromere. These are especially applicable to cases with numerical abnormalities.
2. Hybridizable to multiple sequences from a single chromosome (chromosome painting). These are particularly suitable for structural rearrangements (translocation). Examples include Philadelphia chromosome translocation t(9;22) of CML, the t(8;14), t(2;8) and t(8;22) seen in Burkitt's and 11q23 seen in ALL.
3. Specific to a unique sequence.

B. Application of FISH

1. Application in Acute Leukemias

In B-cell ALL, FISH detects translocation and numerical chromosomal abnormalities (39). Since hyperdiploid karyotype (>50) is the most common cytogenetic abnormality in childhood ALL, centromere-specific probes (for chromosomes 1, 6, 8, 12, 17, 18, X, and Y) detect numerical abnormalities (40). Although this finding carries a beneficial prognostic value, it is not associated with a specific phenotype. In AML, numerical chromosomal abnormalities occur with some frequency. The finding of a trisomy, as in the case of trisomy 8 (41) allows the documentation of clonal response to therapy (42). In addition, as in trisomy 8, FISH allows discrimination between a reactive and a neoplastic myeloid process in cases with questionable diagnosis. Similarly, the availability of centromeric and regional probe sets for chromosome 5 and 7 detect −7/del(7q) and 5q− and assist in determining the presence of MDS, therapy-related MDS, and evaluation of these patients for minimal residual disease (43).

Probe sets for chromosomes 15 and 17 identify the characteristic translocation t(15,17) of acute promyelocytic leukemia (APL) FAB M3. Although the diagnosis of APL can be made by morphology, in some cases a rapid confirmation of the diagnosis may be indispensable to definitively establish the diagnosis before starting the patient on a specific therapeutic regimen. In addition, FISH can detect inversion of chromosome 16 in AML FAB M4 Eo variant.

2. *Application in Chronic Leukemia*

Two-color FISH analysis, using probes for BCR and ABL genes, can detect the doublet signal characteristic of *BCR-ABL* translocation of CML in interphase cells (44). This technique can help (1) to confirm the diagnosis of CML in Ph-negative cases when the conventional karyotype analysis is normal, (2) differentiate between leukemoid reaction and CML, and (3) detect the complex karyotype associated with Ph chromosome.

Finally, since 50% of CLL patients have cytogenetic abnormalities, FISH is much more sensitive than karyotyping analysis to detect MRD. Karyotypic evolution occurs in 15–40% of these patients and is usually associated with disease progression.

Figure 4 depicts how chromosomal aberrations can be detected in interphase nuclei by FISH.

CASE STUDY

Patient

Sixty-three-year-old man.

Chief Complaint

A few weeks of intermittent weakness. The patient consulted his family physician.

Medical History

No previous medical history of hematologic disorder.

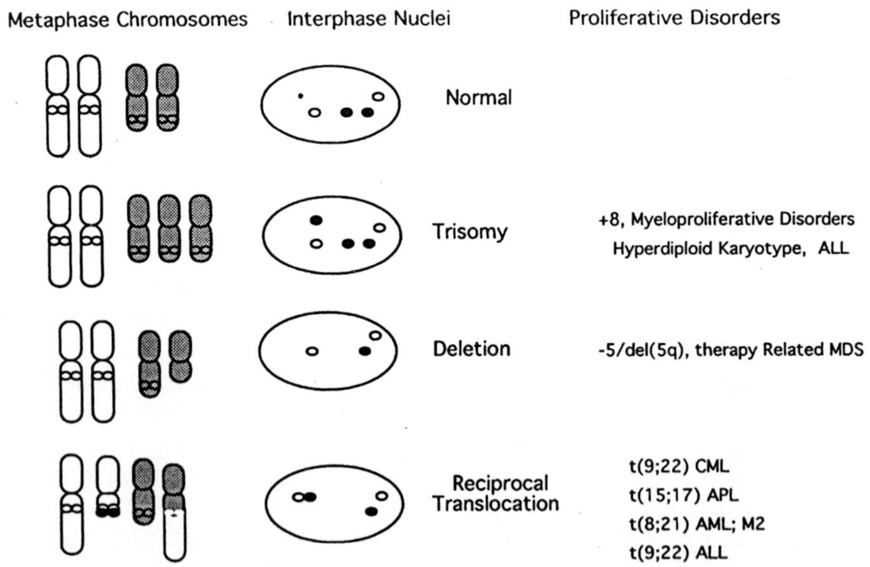

Figure 4 Schematic representation how genomic features on metaphase chromosomes can detect interphase nuclei by FISH. The metaphase chromosomes and their corresponding interphase nuclei are shown using chromosome-specific probes. The signals detected by FISH are shown in the nuclei as circles.

Physical Examination

Splenomegaly (3–4 cm below the left costal margin), no lymphadenopathy or hepatomegaly.

Laboratory Results

WBC	216×10^9/L
Polymorphs	48%
Bands	24%
Lymphs	2%
Monos	2%
Eosinophils	5%
Basophils	3%
Metamyelocytes	9%
Myelocytes	3%
Blasts	3%
Nucleated red cells	1%
Hemoglobin	11.7 g/dL
Platelet count	420×10^9/L

After admission, the patient underwent a bone marrow biopsy, followed by cytogenetic studies.

Bone marrow examination: hypercellular bone marrow, severe granulocytic hyperplasia and mild eosinophilia.

Cytogenetic studies: abnormal karyotype consisting of two clones: one clone with t(9;22) and a second clone with t(9;22) and trisomy 8.

Molecular genetics: showing *BCR* gene rearrangement (Fig. 5).

Diagnosis

Chronic myelogenous leukemia.

Questions

1. Can the diagnosis be suspected from the peripheral blood film examination?
2. What tests firmly establish the diagnosis?
3. How would Southern blot analysis help the diagnosis?

Discussion

Chronic myeloid leukemia is a neoplasm of the pluripotent hematopoietic stem cell characterized by the accumulation of mature granulocytes and their precursors in the bone marrow and the blood. The diagnosis can be made from the results of the peripheral blood cell counts and examination of the blood film. A total leukocyte count is always elevated and is nearly always over 25×10^9/L. The disease eventually transforms into an acute leukemia in which the dominant cells are usually myeloblasts but can instead be pre-B cells or, more rarely, T lymphoblasts. The lymphoid blast crisis of the CML is very similar to de-novo acute lymphoblastic leukemia.

The hallmark of CML is a shortened chromosome 22 (Philadelphia chromosome), which results from a reciprocal translocation involving the long arm of chromosomes 9 and 22. It can be demonstrated in >90% of patients with CML and in 10–25% of patients with ALL.

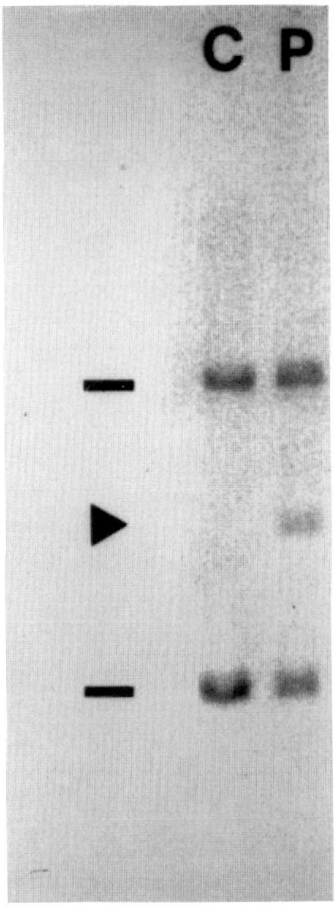

Figure 5 Southern blot phosphoimage of *Hind*III-cleaved genomic DNA probed with ^{32}P-labeled *bcr* DNA (Transprobe-1, Oncogene Science, Inc.) C, negative control; P, patient with chronic myelocytic leukemia. Dashes indicate germline bands; the arrowhead denotes a *bcr* gene rearrangement.

Although this case demonstrates a classic Ph chromosome, in about 20% of patients, banding cytogenetic studies may demonstrate a missing Y chromosome, an additional C group (chromosome 8), an additional chromosome 22q− without 9q+, another stable translocation, or a minor clone. Variant Ph chromosome translocation occurs in about 5% of CML patients and involves complex rearrangement (three chromosomes).

In a small proportion of patients, banding cytogenetic studies do not detect the classic, variant, or masked Ph chromosome. In these cases, Southern blot analysis with probes from the breakpoint cluster region detects rearrangement. In addition, Ph-negative CML patients with BCR rearrangement can express p210(bcr-abl) tyrosine kinase, and such patients have a clinical course similar to Ph-positive CML. Southern blot can be used as a diagnostic test to supplement the cytogenetic analysis.

Bibliography

1. Dewald GW, Schad CR, Christensen ER, et al. The application of fluorescent in situ hybridization to detect *Mbcr/abl* fusion in variant Ph chromosomes in CML and ALL. Cancer Genet Cytogenet 1993; 71:7–14.
2. Kantarjian HM, Deisscroth A, Kurzrock R, et al. Chronic myelogenous leukemia: a concise update. Blood 1993; 82:691–703.

3. Mattson JC, Crisan D, Wilner F, et al. Clinical problem solving using bcl/2 and bcr gene rearrangement analysis. Lab Med 1994; 25(10):648–653.

REFERENCES

1. Matsuda M, Honjo T. Organisation of human immunoglobin heavy-chain locus. Adv Immunol 1996; 6 2:1–29.
2. Roitt I. Antibodies. In: Essential Immunology. 8th ed. Blackwell, 1994:43–63.
3. Lewin J. Rearrangements and the generation of immune diversity. Generation of immune diversity by gene reorganisation. In: Genes V. 1994. Oxford: Oxford University Press, 1994:1103–1135.
4. Roitt I. Membrane receptors for antigen. In: Essential Immunology. 8th ed. Blackwell, 1994:64–80.
5. Leider JM. Transcriptional regulation of T cell receptor genes. Annu Rev Immunol 1993; 11:539–570.
6. Paul W. T lymphocyte receptors. In: Fundamental Immunology. 3d ed. New York: Raven Press, 1991:383–420.
7. Siminovitch KA, Bakhshi A, Goldman P, et al. A uniform deleting element mediates the loss of κ genes in human B cells. Nature 1985; 316(6025):260–262.
8. Hanson CA, Thamilarasan M, Ross CW, et al. Kappa light chain gene rearrangement in T-cell acute lymphoblastic leukemia. Am J Clin Pathol 1990; 93:563–568.
9. Raghavachar A, Thiel E, Hansen-Hagge TE, et al. Rearrangement of T-cell receptor β, γ, δ gene loci in human pre-T cell acute lymphoblastic leukemia. Leukemia 1989; 3:413–418.
10. Loughran TP Jr, Starkebaum G, Aprile JA. Rearrangement and expression of T-cell receptor genes in large granular lymphocytic leukemia. Blood 1988; 71:822–824.
11. Willman Cl. Molecular diagnostics. In: Fenoglio Preiser CM, Willman CL, eds. Pathology. Baltimore: Williams & Wilkins, 1991:118–119.
12. Ayscue LH, Ross DW, Ozer H, et al. bcr/abl Recombinant DNA analysis versus karyotype in the diagnosis and therapeutic monitoring of chronic myeloid leukemia. Am J Clin Pathol 1990; 94: 404–409.
13. Schumacher HR, Cotelingam JD. Gene rearrangement and polymerase chain reaction. In: Chronic Leukemia. Approach to Diagnosis. New York: Igaku-Shoin, 1993:143–161.
14. Cossman J, Uppenkamp M, Sundeen J, et al. Molecular genetics and the diagnosis of lymphoma. Arch Pathol Lab Med 1988; 112:117–127.
15. Crisan D, Mattson JC. Discordant morphologic features in bone marrow involvement by malignant lymphomas: use of gene rearrangement patterns for diagnosis. Am J Hematol 1995; 49:299–309.
16. Griesser H. Gene rearrangement and chromosomal translocation in T cell lymphoma—diagnostic applications and their limits. Virchows Arch 1995; 426:323–338.
17. Arnold A, Cossman J, Bakkshi A, et al. Immunoglobulin gene rearrangements as unique clonal markers in human lymphoid neoplasms. N Engl J Med 1983; 309:1593–1599.
18. Cossman J, Zehnbauer B, Garrett CT, et al. Gene rearrangements in the diagnosis of lymphoma/leukemia: guidelines for the use based on a multi-institutional study. Am J Clin Pathol 1991; 95: 347–354.
19. Gulley ML, Dent GA, Ross DW, et al. Classification and staging of lymphoma by molecular genetics. Cancer 1992; 69(suppl):1600–1606.
20. Chen Z, Le Paslier D, Dausset J, et al. Human T cell gamma genes frequently rearranged in B-lineage acute lymphoblastic leukemias, but not in chronic B cell proliferations. J Exp Med 1987; 165:1000–1015.
21. Weiss LM, Picker LJ, Grogan TM, et al. Absence of clonal beta and gamma T-cell receptor gene rearrangements in a subset of peripheral T-cell lymphoma. Am J Pathol 1988; 130:436–442.
22. Knowles DM. Immunophenotype and antigen receptor gene rearrangement analysis in T cell neoplasia. Am J Pathol 1989; 134:761–785.
23. Waldmann TA, Davis MM, Bongiovanni KF, et al. Rearrangements of genes for the antigen recep-

tor on T cells as a markers of lineage and clonality in human lymphoid neoplasms. N Engl J Med 1985; 313:776–783.
24. Weiss LM, Picker LJ, Copenhaven CM, et al. Large-cell hematolymphoid neoplasms of uncertain lineage. Hum Pathol 1988; 19:967–973.
25. Pelicci P-G, Knowles DM, Dalla-Favera RD. Lymphoid tumors displaying rearrangements of both immunoglobulin and T-cell receptor genes. J Exp Med 1985; 162:1015–1024.
26. Greenberg SJ, Choi Y, Ballow M, et al. Profile of immunoglobulin heavy chain variable gene repertoire and highly selective detection of malignant clonotype in acute lymphoblastic leukemia. J Leuk Biol 1995; 57:856–864.
27. Seriu T, Hansen-Hagge TE, Erz DH, et al. Improved detection of minimal residual leukemia through modifications of the polymerase chain reaction based clonospecific T cell receptor junctions. Leukemia 1995; 9:316–320.
28. Breit TM, Beishaizen A, Ludwig WD, et al. Tal-1 deletions in T-cell acute lymphoblastic leukemia as PCR target for detection of minimal residual disease. Leukemia 1993; 7:2004–2011.
29. Jonsson OG, Kitchens RL, Baer RJ, et al. Rearrangements of the tal-1 locus as clonal markers for T cell acute lymphoblastic leukemia. J Clin Invest 1991; 87:2029–2035.
30. Huang W, Kuang SQ, Huang QH, et al. RT/PCR detection of SIL-tal-1 fusion m-RNA in chinese T cell acute lymphoblastic leukemia (T-ALL). Cancer Genet Cytogenet 1995; 81:76–82.
32. Cline MJ. Molecular basis of leukemia (review article). N Engl J Med 1994; 330:328–336.
35. Garcia A, Roman J, Brunet S, et al. Minimal residual disease in chronic myeloid leukemia in patients with long survival after allogeneic bone marrow transplantation. Med Clin 1995; 104: 401–406.
36. Lion T. Clinical implications of qualitative and quantitative polymerase chain reaction analysis in the monitoring of patients with chronic myelogenous leukemia. The European Investigators on Chronic Myeloid Leukemia Group. Bone Marrow Transplant 1995; 14:505–509.
37. Gaiger A, Henn T, Horth E, et al. Increase of BCR-ABL chimeric mRNA expression in tumor cells of patients with chronic myeloid leukemia precedes disease progression. Blood 1995; 86: 2371–2378.
38. Crisan D, Anstett MJ. *Bcl/2* gene rearrangements in follicular lymphomas. Clin Chem 1993; 39: 1980–1982.
39. Anastasi J, Thangavela M, Vardiman JW, et al. Interphase cytogenetic analysis detects minimal residual disease in acute lymphoblastic leukemia and resolves the question of origin of relapse after allogeneic bone marrow transplantation. Blood 1991; 77:1087–1091.
40. Berger A, Strehl S, Hekele A, et al. Interphase cytogenetic study of childhood acute lymphoblastic leukemia. Med Pediatr Oncol 1994; 23:413–421.
41. Pagliaro LC, Stanley WS. Interphase FISH and morphologic analysis of AML. Cancer Gene Cytogenet 1993; 67:95–100.
42. Jenkins RB, Le Beau MM, Kraker WJ, et al. Fluorescence in situ hybridization: a sensitive method for trisomy 8 detection in bone marrow specimens. Blood 1992; 79:3307–3315.
43. Kibbelaar RE, Vankamp H, Dreef EJ, et al. Combined immunophenotyping and DNA in situ hybridization to study lineage involvement in patients with myelodysplastic syndromes. Blood 1992; 79: 1823–1828.
44. Tkachuk DC, Westbrook CA, Andreeff M, et al. Detection of BCR-ABL fusion in chronic myelogenous leukemia by in situ hybridization. Science 1990; 250:559–562.
45. Van Dongen JJ, Breit TM, Adriaansen JH, et al. Detection of minimal residual disease in acute leukemia by immunological marker analysis and polymerase chain reaction. Leukemia 1992; 6(suppl 1):47–59.
46. Felix CA, Reaman GH, Korsmeyer SJ, et al. Immunoglobulin and T-cell receptor gene configuration in acute lymphoblastic leukemia of infancy. Blood 1987; 70:536–541.
47. Felix Ca, Poplack DG, Reaman GH, et al. Characterization of immunoglobulin and T-cell receptor gene patterns in B-cell precursor acute lymphoblastic leukemia of childhood. J Clin Oncol 1990; 8: 431–442.

48. Schumacher HR. Molecular diagnosis. In: Internal Medicine. Stein et al., St. Louis, Mosby, 1998, 11:559–564.
49. Chan A, Mak TW. Genomic organisation of the T cell receptor. Cancer Detect Prev 1989; 14: 261–267.
50. Brauninger A, Hansmann Martin-Leo, Strickler JG, et al: Identification of common germinal-center B-cell precursors in two patients with both Hodgkin's disease and non-Hodgkin's lymphoma. N Engl J 1999; 340:1239–1247.
51. Busson-Le Coniat M, Salomon-Nguyen F, Hillion J, Bernard OA, Berger R. MLL-AF1q fusion resulting from t(1;11) in acute leukemia. Leukemia 1999 2; 13(2):302–306.
52. Fais F, Ghiotto, F, Hasimoto S, Sellars B, Valetto A, Allen SL, Schulman P, Vinciguerra VP, Rai K, Rassenti LZ, Kipps TJ, Dighiero G, Schroeder HW, Jr., Ferrarini M, Chiorazzi N. Chronic lymphocytic leukemia B cells express restricted sets of mutated and unmutated antigen receptors. J Clin Invest 1998; 102(8):1515–1525.
53. Hilden JM, Chen CS, Moore R, et al. Heterogeneity in MLL/F-4 fusion messenger RNA detected by the polymerase chain reaction in t(4;11) acute leukemia. Cancer Res 1993; 53:3853–3856.
54. Kozu T, Miyoshi H, Shimizu K, et al. Junctions of the AML1/MTG8(ETO) fusion are constant in t(8;21) acute myeloid leukemia detected by reverse transcription polymerase chain reaction. Blood 1993; 82:1270–1276.
55. Miyamoto, T, Nagafuji K, Akashi K, et al. Persistence of multipotent progenitors expressing AML1/ETO transcripts in long-term remission patients with t(8;21) acute myelogenous leukemia. Blood 1996; 87:4789–4796.
56. Pongers-Willemse MJ, et al. Primers and protocols for standardized detection of minimal residual disease in acute lymphoblastic leukemia using immunoglobulin and T cell receptor gene rearrangements and TAL1 deletions as PCR targets: report of the BIOMED-CONCERTED ACTION: investigation of minimal residual disease in acute leukemia. Leukemia 1999 13(1):110–118.
57. Rowley JD, Reshmi S, Sobulo O, et al. All patients with the T(11;16)(q23;p13.3 that involves MLL and CBP have treatment-related hematologic disorders. Blood 1997; 90:535–541.
58. Schultze JL, Donovan JW, Gribben JG. Minimal residual disease detection after myeloblative chemotherapy in chronic lymphatic leukemia. J Mol Med 1999; 77(2):259–265.
59. Shurtleff SA, Meyers S, Heibert SW, et al. Heterogeneity in CBF beta/MYH11 fusion messages encoded by the inv(16)(p13q22) and the t(16;16)(p13;q22) in acute myelogenous leukemia. Blood 1995; 85:3695–3703.

24

Coagulation Theory, Principles, and Concepts

Robert F. Baugh
Medtronic Blood Management, Parker, Colorado

I. INTRODUCTION

The past two decades have witnessed an "explosion" in basic, applied, and clinical knowledge in the field of blood coagulation. Keeping track of this explosion is now a major undertaking. Although much more is known about the components involved and how they relate to specific pathologic disease states, integrating all the findings into a comprehensive understanding is becoming extremely difficult.

The "explosion" in the field has resulted in a large increase in the number of clinicians, engineers, and scientists who have more than a rudimentary knowledge of coagulation. In part, this has been driven by necessity. As thrombolytic drugs, cardiovascular surgery, and interventional cardiology have developed, the need to understand coagulation processes has become more critical. We must now deal not only with the hemorrhagic side of hemostasis, but also with the thrombotic side. Understanding coagulation is no longer just the charge of someone buried deep in the clinical or research laboratory. Some of the drugs and devices being used are challenging our understanding of coagulation mechanisms. Clinical treatments have been developed and applied before the biochemical and physiologic mechanisms are understood. In some sense these adventures into the "unknown" are forcing us to reevaluate and revise our concepts of coagulation processes on the fly.

Another contributor to the "explosion" has been the integration of plasma-based coagulation with the rest of the vascular system. Coagulation research now recognizes the importance of the cellular components of the vascular system. Although this is recognized, it is fair to say that only the tip of the iceberg has been touched with respect to our understanding of these interactions. the expansion of coagulation beyond plasma-based clotting has generated modified cascade hypotheses. Original cascade hypotheses were based on test tube results working with plasma or plasma fractions from patients with known hemorrhagic complications. As the cellular nature of coagulation was recognized, the vascular endothelium and cells of blood had to be taken into account if in-vivo thrombotic or hemorrhagic events were to be interpreted correctly. This enlargement of the scope of "coagulation" has led to the development of a new field. In the past, individuals with an extensive knowledge of coagulation were referred to as "clotters." This terminology is now considered too limiting. Today the specialist is referred to as a "vascular biologist." The past two decades have turned a rather esoteric, small discipline into one of the major multidiscipline fields in medicine.

II. CASCADE HYPOTHESES

The concept of a cascade for explaining the biochemistry of blood coagulation was developed during the 1960s. Since that time cascade theories have been refined, extended, and continually modified. The development of these theories was the result of biochemical and clinical studies which attempted to present a rational, clarified view of the complex nature of coagulation. Envisioning coagulation as a cascade explains how a small stimulus can evoke a response that is out of proportion to the size of the stimulus.

The original cascade hypothesis was developed almost simultaneously in the 1960s by Davie and Ratnoff in the United States (1,2) and MacFarlane in England (3). These cascades were relatively simple and used the nomenclature prevalent at the time (Fig. 1). The cascades were "intrinsic" coagulation, and included what is now referred to as "contact activation." The "intrinsic" terminology pertained to the observation that all the necessary components for coagulation were present, or intrinsic, to blood. As more information became available, the cascades were modified. The recognition of the tissue factor/factor VII component gave birth to the concept of two separate pathways, an "intrinsic" system and an "extrinsic" system, since tissue factor was not an intrinsic blood component (Fig. 2).

Although the coagulation cascade could be divided into intrinsic and extrinsic systems,

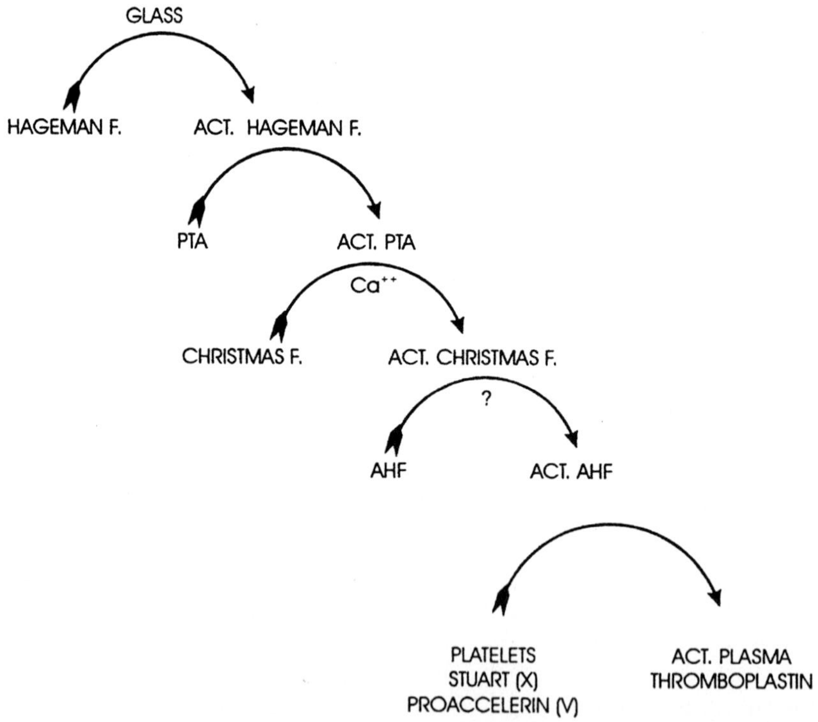

Figure 1 The first use of the concept of a coagulation cascade as present by Davie and Ratnoff in 1962. (Adapted from Ref. 1.)

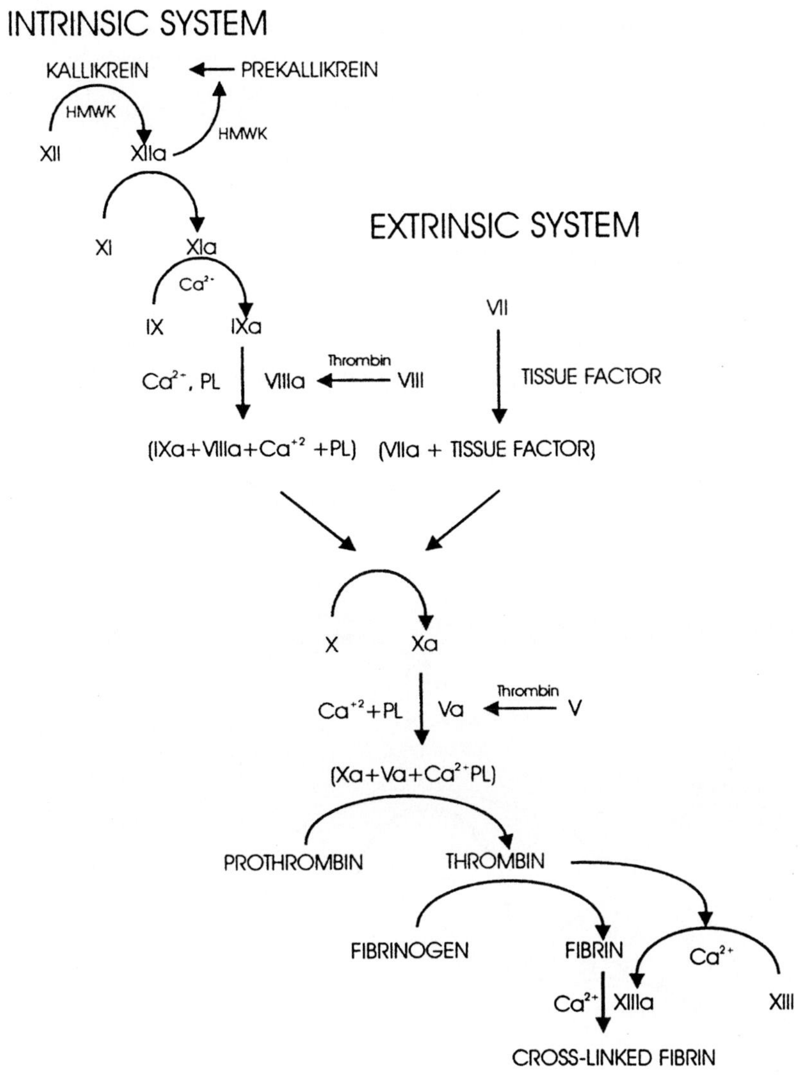

Figure 2 Coagulation cascade incorporating the concepts of an extrinsic and an intrinsic pathway. The two pathways converge at the level of factor X. This particular pathway was presented in a review in 1981 (122).

various clinical observations could not be explained by the hypotheses, although test tube results supported the hypotheses. Intrinsic coagulation was initiated by a series of components referred to as the "contact phase" of coagulation, yet patients defective in these components did not have bleeding problems; in fact, they frequently were prone to episodes of thrombosis (4). Only one "contact factor," factor XI, was associated with bleeding problems, but these were variable (5). Further down the intrinsic pathway, deficiencies in factor VIII and factor IX were always associated with bleeding.

In the last decade there have been a number of attempts to resolve some of the problems created by diagramming coagulation as a "plasma" process. This has led to the conclusion that intrinsic coagulation via "contact activation" is not a significant component of in-vivo coagulation. Extrinsic coagulation, in which the middle components of intrinsic coagulation are part of the general clotting process, must be the way in which in-vivo clotting proceeds (Fig. 3). These recent modifications to coagulation pathways have tried to address clinical findings, but the acceptance of the latest revisions has proceeded slowly (6–8).

III. EXTRINSIC/INTRINSIC COAGULATION

Although the latest views on the processes of clot formation have led to the combination of intrinsic coagulation with extrinsic coagulation, recent whole-blood coagulation experiments have suggested that there still are "intrinsic" and "extrinsic" pathways for coagulation (9,10).

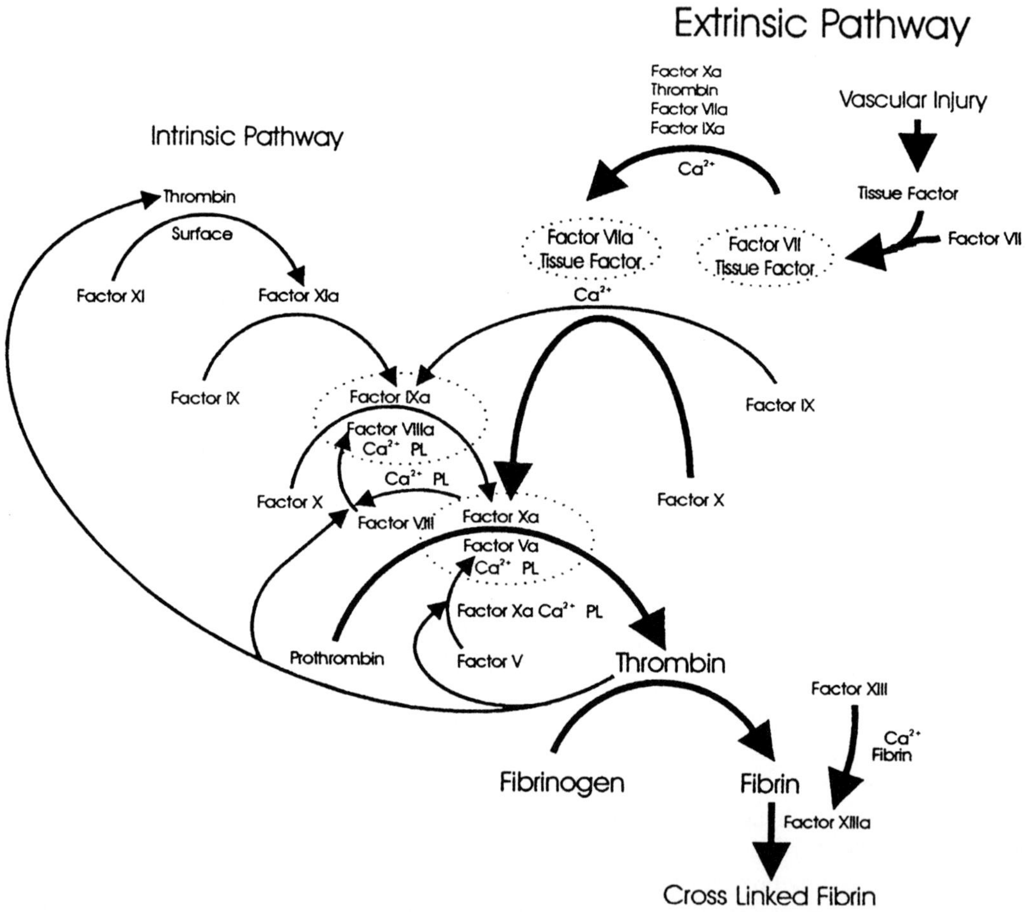

Figure 3 A revised coagulation cascade, circa 1991, which drops classical contact activation. Activation of factor XI is accomplished via the generation of thrombin from the initial pulse of thrombin formed by the extrinsic system (indicated by the heavy arrows). In this adaptation of the pathways, the complexes are indicated by dotted lines. (Adapted from Ref. 123.)

The original meaning of "intrinsic" and "extrinsic" have been lost, but a division remains. Coagulation is initiated via the tissue factor–factor VII link, be it via intrinsic (in this case the factor VIII–factor IX pathway) or via classical extrinsic coagulation. If the medium is whole blood, it has been postulated that the two pathways serve different purposes (11). The intrinsic pathway is concerned with the generation of fluid-phase thrombin and fibrin formation, while the classic extrinsic pathway is concerned with the generation of thrombin, which activates platelets (Fig. 4). If this is true, standard coagulation assays such as the prothrombin time and activated partial thromboplastin time are misleading, and the role of contact activation is unresolved.

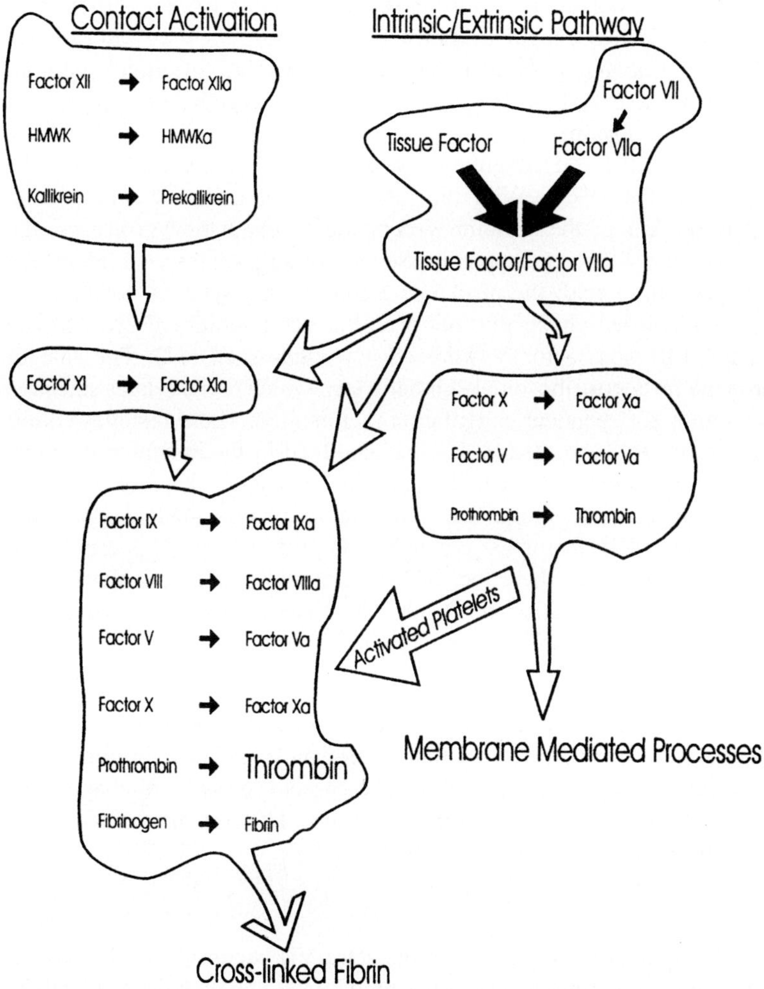

Figure 4 Hypothetical cascade. This is based on information and observations that have yet to be fully substantiated. The process of two distinct pathways relates more to the generation of coagulant activities in different microenvironments. In this hypothesis, the primary trigger for coagulation is still tissue factor, while contact activation occupies a somewhat less important aspect of coagulation.

A. Coagulation Factors

The process by which a clot is formed depends on the interactions of a large number of individual components. Basic components are proteins, phospholipids, metal ions, and carbohydrates. In the case of coagulation, proteins are the most significant elements. The genetic abnormalities of coagulation are deficiencies in proteins, and the product of the coagulation process is a polymerized protein.

1. Serine Proteases and Vitamin K

The enzymes of coagulation are generally serine proteases (proteins which catalyze the modification of other proteins by breaking the links which hold a protein together). The term refers to the fact that each has a serine (an amino acid) present in what is referred to as the active site. Most of the proteases of coagulation are based on the structure of trypsin, the protease found in the stomach. The ability to obtain specificity is related to the remaining structure of the enzyme. Thus, the reason a particular coagulation protease does not "chew up" all proteins is due to its three-dimensional structure. Although there is considerable specificity demonstrated by the coagulation proteases, several are noted for their ability to catalyze the hydrolysis of proteins other than their classic substrates.

For years the impact of vitamin K on coagulation was known, but the reasons for the impact were not unraveled until the 1970s. With the discovery that a unique amino acid, γ-carboxyglutamic acid, was present in the vitamin K-dependent coagulation proteases, the biochemical significance of vitamin K became apparent. Several other proteins were identified that also contained this unique amino acid; the most interesting, with respect to coagulation, was protein C. Protein C was identified physically, but it took several additional years before its role in inactivating factor VIII and factor V were clearly established (12). The role of vitamin K is that of a coenzyme for a postribosomal synthetic step which carboxylates selective glutamate residues in the vitamin K-dependent coagulation factors (13). These residues confer special calcium-binding properties to these factors. Each is involved in the assembly of phospholipid–calcium–protease–cofactor complexes which confers a substantial increase in the activity of the protease to hydrolyze its substrate. The four factors of coagulation containing these specialized residues are factor VII, factor IX, factor X, and prothrombin. This carboxylation mechanism is also the explanation for the effect of Warfarin on coagulation. Warfarin is an antagonist of vitamin K, and carboxylation does not take place, leading to coagulation factors, which cannot assemble in the proper enzymatically active complexes.

2. Structural and Cofactor Proteins

A number of structural proteins are involved in coagulation. A structural protein is required to build something, which has mass. The classic structural protein of coagulation is fibrinogen, which after conversion to fibrin, results in clot formation. The cofactor proteins of coagulation are those which enhance the activity of the coagulation proteases. The primary cofactors are factor VIII, factor V, and high-molecular-weight kininogen.

B. Factor VII

In present-day hypotheses of coagulation, the activation of factor VII is considered the "initiation" of coagulation (14–16). Factor VII circulates in the blood as a single-chain zymogen or precursor that has no activity. Upon tissue injury and the exposure of tissue factor, factor VII is rapidly converted to factor VIIa. This activation occurs when factor VII binds to tissue factor and forms a 1:1 complex. The activation occurs via cleavage of a single arginine–isoleucine bond with factor VII. It is still not known what protease is responsible for the cleavage, but both factor Xa and factor VIIa will activate factor VII experimentally (14,17). These activities are probably important in the acceleration of coagulation, but it cannot yet be determined if they are important in the initial formation of factor VIIa.

Factor VII is synthesized in the liver, and elevated plasma levels of factor VII have been associated with increased thrombotic risk (18–20). Decreased levels of factor VII are associated with bleeding and in some cases an increased risk of thrombosis (21), although the evidence for this is limited. Inherited factor VII deficiencies are extremely rare. The deficiency is transmitted as an autosomal recessive trait. A number of genetic mutations have been identified, and the resulting structural alterations in the factor VII molecule have been identified. The molecular variants generally have decreased activity, although it has been difficult to establish a link between structural variants and clinical prognosis due to the limited number of carriers identified (22–24). The synthesis of factor VII requires vitamin K and, of the common coagulation factors, it is present in plasma at the lowest levels (0.5 μg/mL). It has a turnover rate of about 3–4 hr.

For a good number of years it was believed that the natural substrate for the tissue factor–factor VIIa complex was factor X, but a large amount of experimental data now shows that factor IX may be a more important substrate than factor X (25). The activated form of factor VII is believed to have no activity in the absence of tissue factor. Factor VIIa is not rapidly inactivated once formed, and has a plasma circulating half-life of about 2 hr. It has been suggested that circulating factor VIIa could be the trigger for the initiation of coagulation once tissue factor is exposed (26,27). Tracking baseline levels of factor VIIa in different populations has produced some intriguing findings. In hemophilia A the baseline levels appear to be about 60% of the normal level, while in hemophilia B the levels are only 10%. Upon placing patients with deep vein thrombosis on Warfarin therapy, the levels drop (28). These observations continue to suggest that factor VIIa is critical to the initiation of coagulation.

C. Tissue Factor

Tissue factor, or thromboplastin, is a trigger for coagulation. It is thought to be a specific trigger, as opposed to the nonspecific triggers of classic intrinsic coagulation (negatively charged surfaces). Although it is the trigger, the difficulty remains in determining how factor VII is converted to factor VIIa. Tissue factor has no proteolytic activity; thus, just the combination of tissue factor with factor VII is not sufficient to initiate clotting. Tissue factor is a protein–lipid complex that requires both components for its activity. The apoprotein has been purified, sequenced and cloned. Its interactions with both phospholipids and with factor VII have been studied extensively, and the location of tissue factor in cells, atherosclerotic lesions, and on the surface of activated monocytes has been well documented (29,30). Tissue factor is one of the "reconstituted" components of coagulation. The apoprotein, devoid of any lipid constituents, can be reconstituted by combining the apoprotein with lipid, specifically phosphatidyl choline or phosphatidyl choline-phosphatidyl serine vesicles. The result is tissue factor that has full activity.

The apoprotein portion of tissue factor has a molecular weight of about 46,000. Tissue factor is a membrane or vesicular complex, which is not truly soluble. The types of tissue factor (frequently referred to as thromboplastins) used in coagulation assays are colloidal in nature. A truncated version of the apoprotein can be produced which is soluble. It has been shown to have activity in the presence of phospholipids (31). This form of tissue factor is referred to as sTF. sTF has been crystallized, not only individually, but also complexed with factor VIIa. The molecular coordinates have been determined by x-ray crystallography, and the structure determined (32). Structurally, tissue factor resembles other cell membrane cytokine receptors. If there are any known genetic defects with respect to tissue factor, they have not been well documented.

D. Factor XI

Whereas the other factors of contact activation are left out of current coagulation schemes, factor XI is still included. Since only some patients with a genetic deficiency bleed, it occupies a gray area in current coagulation hypotheses (33,34). Factor XI is a two-chained serine protease precursor that circulates at a plasma concentration of about 4 μg/mL. It has a molecular weight of 160,000, and the two chains are linked by disulfide bonds. The two chains are identical, and each contains a serine protease active site. Factor XI circulates in blood complexed with high-molecular-weight kininogen (35). The stoichiometry of this complex is 1:2, where a high-molecular-weight kininogen is associated with each chain of the factor XI zymogen. During activation by factor XIIa, each chain is cleaved at the same site to produce a molecule with four disulfide-linked chains (two light and two heavy chains). The active serine sites are located in the light chains. This activation sequence does not require either the presence of calcium or phospholipid, but a platelet interaction has been suggested (36,37).

The revised concepts of coagulation place an emphasis on the activation of factor XI by means other than factor XIIa. In these hypotheses, since the generation of factor Xa by tissue factor/VIIa is rapidly quenched by TFPI, the factor IXa–factor VIIIa pathway must be the manner in which clot formation is sustained. The activation of XI is then accomplished by the initial amounts of thrombin formed by extrinsic coagulation and by factor XIa as it is generated (38,39). Although these reactions have been demonstrated experimentally, it is not known if they represent in-vivo coagulation. The possibility also exists that an as yet identified protease takes part in the activation of factor XI.

Factor XIa converts factor IX to factor IXa. The reaction requires calcium, but it has no requirement for phospholipid or for a cofactor similar to factor V or factor VIII. This is the only activation step in coagulation for which a cofactor requirement has not been demonstrated.

E. Factor IX

The recognition that occasionally the plasmas from two hemophiliacs corrected clotting times when mixed led to the discovery that at least two forms of hemophilia exist. It is now well known that the deficiencies noted above were due to factor VIII and factor IX (hemophilia A and hemophilia B). Human factor IX is synthesized in the liver, has a molecular weight of approximately 54,000, and circulates at a plasma concentration of about 5 μg/mL. In normal individuals the plasma concentration of factor IX varies from 50% to 150% of that of a normal plasma pool. The turnover of factor IX is on the order of 2 hr. In addition to genetic abnormalities, a number of acquired disorders affecting factor IX have been described. Liver disease lowers factor IX plasma levels, and Warfarin reduces plasma factor IX activity. An acquired factor IX deficiency occurs in nephrotic syndromes, and reduced levels have been reported in hypothyroidism, Gaucher disease, and amyloidosis (40).

Factor IX circulates as a single-chain glycoprotein with four distinct structural domains. These include the Gla domain (calcium binding γ-carboxyglutamic acid region), two epidermal growth factor regions, an activation peptide, and the catalytic site. The activation of factor IX to produce factor IXa is a two-step process. The single-chain zymogen is first cleaved to produce a two-chain molecule in which the chains are connected by disulfide bonds. This intermediate is functionally inactive until a second cleavage occurs, which releases the activation peptide (41). This sequence can be modified by using Russell's viper venom. Russell's viper venom cleaves at a slightly different initial site, which produces a factor IXa with an activity of about half that of normally activated factor XIa. In certain mutations of factor IX, normal activation produces a similar product and in some individuals leads to hemophilia.

Normal activation of factor IX occurs either via factor XIa or by the factor VIIa/TF complex (42,43). Activation by factor XIa is enhanced by the presence of calcium ions and does not appear to require the presence of a phospholipid membrane surface. The activation by the factor VIIa–tissue factor complex does require phospholipid. Activation of factor IX has also been shown with factor Xa and with trypsin, while it is notably not activated by elastase, kallikrein, factor XIIa, thrombin, or plasmin. Factor IXa is the primary protease in the factor X-activating complex. This complex requires activated factor VIIIa, phospholipid, and calcium.

F. Factor VIII/von Willebrand Factor

The severity of hemophilia illustrates the importance of the role of cofactors in coagulation. Factor VIII is a large protein, and it is one of the least stable of the coagulation factors. It circulates at a concentration of around 150 ng/mL complexed with the von Willebrand factor.

Due to in-vivo proteolysis, it was extremely difficult to identify the "structure" of factor VIII. Using molecular biology techniques, the structure was shown to consist of a variable-length heavy chain linked noncovalently to a light-chain polypeptide (44,45). The combined molecular weight is 290,000. Factor VIII is stabilized by metal ions, in particular calcium. Removal of calcium results in the dissociation of the chains and the loss of activity.

The relationship between factor VIII and von Willebrand factor was known long before factor VIII was characterized structurally. The relationship was so close, in fact, that for a good number of years there existed a "factor VIII-related antigen," which in reality was the von Willebrand factor. It is now accepted that the von Willebrand factor stabilizes factor VIII by forming a noncovalent complex with factor VIII (46). The half-life of highly purified factor VIII is significantly longer (12 hr) in hemophiliacs than it is in patients with homozygous von Willebrand's disease (2–3 hr). To function in the activation of factor X, factor VIII must be activated. This activation, which involves limited proteolysis of factor VIII, can be accomplished either by factor Xa or by thrombin (47). In this scheme, it is thought that activation of factor VIII is accomplished initially by thrombin or factor Xa that is generated by the tissue factor–factor VIIa extrinsic pathway before TFPI shuts down extrinsic coagulation. Once formed, the factor Xa generated by the intrinsic pathway is sufficient to maintain activation of factor VIII. Factor VIIIa is now known to be a heterotrimer (three different chains) which is produced when thrombin activates factor VIII, releasing it from the von Willebrand factor. The resulting trimer is unstable, dissociating and losing activity. Activated protein C hastens the loss of activity by limited proteolysis.

The von Willebrand factor (vWf), which has been so intimately linked with factor VIII, is also involved in platelet adhesion. vWf is a series of multimers that show an impressive range in sizes, anywhere from 500,000 to 20,000,000 in molecular weight. These multimers are formed from a subunit that has a molecular weight of 270,000. The variety of multimers exist due to in-vivo proteolysis of disulfide-linked subunits. There are a number of genetic molecular defects of the von Willebrand factor, ranging from complete absence to multiple molecular variations. In general these can be broken down into three broad classifications: type I, in which there is a partial deficiency of the native species; type II, in which there are qualitative abnormalities in the structure; and type III, in which no plasma vWf can be detected (48). The primary platelet membrane receptor for vWf, GP Ib, apparently binds to vWf after vWf has bound to another surface, such as a vessel wall. Experimentally, it appears that platelet adhesion mediated through vWf occurs only at high shear stresses, but these particular experimental studies do not address all the issues of in-vivo platelet adhesion (49,50).

G. Factor X

Factor X is the protease component of the complex that converts prothrombin to thrombin. Factor X circulates as a two-chain, disulfide-linked precursor (MW = 59,000) which is activated to factor Xa by either the intrinsic or extrinsic blood coagulation systems. It is produced in the liver, and circulates at a plasma concentration of about 8 μg/mL. The half-life appears to be on the order of 24–40 hr (51).

The conversion of factor X to factor Xa involves the removal of an activation peptide which is located in the heaviest of the two chains (MW = 43,000 and 16,000). This is accomplished by either the factor IX complex or the tissue factor–factor VIIa complex. In both cases, a phospholipid membrane enhances activation. Several studies have indicated that factor X can be activated by other proteases (52,53).

The assembly of the complex between factor Xa, factor Va, prothrombin, phospholipid, and calcium has been studied in detail. Models of the complex have been generated based on kinetic and chemical data. Assembly of the complex takes place on the surface of activated platelets and monocytes. This complex appears to consist of a 1:1:1 ratio of factor Xa/factor Va/prothrombin, where the factor Va is bound hydrophobically to the membrane while the vitamin K-dependent proteins are bound via calcium bridges (54).

Factor Xa has several demonstrated activities, other than the conversion of prothrombin to thrombin. Factor Xa activates both factor VII and factor VIII. Factor Xa can also activate protein C in the presence of thrombomodulin. Genetic abnormalities of factor X are relatively rare.

H. Factor V

Factor V is a large, single-chain plasma protein (MW = 330,000) that circulates in human plasma at a concentration of about 7–10 μg/mL. Structurally the molecule is very similar to factor VIII, being comprised of similar domains, even to the extent of sharing the same similarities to ceruloplasmin.

The activation of factor V by thrombin results in the production of four products. Two remain noncovalently linked by the presence of calcium and provide the active cofactor activity, while the two remaining chains appear to have no role in the activity of factor Va. It is hypothesized that the initial factor Xa generated in the absence of factor Va is sufficient to activate factor V. It has also been suggested that platelets and plasmin may be capable of activating factor V.

The genetics of factor V occupy a unique position. A deficiency of factor V is associated with increased bleeding; recently, however, a genetic mutation of factor V, factor V Leiden, has been associated with an increased risk for thrombosis. This relates to a mutation in factor V that makes it resistant to hydrolysis by activated protein C. The prevalence of this mutation is such that it currently is considered the most common hyperthrombotic condition to exist in the general population. This discovery, coupled with defects in the protein C pathway, account for a large number of patients with known thrombotic conditions.

I. Prothrombin/Thrombin

Although most of the other members of the coagulation cascade are now referred to using the standardized nomenclature system, prothrombin and thrombin are more likely to be referred to using their classical names. This is related to the early identification of the importance of prothrombin/thrombin in coagulation.

Prothrombin (factor II) is the zymogen, inactive form of thrombin. It is converted to thrombin by the action of the prothrombinase complex (factor Xa, factor Va, calcium, and phospholipid). This activation involves two proteolytic cleavages, which release an activation peptide referred to as Fragment 1•2. The thrombin formed is autocatalytic, and several variant forms of thrombin can be found. The active form is referred to as α-thrombin. The other forms of thrombin are not known to have an significant physiologic functions.

Prothrombin is a single-chain glycoprotein with a molecular weight of 71,600. About 8% of the molecule is carbohydrate. The studies on the structure–function relationships of the prothrombin molecule have led to it being the model on which other serine proteases of coagulation and fibrinolysis are based. The structure has several unique features that segregate the general structure from other serine-type proteases such as trypsin.

Thrombin is the essential intermediate in the formation of fibrin. Studies of its structure (both prothrombin/thrombin) have led to a better understanding of each of the coagulation proteases, and it was unraveling the structure anomalies in prothrombin which led to understanding the biochemical significance of the vitamin K-dependent clotting factors. Thrombin also has a significant number of other biologic activities (55,56).

J. Fibrinogen/Fibrin

The purpose of the blood-clotting enzymes is the conversion of fibrinogen to fibrin, the basis of clot formation. This event, which is so simple in concept, is one of the most fascinating processes in biology. Fibrinogen is a large, complex molecule that under normal circumstances is soluble. Minor proteolysis leads to the formation of a soluble product that polymerizes spontaneously to form an insoluble mesh composed of fibrils. The nature of this change is subtle. The basic structure is a fibrous molecule that shares many characteristics with other fibrous molecules. It has a molecular weight of 340,000 and consists of three pairs of nonidentical peptide chains denoted as α, β, and γ, which are covalently linked by a series of disulfide bonds. The structure has been well characterized. It is a long chain characterized by a "dumbbell shape," with a central globular mass at its center. Thrombin cleaves two pairs of peptide chains releasing fibrinopeptides A and B yielding fibrin monomer (57,58).

Fibrin monomer polymerizes spontaneously in an organized fashion. For a number of years it could not be demonstrated with available techniques that there was any difference between fibrinogen and fibrin. The actual loss in mass is about 3%, and it was only with the advent of better technology that the events could be worked out. The transformation can only be considered in terms of a structure that has specific polymerization sites that are uncovered by the removal of the fibrinopeptides. This suggests a lock-and-key type of assembly of the monomers into a fibrin mesh. The mesh forms in an organized fashion, proceeding through dimers, trimers, oligomers, protofibrils, and fully developed fibers (59,60).

Fibrinogen participates in other coagulation processes. Platelet–platelet coupling in platelet aggregation occurs via fibrinogen linkages, and low-shear platelet adhesion occurs via fibrinogen bridges between the platelet membrane and the vascular surface. Immobilized fibrinogen will irreversibly bind and activate platelets. Although the receptor sites for fibrinogen on the platelet membrane are known, it is unclear as to all the relevant fibrinogen structural features required for platelet–fibrinogen interactions (62,63).

K. Factor XIII

Factor XIII is a transglutaminase that catalyzes the formation of intermolecular ε-(γ-glutamyl) lysine bonds. Plasma factor XIII consists of four subunits, two a and two b subunits. Patients deficient in factor XIII are characterized by bleeding tendencies, abnormal wound healing, and spontaneous abortions (64–66).

The tetramer circulates at plasma concentrations of about 20 μg/mL, with a dimer of the b subunits having a plasma concentration of 10 μg/mL. The tetramer has a molecular weight of 320,000. The subunits are held together by noncovalent bonds. Factor XIII appears to circulate complexed with fibrinogen. Factor XIII is also found in platelets and placenta, but these forms consist only of the a dimers having a molecular weight of 160,000. The active enzymatic site of factor XIII is located in the a subunits.

Activation of factor XIII occurs through limited proteolysis of the a subunits by thrombin. Following this activation, the b subunit dimer dissociates from the tetramer and the activated a dimer begins cross-linking polymerized fibrin. Cross-linking initially occurs between γ chains in adjacent fibrin molecules, followed by a slower cross-linking occurring between α chains. In addition to cross-linking adjacent fibrin molecules, factor XIII been shown to cross-link α_2-plasmin inhibitor, fibronectin, collagen, von Willebrand factor, thrombospondin, plasminogen, and apolipoprotein a to a fibrin matrix. Inhibitors of factor XIII have not been well characterized. If factor XIII is incubated with thrombin, factor XIII activity is slowly lost and smaller-molecular-weight fragments of factor XIII are formed.

IV. CONTACT ACTIVATION

Contact activation is linked to the coagulation system, fibrinolytic system, kinin system, complement system, and possibly the renin system, and provides one of the primary links between the coagulation system and other biologic defense mechanisms (Fig. 5).

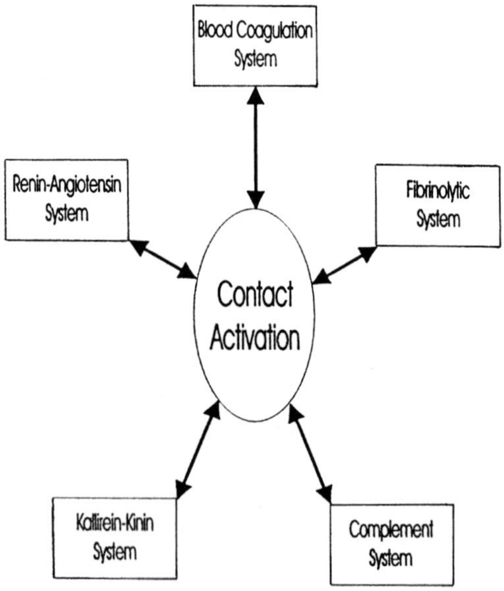

Figure 5 Systems with which the components of contact activation have been demonstrated to interact. The two-way arrows indicate that communication goes both ways via the contact system. Thus any one of the five indicated systems is capable of influencing any of the other systems.

A. Factor XII

The lack of factor XII does not predispose a patient to even a modest bleeding risk, but rather a thrombotic risk. This observation, coupled with the fact that it has been very difficult to describe an in-vivo system which clearly produces the "surface" activation of factor XII similar to the artificial activation seen in vitro, continually questions the relevance of factor XII to normal in-vivo coagulation. It is likely that factor XII activation is important as a general defense mechanism which either preactivates or triggers a number of physiologic, cascade-based defense mechanisms, rather than being a primary event in coagulation (67–69).

Factor XII is a glycoprotein with a molecular weight of about 80,000. It circulates as a single-polypeptide chain zymogen. The average plasma concentration of factor XII is about 30 μg/mL. The activation of factor XII is thought to occur when it binds to a negatively charged surface that exposes sites at which proteolytic cleavage can occur. Several proteases have been shown capable of activating factor XII, plasmin, factor XIa, factor XIIa, and kallikrein. It is thought that the primary mode of activation occurs via kallikrein. The proteolysis of factor XII produces two types of factor XIIa, a single cleavage which results in a two-chain factor XIIa in which the chains are connected by disulfide linkages (α-factor XIIa) and the molecular weight remains unchanged. A second cleavage leads to β-factor XIIa, in which a substantial reduction in molecular weight occurs. β-Factor XIIa is a potent activator of prekallikrein, but it has limited ability to activate factor XI (it does not readily bind to surfaces) (70,71).

B. Prekallikrein/Kallikrein

Plasma prekallikrein was a late-comer to coagulation. Its discovery was by chance. It was originally referred to as the Fletcher factor, which related to the family surname in which the trait was studied. It was later identified as prekallikrein and its role in contact activation was confirmed using antikallikrein serum. Prekallikrein has a molecular weight of about 85,000 and circulates in plasma at a concentration of about 50 μg/mL. Similar to factor XI, prekallikrein circulates in plasma complexed with high-molecular-weight kininogen. Prekallikrein is activated to kallikrein by factor XIIa by limited proteolysis. This results in a two-chained, disulfide-linked protease composed of a light and a heavy chain. The active site serine is located in the light chain. The complex of prekallikrein:high-molecular-weight kininogen binds to negatively charged surfaces. This binding enhances the activation process. Kallikrein is autocatalytic, in which an additional proteolytic cleavage leads to β-kallikrein, which is thought to be involved in generalized inflammatory responses (72–74).

C. High-Molecular-Weight Kininogen

High-molecular-weight kininogen was originally discovered, not by a clinical manifestations of either a thrombotic or hemorrhagic condition, but rather through a prolonged activated partial thromboplastin time. Human plasma contains two different types of kininogens, high-molecular-weight kininogen (HMW) and low-molecular-weight kininogen (LMW). Low-molecular-weight kininogen has no known function in blood coagulation. High-molecular-weight kininogen is much like factor VIII and factor V: It functions as a cofactor. Both types of kininogens are single-chained polypeptides that contain a bradykinin sequence in the center of the chain. High-molecular-weight kininogen has a molecular weight of 120,000 and circulates with an average plasma concentration of 70 μg/mL. The molecule circulates complexed to both factor XI and prekallikrein. It appears that prekallikrein has a higher affinity for HMW kininogen than does factor XI. HMW kininogen binds to negatively charged surfaces, where it facilitates the binding of both factor XI and prekallikrein to the surface where surface bound factor XIIa activates both. HMW kininogen also enhances the activation of factor XII (75).

Kallikrein enhances the activity of HMW kininogen by cleaving the single-chained molecule twice, releasing bradykinin. The resulting two-chained molecule is held together by disulfide linkages, and this results in an apparent enhancement of its cofactor activity in contact activation. Several HMW kininogen-deficient patients have been described, but to this point it is not clear what the main clinical symptoms are. The only notable abnormality is the prolonged clotting test.

V. NATURAL OCCURRING INHIBITORS OF COAGULATION

A number of clinical studies have examined the relationships between clotting factor activities and the risks of abnormal bleeding or clotting. The results indicate that risk profiles are highly influenced by either diminished or excessive activity of coagulation factors. Since the inhibitors play a significant role in the expression of clotting factor activity, abnormalities in either quantity or function will influence the risk of either bleeding or thrombosis, depending on the nature of the imbalance (76).

A. Protein C/Protein S/Thrombomodulin/PCI

Protein C inhibitory activity in blood is the result of a small cascade system (Fig. 6). Protein C, like the coagulation proteases, circulates in an inactive form, which has to be activated. This activation requires cofactors, lipids, and calcium. The mechanism involves thrombomodulin, thrombin, protein C, and protein S (77–80). The protein C pathway involves the formation of a complex between thrombin and thrombomodulin (located in vascular endothelial cell membrane). This complex activates protein C to its active form by limited proteolysis. The activated protein C then inactivates factor Va and factor VIIIa by limited proteolysis in which the cofactor protein S enhances the reaction.

Protein C was originally described in the 1960s as autoprothrombin II-A. Protein C circulates at a plasma concentration of about 5 μg/mL, consisting of two polypeptide chains linked via disulfide bridges. The molecular weight is about 62,000 and the protein has a carbohydrate content of about 23%. Thrombin activates protein C via a single proteolytic cleavage that

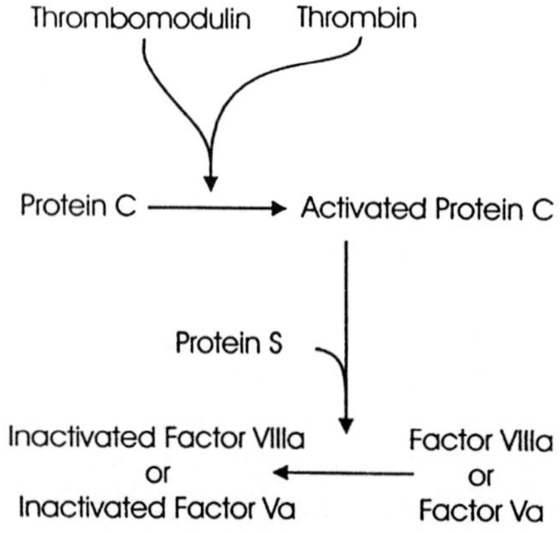

Figure 6 The natural protein C anticoagulant system.

releases an activation peptide. Activated protein C cleaves activated factor V and activated factor VIII very rapidly, but has little activity toward the unactivated forms of the cofactors. Homozygous protein C deficiencies are accompanied by massive thrombotic complications, so this pathway is key to maintaining a hemostatic balance.

Thrombomodulin was the missing key in the protein C-inhibitory pathway. It was not until its discovery that the protein C-inhibitory pathway became kinetically feasible as an in-vivo inhibitory mechanism. Thrombin slowly activates protein C, but when it binds to thrombomodulin its specificity is changed and it rapidly activates protein C. When thrombin is bound to thrombomodulin, it is no longer capable of converting fibrinogen to fibrin; thus it loses its coagulant activity and participates only as a component of an anticoagulation pathway. Thrombomodulin is an integral membrane protein and is found in the membranes of a large number of different cell types. In coagulation, its presence in the vascular endothelium affects coagulation most significantly. The apoprotein has a molecular weight of about 60,300. The structure is characterized by a cytoplasmic C-terminal tail region, a transmembrane section, a glycopeptide-like region, followed by several epidermal growth factor-like regions, a hydrophobic region, and terminates in the N-terminal lectin-like region. In this respect, it is similar to a number of other membrane receptor proteins.

Protein S is also a vitamin K-dependent protein. It circulates in plasma at about a concentration of 20 μg/mL as a single peptide chain having a molecular weight of 70,690. Protein S appears to form a 1:1 complex with activated protein C on lipid surfaces. Exactly how protein S accelerates the inactivation of factor Va and factor VIIIa is not known. Genetic deficiencies in protein S also cause a predisposition toward thromboembolic events.

Protein C inhibitor (PCI) is one of the serine protease inhibitors of activated protein C. PCI is similar to other substrate-type inhibitors (i.e., antithrombin III). It is a single-chain glycoprotein with a molecular weight of 57,000 and circulates at a plasma concentration of about 5 μg/mL. The structure of the molecule is similar to that of other serpins (81,82).

B. Tissue Factor Pathway Inhibitor (TFPI)

Tissue factor pathway inhibitor (TFPI) has been referred to as LACI (lipoprotein-associated coagulation inhibitor) and EPI (extrinsic pathway inhibitor). Although a significant number of early studies suggested the existence of an extrinsic pathway inhibitor, it was not until the 1980s that serious work began on clarifying this activity. TFPI has generated considerable interest in the last several years due to its ability to shut down extrinsic coagulation. This led to the conclusion that extrinsic coagulation could not be the primary pathway for the generation of a fibrin clot. TFPI is what is known as a Kunitz-type inhibitor. Genetic engineering experiments have worked out the basic structure of TFPI. By modifying the structure, the important structural components have been identified. TFPI inhibits both the tissue factor–factor VIIa catalytic complex and can inhibit factor Xa directly. TFPI is a potent inhibitor of trypsin. Heparin has been noted to enhance the factor Xa inhibition as well as increase plasma concentrations of TFPI (83,84).

The mechanism of inhibition of the tissue factor–factor VIIa complex is unique. The process involves not only TFPI, but also factor Xa. The inhibitor complex is a quaternary complex of the four components. Factor Xa is not an absolute requirement, but the inhibitory activity is significantly higher when factor Xa is present.

TFPI circulates in plasma bound to lipoproteins. The molecular size is heterogeneous, with the predominant forms having molecular weights of 34,000 and 40,000. There are other forms of higher molecular weight, and the reasons for this heterogeneity are thought to be due to disulfide links with other plasma proteins. Platelets also contain TFPI and release this TFPI when stimulated with thrombin. The mean normal concentration of TFPI in plasma is around 100 ng/mL, but there appears to be a wide variation in individual plasma levels. To date, no prothrombotic state has been identified due to a lack of TFPI (85).

C. Antithrombin III

Antithrombin III is the classic inhibitor of thrombin. Functionally it appears to be the most important inhibitor of not only thrombin, but also several other serine proteases of coagulation. The structure of antithrombin III is that of standard serine protease inhibitors which are lumped together under the term serpins (SERine Protease INhibitor). Antithrombin III is a single-chain glycoprotein having a molecular weight of 58,200. In the inhibition of thrombin by antithrombin III, a covalent bond is established between the reactive site on antithrombin III and the active site serine in thrombin (86,87).

The most interesting aspect of inhibition by antithrombin III is the impact of heparin. Heparin accelerates the rate of inhibition over 2000-fold. With most proteases this involves a binary complex between heparin and antithrombin III in which the antithrombin III undergoes a conformational change that enhances its ability to interact with the protease; with thrombin, however, a ternary complex is formed in which the thrombin also binds to the heparin polysaccharide chain at sites adjacent to the antithrombin III-binding site. It appears that this is almost a prerequisite for the heparin acceleration of antithrombin III inhibition of thrombin. With the other coagulation proteases, i.e., factor X and factor IX, this does not happen, and neither has a high affinity for heparin. This difference is what distinguishes high-molecular-weight heparins from low-molecular-weight heparins. The low-molecular-weight heparins have decreased ability to accelerate the inhibition of thrombin, yet retain their ability to inhibit factor Xa and factor IXa. The clinical utility of this type of inhibition, i.e., being able to inhibit the activity of factor Xa but not thrombin, has been the subject of a large number of clinical studies, which have yet to show that this confers a significant effect on clinical outcomes. It remains to be established that the inhibition of factor Xa reduces thrombotic risks while lessening the risks of bleeding.

D. Heparin Cofactor II

Heparin cofactor II is another plasma protein inhibitor of thrombin. Like antithrombin III, its activity as an inhibitor is enhanced by the presence of heparin. Unlike antithrombin III, it does not have a high-affinity binding site for heparin, i.e., the pentasaccharide site for antithrombin III binding. It therefore requires higher concentrations of heparin to achieve the same degree of thrombin inhibition. Heparin cofactor II activity is also enhanced by several other polyanionic compounds, including heparan and chondroitin sulfates. Dermatan sulfate, on the other hand, seems to possess a specific binding site for heparin cofactor II. This does not, however, offer any significant advantages over heparin. On a weight basis, considerably less heparin is required than dermatan sulfate to achieve the same degree of thrombin inhibition. Recently, dermatan disulfates have been found to enhance heparin cofactor II's activity even more than dermatan sulfate. There has been some interest in using dermatan-like compounds in place of heparin in such areas as cardiovascular surgery, where it has been reported that bleeding problems occur less frequently with dermatans than with heparins (88–91).

VI. FIBRINOLYSIS AND THE DISSOLUTION OF FIBRIN CLOTS

Fibrinolysis is the dissolution of the fibrin network that forms a fibrin-based blood clot. A system of enzymes, inhibitors, and activators exist which closely parallels the system of enzymes, inhibitors, and activators of the blood-clotting system. In some instances components are common to both systems. Figure 7 illustrates the components of the fibrinolytic system.

A. Plasmin

Just as thrombin is the primary proteolytic enzyme of fibrin formation, plasmin is the primary enzyme of fibrin dissolution. Plasmin exists as an inactive proenzyme (plasminogen) until it is activated to plasmin by limited proteolysis. Plasminogen binds to fibrin, providing a basic control mechanism in fibrinolysis. This localizes the inactive form of the enzyme on the surface of a fibrin clot (92–94).

The activation of plasminogen to plasmin occurs several different ways. The normal form of plasminogen found in plasma has an N-terminal amino acid of glutamine. The active form of the enzyme, plasmin, can cleave plasminogen such that the N-terminal is lysine. Lys-plasminogen has a higher affinity for fibrin and a much shorter half-life than does Glu-plasminogen. The activators of plasminogen can convert either the Glu or Lys form to the respective Glu- or Lys-plasmins. Although the primary substrates for plasmin are fibrin and fibrinogen, plasmin has been demonstrated to hydrolyze a number of other plasma proteins (95–97).

B. Tissue Plasminogen Activator

Tissue plasminogen activator (tPA) is an enzyme released from cells which activates plasminogen to plasmin. The tPA secreted by cells is a single-chain protease. This single-chain form of tPA can be converted to a two-chain form by plasmin, kallikrein, or factor Xa. The conversion of plasminogen to plasmin by tPA is accelerated by the presence of fibrin. Both forms of tPA bind to fibrin, and it has been reported that single-chain tPA binds to fibrin better than two-chained tPA. This was thought to give single-chained tPA better clot selectivity than two-chained tPA, but this observation has been questioned recently. The two-chained form of tPA

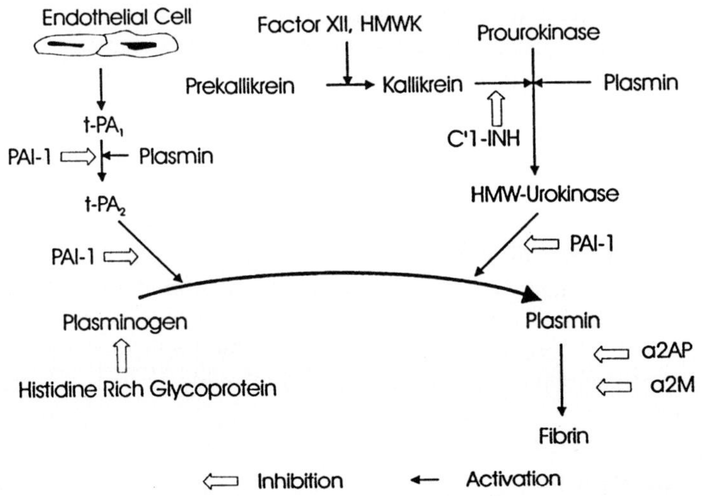

Figure 7 Fibrinolysis. In the diagram, the subscripts on t-PA (tissue plasminogen activator) indicate the single-chain or two-chain form of t-PA. The open arrows indicate the point of action of an inhibitor, while the solid arrows indicate an activation process. C′1-INH is C1 esterase inhibitor, HMW is high-molecular-weight, a2AP is alpha-2-antiplasmin, a2M is alpha-2-macroglobulin, HMWK is high-molecular-weight kininogen.

is more active in converting Glu-plasminogen to plasmin and is inactivated much more rapidly by inhibitors than is the single-chained tPA.

C. Urokinase

Urokinase (u-PA) is a plasminogen activator that is found in both urine and plasma. Urokinase can exist as either a single chain (prourokinase) or in several versions of a two-chain enzyme. Prourokinase exhibits fibrin-specific conversion of plasminogen to plasmin, while the two-chain versions do not. Interestingly, prourokinase does not appear to bind to fibrin, and the mechanism by which prourokinase expresses fibrin specificity is not yet known. It appears that prourokinase is a true zymogen, i.e., it must be activated to urokinase before it can activate plasminogen to plasmin. In some way this activation mechanism must confer the fibrin specificity exhibited by prourokinase (98).

D. Prekallikrein Factor XII

As mention earlier, prekallikrein is a component of the contact activation system of blood clotting. Kallikrein will rapidly convert single-chained tPA to two-chained tPA, and is thought to be involved in the conversion of prourokinase to urokinase. In the test tube, factor XII activation is accompanied by the formation of plasmin. This activation of fibrinolysis depends on the presence of both urokinase and kallikrein. There has been some speculation as to whether this mechanism of plasmin formation has any significance in in-vivo fibrinolysis.

E. Alpha-2-antiplasmin

Alpha-2-antiplasmin is the principal inhibitor of plasmin and is structurally related to antithrombin III. It has three major functional properties: (a) the inhibition of plasmin, (b) interference with the binding of plasminogen to fibrin, and (c) incorporation into a fibrin clot by cross-linking to the alpha chains of fibrin by the action of factor XIIIa (99–101). During clot formation approximately 20% of the alpha-2-antiplasmin cross-links to fibrin. Because of this a normal blood clot will not lyse spontaneously, despite the presence of clot-bound tPA. Clot bound alpha-2-antiplasmin is more effective in preventing clot dissolution than is the free plasma alpha-2-antiplasmin.

F. Alpha-2-macroglobulin

Alpha-2-macroglobulin is a plasma proteinase inhibitor with wide specificity. Structurally alpha-2-macroglobulin is composed of four identical subunits arranged as a pair of dimers. Alpha-2-macroglobulin is an inhibitor of many of the components of the fibrinolytic system. It inactivates plasmin, kallikrein, two-chain urokinase, tPA, and the streptokinase–plasminogen complex (102). Alpha-2-macroglobulin is not related to the typical serine protease family of inhibitors referred to as "serpins." Structurally it is related to the complement proteins C3 and C4.

G. Plasminogen Activator Inhibitor

A number of inhibitors have been identified which inhibit the activity of tPA and urokinase. These inhibitors are related to antithrombin III and are classified as serpins. Plasminogen activator inhibitor 1 (PAI-1) is found in plasma and platelets, and is produced by endothelial cells, hepatocytes, smooth muscle cells, fibroblasts, and various malignant cell types. PAI-1 inhibits the activity of both forms of tPA, and two-chained urokinase, but not prourokinase or the streptokinase–plasminogen complex (103,104).

PAI-2 was originally discovered in extracts from human placenta. PAI-2 is produced by monocytes, granulocytes, and various malignant cell types. PAI-2 is not measurable in normal human plasma; however, measurable plasma levels develop during pregnancy, peaking in the third trimester. PAI-2 inhibits the activity of the two-chained forms of urokinase and tPA, but has little activity with the single-chain forms of either activator (105).

H. C′1-Inhibitor

C′1 inhibitor inhibits activated components of the complement system, factors XIIa and XIa, kallikrein, and plasmin. Its primary effect on fibrinolysis is probably the inhibition of the conversion of single-chain urokinase to the two-chain version (106).

I. Histidine-Rich Glycoprotein

Histidine-rich glycoprotein (HRG) is a plasma protein that acts as a competitive inhibitor of plasmin. HRG forms a reversible complex with plasminogen, lowering the plasma concentration of free plasminogen. HRG plasma levels will determine how much free plasminogen is available for binding to fibrin during and after coagulation.

J. Streptokinase

Streptokinase is not a normal component of human blood; however, it has been used for many years as a drug to induce fibrinolysis. Streptokinase is secreted by group C hemolytic streptococcus. The mechanism by which streptokinase induces fibrinolysis is unique. Streptokinase forms an equimolar complex with plasminogen. This complex activates plasminogen to plasmin and is converted to a streptokinase–plasmin complex by plasmin. Both complexes are potent activators of plasminogen, but are themselves incapable of direct fibrinolytic activity. Since streptokinase is a bacterial origin, one the drawbacks in its use is its antigenicity. High titers of antistreptokinase antibodies due either to recent streptococcal infections or previous exposure to streptokinase can limit the effectiveness of streptokinase treatment (107).

K. Disorders of Fibrinolysis

A number of disease states are characterized by defective fibrinolysis. This can lead either to thrombotic or hemorrhagic states. Defects characterized by lowered or nonfunctional levels of plasminogen or the plasminogen activators clinically present patients who have thrombotic disorders. Conversely a defect in the inhibitors of fibrinolysis, e.g., the plasminogen activator inhibitors or the plasmin inhibitors, can lead to a hemorrhagic state in which formed clots are lysed too rapidly or fibrinogen levels are lowered. Undesired fibrinolysis can present two problems, localized fibrinolysis at the site of a wound in which clot formation is required, or generalized systemic fibrinolysis in which the patient's fibrinogen level is lowered. Although there may not appear to be much difference between the two states, treatment regimens for hemorrhaging generally have to be more drastic if systemic fibrinolysis is present. It presently is not clear if fibrinolysis can deplete coagulation factors other than fibrinogen. Recent reports indicate that thrombin formation may occur via a plasmin-initiated conversion of prothrombin to thrombin, and both the activation and destruction of factor V by plasmin have been reported (108,109).

VII. CELLULAR AND OTHER COMPONENTS OF COAGULATION AND FIBRINOLYSIS

A. Platelets

Platelets have been somewhat of an anomaly in coagulation. Their effect on coagulation has been known for years, yet due to the way in which research has been performed, this effect is slighted. As more has been learned on the clinical front, the impact of platelets on in-vivo thrombosis and bleeding is becoming even more apparent. At some point this should lead to a better presentation of the platelet's contribution to coagulation in coagulation hypotheses.

The primary coagulation activities of platelets are what have been referred to as platelet factor 3 and platelet factor 4 activities. Platelet factor 3 refers to the "lipid" surface that is required for the assembly of coagulation factors. Platelet factor 4 is a platelet component that is released when platelets are activated. It neutralizes the anticoagulant activity of heparin or heparans. For several years there has also been the suggestion that platelets providing a binding site for factor XI, but this remains a debatable issue (110–113).

The platelet factor 3 (PF3) activity is thought to involve the binding of factor V, which leads to the assembly of the prothrombinase complex with factor X. This can be satisfied with various lipids. This is always shown as "PL" (phospholipid) in coagulation diagrams. It is thought that the PF3 activity of platelets is not exposed in a normal resting platelet, however, it appears that the factor V-binding site and platelet factor V are exposed. This suggests that at least two distinct sites are involved in assembling coagulation complexes on platelet membranes. Although factor V may be bound to the platelet membrane, a membrane change is still required to expose classic PF3 activity.

Clotting tests which are sensitive to platelets in whole blood are intrinsic coagulation tests, i.e., the partial thromboplastin time and the activated clotting time. Thus intrinsic coagulation in whole blood seems to depend on platelets, and it is with variations on these tests that it appears that platelets need to be activated before full PF3 activity is exposed. In this case, the PF3 activity is that which clearly accelerates the coagulation reaction (114).

The importance of platelets in in-vivo coagulation processes has been indicated from recent clinical studies in which platelet inhibitors have been shown to have a favorable impact on acute reocculsion rates following interventional cardiology procedures and on myocardial infarctions. These studies point clearly to a significant role for platelets, to the extent that some recent clinical interpretations suggest that platelets are the primary target for preventing adverse thrombotic complications (115–117).

B. White Blood Cells

Various white blood cells have been shown to have procoagulant activity. The most notable are monocytes, in which the exposure of tissue factor in response to activation of the monocytes may be the primary mechanism of septic-induced disseminated intravascular coagulation (118,119). Various forms of cancer also result in the exposure of tissue factor on the surface of monocytes. This exposed tissue factor binds factor VII/VIIa and leads to the assembly of the prothrombinase complex on the surface of the cell. One of the differences between monocytes and tumor cells is that monocytes must express this activity in response to a challenge, whereas tumor cells already express the tissue factor activity. Although the expression of tissue factor on the surface of monocytes/tumor cells is generally viewed as a pathologic process, it is not known whether white blood cells have a role in normal coagulation processes.

Table 1 Coagulation and Fibrinolytic Components

Factor	Common name	Activated product	Molecular weight	Concentration/ plasma
I	Fibrinogen	Fibrin	340,000	3 μg/mL
II	Prothrombin	Thrombin	71,600	200 μg/mL
III	Tissue factor	None	33,000–42,000	NA
IV	Calcium	None	40	2.5 μM
V	Proaccelerin	Factor Va	330,000	10 μg/mL
VI	Activated V	Dropped	NA	NA
VII	Proconvertin	Factor VIIa	63,000	0.5 μg/mL
VIII	Antihemophilic factor	Factor VIIIa	290,000	0.2 μg/mL
IX	Christmas factor	Factor IXa	54,000	5 μg/mL
X	Stuart factor	Factor Xa	59,000	8 μg/mL
XI	Plasma thromboplastin antecedent	Factor XIa	160,000	4 μg/mL
XII	Hageman factor	Factor XIIa	80,000	30 μg/mL
XIII	Fibrin-stabilizing factor	Factor XIIIa	320,000	20 μg/mL
	Prekallikrein	Kallikrein	85,000	50 μg/mL
	HMW kininogen	Bradykinin	120,000	70 μg/mL
	Protein C	Activated protein C	62,000	5 μg/mL
	Protein S	Activated protein S	70,690	20 μg/mL
	Thrombomodulin	None	60,300	NA
	Antithrombin III	None	58,200	125 μg/mL
	Protein C inhibitor	None	57,000	5 μg/mL
	Heparin cofactor II	None	66,000	60 μg/mL
	Tissue factor pathway inhibitor	None	34,000–42,000	100 ng/mL
	von Willebrand factor	None	$0.5–20 \times 10^6$	
	Plasminogen	Plasmin	92,000	200 ng/mL
	α_2-Antiplasmin	None	70,000	70 μg/mL
	PAI-1	None	50,000	20 μg/mL
	C1 esterase inhibitor	None	105,000	0.2 μg/mL
	α_2-Antitrypsin	None	55,000	1.3 μg/mL
	Tissue plasminogen activator	None	69,000	1 μg/mL
	PAI-2	None	48,000	Pregnancy—105 μg/mL
	Histidine-rich glycoprotein	None	75,000	100 ng/mL
	Streptokinase	None	47,000	NA
	α_2-Macroglobulin	None	740,000	2.2 μg/mL
	Prourokinase	Urokinase	54,000	5 ng/mL

C. Phospholipids

In plasma-based coagulation systems, various phospholipids have been known to substitute for what is thought to be the platelet requirement of coagulation. Generally, these phospholipids can be extracted from the membranes of platelets and vascular endothelial cells. It is assumed these must be the naturally occurring components of coagulation. There are several areas in which phospholipids or sulfatides participate in coagulation. These are the assemblies of the complexes involving the vitamin K-dependent clotting factors. This includes the prothrombinase complex, the factor IX–factor VIII complex, and the phospholipid component of tissue factor.

D. Metal Ions

Calcium takes part in a number of different reactions of coagulation, stabilizes certain coagulation factors, and is involved in the functioning platelets and other cellular components of coagulation (120,121). The gamma carboxyglutamic acid component of the vitamin K clotting factors chelate calcium. This simple mechanism is one of the mainstays of the coagulation process. Remove calcium and coagulation no longer takes place. Replace the calcium and coagulation proceeds. Although other divalent metal ions can substitute, the activities of coagulation are only modestly restored. To some extent, the actual contribution of calcium to coagulation is again understood only at the test tube level. What happens in vivo is only a guess. One of the components released by platelets is calcium. This occurs in the microenvironment where the clot is being formed. Since this released calcium must affect the local concentration of calcium, it is interesting to surmise what the real calcium level must be when coagulation is taking place.

VIII. SUMMARY

Coagulation mechanisms continue to get more complex as the scope of interactions of the clotting factors is extended. Although we are still hampered by having to study many of the reactions under "artificial" conditions, the advances which have been made during the past 20 years still show that test tube studies can provide answers and can provide us with predictive value. These types of studies are still open to criticism on a number of different points, but the successes have far outweighed the failures. Efforts must continue to find ways to carry the molecular discoveries into clinical realities. Frequently we find that the molecular understanding does not hold up in the clinical arena, not because the molecular understanding is wrong, but due to the fact that the scope of molecular studies is too limited.

NOTE ADDED IN PROOF

Recent advances in coagulation theory and concepts have concentrated on thrombophilic states (124–127) and modifying current cascade hypotheses to fit clinical observations (128–134). There is still an unclear relationship between classic extrinsic coagulation and intrinsic coagulation, nor is there a clear indication on how blood clotting is initiated. Current focus is concentrating on factor VII/tissue factor and factor XI. The articles cited above indicate this area is still under active investigation and that current hypotheses have yet to fully explain in vivo coagulation mechanisms.

REFERENCES

1. Ratnoff OD, Davie EW. The activation of Christmas factor (factor IX) by activated plasma thromboplastin antecedent (activated factor XI). Biochemistry 1962; 1:677–685.
2. Davie EW, Ratnoff OD. Waterfall sequence for intrinsic blood clotting. Science 1964; 145:1310–1312.
3. MacFarlane RG. An enzyme cascade in the blood clotting mechanism, and its function as a biochemical amplifier. Nature 1964; 202:498–499.
4. Halbmayer W-M, Mannhalter C, Feichtinger C, Rubi K, Fischer M. The prevalence of factor XII

deficiency in 103 orally anticoagulated outpatients suffering from recurrent venous and/or arterial thromboembolism. Thromb Haemost 1992; 68:285–290.
5. Colman RW, Rao AK, Rubin RN, Walsh PN. Factor XI deficiency and hemostasis. Am J Hematol 1994; 45:73–78.
6. Gailani D, Broze GJ Jr. Factor XI activation in a revised model of blood coagulation. Science 1991; 253:909–912.
7. Broze GJ Jr. The role of tissue factor pathway inhibitor in a revised coagulation cascade. Semin Hematol 1992; 29:159–169.
8. Broze GJ Jr. Tissue factor pathway inhibitor and the revised hypothesis of blood coagulation. Trends Cardiovasc Med 1992; 2:72–77.
9. Tijburg PNM, Ryan J, Stern DM, et al. Activation of the coagulation mechanism on tumor necrosis factor-stimulated cultured endothelial cells and their extracellular matrix. The role of flow and factor IX/IXa. J Biol Chem 1991; 266:12067–12074.
10. Hoffman M, Monroe DM, Roberts HR. Coagulation factor IXa binding to activated platelets and platelet-derived microparticles: a flow cytometric study. Thromb Haemost 1992; 68:74–78.
11. Hoffman M, Monroe DM, Roberts HR. Cellular interactions in hemostasis. Haemostasis 1996; 26: 12–16.
12. Esmon CT, Johnson AE, Esmon NL. Initiation of the protein C pathway. Ann NY Acad Sci 1991; 614:30–43.
13. Suttie JW. Synthesis of vitamin K-dependent proteins. FASEB J 1993; 7:445–452.
14. Rao LVM, Rapaport SI. Activation of factor VII bound to tissue factor: a key early step in the tissue factor pathway of blood coagulation. Proc Natl Acad Sci USA 1988; 85:6687–6691.
15. Sakai T, Lund-Hansen T, Paborsky L, Pedersen AH, Kisiel W. Binding of human factors VII and VIIa to a human bladder carcinoma cell line (J82). Implications for the initiation of the extrinsic pathway of blood coagulation. J Biol Chem 1989; 264:9980–9988.
16. Nakagaki T, Foster DC, Berkner KL, Kisiel W. Initiation of the extrinsic pathway of blood coagulation: evidence for the tissue factor dependent autoactivation of human coagulation factor VII. Biochem J 1991; 30:10819–10824.
17. Wildgoose P, Kisiel W. Activation of human factor VII by factors IXa and Xa on human bladder carcinoma cells. Blood 1989; 73:1888–1895.
18. Mann KG. Factor VII assays, plasma triglyceride levels, and cardiovascular disease risk. Arteriosclerosis 1989; 9:783–784.
19. Sousa JC, Soria C, Bruckert E, Tobelem G, Soria J, Caen JC. Fibrinogen and factor VII: Two risk factors for arterial thrombosis. Presse Med 1989; 18:799–800.
20. Poller L, MacCallum PK, Thomsom JM, Kerns W. Reduction of factor VII coagulant activity (VIIC), a risk factor for ischaemic heart disease, by fixed dose Warfarin: a double blind crossover study. Br Heart J 1990; 63:231–233.
21. Green F, Kelleher C, Wilkes H, Temple A, Meade T, Humphries S. A common genetic polymorphism associated with lower coagulation factor VII levels in healthy individuals. Arteriosclerosis 1991; 11:540–546.
22. Weisdorf D, Hasegawa D, Fair DS. Acquired factor VII deficiency associated with aplastic anaemia: correction with bone marrow transplantation. Br J Haematol 1989; 71:409–413.
23. Neuenschwander PF, Morrissey JH. Deletion of the membrane anchoring region of tissue factor abolishes autoactivation of factor VII but not cofactor function. Analysis of a mutant with a selective deficiency in activity. J Biol Chem 1992; 267:14477–14482.
24. Bernardi F, Patracchini P, Gemmati D, et al. Molecular analysis of factor VII deficiency in Italy: a frequency mutation (FVII Lazio) in a repeated intronic region. Hum Genet 1993; 92:446–450.
25. Komiyama Y, Pedersen AH, Kisiel W. Proteolytic activation of human factors IX and X by recombinant human factor VIIa: effects of calcium, phospholipids, and tissue factor. Biochemistry 1990; 29:9418–9425.
26. Bauer KA, Eichinger S, Mannucci PM, Rosenberg RD. Determinants of coagulation activation in humans. Haemostasis 1996; 26:72–75.

27. Morrissey JH. Plasma factor VIIa: measurement and potential clinical significance. Haemostasis 1996; 26:66–71.
28. Sakata T, Kario K, Matsuo T, et al. Suppression of plasma-activated factor VII levels by warfarin therapy. Arterioscler Thromb 1995; 15:241–246.
29. Del Zoppo GJ, Yu J-Q, Copeland BR, Thomas WS, Schneiderman J, Morrissey JH. Tissue factor localization in non-human primate cerebral tissue. Thromb Haemost 1992; 68:642–647.
30. Landers SC, Gupta M, Lewis JC. Ultrastructural localization of tissue factor on monocyte-derived macrophages and macrophage foam cells associated with atherosclerotic lesions. Virchows Arch Int J Pathol 1994; 425:49–54.
31. Stone MJ, Ruf W, Miles DJ, Edgington TS, Wright PE. Recombinant soluble human tissue factor secreted by *Saccharomyces cerevisiae* and refolded from *Escherichia coli* inclusion bodies: glycosylation of mutants, activity and physical characterization. Biochem J 1995; 310:605–614.
32. Banner DW, D'Arcy A, Chène C, et al. The crystal structure of the complex of blood coagulation factor VIIa with soluble tissue factor. Nature 1996; 380:41–46.
33. Seligsohn U. Factor XI deficiency. Thromb Haemost 1993; 70:68–71.
34. Peter MK, Meili EO, Von Felten A. Factor XI deficiency: do patients with a bleeding tendency have other hemostatic defects. Schweiz Med Wochenschr 1996; 126:999–1005.
35. Baglia FA, Jameson BA, Walsh PN. Fine mapping of the high molecular weight kininogen binding site on blood coagulation factor XI through the use of rationally designed synthetic analogs. J Biol Chem 1992; 267:4247–4252.
36. Brennée T, La Porta C, Reddigari SR, Salerno VM, Kaplan AP, Silverberg M. Activation of factor XI in plasma is dependent on factor XII. Blood 1993; 81:580–586.
37. Baglia FA, Seaman FS, Walsh PN. The Apple 1 and Apple 4 domains of factor XI act synergistically to promote the surface-mediated activation of factor XI by factor XIIa. Blood 1995; 85: 2078–2083.
38. Gailani D, Broze GJ Jr. Factor XI activation by thrombin and factor XIa. Semin Thromb Hemo 1993; 19:396–404.
39. Von dem Borne PAK, Koppelman SJ, Bouma BN, Meijers JCM. Surface independent factor XI activation by thrombin in the presence of high molecular weight kininogen. Thromb Haemost 1994; 72–397–402.
40. High KA. Factor IX: molecular structure, eptiopes, and mutations associated with inhibitor formation. Adv Exp Med Biol 1995; 386:79–86.
41. Astermark J, Hogg PJ, Björk I, Stenflo J. Effects of gamma-carboxyglutamic acid and epidermal growth factor-like modules of factor IX on factor X activation. Studies using proteolytic fragments of bovine factor IX. J Biol Chem 1992; 267:3249–3256.
42. Bom VJJ, Reinalda-Poot JH, Cupers R, Bertina RM. Extrinsic activation of human blood coagulation factors IX and X. Thromb Haemost 1990; 63:224–230.
43. Lawson JH, Mann KG. Cooperative activation of human factor IX by the human extrinsic pathway of blood coagulation. J Biol Chem 1991; 266:11317–11327.
44. Lollar P, Parker CG. Subunit structure of thrombin-activated porcine factor VIII. Biochemistry 1989; 28:666–674.
45. Fowler WE, Fay PJ, Arvan DS, Marder VJ. Electron microscopy of human factor V and factor VIII: correlation of morphology with domain structure and localization of factor V activation fragments. Proc Natl Acad Sci USA 1990; 87:7648–7652.
46. Lollar P. The association of factor VII with von Willebrand factor. Mayo Clin Proc 1991; 66: 524–534.
47. Donath M-JSH, Lenting PJ, Van Mourik JA, Mertens K. The role of cleavage of the light chain at positions Arg^{1689} or Arg^{1721} in subunit interaction and activation of human blood coagulation factor VIII. J Biol Chem 1995; 270:3648–3655.
48. Sadler JE, Ginsburg D. A database of polymorphisms in the von Willebrand factor gene and pseudogene. Thromb Haemost 1993; 69:185–191.

49. Hantgan RR, Hindriks G, Taylor RG, Sixma JJ, De Groot PG. Glycoprotein Ib, von Willebrand factor, and glycoprotein IIb:IIIa are all involved in platelet adhesion to fibrin in flowing whole blood. Blood 1990; 76:345–353.
50. Weiss HJ. von Willebrand factor and platelet function. Ann NY Acad Sci 1991; 614:125–137.
51. Hertzberg M. Biochemistry of factor X. Blood Rev 1994; 8:56–62.
52. Hultin MB, Hennessey J, Morrison SA. Dibucaine elicits platelet procoagulant activity in factor VIII and factor X activation by a mechanism involving a sulfhydryl-dependent enzyme. Thromb Res 1992; 68:399–407.
53. Hoffman M, Monroe DM, Roberts HR. Human monocytes support factor X activation by factor VIIa, independent of tissue factor: Implications for the therapeutic mechanism of high-dose factor VIIa in hemophilia. Blood 1994; 83:38–42.
54. Krishnaswamy S, Nesheim ME, Pryzdial ELG, Mann KG. Assembly of prothrombinase complex. Meth Enzymol 1993; 222:260–280.
55. Suidan HS, Niclou SP, Monard D. The thrombin receptor in the nervous system. Semin Thromb Hemo 1996; 22:125–133.
56. Winking M, Heldt RM, Simmet T. Thrombin stimulates activation of the cerebral 5-lipoxygenase pathway during blood-brain cell contact. J Cereb Blood Flow Metab 1996; 16:737–745.
57. Huang S, Mulvihill ER, Farrell DH, Chung DW, Davie EW. Biosynthesis of human fibrinogen. Subunit interactions and potential intermediates in the assembly. J. Biol Chem 1993; 268:8919–8926.
58. Blombäck B. Fibrinogen structure, activation, polymerization and fibrin gel structure. Proceedings of the IVS's meeting in Paris, 17th December, 1993. Thromb Res 1994; 75:327–328.
59. Weisel JW, Nagaswami C. Computer modeling of fibrin polymerization kinetics correlated with electron microscope and turbidity observations: clot structure and assembly are kinetically controlled. Biophys J 1992; 63:111–128.
60. Kini RM, Evans HJ. Prediction of potential protein-protein interaction sites from amino acid sequence—identification of a fibrin polymerization site. FEBS Lett 1996; 385:81–86.
61. Frojmovic MM, Mooney RF, Wong T. Dynamics of platelet glycoprotein IIb-IIIa receptor expression and fibrinogen binding. I. Quantal activation of platelet subpopulations varies with adenosine diphosphate concentration. Biophys J 1994; 67:2060–2068.
62. Frojmovic MM, Mooney RF, Wong T. Dynamics of platelet glycoprotein IIb-IIIa receptor expression and fibrinogen binding. II. Quantal activation parallels platelet capture in stir-associated microaggregation. Biophys J 1994; 67:2069–2075.
63. Ruggeri ZM. The role of von Willebrand factor and fibrinogen in the initiation of platelet adhesion to thrombogenic surfaces. Thromb Haemost 1995; 74:460–463.
64. Greenberg CS, Enghild JJ, Mary A, Dobson JV, Achyuthan KE. Isolation of a fibrin-binding fragment from blood coagulation factor XIII capable of cross-linking fibrin(ogen). Biochem J 1988; 256:1013–1019.
65. Uchino R, Cardinali M, Chung SI. Regulation of extravascular fibrinolysis by factor XIII. Fibrinolysis 1991; 5:93–98.
66. Yee VC, Pedersen LC, Le Trong I, Bishop PD, Stenkamp RE, Teller DC. Three-dimensional sturcture of a transglutaminase: human blood coagulation factor XIII. Proc Natl Acad Sci USA 1994; 91:7296–7300.
67. Halbmayer W-M, Haushofer A, Radek J, Schön R, Deutsch M, Fischer M. Prevalence of factor XII (Hageman factor) deficiency among 426 patients with coronary heart disease awaiting cardiac surgery. Coronary Artery Dis 1994; 5:451–454.
68. Jansen PM, Pixley RA, Brouwer M, et al. Inhibition of factor XII in septic baboons attenuates the activation of complement and fibrinolytic systems and reduces the release of interleukin-6 and neutrophil elastase. Blood 1996; 87:2337–2344.
69. Shibayama Y, Reddigari S, Kaplan AP. Interactions of factor XII with platelets and endothelial cells. Immunopharmacology 1996; 32:24–27.

70. Briseid K, Hoem N-O, Johannesen S, Marthinsen K. Functional correlation between kallikrein and factor XII activated in human plasma. Thromb Res 1990; 57:945–956.
71. Pixley RA, Colman RW. Factor XII: Hageman factor. Meth Enzymol 1993; 222:51–65.
72. McMullen BA, Fujikawa K, Davie EW. Location of the disulfide bonds in human plasma prekallikrein: the presence of four novel apple domains in the animo-terminal portion of the molecule. Biochemistry 1991; 30:2050–2056.
73. Page JD, Colman RW. Localization of distinct functional domains on prekallikrein for interaction with both high molecular weight kininogen and activated factor XII in a 28-kDa fragment (amino acids 141–371). J Biol Chem 1991; 266:8143–8148.
74. Veloso D, Colman RW. Western blot analyses of prekallikrein and its activation products in human plasma. Thromb Haemost 1991; 65:382–388.
75. Hasan AAK, Cines DB, Herwald H, Schmaier AH, Müller-Esterl W. Mapping the cell binding site on high molecular weight kininogen domain 5. J Biol Chem 1995; 270:19256–19261.
76. Pabinger I, Schneider B. Thrombotic risk in hereditary antithrombin III, protein C, or protein S deficiency—a cooperative, retrospective study. Arterioscler Thromb Vasc Biol 1996; 16:742–748.
77. Miletich JP. Endothelial cell-mediated inhibition of procoagulant proteins. Coronary Artery Dis 1991; 2:141–145.
78. Esmon CT. The protein C anticoagulant pathway. Arterioscler Thromb 1992; 12:135–145.
79. Walker FJ, Fay PJ. Regulation of blood coagulation by the protein C system. FASEB J 1992; 6: 2561–2567.
80. Dahlbäck B. The protein C anticoagulant system: Inherited defects as basis for venous thrombosis. Thromb Res 1995; 77:1–43.
81. España F, Berrettini M, Griffin JH. Purification and characterization of plasma protein C inhibitor. Thromb Res 1989; 55:369–384.
82. España F, Griffin JH. Determination of functional and antigenic protein C inhibitor and its complexes with activated protein C in plasma by ELISA's. Thromb Res 1989; 55:671–682.
83. Abildgaard U. Tissue factor pathway inhibitor and heparin. Adv Exp Med Biol 1992; 313:199–204.
84. Jesty J, Wun T-C, Lorenz A. Kinetics of the inhibition of factor Xa and the tissue factor-factor VIIa complex by the tissue factor pathway inhibitor in the presence and absence of heparin. Biochemistry 1994; 33:12686–12694.
85. Enjyoji K, Emi M, Mukai T, et al. Human tissue factor pathway inhibitor (TFPI) gene: complete genomic structure and localization on the genetic map of chromosome 2q. Genomics 1993; 17: 423–428.
86. Petitou M, Lormeau J-C, Choay J. A new synthetic pentasaccharide with increased anti-factor Xa activity: possible role for anionic clusters in the interaction of heparin and antithrombin III. Semin Thromb Hemost 1991; 17(suppl)2:143–146.
87. Hamano S, Nishiyama M, Kikuchi S, et al. Study of low molecular weigth heparin effect on the relation between anticoagulant activity and antithrombin III affinity. Thromb Res 1992; 66: 299–307.
88. Kim YS, Linhardt RJ. Structural features of heparin and their effect on heparin cofactor II mediated inhibition of thrombin. Thromb Res 1989; 53:55–71.
89. Tollefsen DM, Maimone MM, McGuire EA, Peacock ME. Heparin cofactor II activation by dermatan sulfate. Ann NY Acad Sci 1989; 556:116–122.
90. Stuss D, Storck J, Zimmermann RE. The inhibition of thrombin and chymotrypsin by heparin-cofactor II. Thromb Res 1992; 68:45–56.
91. Brister SJ, Ofosu FA, Heigenhauser GJF, Gianese F, Buchanan MR. Is heparin the ideal anticoagulant for cardiopulmonary bypass? Dermatan sulphate may be an alternate choice. Thromb Haemost 1994; 71:468–473.
92. Mayer M. Biochemical and biological aspects of the plasminogen activation system. Clin Biochem 1990; 23:197–211.

93. Henkin J, Marcotte P, Yang H. The plasminogen-plasmin system. Prog Cardiovasc Dis 1991; 34: 135–164.
94. Thompson WD, Stirk CM, Melvin WT, Smith EB. Plasmin, fibrin degradation and angiogenesis. Nature Med 1996; 2:493.
95. Gao S, Morser J, McLean K, Shuman MA. Differential effect of platelets on plasminogen activation by tissue plasminogen activator, urokinase, and streptokinase. Thromb Res 1990; 58:421–433.
96. Wu H-L, Chang B-I, Wu D-H, et al. Interaction of plasminogen and fibrin in plasminogen activation. J Biol Chem 1990; 265:19658–19664.
97. Lijnen HR, Bachmann F, Collen D, et al. Mechanisms of plasminogen activation. J Intern Med 1994; 236:415–424.
98. Fox D, Ouriel K, Green RM, Stoughton J, Riggs P, Cimino C. Thrombolysis with prourokinase versus urokinase: an in vitro comparison. J Vasc Surg 1996; 23:657–666.
99. Williams EC. Plasma α_2-antiplasmin activity. Role in the evaluation and management of fibrinolytic states and other bleeding disorders. Arch Intern Med 1989; 149:1769–1772.
100. Declerck PJ, Lijnen HR, Verstreken M, Collen D. Role of α_2-antiplasmin in fibrin-specific clot lysis with single-chain urokinase-type plasminogen activator in human plasma. Thromb Haemost 1991; 65:394–398.
101. Robbie LA, Booth NA, Croll AM, Bennett B. The roles of α_2-antiplasmin and plasminogen activator inhibitor 1 (PAI-1) in the inhibitiion of clot lysis. Thromb Haemost 1993; 70:301–306.
102. Anonick PK, Gonias SL. Soluble fibrin preparations inhibit the reaction of plasmin with α_2-macroglobulin. Comparison with α_2-antiplasmin and leupeptin. Biochem J 1991; 275:53–59.
103. Booth NA, Simpson AJ, Croll A, Bennett B, MacGregor IR. Plasminogen activator inhibitor (PAI-1) in plasma and platelets. Br J Haematol 1988; 70:327–333.
104. Lindahl TL, Sigudardottir O, Wiman B. Stabiltiy of plasminogen activator inhibitor 1 (PAI-1). Thromb Haemost 1989; 62:748–751.
105. Lecander I, Martinsson G, Casslén B, Andreasen PA, Åstedt B. Occurrence of the specific plasminogen activator inhibitor of placemtal type, PAI-2 in ascitic fluid and tumour vessel blood from patients with ovarian carcinoma. Fibrinolysis 1990; 4:221–224.
106. Huisman LGM, Van Griensven JMT, Kluft C. On the role of C1-inhibitor as inhibitor of tissue-type plasminogen activator in human plasma. Thromb Haemost 1995; 73:466–471.
107. Collen D, Van Hoef B, Schlott B, Hartmann M, Gührs K-H, Lijnen HR. Mechanisms of activation of mammalian plasma fibrinolytic systems with streptokinase and with recombinant staphylokinase. Eur J Biochem 1993; 216:307–314.
108. Takahashi H, Tatawaki W, Wada K, Hanano M, Shibata A. Thrombin vs. plasmin generation in disseminated intravascular coagulation associated with various underlying disorders. Am J Hematol 1990; 33:90–95.
109. Kario K, Matsuo T, Kodama K, Matsuo M, Yamamoto K, Kobayashi H. Imbalance between thrombin and plasmin activity in disseminated intravascular coagulation. Assessment by the thrombin-antithrombin-III complex/plasmin-alpha-2-antiplasmin complex ratio. Haemostasis 1992; 22: 179–186.
110. Vicic WJ, Ratnoff OD, Saito H, Goldsmith GH. Platelets and surface-mediated clotting activity. Br J Haematol 1979; 43:91–98.
111. Rawala-Sheikh R, Ahmad SS, Ashby B, Walsh PN. Kinetics of coagulation factor X activation by platelet-bound factor IXa. Biochemistry 1990; 29:2606–2611.
112. Zucker MB, Katz IR. Platelet factor 4: production, structure, and physiologic and immunologic action. Proc Soc Exp Biol Med 1991; 198:693–702.
113. Zwaal RFA, Comfurius P, Bevers EM. Platelet procoagulant activity and microvesicle formation. Its putative role in hemostasis and thrombosis. Biochim Biophys Acta Mol Basis Dis 1992; 1180:1–8.
114. Moorehead MT, Westengard JC, Bull BS. Platelet involvement in the activated coagulation time of heparinized blood. Anesth Analg 1984; 63:394–398.

115. Murray JC, Kelly MA, Gorelick PB. Ticlopidine: a new antiplatelet agent for the secondary prevention of stroke. Clin Neuropharmacol 1994; 17:23–31.
116. Rajah SM, Nair U, Rees M, et al. Effects of antiplatelet therapy with indobufen or aspirin-dipyridamole on graft patency one year after coronary artery bypass grafting. J Thorac Cardiovasc Surg 1994; 107:1146–1153.
117. Frishman WH, Burns B, Atac B, Alturk N, Altajar B, Lerrick K. Novel antiplatelet therapies for treatment of patients with ischemic heart disease: inhibitors of the platelet glycoprotein IIb/IIIa integrin receptor. Am Heart J 1995; 130:877–892.
118. Gregory SA, Morrissey JH, Edgington TS. Regulation of tissue factor gene expression in the monocyte procoagulant response to endotoxin. Mol Cell Biol 1989; 9:2752–2755.
119. Jude B, Susen S, Flan B, et al. Detection of monocyte tissue factor after endotoxin stimulation: comparison of one functional and three immunological methods. Thromb Res 1995; 79:65–72.
120. Gear ARL, Raha S. Calcium signalling and phosphoinositide metabolism in platelets: subsecond events revealed by quenched-flow techniques. Adv Exp Med Biol 1993; 344:57–67.
121. Yamamoto C, Kaji T, Sakamoto M, Kozuka H, Koizumi F. Calcium regulation of tissue plasminogen activator and plasminogen activator inhibitor-1 release from cultured human vascular endothelial cells. Thromb Res 1994; 74:163–168.
122. Baugh RF, Hougie C. Structure and function in blood coagulation. In: Poller L, ed. Recent Advances in Blood Coagulation. Edinburgh, London, Melbourne, New York: Churchill Livingston, 1981:81–107.
123. Davie EW, Fujikawa K, Kisiel W. The coagulation cascade: initiation, maintenance, and regulation. Biochemistry 1991; 30:10363–10370.
124. Bertina RM. Factor V Leiden and other coagulation factor mutations affecting thrombotic risk. Clin Chem 1997; 43:1678–1683.
125. Schuster KL, Jentschura D. Activated protein C resistance: the commonest hereditary hypercoagulation disorder. Br J Surg 1997; 84:1633–1635.
126. Zöller B, De Frutos PG, Hillarp A, Dahlbäck B. Thrombophilia as a multigenic disease. Haematologica 1999; 84:59–70.
127. Giesen PL, Rauch U, Bohrmann B, Kling D, Roque M, Fallon JJ, Badimon JJ, Himber J, Reiderer MA, Nemerson Y. Blood-borne tissue factor: Another view of thrombosis. Proc. Natl. Acad. Sci. USA 1999; 96:2311–2315.
128. Pyrzdial EL, Lavigne N, Dupuis N, Kessler GE. Plasmin converts factor X from coagulation zymogen to fibrinolysis cofactor. J Biol Chem 1999; 274:8500–8505.
129. Pokhilko AV, Ataullakhanov FI. Contact activation of blood coagulation: Trigger properties and hysteresis—Kinetic recognition of foreign surfaces upon contact activation of blood coagulation: A hypothesis. J Theor Biol 1998; 191:213–219.
130. Schmaier AH. Contact activation: A revision. Thromb Haemost 1997; 78:101–107.
131. Wolberg AS, Stafford DW, Erie DA. Human factor IX binds to specific sites on the collagenous domain of collagen IV. J Biol Chem 1997; 272:16717–16720.
132. Oliver JA, Monroe DM, Roberts HR, Hoffman M. Thrombin activates factor XI on activated platelets in the absence of factor XII. Arterioscler Thromb Vasc Biol 1999; 19:170–177.
133. Bajzar L, Morser J, Nesheim M. TAFI, or plasma procarboxypeptidase B, couples the coagulation and fibrinolytic cascades through the thrombin-thrombomodulin complex. J Biol Chem 1996; 271: 16603–16608.
134. Monroe DM, Hoffman M, Oliver JA, Roberts HR. A possible mechanism of action of activated factor VII independent of tissue factor. Blood Coagul Fibrinolysis 1998; 9:S15–S20.

25

Laboratory Instrumentation, Reagents, Methods, and Patient Sample as Variables in Coagulation

James W. Cook and William A. Rock, Jr.
University of Mississippi Medical Center, Jackson, Mississippi

I. INTRODUCTION

The ultimate function of any reportable test in coagulation is to reflect the actual value of the parameter under investigation in meaningful and useful terms. This pathway, from specimen to final result, is fraught with many pitfalls; for the unwary, it can potentially produce results that are catastrophic and even life threatening.

Measurement in the coagulation laboratory is a multiparameter cornucopia of end points. The end points of the past were often functional and intensely driven by the operator's skill (tilt tube visual end point, bleeding time, etc.). Likewise, reference ranges reflected these variables. The body of interpretive knowledge reflected these numbers and dependency on the human element. A laboratory technician who could consistently perform that important coagulation test was revered and had a unique place in the coagulation laboratories armormentarium. We have all heard that "if Tech 'A' didn't perform that test, I don't believe the results." This reflects a dependency on one person's lab skills and a physician's body of knowledge and experience developed over the years.

With electronics and automation, an unreasonable reliance on the implied accuracy of instrumentation emerged which made the result the "truth" without an understanding as to how that value was achieved. In this chapter we discuss the variability of coagulation testing with a majority of the current instrumentation. This approach will help the reader analyze an electronic and automated system with an eye for what can go wrong. We anticipate that the reader will then be able to ask the right questions when reviewing the results, to assure the best interpretation.

A mathematical model employing the systems concept is developed. Preanalytic variables, analytic variables, and postanalytic variables will be defined, and the system will be analyzed to show the complex interrelationships among these system parameters. Next, instrumentation methodologies will be discussed based on whether or not the system activates the coagulation cascade. Preanalytic, analytic, and postanalytic specimen flow patterns for specific instruments will be developed, employing the model, from which potential sources of error will be defined. The effects of these errors on the final, postanalytic results will then be discussed, and troubleshooting tables will be presented.

II. THE SYSTEMS APPROACH

Any measurement system is a complex set of interrelationships involving the human equation, physical, biologic, immunologic, and biochemical processes, and the interaction of these set members with advanced instrumentation techniques. Within the confines of monitoring the parameters of a physical phenomenon, it is the goal of the measurement system to:

1. Probe the event in an unobtrusive manner as possible
2. Store and deliver this test information to an instrument designed to produce results in a useful and acceptable manner
3. Interpret the results.

Although these are ideal goals to pursue, they are for all practical purposes impossible to attain. As an example, consider the problem of measuring the field strength of a radiated electromagnetic wave. We first must design a probe which will have minimal effect on the distribution of the electric and magnetic fields. The output of this probe must then be transported to the measuring instrumentation with minimal alteration. The measurement technique, with specified sensitivity and selectivity, then operates on the received signal to produce a result which is meaningful to the interpreter. By the time the result is finalized and ready for reporting, it has been altered by the process just described, and the result, no longer exact, represents trade-offs among many variables. Furthermore, without precise knowledge of other variables such as radiation source characteristics, distance from the source, possible interfering radiation, weather conditions, etc., interpretations may be difficult if not impossible.

The same tenets hold for the measurement of biologic analytes. When drawing a blood sample, one must be as unobtrusive as possible. The sample must be collected and stored in a proper and timely fashion with the goal of altering the sample as little as possible. The measurement methodology must meet specifications set by the laboratory. The reagents must be stable. The system errors must be defined, and results must be interpreted within the confines of the clinical history and physical findings.

Within any measurement system, three basic phases of the measurement may be defined:

1. The preanalytic phase consists of those factors which act on the parameter to be measured prior to the time the parameter reaches the measuring instrumentation.
2. The analytic phase represents the measurement of the parameter.
3. The postanalytic phase includes interpretation of the results within the confines of other known factors which may have a bearing on the final outcome.

A diagram of such a system is shown in Fig. 1. A coagulation measurement system must also include these basic components, which can be further broken down into many subsystems. The preanalytic subsystem components consists of:

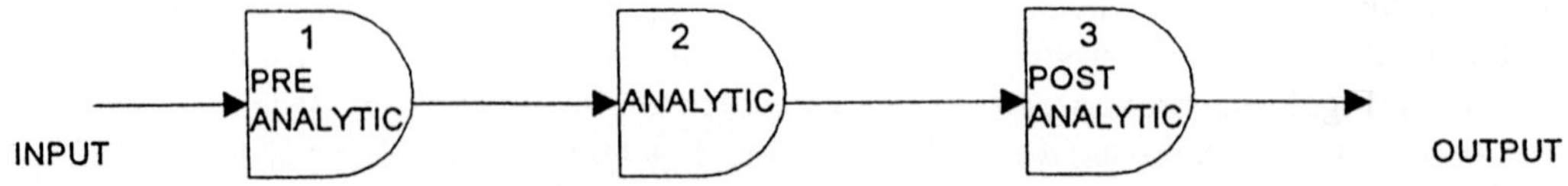

Figure 1 Basic components of a measurement system.

1. The steady-state condition of the patient
2. The process involving the collection, transport, and storage of the sample
3. The instantaneous condition of the patient

The analytic subsystem components include:

4. The measurement methodology (immunologic, biochemical) and the instrumentation

The postanalytic phase subsystem components include:

5. Result interpretation

Many variables, both defined and undefined, known and unknown, will affect each subsystem component. For example, the steady-state condition of the patient will be affected by long-term factors such as age, sex, race, lifestyle, and heredity. The instantaneous condition of the patient is affected by short-term factors which cumulatively determine the current state of health of the patient and might include recent diet, emotional stress, acute illness, medications, current medical history and physical findings, etc. The collection, transport, and storage of the sample are biased by factors which could change the final result. These factors cumulatively make up a portion of the preanalytic variables. The preanalytic variables affecting the final result also include the skill and emotional state of the technician, the proper mixing of the collected specimen with the appropriate additive in the correct amount, the elapsed time between collection and storage, and the storage of the sample. The analytic variables are those which affect the final result by influencing the instrumentation results directly, and include system error, system noise, and the reagents utilized. Among the variables affecting the final results are the experience of the interpreter, the emotional state of the investigator, and unknown and undefined factors.

III. DEVELOPMENT OF THE COAGULATION TEST RESULT MODEL FOR VARIABILITY

The construction of the model is subject to the following assumptions:

1. The multiple variables affecting each subsystem component have an additive (or subtractive) effect on the expected outcome.
2. The output of each subsystem has a definite effect on the following sub system.
3. There are undefined and unknown variables which can affect the outcome of each subsystem component. These factors will be represented by a gain function which is assumed to be linear.

The model for a coagulation measurement system is shown in Fig. 2. Vertical lines separate the different phases of the measurement system. The subsystem components are identified by the gain functions A1 through A5. The input variables are identified by E1 through E17. The output of each subsystem component is identified by Eo1 through Eo5.

From Fig. 2, the preanalytic factors are represented by

1. Component 1—the steady-state condition of the patient with gain function A1. The input variables to component 1 include

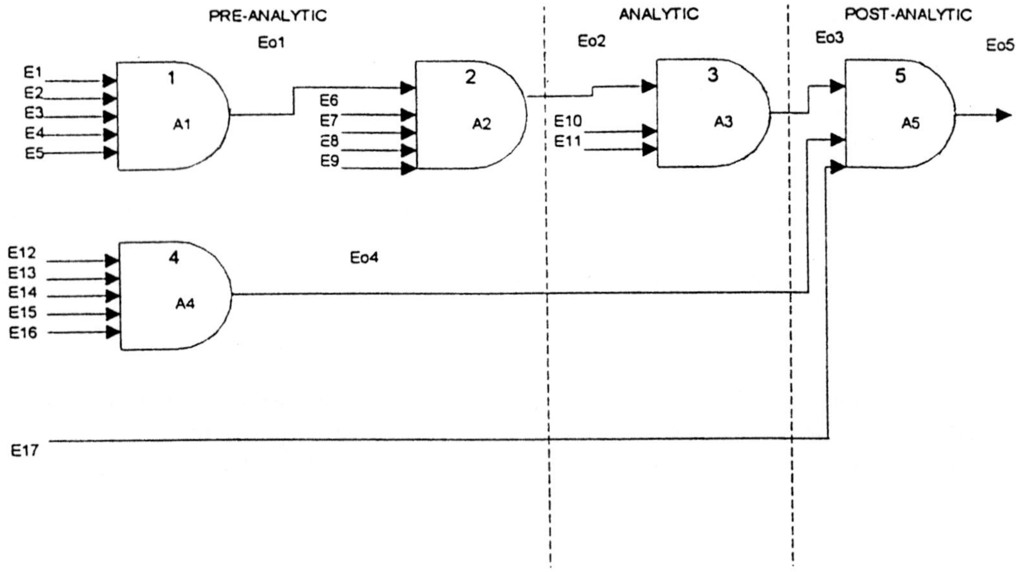

THE SYSTEM PARAMETERS ARE DEFINED AS FOLLOWS:

COMPONENT DEFINITION.

A1 is the "gain" of component 1, "THE STEADY-STATE CONDITION OF THE PATIENT".
A2 is the "gain" of component 2, "SAMPLE COLLECTION, STORAGE, AND TRANSPORT".
A3 is the "gain" of component 3, "INSTRUMENTATION METHODOLOGY".
A4 is the "gain" of component 4, "THE INSTANTANEOUS STATE OF THE PATIENT".
AND
A5 is the "gain" of component 5, "THE INTERPRETATION OF RESULTS".

VARIABLE DEFINITION

E1, E2, E3, ...En, represents variables which affect their corresponding system component.

Figure 2 Systems measurement model illustrating the complex interrelationships between reported analyte values and the corresponding independent variables.

E1 = age
E2 = sex
E3 = lifestyle
E4 = race
E5 = heredity

The gain function A1 represents events which are random or unexpected variables which could affect the outcome of the final result by influencing the output of component 1.

2. Component 4—the instantaneous state of health of the patient with gain function A4. The input variables to component 2 include

E12 = recent diet
E13 = emotional stress
E14 = acute illness
E15 = medications
E16 = current medical history and physical examination findings

The gain A4 represents unrecognized factors which can affect the instantaneous state of health of the patient, such as diurnal rhythms, menstrual cycle irregularities, etc.

3. Component 2—sample collection, storage, and transport of the specimen with gain A2. The variables affecting this subsystem component are, to name a few,

E6 = the skill and emotional state of the technician
E7 = proper mixing of the collected specimen with the appropriate additive in the correct amount
E8 = elapsed time between collection and storage
E9 = collection storage

The gain A2 could include inadvertent stimulation of the clotting system with small-bore needles and expired collection tubes.

From Fig. 2, the analytic phase (the actual instrumentation used) is represented by component 3 with gain function A3. The variables affecting the analytic phase include

E10 = reagents and biologic method used
E11 = instrument sensitivity and selectivity

The gain function a3 could include random failures, system noise, and bias.

The postanalytic phase is shown in component 5, the interpreted results. The input variables could include

E17 = the skill of the interpreter

IV. MODEL ANALYSIS

From Fig. 2, the output of component 1, at node 1, is

$$\mathrm{Eo1} = \mathrm{A1V1} \tag{1}$$

where A1 is the "gain" of component 1, and V1 is the summation of all input variables affecting the output of component 1, that is,

$$\mathrm{V1} = \mathrm{E1} + \mathrm{E2} + \mathrm{E3} + \mathrm{E4} + \mathrm{E5}$$

The output of component 2, at node 2, is

$$\begin{aligned}\mathrm{Eo2} &= \mathrm{A2(Eo1 + V2)}\\ &= \mathrm{A2(A1V1 + V2)}\end{aligned}$$

$$= A2[A1(E1 + E2 + E3 + E4 + E5) + E6 + E7 + E8 + E9]$$
$$= A1A2(E1 + E2 + E3 + E4 + E5) + A2(E6 + E7 + E8 + E9) \quad (2)$$

Likewise, the output at node 5, Eo5 (the final interpreted result), is

$$Eo5 = A1A2A3A5(E1 + E2 + E3 + E4 + E5) + A2A3A5(E6 + E7 + E8 + E9) + A3A5(E10 + E11) + A4A5(E12 + E13 + E14 + E15 + E16) + A5(E17) \quad (3)$$

As is readily apparent from Eq. (3), the final interpreted result is a complex expression reflecting the possible magnification of errors induced by both defined and undefined variables within the general measurement system. The expression could be nonlinear and represented by a polynomial whose order is determined by the number of defined components, variables, and whether or not they are nonlinear. Note that there are five terms in the output expression, one for each system component. Note also that the expression predicts that the final result is dependent on the multiple gain functions of the model, and those variables modifying the output of the various components are themselves modified by gains of the other system components. For example, the first term in the output expression consists of the summation of the variables affecting the "steady-state" condition of the patient multiplied by the "gain" A5 (as well as A1, A2, A3, A4). This in effect says that the interpretation (A5) has an effect on the output of the "steady-state" condition of the patient. Indeed, if the results of the test are abnormal, the interpreter could review the chart again and make a decision which could change the "steady-state" amplifier output—In essence, a type of feedback.

If a measurement system were modeled as above, a sample flow chart could be developed for each instrumentation methodology. The various decision points could be defined and they could represent sources of error to be investigated. Also, their effects on the final result could be predicted.

V. INSTRUMENTATION METHODOLOGIES

During the first half of this century, laboratory assessment of the coagulative properties of blood consisted largely of the evaluation of patient bleeding times, whole-blood clotting time, and later the prothrombin time (PT) as well as the activated partial thromboplastin time (APTT). During this time period, the methods employed were labor intensive and the technicians utilized visual end points of clot formation in an attempt to describe the coagulation process. Needless to say, results varied between laboratories and between technicians. The first breakthrough in standardizing the detection of the coagulation end point came in the 1950s and 1960s, when BBL, a division of the Becton and Dickinson Company automated the manual wire loop method of determining the critical clotting end point with the development of the fibrometer. This instrument, still found in many laboratories today, utilizes an electromechanical technique to detect formation of the first fibrin strand and hence establish an objective end point for clot formation.

In the 1960s and 1970s, as a result of research spin-offs from America's effort to land a man on the moon, tremendous advances occurred in electronic computers and instrumentation technologies. During this same time period, an information explosion was also taking place within the biologic sciences. With the advent of more advanced electronics allowing sophisticated measurement techniques and the rapid advancement of our knowledge of the coagulation process, automated instrumentation has been developed to perform the many tests in the armamentarium of the coagulation specialist.

The instruments which are commercially available today utilize various physical and biochemical techniques to quantitate the spectrum of tests required by clinicians to evaluate the dynamics of coagulation adequately. An excellent discussion outlining the properties of the various instruments utilized in present-day hemostasis laboratories can be found in Schoeff and Williams' text, *Principles of Laboratory Instrumentation* (St. Louis, Mosby: 1993). In the evaluation of the "secondary hemostatic" process, consisting of the activation of the coagulation cascade, the various tests are categorized by (a) those which depend on the detection of the clot end point and (b) those which quantitate the desired analyte directly, without activation of the clotting cascade.

VI. "SECONDARY HEMOSTASIS"—THE ACTIVATION OF THE COAGULATION CASCADE

A. Measurement of Desired Analytes Using End-Point Clot Detection

In this technique, the parameters measured include:

1. Whole-blood clotting time
2. PT
3. APTT
4. Factor assays (PT and APTT based)
5. Mixing studies

The method utilizes the electromechanical fibrometer.

The BBL fibrometer is an electromechanical instrument which samples the coagulum at a rate of 2 times per second. To perform the clot analysis, the technician must manually pipette a reagent into the fibrometer cup and incubate the reagent at 37°C for at least 4 min. Next, the cup is placed in the reaction well and the preheated patient specimen is added. At precisely the same time, a stopwatch must be started manually (unless an available option to start the timer automatically has been purchased). With the addition of the patient sample, the stainless steel probe begins to move in an elliptical pattern in the vertical plane, alternately entering and leaving the fluid of the sample. The small hook at the end of the movable probe enters the solution 2 times per second and the electrical resistance is monitored. When there is no fibrin strand and the probe is out of the solution, the resistance between the fixed and movable probes is infinite and the end point has not been detected. When the first fibrin strand is formed, an electrical circuit between the fixed and movable probes is completed, and the "out of solution" resistance is sharply decreased. This represents the "end of clot detection" point and the timer is stopped.

The specimen flow pattern is shown in Fig. 3, where each component of the block diagram represents a point of potential error. If the patient's hematocrit is not examined during the preanalytic phase, we could have an improper blood-to-anticoagulant ratio. The 9:1 ratio of blood to sodium citrate is valid only for hematocrits >25% and <50%. With higher hematocrits, plasma is proportionally less, and if one uses the normal amount of sodium citrate to anticoagulate the specimen, the calcium in the smaller amount of plasma will be reversibly bound by the "excess" citrate. After the plasma calcium is reversibly bound, excess unbound sodium

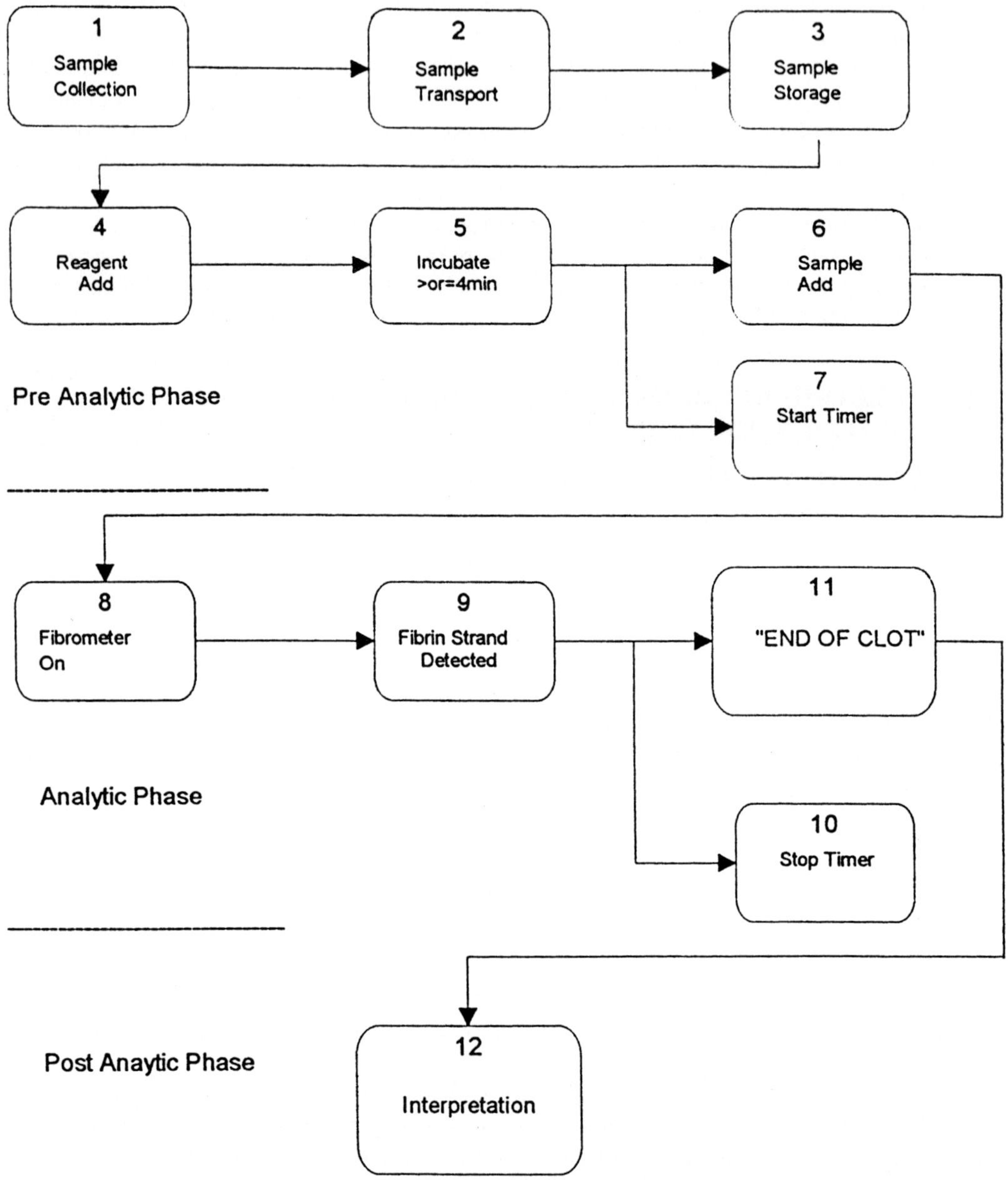

Figure 3 Sample flow pattern for the BBL fibrometer.

citrate is present. During the analytic (measurement) phase, when the "normal" amount of calcium is added to induce the clotting cascade, a portion of this calcium is bound by the unused portion of the sodium citrate and it is possible that the clotting factors do not have enough calcium to activate the clotting cascade properly. In this case, the clot end point will never be seen. During the postanalytic (interpretative) phase, the interpreter will have to report/interpret the result as a prolonged test result.

In a similar manner, if the hematocrit is too low, the corresponding portion of plasma is too large. If the "normal" amount of citrate is added to anticoagulate the specimen, it will quickly bond, leaving "excess" calcium yet to be bound and hence the coagulation cascade can still proceed to completion. We will in effect receive a specimen whose cascade has already been actived. Even if the specimen is delivered to the lab quickly and the calcium then added, the true value will be shortened. Again, the interpreter can be misled into misinterpreting a true value. The variables introduced during the preanalytic phase thus have a profound effect on both the analytic phase and the postanalytic phase.

Another preanalytic variable is improper storage of the sample, which could cause the loss of heat-labile factors V and VIII. Again the sample would fail to clot, leading to a prolonged test.

Other sources of identifiable error include:

Defective aspirators, dirty or faulty pipette tips, and faulty O-rings associated with automated systems.

Poor pipetting techniques will introduce errors relating to improper ratios for the sample + anticoagulant to the calcium added. This could lead to a prolonged end clot detection and incorrect results.

Reagent deterioration could cause a reduction in the amount of thromboplastin, partial thromboplastin, or calcium available to reactivate the sample, again resulting in a prolonged test.

The collected sample could be contaminated with heparin (drawn through heparinized lines), causing a prolonged test result.

A dirty fibrometer probe could cause an increase in electrical resistance, prolonging the end clot point detection time.

Incorrect incubation temperature, $>37°C \pm 5°C$, could destroy heat-labile factors, prolonging the time to clot detection, or not bringing the temperature to the established $>37°C \pm 5°C$, resulting in a deficient incubator temperature with decreased activation of clotting factors and a prolonged test result.

The discrepancies associated with the manual method of starting the timer at the same time the sample is added, and defective timers, will lead to timing errors.

Table 1 illustrates the possible errors associated with the fibrometer and the sample preparation technique utilized, and the effects on the various phases of the methodology.

B. Electronic Derivation of "End of Clot" Utilizing Optical Density

Instrumentation measuring the "clot end point" by monitoring the optical density of the coagulum as a function of time occupies a prominent position in today's modern coagulation laboratory. At the heart of the system is the methodology utilized to detect this phenomenon, which in the most simple terms consists of a light source and a light detector. The sample to be investigated is placed between the source and the detector, and the intensity of the electromagnetic light wave is modulated by the coagulation process as it proceeds to completion. Figure 4 represents such a system, and Figs. 5 and 6 illustrate the waveforms associated with each component.

The exponential rise in the optical density of the coagulum as a function of time, as depicted in Fig. 5, can be represented by

Table 1 Errors and Solutions for the Electromechanical "End of Clot" Instrument (Fibrometer)

Observed errors	Possible cause and solution
Prolonged test	Improper amount of anticoagulant added to sample tube—Calculate correct amount and redraw.
	Improper amount of sample or reagent added to well—Correct and rerun.
	Improper storage of sample prior to testing can result in loss of heat-labile factors—Redraw and rerun.
	A prolonged "normal" sample can be contaminated by anticoagulants during the draw—Redraw from "clean" line and rerun.
	Improper instrument temperature—Reset temperature and rerun.
	Dirty probes can increase the electrical resistance and hence increase the clotting time—Clean probes and rerun.
	Delay in starting the stopwatch—Coordinate with the addition of sample and rerun.
	Clotted sample—Redraw and rerun.
	Bent electrode—Straighten and rerun.
	Dirty pipettes—Clean and rerun.
Shortened test	Probes—See manual.
	Incorrect sample volume—Correct and rerun.
	Bubbles in sample—Correct and rerun.
	Lengthened electrodes (occurs during cleaning)—Correct and rerun.

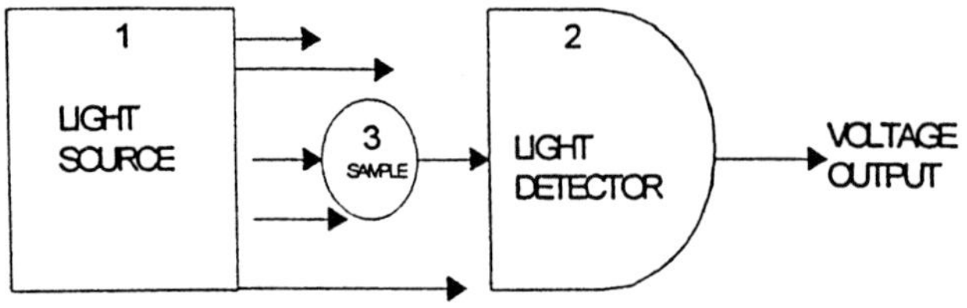

Figure 4 Basic system for detection of optical density.

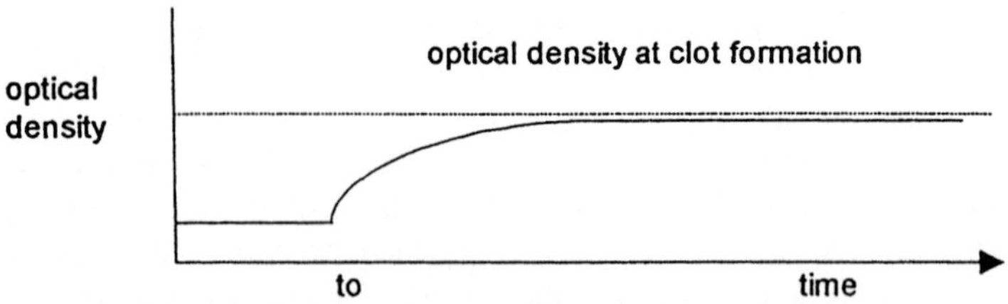

Figure 5 Optical density of clot formation as a function of time.

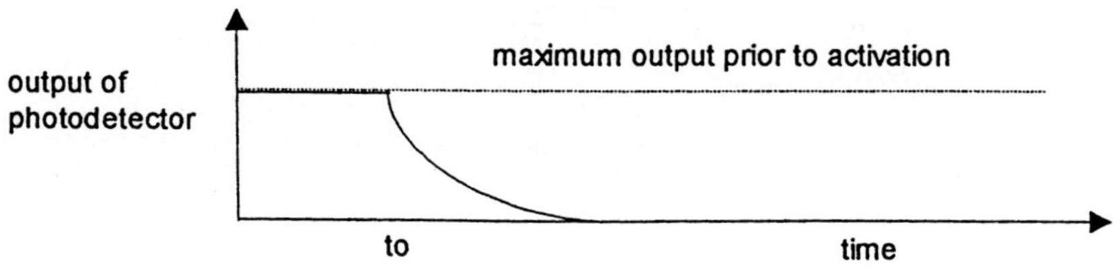

Figure 6 Voltage output of the photodetector as a function of time.

$$\mathrm{OD}(t) = \mathrm{OD}_{\max}(1 - \varepsilon^{-t/RC}) \tag{4}$$

where

OD = optical density
$\mathrm{OD}_{\max}$ = maximum optical density occurring at "end of clot"
RC = "time constant" of the coagulum
t = time

From Eq. (4) it can be seen that the rate of increase of optical density is a function of the coagulum "time constant" *RC*, and that *RC* must be a function of the entire coagulation cascade; that is, if there are factor deficiencies, the mathematical product *RC* is increased, and the amount of time required for the coagulum to reach maximum optical density is lengthened.

The actual output of the photodetector is depicted in Fig. 6. The exponential fall in the detector output can be represented by Eq. (5):

$$\mathrm{Eo}(t) = E_{\max}(\varepsilon^{-t/RC}) \text{ volts} \tag{5}$$

where

Eo = voltage output of the detector at any instant of time
$E_{\max}$ = maximum value of voltage obtained prior to activation of the coagulation cascade, where light transmission through the sample is at a maximum
RC = the same "time constant," a number associated with the integrity of the sample's coagulation system
t = time

It may be seen from Eq. (5) that if factor deficiencies are present in a sample, then again, the mathematical product *RC* is lengthened and the amount of time for the detector output to fall to zero ("clot end-point detection") is increased.

Thus, all the information required to identify the clotting end point is found in this basic detection system. One other point of interest is that this system can be modeled electronically using a simple electrical circuit as shown in Fig. 7, where the output of the resistor (Vr) corresponds to the output of the photodetector, the output of the capacitor (Vc) corresponds to the optical density, and $t = 0$ corresponds to the time at which the coagulation cascade is activated.

The Electra model 1000C, .1400,1800 manufactured by Medical Laboratory Automation, Inc. (Pleasantville, NY), is a versatile system, performing either "clot end point" assays or

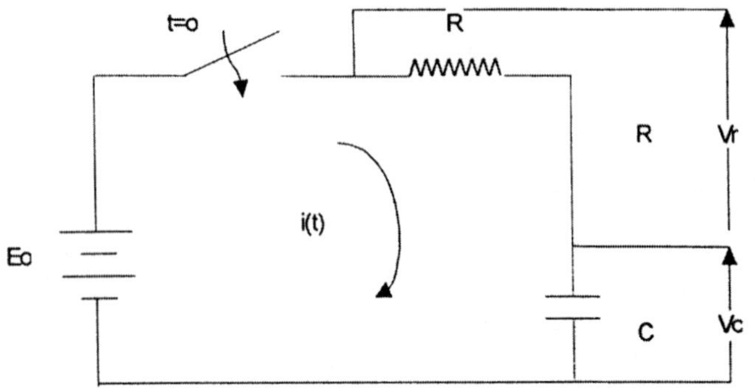

Figure 7 An electronic model for the activation of the coagulation cascade and monitoring of the optical density.

chromogenic assays. The model 1000C incorporates the above-discussed technology in determination of the "clot end point," and a complete discussion of their methodology is found in the theory of operation section of the operator's manual. The model 1000C derives the second mathematical derivative from the output of the photodetector and utilizes this pulse to determine the "end of clot point." The first derivative of the optical density represents the velocity of clot formation. The second derivative of the optical density represents the acceleration of clot formation as a result of activation of the cascade. When the amplitude of the second derivative exceeds the acceptance level, then "end of clot" is detected. These events are illustrated in Fig. 8. The timing sequence for the process is as follows:

1. The reagent is added, and this begins the timing for clot formation at time $t = t_0$.
2. The addition of the reagent creates turbulence, which could be interpreted as the clot end point. Hence a guard interval is established to prevent the detector from "seeing" this turbulence. Their guard interval is $(t_1 - t_0)$.
3. At time $t = t_1$, the detector output is enabled and the second derivative of the detector output is obtained electronically and defined as the clot detection end point.
4. The clotting time is defined as $t_2 - t_0$.

The model 1000C, in the "clot end point" mode, can determine

1. PT
2. APTT
3. Fibrinogen
4. Thrombin time
5. Factor assays
6. Protein C

and any other assay requiring clotting. To run assays, the operator:

1. Loads consumables
2. Creates a patient list
3. Inserts collection tubes containing patient samples

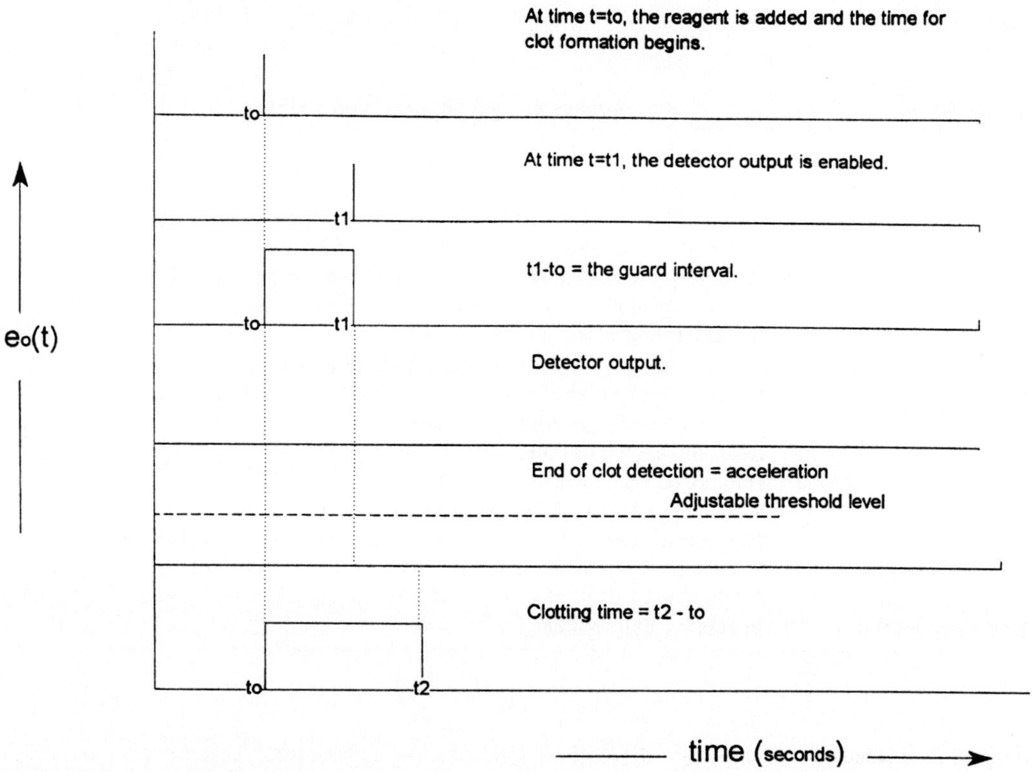

Figure 8 Timing diagram for the Medical Laboratory Automation Electra model 1000C. (Courtesy of Medical Laboratory Automation, Inc., Pleasantville, NY.)

4. Identifies samples using the bar-code reader
5. Selects tests to be run

The model 1000C than runs these tests automatically.

The patient sample flow diagram is shown in Fig. 9. The diagram shows only those variables for the analytic and postanalytic phases, as the steps for the preanalytic flow are the same as shown in Fig. 3.

Possible errors associated with the use of MLA Electra 1000C are listed in Table 2.

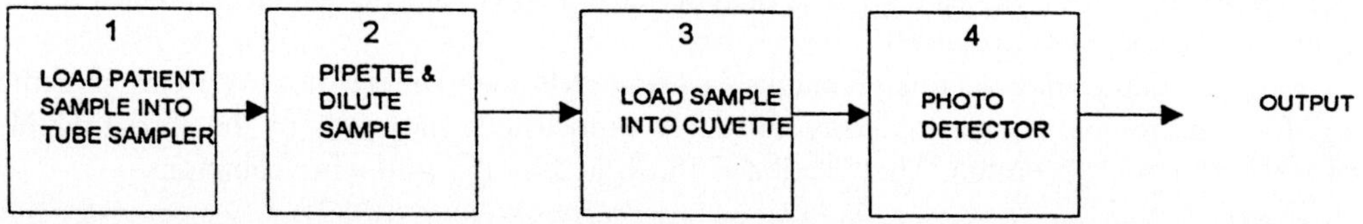

Figure 9 Schematic block diagram for the Medical Laboratory Automation Electra model 1000C.

Table 2 Errors Associated with Use of the MLA Electra Model 1000C for Clot Detection

Possible errors in the Electra 1000C	Applies to "end clot detection" mode
Prolonged clotting time	All preanalytic variables will be the same.
	The patient is anticoagulated and the "clot end point" is not reached during the instrument observation time—Must use the "long" test method.
	Bubbles present in sample (probe will sense bubbles as a liquid, move in another 0.12 in., and begin to aspirate air.)
	Incorrect fluid level.
	Lipemic sample—Must run by alternate technique.
	Signal generated by photodetector output is too weak to be detected—Bad light source, detector, etc.
	Reagents are out of date.
	Hemolized specimen.
	Very clear plasma—OD change not seen.
	Clot formed during the guard interval and therefore not detected.
Shortened clotting time	The "acceptance level" is too low and electronic noise triggers "end clot."
Poor reproducability	Flickering light source.

C. Measurement of Desired Analyte by Direct Quantitation Without Activation of the Coagulation Cascade

Desired analytes can be measured by direct quantitation, without activation of the coagulation cascade. With this technique, the following parameters can be measured:

1. Factor assays
2. Protein C
3. Plasminogen
4. Heparin
5. Antithrombin III
6. PT and APTT

The method utilizes a chromogenic assay, a technique which quantitates the amount of chromophore produced as a result of a reaction between the analyte to be measured and a synthetic substrate. In particular, a specific enzyme–substrate reaction is monitored for color produced at a particular wavelength. The quantity of unknown analyte can be derived from the amount of chromophore produced.

A typical application of this technique is Dade's (Baxter Diagnostics AG) chromogenic assay for antithrombin III. In this assay, the ATIII is measured indirectly by the partial inhibition of an excess of thrombin. The reaction is illustrated by the following equations.

$$\text{ATIII} + \text{thrombin} + \text{heparin} \rightarrow (\text{ATIII–heparin–thrombin})\ \text{complex} + \text{residual thrombin} \quad (6)$$

where ATIII is the sample to be measured, thrombin is a reagent to be added in excess in a known amount, and heparin activates the sample ATIII. The result of this chemical reaction is the ATIII–heparin–thrombin complex and residual thrombin.

The residual thrombin is now allowed to react with a synthetic substrate reagent. This substrate is a lyophilized preparation of H-D-CHG-GLY-ARG-*p*NA, corresponding to amino acid sequences representing the enzyme substrate with an attached chromophore tag, *p*-nitroaniline (*p*NA). The reaction is

$$\text{Residual thrombin} + \text{synthetic substrate} \rightarrow \text{H-D-CHG-Arg-OH} + p\text{NA} \qquad (7)$$

The *p*NA that is produced can now be measured by a spectrophotometer which operates at 405 nm, at a path length of 1.0 cm.

Figure 10 shows a configuration block diagram of the instrumentation required to perform chromogenic analysis of a sample analyte. From Fig. 10, the light source is filtered to a frequency which is predicated on the chromophore used in the measurement. This filtered light then passes through the sample and falls on the photodetector. To quantitate the sample, reagent is introduced to the sample and chromophore production begins in a manner similar to that shown in Eqs. (6) and (7). Filtered light at the predetermined frequency passes through the sample, is absorbed by the chromophore, and the optical density of the sample changes in proportion to the amount of chromophore present.

The MLA Electra 1000C utilizes the chromphore *p*-nitroaniline, which has an optical absorbance peak at 405 nm, after it is hydrolyzed. The 1000C bases results on the rate of optimal density change, rather than utilizing the quenched reaction method. During operation, light is passed through the sample at 405 nm, and the substrate reagent (containing *p*NA) is added. Reaction between the reagent substrate and the measured analyte ensues and the chromophore *p*NA is released. The optical density of the mixture now changes with the production of *p*NA. The optical density as a function of time is monitored, and the voltage output of the photodetector is described as the change in absorbance, termed "delta absorbance" by MLA. A predetermined sampling interval is defined for each analyte and during this observation time, measurements of changing optical density are taken. After the timing interval has ended, the 1000C determines the linearity of the data just gathered, and prints the results in "delta absorbance" per minute. These "delta absorbance" data are now compared to a stored reference curve for that assay, and the machine automatically calculates the percent activity of the analyte in the sample. A sample flow diagram is shown in Fig. 11 for the measurement of antithrombin III using the Dade chromogenic assay and the MLA Electra 1000C system. Once again, the steps in the procedure are identified as preanalytic, analytic, and postanalytic. Errors can occur with each step. Table 3 lists possible errors in results using the MLA Electra 1000C while operating in the chromogenic assay mode.

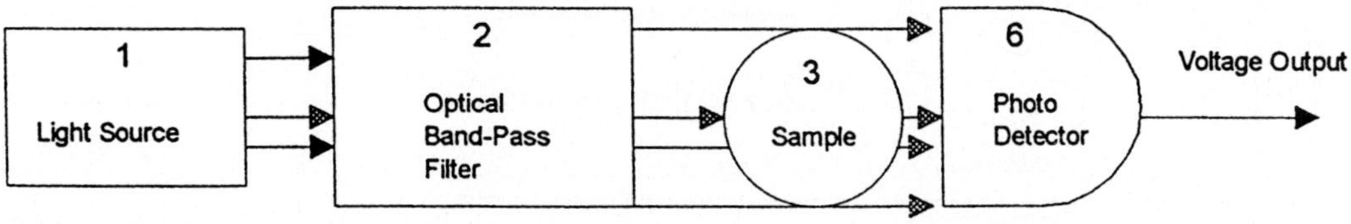

Figure 10 Block diagram for a chromogenic assay instrumentation system.

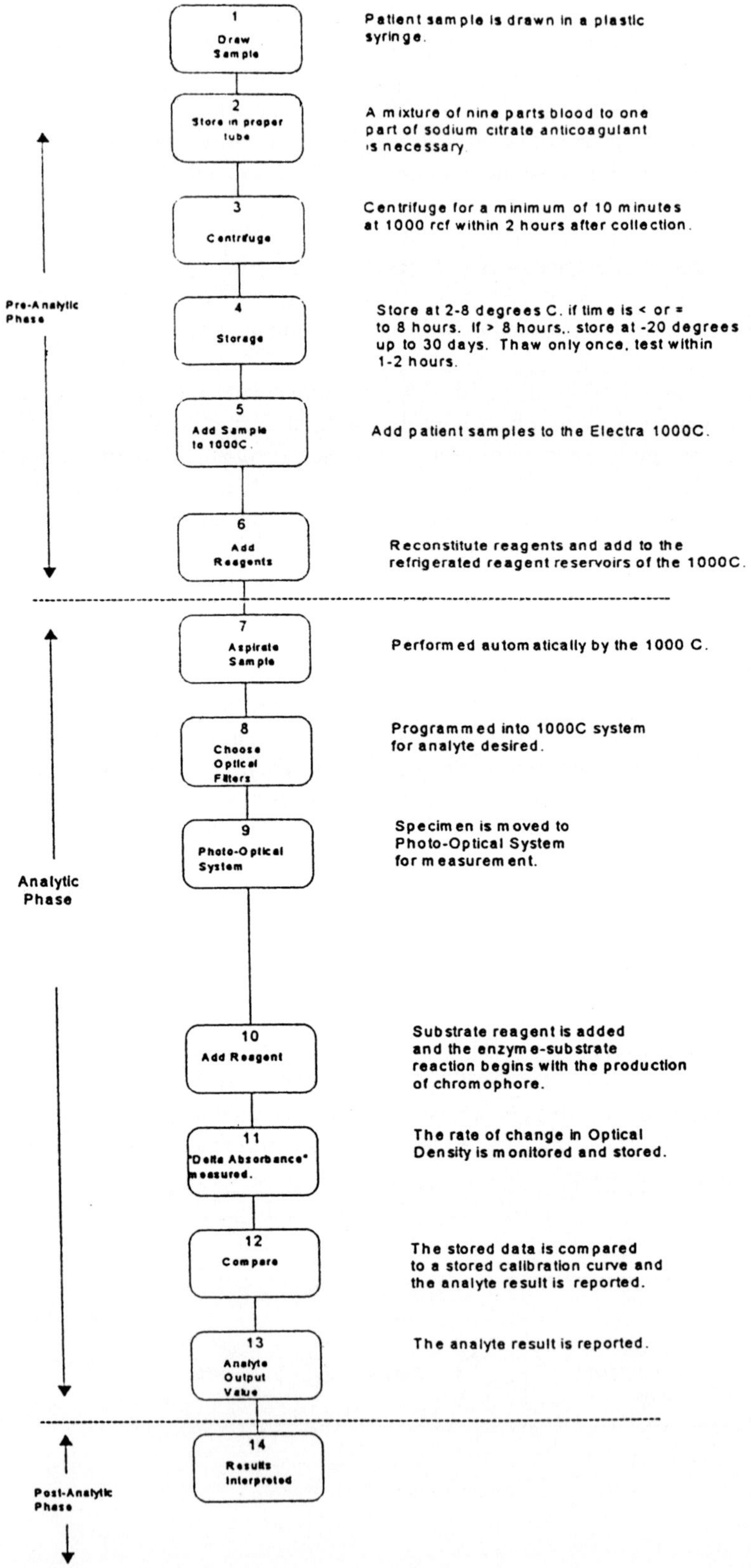
1
Draw Sample
Patient sample is drawn in a plastic syringe.
2
Store in proper tube
A mixture of nine parts blood to one part of sodium citrate anticoagulant is necessary.
3
Centrifuge
Centrifuge for a minimum of 10 minutes at 1000 rcf within 2 hours after collection.
Pre-Analytic Phase
4
Storage
Store at 2-8 degrees C. if time is < or = to 8 hours. If > 8 hours,. store at -20 degrees up to 30 days. Thaw only once, test within 1-2 hours.
5
Add Sample to 1000C.
Add patient samples to the Electra 1000C.
6
Add Reagents
Reconstitute reagents and add to the refrigerated reagent reservoirs of the 1000C.
7
Aspirate Sample
Performed automatically by the 1000 C.
8
Choose Optical Filters
Programmed into 1000C system for analyte desired.
9
Photo-Optical System
Specimen is moved to Photo-Optical System for measurement.
Analytic Phase
10
Add Reagent
Substrate reagent is added and the enzyme-substrate reaction begins with the production of chromophore.
11
"Delta Absorbance" measured.
The rate of change in Optical Density is monitored and stored.
12
Compare
The stored data is compared to a stored calibration curve and the analyte result is reported.
13
Analyte Output Value
The analyte result is reported.
14
Results Interpreted
Post-Analytic Phase

Table 3 Possible Errors Associated with the MLA Electra 1000C Using the Dade ATIII Chromogenic Assay

Possible errors in the Electra 1000C	Applies to chromogenic assay mode using Baxter's Dade ATIII chromogenic assay
Reported quantity of analyte greater than expected	Increased concentration of reagents due to evaporation—Check lid on reagents. Increased reagent concentration due to improper reconstitution. Short centrifuge time resulting in platelet-rich plasma—Could increase optical density. Increased volume of thrombin reagent pipetted into sample—Resulting in increased chromophore production. Check tubing, pipette. Improper stored calibration curve. Reagent contamination or change in lot numbers. Incorrect anticoagulant—Oxalate could precipitate under certain conditions increasing optical density. Check pH of water.
Reported quantity of analyte less than expected	Deceased reagent concentration due to decreased volume of reagent pipetted into sample—Misaimed nozzel or contaminated tubing. Increased centrifuge time can destroy factors. Improper reconstitution of reagents. Stretched or leaking tubing. Reagent contamination. Expired reagents or change in lot numbers. Check pH of water.

VII. "PRIMARY HEMOSTASIS"—FORMATION OF THE PRIMARY HEMOSTATIC PLUG

The normal hemostatic mechanism is the body's response to blood loss. Three components are necessary for adequate hemostasis: (a) vascular components, (b) platelets, and (c) soluble coagulation proteins. A primary hemostatic plug is first formed by the action of platelets; in the process, the coagulation cascade is activated, with the formation of fibrin as the end result. Evaluation of the parameters of the cascade were discussed in the previous section. Now, the primary hemostatic mechanism and associated variables are addressed.

Adequate and timely formation of the primary hemostatic plug is dependent on both the number and the functional properties of the patient's platelets. Postinjury, effective formation of the primary hemostatic plug begins when the platelets are exposed to the underlying collagen in the vascular endothelium. The platelets, through the adhesion molecules glycoprotein IA, IIA, GpIb, and von Willebrand factor (see Chapter 28 by J. L. Miller, as listed in the Bibliography) adhere to the vascular collagen. The plasma von Willebrand factor, an adhesive glycopro-

FACING PAGE

Figure 11 Patient sample flow diagram for the MLA Electra 1000C, utilizing Baxter's Dade ATIII chromogenic assay.

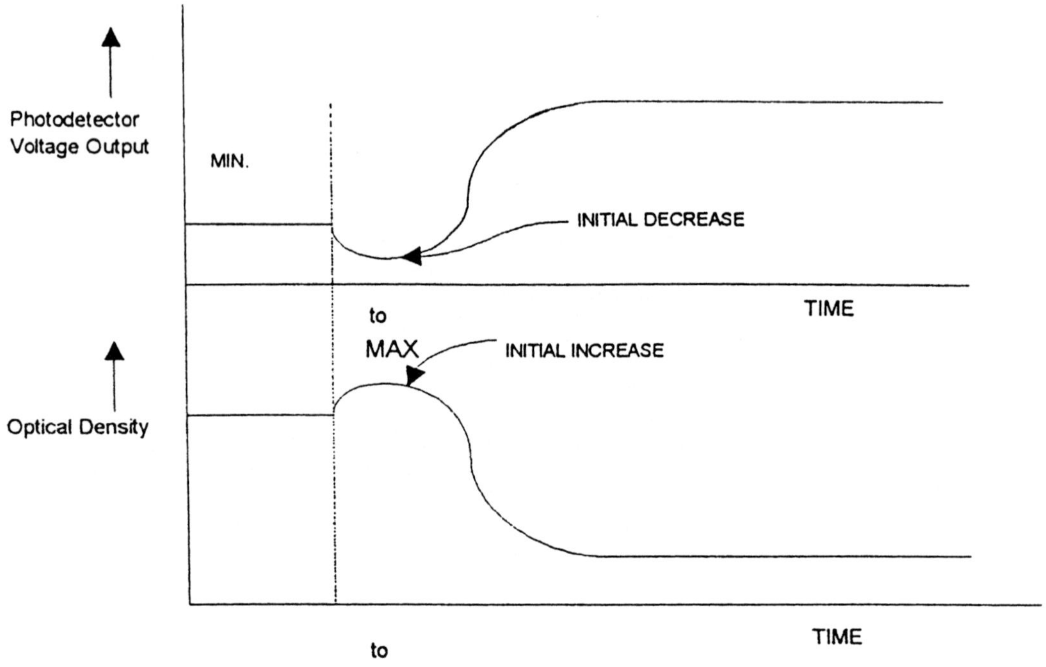

Figure 12 Platelet aggregation curve after stimulation with ADP.

tein molecule which forms a link between the platelet receptor site on glycoprotein IB and the subendothelial collagen, anchors the platelets to the collagen. After adhesion, the platelets are activated, undergo shape change, release their granules, and, through the activation of the cyclooxygenase pathway within the vascular endothelial cells, produce arachidonic acid products such as thromboxane A2 and prostacyclin PGI2. Platelet granule release is from dense granules (calcium, serotonin, and ADP) and alpha granules (among other proteins, von Willebrand factor, and platelet factor 4). Aggregation of platelets then occurs to form the primary hemostatic plug. At the same time, the coagulation cascade is activated and the clot is stabilized with the formation of fibrin. During the time interval when the clot is being formed, the fibrinolytic system is activated to dissolve the clot. It can thus be seen that in order for adequate primary hemostatis to occur, adhesion, activation, and then aggregation must occur. A delicate balance exists between the tendency to bleed and that to clot. Disorders of any of these necessary sequential steps can result in either bleeding or thrombotic tendencies.

In the laboratory evaluation of platelets, we are concerned with both platelet number and platelet functional activity. Consequently, our first indication of a possible primary hemostatic abnormality is in the Coulter counter's CBC with platelet count. If the platelet count is low, the patient may have an increased tendency to bleed. If the number is high, the trend may be toward thrombosis. If the count is normal and the patient bleeds, then we suspect a functional abnormality.

The bleeding time is a semigross measure of the function of platelets. It is highly labor intensive and fraught with opportunities for inter- and intraoperator variability. It is not indicated as a screening test for the risk of surgical bleeding. The technician must be skilled in the manner in which the test is administered; when the test is performed properly and the result

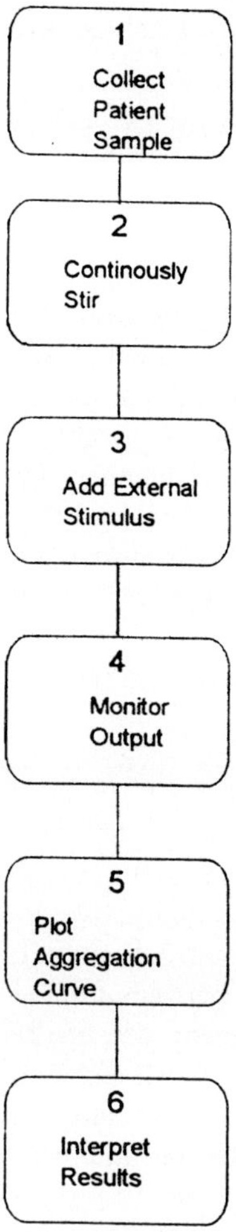

Figure 13 Patient sample flow chart for platelet aggregation.

exceeds 9–10 min, more elaborate testing methods are required to ascertain the precise etiology of the platelet functional abnormality. One of these methods is whole-blood platelet aggregation. When citrated platelet-rich plasma is continuously stirred in a platelet aggregometer and energy from a light source is passed through the coagulum, the platelet response to an external stimulus can be monitored as a change in optical density or electrical impedance. Currently, external reagents, including collagen, ADP, epinephrine, and arachidonic acid, are used to precipitate aggregation. Ristocetin causes platelet agglutination.

Some aggregometers allow the simultaneous sampling of ADP as the platelet-rich mixture is activated by an external stimulus. This dual sampling technique allows measurement of both platelet aggregation and platelet release activities.

Dade International, Incorporated, has developed new Dade PFA Reagents to aid in the detection of platelet dysfunction in citrated human whole blood. The PFA-100 instrument and test cartridge system simulates the process of platelet adhesion and aggregation in vitro. The system determines the time from the start of the test until the platelet plug covers an aperture, hence automating and standardizing the bleeding time.

A. Aggregometer Studies Utilizing Photogrammetric Techniques

A typical aggregometer setup which monitors optical density is similar to that shown in Fig. 4. The voltage output curve from the photodetector, representing platelet aggregation after stimulation by an external source, is shown in Fig. 12. The external stimulus is added at time t_0. The initial platelet change in shape from diskoid to spherical increases the optical density and decreases the light transmittance. The subsequent formation of platelet clumps decreases the optical density and increases the light transmittance, both in an exponential manner. The change in optical density is also shown in Fig. 12. If the platelets fail to adhere, release their granules, or aggregate properly, then the aggregation response is abnormal. This is reflected in a less than optimal change in optical density, and a diminished response to the external stimuli is observed.

Figure 13 outlines the patient sample flow diagram, where each node represents a possible source for error. Possible errors are shown in Table 4.

VIII. THE IMMUNOASSAY

The immunoassay is an immuno/biochemical technique utilized for the direct qualitative and quantitative determination of the chemical substance under investigation, without activation of the coagulation cascade. This technique relies on the highly specific binding between an antigen and its corresponding antibody. The reaction is monitored by the attachment of a marker substance to either the antigen or the antibody and can consist of a radioactive label, a chemophor, a flourophor, or an enzyme. Figure 14 shows various types of immunoassays and their classification based on procedural differences. A type of immunoassay of particular interest is the enzyme-linked immunosorbant assay or ELISA (sandwich) assay.

The enzyme-linked immunosorbant assay (ELISA) is a technique utilized for the determination of an analyte which exhibits high sensitivity and specificity. At the heart of the ELISA is the "solid phase," a support component whose sole function is to bind protein (either antigen or antibody) such that bound enzyme can be separated from free enzyme. Solid phases presently in use include plastic plates with wells, plastic beads, plastic test tubes, polymer coated metals, etc.

Figure 15 shows the development of the ELISA sandwich. In Fig. 15a, the solid-phase component is shown. Analyte antibody is attached to the solid phase by irreversibly absorbing or covalently binding the protein (Fig. 15b). A substance must now be added to mask the remainder of the exposed solid-phase surface (Fig. 15b). The analyte (antigen) to be measured is now added and allowed to react with the antibody to the antigen (Fig. 15c). The mixture is allowed to incubate and is then washed. In the next step (Fig. 15d), a second analytic antibody, conjugated to an enzyme, is added and allowed to react with the antigen sites. This mixture is then incubated and washed. At this point, the ab-an-ab-enzyme "sandwich" has been formed. Enzyme substrate is now added, and as it acts on the enzyme, chromophores are produced, the number of which is directly proportional to the quantity of the analyte (antigen) present in the sample. The chromophores can now be measured by electronic instrumentation.

Table 4 Possible Errors Associated with Platelet Aggregometer Studies

Possible aggregometer error	Platelet function studies
Plot shows longer time or smaller change in optical density than expected.	1. Expired reagents (external stimuli). 2. Collection problems—Check tubes. 3. Sample contaminated.
Plot shows shorter time than expected.	1. Platelets already stimulated.
Aggregation changes are altered.	1. Aggregation is less using anticoagulant solutions which excessively bind calcium. (EDTA and high-sodium citrate inhibit aggregation.) 2. Contamination of sample with RBCs can mask existing aggregation responses; abnormally depressed curves can result. 3. With low platelet counts, the secondary phase, because of its diminished slope, tends to be obscured by the primary wave of aggregation and thus appears to be absent. 4. Prolonged time interval after venipuncture produces a variable response depending on aggregating agent used. 5. Changes in pH of platelet-rich plasma have a profound effect on aggregation. No aggregation occurs below a pH of 6.4 or above a pH of 10, with maximal aggregation thought to occur at a pH of 8.0. 6. The temperature at which the sample is stored and temperature at which the sample is run has a significant effect on the rate and extent of aggregation. 7. Stir speed can have an effect on aggregation. Generally, no significant changes occur as the stir speed varies from 600 to 1200 rpm. 8. Exercise and mental stress can effect aggregation. 9. Ethanol ingestion can markedly alter both the primary and secondary aggregation curves.

In our laboratory, Asserchrom (a trademark of Diagnostica Stago, in France) provides the ELISA assay used to determine protein S and protein C. From Asserchrom product information, the solid phase consists of two strips of 16 wells each, coated with rabbit antihuman protein C or protein S f(ab′) fragments. The enzyme utilized is peroxidase, and the substrate is *ortho*-phenylenediamine (OPD). The process is partially automated by the Dynatech MR700-DIAS measurement system.

In essence, a plastic support coated with rabbit anti-human protein C antibodies captures the protein C to be measured. Then, rabbit anti-protein C antibody, coupled with peroxidase, binds to the remaining free antigenic sites of the protein C. This forms the ELISA "sandwich." The bound chromophore peroxidase (the enzyme) reacts with the substrate OPD in the presence of hydrogen peroxide. After a predetermined time, the reaction is stopped with a strong acid. The amount of color which has been produced is related to the concentration of the protein C that was present initially.

The Dynatech system is a microprocessor-controlled instrument consisting of interchangeable modules designed to wash, aspirate, incubate, dispense reagents, then measure absorbance

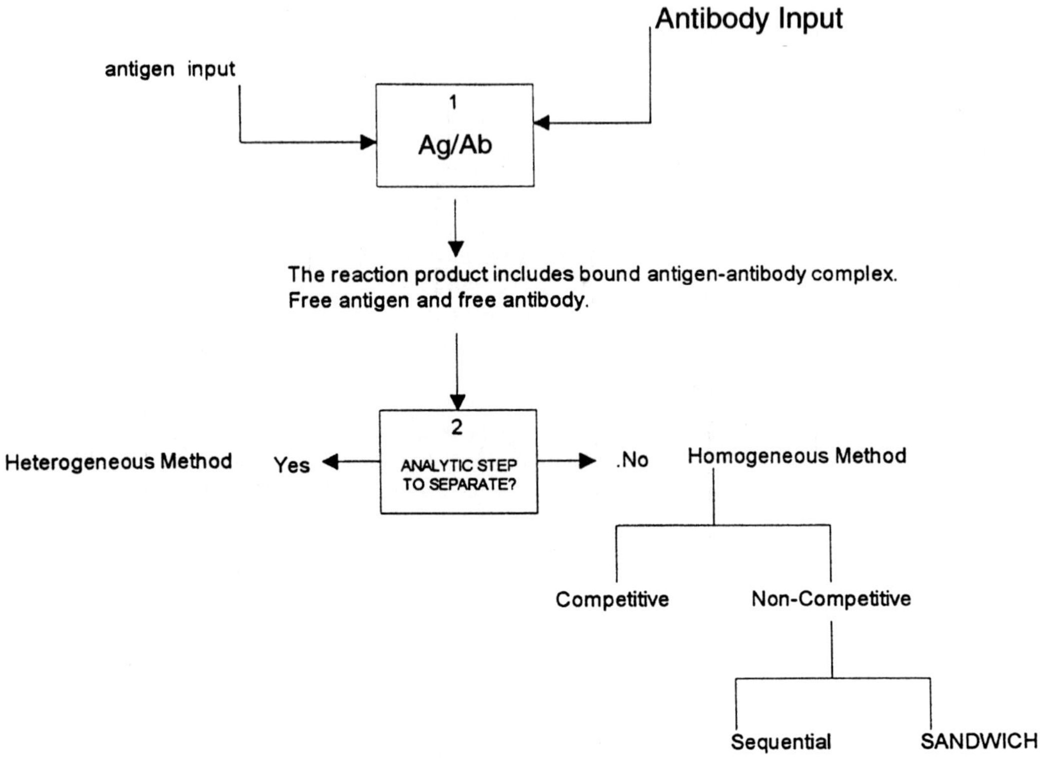

Figure 14 Immunoassay methodologies.

by the chromophore in either single or dual wavelengths. Figure 16 illustrates the steps in the movement of the patient sample through the Asserchrom-Dynatech system. Possible errors in the assay are listed in Table 5.

IX. SUMMARY

In this chapter, a generalized approach to the development of system error algorithms has been developed. A model of a measurement system was developed which defined preanalytic, analytic, and postanalytic variables, and illustrated the complex interrelationship among the variables. The expression for the model output suggested that the final result is the product of all of the considered variables. Indeed, in the real world, it is evident that errors can be compounded throughout a measurement system, and an error made in collection can modify the analytic and the postanalytic phases of any analyte determination. The hemostatic mechanism was used as the basis for discussion of the evaluation of coagulation system parameters. The "secondary hemostatic" process was discussed first. The biophysical principles underlying each measurement process was discussed, and a specific instrument was chosen to illustrate the principle involved. A patient sample flow diagram was developed for the instrument and the specific test reagent package. Potential errors were defined and listed in tables.

In the evaluation of any coagulation analyte, it is mandatory that the patient history and the present physical findings be available. Without this information, it is impossible to deter-

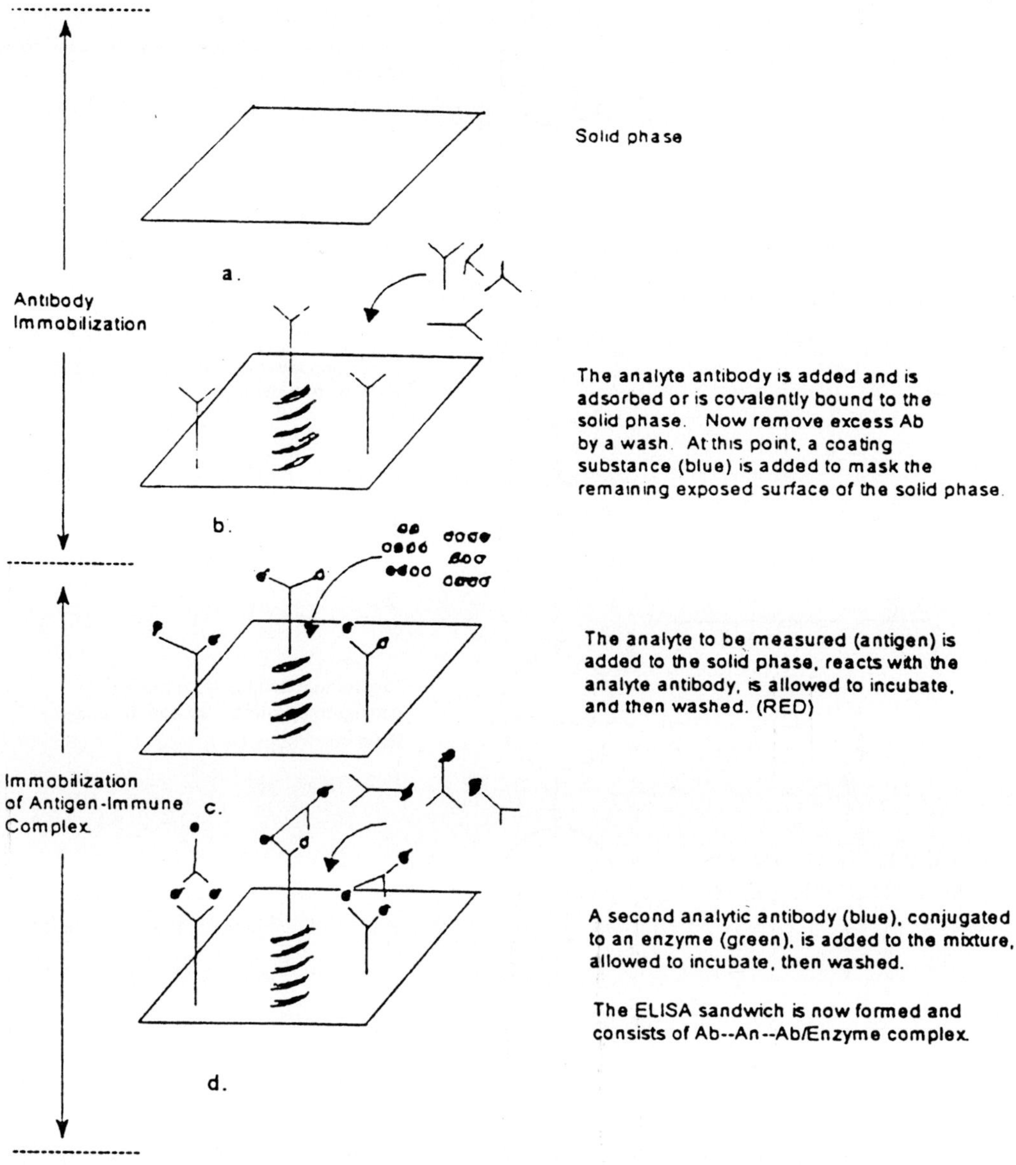

Figure 15 Development of the ELISA sandwich.

mine whether the results are acceptable. One must be aware of the limitations of the individuals collecting the samples and ensure their optimal performance with continued education. In order to interpret results correctly, the individual responsible should be intimately aware of instrument operation. For this, patient sample flow charts can be developed to help pinpoint error sources. Finally, once all of the above factors have been defined, a permanent error table can be devised and referred to as necessary. Present instruments are becoming more self-sufficient, and many produce error messages to allow the operator to be aware of pending problems.

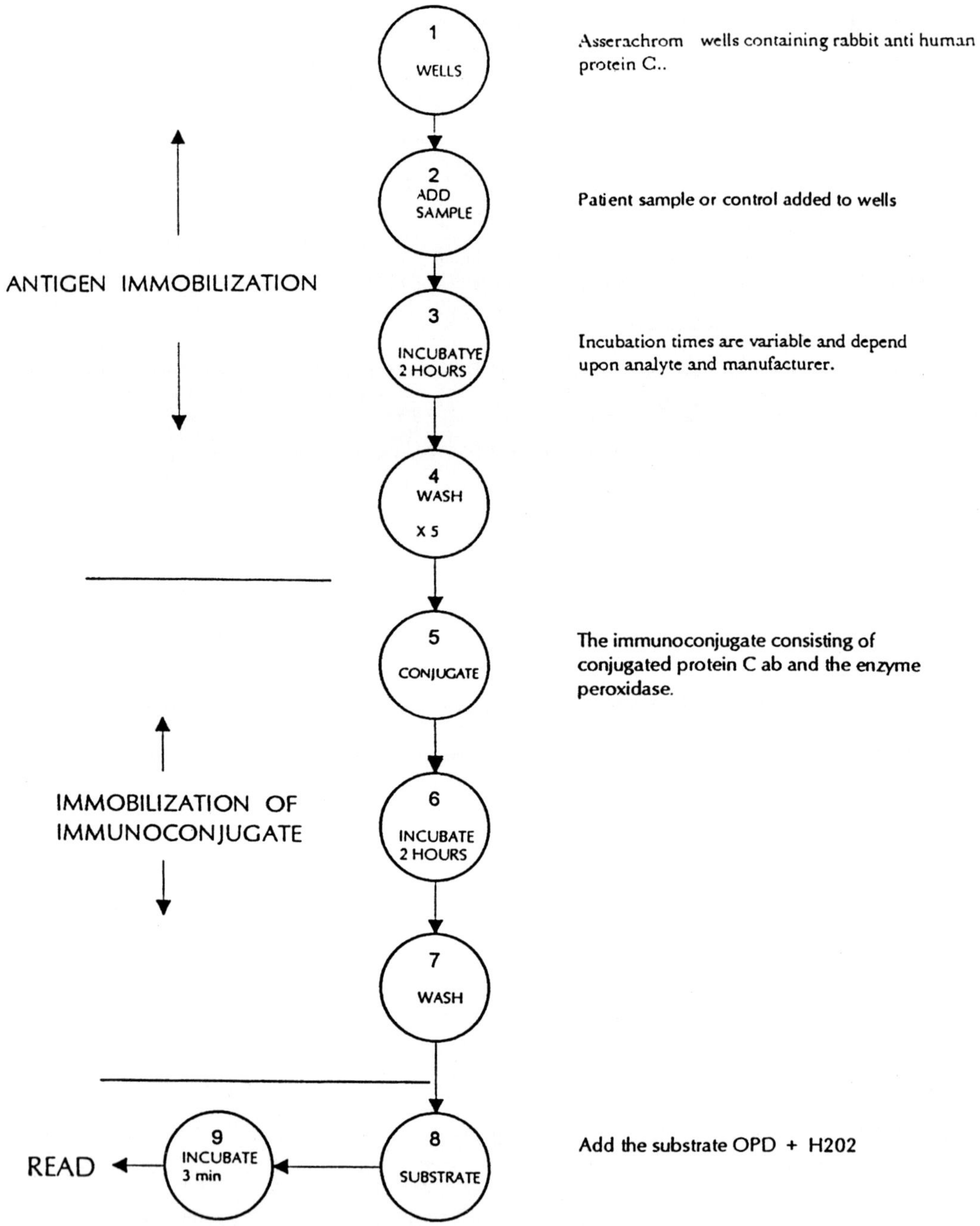

Figure 16 Patient sample flow diagram for Asserchrom ELISA assay.

Table 5 Possible Errors in Utilizing the Dynatech-Asserchrome ELISA Assay

Possible errors in the Dynatech system	Applies to the ELISA assay mode using the Asserachrom protein C assay
Reported quantities greater than expected	1. All errors reported in Table 3 apply here, since both instruments operate as spectrophotometers.
	2. Incorrect amount of reagents pipetted.
	3. Improper wash.
	4. Contaminated reagents.
Reported quantities less than expected	1. All errors reported in Table 3 apply here, since both instruments operate as spectrophotometers.
	2. Incorrect amount of reagents pipetted.
	3. Contaminated reagents.
	4. Plastic wells exposed too long to light.
	5. Expired reagents.
	6. Improperly stored reagents and wells.

However, these systems are not all inclusive, and the methodology outlined in this chapter will continue to be a primary source of error definition.

BIBLIOGRAPHY

1. Baster Diagnostics. Antithrombin III Chromogenic Assay. Deerfield, IL: Baxter Diagnostics AG, Dade, Technical Product Information, 1984.
2. Becton, Dickerson, and Company. The Fibro System Manual. BBL Division of Becton, Dickerson, and Company, 1977.
3. Diagnostica Stago. Stachrom Protein C, Colorimetric Assay. France: Diagnostica Stago, 1994.
4. Dynatech. MR700 DIAS ImmunoAssay System Operators Manual, rev. JF2/0595. Dynatech Laboratories, 1995.
5. Groner W, Simpson E. Practical Guide to Modern Hematology Analyzers. New York: Wiley, 1995.
6. Medical Laboratory Automation. MLA Electra 1000C, Automatic Coagulation Timer Operators Manual. Pleasantville, NY: Medical Laboratory Automation, Inc., 1993.
7. Miller JL. Blood platelets, blood coagulation and fibrinolysis. In: Henry JB, ed. Clinical Diagnosis and Management by Laboratory Methods. 19th ed. Philadelphia: Saunders, 1996.
8. Newhouse P, Clark C. The variability of platelet aggregation. In: Triplett DA, ed. Platelet Function. Education Products Division, American Society of Clinical Pathologists, 1978.
9. Walenga JM. Automation in hemostasis. In: Shoeff LE, Williams RH, eds. Principles of Laboratory Instruments. St. Louis, Mosby, 1993.

26

The Decision Process in the Laboratory Diagnosis and Management of Bleeding and Clotting Disorders

William A. Rock, Jr.
University of Mississippi Medical Center, Jackson, Mississippi

I. INTRODUCTION

The successful resolution of a bleeding or clotting emergency reflects the diagnostic skills of the physician, the interpretation of all available information, application of previous experience, and the actions taken to stop bleeding or prevent thrombosis. In this chapter we address those issues the physician is called upon to address in the diagnosis and management of the bleeding problem or clotting problem. These are (a) the decisions to make a diagnosis based on history, (b) the decisions to select the appropriate coagulation tests to identify or confirm the diagnosis, and (c) the decision on what will be the management of the bleeding or clotting problem. What is most challenging and difficult about decision making in bleeding or clotting is the accurate assessment of the multiple processes intrinsic to coagulation. It is the sum of these variables that affect the risk assessment for bleeding or clotting and the success or failure of management. The diagnosis is the first step and an enormous one at that.

Many approaches have been published as to the diagnosis of the cause of inappropriate bleeding or clotting (1–6). One aspect of the diagnostic process is the history of the patient, followed by the selection of laboratory tests to "construct" a diagnosis objectively. The taking of history should not be arduous, and should be succinct and to the point.

One of the more successful tools we have used in the assessment of a bleeding or clotting disorder is to ask questions, *lots of questions*. These are often questions for which there is no clear-cut answer, but the thought process humbles one immediately from both the ability to "construct" a diagnosis and to manage the disorder. The limitations of our ability to diagnose and manage a particular case will become clearer as we ask the questions. As a result we will also be motivated to think clearer, know our limitations, and better define our expectations. In the new world of limited resources, our skill development is essential to the survival of quality medicine. Asking questions, the *tough questions* has the capability of keeping us on target with our management.

In this chapter the history questions have been organized around acute versus chronic bleeding or thrombosing events. This is intended to provide a baseline from which to develop additional and perhaps more specific questions as experience with asking questions develops. Regional, ethnic, age-specific, and gender-specific questions over time will be developed for the population questioned.

II. THE DIAGNOSIS OF BLEEDING AND INAPPROPRIATE CLOTTING DISORDERS: A WORKING OUTLINE

A. Portraying the Bleeding Disorder with the Patient's History

The first natural division of this process is the status of the patient when first seen. Is this an acute bleeding problem, or a chronic bleeding problem? We begin with the chronic bleeding problem.

1. Chronic Bleeding Problem

Hospital inpatient or outpatient:
- Presenting symptoms: How long has the patient had the symptoms?
  - Incision versus mucosal bleeding versus joint bleeding?
  - Bruising; where, how frequent, what parts of the body?

When did the bleeding start in the past; this time?
Has there been a previous history of this exact kind of event; similar?
Is there a family history of this problem or a similar problem?
Describe all invasive procedures however minimal and associated bleeding if any:
- Minor lacerations, fall abrasions, kitchen knife laceration
- Minor surgery: teeth pulled, tonsils
- Pregnancy and childbirth
- Surgery: appendectomy, hysterectomy, hemorrhoidectomy, etc.
- Accidents: automobile accident, gunshot wound, other trauma
- Physiologic bleeding as in menstrual pattern, easy bruising during menses or hormone therapy, pattern of menstrual bleeding after menarche
- Blood in body fluids; urine, stool, vomitus, cough, expectoration
- List all medications, particularly those related to clotting or thrombosis:
  - Those medications taken currently
  - Those medications taken when bleeding was a problem
- Has medication been associated with bleeding or bruising in the past; blood in urine or stool?
  - What medications do you take at home for pain, headache?

Describe those illnesses the patient has now or has had in the past:
- Liver disease, hepatitis, ethanol abuse
- Renal disease
- Hypertension, heart disease, pulmonary disease, stroke
- Diabetes mellitus, peripheral vascular disease, management difficulty
- Cancer, chemotherapy, radiation therapy, surgery

Additional information is obtained with observation
- Age: relatively unlikely to have a congenital cause
- Sex: sex-linked bleeding disorders
- Socioeconomic situation: diet, nutrition, ability to purchase medications
- External scars: previous surgery, location of scars
- Teeth status: all teeth present, or some or all pulled

2. Acute Bleeding Problem

Obviously, the assessment and management sequences in the midst of an acute bleeding diathesis does not provide the time to initiate the history assessment. However, the information can be useful in the postintervention period, whether for an invasive procedure performed in a physician's office or clinic or in the operating room surgical situation.

Hospital outpatient: Determine the severity of the problem and its risk for death. As quickly as possible, proceed through the above list for chronic bleeding problems. Continued bleeding can be the result of a disease or medication known to the patient or family, but the information has to be requested.

Hospital inpatient/emergency room: From the time of trauma to the time you see the patient allows you to interpret physical findings and laboratory studies as do to acute or blood loss over several hours with fluid replacement.

With trauma, all of the above plus evidence of ongoing clots identified at wound sites and thrombosed veins or arteries equates with the ability to clot.

Absence of any clots suggests medication effects, and or the amount of blood lost with fluid replacement.

The application of these elements to the bleeding patient will direct the physician to the selection of laboratory tests. This can be difficult and expensive. The patient's complete history and the physician's experience are invaluable in making productive choices. For bleeding disorders, the list of possibilities, medications, or situations is obviously endless and so cumbersome as to be useless. However, asking questions of the patient and family from a short list of primary concerns will initiate the patient and often the family as well into thinking about past history corresponding to the questions being asked. Informed and interested patients and family can make a significant contribution in identifying possible disorders and assisting in the selection of laboratory or other tests. Many patients carry a list of their medications with them at all times.

B. Associating the Inappropriate Clotting Disorder with the Patient's History

The first natural division of this process is the initial presentation of the patient. This problem may be acute, or a clotting problem with a long history of ischemic events. We begin this outline with the chronic inappropriate clotting problem.

1. *Chronic Inappropriate Clotting Problem*

The history is directed toward ascertaining the time intervals and possible mechanisms related to activities that create a hypercoagulable state.

Hospital inpatient or outpatient

Presenting symptoms

When did the history of clotting problems start, this time?

Has there been a previous history of this exact kind of event, similar?

Is there a family history of this problem or a similar problem?

Are there any activities or procedures that preceded the event, or what were you doing the day before the event? Were you doing anything such as picking up heavy boxes, or other strenuous exercise? Were you under any stress the day before? The following events may be associated with an acute-phase type of response:

Pregnancy and childbirth

Surgical procedures: appendectomy, hysterectomy, hemorrhoidectomy, back surgery

Accidents: automobile accident, fractured femur

Emotional: family conflicts, stresses, work-related stress

Describe all medications, particularly those associated with an increased risk for thrombosis
  Those medications taken currently as well as those taken when the patient had the past event. Examples include oral birth control pills, and rebound from warfarin therapy. Was the patient on any anticoagulant medication during this episode or previous episodes?
  Has any medication been associated with clotting problems in the past?
  Describe those illnesses the patient has now or has had in the past:
    Liver disease
    Renal disease
    Hypertension, heart disease, pulmonary disease
    Diabetes mellitus
    Cancer
Occupation, sedentary, immobilization of extremities, stress

2. *Acute Inappropriate Clotting Problem*

In many instances the patient is too ill to be able to provide a history. The only history source becomes the medical record or family members. These sources should be investigated with the same intensity as with the patient. With an acute problem such as a stroke, myocardial infarction, pulmonary embolus, or sudden loss of lower leg circulation, the patient is most likely or soon to be an inpatient. Therefore there will usually be no distinction as to how these cases are initially studied.

Outpatient, hospital inpatient, or emergency room: Determine the severity of the problem and its risk for death
As quickly as possible, proceed through the above list
Additional information is obtained with observation
  Age: relatively unlikely to have a congenital cause in the elderly with no previous history, but the elderly are more likely to have acquired causes
  Sex: Hormone-related frequency of thrombotic events
  Race: Some congenital causes for thrombosis are rare or prevalent in specific racial or ethnic groups
  Obesity: morbid, endocrine etiology

The application of these historical elements to the patient will direct the laboratory investigation into a mechanism related to inappropriate blood clotting. As in the case of an investigation of bleeding disorders, the laboratory assessment can be expensive. The identification of some of the more common causes or risk factors, such as stasis, abnormal blood circulation, accelerated atherosclerosis, and/or atrial fibrillation, should be part of the patient's workup. The laboratory investigation will complement the blood flow and visualization assessment. Often an additional ingredient such as a congenital defect in coagulation regulation will be a contributor to the cause of the clot ("the second hit"), and is why the inappropriate clotting occurred.

III. ASSOCIATING THE PATIENT'S BLEEDING OR INAPPROPRIATE CLOTTING DISORDER WITH LABORATORY TESTING AND USING THE INFORMATION TO MODIFY YOUR MANAGEMENT

As our knowledge of coagulation escalates each year, we find ourselves inundated with new assessments of data which tell us that substance "xyz" is probably associated with bleeding or thrombosis seen in disease or condition A. But what do we do with this new information? How can we use the information to effect a change in the treatment or management of a disease process? Not all studies are randomized, with good statistics on the differences between different test methods or treatments. Many such reports make no attempt to guide the reader as to how to apply this new information in a practical manner to stop bleeding or inappropriate clotting. Practical application is left to the reader's imagination and creativity. In addition, many diseases that can affect coagulation involve multiple organs, such as liver, renal, cardiac, and pulmonary disease. It also follows, therefore, that treatment is also complex and must address many different aspects of the patient's disease. This compounds the difficulty in evaluating coagulation studies, and how the coagulation studies are affected by the many disease processes.

The value of laboratory tests also changes with time. Recent synopses of bleeding time demonstrated the bleeding time test's inability to predict surgical bleeding (7–11). However, bleeding time still has value in assessing platelet function for management in uremia, and in screening for suspected von Willebrand's disease, or other congenital causes for a platelet defect. A test that has heretofore been used without questioning to predict surgical bleeding has been shown to have little real value for that purpose today. As a screening test, the bleeding time continues of demonstrative limited value as a preoperative test to predict surgical bleeding (11).

As part of our effort to be accurate and yet reasonably practical in reaching a decision and effecting therapy that addresses the many variables noted above, we developed five questions that can help place the problem/situation in a realistic perspective (see Table 1). However, before we start thinking about applying theory to ordering and interpreting laboratory studies for bleeding and clotting disorders, we should address some issues of supporting infrastructure and practicality.

Baseline studies or preoperative studies do have value in assessing changes, the severity of losses, and providing a basis for corrective action. Rarely will the screening tests have predictive value as to who will bleed or clot inappropriately. Those situations that require preprocedure baseline studies are determined by experience, the availability and turnaround time of laboratory testing, and the specifics of the procedure or disease and its customary risk for bleeding/inappropriate clotting problems. It is obvious that a change in platelet count from 350,000 mm^3 to 60,000 mm^3 is not the same as drop from 175,000 mm^3 to 60,000 mm^3. The risk for bleeding may be the same, but the mechanisms by which you got to the 60,000 mm^3

Table 1 Five Questions To Ask Before You Start Ordering or Interpreting Laboratory Tests or Begin Treatment of a Bleeding or Inappropriate Clotting Disorder

Are the coagulation values truly abnormal for the patient?

Are the measured coagulation abnormalities amenable to therapy that will stop bleeding or prevent thrombosis?

When therapy is begun, does the patient respond either clinically and/or with regard to the laboratory tests?

Is there a less than perfect threshold for effective hemostasis or anticoagulation, and do multiple minor defects in the coagulation system add their potential to result in bleeding or thrombosis?

Are coagulation or anticoagulation replacement therapies and procedures worth continuing, based on what criteria?

Table 2 Baseline Coagulation Studies that Should Be Available on a Routine Basis for the Assessment of Bleeding and Clotting Disorders

Complete blood count
Platelet count
Prothrombin time
Activated partial thromboplastin time
Fibrinogen
Bleeding time (for nonsurgical bleeding)

are potentially different processes with potential for completely different outcomes and requirements for therapy. The same goes for prothrombin time, partial thromboplastin time, fibrinogen, or other clotting assay.

The baseline studies should be routine enough to be repeated 24 hours a day, 7 days a week. Esoteric lab testing is of little value at 2:00 a.m. Sunday morning in assessing the patient and selecting medication or blood/blood component therapy. Certainly, selected specialized testing is appropriate. However, it is difficult to build from experience and develop treatment algorithms on unavailable testing. This is not to say that more complex testing is not important. Our laboratory does its share. Save portions of the sample in 1-mL aliquots in plastic and securely capped tubes at −70°C for processing the next day.

The selection of tests required for the assessment of bleeding or clotting will reflect the commitment and interest in making the diagnosis and the best management. A minimal selection (see Table 2) is needed for the initial assessment. In addition, the hospital that can be expected to fully support a surgery service and patients with GI bleeding from any cause, and the accurate management of thrombotic events, will need additional tests tailored to address the diagnosis and the success of management (see Table 3).

There has to be a reliable means to get the necessary tubes of blood to the laboratory for testing purposes, and the results to where you and the patient are located. Laboratory studies that are 3 hr old are *cold* and are most likely of no value in assessing the situation or making a decision. You should not ask your colleagues to test before, during, and after therapy if the laboratory test results will be too late or too old to make any difference.

The selection of instrumentation and reagents must be based on solid principles of accu-

Table 3 Examples of Coagulation Profiles that Can Be Used in Assessing Specialized Bleeding and Clotting Disorders

Liver disease	Hypercoagulable state
Baseline coagulation profile	Baseline coagulation profile
Factors V, VII, VIII, IX	Factors VII, VIII
Plasminogen, antithrombin III	Antithrombin III
Euglobulin clot lysis	Euglobulin clot lysis
	Protein C, protein S (total and free)
	Kaolin clotting time, lupus anticoagulant studies
	Anticardiolipin antibodies
	Factor V Leiden (APC resistance)

racy and precision. An insensitive PT or aPTT reagent will not keep you out of trouble by not detecting a low level of a particular clotting factor. The patient will continue to bleed, use ungodly amounts of blood, may bleed to death, and you will never know why. The most expensive system is of course not necessarily the best, but your understanding of what the instrument and reagents will do will determine whether the best decisions are being made.

The sensitivity of your instrument/reagent system to detect deficiencies and diseases ought to be as high as possible. If, for instance, the lower end of your reference range for the prothrombin time detects a factor VII level at 45% of normal rather than the usual 30%, expect to have to work up a lot of falsely significant prothrombin times. If the aPTT reagent is insensitive to the lupus anticoagulant, or heparin, plan on missing a lot of lupus anticoagulants that would explain a thrombotic event and difficulty managing heparin therapy.

The laboratory staff must have skill and personnel depth in what tests they are asked to perform. Often, advanced instrumentation along with on-board computers will be touted as the painless way to overcome the tedium of factor assays. However, when the medical technologist first performs the assays by plotting each point and drawing the line, the sources of error are learned and appreciated. There are clotting times that do not fit the dilutions, and curves that "just do not look right." In addition, the direct observation of a clot and its lysis has a unique visual impact of what fibrinolysis is all about that cannot be appreciated from a number or picture.

Absenteeism due to vacation, illness, unplanned vacancy, or unavailability because of excessive workload are not acceptable reasons for delayed or absent results. The laboratory must be as dependable as possible in order to obtain data for decision making. When the data are absent, informed management will be lacking, and management decisions will be without clarity or validity. With these practical support questions discussed, the asking of purposeful questions is the next useful and practical step.

A. Are the Coagulation Values Truly Abnormal for the Patient?

An abnormal coagulation lab test does not necessarily predict who will bleed or thrombose.

1. What are the mechanisms or causes for these abnormal results? Make sure the results are real, and not due to heparin contamination via A-line or pseudothrombocytopenia (platelet clumping), for example. Ask questions about the time intervals between what is happening to the patient, what has been done to the patient, and the coagulation results. Coagulation is a dynamic process that changes with time; physical intervention and therapy have direct effects on laboratory results. The medical chart will provide information on medications given and when. When exactly was the blood collected, and from where?

2. Are the abnormalities significant in that they can predict or result in clotting or bleeding? Certainly, a platelet count of 10,000 mm^3 can pose an increased risk for spontaneous bleeding, but what about 25,000 mm^3, 45,000 mm^3, 80,000 mm^3, or 120,000 mm^3? The unique circumstances of the patient must be reviewed in concert with experience, the experience of others, and recommendations from the literature. What about an aPTT of 45 sec versus 55 sec versus 70 sec? Which will more likely bleed? This depends on why the aPTT is prolonged: Heparin? Factor VIII deficiency? Factor XII deficiency? A combination of factor deficiencies? Inhibitor? Factor VIII inhibitor? Lupus anticoagulant? The point is that a prolonged aPTT has no value unless you have an idea as to why it is prolonged. Degree of prolongation will mean different effects in different patients depending on one or multiple diseases, medications, and on and on. Take the time to learn the uniqueness of each patient, and understand how the

patient's coagulation system is responding to his or her disease, and what intervention has accomplished with the disease process as well as the patient's coagulation system. These concepts may seem somewhat lofty, but to have any real impact on what is affecting the patient, you must know the patient.

B. Are the Measured Coagulation Abnormalities Amenable to Therapy That Will Stop the Bleeding or Prevent Thrombosis?

This question is one of the most difficult to answer. When there is difficulty in predicting a propensity to bleed from an abnormal test, how do you determine if the abnormality is amenable to therapy? You will develop criteria for that answer with time and experience—criteria built on what you have been taught, your experience with the coagulation numbers, experience with the numbers from the laboratory (instrumentation, reagents, and technical staff), or from other laboratories. There are no tables or systems that will address or predict patient response to therapy. A trial of a particular therapy with a means to assess or document improvement is a very practical way to define the processes as well as ascertain the value of therapy.

1. *What are your criteria for answering the above question?* Look at all the tests you use to assess a bleeding or inappropriate clotting problem along with the history. A single abnormal test may suggest a single system defect (deficiency or inhibitor), where multiple abnormal tests may suggest a system disorder with multiple diseases or processes occurring at once. Look for combinations of medications, blood/component replacement, and other forms of therapy to have an effect. Excessive use of plasma expanders, >2 L, may give you an artifactual prolongation of the PT and aPTT, and dilute your platelet count. In a patient who has no risk factors for sepsis, this is likely a therapy and dilution effect. Sepsis may come later, but in the acute aspect of this patient, consumption is unlikely. Therapy is then based on compensating for the dilutional effect, and not the use of antibiotics or antifibrinolytic agents.

2. *How do you test your hypothesis in this particular patient?* Establish a working diagnosis on which therapy is initiated. Repeat key coagulation tests that are most likely to be directly modified by the therapy. One of the most difficult tasks is to determine what amount or volume of FFP in a 4-kg child or an 80-kg woman will be required to alter or correct the dynamic process. Start with a formula such as millimeters per kilogram or units of FFP per units of estimated blood loss or replacement, and modify as needed as the response and complications of the intervention develop. The dynamics of the disease or process may not be amenable to therapy despite your correct diagnosis. Or is the diagnosis incorrect? After you initiate your therapy, monitor again. The process of treatment followed by specific coagulation testing will build a knowledge base as to how the patient responds, and will serve as a correlation dynamic for diagnosis—laboratory testing—and the response to therapy for this case and possibly the next case. With regularly scheduled monitoring, the earliest correction of the defects is identified, and if bleeding continues or thrombosis continues, other mechanisms for the problem can be investigated in a timely manner.

C. When Therapy Is Begun, Does the Patient Respond Either Clinically and or with Regard to the Laboratory Tests?

The clinical response in the long run will be more important than a number change. However, the mere fact that you observe a significant change in your monitored variables is encouraging. This is a most intense part of the management process. Aggressive use of your chosen approach with sufficient monitoring (a minimum of every 2 hr in an acute process, perhaps within 30 min of completion of therapy, will tell you the status of the coagulation system. Increasing the quantity of a particular therapy, such as a trial of 6 units of FFP over 6 hr with no change or even worsening of your tested parameters, is good evidence that further therapy will most likely have limited success in correcting any deficiencies, much less stop the bleeding. As you document the improvement in coagulation studies, the frequency of laboratory monitoring may be reduced to 4 or 6, 8, or 12 hr depending on the clinical response. If this is a case of a well-established problem such as factor VIII replacement in a hemophiliac, the dosage and frequency may not require frequent or specific monitoring. However, with an inhibitor you can certainly know via the aPTT or factor VIII:C assay within 2 hr or less in most cases. One of the more frequent restrictions to sufficient monitoring is availability. Again, common tests performed 24 hours a day are the minimum requirement. Over a period of days or weeks, the aPTT value in a specific hemophiliac patient will tell you where the factor VIII assay will be for that particular patient. Build a file for that patient. At the next admission you can compare aPTT and factor VIII values for changes.

Resistance to heparin therapy in the patient with clinical thrombosis may reflect several different aberrations, which must be addressed one at a time: inadequate maintenance heparin, interruption in therapy (>30 min), absent heparin rebolusing while increasing the maintenance heparin, decreased AT-III, previous doses of heparin in the CCU prior to a coronary bypass procedure, and elevated factor VIII and fibrinogen reducing the aPTT response to heparin. It is important to develop a step-by-step approach that will eliminate the more common causes of the bleeding or clotting problem. After this analysis (collect the blood you need at the first phlebotomy), follow with testing for the less frequent causes.

D. Is There a Less-Than-Perfect Threshold for Effective Hemostasis or Anticoagulation, and Do Multiple Minor Defects in the Coagulation System Add Their Potential to Result in Bleeding or Thrombosis?

For this question, reference ranges (normality?) and evidence for bleeding or inappropriate clotting will conflict. Defining the parameters of your deficiency(ies) is important to correlate numbers with the clinical situation. The reference ranges reflect the normal population. The thresholds for bleeding reflect the level and significance of the deficiency(ies) in that patient. Typically bleeding does not occur at or just below the reference range, but usually much lower. Decreased levels do not necessarily mean that there is a risk for bleeding. Low factor VII:C and dysfibrinogenemias can be associated with both bleeding and inappropriate clotting. Take the time to study the patient, learn what tests to order, and study the results on this particular patient with an eye to what to expect and the actual results. Be ready to change testing and management directions. Stay with the problem. Broaden your approach, and expect to do some nonproductive, unsuccessful fishing. You may find the answer in returning to the patient to ask to see the medications bottles, because the tests tell you the patient's bleeding may be caused by a medication. The pharmacy has dispensed the wrong medication on occasion. An additional $400 worth of testing can quickly equal the cost of 4 units of blood without the risks of a blood transfusion.

Do multiple minor defects add their potential to result in bleeding or thrombosis? They often do in unanticipated ways. The history should clue you in to this problem. The patient may deny taking aspirin, but takes an antacid with aspirin. Over-the-counter medications are taken by patients without their realizing that they are taking medication that can affect bleeding. The patient with chronic alcoholism or hepatitis may have liver dysfunction to the degree that all the clotting factors, modulators, and protease inhibitors will be functionally or qualitatively abnormal, affecting all aspects of coagulation. Screening tests such as PT and aPTT do not always become more prolonged with multiple deficiencies. Factor assays for specific vitamin K versus non-vitamin K-dependent factors can be helpful in determining single or multiple deficiencies. The patient's diet may also contribute to a lack of vitamins and calories, which can have an effect on total protein and albumin as well as detoxifying liver enzyme systems.

E. Are Coagulation Replacement Therapies and Procedures Worth Continuing, Based on What Criteria?

We have to come to grips with the realities of the collapse of therapy in some patients. This realization should be the result of the assessment of the nature of therapy, the quantity of therapy, was the therapy enough, and the conclusion that the bleeding or thrombotic problem will not be fixed with the current therapy. This realization is often difficult to accept. An attempt to reach this realization as accurately, reasonably, and quickly as possible will not only improve the status of those who do respond, but will also determine which are hopeless or amenable to an organ transplant or other, more invasive attempt to resolve the problem.

Asking these questions when an abdominal aortic aneurysm ruptures minutes before cross clamping in the resection in the operating room does not make a lot of sense. In the immediate situation it may not solve the more pressing urgency, but later, when the patient is in SICU with a continued ooze, the questions have merit. So where do you start? Start by documenting a good history as soon as you can, and order those tests which can give you the most information in the most expedient manner. Continue to monitor what you do for the patient. Seek assistance with the tough ones, learn from your experience, and whatever you do, don't lose your intensity.

IV. SUMMARY

Bleeding and inappropriate clotting disorders are often unique in every patient, and demand an intense consideration of all the information practical and possible. Experience will teach you even more. The laboratory, when properly organized, planned, and supported, will provide timely information needed to make the diagnosis, monitor intervention, and provide objective evidence of your frustration or success. The absence of a history, inappropriate test monitoring, and not understanding fundamentally what the history and laboratory information tells you about the situation is often the mechanism whereby a correct diagnosis cannot be made and intervention becomes costly and nonproductive.

REFERENCES

1. Grabowski EF, Corrigan JJ. Homeostasis: general considerations. In: Miller DR, Bachner RL, eds. *Blood Diseases of Infancy and Childhood*. 7th ed. New York: Mosby-Year Book, 1995:849–865.
2. Burns ER. Clinical Management of Bleeding and Thrombosis, Part II: Diagnosing Bleeding Disorders. London: Blackwell Scientific, 1987:43–107.
3. Kitchens CS. Approach to the bleeding patient. In: Penner JA, Hassouna HI, eds. Coagulation Disorders I. Philadelphia: Saunders, 1992:983–989.
4. Bowie EJW, Owen CA. The clinical and laboratory diagnosis of hemorrhagic disorders. In: Ratnoff OD, Forbes CD, eds. Disorders of Hemostasis. 3d ed. New York: Grune & Stratton, 1996:53–78.
5. Beal RW, Isbister JP. History, philosophy and ethics of blood component therapy. In: Blood Component Therapy in Clinical Practice. London: Blackwell Scientific, 1985:1–10.

6. McLoughlin TM, Greilich PE. Preexisting hemostatic defects and bleeding disorders. In: Blood: Hemostasis, Transfusion, and Alternatives in the Perioperative Period. New York: Raven Press, 1995:25–70.
7. De Caterina R, Lanza M, Manca G, et al. Bleeding time and bleeding: an analysis of the relationship of the bleeding time test with parameters of surgical bleeding. Blood 1994; 84:3363–3370.
8. Gewirtz AS, Miller ML, Keys TF. The clinical usefulness of the preoperative bleeding time. Arch Pathol Lab Med 1996; 120:353–356.
9. Rodgers RPC, Levin J. A critical reappraisal of the bleeding time. Semin Thromb Haemost 1990; 16:1–20.
10. Lind SE. The bleeding time does not predict surgical bleeding. Blood 1991; 77:2447–2567.
11. Peterson P, Hayes TE, Arkin CF, Bovill EG, Fairweather RB, et al. The preoperative bleeding time test lacks clinical benefit, College of American Pathologists and American Society of Clinical Pathologist's Position Article. Arch Surg 1998; 133:134–139.

27

Concepts of Replacement Therapy: Blood Components, Blood Derivatives, and Medications

Francis R. Rodwig, Jr.
Ochsner Medical Institutions, New Orleans, Louisiana

A basic understanding of the concepts of blood component therapy is needed to select the appropriate product for patients with hematologic disorders that require transfusions. In early transfusion medicine practice, all patients requiring a transfusion, regardless of their physiologic defect, were transfused with whole blood. Over time, especially with the development of plastic bags and appropriate preservative solutions, a unit of donated whole blood could be separated into red blood cells, platelets, plasma, cryoprecipitate, and other blood components and derivatives. This process allows patients to receive components to target their particular needs, and, since one unit will benefit several patients, the most efficient use of this scarce resource.

I. BLOOD COMPONENTS

A. Whole Blood

Whole blood represents the blood collected from a standard blood donation. The whole blood unit contains approximately 450 mL of blood and 63 mL of an anticoagulant/preservative solution, resulting in a hematocrit of about 40%. The product has a shelf life of 21–35 days, depending on the type of anticoagulant, and is stored at 1–6°C. While a unit of whole blood does contain all the cellular and plasma constituents present in the circulating blood, this product cannot provide an adequate source of all these components. Specifically, refrigerated whole blood is quickly depleted of viable platelets and leukocytes, and there is a decrease in the activity of the labile clotting factors (factors V and VIII).

1. Indications

Whole blood provides the oxygen-carrying capacity of the red blood cells as well as the intravascular volume expansion properties of plasma. In addition, the hemostatic effect of the more stable clotting factors may be beneficial. The only indication for the use of whole blood is an actively bleeding patient with significant blood loss (>20–25% of the total blood volume).

Patients with symptomatic anemia who are normovolemic, especially pediatric patients and adults with compromised cardiac and renal function, are at risk of developing circulatory overload from whole blood.

2. Dosage/Administration

One unit of whole blood should increase the hemoglobin by 1 g/dL, or the hematocrit by 3–4%. To increase the hemoglobin by 1 g/dL in a pediatric patient, the dosage is 8–10 mL/kg. Whole blood can be administered as rapidly as tolerated by the patient's condition, but the time period should not exceed 4 hr.

B. Red Blood Cells

Red blood cells (commonly called packed red blood cells) are prepared by centrifugation of a unit of whole blood, followed by the removal of 200–250 mL of platelet-rich plasma. This product is stored at 1–6°C with a hematocrit of approximately 70%, and has a shelf life of 21–35 days. An additive solution may be added to the red cells, extending the shelf life to 42 days, with a hematocrit of 50–60%.

1. Indications

Red blood cells are indicated for the treatment of symptomatic anemia in patients who require an increase in oxygen-carrying capacity and red blood cell mass. Few topics in the field of transfusion medicine have received as much attention over the last decade as the decision process as to when a patient should receive a red blood cell transfusion, and the appropriate dose. The assessment of data used to make the transfusion decision has been termed the "transfusion trigger." The traditional principle of transfusing all patients with a hemoglobin level less than 10 g/dL (or hematocrit <30%, the so-called "10/30" rule) is now outdated. The topic of red blood cell transfusions was addressed by a National Institute of Health Consensus Conference (1), with a number of additional reports in the literature over the last few years. In general, the data in these reports suggest that many patients receive little benefit from a red blood cell transfusion unless the hemoglobin is less than 8 g/dL, and in some cases less than 7 g/dL. One significant benefit of the effort to prevent transfusion-transmitted disease has been the change in the transfusion trigger from a laboratory value to a thorough evaluation of the patient, including patient history, cardiac status, oxygen delivery, consumption, and extraction ratios (2). Careful consideration of the cost–benefit ratio has reduced the number of transfusions in most centers, with an overall improvement in transfusion practices (3).

2. Dosage/Administration

The dosage and administration of packed red blood cells are similar to that described by whole blood (above). Slow rates of transfusion may be needed for patients with compromised cardiac and/or pulmonary function.

Several varieties of red blood cells other than the standard packed red blood cells are available. While the preparation methods and indications are different, the dosage, administration, and expected outcome are similar to a packed red blood cell transfusion. Since these products are costly, and the extra manipulation increases the chances of error or contamination, they should be used judiciously, and only for the proper indications.

a. Washed Red Blood Cells. Red blood cells can be "washed" of plasma and leukocytes by the addition of saline, utilizing automated methods. Once washed, the shelf life of this product is reduced to 24 hr. Plasma and plasma proteins are responsible for allergic and anaphylactic transfusion reactions. Other "storage lesion" defects, such as extracellular potassium and cytokines, can lead to other transfusion-related complications (4). The primary indication for washed red blood cells is for patients who have experienced recurrent allergic or urticarial reactions which do not respond to simple antihistamine therapy. In addition, patients who may have difficulty with the transfusion of certain plasma products, such as complement (paroxysmal nocturnal hemoglobinuria), IgA (congenital IgA deficiency), and potassium (neonatal exchange transfusions or intrauterine transfusions) should receive washed red blood cells.

b. Frozen/Deglycerolized Red Blood Cells. The shelf life of red blood cells can be extended to 10 years by the addition of a cryopreservative solution (glycerol) followed by freezing (<–65°C). When needed, the unit is thawed and the glycerol is removed by a variant of the washing procedure (deglycerolization). Frozen/deglycerolized red blood cells are needed for long-term storage of rare or special units (e.g., special antigen typings or IgA-deficient donors). Also, autologous units can be frozen if the day of surgery is delayed. Once thawed and deglycerolized, these products must be used within 24 hr.

c. Leukocyte-Reduced Red Blood Cells. Before the development of leukocyte-removal filters, both washed and frozen/deglycerolized red blood cells were used for the prevention of febrile, nonhemolytic transfusion reactions. This relatively common reaction was in part due to leukoagglutinins in the recipient plasma that reacted with the passenger leukocytes in red blood cell (and platelet) transfusions (5). These white blood cells, which contribute little benefit in a transfusion, have also been implicated in many of the other adverse effects of transfusion, including HLA alloimmunization (6), immunomodulation, and transmission of certain viruses (7). Recent evidence has become available that the production of cytokines by these leukocytes may contribute significantly to febrile reactions (8). Several methods have been used to reduce the number of leukocytes in red blood cell and platelet transfusions, with varying degrees of effectiveness. Modern, third-generation filters are now available that are extremely efficient in removing the number of leukocytes (>99.9%, or 3 log removal) (9). The red blood cell or platelet product can be rendered leukocyte reduced either at the time of transfusion (bedside filtration) or prior to storage by the blood collection facility.

C. Platelets

Platelets are minute fragments of megakaryocyte cytoplasm that are responsible for primary hemostasis. Platelets are usually prepared from whole blood by centrifugation, removing the platelet-rich plasma, followed by an additional centrifugation step to concentrate the platelet product. Platelet concentrates, which have a volume of 50–70 mL, are stored at room temperature (20–24°C), with a shelf life of 5 days. An average platelet concentrate contains approximately 5.5×10^{11} platelets. Typically, these individual units are pooled prior to use to provide an appropriate dose. An increasingly popular method for obtaining platelets utilizes apheresis technology. Here, whole blood is removed from a donor and separated into its components by the apheresis equipment. The platelets are then directed into a collection bag, and the remaining components are returned to the donor. This technique provides a product equivalent to 6–10 units of pooled platelets in a plasma volume of 200–300 mL. The storage requirements and shelf life are identical to platelet concentrates. The advantages of this product include the reduced number of donor exposures to decrease the risk of transfusion-transmitted diseases and alloimmunization. The disadvantages include the need for specialized equipment and personnel, the requirement of two venipunctures, and the time commitment made by the donor.

1. Indications

Like red blood cell transfusion decisions, there has been extensive debate about the decision to transfuse platelets and the appropriate dosage and expected benefit (10). Platelets are commonly transfused to patients with primary disorders of the bone marrow, including the sequelae of chemotherapy and radiation therapy. The decision to transfuse platelets is made by a clinical evaluation of the patient and the patient's platelet count. Patients with a platelet count less than 10,000/μL are at increased risk for spontaneous hemorrhage, and at significant risk for bleeding with trauma, invasive procedures, or ulceration. These patients should receive a platelet transfusion regardless of apparent bleeding. Patients with platelet counts between 10,000 and 30,000/μL are at slight risk for spontaneous hemorrhage, and may be candidates for transfusion in the absence of bleeding. However, the traditional "trigger" of 20,000/μL for prophylactic platelet transfusion has been questioned (11). Patients with platelet counts between 10,000 and 50,000/μL are at variable risk for bleeding with trauma, invasive procedures, or ulceration. Transfusion of platelets is indicated for these patients if bleeding is apparent, or prior to an invasive procedure. For major surgeries, the platelet count should be increased to above 50,000/μL. Platelet transfusion therapy is more difficult in patients with thrombocytopenia secondary to enhanced destruction of platelets by immunologic mechanisms or consumption, since therapeutic levels are more difficult to attain (see below).

2. *Dosage/Administration*

A recommended dosage for platelet transfusion is one that will increase the platelet count to above 50,000/μL. An often-used calculation is 1 unit/10 kg of body weight, or one apheresis product for an adult. Some centers provide a standardized, pooled dose for adults (e.g., 6 units). An increase of 5,000–10,000/μL is expected for every unit of platelets transfused. Such increments are often not reached because of a number of conditions common to hospitalized patients, including fever, sepsis, splenomegaly, ongoing bleeding, and interaction with medications, among others. In some patients who have received multiple transfusions, the development of human leukocyte antigen (HLA) or platelet-specific antibodies may lead to refractoriness to platelet transfusions. If this is suspected, a platelet count can be obtained 10 min to 1 hr after transfusion. The corrected count increment (CCI) can then be obtained by the following formula:

$$\mathrm{CCI} = \frac{(\text{posttransfusion platelet count} - \text{pre-count})}{\text{no. of platelets transfused } (10^{11})} \times \text{body surface area } (\mathrm{m}^2)$$

If the CCI is <7,500–10,000/μL, alloimmunization is likely. These patients may require apheresis platelets that are crossmatched or HLA matched. While platelets can be infused rapidly, routine transfusions are usually given at 5–10 mL/min.

D. Fresh Frozen Plasma

A unit of fresh frozen plasma (FFP) consists of plasma that is separated from whole blood and frozen within 8 hr of collection. FFP is stored at −18°C or less for up to 1 year, with an average volume of 200–250 mL. Like platelets, apheresis techniques can be used to produce larger volume of FFP from a single donor (500–600 mL, the equivalent of 2–3 units of FFP). FFP contains all the components of the coagulation, fibrinolytic, and complement systems. Timely preparation and freezing of the plasma is needed to ensure adequate levels of the labile clotting factors V and VIII, which decay with refrigerated or room-temperature storage. Each milliliter of FFP contains approximately 1 unit (100% activity) of each coagulation factor.

1. *Indications*

The primary indication for the use of FFP is a history or clinical course consistent with a congenital or acquired deficiency of coagulation factors, with active bleeding, or prior to an operative or other invasive procedure. It is recommended that the coagulation defect be documented by at least one of the following: (a) prothrombin time (PT) greater than 1.5 times the midpoint of the normal range (usually >18 sec); (b) activated partial thromplastin time (aPTT) greater than 1.5 times the top of the normal range (usually >55–60 sec); and (c) coagulation factor assay of less than 25% activity. Patients with congenital factor deficiencies for which factor concentrates are not available (e.g., factors V or XI), are occasionally candidates for FFP transfusion. Patients with certain acquired coagulation factor deficiencies, such as seen following massive transfusion, or reversal of warfarin anticoagulation, are appropriate candidates for FFP transfusion. Patients undergoing plasma exchange therapy for certain disease states such as thrombotic thrombocytopenic purpura (TTP) or the hemolytic uremic syndrome (HUS) should receive FFP as the replacement fluid.

2. *Dosage/Administration*

The usual starting dose of FFP is 5–10 mL/kg of body weight [400–500 mL, or 2 units (bags) of FFP, or one plasmapheresis unit]. Some patients, especially those with consumptive coagulopathies, may need 10–15 mL/kg. The decision to transfuse additional units of FFP depends on the underlying disease, extent of active bleeding, half-life of the deficient clotting factor, and lab parameters. Since this product is frozen, adequate time must be allowed for thawing prior to transfusion. Like platelet transfusion, rapid transfusions are acceptable for seriously volume-depleted patients, and with a routine infusion rate of 5–10 mL/min.

E. Cryoprecipitate

Cryoprecipitate is a concentrated source of specific plasma proteins (12). Thawing FFP at 1–6°C (instead of 37°C) produces a small volume of precipitate that can be removed and refrozen. The 10–15 mL of cryoprecipitate is stored at −18°C or less for up to 1 year. This product is also called cryoprecipitate AHF (antihemophilic factor), since it contains 80–120 units of FVIII:C (approximately 50% of the FVIII:C content of a unit of FFP). The other important components of cryoprecipitate are fibrinogen (150–250 mg/unit), von Willebrand factor (FVIII:vWF, 40–70% of the original FFP), factor XIII, and fibronectin.

1. *Indications*

The most common indication for the use of cryoprecipitate in the United States today is hypofibrinogenemia. Other derivatives that contain fibrinogen in a concentrated form are not approved for use by the Food and Drug Administration. Most cases of hypofibrinogenemia are associated with patients with a consumptive coagulopathy, who should receive other blood components. Cryoprecipitate can provide an appropriate concentration of fibrinogen in the smallest volume possible. Fibrinogen levels above 100 mg/dL are usually adequate for hemostasis. Cryoprecipitate can also be used for patients with von Willebrand's disease, but this product should be reserved for those cases that are unable to receive or unresponsive to DDAVP, or when a factor VIII product that contains vWF is not available. The same rule should apply to patients with hemophilia A when factor VIII concentrates are not available. A growing use of cryoprecipitate is as the source of fibrinogen and fibrin-stabilizing factor (factor XIII), which is mixed with bovine thrombin to produce a surgical adhesive, commonly called fibrin glue (13).

2. *Dosage/Administration*

The dosage of cryoprecipitate is dependent on the clinical need.

In hypofibrinogenemia, the dosage can be calculated by the following formula:

$$\text{Fibrinogen (mg) required} = \text{plasma volume (mL)} \times [\text{desired} - \text{initial fibrinogen level (mg/dL)}]$$

Since each bag (unit) of cryoprecipitate has approximately 250 mg, the number of units needed is determined by the fibrinogen required (mg)/250.

The plasma volume can be estimated by (a) [70 mL/kg × weight (kg)] × (1 − hematocrit), or (b) 40–50 mL/kg × weight (kg).

An empirical rule is to give 1 unit of cryoprecipitate for every 5 kg of body weight.

In von Willebrand's disease, the standard dose is 1 unit/10 kg of body weight. In the event that FVIII concentrates are not available, the dosage of cryoprecipitate for a patient with hemophilia A can be determined from the following formula:

$$\text{Units of FVIII} = (\text{desired FVIII level} - \text{initial FVIII level}) \times \text{plasma volume}$$

Since each bag (unit) of cryoprecipitate has approximately 80 mg of factor VIII, the number of units needed is determined by the units required/80.

As with FFP, the need for repeat infusions varies with the deficient factor, its transfusion half-life, whether consumption is present, and the patient's previous response to therapy. The products are usually pooled, with similar administration guidelines to fresh frozen plasma.

F. Granulocytes

Granulocytes can be provided as a transfusion product for patients with severe neutropenia by cytapheresis of a single donor or removal of the buffy coat from units of fresh whole blood for use in neonates. Granulocyte transfusions are used infrequently today. The use of recombinant growth factors to speed marrow recovery (see below), newer antibiotics, and the common adverse effects of granulocyte transfusion have all contributed to the decline in use. In addition, there is controversy as to the therapeutic effectiveness of granulocyte transfusions. A major factor is the difficulty of obtaining an adequate dose from a donor. There has been renewed interest in this therapy with recent data that much larger yields of granulocytes can be obtained from donors stimulated with granulocyte colony-stimulating factor (G-CSF) (14).

1. Indications

The indications for granulocyte transfusions are not well established. In general, the patient should be severely neutropenic (absolute granulocyte count <500/mL), fever for 24–48 hr, or sepsis unresponsive to other modes of therapy, myeloid hypoplasia, and a reasonable chance for recovery (15).

2. Dosage/Administration

The yield of a granulocyte preparation can vary widely, and cannot be standardized. The transfusion should be transfused as quickly as possible following collection, since granulocytes have a short half-life. Often, there is insufficient time to perform the required testing for infectious diseases, and the ordering physician must indicate that the benefits of the transfusion outweigh the risk. The therapy should continue for 3–4 days. Reactions to granulocytes are common and can be severe. Premedication with antihistamines, acetaminophen, or corticosteroids may be needed. Leukocyte removal filters should not be used, and the product should be irradiated to prevent graft-versus-host disease. The peripheral white blood cell count will not increase following transfusion, since the cells will quickly leave the circulation. Therefore, a resolution of the infection or clinical improvement would indicate success.

II. BLOOD DERIVATIVES

Blood plasma derivatives are plasma protein concentrates prepared from large pools of human plasma. Cohn fractionation, a manufacturing process that precipitates and collects specific plasma proteins in cold ethanol mixtures, is the primary method used to prepare these products. Other processes, such as immunoaffinity chromatography, adsorption/elution techniques, or monoclonal antibodies allow purification of these products. Viral inactivation procedures include heating, detergent-solvent techniques, and affinity column purification. Recently, recombinant DNA-produced factor VIII concentrates have been licensed.

A. Factor VIII Concentrates

Hemophilia A is a congenital (X-linked recessive) disorder, with a deficiency of the coagulant portion of the factor VIII molecule (FVIII:C). This deficient factor affects the mechanism of fibrin clot formation and can lead to clinical bleeding, especially in the joints and soft tissues. Infusions of factor VIII may be necessary to prevent or control bleeding episodes. While plasma and cryoprecipitate contain this factor, lyophilized concentrates that can be easily stored, reconstituted, and infused have dramatically changed the management of patients with hemophilia. Many different FVIII products are available, with different methods of production, purity, concentration, viral inactivation processes, and cost (Table 1) (16). The porcine-derived

Table 1 Factor VIII Products

Product name	Manufacturer	Method of viral inactivation	Hepatitis safety studies in humans
Intermediate- and high-purity factor VIII products derived from human plasma			
Profilate OSD	Alpha	SD (TNBP & polysorbate 80)	No
Koate-HP	Miles	SD (TNBP & polysorbate 80) 27°C, 6 hr	No
New York Blood Center FVIII-SD	New York Blood Center	SD (TNBP & cholate) ≥ 24°C, 6 hr	Yes
Humate-P	Behringwerke	Heated in solution (pasteurized), 60°C, 10 hr	Yes
Immunoaffinity-purified factor VIII products (ultrapure) derived from human plasma			
Monoclate P	Armour	Pasteurized (60°C, 10 hr)	Yes
Hemofil M	Baxter-Hyland	Solvent-detergent (TNBP/Triton-X100) ≥ 25°C, ≥10 hr	Yes
Coagulation FVIII Method M	Baxter-Hyland (for American Red Cross)	Solvent-detergent (TNBP/Triton-X100) ≥ 25°C, ≥10 hr	No
Recombinant DNA-produced factor VIII products			
Recombinate	Baxter-Hyland	None	Yes
Bioclate	Armour	None	Yes
Kogenate	Miles	None	Yes
Helixate	Armour	None	Yes
Porcine factor VIII			
Hyate C	Porton Products	None	Yes

Abbreviations: SD, solvent-detergent; TNBP, tri(*n*-butyl)-phosphate.

FVIII preparation has been shown to be effective in the management of patients with FVIII inhibitors (17).

1. Indications/Dosage

The dose of FVIII depends on the therapeutic need. Infusions may be given prophylactically to prevent bleeding episodes. If bleeding has occurred, the nature of the bleeding, severity of the factor deficiency, and the patient's previous response to treatment determine the dosage. One unit of factor VIII/kg of body weight will increase the patient's factor VIII level by approximately 2% (0.02 U/mL) (18). If time allows the FVIII:C level to be determined, a target level can be identified. The number of units required can then be calculated as described above (section on cryoprecipitate).

Since FVIII has a half-life of 8–12 hr, repeat doses may be needed at reduced dosage to maintain clot stability and promote healing. FVIII assays should be used to monitor the therapy.

B. Factor IX Concentrates

Early factor IX concentrates were prothrombin complex concentrates because they also contained considerable amounts of the vitamin K-dependent factors II, VII, and X. This product was associated with an increased risk for developing thrombosis. Newer factor IX concentrates have a higher degree of purity, with less risk of thrombogenicity. These products are listed in Table 2 (16).

1. Indications/Dosage

The indications for factor IX infusion in patients with a congenital deficiency of this protein (hemophilia B) are similar to those of patients with hemophilia A (above). Factor IX concentrates may be useful in patient with low-titer factor VIII inhibitors (<10 Bethesda units). Higher loading doses may be needed because of reduced in-vivo recovery.

Table 2 Factor IX Products

Product name	Manufacturer	Method of viral inactivation	Hepatitis studies in humans
Coagulation factor IX			
AlphaNine-SD	Alpha	SD TNBP/Polysorbate 80 24–30°C, ≥6 hr	No
Mononine	Armour	Ultrafiltration sodium thiocyanate	Yes
Factor IX complex concentrates			
Konyne 80	Miles	Dry heat, 80°C, 72 hr	No
Proplex T	Baxter-Hyland	Dry heat, 68°C, 14 hr	No
Profilnine HT	Alpha	Heated in *n*-heptane solution 60°C, 20 hr	No
Bebulin	Immuno	Vapor heated (10 hr, 60°C, 1190 mbar + 1 hr, 80°C, 1375 mbar)	Yes
Activated factor IX complex concentrates (inhibitor treatments)			
Autoplex	Baxter-Hyland	Dry heat, 68°C, 144 hr	No
FEIBA	Immuno	Vapor heated (10 hr, 60°C, 1190 mbar + 1 hr, 80°C, 1375 mbar)	No

Abbreviations: TNBP, tri(*n*-butyl)-phosphate.

C. Anti-Inhibitor Coagulation Complex

Anti-inhibitor coagulation complex (AICC) is essentially a prothrombin complex concentrate in which the factors are activated during the manufacturing process. The risk of thrombosis or disseminated intravascular coagulation (DIC) is increased with their use.

1. Indications/Dosage

AICC infusion is indicated for patients with high-titer factor VIII inhibitors (>10 Bethesda units). Its use should be reserved for individuals who are experienced with the product because of its expense and risks. These products are standardized by their ability to correct the clotting time (aPTT) in factor VIII inhibitor patients. The manufacturer's package insert will provide the appropriate dose required.

D. Antithrombin III

Antithrombin III (ATIII) is a naturally occurring serine protease inhibitor which is synthesized in the liver. Patients with hereditary ATIII deficiencies do not effectively inhibit thrombin activation and are subject to thromboembolic disease. ATIII concentrates, which are produced in a manner similar to factor VIII and IX concentrates, are now available.

1. Indications

ATIII concentrates are approved for replacement of ATIII as prophylaxis against thrombosis perioperatively, or as therapy for thromboembolic events. The use of this product is being studied in a number of other diseases that can lead to an acquired ATIII deficiency, including disseminated intravascular coagulation (DIC) (19).

E. Colloid Solutions

Human albumin and plasma protein fraction (PPF) are also prepared by fractionation of pooled human plasma. These products are heat treated, and are generally accepted to be virally safe. Albumin is available as a 5% or 25% solution, in which 96% of the total protein is albumin. PPF is a 5% solution with albumin comprising 83% of the total protein. These products provide volume expansion and colloid (oncotic) replacement in hypovolemic states.

F. Immune Globulin

Immune globulin was introduced as a plasma derivative in the 1950s as an intramuscular preparation as a mode of therapy for patients with a primary humoral immune deficiency. An intravenous form (IVIg) became available in the 1980s to circumvent the limitations of the intramuscular preparation, including pain of injection, limited volume of injections with reduced dosage, inconsistent absorption, and anaphylactic reactions. These products are also prepared by fractionation of pooled human plasma.

1. Indications

Intramuscular preparations are rarely used for patients with hematologic disorders. However, there has been a considerable increase in the number of clinical indications for the use of intravenous immune globulin over the past several years. In general, the indications for IVIg can be listed into four categories (20).

1. Replacement therapy for patients who have a defined inability to make antibody to a specific challenge.
2. Immune system augmentation in patients who have normal or relatively normal im-

mune systems but require additional support because of an underlying condition—for example, to augment the immune response to prevent sepsis in patients who undergo multiple surgical procedures.
3. Immune system supplementation, such as for patients who undergo bone marrow transplantation and whose ability to make specific antibody is compromised by the preoperative regimen, use of other drugs, or viral infections.
4. Immune-mediated disease, which represents the largest group of IVIg patients.

A recent consensus conference addressed many of the issues of off-label uses (21).

G. Rh Immune Globulin

Rh immune globulin (RhIg) is a concentrate of primarily IgG anti-D prepared from selected donors who have become immunized to the D antigen (the major antigen of the Rh system) by transfusion or pregnancy.

1. Indications

RhIg is used primarily as a prophylactic measure against the development of anti-D in Rh-negative patients, especially females of child-bearing years, to prevent hemolytic disease of the newborn. Another use is to prevent Rh immunization in Rh-negative individuals who have received platelet concentrate from Rh-positive donors. The recently licensed intravenous preparation of RhIg has also been shown to be an effective treatment for idiopathic thrombocytopenia purpura (ITP) or thrombocytopenia in human immunodeficiency virus (HIV)-infected patients (22).

2. Dosage

The standard dose of intramuscular or intravenous RhIg is 300 μg, which will counteract 15 mL of Rh-positive red blood cells. A smaller intramuscular (50 μg) or larger intravenous (600 μg) dose is available. Preferably, the dose should be administered within 72 hr of the exposure (or potential exposure) to Rh-positive (or unknown) red blood cells.

III. PHARMACOLOGIC AGENTS

Medications have become increasingly important as an adjunct or alternative to traditional transfusion therapy. These are usually divided into two categories: hematopoietic growth factors and agents to reduce acute blood loss.

A. Hematopoietic Growth Factors

Hematopoietic growth factors are one class of biologic response modifiers (cytokines), regulatory proteins, and glycoproteins secreted by cells that control the biologic behavior of other cells (23). Recombinant technology has resulted in the development of several of these proteins for therapeutic use. Since the dosages vary with each indication, it is recommended that the package insert be reviewed prior to the use of these agents.

Erythropoietin is a glycoprotein produced primarily in the kidney when specialized cells detect reduced oxygen concentrations in the circulating blood. This growth factor works by stimulating intermediate (erythroid-committed) stem cells (both the blast-forming unit-erythrocyte {BFU-E} and the colony-forming unit-erythrocyte {CFU-E}) to induce proliferation and differentiation of red blood cells. Currently, the use of recombinant erythropoietin has been approved for anemia in patients with (a) chronic renal failure, (b) human immunodeficiency virus (HIV) infection on zivoudine therapy, and (c) malignancies undergoing chemotherapy. Many other disease processes are being investigated, including the anemia of prematurity, and in Jehovah's Witness patients. In addition, several studies have been completed to evaluate erythropoietin to increase the number and red cell volume of autologous blood donations.

Two other cytokines, granulocyte colony-stimulating factor (G-CSF) and granulocyte-macrophage colony-stimulating factor (GM-CSF) are commercially available. G-CSF and GM-CSF stimulate myeloid cell proliferation and differentiation, and are used to supplement endogenous myeloid cytokines to reduce the severity and duration of neutropenia following chemotherapy. GM-CSF has been approved for the acceleration of myeloid recovery during autologous bone marrow transplantation for lymphoma, and G-CSF has been approved to treat neutropenia in patients with nonmyeloid malignancies after chemotherapy. These cytokines show marked promise for other forms of neutropenia (AIDS-related, and congenital), and to enhance the recovery of peripheral blood stem cells in allogeneic and autologous donors (14).

The control and prevention of bleeding secondary to thrombocytopenia following chemotherapy has been the primary reason for the extensive growth in the number of platelet transfusions utilized over the past several decades. However, the expense of these products (including HLA-matched or crossmatched platelets), their complications (alloimmunization, infectious diseases), and the logistics of recruiting and maintaining a ready supply of platelet donors are significant issues. A biologic response modifier for platelets has long been postulated. Recently, several groups have identified a polypeptide similar to erythropoietin that appears to stimulate the proliferation and differentiation of megakaryocytes (24–26). If recombinant therapy becomes available in the near future, there will be a significant benefit to patients with thrombocytopenia, and will reduce the burden of increased platelet collections.

B. Pharmacologic Agents to Reduce Blood Loss

DDAVP (1-deamino-8-D-arginine vasopressin) is a synthetic analog of the pituitary antidiuretic hormone vasopressin. This hormone stimulates the release of FVIII:vWF and FVIII:C from vascular endothelial cell storage. DDAVP has been used for mild hemophilia A and von Willebrand's disease, and may have benefit in a number of platelet disorders, including the platelet dysfunction associated with anemia, and myelodysplastic syndromes, among others (27). DDAVP can be administered subcutaneously or intravenously. The therapeutic dosage is 0.3–0.4 μg/kg of body weight, which results in 2–4× increase in factor VIII and vWF. Single doses are commonly used prophylactically or during bleeding episodes. Repeat doses must be used with caution, since side effects, including tachyphylaxis, hyponatremia, and fluid retention can be seen. DDAVP is contraindicated in the rare type IIb von Willebrand syndrome, where platelets have abnormally sensitive responsiveness to vWF.

Episilon-aminocaproic acid and tranexamic acid are synthetic analogs of lysine which inhibit fibrinolysis by saturating the lysine-binding sites on which plasminogen and plasmin bind to fibrinogen and fibrin (28). The drugs can be used both systemically and locally. Their use is indicated for the treatment of fibrinolysis, especially in cardiac bypass operations and liver transplantation. Tranexamic acid is 7–10 times as potent as episilon-aminocaproic acid, and may be most useful as a single bolus agent (10 mg/kg) prior to a skin incision. Caution should be used in patients with DIC, since the coagulation proteins may be activated excessively.

Aprotinin is a proteinase inhibitor with anti-inflammatory properties and additional effects on platelet function. It inhibits plasmin, kallikrein, and trypsin. In addition, it may have some activity against urokinase. This drug has been shown to reduce surgical blood loss significantly during a number of clinical trials, and was recently approved for use in this setting. Anaphylaxis and hypotension have been associated with the use of aprotinin, but the risk of thrombosis appears low (25). Protocols for use may vary, and the package insert should be consulted before use.

C. Blood Substitutes

Since no blood substitute is currently available, only a brief mention will be made here. Stroma-free hemoglobin solutions, in which free hemoglobin (obtained from outdated human or porcine red blood cells) has been separated from red blood cell membranes, must be modified to prevent the significant side effects associated with its use. However, the efficient oxygen-carrying capabilities of this product hold great promise. Several manufacturers have products now in advanced clinical trials. Hemoglobin produced by recombinant DNA techniques is also under investigation. Perflourochemicals have also been studied as a plasma oxygen carrier. It should be noted that these products can only serve to substitute for one function of blood, oxygen transport, and will not replace red blood cell transfusions in most settings (29).

IV. BASIC PRINCIPLES OF TRANSFUSION PRACTICE

Donations are carefully screened by questioning the donor for high-risk behavior and by testing for infectious diseases. However, there is a small risk of disease transmission with most blood components.

All blood components must be transfused through a blood filter.

Transfusions should be completed within 4 hr. Careful attention should be paid to the first 15 min of the transfusion, since most adverse effects will be noted during that time period.

Compatibility testing (crossmatching) is required for whole blood, red blood cells, and granulocyte transfusions.

Type O red blood cells can be released prior to determination of ABO-Rh in an acute emergency.

Since clerical error is the most common cause for incompatible transfusions, rigid blood administration policies should be followed, especially the careful identification of the recipient.

Blood and components should be transfused through a 19g or larger needle (23g for pediatric patients).

Only 0.9% saline should be added to blood. Drugs should not be added.

Blood warmers are available for exchange transfusions, patients with cold hemagglutin disease, and when rapid infusion of cold blood may lead to cardiac arrhythmias.

All hospitals are required by accrediting bodies to develop transfusion guidelines and standards for transfusion practice. This is usually accomplished with the help of the medical staff in a transfusion committee.

V. ADVERSE EFFECTS OF TRANSFUSION

The transfusion of blood and blood components can be an integral part of patient care. However, there can be serious adverse effects associated with transfusion. One method of organizing these problems is to divide them into acute reactions, which occur during or within 24 hr of the transfusion, and delayed reactions, which occur days, or even years, following the transfusion.

A. Acute Transfusion Reactions

1. Acute Hemolytic Transfusion Reactions

Acute hemolytic reactions can be the result of either immune or nonimmune mechanisms. Immune-mediated hemolytic reactions usually occur when incompatible red blood cells are transfused into a patient with a preexisting antibody. These antibodies, usually a naturally occurring IgM antibody to the group A or B antigens, fix and activate the complement cascade, resulting in intravascular lysis of the red blood cell membrane. Free hemoglobin is released, leading to hemoglobinemia and hemoglobinuria. The potent antigen–antibody interaction also leads to other metabolic pathways that can result in serious clinical effects. These include activation of the coagulation cascade, a neuroendocrine response, and release of complement-derived anaphylatoxins and cytokines. The manifestations of these reactions can result in fever, hypotension and shock, bronchospasm, DIC, and renal failure. Table 3 illustrates the management of a patient when an acute hemolytic reaction is suspected (30).

2. Non-Immune Hemolysis

Hemolysis can occur by several mechanisms other than an antigen–antibody reaction, although the clinical symptoms are similar. Mechanical damage can occur because of a mechanical or diseased heart valve, extracorporeal circuit (e.g., cardiac bypass), or other reasons for increased shear stress. Intravenous fluids other then normal saline or other approved fluids can result in osmotic lysis of the transfused cells. Inappropriate heating or cooling of blood can also result in red cell hemolysis. Finally, bacterial contamination of blood during storage can lead to lysis.

3. Febrile, Nonhemolytic Reactions

Fortunately, the fever seen with hemolytic reactions is rarely seen. However, fever responses to transfusion are relatively common. The fever is usually the result of antibodies directed

Table 3 Workup of an Acute Intravascular Hemolytic Transfusion Reaction

If an acute transfusion reaction occurs:

1. Stop blood component transfusion immediately
2. Maintain IV access with an appropriate crystalloid or colloid solution
3. Maintain blood pressure, pulse
4. Maintain adequate ventilation
5. Give a diuretic and/or institute fluid diuresis
6. Obtain blood/urine for a transfusion reaction workup

Blood Bank workup of suspected transfusion reaction

- a. Check paperwork to ensure correct blood component was transfused to the right patient
- b. Evaluate plasma for hemoglobinemia
- c. Perform direct antiglobulin test
- d. Repeat compatibility testing (crossmatch)
- e. Repeat other serologic testing as needed (ABO, rh)
- f. Analyze urine for hemoglobinuria

If intravascular hemolytic reaction is confirmed:

7. Monitor renal status (BUN, creatinine)
8. Monitor coagulation status (prothrombin time, partial thromboplastin time, fibrinogen)
9. Monitor for signs of hemolysis (LDH, bilirubin, haptoglobin)
10. If sepsis is suspected, culture as appropriate

against leukocytes and platelets (5), and the infusion of cytokine pyrogens (8). A diagnosis of a febrile, nonhemolytic transfusion reaction can be made only when other causes of fever are ruled out. The temperature increases ≥1°C, and is often associated with chills. Symptomatic therapy, including the use of oral antipyretics, is usually sufficient. If a patient has recurrent febrile reactions, leukodepleted blood may be useful in preventing such responses.

4. *Urticaria/Anaphylaxis*

Another common response to transfusion is an allergic reaction, with rash and/or hives and itching, usually without fever. This recipient immune response is directed against soluble proteins in the donor plasma. If urticaria is the only symptom noted, the transfusion can be temporarily discontinued while an antihistamine (e.g., diphenhydramine, 25–50 mg, either orally or intravenously) is administered. If the symptoms are resolved quickly, the transfusion can be restarted. Pretreatment with an oral antihistamine can usually prevent such reactions in susceptible patients. Washed red blood cells may be needed in patients who are refractory to these measures. Anaphylactic reactions can occur, with the classic symptoms of a severe allergic reaction, including apprehension, laryngeal and facial edema with respiratory compromise, nausea, vomiting, loss of consciousness, and shock. This reaction is most often seen in patients with a congenital IgA deficiency, but may be seen in other conditions (31). Aggressive treatment of the anaphylaxis is needed, which includes stopping the transfusion, establishing or maintaining intravenous access, and the use of epinephrine. Airway protection and the use of corticosteriods may be needed. Preventative measures should include the use of blood products with the plasma removed, or blood or components from IgA-deficient donors.

5. *Hypervolemia*

Circulatory overload, resulting in congestive heart failure and pulmonary edema, is one of the more common adverse effects of transfusion, usually in elderly patients with compromised cardiac or pulmonary function. Standard therapy may be needed, including oxygen and diuretics. Smaller-volume transfusions, administered slowly, should prevent hypervolemia in these patients.

6. *Transfusion-Related Acute Lung Injury*

Antibodies directed against HLA or neutrophil antigens may be present in the plasma of donors. In rare cases, these antibodies react with the recipient's leukocytes, which can lead to increased endothelial permeability in the pulmonary circulation. Other causes have also been implicated in this reaction (31). Noncardiogenic pulmonary edema can result, with clinical findings such as dyspnea, fever, chest pain, cough, hypoxemia, and hypotension. Respiratory support should include oxygen and/or mechanical ventilation. Corticosteroids may be helpful. These reactions are often self-limited. Prevention involves the identification of an implicated donor, from whom plasma products must not be used.

7. *Bacterial Sepsis*

Bacteria can be introduced into blood during collection (either asymptomatic bacteremic donors, or from skin contamination) or during component preparation and handling. Such contamination is more common in platelet components, which are stored at room temperature, but has been documented in refrigerated blood. The infusion of bacteria and endotoxins can result in a significant, even fatal reaction. Clinically, the patient exhibits a rapid onset of chills, rigors, fever, nausea and vomiting, and hypotension, which may progress to shock, renal failure, and DIC. Aggressive supportive therapy and intravenous antibiotics are required. Meticulous attention to the collection, manipulation, and storage of blood in the most sterile manner is needed to prevent such occurrences.

8. Metabolic Complications

Small-volume transfusions under normal circumstances have minimal metabolic effects. However, rapid infusion of large volumes or massive transfusion (more than one blood volume transfused within 24 hr) can lead to a number of metabolic abnormalities. Hypothermia can occur with the transfusion of refrigerated blood or freshly thawed plasma, which can precipitate ventricular arrhythmia. A significant amount of the anticoagulant sodium citrate may be transfused in these settings, which can lead to hypocalcemia. Hyperkalemia as a metabolic byproduct during storage may occur in patients with renal failure, and rarely in neonates. Dilution of both platelets and clotting proteins can occur during massive transfusion episodes. These deficits should be documented by laboratory testing prior to additional ordering of these components.

B. Delayed Reactions

1. Delayed Hemolytic Transfusion Reactions

Delayed hemolytic transfusion reactions are the result of alloimmunization to red blood cell antigens. These antibodies, either newly developed or from an anamnestic response to transfusion, can become attached to transfused red blood cells. Complement is rarely activated, but these cells are cleared by the reticuloendothelial system. This extravascular hemolysis is usually mild, but can be severe. The patients exhibit mild symptoms such as fever and malaise. The diagnosis is often made when additional blood is ordered for recurring anemia. Acute therapy is rarely required. All subsequent red blood cell transfusions must lack the specific antigen, which can lengthen the time required to find compatible blood.

The alloimmunization to leukocyte antigens and platelet refractoriness was discussed earlier.

2. Graft-Versus-Host Disease

Graft-versus-host disease (GVHD) occurs when viable T lymphocytes in cellular blood components engraft in the recipient, eliciting a severe immune response. This rare complication occurs in immunocompromised patients who cannot mount an adequate immune defense, or immunocompetent patients who do not recognize specific HLA haplotypes. The diagnosis of GVHD is difficult, and the patients exhibit a wide range of clinical symptoms, including fever, dermatitis, hepatitis, diarrhea, and pancytopenia. Unfortunately, most cases of transfusion-associated GVHD are fatal, since no effective treatment exists. Gamma-irradiation of cellular blood products inhibits the T lymphocytes from replication, and thus prevents GVHD. Irradiation is recommended for: (a) blood received from blood relatives, (b) intrauterine transfusions, (c) immunodeficient recipients, and (d) bone marrow transplant recipients (31).

3. Posttransfusion Purpura

Posttransfusion purpura is a rare disorder characterized by a rapid decline in the patient's platelet count 7–10 days following a blood transfusion, with little benefit from platelet transfusions (32). The affected patients are usually multiparous females. A platelet specific alloantibody (usually anti-HPA-la, formerly anti-PL^{A1}) is responsible for the thrombocytopenia, although the mechanism for the destruction of autologous platelets is poorly understood. Therapy includes plasma exchanges and intravenous immunoglobulin.

4. *Iron Overload*

Chronically transfused individuals, especially those with hemoglobinopathies, continually accumulate iron from the red blood cell units (200–250 mg of iron in each unit). Iron deposition in the heart, liver, and endocrine glands will eventually compromise their function. Treatment with desferrioxamine, an iron-chelating agent, is difficult and often unsuccessful.

5. *Transfusion-Transmitted Disease*

Although infectious diseases transmitted by the transfusion of blood and blood components are relatively uncommon, both recipients and physicians view this complication as the most important. An extensive review of this topic is not possible in this chapter, and only a brief synopsis of the significant infections and their current risks will be presented. The process of transfusion-transmitted disease prevention begins with the careful selection of donors, who must answer an extensive list of questions to identify those at risk for disease transmission. Laboratory testing for hepatitis B and C, human immunodeficiency virus (HIV), human T-cell lymphotropic virus (HTLV), and syphilis are performed on a sample from each donation. While these two sections of the screening process have been improved continuously, the risk of disease transmission is not zero; "window period" donations are still a concern, and screening for certain known (and unknown) diseases can be difficult. However, it is clear that the blood supply is now as safe as it has ever been (Table 4).

a. Hepatitis. A number of measures has drastically decreased the risk of posttransfusion hepatitis, including an all-volunteer blood supply, hepatitis B surface antigen testing, the availability of the hepatitis B vaccine, improved donor questioning, and the development of a screening antibody test for hepatitis C.

b. Human Immunodeficiency Virus (HIV). HIV infection (and AIDS) is the most feared complication of transfusion. The devastating effects of this disease has changed the practice of transfusion medicine. First reported in a transfusion recipient in 1982, this disease has affected thousands of patients who have received transfusion therapy. The hemophilia population has

Table 4 Adverse Effects of Blood Transfusion

	Incidence per unit transfused
Acute reaction	
Acute hemolytic	1:25,000
Febrile, non-hemolytic	1:200
Allergic	1:1000
Anaphylaxis	1:150,000
Hypervolemia	1:200
Bacterial contamination	1:1,000,000
Delayed reaction	
HIV	1:562,500–1:825,000
HTLV	1:625,000
Hepatitis B	1:200,000
Hepatitis C	1:103,000
Syphilis	Unknown (extremely rare)
Malaria	Unknown (extremely rare)
Graft-versus-host disease	Unknown (extremely rare)

been dramatically affected, since approximately 50% of hemophiliacs receiving clotting factor concentrates (and, thus, markedly increased donor exposures) were infected during the early 1980s. The donor screening process, including improved testing for antibodies to both HIV-1 and HIV-2, as well as the recently licensed HIV-1 antigen test, have reduced the risk of transmission significantly.

c. Human T-Cell Lymphotropic Virus (HTLV). HTLV-I is a retrovirus that has been associated with adult T-cell leukemia-lymphoma and a neurologic disease termed the HTLV-associated myelopathy (HAM). A closely related virus, HTLV-II, has been rarely associated with HAM. Persons infected with these viruses have life-long infections. HTLV is endemic in parts of Japan, Africa, Brazil, and the Caribbean basin. These viruses are strongly cell associated.

d. Cytomegalovirus. Cytomegalovirus (CMV) infections associated with transfusion are uncommon, but can lead to serious morbidity in premature infants and recipients of organ or bone marrow transplants. Clinically, a number of symptoms can be seen, including pharyngitis, lymphadenopathy, and hepatitis. These patients, and seronegative pregnant females, should receive blood that is seronegative for CMV. Recent data supports the use of leukodepletion by filtration to render cellular components CMV "safe" (7).

e. Syphilis. Syphilis is a rare complication of transfusion, since the phase of spirochetemia is transient, a serologic test for syphilis is done on each donation, and the spirochetes cannot survive refrigerated temperature.

f. Parasites. Transmission of malaria, although rare, is the most common parasite-borne disease associated with transfusion. Other rare parasitic infections include babesiosis and Chagas' disease. Prevention involves the deferral of donors with these infections (or at increased risk for them).

NOTE ADDED IN PROOF

Since this manuscript was completed there have been several advances in the practice of transfusion medicine. Two new plasma products are now being used in some centers. The first employs a solvent–detergent treatment that inactivates enveloped viruses such as hepatitis B, hepatitis C, and HIV (33–34) in a pooled product. The second involves placing a unit of plasma in quarantine until the donor is retested for the standard screening tests at a later date. If the tests are negative the unit is released for use. Finally, the use of a polymerase chain reaction process for nucleic acid detection hepatitis C and HIV is being investigated on a national level in the United States (35).

REFERENCES

1. Perioperative red cell transfusion. NIH Consensus Development Conference Statement. 7:1, 1988.
2. Wilkerson DK, Rosen AL, Gould SA, et al. Oxygen extraction ratio: a valid indicator of myocardial metabolism in anemia. J Surg Res 1987; 42:629–634.
3. Welch HG, Meehan KR, et al. Prudent strategies for elective red blood cell transfusion. Ann Intern Med 1992; 116:402–406.
4. Vengelen-Tyler, ed. Noninfectious Complications of Blood Transfusion. Technical Manual. 12th ed. Bethesda, MD: American Association of Blood Banks, 1996.
5. Brubaker DB. Clinical significance of white cell antibodies in febrile transfusion reactions. Transfusion 1990; 30:733–737.

6. Meryman HT. Transfusion-induced alloimmunization and immunosuppression and the effect of leukocyte depletion. Transfusion Med Rev 1989; 3:180–193.
7. Bowden RA, Slichter SJ, Sayers M, et al. A comparison of filtered leukocyte-reduced and cytomegalovirus (CMV) seronegative blood products for the prevention of transfusion-associated CMV infection after marrow transplant. Blood 1995; 86(9):3598–3603.
8. Muyelle L, Joos M, Souters E, et al. Increased tumor necrosis factor α (TNF α), interleukin 1, and interleukin 6 (IL-6) levels in plasma of stored platelet concentrates: relationship between TNFα and IL-6 levels and febrile transfusion reactions. Transfusion 1993; 33:195–199.
9. Dzik S. Leukoreduction blood filters: filter design and mechanisms of leukocyte removal. Transfusion Med Rev 1993; 7:65–77.
10. Development Task Force of the College of American Pathologists. Practice parameter for the use fresh frozen plasma, cryoprecipitate, and platelets. JAMA 1994; 271:777–781.
11. Beutler E. Platelet transfusions: The 20,000/μl trigger. Blood 1993; 81(6):1411–1413.
12. Poon M. Cryoprecipitate: uses and alternatives. Transfusion Med Rev 1993; VII(3):180–192.
13. Givvle JW, Ness P. Fibrin glue: the perfect operative sealant? Transfusion 1990; 30:741–747.
14. Caspar CB, Seger RA, Burger J, et al. Effective stimulation of donors for granulocyte transfusions with recombinant methionyl granulocyte colony stimulating factor. Blood 1993; 81:2866.
15. Vengelen-Tyler V, ed. Blood Transfusion Practice. Technical Manual. 12th ed. Bethesda, MD: American Association of Blood Banks, 1996.
16. Goldsmith JC. The coagulation cascade and coagulation factor replacement in hemophilia. In: Petz LD, Swisher SN, Kleinman S, et al., eds. Clinical Practice of Transfusion Medicine. New York: Churchill Livingstone, 1996:191.
17. Kessler CM. Factor VIII inhibitors—an algorithmic approach to treatment. Semin Hematol 1994; 31(234):33–36.
18. Lusher JM. Congenital coagulopathies and their management. In: Rossi EC, Simon TL, Moss GS, et al., eds. Principles of Transfusion Medicine. Baltimore, MD: Williams & Wilkins, 1996:426.
19. Kurtz SR. Coagulation factor replacement for patients with acquired coagulation disorders. In: Petz LD, Swisher SN, Kleinman S, et al., eds. Clinical Practice of Transfusion Medicine. New York: Churchill Livingstone, 1996:433–450.
20. Gelfand E. Current status of IVIg therapy. Pharm Therapeut 1996; 21(4S):4.
21. Ratko TA, Burnett DA, Foulke GE, et al. Recommendations for off-label use of intravenously administered immunoglobulin preparations. JAMA 1995; 273(23):1865–1870.
22. Bussel JB, Graziana JN. Intravenous anti-D treatment of immune thrombocytopenic purpura: analysis of efficacy, toxicity, and mechanism of effect. Blood 1991; 77(9):1884–1893.
23. Kruskall MS. Biologic response modifiers—hematopoietic growth factors. In: Petz LD, Swisher SN, Kleinman S, et al., eds. Clinical Practice of Transfusion Medicine. New York: Churchill Livingstone, 1996:1023–1039.
24. Lok S, Kaushansky K, Holly RD, et al. Cloning and expression of murine thrombopoietin cDNA and stimulation of platelet production in vivo. Nature 1994; 369:568.
25. Wendling F, Maraskovsky E, Debili N, et al. c-mpl Ligand is a humor regulator of megakaryocytopoiesis. Nature 1994; 369:571.
26. De Sauvage FJ, Hass PE, Spencer SD, et al. Stimulation of megakaryocytopoiesis and thrombopoiesis by the c-mpl ligand. Nature 1994; 369:533.
27. Schulman S. DDAVP—the multipotent drug in patients with coagulopathies. Transfusion Med Rev 1991; V(2):132–145.
28. Spence RK. Blood saving strategies in surgical patients. In: Petz LD, Swisher SN, Kleinman S, et al., eds. Clinical Practice of Transfusion Medicine. New York: Churchill Livingstone, 1996: 521–537.
29. Spence RK. Blood substitutes. In: Petz LD, Swisher SN, Kleinman S, et al., eds. Clinical Practice of Transfusion Medicine. New York: Churchill Livingstone, 1996:967–984.
30. Pisciotto PT, ed. Blood Transfusion Therapy: A Physicians Handbook. 4th ed. Bethesda, MD: American Association of Blood Banks, 1993.

31. Vengelen-Tyler V, ed. Non-Infectious Complications of Blood Transfusion. Technical Manual. 12th edition. Bethesda, MD: American Association of Blood Banks, 1996.
32. McFarland JG. Alloimmune thrombocytopenias. In: Rossi EC, Simon TL, Moss GS, et al., eds. Principles of Transfusion Medicine. Baltimore, MD: Williams & Wilkins, 1996:426.
33. Horowitz B, Bonomo R, Prince AM, et al. Solvent/detergent–treated plasma: a virus inactivated substitute for fresh frozen plasma. Blood 1992; 79:826–831.
34. Bianco, C. Choice of human plasma preparations for transfusion. Transfusion Med Rev 1999; 13(2): 84–88.
35. Hewlett IS, Epstein JS. Food and Drug Administration conference on the feasibility of genetic technology to close the HIV window in donor screening. Transfusion 1997; 37:346–351.

28

Hereditary Causes for Plasma Clotting Bleeding

Aubrey A. Lurie
Louisiana State University Medical Center, and Overton Brooks VA Medical Center, Shreveport, Louisiana

I. INTRODUCTION

Mutations of the plasma coagulation proteins may be associated with bleeding, ranging from severe and debilitating hemorrhages to mild hemorrhage induced by trauma. This range of clinical manifestation may be correlated, in part, with the concentration of the clotting factor in circulating plasma, and also with the role the clotting factor plays in the coagulation cascade. For example, lower levels of factors VIII and IX functional activity are associated with more bleeding than higher levels, and severe deficiencies of factors VIII and IX functional activity lead to more hemorrhages and are more difficult to control than deficiencies of other factors, indicating the impact of factors VIII and IX on the amplification of enzyme activity required to convert fibrinogen to fibrin (1,2).

The hereditary causes of inappropriate bleeding are rare, yet their impact on health costs, blood transfusion practice, and knowledge of normal coagulation is large. Their study has justified the attention and expense spent, apart from the sociopolitical impact of their management on individuals, society, and national blood transfusion services, and on health legislation worldwide.

Molecular biology advances have contributed greatly to the understanding of the structure and genetics of these inherited disorders (3), as well as in the production of recombinant therapeutic products, or transgenic animals. The hope is that products used for therapy may be produced synthetically, and not transmit diseases nor induce refractory states. It is also hoped that genetic manipulation may correct the abnormal genes to produce normal functioning products.

The most common of these (rare) inherited conditions is von Willebrand's disease, with an estimated prevalence as high as 1% (4), followed by hemophilia A (classical hemophilia; factor VIII:C clotting factor deficiency) and hemophilia B (Christmas disease, factor IX deficiency).

As the prototype bleeding disorder is hemophilia A, the discussion of clinical presentation, diagnosis, and management will center on this disorder, and differences to the others will be described later.

II. HEMOPHILIA A (CLASSICAL HEMOPHILIA; FACTOR VIII:C DEFICIENCY)

Hemophilia A is an X-linked, recessively inherited disorder affecting 1 in 5000 males (5). Because of its rarity, it is unusual for a physician to encounter more than an occasional patient, unless he or she is associated with a specialized hemophilia clinic. Therefore, for optimum management these patients are best treated in specialized centers, where collective experience will ensure adequate therapy with replacement factors, supervised rehabilitation, management of complications, and instruction in and supervision of home or self-treatment programs. Such centers provide genetic counseling and often receive state assistance for the purchase of the expensive factor concentrates.

A. Clinical Presentation

Clinical presentation is correlated with the level of functioning factor VIII clotting activity (factor VIII:C) in the circulating plasma (2). Patients with <1% factor VIII:C (<0.01 μ/mL) are *severely affected*, and hemorrhage easily, often unprovoked. The possession of 1–5% (0.01–0.05 μ/mL) factor VIII:C accords some protection from bleeding, and these patients are considered to be *moderately severely* affected hemophiliacs. This subgrouping is somewhat arbitrary, as these individuals still have severe bleeding episodes. However, possessing >5% factor VIII:C (>0.05 μ/mL) protects the patients from spontaneous or unprovoked hemorrhage, although surgical hemostasis requires >30% (>0.3 μ/mL) factor VIII. Thus, patients with less than 20–30% factor VIII:C (0.2–0.3 μ/mL) may bleed excessively after surgical procedures, unless treated. Nevertheless, these patients are considered clinically to be *mildly affected hemophiliacs*.

In severely and moderately severely affected patients, unprovoked or "spontaneous" hemorrhages occur most frequently into joints, especially the knees, elbows, and ankles (1). Hip and shoulder joint bleeds are less frequent. The knee joint is particularly vulnerable, as it is not protected by large muscle groups and has only its capsule and ligamentous extensions from the thigh to provide stability. Bleeds into knees may occur even during sleep, when patients turn. The elbow joint is frequently leaned on, which may account for its vulnerability. The ankle is a complex and unstable joint, and easily traumatized. Hemorrhages into joints are painful, and may be so even without clinical swelling. This may cause difficulties for the patient, who "feels" that a bleed is occurring but is unable to convince his physician that this is so if there is no clinical swelling. Treatment may be delayed. As each intraarticular bleed is associated with articular damage, the early institution of therapy is one of the advantages of patient self-treatment. A vicious cycle of bleeds, swelling, muscle wastage due to pain and immobilization, further joint destablization, and recurrent hemorrhages may ensue. Articular destruction can be severe, resulting in crippling deformity (6,7). Thus, early treatment is encouraged, usually with factor replacement, despite all of the latter's attendant hazards. Rehabilitation includes initial immobilization, then careful mobilization and muscle-strengthening exercises. Guidance by a physical therapist is useful, and it may be prudent to mobilize under the protection of factor replacement therapy.

Intramuscular hemorrhages also occur frequently (2). These are clinically not as painful as joint bleeds, and a significant volume of blood may seep into the muscle compartment before clinical swelling is noted. As these hemorrhages are not painful, they may be disregarded by patients and attendants, which may have dire consequences, due to compartment muscle compression necrosis or pressure on nerves with consequent neuropraxias in the form of loss of sensation and contracture deformities. Muscle groups commonly involved are the gastrocnemii, hamstrings, and ilio-psoas muscles. Hemorrhages into the ilio-psoas muscles may manifest as lower abdominal pain, which, if occurring on the right side, may clinically resemble acute appendicitis. Loss of sensation on the inner aspect of the thigh may be the only clinical manifestation of an ilio-psoas hemorrhage. If treated early, raising the clotting levels to 20–30% for several days may be sufficient. However, if hemorrhages are large or compromised, higher levels should be aimed for and should be maintained for several days to allow resorption of blood and to prevent rebleeding.

Other sites of hemorrhage may occur, and no site is immune. Hemorrhages have been seen in the throat, chest, abdomen, wall of intestines, testes, kidneys, and brain. Hematuria may be particularly perplexing and resistant to factor replacement (1). Adequate hydration is important, and corticosteriods may help stop the hemorrhage. Epsilon-aminocaproic acid (EACA) should not be used to treat hematurias for fear of causing lytic-resistant clots in the renal collecting system with subsequent renal shutdown. If hematuria is persistent, it may be worthwhile investigating the urinary tract for causes other than the hemophilia. This need be done only if the hematuria is persistent. Analgesic nephropathy may occur if analgesics are abused and was a common complication in hemophiliacs in the past.

Gastrointestinal hemorrhages are unusual (5) and may have an underlying cause, such as peptic ulceration, which is compromised further by the hemophilia. The amount of diagnostic testing necessary should be assessed clinically.

Lacerations, if severe, may require factor replacement besides the local measures applied. Mouth lacerations are common and are managed effectively with EACA or tranexamic acid for several days, after initial factor replacement. One dose of factor VIII infusion followed by 5 days of antifibrinolytic therapy is often effective.

Intracerebral hemorrhages are true emergencies (5) and should be treated aggressively with large doses of factor VIII to raise levels to 50–100%. Thus, any head trauma, especially if accompanied by headache, reduced cognition, or limb weakness, should be managed seriously. Treatment should be instituted before ancillary investigations such as CAT or MRI scans are taken. If these confirm an intracerebral hemorrhage, aggressive treatment to raise factor levels to 100% should be maintained until resolution.

Patients with >5% factor VIII:C (>0.05 μ/mL) levels (mildly affected hemophiliacs) may be diagnosed later in life and only when challenged with trauma induced by sport, dentists, or surgeons. These patients do not have unprovoked hemorrhages and may bleed excessively only after the induced trauma. The sex-linked inheritance is similar to that in severe patients. Interestingly, female carries often have reduced factor VIII:C levels and may be inconvenienced by heavy menses.

Management of patients in the Emergency Room may be problematic, in the event, for example, of a motor vehicle accident, and if the patient knows only that he is a "a bleeder," without knowledge of which factor is deficient or the degree of deficiency. Clinical examination may give an indication of the severity if, for example, swollen or contracted joints are found. Fresh frozen plasma (FFP) should be started until a more precise diagnosis is available. FFP contains all the clotting factors including the von Willebrand factor and can effectively raise factor levels to 20–30%. Higher levels will necessitate factor concentrates. The dose of FFP is 20 mL/kg body weight (B.Wt). FFP is available in most hospitals, whereas the factor concentrates may not be.

B. Pathophysiology

Much progress has been made in determining the underlying molecular abnormalities of all of the inherited bleeding disorders. The structure of the factor VIII gene is now known. The factor VIII gene is large (186 kb and 26 exons) and situated at Xq28 (6). Forty percent of patients with severe hemophilia have an inversion mutation in intron 22 between exons 22 and 23 (5,8,9). Other patients have been shown to have specific point or missense mutations, gene deletions, insertions, or complex rearrangements (10). If the genetic abnormality can be established in a particular family, genetic counseling may be more exact, especially if performed on parental and fetal DNA.

C. Laboratory Diagnosis

The diagnosis of hemophilia A is now well established. A family history of a sex-linked inheritance is useful, but 30% of patients may not have this available, either due to a new mutation, or inheritance through several generations of females with no male expression.

The laboratory diagnosis is made on finding a normal prothrobin time (PT) and prolonged activated partial thromboplastin time (PPT). Factor VIII:C levels are reduced. Important laboratory differentiation is from von Willebrand's disease and so a bleeding time, and von Willebrand assay (ristocetin cofactor), will be normal. Previously, the factor VIII antigen was measured, which is normal in hemophilia A and reduced to levels similar to that of the factor VIII: C in von Willebrand's disease. It is not usual to measure this antigen level nowadays. If the factor VIII:C level is <1%, it is important to screen for a factor VIII:C inhibitor (antibody), as its presence may compromise treatment considerably. The detection of inhibitors together with significant plasma factor VIII:C has been described but is rare.

D. Management

Management is primarily with factor replacement and is dealt with more fully in other chapters. Ancillary pharmacologic agents may be used to support and reduce the amounts of factor replacement products infused. These include agents such as 1-amino-8-D-arginine vasopressin (DDAVP) and EACA or tranexamic acid.

Two considerations should govern the amount of replacement factor given: the type of hemorrhage being treated, and the half-life of the infused clotting factor. For example, in nonsurgical or nondangerous bleeds, the aim of therapy is to raise and maintain the factor level above 5%. As the half-life of factor VIII is 12 hr, the factor VIII level could be raised and maintained to 20–30% by daily or twice-daily infusions, until the bleed is controlled. If caught early, 1–2 days' treatment may suffice. The dose given is adjusted for the weight of the patient. The average response of factor VIII:C infused in concentrate form is 1.5% rise per unit of factor per kg. B.Wt. This can be resolved into an algebraic formula of (Rise × wt/kg)/dose = 1.5 or expressed as dose required = (rise × wt/kg)/1.5 (1). For example, to treat a simple hemarthrosis, the aim is to raise the factor from <1% to >5%. The level usually aimed for is 20–30%. The amount of factor VIII:C concentrate required to achieve 30% in an 80-kg person is 1600 units. In 12 hr this should fall to 15%, at which time the dose may be repeated, giving 800 units b.i.d., or 1600 units infused per day until the bleeding has stopped.

Surgical procedures require higher levels and these need to be maintained above 30%. Using the same formula, a level of 100% would be achieved in an 80-kg patient with 5300 units. In managing patients undergoing surgery, it is important to monitor the response to the infusion given by measuring the factor VIII:C levels pre- and postinfusion. This will ensure that the observed response is close to the calculated response, and will guide the time for, and the amount of, the next dose. Also, monitoring plasma factor levels will determine if the half-life of the commercial factor concentrate is less than 12 hr. If so, the next dose may be given at a shorter interval. Rationalizing treatment in this manner will individualize the treatment to each patient and surgical procedure (2). The factor replacement should continue until surgical healing is complete. Use of EACA to inhibit fibrinolysis may reduce the amount of concentrate required (11), but has the theoretical possibility of being associated with thrombosis.

E. Laboratory Diagnosis of Factor VIII:C Inhibitors

About 10–15% of severe hemophiliacs will develop antibodies to the replacement factor VIII infused (12–14). These antibodies destroy functional activity of the factor VIII:C. They were considered enzyme inhibitors in the 1950s, hence the name. However, they are IgG antibodies, predominantly subclass IgG_4 (15).

The reasons why only a minority of these (factor-deficient) patients develop inhibitors (antibodies) is not clear. Severely affected hemophiliacs are more likely to develop inhibitors than those who are mildly affected, as are the young (16,17). Previously untreated patients (PUPS) may have a higher rate of inhibitor development (17), which implies that repeated treatment induces some immune tolerance. No genetic prediction on who will develop an inhibitor is possible as yet. There are concerns, too, that the more purified and recombinant therapy products may be more immuno-stimulating (13,18).

Clinical suspicion for the development of an antibody to factor VIII:C should arise if a patient fails to respond as expected to the material infused. Also, if the rise to the infusion or the half-life ($T_{1/2}$) of the infused factor is being followed, failure to reach the expected rise, or a more rapid $T_{1/2}$, may indicate an inhibitor/antibody to the clotting factor.

Laboratory conformation of the inhibitor requires factor VIII:C assays be performed on the patient's plasma after a known amount of factor VIII is added. The inhibitor may be time dependent, i.e., take several hours to inactivate the clotting factor, so repeat factor assays are performed after incubating the mixture of patient's plasma with added factor VIII at 37°C for 2 hr. The assay is run in parallel with a known factor VIII:C-deficient plasma without an inhibitor, to which is added the same amount of factor VIII:C.

The amount of inhibitor present in a milliliter of plasma can be quantified. In the United States this is usually done by a calculation decided at a consensus conference held in Bethesda and called the Bethesda unit (12). Although the kinetics of the interaction between the inhibitor and factor VIII:C is complex, quantifying by a widely accepted method such as the Bethesda unit is useful for following the progression of the inhibitor concentration.

The management of patients with inhibitors has two goals (13). The first and immediate goal is to stop hemorrhages or provide hemostasis at surgery. A longer-term goal is to reduce the titer of antibody detected and to induce immune tolerance. Low titers (<3 Bethesda units) may be managed by neutralizing the inhibitor with large doses of factor VIII:C concentrate, or using xeno-factor VIII:C, for example, as a porcine factor VIII:C concentrate, which may have less cross reactivity with the factor VIII:C antibody than human factor VIII:C. Immunosuppressants such as cyclophosphamide or steroids may be given concomitantly to reduce an anamnestic response. Other products used are nonactivated or activated factor IX:C concentrates; plasmapharesis; absorption of the inhibitor on affinity columns, recombinant factor VIIa (rVIIa) (19); or continuous infusion of a monoclonal antibody-purified factor VIII concentrate (20). These more heroic procedures are used with high titers (>10 BU) for life-threatening hemorrhages.

The diagnosis and management of hemophilia A and the other congenital deficiency disorders is not confined to the coagulation laboratory. The lives of severely affected individuals are torrid. They face repeated painful hemorrhages, which result in crippling deformities. Normal activities need to be circumspect, and seemingly simple experiences, such as dental extractions, can be hazardous. There is the constant fear of the development of inhibitors, and of contracting hepatitis C or HIV. In countries with sophisticated medical care, quality and length of life have been prolonged by grouping patients into specialized centers, which are able to provide care by knowledgeable physicians, nurses, physical therapists, social workers, genetic counselors, dentists, orthopedists, coagulation laboratory support, blood transfusion services, pharmacies, and, in the last decade, infectious disease specialists. Replacement infusions in the form of dried concentrates, and prophylactic use, allow hemophiliacs to be fully mobile, and to fulfill professional, business, and social aspirations. The outlook from the 1950s until the 1980s was that the hemophiliacs should consider themselves no worse off than insulin-dependent diabetics, or sickle-cell patients. Then the AIDS epidemic struck, hitting this patient group very severely. In an abstract submitted to the 22nd International Congress of the World Federation of Hemophilia, held June 23–28, 1996, in Dublin, Ireland, I. Walker of the Association of Hemophilia Clinic Directors of Canada reported on the causes of death in Canadian hemophiliacs from 1980 to 1995 (21). In this period, 359 of 2038 (18%) of patients registered died. The causes of death were HIV related (62%), hemorrhages (9%), hepatic failure (8%), cardiovascular (5%), cancer other than lymphoma or Kaposi's sarcoma (4%), accidents (4%), miscellaneous (4%), non-HIV-related infections (1%), and unknown (3%). Of 219 HIV-related deaths, 13 were lymphoma, and 1 Kaposi's sarcoma. Hepatic failure occurred in 46 cases, 41 of whom were HIV positive. Fifty-six percent of HIV-negative individuals were seropositive for the hepatitis viruses. Thus a sophisticated microbiology laboratory is an important commitment in the management of these patients. Similar causes of death were found in U.S. hemophiliacs in a study from the National Institutes of Health (NIH) and the Centers for Disease Control (CDC) (22).

III. HEMOPHILIA B (FACTOR IX DEFICIENCY)

The clinical manifestations of hemophilia B or factor IX deficiency are identical to those of factor VIII:C deficiency, except that the abnormality is in the factor IX gene and plasma protein. This form, too, is sex-linked and shows a correlation between factor IX:C levels and clinical expression (1,2). Laboratory diagnosis is based on finding a prolonged PTT and decreased factor IX:C level. Factor VIII:C and the von Willebrand factor are normal. The other vitamin K-dependent factors are normal as well.

Treatment is with factor IX:C concentrate. An important difference from the factor VIII:C concentrates is that the rise/μ/kg is closer to 1% with factor IX:C concentrates, in contrast to 1.5% seen with the factor VIII:C concentrates (1,2). The half-life of factor IX:C is 24 hr, however, so theoretically, this disorder should be easier to treat. In practice, though, both factors VIII:C and IX:C deficiency states are treated in similar fashion, with concentrates been given once daily, or more frequently, depending on the lesion being treated. Thus, surgical hemostasis may require twice or thrice-daily infusions in the operative and postoperative stages, while hemarthroses may require one dose only or daily doses for a few days.

Factor IX:C inhibitors are rare, and would be detected in a similar Bethesda-type assay.

IV. von WILLEBRAND'S DISEASE

A. Clinical Features and Laboratory Diagnosis

von Willebrand's disease (vWD) is an inherited disorder that occurs more frequently than hemophilia A or B (23). Its biology is complex because the von Willebrand factor (vWF), synthesized in endothelial cells and megakaryocytes, combines and stabilizes, in the circulation, clotting factor VIII (factor VIII:C), protecting it from inactivation by activated protein C or activated factor X (24,25). vWF also binds to receptors on subendothelial collagen and activated platelet membranes. Defects of vWF result both in abnormal platelet function and coagulation (clotting) defects. The pattern of bleeding tends to involve skin and mucus membranes, although if the clotting component is reduced to very low levels, joint and muscle hemorrhages may occur as well, similar to classical hemophilia.

As the understanding of the vWF genetics, structure and function has increased, so has the subclassification of the types of von Willebrand's disease. As many as 28 subtypes were described until, in 1993, a revised classification was developed and endorsed by the Subcommittee on von Willebrand Factor of the International Society on Thrombosis and Haemostasis (ISTH) (23,25). In essence, there are three main types of vWD, based on the pattern of molecular weight (M.Wt.) multimer bands of the plasma vWF detected after electrophoresis on SDS-agarose gel electrophoresis. Normal vWF in plasma separates into many bands of high, intermediate, and low M.Wt. The larger vWF multimers bind platelets to subendothelial collagen.

Type 1 vWD has a normal distribution of M.Wt. bands, but decreased amounts, i.e., a quantitative reduction of vWF. This is the most frequent type of vWD; it is autosomal dominant in inheritance, and is most frequently a *mild* disorder. It is possible that as many as 1% of the population are heterozygous for this deficiency (4).

Diagnosis is made by finding a prolonged bleeding time with a normal platelet count, normal PT, and prolonged PTT due to decreased factor VIII:C levels, usually ranging from 15% to 50%. Factor VIII:C levels are labile in these patients, and assays on specimens taken at different times may need to be performed to detect the nadir of factor VIII functional activity. von Willebrand antigen levels, if measured, are similar to the factor VIII:C level. The diagnosis is confirmed by measuring the von Willebrand factor activity, such as with a Ristocetin-induced platelet aggregation test. Ristocetin, an antibiotic, potentiates the attachment of the vWF to a platelet membrane receptor, glycoprotein Ib/IX. This platelet aggregation test is commercially available. The vWF levels are usually at 15–50%.

Type 2 vWD shows abnormal patterns of M.Wt. bands of the vWF, i.e., qualitative and functional defects of vWF. There are several subtypes: types 2A, 2B, 2M, and 2N (26).

Type 2A vWD is caused by decreased high-M.Wt. multimers resulting in decreased interaction of the vWF and the platelet receptor glycoprotein 1B/IX. Mutations have been described in the A2 domain of the vWF molecule (27).

Type 2B vWD also shows decreased high-M.Wt. bands, but there is increased affinity of the vWF for the platelet receptor glycoprotein 1b/IX. This is demonstrated in the laboratory by an exaggerated response of platelet aggregation to *low* doses of Ristocetin. Mutations occur in the A1 domain of the vWF that normally represses GP1b binding (25). The significance of this type 2B subtype is that, if treated with DDAVP, severe thrombocytopenia may ensue.

Type 2M vWD shows a normal multimer pattern but decreased Ristocetin-induced binding of the vWF with platelet receptor glycoprotein 1B/IX (25). Botrocetin, derived from the venom of *Bothrops jararaca*, also facilitates the binding of vWF to GP1b. The sites of binding for Ristocetin and Botrocetin to the vWF differ. Ristocetin binds to amino acid sequences outside the A1 loop of the vWF molecule, whereas Botrocetin binds to amino acid sequences within the A1 loop. In the type 2M variant, Botrocetin binding of vWF to GP1b is normal, whereas Ristocetin binding is absent.

Missense mutations have been identified in the A1 domain of the vWF. This subtype is difficult to diagnose (26,28).

Type 2N vWD shows a normal multimer pattern but decreased affinity of vWF for binding with factor VIII:C. As a result, factor VIII:C is not stabilized, and has a short survival. These patients, therefore, have decreased factor VIII:C levels, and mimic hemophilia A (29). Inheritance is, however, autosomal and not sex-linked, as in hemophilia A. Mutations have been identified in the FVIII:C-binding domain of the vWF molecule, at exons 18 through 24 (30). Diagnosis is by a factor VIII:C binding assay or molecular analysis. It is possible that patients previously classified as mild hemophilia A may have this subtype of vWD. When the binding assay becomes more available, mildly affected hemophilia A patients should be reexamined (31).

Type 3 vWD is autosomal recessive in inheritance, and is associated with severe hemorrhages of all types (25). Factor VIII:C and vWF levels are very low or undetectable, as are the factor VIII multimers. Joint and muscle hemorrhages are frequent, and if the patient is female, she may have severe menorrhagia. Being female, she may have great problem convincing physicians that she is a congenital bleeder, as most physicians have read or encountered bleeders in males only.

Thus, despite the efforts to simplify the classification of vWD, it is likely, as the molecular mutations are identified further, that the subtypes will proliferate once again.

Also to be considered is a platelet-type vWD (32). This not due to an abnormality of the plasma vWF but rather of the platelet glycoprotein receptors. This variant has been called "pseudo-vWD." In the patients described so far, the abnormal platelet receptors interact more avidly with the vWF. This subtype is detected in the laboratory as an exaggerated response to Ristocetin similar to that seen in the type 2B variant.

Compound heterozygotes occur, which may make genetic counseling as difficult as it is in the hemoglobinopathies and thalassemias.

The use of DDAVP in the treatment of vWD has been of great benefit, as it reduces or obviates the use of plasma products, with all of their potential infectious agents. Most responders to DDAVP will have type 1 vWD, some will have type 2A or 2M, and very few will have 2N or type 3 vWD (23). The dangers of the use of DDAVP in type 2B have been emphasized, although it has been useful in some patients. It is also important, if using factor VIII concentrate preparations, to be sure that those preparations also contain the vWF to stabilize the infused factor VIII. Many purified factor VIII concentrates lack significant amounts of vWF.

V. UNCOMMON HEREDITARY CAUSES OF INAPPROPRIATE BLEEDING

A. Deficiency of Factor II, V, VII, X, or XI

Deficiencies of factors II, V, VII, X, or XI are rare, and are associated with excess bleeding rarely, following trauma or surgery. The reason for this is that patients usually have >10% of clotting activity, and the hemostatic level for these factors is about 10%. Only factor XI deficiency is the exception, in that patients with mildly subnormal levels, e.g., 40%, may have hemorrhages, while others, with low levels, do not bleed (2). Most bleeding episodes follow trauma or surgery, and spontaneous hemorrhages seldom occur. Treatment is therefore fairly easy. If the level of coagulation factor is >10%, it may not be necessary to give FFP prophylactically at surgery. Rather, it is prudent to wait and see whether excess bleeding occurs during or following surgery, at which time FFP may be given. A dose of EACA may be given at the time of surgery to prevent clots from being lysed, although this should be weighed against the possibility of developing postoperative deep vein thrombosis resistant to lysis. Exceptions to the above occur, and the author has encountered patients with <1% factor X who bled extensively; as well as a family with severe combined factor V and factor VIII:C deficiency whose hemorrhages correlated with the factor VIII:C level. Management of this family was achieved by elevating the factor VIII:C to hemostatic levels. Also, patients with factor VII:C deficiency may have a variable expression, with little correlation between factor VII:C levels and hemorrhages, and even thromboses (33).

Laboratory diagnosis is made on finding a prolonged PT or PTT and then confirming with the appropriate specific assay.

Deficiencies of factors XII, pre-kallikrein, or HMW-kininogen are not associated with excess bleeding. Diagnosis is made by finding a very prolonged PTT (>100 sec), which corrects to normal on mixing studies. Specific assays will clinch the diagnosis. No treatment is required.

CASE STUDY

The patient is a 20-year-old female who is referred by a dentist. She is to have a third molar extraction, and noted easy bruising, especially after taking several aspirins for her toothache. She had also bled excessively previously after a dental extraction. In the laboratory, you question her and find that she has always had menorrhagia, and at junior high school was susceptible to nose bleeds. She participated on the swim team. She has one healthy brother with no bleeding problems, but seems to recall a cousin on the West Coast who was a "bleeder."

Question 1. What screening tests would you do?

Answer: The following tests and results were obtained.

CBC and platelet count: normal values, and normal morphology
Bleeding time: 8 min ($N = 2$–9 min)
PT/PTT = 12/34 (N. plasma control = 11.6/25.0)
PTT mix (N + PT) = 26.0 sec

Question 2. What further tests would you order?

Answer:

Factor VIII:C assay (%):20 (N 50–150)
von Willebrand factor activity (%):90 (N 50–150)
von Willebrand multimer pattern: normal

Question 3. What is your diagnosis?

Answer: Carrier for hemophilia A. The decreased factor VIII:C is due to inactivation of the normal X gene (Lyon effect).

Question 4. How should the patient be treated to ensure adequate hemostasis at dental extraction?

Answer: It should be easy to raise the factor VIII:C levels to adequate levels for dental hemostasis with DDAVP, or small doses of factor VIII replacement. For example, DDAVP in the dose of 0.3 μ/kg effects a three- to fourfold increase in factor VIII:C. This should be given 30–60 min before the surgery begins. Specimens for factor VIII:C assays should be taken before the dose of DDAVP and then at the time of commencement of the extraction. This will give information on the response of factor VIII:C to the infusion of DDAVP. The difference between the postinfusion factor VIII:C level and the preinfusion factor VIII:C level is the rise achieved by the dose of DDAVP given. The postinfusion level will indicate whether a hemostatic level has been obtained (>30%). The anticipated response to DDAVP is expected to be a factor VIII:C level of 60–70%. Breakdown of clots may be inhibited by infusing EACA (0.1 mg/kg) after the DDAVP has completed and then continued 6 hr orally postextraction at the same dose for 5 days. Aspirin-containing analgesics should be avoided postextraction. Gentle mouthwashes and soft foods should be given, as is customary after such extractions. Excess blood loss is easily monitored with dental extractions, merely by looking at the tooth socket. No further hemostatic treatment should be necessary.

The patient has an uneventful recovery. Several months later, she informs you that she plans to marry and wishes to know if she is an obligatory carrier for hemophilia A.

Question 5. Is this patient an obligatory carrier for the hemophilia A gene?

Answer: If the male relative has been identified as having factor VIII:C deficiency, then, by virtue of the patient having a decreased factor VIII:C level, she is most likely to be an obligatory carrier. This could be proved by demonstrating the same chromosomal aberration in the patient's DNA and male relative. If that relative is not available for study, an inversion mutation of the factor VIII gene should be sought, as this occurs in 50% of cases (34). The patient marries and presents to you for consultation when she is 2 months pregnant.

Question 6. Is her fetus likely to be a hemophiliac, and what is her management during pregnancy and delivery?

Answer: Amniotic villi fetal DNA should be analyzed by PCR probing for the same chromosomal abnormality of the factor VIII:C gene as occurs in the mother's DNA. The sex of the fetus should be identified. The management of the patient's pregnancy should be the same as for a normal individual. It is expected that the factor VIII:C level will elevate to normal levels during the pregnancy, and that no hemostatic difficulty will occur at delivery, either by vaginal or caesarean delivery. Should hemorrhage be excessive, this may be managed with infusions of FFP, or administration of DDAVP. It should not be necessary to administer factor VIII concentrates.

REFERENCES

1. Duthie RB, Mathews JM, Rizza CR, Steel WM. The Management of Muscular-Skeletal Problems in the Haemophilias. Blackwell Scientific, Oxford, London, Edinburgh, Melbourne, 1972.
2. Biggs R. Treatment of Haemophilia A & B and von Willebrand's disease. Blackwell Scientific, Oxford, London, Edinburgh, Melbourne, 1978.
3. Naylor J, Nichelson P, Goodeve A, Hassock S, Peake I, Giannelli F. A novel DNA inversion causing severe hemophilia A. Blood 1996; 87:3255–3261.
4. Rodeghiero F, Castaman G, Dini E. Epidemiological investigation of the prevalence of von Willebrand's disease. Blood 1987; 69:454–459.
5. Furie B, Limentani SA, Rosenfield CG. A practical guide to the evaluation and treatment of hemophilia. Blood 1994; 84:3–9.
6. Hoyer LW. Hemophilia A. N Engl J Med 1994; 330:38–47.
7. Rippey JJ, Hill RRH, Lurie A, Sweet MBE, Thonar AJ-MA, Handelsman JE. Articular cartilage degradation and the pathology of haemophilic arthropathy. S Afr Med J 1978; 54:345–351.
8. Lakich D, Kazazian H Jr, Antonarakis SE, Gitschier J. Inversions disrupting the factor VIII gene are a common cause of severe haemophilia A. Nature Genet 1993; 5:236–241.
9. Antonarakis SE, Rositter JP, Young M, et al. Factor VIII gene inversions in severe hemophilia A: results of an international consortium study. Blood 1995; 86:2206–2212.
10. Peake I. Molecular genetics and counseling in haemophilia. Thromb Haemost 1995; 74:40–44.
11. Lurie A, Silverman NH, Jackson FR. An approach to dental extractions in haemophilia and related bleeding disorders in children. S Afr Med J 1972; 46:1743–1746.
12. Kasper CK. Laboratory diagnosis of factor VIII inhibitors. In: Kessler CM, ed. Acquired Hemophilia. Princeton, NJ: Excerpta Medica, 1995:9.

13. Aledort LM. Inhibitors in hemophilia patients: current status and management. Am J Hematol 1994; 47:208–217.
14. Aledort LM. A Perspective on Inhibitor Development and Factor VIII Concentrates (Monograph). Washington DC: American Red Cross, 1992.
15. Hoyer LW. Recent Developments in the Study of Inhibitors to Factor VIII Therapy (Monograph). Washington DC: American Red Cross, 1993:5–8.
16. Schwarzinger I, Pabinger I, Korninger C, et al. Incidence of inhibitors with severe and moderate hemophilia A treated with factor VIII concentrates. Am J Hematol 1987; 24:241–245.
17. Ehrenforth S, Krenz W, Scharrer I, et al. Incidence of development of factor VIII and factor IX inhibitors in haemophiliacs. Lancet 1992; 339:594–598.
18. Lusher JM, Salzman PM, Monoclate® Study Group: viral safety and inhibitor development associated with factor VIII:C concentrate ultra-purified from plasma in hemophiliacs previously unexposed to factor VIII:C concentrates. Semin Hematol 1990; 27:1–7.
19. Seremetis SV. The clinical use of factor VIIa in the treatment of factor VIII inhibitor patients. Semin Hematol 1996; 1(suppl 4):53–55.
20. Gordon EM, al-Batniji F, Goldsmith JC. Continuous infusion of monoclonal antibody-purified factor VIII: rational approach to serious hemorrhages in patients with allo/autoantibodies to factor VIII. Am J Hematol 1994; 45:142–145.
21. Walker I. Causes of death in Canadians with hemophilia 1980–1995 (abstr). 22nd International Congress of the World Federation of Hemophilia, Dublin, Ireland, 1996.
22. Chorba TL, Holman RC, Strine TW, Clarke MJ, Evatt BL. Changes in longevity and causes of death among persons with hemophilia A. Am J Hematol 1994; 45:112–121.
23. Sadler JE, Gralnick HR. Commentary: a new classification for von Willebrand disease. Blood 1994; 84:676–679.
24. Girma JP, Ribba AS, Meyer D. Structure function relationship of the A1 domain of von Willebrand factor. Thromb Haemost 1995; 74:156–160.
25. Sadler JE, Matsushits T, Dong Z, Tuley EA, Westfield LA. Molecular mechanism and classification of von Willebrand disease. Thromb Haemost 1995; 74:161–166.
26. Ginsberg D, Sadler JE. von Willebrand disease: a database of point mutations, insertions and deletions. Thromb Haemost 1993; 69:177–184.
27. Rabinowitz I, Tuley EA, Mancuso DJ, et al. von Willebrand disease type B: a missense mutation selectively abolishes Ristocetin-induced von Willebrand factor binding to platelet glycoprotein 1b. Proc Natl Acad Sci USA 1992; 89:9846–9849.
28. Schneppenheim R, Budde U, Krey S, et al. Results of a screening for von Willebrand disease type 2N in patients with suspected haemophilia A or von Willebrand disease type 1. Thromb Haemost 1996; 76:598–602.
29. Nebitt IM, Goodeve AC, Guilliatt AM, Makris M, Preston, FE, Peake IR. Characterisation of type 2N von Willebrand's disease using phenotypic and molecular techniques. Thromb Haemost 1996; 76:959–964.
30. Mazurier C, Meyer D. Factor VIII binding assay of von Willebrand factor and the diagnosis of type 2N von Willebrand disease—results of an international survey. Thromb Haemost 1996; 76:270–274.
31. Miller JL, Cunningham D, Lyle VA, Finch CN. Mutation in the gene encoding the α chain of platelet glycoprotein 1b in platelet type von Willebrand disease. Proc Natl Acad Sci USA 1991; 88: 47–61.
32. Biggs R, Macfarlane RG. Treatment of Haemophilia and other Coagulation Disorders. Blackwell Scientific, Oxford, UK, 1966:245.
33. Triplett DA. Symposium on Coagulation in Clinics in Laboratory Medicine. 1984; 4:234–244.
34. Jenkins PV, Collins PW, Goldman E, et al. Analysis of intron 22 inversions of the factor VIII gene in severe hemophilia A: implications for genetic counseling. Blood 1994; 84:2197–2201.

29

Congenital Platelet Dysfunction and von Willebrand Disease

Jonathan L. Miller
State University of New York Health Science Center at Syracuse, Syracuse, New York

I. INTRODUCTION

Patients who have either a congenital disorder of platelet function or von Willebrand's disease (vWD) are at risk for a heightened bleeding tendency. The initial arrest of bleeding following injury, termed primary hemostasis, is dependent on the adhesion of platelets to exposed subendothelium, with von Willebrand factor (vWF) serving as an adhesive ligand mediating this process. To a very large extent, a quantitative or qualitative deficiency of either platelets or of vWF will produce the same clinical findings. These include easy bruising and an increased tendency to bleed from a variety of mucosal surfaces. Epistaxis, bleeding from oral mucosa, increased bleeding following dental procedures, menorrhagia, and bleeding from the gastrointestinal mucosa are particularly common. Additionally, since vWF functions as the carrier protein for circulating factor VIII, a severe deficiency of vWF or a mutation compromising functionality of the binding site for factor VIII (the Normandy variant of vWD) may also impair secondary hemostasis, resulting in the deep tissue bleeds (e.g, in brain, muscle, and joints) typically seen in hemophilia. Since the approach to treatment will vary enormously according to the specific etiology underlying highly similar clinical findings, a carefully performed laboratory evaluation is critical to successful patient management.

II. EVALUATION OF PATIENTS

A. Initial Clinical Presentation

A patient initially presenting with a suspected disorder of primary hemostasis will typically have experienced one or more episodes of bleeding or bruising felt to be disproportionate to the inciting injury. Other patients without complaints of an increased bleeding tendency may present for further evaluation of a prolonged bleeding time that was discovered in the course of preoperative testing. Still other patients without clear-cut bleeding symptoms, but who are close relatives of patients diagnosed as having vWD or a congenital platelet disorder, may present for determination of whether or not they too have inherited such a disorder.

B. Clinical History

One cannot emphasize too strongly the importance of a carefully obtained, interactive bleeding history. Reliance on questionnaires filled in by patients can result in greatly divergent characterizations of similar degrees of actual bleeding severity. Moreover, due to the often confusing names and actual compositions of many over-the-counter medications, it is not at all unusual for a patient initially to deny taking a nonsteroidal anti-inflammatory agent, yet for a more persistent questioning of the details of all medications actually taken recently to uncover such an occurrence. Since acquired abnormalities of platelet function secondary to drugs having antiplatelet actions are far more common than inherited disorders of platelets, or of vWF, it is critical to try to identify such a possibility very early on in the evaluation. This is particularly true in the case of a patient with a generally negative bleeding history, in whom a prolonged bleeding time was the primary basis for referral. In fact, since bleeding time determinations in individuals without a positive bleeding history have been found to lack predictive value with respect to the degree of operative blood loss (1), it may be questioned whether the bleeding time should even be used as a screening test in patients lacking a personal or family history of bleeding—and thus whether this should form the point of entry for more involved laboratory evaluation. This issue does, however, remain controversial (e.g., see Ref. 2).

C. Initial Laboratory Evaluation

The clinical history provides the single most important guide for developing a laboratory testing strategy in the individual patient. In instances where neither the personal nor the family bleeding history is particularly impressive, and only an incidentally performed bleeding time has contributed abnormal results to the record, only minimal further testing may be in order. This should certainly include a CBC with platelet count, if not already performed. Performing yet another bleeding time test is difficult to recommend in this context; however, if there is reason to believe that a previously performed bleeding time may have been prolonged because of technical error or because of a drug that has since been discontinued, a repeat bleeding time test may sometimes be useful. This is particularly true in those cases where an anticipated normal result may be expected to reduce anxiety associated with the previously reported result.

Unless there is a family history of a congenital platelet disorder, an urgent need for a definitive diagnosis, or an unusual situation in which a subsequent patient visit would be quite difficult to arrange, platelet function studies are often not included at the time of the initial patient visit. By this approach, one has the practical advantage of working principally with citrated platelet-free plasma, which may be readily transported, frozen, and tested subsequently in a batched mode. Platelet function testing, in contrast, requires highly trained personnel to be available to perform these studies at the time of the blood drawing.

In patients presenting with a convincing history of a primary hemostatic disorder, assay of vWF level is ordinarily performed on a plasma sample obtained at the initial patient visit. Both antigenic and functional assays of plasma vWF are performed (see below); additionally, it is useful to perform a factor VIII assay on this sample. In view of the considerably greater effort and expense involved in performing studies of platelet function, as opposed to assay of vWF, together with the fact that the incidence of vWD is far greater than that of the congenital platelet disorders, arranging the testing sequence in this fashion is advantageous. In those cases where a comparable decrease in the levels of vWF antigen and vWF functional activity is observed, vWF attributable to a quantitative decrease in vWF is most likely, and further testing of platelets is unlikely to be contributory. In instances where vWF functional activity appears to be significantly lower than that of vWF antigen, the possibility of a hyperresponsive type

2b or platelet-type vWD may need to be considered; in some instances this may involve further testing of the patient's platelets.

D. Definitive Laboratory Diagnosis and Treatment Management

Beyond the initial evaluation, more advanced tests of vWF or of platelet function, biochemistry, or structure may be required to reach a definitive diagnosis. These are detailed in conjunction with the discussion of individual diseases below. Treatment in most instances consists of replacement therapy with exogenous platelets or vWF, or stimulation of the release of endogenously stored vWF with desmopressin (DDAVP). While of controversial value in an asymptomatic patient, the bleeding time test may be of value for monitoring the response over time to treatment in the individual patient. Additionally, direct measures of vWF level and of platelet functional activity may of course be used to follow the response to therapy.

III. CONGENITAL PLATELET DISORDERS (SEE TABLE 1)

A. Surface Membrane Abnormalities

1. Glanzmann Thrombasthenia

In Glanzmann thrombasthenia, the platelet count is normal, and platelets are normal in appearance on the peripheral blood film. Clumping of platelets may not be observed even in a blood film prepared from nonanticoagulated blood. There is little or no aggregation or dense granule secretion in response to most platelet stimuli, including ADP, epinephrine, thrombin, or collagen. Clot retraction is typically decreased also. Ristocetin, in contrast, does stimulate an initial agglutination response and a normal degree of dense granule secretion.

Nurden and Caen (4) and Phillips et al. (5,6) demonstrated that the underlying abnormality in Glanzmann thrombasthenia was a decrease in the content of surface membrane glycoproteins (GP) IIb and IIIa. In the laboratory this can be demonstrated most conveniently by flow cytometry, using monoclonal antibodies (MABs) directed against epitopes within the GP IIb/IIIa complex (7–9). Although the technique is restricted largely to research laboratories, more precise quantitation of GP IIb/IIIa receptor molecules may be obtained by studying the binding of radiolabeled monoclonal antibodies to this complex (10). Additionally, detailed characterization of the individual chains comprising the receptor complex is possible through a variety of glycoprotein analyses (8,11,12).

Since the GP IIb/IIIa complex functions as a receptor for fibrinogen, the absence or malfunctioning of this receptor impairs the ability of fibrinogen to link platelets together following platelet activation, thus explaining the poor aggregation responses observed following challenge of platelets with a variety of stimuli. A large number of specific deletions and point mutations in the DNA coding for glycoproteins IIb and IIIa have in fact recently been reported (13). Symptomatic patients typically show either homozygous or doubly heterozygous expression of such defects, while singly heterozygous individuals are usually free of bleeding manifestations.

2. Bernard-Soulier Disease

The hallmark of Bernard-Soulier disease is the combination of giant platelets, thrombocytopenia, and a selective impairment of aggregation induced by the agonist ristocetin. Whereas in the case of a deficiency of plasma vWF (i.e., vWD) the addition of exogenous vWF prior to

Table 1 Inherited Platelet Disorders

Major categories	Aggregation pattern in platelet-rich plasma	Release of ATP and serotonin	Inheritance	Other characteristic abnormalities
I. Surface membrane defects				
Glanzmann thrombasthenia	Markedly decreased with all agents except ristocetin (which may show a reversible single wave)	May be decreased with collagen, ADP, and epinephrine; normal with thrombin and calcium ionophore	Autosomal recessive	Glycoproteins IIb and/or IIIa decreased, absent, or functionally abnormal; platelet fibrinogen may be decreased; decreased clot retraction; decreased platelet clumping on blood film
Bernard-Soulier disease	Markedly decreased with ristocetin, without correction by von Willebrand factor; may be decreased with thrombin; normal response to other agents	Decreased with ristocetin (or with the snake venom botrocetin)	Usually autosomal recessive; rare variant autosomal dominant	Platelets appear large on blood film and are frequently decreased in number; glycoproteins Ib and/or IX decreased, absent, or functionally abnormal; decreased adhesiveness to subendothelium or to glass beads; decreased receptor for quinidine-dependent antibodies
Platelet-type von Willebrand disease	Increased with low ristocetin concentrations; uniquely agglutinated by asialo-von Willebrand factor; normal responses to other agents	Cryoprecipitate by itself produces release; normal with other agents	Autosomal dominant	Borderline thrombocytopenia; selective decrease of higher-molecular-weight von Willebrand factor multimers in plasma; increased platelet binding of normal von Willebrand factor
Collagen receptor defect	Markedly decreased or absent with collagen; normal resposne to other agents	Decreased with collagen		Decreased adherance to collagen both at low and high shear rates; may be associated with deficiency of platelet thrombospondin; may revert to normal at menopause

(continued)

II. *Granule defects*				
Dense granule deficiencies (Hermansky-Pudlak, Chediak-Higashi, Wiskott-Aldrich, and thrombocytopenia with absent radii syndromes) or as an isolated abnormality	Decreased aggregation, particularly of second phase, with weak agents; usually normal response to arachidonic acid, calcium ionophore, and high concentration of weaker agents	Decreased	Autosomal (except for Wiskott-Aldrich syndrome, which is sex-linked)	Decreased dense granule content of ADP, ATP, 5-HT, and calcium; increased total platelet ATP:ADP ratio; oculocutaneous albinism and reticuloendothelial ceroid deposition in Hermansky-Pudlak; thrombocytopenia associated with Chediak-Higashi, Wiskott-Aldrich, and thrombocytopenia with absent radii; decreased autologous platelet survival and an increase in platelet-associated IgG is seen in Wiskott-Aldrich syndrome
Alpha granule deficiencies (gray platelet syndrome)	Decreased with all agents	Decreased with all agents	Autosomal	Large, pale-appearing platelets on blood film, accompanied by thrombocytopenia; decreased alpha granules by electron microscopy; decreased cellular content of platelet fibrinogen, platelet factor 4, and platelet-derived growth factor; possible marrow fibrosis
Combined dense and alpha granule deficiencies	Decreased	Decreased		Heterogeneity of granule deficiencies reported

(continued)

Table 1 Continued

Major categories	Aggregation pattern in platelet-rich plasma	Release of ATP and serotonin	Inheritance	Other characteristic abnormalities
III. Defects in signal transduction				
Defects in calcium mobilization	Decreased with ADP, epinephrine; normal response to collagen, thrombin, or other strong agonists	Decreased with ADP, epinephrine; normal response to collagen, thrombin, or other strong agonists		Exact molecular mechanisms underlying defects still unknown
Defects in arachidonic acid mobilization	Decreased with ADP, epinephrine, collagen; normal response to arachidonic acid	Decreased with ADP, epinephrine, collagen; normal response to arachidonic acid		Normal dense granule content of ADP and ATP
Defects in arachidonic acid metabolism	Decreased with weak agents; unresponsive to arachidonic acid but normal response to platelet endoperoxides	Decreased with weak agents; normal response to platelet endoperoxides		Formation of lipoxygenase products from exogenous ^{14}C-arachidonic acid appears to be normal
IV. Miscellaneous				
Isolated disorders of aggregation and release as a concomitant finding in a variety of pathologic states including Epstein syndrome, the May-Hegglin anomaly, Down syndrome, inherited connective tissue disorders, and congenital heart disease	Variable	Variable		Heterogeneity of defects

Source: Modified from Ref. 3.

stimulation with ristocetin restores the aggregation response, comparable improvement is not observed with Bernard-Soulier disease.

The underlying problem in Bernard-Soulier disease is a quantitative or qualitative abnormality in the platelet GP Ib/IX/V receptor complex for vWF. A single mutation in any of the individual glycoprotein chains comprising the receptor can result in a failure of the receptor to insert in the platelet membrane. Specifically, the Bernard-Soulier phenotype may result from either a homozygous or a doubly heterozygous mutation in GP Ib alpha, GP Ib beta, GP IX, or GP V. Additionally, a mutation in the leucine-rich region of GP Ib alpha expressed in an autosomal dominant fashion may result in a Bernard-Soulier phenotype (14,15). Preparation of platelet-rich plasma may be unusually difficult in Bernard-Soulier disease, since the platelets in this disorder are characteristically of increased size and tend to be spun down with the leukocytes. Whole blood flow cytometric analysis may accordingly be of particular utility in the diagnosis of Bernard-Soulier disease (9).

3. Platelet-Type von Willebrand Disease

In the autosomal dominant disorder termed platelet-type vWD, a mutation in GP Ib alpha results in an increase-of-function abnormality of the platelet. In this disorder, only minimal stimulation is required to produce vWF binding to the platelet. In the laboratory, such heightened interaction between vWF and platelets can be demonstrated by stimulating platelets with quite low concentrations (≤0.5 mg/mL) of ristocetin (16,17). In those laboratories where equipment is available for inducing aggregation by imposition of shear force, a lower shear force is required than to aggregate normal platelets (18). Recent studies at the molecular level have identified mutations within the GP Ib alpha chain occurring in a heterozygous fashion in patients with this disorder (17,19,20). Because this disorder in many ways mimics the type 2B variant of vWD (see below), it has also been termed pseudo-vWD (21). Distinguishing between platelet-type and type 2B vWD can be difficult; several strategies for accomplishing this distinction have been published (22,23).

4. Collagen Receptor Defect

There have been several reports suggesting that an abnormality of a platelet collagen receptor might be responsible for a platelet-associated bleeding disorder. Several reports have identified a deficiency of platelet GP Ia in female patients with mild bleeding disorders (24–26). Additionally, abnormalities involving platelet GP VI and GP IV have been described. However, the number of patients characterized to date has been small, and it is difficult to be certain whether the observed glycoprotein abnormality is in fact the key determinant underlying the bleeding disorder. In particular, it is difficult to assess the role of GP IV, since many patients who apparently lack this glycoprotein are actually asymptomatic.

B. Storage Granule Abnormalities

Deficiencies in platelet granule content may occur as manifestations of other disorders. There is characteristically a deficiency of platelet dense granules in the Hermansky-Pudlak syndrome. If giant inclusion granules are seen within the platelet cytoplasm, the possibility of the Chédiak-Higashi syndrome should be considered. In patients who have the sex-linked Wiskott-Aldrich syndrome, there is typically a decrease not only in platelet numbers, but also in platelet size. This disorder is associated with a deficiency in a platelet membrane glycoprotein of 115,000-Da molecular weight. However, it remains uncertain whether this glycoprotein deficiency actually plays a critical role in the pathogenesis of the Wiskott-Aldrich syndrome.

In patients who truly have a deficiency of dense granules, stimulation of platelets even

Table 2 Disorders Involving von Willebrand Factor

	von Willebrand disease subtypes						Platelet-type (pseudo) vWD
		Qualitative vWF abnormality					
	1	2A	2B	2M	2N	3	
Defining attribute	vWF partial quantitative deficiency	↓HMW multimers, ↓function	↓HMW multimers, ↑function	Despite all multimers, ↓function	↓vWF affinity for factor VIII	vWF Full quantitative deficiency	Platelet GPIbα mutations
Most common genetics	Autosomal dominant	Autosomal dominant	Autosomal dominant	Autosomal dominant	Autosomal dominant	Autosomal recessive	Autosomal dominant
Bleeding time	Often increased	Usually increased	Usually increased	Often increased	Usually normal	Markedly increased	Usually increased
Platelet count	Normal	Normal	Decreased	Normal	Normal	Normal	Decreased
Factor VIII	Often decreased	May be decreased	May be decreased	May be decreased	Markedly decreased	Markedly decreased	May be decreased

vWF antigen	Usually decreased	Usually decreased	Often decreased	Usually decreased	Usually normal	Markedly decreased	Often decreased
Ristocetin cofactor	Usually decreased	Decreased	Decreased	Usually decreased	Usually normal	Markedly decreased	Decreased
vWF binding to platelets	Decreased	Decreased	Increased due to abnormal vWF	Decreased	Usually normal	Markedly decreased	Increased due to abnormal platelet GPIbα
vWF multimer pattern	Normal	HMW multimers absent	HMW multimers may be absent	Abnormal structure, but all HMW multimers present	Normal	All multimers markedly decreased	HMW multimers absent
vWF binding to factor VIII	Normal	Normal	Normal	Usually normal	Markedly decreased	Presumably normal	Normal

Source: Modified from Ref. 3.

with strong agonists such as thrombin or the calcium ionophore A23187 will fail to result in a normal secondary wave of aggregation. Lack of released ADP from the dense granules most likely underlies this phenomenon. In clinical practice, however, it is difficult to measure released ADP directly. In contrast, it is relatively easy to measure the ATP that is released from dense granules concurrently with the ADP, using the firefly luciferin-luciferase technique (27), so that measurement of ATP release functions in the clinical laboratory as a surrogate measure for the release of ADP. Definitive diagnosis of a deficiency of platelet dense granule content is difficult, due to the significant adenine nucleotide content present within the platelet apart from that actually contained within the dense granules. This problem has been approached, however, through measurement of not only the absolute amounts, but also the ratio, of ATP to ADP contained within patient platelets. In patients who have decreased adenine nucleotides in the dense granular storage pool, assay of the total cellular content of ATP and ADP reveals a characteristic increase in the ratio of ATP to ADP, since the storage pool ATP:ADP ratio is approximately 2:3, whereas the cytoplasmic metabolic pool ATP:ADP ratio is in the range of 8:1 to 10:1 (28).

A selective deficiency of platelet alpha granules, in which patients have platelets that are deficient in their cellular content of platelet fibrinogen, platelet factor 4, β-thromboglobulin, and platelet-derived growth factor, has also been described. Due to the appearance of these large platelets on peripheral blood films, this disorder is known as the gray platelet syndrome. Platelet function is abnormal with respect to both aggregation and secretion.

C. Signal Transduction Abnormalities

For patients who show a poor aggregation and secretion response to multiple agonists, the first consideration should always be an acquired disorder secondary to ingestion of aspirin or another medication having antiplatelet activity. As discussed above, rare patients may actually have a deficiency of stored granular material. In patients for whom these explanations appear unlikely, a defect in the mechanism transducing the platelet stimulus may be considered. Since the metabolism of the platelet is in fact quite complex, there are a variety of potential defects in this process. This includes abnormalities of the arachidonic acid pathway (29–33), of events leading to calcium mobilization (34–36), and undoubtedly a variety of molecules involved in platelet activation that are still being characterized. Clearly, very few laboratories, except specialized laboratories in research institutions, are prepared to pinpoint the specific abnormality underlying aberrant signal transduction in an individual patient.

IV. von WILLEBRAND'S DISEASE (SEE TABLE 2)

von Willebrand's disease is characteristically transmitted in an autosomal dominant fashion. Rarer autosomal recessive variants have, however, been described. von Willebrand's disease may broadly be divided into quantitative and qualitative abnormalities. A decreased rate of synthesis of structurally normal vWF molecules is termed type 1 vWD. A variety of mutations produce structurally abnormal vWF, constituting the type 2 disorders. In a rough sense, this may be thought of similarly to the thalassemias and the hemoglobinopathies in the context of disorders of hemoglobin. Most structural abnormalities of vWF lead to a decrease of function. If there is a demonstrated alteration of the normal multimerization of the vWF molecule (typically requiring gel electrophoresis to separate the polydisperse-molecular-weight forms of vWF, followed by immunostaining), then the disorder is called a type 2A vWD. If a decrease of function of vWF is not associated with a demonstrable absence of high-molecular-weight vWF multimers, it is termed a type 2M vWD. Rare patients who possess a vWF molecule that binds to platelets under conditions of only minimal stimulation [with low (≤0.5 mg/mL) concentrations of ristocetin, low concentrations of the snake venom protein botrocetin, or imposition of a quite low shear force] are said to have type 2B vWD. Usually these patients will show an absence of the highest-molecular-weight vWF multimers, although by the current classification of vWD, patients who have vWF showing gain-of-function properties are considered to have type 2B even if there is not a demonstrable abnormality of the vWF multimeric pattern (37,38).

Mutations affecting the ability of vWF to bind circulating factor VIII result in a phenotype bearing a strong similarity to hemophilia A, except that the inheritance pattern is autosomal rather than sex-linked. Patients who have vWF mutations of this type are classified as having type 2N vWD, reflecting the first characterization of such a disorder in a patient from Normandy, France.

Finally, the term type 3 vWD has been applied to the most severely affected vWD patients, who have been considered to have a autosomal recessive form of the disorder. These patients are either doubly heterozygous or truly homozygous for severe vWF mutations. They have a markedly reduced or absent level of ristocetin cofactor activity, and vWF antigen may be undetectable. Since these patients additionally have a moderate to severe reduction of their circulating factor VIII levels, they also may manifest bleeding symptoms characteristic of hemophilia.

In the clinical laboratory, evaluation of circulating vWF is typically performed in both an immunologically based assay and in a functional assay. In the former, vWF antigen is determined using immunoelectrophoretic, ELISA, or other methodologies. The functional activity of vWF is usually measured by incubating formalin-fixed normal platelets with patient plasma, adding ristocetin, and then quantitating the extent or rate of the resulting platelet aggregation to give the amount of "ristocetin cofactor" activity. Since vWF is normally complexed with factor VIII in the circulation, assay of the plasma factor VIII level has also proved to be useful in the evaluation of vWD. In particular, a commensurate decrease in the levels of vWF antigen, ristocetin cofactor activity, and factor VIII constitutes the prototypical pattern anticipated in a type 1 vWD, although many patients diagnosed with type 1 vWD may actually deviate appreciably from this pattern. In most patients with a type 2 variant (except the type 2N "Normandy" subtype), immunologic assay of vWF would not be anticipated to result in as low a value as seen in a functional assay of the patient's vWF. While this follows logically for the decrease-of-function mutations, it is a less intuitive finding for the gain-of-function 2B variants. However, due to the increased in-vivo reactivity with platelets of the higher-molecular-weight vWF multimers and subsequent loss of this bound vWF from the circulation in type 2B vWD, patients with this disorder essentially have an "acquired" deficiency in the plasma of these highly active multimers. While the lower-molecular-weight multimers continue to be detected in immunologic assays, these relatively impotent forms of the molecule contribute much less to functional assays.

For patients who have a classic 2N subtype, in which alteration of function exerted by a mutation is restricted to the binding site for factor VIII, both the immunologic and functional assays for vWF may be anticipated to be normal. The hallmark of this disorder, of course, is the resulting decrease in the level of circulating factor VIII. The key features of abnormalities involving the vWF molecule are summarized in Table 2.

ABO blood type considerations may complicate diagnosis of vWD, particularly for mild type 1 patients. The level of plasma vWF tends to be lower in patients with blood group O and higher in patients with blood group AB. Accordingly, individuals who actually possess a genetic defect for vWF may incorrectly be presumed not to have this gene; and conversely, occasional patients whose relatively low level of vWF may be due in part to their group O status may incorrectly be thought to have a genetic abnormality of the vWF gene itself (39). Due to the great diversity of mutations capable of producing a vWD phenotype, tests at the protein level, rather than the DNA level, remain the mainstay for diagnosis of vWD. Modulating influences such as ABO blood type accordingly to make it difficult to sort out such issues at the present time.

CASE STUDY 1

A 19-year-old woman has had a life-long history of easy bruising. When she was younger, she experienced frequent nosebleeds, although these have been occurring less frequently over the past 5 years. Menses have been quite heavy, to the point that they are of concern both to the patient and to her primary care physician. The most immediate concern, however, is an impacted wisdom tooth that her dentist would like to see extracted. The patient was adopted shortly after birth, and virtually no medical history pertaining to her biologic relatives is available.

An initial hemostatic evaluation revealed a normal prothrombin time and a normal thrombin time, but a partial thromboplastin time prolonged 10 sec above the upper limit of normal. A CBC showed a normal WBC; an RBC, hemoglobin, and hematocrit all at or just above the lower limit of normal; and, a platelet count in the center of the normal range. On the peripheral blood film, platelets appeared present in normal numbers, showed a normal size distribution, appeared to exhibit a normal clumping tendency, and appeared to be of normal granularity. A template bleeding time had previously been performed on two separate occasions, and in each case was moderately prolonged at 14–16 min (normal range 2–8 min).

Discussion of Diagnostic Evaluation

From the history, there was strong suspicion of a congenital disorder of primary hemostasis, since epistaxis, easy bruising, and menorrhagia are classic hallmarks of this group of bleeding disorders. The severity of the presumed bleeding disorder remains difficult to gauge from the history as given. In the absence of a need for transfusions, or of experiences such as an episode of epistaxis so severe that a sheet or pillow was literally drenched in blood, one may tentatively postulate that a bleeding disorder is more likely to be of only moderate, rather than marked, severity. Clearly, the opportunity to determine a possible familial pattern of an increased bleeding tendency would be of major value, although it is not possible in the present case.

The initial laboratory data provide a starting point for further laboratory evaluation. Clearly there is not a quantitative platelet disorder. The borderline anemia appears consistent with the patient's history of menorrhagia. The bleeding time is elevated, but interpretation of this must be done with caution, since it is entirely possible that even the prolongation on two separate occasions could reflect the acquired effects of medications, rather than providing clues about an underlying hemostatic disorder. While the patient could not recall whether or not she had taken medications prior to the first bleeding time test, she insisted that she had not taken aspirin, other nonsteroidal anti-inflammatory agents, or, for that matter, any other prescription or over-the-counter drugs for the week prior to the second bleeding time test.

In the screening tests of secondary hemostasis, only the partial thromboplastin time was abnormal. This information is extremely helpful. The observed pattern of results provides no suggestion for a deficiency of coagulation factors participating in the extrinsic pathway or in the common pathway. The normal thrombin time confirms that the patient's fibrinogen is likely to function normally in coagulation. Certainly the combination of a prolonged bleeding time and a prolonged PTT should immediately raise the question of vWD because, since vWF serves both as a participant with platelets in primary hemostasis and as a carrier for the factor VIII that is critical to secondary hemostasis, a deficiency of vWF would appear capable of explaining all the available findings.

A very simple test that can provide considerable power in a setting such as this is the performance of an equal-parts mixture of the patient's plasma with normal control plasma, followed by a repeat determination of the PTT. Due to limitations in sensitivity of the PTT to individual factor deficiencies, a factor VIII level of 50% (50 U/dL) would not typically be low enough to bring the PTT into the abnormal range. Thus, even if the patient had virtually no circulating factor VIII, mixture with normal control plasma (that has previously been confirmed to have a factor VIII level of approximately 100%) should correct the PTT. If the PTT of the mixture is no more than 5 sec longer than that of the normal control plasma itself, mixing may be said to have corrected the abnormality. Conversely, if this degree of correction is not observed, then the possibility of an inhibitor should be considered.

When a PTT mixing test as described above was performed on the patient's plasma, virtually no correction was observed. The PTT remained 9 sec beyond that of the upper limit of the normal range, and in fact 15 sec beyond that of the normal control plasma itself.

It is important to consider what this new information did and did not imply about the pathogenesis of the patient's presumed bleeding disorder. Although some sort of circulating inhibitor of coagulation did appear to be present, this would not at all eliminate the original hypothesis of vWD. Thus, although one must always strive to find the fewest explanations that will satisfy all of the clinical and laboratory observations, one must constantly remember that multiple processes may be operative. While investigation of a possible vWD diagnosis remained central to the evaluation, it became necessary also to characterize the inhibitory factor in the patient's plasma.

Evaluation of the vWF/factor VIII complex was undertaken on the patient's plasma. A Laurell "rocket" immunoelectrophoretic analysis revealed a significant decrease, to 24 U/dL. Functional activity of this vWF was assayed at 28 U/dL by the ristocetin cofactor assay, in which the patient's plasma vWF is used to support the aggregation of formalin-fixed normal platelets. Performance of the factor VIII assay was less straightforward, with a significant deviation from linearity with the control plasma at all but the greatest dilutions of patient plasma; at these latter dilutions, however, the factor VIII activity did appear to be in the 25–35 U/dL range. A confirmatory chromogenic factor VIII assay gave a value of 27 U/dL. On a return visit, platelet-rich plasma was obtained from the patient, and ristocetin-induced platelet aggregation (RIPA) was studied using ristocetin concentrations ranging from 0.5 to 1.2 mg/mL. There was no aggregation in response to 0.5 mg/mL ristocetin (normal findings), and suboptimal responses to 0.9, 1.0, and 1.2 mg/mL ristocetin. The addition of exogenous vWF (in the form of cryoprecipitate) prior to the addition of the 1.2 mg/mL ristocetin concentration fully normalized the aggregation response.

A platelet neutralization procedure in which previously activated platelets are substituted for exogenous phospholipid resulted in significant shortening of the PTT, consistent with the possibility of a lupus-like anticoagulant. The hexagonal phase phospholipid neutralization assay also gave results consistent with the presence of a lupus-like anticoagulant.

Based on all the available data, a reasonable diagnosis would be that this patient does in fact have vWD, most likely a type 1. She additionally probably has a lupus-like anticoagulant. Unlike asymptomatic patients in whom a lupus-like anticoagulant may readily be diagnosed, the situation is a little more complicated here, since the patient does present with a positive bleeding history. Clearly, one would not want to miss the diagnosis of an inhibitor that, unlike a lupus-like anticoagulant, might be capable of impairing in-vivo hemostasis. The available data, however, do appear to support the conclusion that this patient's bleeding tendency may quite reasonably be explained by her decreased level of vWF and of factor VIII.

In preparation for oral surgery, the patient was given a trial administration of desmopressin (DDAVP). Prior to and at 90 min following the DDAVP administration, a bleeding time test was performed, and blood was drawn for coagulation studies. The baseline bleeding time was once again prolonged at 15 min. It did, however, shorten to 9 min following the DDAVP. The factor VIII level rose approximately threefold, to 81 U/dL. The vWF measured either immunologically or functionally rose approximately 2.5-fold, into the low-normal range. The platelet count did not show significant change in response to the DDAVP. These results clearly demonstrated the usefulness of DDAVP in this patient, and provided further support for an underlying vWF deficiency, rather than an inhibitor, being responsible for the decreased factor VIII level. A similar administration of DDAVP was employed in conjunction with extraction of the patient's wisdom tooth. Very little bleeding was observed, and the patient's recovery was uneventful.

The question did arise in the course of the evaluation of whether or not to pursue further studies, such as vWF multimeric analysis, in order to obtain a more definitive characterization of vWD subtype. In view of the commensurate decrease of all assayed components of the vWF/factor VIII complex, type 1 vWD appeared most likely. Even if the patient did have a qualitative abnormality of vWF, treatment would not have differed, particularly since the RIPA study excluded the possibility of a type 2B increase-of-function subtype. The patient was informed that she did carry a diagnosis of vWD, and that this disorder was most likely to follow an autosomal dominant pattern of transmission. She continues to be seen regularly by her primary care physician.

CASE STUDY 2

A 52-year-old man has had a life-long history of easy bruising. As a child, he recalls excessive bleeding following relatively minor cuts and scratches, and nosebleeds often requiring more than 30 min to stop. The epistaxis was bilateral, and was treated multiple times by cauterization. The patient frequently experiences bleeding of the gums in association with tooth brushing, and occasionally even from eating. Gastrointestinal bleeding has been documented, and colonoscopy is planned. The patient relates that he has had a blood transfusion at least one time in the past, in conjunction with orthopedic surgery performed on his ankle. Neither of his parents, nor any of his three sisters, are known to have had a significant bleeding disorder. At the time of his visit, the patient stated that he had refrained from taking any medications for the past week. In response to a series of follow-up questions, he specifically denied having taken aspirin, other nonsteroidal anti-inflammatory agents, or any of a series of agents known to have antiplatelet activity.

Hemostatic evaluation in the laboratory revealed a prothrombin time, partial thromboplastin time, and thrombin time all well within their respective normal reference intervals. The platelet count was in the lower normal range, at 189,000/μL, and the mean platelet volume was normal. Platelets appeared normal in number, size, and granularity on the peripheral blood film, although the degree of platelet clumping was noted to be only minimal. In a template bleeding time study, bleeding had still not stopped at either of two sites at 20 min following the initial incisions.

Discussion of Diagnostic Evaluation

This gentleman presents with an impressive history of excessive bleeding that emphasizes, although is not necessarily restricted to, bleeding from mucosal surfaces. The past transfusion requirement is noteworthy, although without more detail as to the extent of bleeding that may have occurred in relationship to the degree of tissue injury, this information remains difficult to interpret. The apparently life-long history of bleeding certainly suggests a congenital disorder. The available family history, however, appears to exclude any autosomal-dominant bleeding diathesis.

The most striking finding in the initial laboratory studies was the prolonged bleeding time. When queried as to any possible technical artifacts or other circumstances that might have contributed to the results, a highly experienced medical technologist who had performed the test confirmed that no technical problems had arisen in conjunction with this test, and that the reported results did appear to be valid.

Although the platelets appeared to show less than the usual amount of clumping on the peripheral blood film, this observation alone is fairly subjective, and is really not sufficient to identify the underlying problem as a platelet disorder. The normal appearance of individual platelets on the smear certainly make a gray platelet syndrome unlikely. Moreover, the normal platelet count, together with a normal mean platelet volume and normal size appearance of platelets on the peripheral blood film, are not suggestive of Bernard-Soulier disease. Glanzmann thrombasthenia deserves further diagnostic consideration, as do other disorders of platelet structure or function. While vWD remains a diagnostic possibility, the family history does not suggest that this would be of the usual autosomal dominant variety. The possibility of an autosomal-recessive type 3 vWD may essentially be excluded, since in this disorder the virtual absence of circulating vWF leads in turn to a severe deficiency of factor VIII, which would have resulted in a significant prolongation of the partial thromboplastin time.

Additional laboratory studies were undertaken. von Willebrand factor assayed both immunologically and functionally, as ristocetin cofactor activity, was well within the normal reference interval. These findings effectively eliminated a diagnosis of vWD.

Platelet lumi-aggregation studies were performed. As may be seen in Fig. 1, addition of a variety of agonists to the platelet-rich plasma (PRP) of a normal individual results in increased light transmission, which is reflected by a downward deflection in the aggregation channel (upper tracing in each panel). Stimulation of platelet secretion results in the release of ATP from the platelet's dense granules. This released ATP then reacts with firefly luciferin and luciferase present in the cuvet in a light-emitting reaction. This light is detected by a second photodetector operating at a wavelength different from that used in the aggregation channel. ATP release is accordingly represented by an upward deflection in the secretion channel (lower tracing in each panel). At the end of each run, a known amount of ATP has been added to the cuvet, providing an internal standard for the secretion channel that may be used in quantitative determinations of the amount of ATP released.

Comparison of the lumi-aggregation patterns observed with PRP from the patient (Fig.2) with the normal series of responses seen in Fig. 1 is informative. The weak agonists ADP and epinephrine are observed to produce virtually no aggregation or secretion. In the case of the stronger agonists collagen, arachidonic acid, calcium ionophore, and thrombin, there is consistently only a very diminutive aggregation response, although an appreciable secretory response is in fact observed. The only agonist that produces a brisk and full aggregatory response is ristocetin at moderate (0.9 mg/mL) and high (1.5 mg/mL) concentrations. (The lack of an aggregatory response to the low (0.5 mg/mL) ristocetin concentration is a normal finding.)

These platelet function studies clearly confirm the absence of Bernard-Soulier disease, in

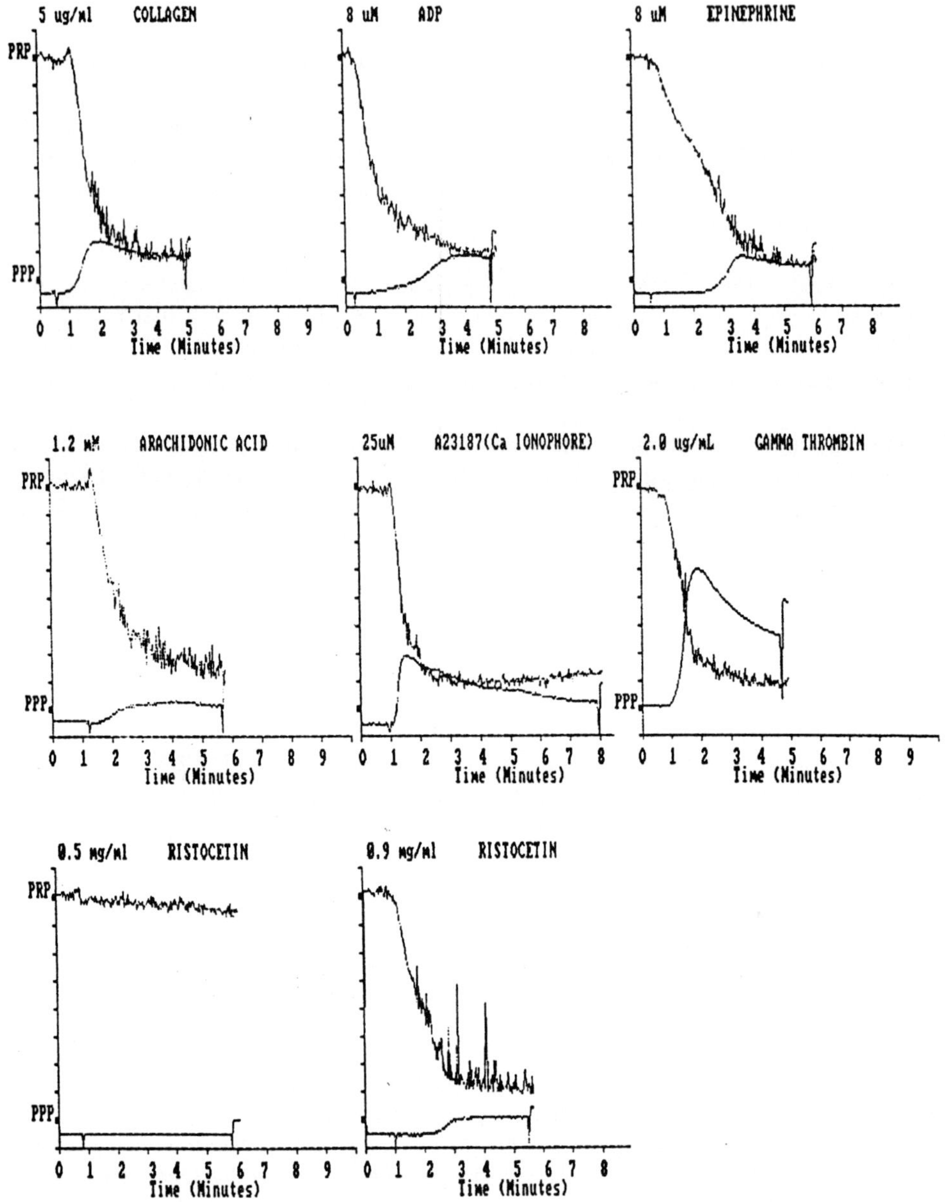

Figure 1 Normal platelet function studies.

view of the strong responses to ristocetin. The observed ATP secretion in response to a variety of strong agonists argues against an underlying dense granual storage pool disorder. Moreover, the ability of arachidonic acid to stimulate dense granule secretion provides laboratory confirmation that the patient indeed did not recently ingest aspirin or other medications capable of inhibiting the arachidonic acid pathway. What does emerge from these studies is a pattern in which virtually all platelet agonists—except ristocetin—produce little or no aggregation,

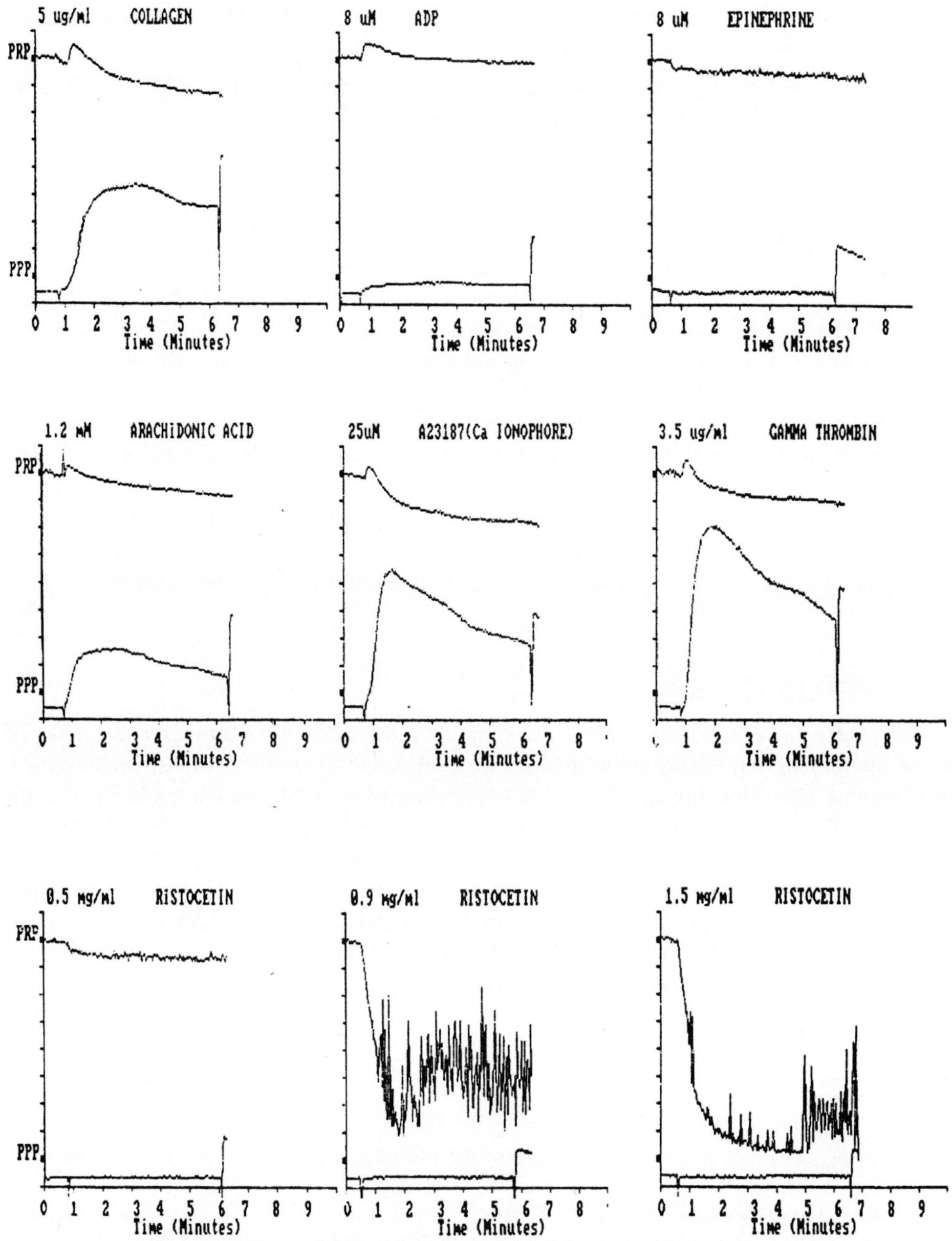

Figure 2 Case 2: Patient's platelet function studies.

accompanied by platelet secretion in response to the stronger agonists. This pattern is virtually diagnostic of Glanzmann thrombasthenia.

Clot retraction at 4 hr after blood clotting was also observed to be only minimal, consistent with Glanzmann thrombasthenia. While it was not performed on this patient, flow cytometry would certainly be anticipated to show a marked decrease in the surface expression of the platelet glycoprotein IIb/IIIa complex, but a normal complement of other platelet markers.

Since Glanzmann thrombasthenia follows an autosomal-recessive transmission pattern, it is not unreasonable that neither of the patient's parents was identified as having a clinical bleeding diathesis. Assuming that the patient has in fact inherited one abnormal gene from each of his parents, and that inheriting only one of these defective genes does not produce bleeding symptoms, then each of the patient's sisters would have a 25% chance of inheriting two normal genes, a 50% chance of inheriting only one affected gene (yet still being asymptomatic), and only a 25% chance of inheriting the two abnormal genes associated with expression of the Glanzmann thrombasthenia phenotype.

The transfusion of normal platelets may be necessary to arrest the bleeding associated with serious injury or major surgery. The decision to transfuse platelets must, however, be balanced by the concern that the normal platelets may elicit an immunologic response by the patient against epitopes within glycoprotein IIb/IIIa that are absent in his own platelets, since effective treatment becomes much more difficult following the formation of such antibodies.

NOTE ADDED IN PROOF

Of particular note since this manuscript was completed, there has been an increased effort on the part of equipment manufacturers to provide instruments to serve as an in vitro replacement for the venerable skin bleeding time test, while avoiding the complexities associated with the more involved functional studies of platelets and of von Willebrand factor. Instruments are now being introduced accordingly for testing in clinical laboratories in which patient blood is drawn and then perfused through a variety of different chambers, where it is subjected to shear stress and/or platelet agonists. Both quantitative and qualitative abnormalities of platelets and of von Willebrand factor may be detected by this approach, thus potentially providing a new in vitro screen for disorders of primary hemostasis.

REFERENCES

1. Rodgers RPC, Levin J. A critical reappraisal of the bleeding time. Semin Thromb Hemost 1990; 16:1–20.
2. Bowie EJW, Owen CA Jr. Clinical and laboratory diagnosis of hemorrhagic disorders. In: Ratnoff OD, Forbes CD, eds. Disorders of Hemostasis. 3d ed. Philadelphia: Saunders, 1996:53–78.
3. Miller JL. Blood platelets. In: Henry JB, ed. Clinical Diagnosis and Management by Laboratory Methods. 19th ed. Philadelphia: Saunders, 1996:701–718.
4. Nurden AT, Caen JP. An abnormal platelet glycoprotein pattern in three cases of Glanzmann's thrombasthenia. Br J Haematol 1974; 28:253–260.
5. Phillips DR, Jenkins CSP, Lüscher EF, Larrieu MJ. Molecular differences of exposed surface proteins on thrombasthenic platelet plasma membranes. Nature 1975; 257:599–600.
6. Phillips DR, Agin PP. Platelet membrane defects in Glanzmann's thrombasthenia. Evidence for decreased amounts of two major glycoproteins. J Clin Invest 1977; 60:535–545.
7. Montgomery RR, Kunicki TJ, Taves C, Pidard D, Corcoran M. Diagnosis of Bernard-Soulier syn-

drome and Glanzmann's thrombasthenia with a monoclonal assay on whole blood. J Clin Invest 1983; 71:385–389.
8. Kempfer AC, Frontroth JP, Lazzari MA. Visualization of platelet glycoproteins Ib and IIIa by immunoenzymatic stain using avidin-biotin peroxidase complex. Thromb Res 1991; 64:395–404.
9. Michelson AD. Flow cytometry: a clinical test of platelet function. Blood 1996; 87:4925–4936.
10. Scudder LE, Kalomiris EL, Coller BS. Preparation and functional characterization of monoclonal antibodies against glycoprotein Ib. Meth Enzymol 1992; 215:295–311.
11. George JN, Nurden AT, Phillips DR. Molecular defects in interactions of platelets with the vessel wall. N Engl J Med 1984; 311:1084–1098.
12. Catimel B, Parmentier S, Leung LLK, et al. Separation of important new platelet glycoproteins (GPIa, GPIc, GPIc*, GPIIa and GMP-140) by f.p.l.c. Characterization by monoclonal antibodies and gas-phase sequencing. Biochem J 1991; 279:419–425.
13. Coller BS. Hereditary qualitative platelet disorders. In: Beutler E, Lichtman MA, Coler BS, et al., eds. Williams Hematology. 5th ed. New York: McGraw-Hill, 1995:1364–1385.
14. Miller JL, Lyle VA, Cunningham D. Mutation of leucine-57 to phenylalanine in a platelet glycoprotein Ib alpha leucine tandem repeat occurring in patients with an autosomal dominant variant of Bernard-Soulier disease. Blood 1992; 79:439–446.
15. Ware J. Russell SR, Marchese P, et al. Point mutation in a leucine-rich repeat of platelet glycoprotein Ib alpha resulting in the Bernard-Soulier syndrome. J Clin Invest 1993; 92:1213–1220.
16. Miller JL, Castella A. Platelet-type von Willebrand's disease: characterization of a new bleeding disorder. Blood 1982; 60:790–794.
17. Miller JL. Platelet-type von Willebrand disease. Thromb Haemost 1996; 75:865–869.
18. Murata M, Fukuyama M, Satoh K, et al. Low shear stress can initiate von Willebrand factor-dependent platelet aggregation in patients with type IIB and platelet-type von Willebrand disease. J Clin Invest 1993; 92:1555–1558.
19. Miller JL, Cunningham D, Lyle VA, et al. Mutation in the gene encoding platelet glycoprotein Ibα in platelet-type von Willebrand disease. Proc Natl Acad Sci USA 1991; 88:4761–4765.
20. Russell SD, Roth GJ. Pseudo-von Willebrand disease: a mutation in the platelet glycoprotein Ibα bene associated with a hyperactive surface receptor. Blood 1993; 81:1787–1791.
21. Weiss HJ, Meyer D, Rabinowitz R, et al. Pseudo von Willebrand's disease: an intrinsic platelet defect with aggregation by unmodified human factor VIII/von Willebrand factor and enhanced adsorption of its high-molecular-weight multimers. N Engl J Med 1982; 306:326–333.
22. Miller JL. Sorting out heightened interactions between platelets and von Willebrand factor: "IIB or not IIB?" is becoming an increasingly answerable question in the molecular era. Am J Clin Pathol 1991; 96:681–683.
23. Scott JP, Montgomery RR. The rapid differentiation of type IIb von Willebrand's disease from platelet-type (pseudo-) von Willebrand's disease by the "neutral" monoclonal antibody binding assay. Am J Clin Pathol 1991; 96:723–728.
24. Nieuwenhuis HK, Akkerman JW, Houdijk WP, Sixma JJ. Human blood platelets showing no response to collagen fail to express surface glycoprotein Ia. Nature 1985; 318:470–472.
25. Nieuwenhuis HK, Sakariassen KS, Houdijk PM, Nievelstein PFEM, Sixma JJ. Deficiency of platelet membrane glycoprotein Ia associated with a decreased platelet adhesion to subendothelium: a defect in platelet spreading. Blood 1986; 68:692–695.
26. Kehrel B, Balleisen L, Kokott R, et al. Deficiency of intact thrombospondin and membrane glycoprotein Ia in platelets with defective collagen-induced aggregation and spontaneous loss of disorder. Blood 1988; 71:1074–1078.
27. Miller JL. Platelet function testing: an improved approach utilizing lumi-aggregation and an interactive computer system. Am J Clin Pathol 1984; 81:471–476.
28. Weiss HJ. Inherited abnormalities of platelet granules and signal transduction. In: Colman RW, Hirsh J, Marder VJ, Salzman EW, eds. Hemostasis and Thrombosis. 3d ed. Philadelphia: Lippincott, 1994:673–684.
29. Nichols WL, Didisheim P, Gerrard JM. Qualitative platelet disorders. In: Pollar L, ed. Recent Advances in Blood Coagulation—3. New York: Churchill Livingstone, 1981:41–80.

30. Defreyn G, Machin SJ, Carreras LO, et al. Familial bleeding tendency with partial platelet thromboxane synthetase deficiency: reorientation of cyclic endoperoxide metabolism. Br J Haematol 1981; 49:29–41.
31. Wu KK, Minkoff IM, Rossi EC, et al. Hereditary bleeding disorder due to a primary defect in platelet release reaction. Br J Haematol 1981; 47:241–249.
32. Mestel F, Oetliker O, Beck E, et al. Severe bleeding associated with defective thromboxane synthetase [letter]. Lancet 1980; 1:157.
33. Rao AK, Koike K, Willis J. Platelet secretion defect associated with impaired liberation of arachidonic acid and normal myosin light chain phosphorylation. Blood 1984; 64:914–921.
34. Lages B, Malmsten C, Weiss HJ, et al. Impaired platelet response to thromboxane-A2 and defective calcium mobilization in a patient with a bleeding disorder. Blood 1981; 57:545–552.
35. Hardisty RM, Machin SJ, Nokes TJC, et al. A new congenital defect of platelet secretion: impaired responsiveness of the platelets to cytoplasmic free calcium. Br J Haematol 1983; 53:543–557.
36. Rao AK, Kowalska MA, Disa J. Impaired cytoplasmic ionized calcium mobilization in inherited platelet secretion defects. Blood 1989; 74:664–672.
37. Sadler JE, Gralnick HR. A new classification for von Willebrand disease. Blood 1994; 84:676–679.
38. Sadler JE. A revised classification of von Willebrand disease. For the subcommittee on von Willebrand factor of the scientific and standardization committee of the International Society on Thrombosis and Haemostasis. Thromb Haemost 1994; 71:520–525.
39. Gill JC, Endres-Brooks J, Bauer PJ, et al. The effect of ABO blood group on the diagnosis of von Willebrand disease. Blood 1987; 69:1691–1695.

30

Acquired Bleeding Disorders Associated with Disease and Medications

William A. Rock, Jr.
University of Mississippi Medical Center, Jackson, Mississippi

Sue D. Walker
Hattiesburg Clinic, Hattiesburg, Mississippi

I. INTRODUCTION

Acquired bleeding disorders are the most common causes for bleeding. There are obviously many classifications and categories of mechanisms depending on interest and usefulness. This chapter reviews some of the more common causes of acquired bleeding. These are the more frequent causes seen in our experience in a large metropolitan hospital. This list makes no pretension to be complete. However, the same basic principles of analyzing patient processes can be applied to almost any situation.

II. ACQUIRED BLEEDING DISORDERS RELATED TO DISEASE

Acquired bleeding disorders related to disease processes are difficult to diagnose in many instances, and even when categorized as to etiology represent one of the more difficult groups to manage. This discussion addresses five of the more prevailing disease processes associated with bleeding problems. This group includes liver disease, renal failure, disseminated intravascular coagulation, cancer, and naturally occurring inhibitors associated with bleeding.

A. Liver Disease

The many mechanisms for bleeding as a consequence of liver disease are difficult to identify correctly and even more difficult to manage. This discussion concentrates on the frequently seen liver diseases such as cirrhosis, viral hepatitis, and poisoning. Conceptually, bleeding in patients with cirrhosis, viral hepatitis, or poisoning is an acute or chronic process. The absent coagulation components are the consequence of the loss of functioning hepatocytes, which means no production of clotting substances or disposal of procoagulants, activators, or metabolic debris. In addition, there can be disruption of the vascular system of the stomach and adjacent structures, as is seen in acute gastritis or ruptured esophageal varices.

1. Hepatitis, Acute Poisoning, and Cirrhosis

Bleeding in patients with liver disease presents many complex alterations of hemostasis. The main alterations are listed in Table 1, together with those tests frequently used to document or quantitate their presence. The acute or chronic liver disease manifestations have mechanisms which are common and mechanisms which are different from each other. The common features include loss of clotting/inhibitor substances, and acute gastritis, and the different features include increased portal pressure, varices, and limited recovery potential of hepatocytes. Nonunique complicating situations such as medications such as aspirin, nonsteroidal anti-inflammatory drugs (NSAIDs), or heparin, and sepsis or renal failure, will make diagnosis and management more difficult (1–7).

Conventional wisdom concerning the treatment of bleeding in liver disease is usually based on two major provisos. The patient with acute viral hepatitis, acute poisoning, or liver cirrhosis is bleeding, has a low hematocrit and abnormal routine coagulation studies such as PT and PTT, and thrombocytopenia. In addition, (a) the patient is bleeding because the coagulation studies are abnormal, or (b) the bleeding is from a vascular tear and is increased due to the coagulation abnormalities. With this common approach there is an implied medical indication to replace any red cell, platelet, or clotting factor deficiency. This results in the persistent use of blood and blood component therapy, often without an achievable goal. To better define the dynamics of bleeding in liver disease, each of the elements involved are reviewed (Tables 1 and 2). In addition, there is a review of the selection of laboratory tests to better define the disease, the risk for bleeding, and the management decisions (Tables 3–5). The parameters which characterize bleeding in these patients are most frequently abnormalities in the vasculature, platelets, plasma clotting proteins, fibrinolysis, inhibitors, and activated procoagulants (8). Diurnal variation in bleeding from esophageal varices (at 0800 and 2000 hr) is a characteristic unique to cirrhosis that may have an influence on success of therapy (9).

a. Vasculature Dysfunction.

i. Mechanism: Vascular damage may result from poor nutrition, excess estrogen, toxic effects of antimetabolites, portal hypertensive gastrophy (10), or vessel rupture from increased portal circulatory pressure.

ii. Laboratory Tests: There are no laboratory tests for evaluating vessel structure; however, gastroscopy and the visual recognition of the sites of bleeding, spider angiomata, and ecchymoses provide objective documentation of vessel fragility and rupture.

Table 1 Systems to Evaluate Before Initiating a Management Approach for Bleeding in Liver Disease

1.	Vascular damage and platelets:
	Observe, visualize bleeding vessels, platelet count
2.	Plasma clotting system:
	Prothombin time, aPTT, fibrinogen, prekallikrein, factors V, VII, VIII, IX
3.	Fibrinolytic system:
	Plasminogen, euglobulin clot lysis, 3-P test, FDP, D-dimer
4.	Clotting inhibitors:
	Antithrombin-III, proteins C and S
5.	Activated procoagulants:
	Euglobulin clot lysis, factor VIII, AT-III, proteins C and S

Table 2 Mechanisms Affecting Liver Function in Liver Disease

- Production of coagulation and inhibitor/modulating factors
  - Factor not produced or increased
  - Inhibitor not produced
  - Activator increased
- Reduced degradation
  - All metabolic toxins degradation
  - Medication
  - Disposal of metabolic waste
- Anatomy alterations from vascular alterations
  - Portal hypertension
    - Dilated portal veins, varices, cholestatic obstruction, ascites
  - Portal vein, hepatic vein thrombosis
- Inability to respond to increased metabolic demands
  - Liver dysfunction: loss of gluconeogenesis
  - Toxic effect on physiologic responses
    - Bone marrow production
    - Protein production and synthesis

iii. Management: Management includes removing alcohol and improving nutrition and liver function. Surgical intervention with shunting, sclerosis of varices, and medication (beta-blockers or estrogen) are beneficial (5,11,12).

b. Platelet Dysfunction and Thrombocytopenia.

i. Mechanism: Thrombocytopenia results from sequestration in the spleen, ongoing consumption, ethanol- or toxic-suppressed marrow, and ethanol destruction of platelets, but probably not a lack of thrombopoietin (13). Platelet dysfunction may be made worse due to a low hematocrit, circulating ethanol, and old, nonfunctioning platelets.

ii. Laboratory Tests: The platelet count documents number. Bleeding time or platelet aggregation studies can safely be assumed to be abnormal in the most severe cases of liver dysfunction. With an abnormal vasculature in liver disease, the bleeding time is not a true measure of platelet function (14–17). Some medications may also add to the platelet defect, such as antibiotic therapy (see below).

Table 3 Conventional Laboratory Testing in the Primary Evaluation of Bleeding in Liver Disease, and Thresholds for Concern

- Complete blood count including platelet count, and peripheral smear examination
  - Elevated WBC: >20,000 mm^3, rule out infection/inflammation
  - Decreased platelet count: <100,000 mm^3, peripheral destruction or lack of marrow production
  - WBC differential: neutrophil left shift, rule out infection or inflammation, or sepsis, DIC
  - Hematocrit: <24%, mechanism of loss; bleeding or destruction
- Prothrombin time: >16 sec
- Activated partial thromboplastin time: >45 sec
- Fibrinogen: <100 mg/dL

Table 4 Coagulation Profile for Assessment of Coagulation Abnormalities in Liver Disease

Automated hematology profile (CBC)
Review of peripheral smear
Platelet count
Prothombin time (PT)
Activated partial thromboplastin time (aPTT)
Fibrinogen
Factors V, VII, VIII, IX
Plasminogen
Antithrombin-III
Euglobulin clot lysis

iii. Management: Management includes improving liver function with support and improved nutrition. Platelet transfusions are of limited value. DDAVP may improve platelet function on a limited basis (18–20).

c. Plasma Clotting Proteins Dysfunction or Absence.

i. Mechanism: Clotting factors II, V, VII, IX, X, XI, XII, XIII, and fibrinogen are all lost due to decreased liver function, with inadequate production and abnormal synthesis. Factors II, VII, IX, X are decreased due to the absence of vitamin K (gamma-carboxylation). An unknown vitamin K deficiency and/or abnormalities of vitamin K utilization may also be the etiology of many bleeding problems in liver disease.

ii. Laboratory Tests: PT, PTT, and fibrinogen (note, 30% of a clotting factor will give a normal PT and aPTT) should be routine. Special studies include assays for factors V, VII, VIII, IX, plasminogen, antithrombin-III, prekallikrein, and euglobulin clot lysis.

iii. Management: Management includes replacement of clotting proteins with fresh frozen plasma (FFP), cryoprecipitate, factor concentrates such as FVII or IX, or Autoplex (19–21). Rarely will correction of the clotting tests stop the bleeding, but the test values before and after therapy are an excellent measure of the magnitude of the liver cell dysfunction and death. For instance, the improvement of the PT from 28 sec to 17 sec demonstrates a dysfunctional liver system that can respond to 6 units of FFP because the liver disease process has been slowed or is less significant than is suggested by the initial coagulation values or liver enzymes. On the other hand, no response or actually worsening of the clotting tests describes a dysfunctional system that is not amenable to therapy, and for which blood and blood component therapy do not offer hope of improvement. The 6-unit trial of FFP, followed by a second 6-unit trial of FFP with no improvement (the second trial being for those who need convincing) provides good objective evidence for the hopelessness of using FFP to stop the bleeding. The in-vivo trial of 6 or 12 units of FFP is preferred to 30 to 40 units of FFP over several days to weeks (22–24).

d. Activation of the Fibrinolytic System.

i. Mechanism: Primary activation of the plasminogen-to-plasmin conversion is due to failure of the liver to detoxify activators as well as decreased alpha-2-antiplasmin synthesis. Secondary activation due to fibrin deposition within the necrotic liver may also contribute to an exaggerated fibrinolytic response.

ii. Laboratory Tests: Tests should include plasminogen, alpha-2-antiplasmin, euglobulin clot lysis, plasma protamine paracoagulation, FDP, and D-dimer. These tests document the presence of pathologic fibrinolysis and the degree of liver dysfunction affecting production and increased utilization of plasminogen and alpha-2-antiplasmin.

iii. Management: Generally, there is no realistic way to reduce ongoing fibrinolysis due to liver dysfunction. A return to improved liver function is probably the best to be hoped for. Antifibrinolytic agents, epsilon-aminocaproic acid, tranexamic acid, and aprotinin have been of limited value (18,25,26).

e. Inhibitors of Clotting.

i. Mechanism: Proteases that normally respond to thrombin formation or fibrin generation are either not produced, are consumed or utilized at an accelerated rate, or do not function. Antithrombin-III (AT-III), proteins C and S (vitamin K dependent) are affected.

ii. Laboratory Tests: Antithrombin-III, proteins C and S.

iii. Management: Like fibrinolysis, there is no realistic way to reduce this process. Very limited intervention success has been achieved with fresh frozen plasma. The infusion of AT-III concentrate has demonstrated some success in acute liver failure as a naturally occurring anticoagulant that will prevent decrease intravascular thrombosis without systemic anticoagulation and its inherent risk for additional bleeding (18,26,27).

f. Pathologically Activated Procoagulants.

i. Mechanism: Protein metabolites which have not been detoxified by the liver are continuously activating the clotting system and consuming both the clotting factors and inhibitors, the raw surfaces of necrotic liver, and supporting tissues that activate the clotting system.

Table 5 Factor Assays Useful in Differentiating Liver Failure, Vitamin K Deficiency, and Disseminated Intravascular Coagulation

Factor V: critical value <30% (50–150%)
Manufactured by hepatocytes, when <30% ominous sign of hepatocyte failure
Not vitamin K dependent for activation
Acute phase responder, acute cholestasis
Factor VII: critical value <10% (50–150%)
Manufactured by hepatocytes
Vitamin K-dependent activation
Short half-life, 4–6 hr; quickly consumed, sensitive measure of vitamin K deficiency and hepatocyte production when factor IX is normal
Factor VIII: critical value <100% [expect >190%] (50–150%)
Manufactured in liver but not by hepatocytes
Not vitamin K dependent for activation
Increased >190% with liver disease (acute phase responder)
Decreased values suggest DIC or total liver failure
Factor IX: critical value <30% (50–150%)
Manufactured by hepatocytes
Vitamin K-dependent activation
Long half-life, 25 hr; therefore if normal reduces significance of vitamin K deficiency or utilization defect

ii. Laboratory Tests: Indirect, euglobulin clot lysis and decrease in specific factors such as F VIII, AT-III, proteins C and S, and fibrinogen that are consumed.

iii. Management: There is no specific intervention. Apheresis is of no value. Improvement in liver function is the best hope for reduction. Liver transplant may be the ultimate solution (28–31).

2. *Coagulation Laboratory Testing in Liver Disease*

In liver dysfunction, any critical alteration in coagulation parameters is usually one of multiple defects as described above. These multiple defects are the result of the liver cell developing altered function in the production of coagulation, fibrinolytic and inhibitor proteins, absent degradation of metabolic wastes, altered liver anatomy creating abnormal circulatory patterns and pressures, and altered physiologic responses to usual demands such as stress, increased production of proteins, or other compounds involved in metabolism. See Table 2 (13,16,18).

Routine testing for liver disease has customarily consisted of a CBC (to determine an elevated white blood cell count, thrombocytopenia, and red cell fragmentation), prothrombin time, partial thromboplastin time, and a quantitative fibrinogen (Table 3). The addition of four factor assays (see Table 4) can provide considerable supplementary insight into the differentiation of a vitamin K deficiency, disseminated intravascular coagulation, and hepatocyte dysfunction as they are related to the cause for bleeding. These are assays for factors V, VII, VIII, and IX. Assays for plasminogen, antithrombin-III, and euglobulin clot lysis time can be added to define the severity of concurrent fibrinolysis and or thrombosis (see Table 4).

A review of routine laboratory testing with a PT and aPTT raises important questions as to the significance of an abnormal result. One issue is the importance of a prolonged prothrombin time. What is the difference between a 15-sec versus a 19-sec prothrombin time as they relate to the cause or risk for bleeding? The importance of this question relates to the use of FFP to correct the PT. Customary thought processes are that the difference, however small, is significance, and the value must be corrected to normal. The difference *might* mean something, but in fact we often do not really know what the difference means in predicting the cause or risk for bleeding (32).

Correction with FFP would begin with 6–12 units of FFP over 12–24 hr. The infusions need to be repeated every 24 hr in most cases of severe liver disease. The gastrointestinal literature reviews the causes of bleeding in liver failure and provides lists of medications and different kinds of invasive shunts to be used (33–39). Blood and blood component transfusions are not the definitive treatment for bleeding in liver disease (19–21,40,41). In practice, however, the hospital blood bank knows when the characteristic liver disease patient with a GI bleeder enters the emergency department. There are demands for packed red cells, multiple units of fresh frozen plasma, and platelets. A common approach is to give large amounts of blood and blood products and observe the patient for cessation of bleeding. If bleeding does not stop, more aggressive procedures are initiated to identify the cause. This process is so pervasive as to suggest that it has real merit, yet I know of no literature as to its usefulness (40). However, bleeding per se has been reported to predict death (42). Mortality was related to the severity of liver failure, magnitude of blood loss, and the inability of therapy to stop bleeding.

The factor assays provide additional information for the assessment of the contribution of plasma clotting to bleeding (see Table 4). The prothrombin time and activated partial thromboplastin time are general tests, whereas the factor assays V, VII, VIII, and IX are specific for the three diagnostic problems in liver dysfunction described above (16,43–45).

First we should differentiate vitamin K deficiency from liver disease. A normal factor V with low factor VII and low-normal factor IX suggest vitamin K deficiency.

When factor V falls below 35%, hepatocyte dysfunction is contributing to the prolonged PT. Low levels of factor V, <30%, suggest major liver cell death/dysfunction and a poor prognosis.

Factor VIII is usually markedly increased, to 200% plus. A low-normal factor VIII level (60–70%) in liver disease suggest the presence of disseminated intravascular coagulation (DIC) as well. Along with the decrease in factor VIII, a drop in fibrinogen below 100 mg/dL, and a dropping or low platelet count below 100,000 mm^3, is added evidence for DIC. Factors V, VII, and IX will also drop to less than 30% with DIC. With the added element of DIC, management will necessarily involve treating the cause of the DIC at the same time. However, note that in complete, total liver failure, all the factors usually fall below 10%. Markedly low levels, <30% of plasminogen, antithrombin-III, and a very short euglobulin clot lysis time, <15 min, confirm the gravity of the liver failure (46–48).

Also note that transfusion of FFP will increase the circulating plasminogen significantly, to levels that permit fibrinolysis, resulting in lysis of some clots. The FFP may therefore actually increase bleeding in some areas of the body.

In practice, the bleeding liver failure patient will often have the PT and APTT treated when bleeding is the result of vascular fragility or the tear of esophageal or gastric vessels. An unending supply of FFP, cryoprecipitate, platelets, or packed red cells cannot repair a laceration. They may improve an ooze or capillary bleeding with low vascular pressure, but not the high pressures seen in the venous portal system around the esophagus and stomach in portal hypertension. A realistic approach to the management of bleeding in liver disease or liver failure would naturally be directed at several levels and might be as follows.

Direct intervention with the bleeding cirrhotic would be a combined effort of aggressive control of the anatomic bleeding site coupled with a controlled trial of component therapy and selected medications. Acute gastritis is the most common cause for bleeding, followed by bleeding esophageal varices. Sclerosis of esophageal varices, treatment with vasoactive drugs, and/or shunting should be implemented immediately once indications are established. The best to be hoped for is a return to the pre-insult/bleeding liver function status and coagulation status, with control of the bleeding varices. In acute liver failure from hepatitis or poisoning, direct intervention would be a supporting role directed at reducing liver toxicity and antacid therapy (49). Component therapy is of very limited value in buying time until liver function returns. Patients with acute viral hepatitis may have very abnormal coagulation studies but may not bleed, and may return to adequate liver and coagulation function. These patients may leave the hospital in relatively good shape. Patients with acute poisoning of the liver, such as from alcohol, acetaminophen, pesticide poisoning with organophosphates, or mushrooms, and in fulminent liver failure, generally have a poor prognosis. The amount of toxin exposure is the determining factor. Death is usually the result, with limited success with any supportive therapy (10,11,20,33–39,50–58). Fulminating liver failure from any cause is not amenable to intervention with medication and blood component therapy. Liver transplant offers the best hope of survival in these cases (see Table 6).

Case Study 1

History. This is the case of a 65-year-old woman with a long history of chronic alcoholism who has had multiple admissions for bleeding esophageal varices, bleeding hemorrhoids, and severe anemia. Multiple attempts at esophageal sclerosis have been unsuccessful in stop-

Table 6 Liver Diseases, Mechanisms, and Management for Bleeding

Liver disease	Usual mechanisms for bleeding[a]	Management of bleeding
Acute liver failure	Acute hemorrhagic gastritis	Gastric icing, antacids
Alcoholic hepatitis (6)	Gastrointestinal/gastric, esophageal varices, gastritis	Nutritional supplementation
Fulminant hepatitis (31)	Multiple organ failure: respiratory, renal, liver, CNS, GI, with GI bleeding	Limited/none/transplant
Cirrhosis (9,10,28,58)	Esophageal, gastric, and rectal varices	Iced lavage, vasopressors, balloon tamponade, sclerotherapy, endoscopic variceal band ligation, esophageal stapling, transection esophagogastric junction, portacaval shunts, transjugular hepatic shunts, liver transplantation
	Portal hypertensive vasculopathy	Supportive
	Factor deficiencies, increased fibrinolysis	Supportive
	DIC, increased consumption	Treat cause of DIC

[a]Obviously, bleeding may be made more significant with hepatocyte dysfunction and absent clotting factors. However, only occasionally will spontaneous hemorrhage from a clotting defect result in GI bleeding. CNS bleeding, however, is a major risk.

ping the esophageal bleeding. The patient is actively bleeding and is scheduled for a porto-caval shunt. The patient denies any personal or family history of a bleeding disorder. Current medications include Intra-lipid, Maalox, Mefoxin, Zantac, Gentamicin, and Aldactone.

Preoperative Laboratory Studies.

Hct 28.5% (39–45%)	Albumin 2.4 g/dL (3.5–5.1 g/dL)
WBC 5600 mm^3 (2,500–10,000 mm^3)	SGOT 33 IU (5–35 IU)
Platelet 265,000 mm^3 (150,000–400,000 mm^3)	SGPT 3 IU (5–35 IU)
Prothrombin time 12.7 sec (10.2–13.3 sec)	LDH 218 IU (70–238 IU)
aPTT 26.5 sec (24–36.8 sec)	Alk PO4 102 IU (43–130 IU)
Fibrinogen 345 mg% (170–410 mg%)	Bilirubin 1.7 mg/dL (0.1–1.3 mg/dL)

Additional Coagulation Studies.

Factor V 150% (50–150%)	Plasminogen 83% (80–120%)
Factor VII 38% (50–150%)	AT-III 77% (80–120%)
Factor VIII 300% (50–150%)	Euglobulin clot lysis 65 min (>60 min)
Factor IX 100% (50–150%)	

The patient had a successful porto-caval shunt several days later. Packed red cells (6 units), fresh frozen plasma (4 units), and platelet transfusions (10 units) were given during surgery. The patient did well postoperatively, with no surgical or bleeding problems. The changes in the coagulation studies were as follows:

	Pre-op	Intra-operative	Immediate post-op	Post-op 2 hr
	Blood components infused: PRBC = 6, FFP = 4, Plt = 10			
Hct	28.5%	28.8%	39.6	35.6
Plt ct	265,000 mm^3	183,000	146,000	156,000
PT	12.7 sec	14.0	15.1	12.5
APTT	26.5 sec	30.8	28.9	32.5
Fibrinogen	345 mg%	205	225	225

Pre-op factor assays	Post-op factor assays
	(Predicted increase in factors is +6%)
F V 150%	F V 84%
F VII 38%	F VII 32%
F VIII 300%	F VIII 130%
F IX 100%	F IX 84%

Question.

1. *How do you explain the changes?* The patient bled from the technical aspects of the surgery. The blood components were given on an empirical basis, and the factor assays demonstrate that the FFP had minimal impact. Certainly there would have been some consumption of clotting factors, particularly the labile factors V and VIII. However, the factor VIII levels of the patient are higher than the levels in FFP. The best you could hope for would be retention of the factor VIII levels in FFP. There was no change in factor VII, and a mild decrease in factor IX was noted. The FFP did not improve factor VII, and factor IX decreased slightly, suggesting some loss through bleeding or increased utilization that neither the patient's liver nor FFP could replace. The hematocrit also increased to a higher level than that seen preoperatively. In summary, the use of component therapy had limited value in this patient with significant liver cirrhosis. The underlying mechanism for bleeding is usually a vascular laceration, for which component therapy is of no value.

Case Study 2

History. This is the case of a 33-year-old woman admitted in hepatic coma. The patient has had a diagnosis of chronic hepatitis B for 10 years. She received multiple blood transfusions for left and right total hip replacements 10 years ago and subsequently developed hepatitis.

The patient is not now actively bleeding from any site or orifice. There is no personal or family history of bleeding disorder.

Current medications include Solumedrol and lactulose.

Laboratory Studies on Admission.

Hct 40.3% (37–47%)	Albumin 2.6 g/dL (3.5–5.1 dL)
WBC 7100 mm^3 (5–10 mm^3)	SGOT 1971 IU (5–35 IU)
Platelet count 359,000 (140–440 × 10^9)	SGPT 1617 IU (5–25 IU)
Prothrombin time 35.6 sec (10.5–13.6 sec)	LDH 509 IU (70–238 IU)
aPTT 92.4 sec (24.5–36.0 sec)	AlkPO4 289 IU (43–130 IU)
Fibrinogen 56 mg/dL (170–410 mg/dL)	Bilirubin 22.3 mg/dL (0.1–1.3 mg/dL)

Additional Coagulation Studies.

Factor V 18% (50–150%)
Factor VII 3% (50–150%)
Factor VIII 160% (50–150%)
Factor IX 8% (50–150%)
Plasminogen 20% (80–120%)
Antithrombin-III 6% (80–120%)
Euglobulin clot lysis 70 min (>60 min)

Question.

1. *How would you manage this patient? Component therapy?* The patient is not bleeding. There were rare petechie around venapuncture sites, but otherwise no bleeding or bruising. The patient was not transfused with blood or blood components. She was given i.v. fluids, and transported to another hospital for a successful liver transplant.

   This case illustrates that, with the very worst clotting studies, abnormal coagulation is not always the cause of bleeding. Spontaneous bleeding is always a risk, but with an intact vascular system and no trauma, bleeding is not necessarily the result.

B. Renal Failure

Bleeding in renal failure can be divided into acute renal failure as seen in acute glomerulonephritis and nephrotic syndrome, and bleeding in chronic end-stage renal failure. Each condition or underlying disease process must be identified and managed along with the risk for thrombosis or bleeding.

1. Acute Renal Failure

a. Acute Glomerulonephritis. In acute renal failure such as acute glomerulonephritis, the clotting system is not usually affected directly by the disease. Blood loss via the kidneys can be extensive, but is not a reflection of an altered coagulation status (59). In acute glomerulonephritis, thrombocytopenia may occur as a result of shortened platelet survival, and antiplatelet therapy may actually reduce the thrombocytopenia (60,61); however, bleeding due to an intrinsic alteration in the plasma clotting system is not usually seen. Other complicating diseases such as sepsis or DIC may complicate the clinical presentation. Acute renal failure can become chronic renal failure resulting in significant bleeding risk; see below (62,63).

b. Nephrotic Syndrome. In nephrotic syndrome the renal tubules cease to function, resulting in the urinary loss of AT-III, F IX, factor XII, and prekallikrein (64). Patients present with thrombosis but rarely with bleeding. Renal vein thrombosis, lower-extremity deep vein thrombosis, pulmonary embolus, stroke, and acute myocardial infarction do occur, but the exact mechanism has not been well defined. Treatment with anticoagulants may be required and may result in a risk for bleeding.

c. Hemolytic Uremic Syndrome (HUS) and Thrombotic Thrombocytopenic Purpura (TTP). These syndromes are identified with defined signs and symptoms such as acute renal failure, thrombocytopenia, hemolytic anemia, and fever (65). The causes of bleeding and death by these two processes are horrific and difficult to manage. The diagnosis is often one of exclusion. These two processes are often (66) described as the same disease process with different manifestations. The etiology is not agreed on, but TTP may be due to decreased prostacyclin or the absence of another platelet inhibitor resulting in intravascular platelet deposition. In HUS, the process may be due to an abnormality in large von Willebrand factor multimers. Both mechanisms can cause platelet deposition on the vessel wall.

Laboratory tests include CBC with platelet count and observation for red cell fragmentation, and von Willebrand multimer analysis.

Management involves treating the underlying infectious disease when present, as well as support in an intensive care unit. Plasmapheresis is the treatment of choice for TTP and is thought to prevent platelet deposition (63,66–69).

2. *Chronic Renal Failure*

Chronic renal failure is associated with a significant chronic bleeding disorder due primarily to marked platelet dysfunction. This is perhaps one of the most common mechanisms for disease-related acquired bleeding disorders. The clinical presentation of bleeding is mucosal bleeding as a result of platelet dysfunction. Spontaneous bleeding as well as postsurgical bleeding can be expected in uremic patients, but they do not always occur (50,70,71). Therefore, another, yet unrecognized compounding cause for bleeding may be present. This may be medication-induced platelet dysfunction, nutritional deficiencies such as of vitamin K, or antibiotics given for infections which may affect platelet function as well as cause a vitamin K deficiency. Heparin required for hemodialysis may also contribute to bleeding problems.

a. Laboratory Testing. Routine coagulation studies usually performed for the initial evaluation of a bleeding uremic patient include the following:

CBC, platelet count
Template bleeding time
PT, PTT, fibrinogen

Since almost every uremic patient does have a platelet defect to one degree or another, the bleeding time will be prolonged in the majority of patients. To obtain better documentation of the platelet dysfunction and demonstrate a response to therapy, the physician may want to consider (a) platelet aggregation studies, which may demonstrate decreased or absent response to collagen, ADP, and epinephrine; and (b) bleeding time before and after DDAVP or cryoprecipitate therapy.

b. Mechanisms. Defects in primary hemostasis (platelet plug formation) are characterized by the inability of platelets to adhere to the vessel disruption, and a failure of interplatelet aggregation leading to the formation of a platelet plug. Platelet dysfunction is documented by a prolonged bleeding time. Metabolic breakdown products such as guanidinosuccinic acids, phenol, and phenolic acids not excreted by the kidney might have a direct effect on platelet interactions (72,73), inhibition of GPIIb-IIIa activation by preventing it binding to fibrinogen (74–77), increased prostacycline release in injury of the vascular endothelium in chronic renal failure patients inhibiting platelet adhesion (78), and parathyroid hormone with a direct effect on the availability of calcium ions (79,80). Also of note is the relationship of chronic renal failure and gastrointestinal bleeding, as in angiodysplasia of the colon and cecum (81–83). Activated fibrinolysis may also play a role in increased bleeding in selected patients (mezzao).

c. Management. Maintain a hematocrit above 30% to maintain nutrition oxygen and ADP to the platelets. Platelet dysfunction improves as documented by a shortened bleeding time, and clinical bleeding is reduced by treatment with DDAVP and cryoprecipitate (84). von Willebrand factor (factor VIII antigen) in cryoprecipitate or released by DDAVP may be reduced in quantity, or become nonfunctional in chronic renal failure. With therapy, the endothelial release of stored von Willebrand multimers increases, which improves platelet adhesion/aggregation. Cryoprecipitate also provides replacement of large multimers, improving platelet adhesion/aggregation as evidenced by reduced bleeding. Dialysis improves platelet function as evidenced by an occasional shortened bleeding time, improved platelet adhesion to glass beads, PF3 availability, and reduced bleeding. Dialysis removes metabolites such as phenol and guanidinosuccinic acid. Always perform dialysis before a surgical procedure to reduce the tendency to bleed.

Miscellaneous effects of chronic renal failure include increased parathyroid hormone levels which increase platelet Ca^{2+} and cyclic AMP-reducing aggregation, and increased endothelial cell production of prostacyclin-inhibiting platelet aggregation. Conjugated estrogen shortens the bleeding time and may reduce GI and CNS bleeding, although the mechanism is not known (85–88).

With defects in secondary hemostasis; general nutrition is important in treating all aspects of the uremic patient. With chronic infections and treatment with antibiotics, a vitamin K deficiency is seen occasionally. The prolonged prothrombin time will suggest a vitamin K deficiency. Confirmation with a factor VII assay and/or treatment with vitamin K are needed.

A comprehensive approach to managing a bleeding patient should include (a) maintaining a hematocrit >30% with blood transfusions and or erythropoietin therapy; (b) dialysis before surgery or other high-risk invasive procedure, leaving all drains in after the next dialysis if possible, and dialysis as needed during bleeding episodes, with full recognition of the relationship of dialysis and heparin; (c) transfusion of cryoprecipitate and or DDAVP (0.3 μg/kg body weight in 50 mL normal saline over 30 min); (d) control of infections with antibiotics and vitamin K therapy with prolonged antibiotic use; and (e) long-term management of bleeding problems with estrogen if clinically indicated (89–93). In managing the chronic renal failure patient who is bleeding, there is often much frustration with continued bleeding when surgical hemostasis is achieved. Bleeding over several days does occur, and with a renal biopsy retroperitoneal hemorrhage is a significant complication. Unfortunately, despite therapy, the best that can be achieved is a slowing and eventual stopping of the bleeding. A sudden or miraculous cessation of all bleeding usually does not occur (Table 7).

Case Study 3

A 36-year-old man on long-term hemodialysis presents with a sudden onset of bleeding into the right orbit. There is no previous history of a bleeding problem. Current drugs do not interfere with coagulation.

Table 7 Strategies for Controlling Bleeding in Chronic Renal Failure

Action	Improves	Complications
Maintain Hct > 30%	Improves platelet function	Thrombosis of access shunts
Red cell transfusion	Nurtures platelets	Infectious disease
Erythropoietin therapy		
Increase Von Willebrand factor	Platelet binding to collagen	Thrombosis, infections
Cryoprecipitate (4–21 hr)		Blood-borne pathogens
DDAVP (24 hr)		Inappropriate thrombosis
Hemodialysis	Reduce uremic poisons	Heparin causes bleeding Damage to platelets, half life or decreased half life
Estrogen	Platelet function	No known complications

Initial Laboratory Studies.

Hct 27.7% (41–46%)	WBC 10,700 mm^3 (3,000–11,000 mm^3)
Template bleeding time 15 min (1–9 min)	Fibrinogen 390 mg/dL (150–400 mg/dL)
PT 20.4 sec (10.5–13.2 sec)	aPTT 38.5 sec (26.3–39.8 sec)

Questions.

1. *Does the coagulation profile identify the most likely possibilities?* The bleeding time indicates poor platelet function. The prolonged PT suggests the possibility of a vitamin K deficiency.
2. *What additional coagulation studies would you order?* The seriousness of the location of the bleed necessitates a more thorough investigation.

Factor VIII 500% (50–150%)	von Willebrand factor 230% (45–185%)
Factor IX 38% (50–150%)	von Willebrand cofactor 240% (45–140%)
Factor VII 11% (50–150%)	Platelet adhesion P = 89%, C = 98% (>75%)
Factor V 90% (50–150%)	Platelet aggregation Normal to epinephrine, and ristocetin, abnormal to ADP and collagen
Inhibitor Screen: Neg	

3. *What are the possibilities?* Possibilities include the platelet defect that is common to uremia, and the vitamin K deficiency that is frequently seen in poor nutrition and long-term antibiotic therapy without vitamin K replacement. Management should be to improve the hematocrit to 30%, add DDAVP and cryoprecipitate to improve bleeding time, and initiate vitamin K therapy. Fresh frozen plasma should be concurrent with the vitamin K therapy, because the location of the bleeding requires rapid correction. On hemodialysis, the use of heparin will still create a risk for bleeding for which there is no recourse except to minimize the circulating heparin during the dialysis, and neutralize the heparin after dialysis.

C. Disseminated Intravascular Coagulation

Disseminated intravascular coagulation (DIC) is not a disease, but rather the manifestation of an underlying disease process. DIC is generally described as *acute* or *chronic* in its relationship to a clinical manifestation. The following disease processes are associated with acute DIC: infections, obstetrical crisis (placenta abruptio, placenta previa, amniotic fluid embolus), acute leukemia (in particular, promyelocytic leukemia), liver failure, trauma, crushing injury. Chronic DIC is associated with metastatic cancers and in particular mucin-producing tumors, and giant cavernous hemangiomas (70,94–96).

Two of the more common causes of acute DIC are bacterial sepsis and placenta abruptio. These require analysis as to mechanism, laboratory testing, and management. The same selection of laboratory tests and intervention concepts will succeed for many of the other possible causes for DIC. Treatment of the underlying cause is fundamental to DIC resolution. The use of blood component therapy and medication in the treatment of DIC is not scientifically established in the literature founded on good clinical trials. Good clinical trials will probably never occur. We are left with personal experience, anecdotal evidence, and small series reports that elaborate one group's experience. Reusing what works is a common personal approach, combined with an occasional addition of new therapy modalities for those cases in which the customary does not work (96–98).

1. Bacterial Sepsis

Bacterial sepsis is the growth of infectious bacteria in the patient's bloodstream. The bacteria actively infiltrate organs and tissues, with an acute inflammatory response resulting in a leukocytosis and granulocytic left shift. In immune-compromised patients the leukocyte response may be meager or nonexistent. Thrombotic thrombocytopenic purpura (thrombocytopenia) and hemolytic uremic syndrome (acute renal failure) may also be manifestations of bacterial or viral sepsis (66).

Mechanism. The Gram-positive or Gram-negative bacteria proliferate in body tissues and can lead to a septic syndrome, septic shock, and multiple-system organ failure. The body defenses and physiologic responses may contribute to the overall changes and breakdown in the body's ability to overcome the proliferation of the bacteria. The bacteria and the reaction of neutrophils produce a necrotic material that stimulates cytokines, extracellular proteases, complement, factor XII, plasminogen, and bradykinin pathways. In TTP and HUS, these changes occur with occlusive thrombi made of platelets in vital organs (66). Multiple-systems organ failure may include septic syndrome plus severe dysfunction of at least two organ systems; cardiovascular failure; acidosis and respiratory failure; acidosis and renal failure; platelet dysfunction and hematologic failure; leukopenia, thrombocytopenia, anemia, neurologic failure, seizures, and hepatic failure; and decreased clotting factors (99). Bacterial endotoxins affect vessel wall integrity directly, with loss of endothelial cells and activation of platelets and contact factors XI and XII. These endotoxins have vasodilatory effects initiating hypotension, inadequate tissue perfusion, tissue damage, and death of tissues and organs (27,97,100,101).

a. Laboratory Tests. Laboratory tests should include confirmatory tests and blood cultures. Baseline screening tests are coagulation profile with CBC, platelet count, PT, aPTT, and fibrinogen. Studies of factors V, VII, and VIII will help differentiate liver dysfunction and vitamin K deficiency from the consumption in DIC. Additional laboratory studies such as AT-III, protein C, and tPA activity may help in the differentiation of bacterial infection from sepsis (98).

Documentation of an accelerated fibrinolytic process can be made with euglobulin clot lysis time, plasma protamine paracoagulation, plasminogen, FDP, and D-dimer.

b. Management. Treat and manage the underlying cause: Drain abscesses, initiate antibiotic therapy, etc. Supportive therapy should include the full range of blood component replacement including AT-III concentrates (27,102). Anticoagulant therapy such as heparin or antifibrinolytic agents such as Amicar are not helpful. Intensive care unit support is also essential to resolution (see Table 8).

2. Placenta Abruptio

Placenta abruptio results from the premature separation of the placenta from the uterus prior to delivery. With the infant still in the uterus, the markedly thrombogenic amniotic fluid enters the maternal circulation, resulting in a consumptive coagulopathy (DIC). Fibrinolysis initiated

Table 8 General Laboratory Test Goals of Blood Component Replacement in Acute Disseminated Intravascular Coagulation with Active Bleeding

Hematocrit:	Maintain >25%
Platelet count:	Maintain >80,000–100,000 mm^3
Prothrombin time:	Maintain within 3 sec of upper limit of reference range
Activated partial thromboplastin time:	Maintain within 5 sec of upper limit of reference range
Fibrinogen:	Maintain >100 mg/dL

by fibrin formation proceeds unchecked until there is no fibrin to lyse. The patient will start to bleed when all the clotting factors and platelets are consumed, and fibrin clots cannot be formed.

a. Mechanism. Amniotic fluid activates the intrinsic and extrinsic clotting systems, consuming clotting factors and platelets.

b. Laboratory Tests. Coagulation profile, fibrinogen (elevated in pregnancy; may be normal during DIC), factors V and VIII (factor VIII elevated in pregnancy; may be normal during DIC), euglobulin clot lysis, plasminogen, AT-III, FDP, D-dimer.

c. Management. Treat and manage the underlying cause; deliver the infant. Until the infant is delivered, the underlying cause will continue to consume clotting factors and platelets. Treatment with blood components, fresh frozen plasma, cryoprecipitate, platelets, or packed red blood cells for identified deficiencies can be used as a time-buying strategy. The blood and blood components will not cure the patient. Anticoagulants and antifibrinolytic agents are generally not successful, and may cause more harm (see Table 8).

Blood component replacement volumes for 70-kg person with constant assessment to prevent fluid overload are as follows:

Packed red cells	1–2 units followed by hematocrit
Platelets	1 apheresed unit or 6 to 10 pooled platelets followed by platelet count
Fresh frozen plasma	2 units of FFP (10 mL/kg), perhaps another 2 units if PT and aPTT changes remain >10 sec over upper limit of reference range
Cryoprecipitate	10 units of pooled cryoprecipitate for fibrinogen for 100–125 mg/dL followed by fibrinogen determination

Monitor at a minimum of every 2 hr, and after blood components are infused. The eventual resolution of bleeding is dependent on removal of the cause. Component therapy may provide a brief time interval until successful treatment is achieved, but blood bank resources will not cure the patient.

3. Chronic Disseminated Intravascular Coagulation

Chronic DIC is the manifestation of the slow, continuous activation of the clotting system. If it is slow enough, the patient's compensatory mechanisms for the ongoing consumptive process may result in a compensated form of DIC with eventual elevations in fibrinogen and clotting factors. However, measures of ongoing fibrinolysis such as FDP, D-dimer, and clot lysis can be the most abnormal values seen.

Mechanism. The continuous infusion of clot-activating/fibrin-generating material such as metastatic tumors and tumor breakdown products initiates consumption followed by fibrinolysis. When the body can no longer compensate, clinical bleeding becomes apparent.

Management. At this point, the management goal becomes supportive or palliative, with no true resolution anticipated. Removing the underlying mechanism such as by more aggressive chemotherapy, or removal of the aneurysm or large AV malformation, will be the ultimate objective (103), but this is often not possible in these patients.

Laboratory Studies. Coagulation profile; CBC, platelet count, PT, aPTT, and fibrinogen, along with documentation of fibrinolysis as described for the acute form.

Case Study 4

A 21-year-old primagravida at 36 weeks gestation presents with severe abdominal pain, hypotension, and signs of fetal distress. While in the emergency room, approximately 150 mL of bright red blood is obtained on vaginal examination.

Initial Laboratory Studies.

Hct 29% (39–45%)	Prothrombin time 18 sec (10.2–13.3 sec)
WBC 19,000 mm^3 (3000–10,000 mm^3)	aPTT 56 sec (24–36.8 sec)
Platelet count 45,000 mm^3 (170,000–400,000 mm^3)	Fibrinogen 250 mg/dL (150–400 mg/dL)
Smear Fragmented RBCs	Bleeding time >15 min (1–9 min)

Questions.

1. *The history and laboratory studies describe what condition?* Placenta abruptio with a DIC syndrome resulting in the consumption of platelets and clotting factors.
2. *What additional tests might be useful?* Tests that would further describe and document the degree of consumption and thereby guide further use of component therapy.

Additional Studies.

Factor VIII C 105% (50–150%)	Euglobulin clot lysis 10 min (>60 min)
Factor V 35% (50–150%)	3-P test Positive (negative)
Factor VII 25% (50–150%)	Antithrombin-III 60% (80–120%)

Questions.

3. *Are there any unusual laboratory findings in this patient?* The normal fibrinogen and Factor VIII C are elevated in pregnancy and may not be as low as anticipated. The marked decreases in factors V and VII with positive studies for ongoing fibrinolysis (euglobulin clot lysis and 3-P test) and decreased AT-III describe a fulminating DIC process.
4. *How should this patient be managed?* The underlying cause is the detached placenta with the infant remaining in the uterus, resulting in continuous infusion of amniotic fluid into the maternal circulation. The infant must be delivered to stop the infusion of amniotic fluid. Component therapy will buy some time until the patient's own liver and bone marrow can replace the consumed clotting elements. Component therapy cannot stop the bleeding.

Case Study 5

A 59-year-old man is admitted from his physician's office with the diagnosis of perinephric abscess treated previously for 10 days with antibiotics for pyelonephritis. The patient has been unable to eat, and has received only oral fluids. On admission the patient had recently begun to bleed from venipuncture sites, and the PT and aPTT are prolonged. There is no personal or family history of a bleeding disorder.

Initial Laboratory Studies.

Hct 31% (39–45%)	Prothrombin time 28.5 sec (10.5–13.8 sec)
WBC 9400 mm^3 (3500–10,000 mm^3)	aPTT 51.5 sec (23–36 sec)
Platelet count 76,000 mm^3 (150,000–400,000 mm^3)	Fibrinogen 68 mg/dL (170–400 mg/dL)
FDP Positive (negative)	Bleeding time 5 min (1–9 min)

Question.

1. *What is the most likely diagnosis?* The clinical signs and symptoms are of an acute infection with probable bacterial sepsis. The prolonged PT, aPTT, decreased fibrinogen and platelet count, and positive FDP suggest disseminated intravascular consumption with secondary fibrinolysis.

Additional Laboratory Tests.

Factor V 25% (50–150%)	Euglobulin clot lysis 15 min (>60 min)
Factor VII 10% (50–150%)	Antithrombin-III 55% (80–120%)
Factor VIII 60% (50–150%)	3-P test Positive (negative)
Factor X 8% (50–150%)	Factor IX 40% (50–150%)

Question.

2. *What diagnosis is most likely? How would you treat this coagulation problem?* The diagnosis of sepsis is most likely, and a positive blood culture would certainly firm up the diagnosis. The reduction of clotting factors suggests consumption and possible vitamin K deficiency as well. Management should consist of support with specific antibiotics, vitamin K therapy, packed red cells to maintain tissue oxygenation, and blood component therapy. The use of FFP, cryoprecipitate, and platelet transfusion will not cure the patient, but will reduce the losses brought about by the sepsis. When bleeding is not a problem, component therapy solely to correct a number may not be productive. Correction to normal coagulation values will be next to impossible until the sepsis is no longer present. Monitoring coagulation status every 4–8 hr will provide evidence of improvement or worsening of coagulation status, regardless of the clinical presentation. Volume overload may be a significant problem in the patients who are not bleeding, and prophalyxis regardless of its desirability may create more problems.

D. Malignant Neoplasms (Cancer): Leukemia and Solid Tumors

Cancer may cause severe bleeding as well as thrombosis. With today's aggressive use of screening tests, aggressive surgery, radiation, and chemotherapy, as well as organ transplantation, patients do not always present with bleeding or thrombosis. However, chemotherapy, radiation, and surgical therapy may create bleeding problems as a result of damage to tumor or healthy tissue (104–110).

1. Leukemias

Leukemias include the malignant proliferation of all the hematopoetic cell lines, including myeloid, erythroid, monocytoid, megakaryocytic, and lymphoid cells from the marrow or lymph nodes.

a. Mechanism. *Untreated*: There may be severe thrombocytopenia (bone marrow infiltration, consumption, splenomegaly, myelofibrosis), qualitative platelet defect, infiltration of liver and vessel wall by leukocytes, DIC, and syndrome from cell breakdown products. Leukemias associated with risk for bleeding in decreasing order of frequency are acute promyelocytic, acute myelomonocytic, acute myeloblastic, chronic myelogenous, chronic lymphocytic, and monocytic leukemia (110,111).

Treated: Thrombocytopenia from chemotherapy and radiation therapy, and immune-compromised status with sepsis inducing a DIC.

b. Laboratory Tests. CBC, platelet count, peripheral smear, bone marrow for diagnosis. *Special testing*: coagulation profile; factors V, VII, and VIII; euglobulin clot lysis; FDP; D-dimer; and inhibitors identified with multiple levels of testing. The value of additional testing over the routine is to document the severity of the deficits at the baseline analysis and subsequently to evaluate failure to respond to cancer therapy and/or blood and component therapy. Sometimes unrecognized vitamin K deficiencies are identified, and the inapparent severity of a factor level is elucidated. In many cases, treated or untreated leukemias can be managed with routine testing (106,107,112–114).

c. Management. Treatment with chemotherapy is indicated. Reduction of the leukemic cell mass before treatment (apheresis) may be required. As therapy progresses, periodic monitoring for loss of platelets and/or consumption of coagulation elements will provide valuable information on the effect of therapy, and when a potentially disastrous coagulation level is reached. This will provide guidance for the management with appropriate blood component replacement therapy, antibiotics, steroids, antifibrinolytic therapy, or AT-III concentrates.

2. *Solid Tumors*

Solid tumors refer to the proliferation of malignant tissue cells resulting in a tumor aggregate that grows locally and spreads or metastasizes to other parts of the body. This is characteristically seen in carcinoma of the breasts, lung, colon, prostate, liver, and pancreas, for instance.

a. Mechanism. Untreated solid tumors: The tumor and tumor substances such as mucin are released into the circulating blood. This material is thrombogenic, leading to the consumption of clotting factors and platelets, and finally to an exaggerated fibrinolytic response seen in DIC, or may present clinically as thrombosis of tissues, vessels, or organs. The tumor substance may also function as a platelet or clotting inhibitor (115). The response to the tumor may result in a compensated, overcompensated, or uncompensated coagulation response. Fibrinogen, factor VIII, and platelet count may be decreased, normal, or increased. As the untreated tumor invades the bone marrow, liver, or other vital organs, the entire coagulation system may be destroyed, leading to massive, uncontrollable hemorrhage. Plasma cell tumors and lymphomas may also produce paraproteins, that inhibit clotting.

Treated solid tumors: In addition to all of the above, tumor necrosis from the chemotherapy or radiation therapy may further induce a DIC-like syndrome. Therapy may cause an immune-compromised patient who develops sepsis or DIC to begin extensive bleeding.

b. Laboratory Tests. Coagulation profile, factors V and VIII, euglobulin clot lysis, plasminogen, AT-III.

c. Management. The management for this group of patients will always be complex, balancing the risk of treatment with the consequences of no treatment (116). The overwhelming majority of patients with cancer undergo surgery or radiation/chemo/immune therapy. Supporting these patients with blood components for specific deficiencies, isolation during increased risk for infection, and the appropriate use of antimicrobials is essential to success. Careful hematologic, coagulation, and immune status monitoring throughout the patient's management for the tumor is essential to identifying the effect of therapy and unanticipated problems.

Case Study 6

A 65-year-old man presents in the emergency room with ecchymoses on both forearms, and bleeding from his gums. The patient has a past history of carcinoma of the prostate, under therapy for 6 years. A prostatectomy 6 years ago revealed metastasis to periprostate tissues and bladder wall.

Initial Laboratory Tests.

Hct 34% (39–45%)	Prothrombin time 16 sec (10.2–13.3 sec)
WBC 12,300 mm^3 (3500–10,000 mm^3)	aPTT 51 sec (24–36.8 sec)
Platelet count 120,000 mm^3 (50,000–400,000 mm^3)	Fibrinogen 40 mg/dL (170–410 mg/dL)
Bleeding time >15 min (1–9 min)	FDP Positive >1:40 (negative)

Questions.

1. *What is the most likely diagnosis?* Carcinoma of the prostate with metastasis.
2. *What additional studies would you order?*

Factor V 30% (50–150%)	Euglobulin clot lysis <10 min (>60 min)
Factor VIII 120% (50–150%)	3-P test 4+ positive (negative)
Plasminogen 40% (80–120%)	
Antithrombin-III 65% (80–120%)	

3. *What do the additional studies describe?* They demonstrate ongoing intravascular fibrinolysis (both chronic and acute), consumption of clotting factors, and loss of natural inhibitors (AT-III).
4. *How would you manage this patient?* If elimination or reduction of the tumor is not possible, blood component or anticoagulant therapy will be of limited value in the prevention of bleeding or thrombosis. Often the use of blood and blood components is used for supportive or palliative purposes, to make the remaining days or weeks as comfortable as possible.

E. Acquired Antibodies or Inhibitors to the Coagulation System Which Result in Bleeding

Acquired antibodies or inhibitors to the coagulation system are not new aspects of acquired bleeding, but are now being more completely identified and characterized. The single most well known inhibitor is the lupus anticoagulant, but this inhibitor is usually associated with thrombosis, not bleeding. Acquired antibodies or inhibitors as a cause for bleeding are seen infrequently, are often difficult to fully characterize, and are usually difficult to manage.

a. Mechanisms. There are two broad groups of inhibitors: (a) Acquired inhibitors are antibodies that neutralize clotting factors (usually IgG antibodies). The inhibitors to factors VIII and IX may be acquired through repeated transfusions with concentrates, as in hemophilia (factor VIII:C), or may be seen spontaneously, particularly with tumors, postpartum patients, and the elderly, but the majority unknown (117,118). Of particular recent interest are the inhibitors associated with the use of topical bovine thrombin (119,120). Recent work suggests that bovine thrombin may not cross-react with human thrombin (121), but has been seen associated with a fatal outcome (124). Nonspecific inhibitors and non-neutralizing antibodies may be involved, such as immunoglobulins or paraproteins with variable specificity for the factor they inhibit (108,122,123). Examples of specific antibodies include antibodies to von Willebrand factor, which have been seen in all of the following diseases: multiple myeloma, systemic lupus erythematosus, chronic lymphocytic leukemia, Waldenstrom's macroglobulinemia, essential thrombocythemia, polycythemia vera, and chronic myelogenous leukemia (122,125, 126). The inhibitors can also be unrestricted, as in myeloma proteins which interfere with the platelet interactions and the formation of the fibrin plug (121,124). There are also rarer IgG specific antibodies to thrombin, factors II, V, VII, XI, XII, and XIII, and prekallikrein (127–131).

b. Laboratory Tests. Suspicion of an inhibitor is traditionally based on the presence of bleeding or bruising with a prolonged aPTT or PT. Mixing studies of patient with control 1 : 1 and 4 : 1 tested immediately and after 2 hr of incubation at 37°C assist in the differentiation of a factor deficiency which shows correction, as opposed to an inhibitor which does not show correction. An inhibitor with the incubation step will demonstrate addition prolongation. Non-neutralizing antibodies are rare and do not follow the usual pattern of prolongation with incubation (122). Evidence of an underlying disease such as hemophilia, or postpartum status, may be a clue to the process. Direct laboratory studies toward a specific deficiency identified in screening testing will help define the inhibitor. Extremely high antibody titers can make the specific diagnosis more difficult, as the inhibitor can affect confirmatory clotting endpoint tests such as factor assays and tests for a lupus anticoagulant.

c. Management. Identify the deficiency, and the underlying disease if possible. In non-surgical cases of bleeding with a low titer inhibitor, the straightforward correction of the inhibitor-induced factor deficiency may stop the bleeding. Each inhibitor behaves differently: Some inhibitors to factor VIII, whether spontaneous or in hemophiliacs, will not respond to factor concentrates, requiring aggressive use of porcine factor VIII concentrates, or immunosuppression as with cyclophosphamide. In addition, trials with bypass concentrates such as prothrombin complex concentrates as in Konyne or FEIBA and most recently factor VII concentrates are sometimes successful. See Chapters 27 (Rodwig) and 28 (Lurie). Inhibitors titers may be required for proper assessment of the inhibitor and defining success of therapy. When the underlying disease is producing a paraprotein, only removal of the protein-producing tumor will stop the bleeding. Loss of factor X due to factor X absorption on to systemic amyloid is not amenable to any known therapy.

Case Study 7

A 72-year-old man presents with hematuria due to bladder stones. There are bruises on his arms and legs that he cannot explain. A preliminary workup demonstrates a prolonged PT and aPTT. There is no personal or family history of bleeding disorders. The patient has had teeth extractions, an appendectomy, and a hernia repair without bleeding problems. He is on no medication.

Initial Laboratory Tests.

Hct 41.7% (39–45%)
WBC 10,000 mm^3 (3500–10,000 mm^3)
Platelet count 108,000 mm^3 (150,000–400,000 mm^3)
Fibrinogen 185 mg/dL (170–410 mg/dL)
Bleeding time 9 min (1–9 min)

Prothrombin time 14.7 sec (10.2–13.3 sec)
aPTT 74.4 sec (24–36.8 sec)

Questions.

1. *What is the significance of the patient's age, and an abnormal aPTT without a history of significant bleeding problems?* The appearance of a prolonged aPTT in a male with

no history of a congenital disorder such as hemophilia A or B is most likely an acquired inhibitor until proven otherwise. Certainly a prekallikrein, factor XI, or factor XII deficiency is possible, but these congenital deficiencies should not present with bleeding problems as seen with factor VIII deficiencies.

2. *What additional laboratory studies would you order to better define the possibilities?*

Factor V 77% (50–150%)	Mixing study using the aPTT:		
Factor VII 100% (50–150%)	P : C	Immediate	37°C for 2 hr
Factor VIII 8% (50–150%)	1 : 1	54	68
Factor IX 53% (50–150%)	4 : 1	61 sec	72 sec
Euglobulin clot lysis >60 min (>60 min)	Control	27 sec	31 sec

The factor studies demonstrate a low factor VIII, and the mixing studies demonstrate no correction with both the 1 :1 and 4 : 1 mixtures with and without incubation.

3. *What is the diagnosis? How would you manage this patient?* The diagnosis is an acquired factor VIII inhibitor. A trial of factor VIII concentrate was initiated because the patient developed hematuria and was successfully managed during the acute process. The patient stopped bleeding but retained a prolonged aPTT and low factor VIII for approximately 3 months. These disappeared and did not return.
4. *How would a patient with hemophilia and a factor VIII antibody differ?* They may, in fact, appear the same. However, the response to factor VIII concentrate may differ and treatment of the hemophiliac may be required until the bleeding site as in surgery is well healed. A high titer antibody could in both cases require similar aggressive approaches, such as immune suppression and bypass concentrates. The hemophiliac will not lose the antibody.

III. ACQUIRED BLEEDING DISORDERS AS A RESULT OF MEDICATION

Medications are one of the largest group of causes for acquired bleeding disorders in this country. The population as a whole partakes freely of over-the-counter medications without conscious thought of the possibility of the medication causing an untoward effect or complication such as a bleeding disorder. In addition, the use of prescribed medication to prevent thrombosis is increasing daily with the aging population in the United States, and large clinical trials are revealing the significantly decreased morbidity/mortality in patients at high risk for thrombosis who are being treated with medications designed to prevent further thrombosis. These medications, in turn, may contribute to an acquired bleeding disorder.

This discussion will attempt to analyze therapies, primarily medications, that affect the hemostatic system directly. We will look at common and a few uncommon therapies and their relationships to acquired bleeding disorders. The following categories of drugs may affect coagulation: antiplatelet drugs; anticoagulants; fibrinolytics; chemotherapy; antibiotics.

A. Antiplatelet Drugs

The antiplatelet drugs include aspirin, nonsteroidal anti-inflammatory drugs, sulfinpyrazone, dextrans, hetastarch, dipyridamole, ticlopidine, abciximab, and calcium channel antagonists. The acquired disorders of platelet functions are the most common of all the hematologic abnormalities. Many drugs are known to affect platelet function (Table 9). Some of these agents are

Table 9 Medications and Chemicals Affecting Platelets by All Mechanisms

Acetaminophen	Acetazolamide	Acetohexamide	Allopurinal
Allylisopropylacetylurea	Allylisopropylbarbiturate	Alpha-methyldopa	Aminophylline
Aminopyrine	Aminosalicylic acid	Amitriptyline	Amobarbital
Amodiaquine	Amphotericin B	Ampicillin	Amrinone
Antazoline	Antidepressants	Antihistamines	Antipyrine
Arsenicals	Arsine	Aspirin	Aureomycin
Azathioprine	Bendroflumethiazid	Benzene	Betamethasone
Butabarbital	Butabarbitone	Calcium channel blockers	Carbamazepine
Carbenicillin	Carbimazole	Carbon tetrachloride	Carbromal
Carphenazine	Cephalothin	Cefazolin	Centalun
Cephalexin	Cephalosporins	Cephaloridine	Cephalothin
Chloramphenicol	Chloral hydrate	Chlorate	Chlordiazepoxide
Chloroguanide	Chlorophenothane	Chloroquine	Chlorothiazide
Chlorpheniramine	Chlorpromazine	Chlorpropamide	Chlortetracycline
Chlorthalidone	Clindamycin	Clofibrate	Clonazepam
Clopamide	Cloxacillin	Colchicine	Copper sulfate
Corticotropin	Cortisone	Cycloserine	Cyproheptadine
Desimipramine	Desipramine	Dexamethasone	Diatrizoate
Diazepam	Diazoxide	Dibenzyline	Dicoumarol
Diethylstilbestrol	Digitoxin	Digoxin	Dihydroergotamine
Diphenhydramine	Diphenylhydantoin	Diflunisal	Diltiazem
Diphenhydramine	Dipyridamole	Disulfiram	Dobutamine
Doxepin	Erythromycin	Ethacrynic acid	Ethambutol
Ethanol	Ethosuximide	Ethyl-allyl-acetylurea	Ethylchlorvinyl
Ethyl-phenylhydantoin	Furadantin	Fenoprofen	Fluorocytosine
Fluphenazine	Furosemide	Gentamicin	Glucocorticoids
Glutethimid	Glyburide	Glymidine	Gold
Griseofulvin	Guanidine	Haloperidol	Heparin
Hydralazine	Hydrochlorothiazide	Hydroxychloroquine	Hydrocortisone
Hypnotics	Ibuprofen	Idoxuridine	Imipramine
Indomethacin	Influenza vaccine	Insecticides	Iodides
Iopanoic acid	Isoniazid	Isoproterenol	Isotretinoin
Isoxicam	Isuprel	Keflin	Levodopa
Lincomycin	Lithium	Marijuana	Measles vaccine
Meclofenemate	Mefenamic acid	Mephenytoin	Meprobamate
Mercurial diuretics	Mercury	Methapyrilene	Methicillin
Methimazole	Methyldopa	Methylthiouracil	Methysergide
Mezlocillin	Moxalactam	Mumps vaccine	Nafcillin
Nalidixic acid	Neomycin	Nifedipine	Nitrofurantoin
Nitroglycerin	Nitroprusside	Novobiocin	Orphenadrine
Oxacillin	Oxazepam	Oxyphenbutazone	Oxytetracycline
Papaverine	Para-aminosalicylate	Paramethadione	Penicillamine
Penicillin	Pentamidine isethionate	Pentazocine	Pentobarbital
Perphenazine	Persantine	Pertussis vaccine	Phenacemide
Phenacetin	Phenformin	Phenindione	Phenobarbital
Phentolamine	Phenylbutazone	Piperacillin	Plaquenil
Poliomyelitis vaccine	Polythiazide	Practolol	Prednisolone
Prednisone	Primidone	Probenecid	Procainamide
Procarbazine	Prochlorperazine	Promethazine	Propoxyphene
Propranolol	Propylthiouracil	Protriptyline	Pyrimethamine

Table 9 Continued

Quinacrine	Quinidine	Quinine	Regitine
Reserpine	Rifampin	Ristocetin	Rubella vaccine
Salicylamide	Salicylazosulfapyridine	Sedatives	Smallpox vaccine
Sodium salicylate	Solvents	Spironolactone	Stibophen
Streptomycin	Sulfadiazine	Sulfadoxine	Sulfamerazine
Sulfamethazin	Sulfamethizole	Sulfamethoxazole	Sulfamethoxydiazine
Sulfamethoxypridazine	Sulfanilamide	Sulfapyridine	Sulfathiazole
Sulfisoxazole	Sulfonamides	Sulindac	Tamoxifen
Tetanus vaccine	Tetracycline	Thallium	Theophylline
Thioridazine	Ticarcillin	Tolazamide	Tolbutamide
Toluene	Triamcinolone	Trichlormethiazide	Trifluoperazine
Trimeprazine	Trimethoprim	Trimethadione	Trimethoprim-
Typhoid vaccine	Urokinase	Valproic acid	Verapamil
Vitamin A	Vitamin K	Xylene	

Source: Modified from Refs. 14 and 154.

used specifically for their antithrombotic activity, with diminished platelet function being the therapeutic goal. Abnormal platelet function, however, is an unwanted side effect with many of the other agents (60,61).

The 1980s witnessed the emergence of a renewed interest in platelet inhibitors, which resulted from a better understanding of the role of platelets and thrombosis in the pathogenesis of coronary artery disease. In addition, information from aspirin trials in patients with cardiovascular and cerebrovascular disease further supported the use of antiplatelet therapy in unstable angina, acute myocardial infarction, chronic coronary disease, coronary revascularization procedures, and cerebrovascular ischemia. Also currently evolving is the role of platelet inhibition for primary prevention of coronary disease and for prevention of stroke in patients with atrial fibrillation.

Aspirin is clearly the most widely used antiplatelet agent. Single doses prolong bleeding time. Aspirin interferes with platelet function by irreversibly acetylating the active site of platelet cyclooxygenase, so that the ability of the platelet to synthesize thromboxane A2, a prostaglandin derivative which is a potent vasoconstrictor and inducer of platelet aggregation and platelet release reaction, is impaired for the life span of the platelet (7–10 days). Since cyclooxygenase is irreversibly acetylated, the platelets are unable to generate new enzyme (132,133).

Combinations of aspirin and *dipyridamole* or aspirin and *sulfinpyrazone* have been recommended for antithrombotic action for prophylaxis in various high-risk situations (coronary bypass and total hip replacement). Patients post-myocardial infarction on aspirin therapy are at reduced risk of subsequent death and nonfatal reinfarction, and aspirin is also used for reducing the risk of transient ischemic attacks (TIAs) and stroke in patients who have had transient ischemia of the brain due to fibrin platelet emboli (134).

Laboratory tests affected include the following.

1. Impaired platelet aggregation with epinephrine, ADP, arachidonic acid, and low concentrations of collagen and thrombin, a direct result of inhibition of cyclooxygenase.
2. Prolonged bleeding time; this effect is less consistent than the platelet aggregation abnormality. The prolonged bleeding time does not consistently indicate that there is an increased risk for bleeding.

Therapeutic aspirin used in combination with oral anticoagulants has an additive hypoprothrombinemic effect. The combination of a platelet defect with a plasma clotting defect will place the patient at significant risk for spontaneous or postoperative bleeding. Aspirin can also increase the risk of bleeding in heparin-anticoagulated patients. Other adverse reactions of aspirin therapy may include thrombocytopenia, purpura, and fecal blood loss (135).

Diflunisal, a salicylic acid derivative, is chemically different from aspirin. Because of the absence of the acetyl group, diflunisal inhibits prostaglandin synthetase in a reversible manner. At 2 g daily, diflunisal inhibits platelet function, and bleeding time is slightly increased. Both aspirin and diflunisal cause significant fecal blood loss in higher doses. Co-administration of diflunisal and oral anticoagulants may also cause increased hypoprothrombinemic effects, as diflunisal competitively displaces coumarins from their protein-binding sites, increasing the availability of the coumarins (134).

Nonsteroidal anti-inflammatory drugs (*Indocin*, *Ibuprofen*, *Naprosyn*), like aspirin, inhibit the activity of platelet cyclooxygenase, and thus aggregation, in a reversible fashion. The effect is quantitatively less and of shorter duration than that seen with aspirin. These agents may prolong the bleeding time within the normal range, and platelet function is restored in 2–3 days when these drugs are no longer in the circulation. Use with caution in patients with intrinsic coagulation defects and in those on anticoagulant therapy such as coumadin. Serious GI toxicity such as ulceration, bleeding, and perforation can occur at any time, without warning (134).

Sulfinpyrazone is a pyrazolidine derivative, and is a potent uricosuric agent which also has antithrombotic and platelet inhibitory effects. It lacks anti-inflammatory and analgesic properties. Sulfinpyrazone competitively inhibits prostaglandin synthesis and thereby prevents platelet aggregation (134).

Dextrans are partially hydrolyzed branched polysaccharides of glucose. Two preparations are used clinically, an average-molecular-weight dextran and a low-molecular-weight dextran. Both are effective plasma expanders and also affect and depress platelet function by physically interfering with platelet collagen and platelet-to-platelet interaction. With this inhibitory capability, dextran has been used as an antithrombotic agent. This therapeutic effect is variable from patient to patient, and may be achieved without a significant increased risk of bleeding. However, dextrans may confuse the significance of a prolonged bleeding time and impair platelet aggregation and platelet procoagulant activity. With systemic dilution the dextrans may also cause a modest reduction in plasma von Willebrand factor concentration, and make worse thrombocytopenia, anemia, or hypofibrinogenemia. In patients with an active hemorrhagic site, the increase in perfusion pressure and improved microcirculatory flow may cause additional blood loss (136).

Hetastarch (hydroxyethyl starch) is a synthetic glucose polymer that is used for plasma expansion. For the same reasons as with dextran, hetastarch may prolong the bleeding time. Volumes exceeding 1 L in an average adult may result in prolongation of the PT and aPTT. This prolongation is not always associated with bleeding, but in surgical or trauma patients the cause for bleeding is not always clear. The prolongation in the PT and APTT is not always associated with bleeding and may occur before an actual defect in coagulation is present (137).

Dipyridamole is a platelet adhesion inhibitor. It appears to inhibit phosphodiesterase, resulting in accumulation of cAMP, and intracellular cAMP reverses and inhibits platelet activation. Dipyridamole is sometimes given in combination with aspirin; the antithrombotic effects are synergistic or additive to the aspirin effect. It is also an adjunct to coumarin anticoagulants in the prevention of postoperative thromboembolic complications of cardiac valve replacement. Daily low-dose aspirin in conjunction with dipyridamole has been used for the prevention of preeclampsia; this is associated with a low risk of maternal hemorrhagic complications, which may be reversed with platelet transfusions (135).

Ticlopidine is one of the most potent antiplatelet drugs available. Ticlopidine inhibits both platelet aggregation and release of platelet granule constituents. The bleeding time is prolonged. Ticlopidine interferes with platelet membrane function by inhibiting ADP-induced platelet–fibrinogen binding and subsequent platelet–platelet interactions. Like aspirin, the inhibitor effect is irreversible, and lasts the life span of the platelet. Platelet aggregation studies are affected, especially ADP-induced aggregation as well as aggregation and release induced by epinephrine, arachidonic acid, collagen, and thrombin (138).

In large clinical trials, Ticlopidine significantly reduced the risk of fatal and nonfatal stroke in patients who had experienced stroke precursors. However, because Ticlopidine is associated with a significant risk of neutropenia and/or agranulocytosis, which may be severe and life-threatening, its use is reserved for patients who are intolerant to aspirin therapy where indicated to prevent stroke (139–142).

Ticlopidine has an increased risk for bleeding with complications such as ecchymosis, epistaxis, hematuria, conjunctival hemorrhage, GI bleeding, and perioperative bleeding. Intracerebral bleeding is rare, but has been reported. Use reasonable caution when the patient may be at risk of increased bleeding from trauma, surgery, etc. Discontinue the drug 10–14 days prior to elective surgery—increased surgical blood loss has occurred in patients undergoing surgery during treatment with Ticlopidine. Ticlopidine should also be used with caution in patients who have lesions with a propensity to bleed, such as GI ulceration, or in patients using drugs that might induce such lesions. In the event of bleeding, platelet transfusions may be used to reverse the effect of Ticlopidine, and a prolonged bleeding time may be normalized within 2 hr after administration of 20 mg methylprednisolone IV.

Coadministration of Ticlopidine and aspirin is not recommended; Ticlopidine potentiates the inhibitory effect of aspirin on collagen-induced platelet aggregation.

The antiplatelet agent *Abciximab* is a Fab fragment which binds to the intact glycoprotein IIb/IIIa receptor of human platelets (134). GPIIb/IIIa is the major platelet surface receptor involved in platelet aggregation. Abciximab inhibits platelet aggregation by preventing the binding of fibrinogen, vWF, and other adhesive molecules to the GPIIb/IIIa receptor sites on activated platelets. It is intended for use with aspirin and heparin as an adjunct to platelet aggregation inhibition, primarily in patients at high risk for closure of treated coronary vessels after coronary angioplasty or removal of an atheroma.

The most common complication of Abciximab is bleeding, and treatment is associated with statistically significant increases in both major and minor bleeding events and in bleeding requiring transfusion. Bleeding sites include GI, GU, retroperitoneum, intracerebral, and arterial access sites.

Calcium channel blockers (*Nifedipine*), alone and in combination with aspirin, cause inhibition of platelet function. This is thought to be a function of inhibition of calcium transport across the platelet membrane. Patients have experienced bruising, petechiae, and bleeding. Nifedipine decreases platelet aggregation in vitro. There may also be an increase in the bleeding time in some patients.

B. Plasma Clotting Anticoagulants

Blood coagulation involving both the intrinsic and the extrinsic pathways and resulting in the formation of a stable fibrin clot involves a cascade of proteolytic reactions involving the interaction of the clotting factors, platelets, and tissue factors. Therapeutic plasma clotting anticoagulation occurs at many different levels of this coagulation cascade. Anticoagulants used therapeutically include warfarin and coumadin (oral coumarin), heparin, low-molecular-weight heparin, anisindione (an indandione derivative), Arvin (ancrod), and hirudin.

The clinical patient under long-term treatment with coumarin is the one who is most likely to develop a significant hemorrhagic problem. A small amount of bleeding into a critical site, e.g., a subdural hematoma or bleeding into the wall of the small intestine with consequent intestinal obstruction, can be more serious than heavy gastrointestinal blood loss.

Coumadin (coumarin, warfarin) is the most commonly used oral anticoagulant and is the agent of choice in long-term anticoagulation. Coumarins and indandiones interfere with the hepatic activation of the vitamin K-dependent procoagulant factors II (prothrombin), VII, IX (Christmas factor), and X (Stuart factor), with the resultant production of proteins that are immunologically similar to the naturally occurring factors but functionally markedly abnormal (PIVKA—proteins induced by vitamin K absence). Vitamin K-dependent proteins possess carboxylglutamyl residues that are crucial for their clotting function by virtue of their ability to bind calcium and phospholipid. Coumadin inhibits the enzyme vitamin K1 reductase, and thereby reduces the generation of the active form of vitamin K which is intimately involved in the gamma carboxylation of the glutamic acid residues (Figure 1). Anticoagulant effects are dependent on the half-lives of these clotting factors, which are II = 50 hr, VII = 6 hr, X = 24 hr, and IX = 36 hr, respectively. The effect of coumadin on the coagulation system is conventionally measured by the prothrombin time, which is sensitive to reductions in factors VII and X and, to a lesser degree, factor II. The early depletion of factor VII after institution of coumadin therapy (because of its short half-life) is reflected in prolongation of the prothrombin time within 8 to 12 hr, but full anticoagulation/antithrombotic effect of therapy might not be achieved for 3–5 days when all of the vitamin K-dependent factor levels have fallen. Optimal anticoagulant control with coumadin is achieved in theory when a complete antithrombotic effect is achieved while exposing the patient to the least risk of hemorrhage. The most useful markers for monitoring the therapeutic effect of the oral anticoagulants are the prothrombin time (PT) and the International Normalized Ratio (INR) (143).

Hemorrhage is the principal adverse effect of the oral anticoagulants, and is a consequence of the intended anticoagulant effect. The risk of hemorrhage is related to the level of intensity and duration of therapy. GI hemorrhage secondary to peptic ulceration or silent neoplasm is responsible for many of the deaths due to oral anticoagulant therapy. Laboratory monitoring of the patient on coumadin therapy is achieved with frequent PTs (usually kept within a range of 1.5–2 times the mean normal) and INRs (between 2.0 and 3.0) but varies according to the clinical diagnosis. Spontaneous bleeding is more likely when the PT or INR are outside of therapeutic range; however, bleeding that occurs when the PT and INR are within the therapeutic range warrants investigation, for a blood vessel defect may be the cause for bleeding.

The frequency of hemorrhage correlates directly with the intensity of coagulation, and occurs more often in elderly patients on large doses. Excessive anticoagulation in the presence of life-threatening hemorrhage requires rapid correction of the excessive depletion of factors II, VII, X, and IX, which can be achieved by the administration of fresh frozen plasma or commercial factor IX complex. Most often, however, the patient on oral anticoagulant is found on follow-up to have an INR outside the therapeutic range, but without obvious bleeding problems. Measures taken depend on the severity of the problem, but may include reduction in the dose, omission of one or more doses, and, if necessary, a small dose (2–5 mg) of vitamin K, which begins to correct the INR within 6–12 hr. Higher doses can make the patient refractory to coumadin for a period of 1–2 weeks. A rebound hypercoagulable state with elevated clotting factors has been described occasionally with the cessation of coumadin. However, the

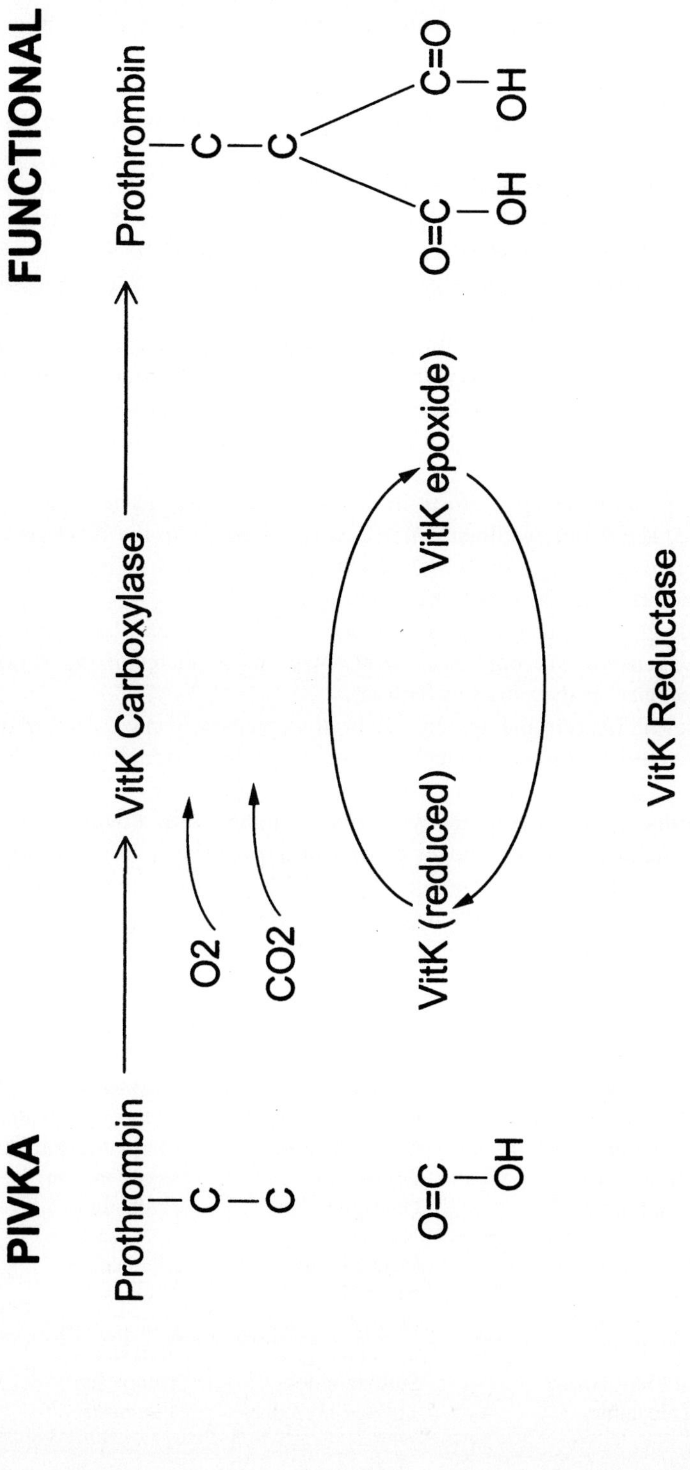
PIVKA
Prothrombin
C
C
O=C
OH
VitK Carboxylase
O2
CO2
VitK (reduced)
VitK epoxide
VitK Reductase
FUNCTIONAL
Prothrombin
C
C
O=C
OH
C=O
OH

Figure 1

actual incidence of the rebound phenomenon is unknown, and its overall clinical significance is also unknown (144).

The risk of hemorrhage is also increased with concomitant use of many drugs, many of which displace coumadin from its protein-binding sites, making more drug available for anticoagulant effect (see Table 10). [*Note*: The INR is the standardization of the sensitivity of the prothrombin time to the effect of coumadin. The patient's PT is divided by the mean normal PT for the laboratory taken to the power of the International Sensitivity Index (ISI). See Chapter 32 by Fink.]

Heparin is a naturally occurring sulfated glycosaminoglycan, and is an important and widely used anticoagulant for several reasons. Heparin is effective in the prevention and treatment of many thromboembolic disorders; in contrast to coumadin, it has a rapid onset of anticoagulant activity. Heparin's therapeutic activity is easily monitored in the laboratory, and it is inexpensive (145). Low-dose heparin is the treatment of choice as prophylaxis for DVT and pulmonary embolism in most in-hospital patients. It is not a homogeneous substance but, rather, a mixture of polysaccharide molecules that vary in molecular weight from 2,000 to 40,000. Experimental data suggest that the low-molecular-weight fractions of heparin (LMWH) are as effective as conventional heparin in preventing thrombosis but may be associated with a lower bleeding tendency (134).

Heparin exerts its anticoagulant action in the presence of the alpha-2-globulin antithrombin-III (AT-III). Heparin's anticoagulant action involves binding to the lysyl groups of AT-III, inducing a conformational change in AT-III which vastly enhances its inhibitory action on the serine centers of factors XIIa, XIa, IXa, Xa, and thrombin (146).

The most commonly used test to monitor heparin effect is the aPTT, because it is routinely available and is inexpensive. The only theoretical objection to this test is that it does not reflect the influence of platelets on the effect of heparin.

Hemorrhage during heparin therapy can occur at virtually any site. A fall in the hematocrit or blood pressure should lead to serious consideration of a hemorrhagic event. Also, thrombocytopenia occurs in patients on heparin with a reported incidence of up to 30% (134). The incidence of heparin-associated thrombocytopenia is higher with bovine than with porcine heparin. Low-dose therapy results in fewer complications, as the severity is dose related. Despite the rarity of thrombocytopenia induced by LMWH, platelet counts must be performed before the start of therapy, on the fifth day, and subsequently two to three times a week as with standard heparin (147). Thrombocytopenia developing within 2–3 days after beginning

Table 10 Drugs that May Increase the Anticoagulant Effect of Warfarin or Anisindione

Acetaminophen	Aminoglycosides	Amiodarone	Androgens
Beta blockers	Cephalosporins	Chloral hydrate	Chloramphenicol
Cimetidine	Clofibrate	Corticosteroids	Cyclophosphamide
Dextrothyroxine	Diflunisal	Disulfiram	Erythromycin
Fluconazole	Gemfibrozil	Glucagon	Hydantoins
Ifosfamide	Influenza virus vaccine	Isoniazid	Ketoconazole
Loop diuretics	Lovastatin	Metronidazole	Miconazole
Mineral oil	Moricizine	Nalidixic acid	NSAIDs
Omeprazole	Penicillins	Phenylbutazones	Propafenone
Quinidine	Quinine	Quinolones	Salicylates
SMZ-TMP	Sulfinpyrazone	Sulfonamides	Tamoxifen
Tetracyclines	Thioamines	Thyroid hormones	Vitamin E

heparin therapy tends to be mild and is due to direct action of heparin on the platelets. Thrombocytopenia developing after a delay of 5–12 days after beginning either low- or high-dose heparin can have serious consequences and may reflect the presence of an antibody against platelets (148). An increased risk of bleeding is possible during concurrent administration of heparin and salicylates.

Enoxaparin sodium and *Dalteparin sodium* are low-molecular-weight (LMW) heparins with antithrombotic properties characterized by a higher ratio of anti-FXa to anti-FIIa activity than unfractionated heparin. These LMW heparins effectively catalyze the inactivation of activated factor X by AT-III, but do not prolong the aPTT or the thrombin time as standard heparin does. This may lead to a more favorable ratio of antithrombotic activity to hemorrhagic risk compared to standard heparin. Enoxaparin prevents postoperative DVT following hip replacement surgery, and Dalteparin is indicated for prophylaxis against DVT in patients undergoing abdominal surgery who are at risk for thromboembolic complications. Like other anticoagulants, these should be used with care in patients with increased risk of hemorrhage, or in patients receiving platelet inhibitors because of the increased risk of bleeding. The incidence of hemorrhagic complications during treatment with heparin has generally been low, however. The most common complication is hematoma at the subcutaneous injection site. In the normal clinical prophylactic use of LMWH, monitoring is not necessary. Hemorrhagic complications associated with heparin therapy may be largely neutralized by the slow i.v. injection of protamine sulfate.

Hirudin, a thrombin inhibitor developed from leeches, is a 65-amino acid polypeptide and is the most potent and selective inhibitor of thrombin known. Through DNA recombinant technology, hirudin is now available in sufficient quantity for testing. Hirudin has high affinity for thrombin and effectively blocks all proteolytic functions of the enzyme. So, hirudin prevents not only fibrin formation but the thrombin-catalyzed hemostatic reactions, such as activation of factors V, VIII, XIII, and the thrombin-induced platelet reactions. Whereas platelet factor 4 is the naturally occurring inhibitor of heparin, there is no natural inhibitor of hirudin, so the only limiting factor for thrombin blockade is the dose of hirudin. Preclinical studies of hirudin in humans are well under way (149).

Ancrod (*Arvin*) is an enzyme purified from the venom of the pit viper. The proteolytic effect of ancrod on fibrinogen, as opposed to thrombin, involves cleavage only of fibrinopeptide A from the fibrinogen molecule. The resultant fibrin is susceptible to fibrinolysis, presumably because it is not cross-linked and contains degraded alpha chains. Ancrod is used as an antithrombotic in patients with heparin-induced thrombocytopenia or thrombosis who require immediate and continued anticoagulation (150).

The use of ancrod does not result in frequent hemorrhagic complications. If complications occur, they can be controlled by replacement of fibrinogen (cryoprecipitate). The effect of ancrod is monitored by measuring the fibrinogen level (134).

C. Fibrinolytics

Commonly used fibrinolytic agents include tissue plasminogen activators (tPA), Alteplase, Anistreplase, streptokinase, and urokinase. Acquired bleeding disorders during therapy with these agents are due predominantly to the effects of significant hypofibrinogenemia, and increased fibrin degradation products on fibrin clot formation. The fibrinolytic agents impair platelet function by two mechanisms: (1) High levels of fibrin degradation products coupled with very low levels of fibrinogen may impair platelet aggregation; and (2) plasminogen can bind to the platelet surface, where it is converted to the proteolytic enzyme, plasmin, by the thrombolytic drug. On the platelet surface, plasmin degrades glycoprotein Ib, impairing the interaction of the platelet with vWF and fibrinogen, thereby dispersing platelet aggregates.

Alteplase is a tPA (serine protease enzyme) produced by recombinant DNA used in the management of acute myocardial infarction and pulmonary embolism. Bleeding from any site is the most common complication. Concomitant use of heparin may contribute to the bleeding. As fibrin is lysed during tPA therapy, bleeding from recent puncture sites may occur. Risks of bleeding is greater in patients with recent surgery, obstetric delivery, organ biopsy, cardiovascular disease, GI or GU bleeding, trauma, etc. The incidence of intracranial bleeding is higher with doses in excess of 100 mg (134). The risk of bleeding is increased if heparin, vitamin K antagonists, aspirin, or dipyridamole is given prior to, during, or after Alteplase therapy.

Anistreplase (anisoylated plasminogen streptokinase activator complex, APSAC) is indicated in the management of acute myocardial infarction in adults, for the lysis of thrombi obstructing coronary arteries (134). The most common complication associated with Anistreplase therapy is bleeding, at any site. The overall incidence of bleeding in clinical trials was 14.6%. Critical location bleeding (intracranial, GI, etc.) should prompt immediate termination of any concomitant heparin, and consideration of protamine to reverse heparinization. If necessary, the bleeding tendency can be reversed with appropriate replacement therapy.

Urokinase and *streptokinase* are thrombolytic enzymes indicated in acute evolving transmural myocardial infarction, pulmonary emboli, coronary artery thrombosis, arterial thrombosis and embolism (except those originating from the left side of the heart), and occluded i.v. catheters and AV cannulae (134). Minor bleeding occurs often, mainly at invaded or disturbed sites, where local pressure may be used to control minor bleeding. Several fatalities due to cerebral and other serious internal hemorrhages have occurred. Discontinue the infusion, as slowing the rate of administration may actually make the bleeding worse. Manage blood loss and reverse the bleeding tendencies using packed red blood cells, cryoprecipitate, and/or FFP. Thrombolytic enzymes alone or in combination with anticoagulants and antiplatelet agents cause bleeding complications.

D. Chemotherapy

Malignancies are associated with an increased risk of thrombosis, but the role of cytotoxic drugs in the development of altered hemostasis is well known (151). Almost all of the antineoplastic agents cause some degree of bone marrow suppression with neutropenia, anemia, and/or thrombocytopenia. Only some are associated with a significant risk for hemorrhagic complications, and this discussion will be limited to these more common complications of chemotherapy.

1. *Antibiotic Antineoplastics (134)*

Mitomycin-C (MTC) is an antimammalian cell antibiotic which induces prolonged thrombocytopenia due to myelosuppression. Bone marrow toxicity occurs in 64% and is the most common and severe toxic effect of mitomycin.

Plicamycin (mithramycin) is another antibiotic antineoplastic. Hemorrhagic tendency, severe thrombocytopenia, and even death may result from its use. Thrombocytopenia may be rapid in onset and may occur at any time during therapy. "Hemorrhagic syndrome," the most important form of toxicity, is most likely due to abnormalities in multiple clotting factors, usually begins with epistaxis, and is dose related. The onset of an overt bleeding episode is not necessarily associated with abnormalities in clotting time or clot retraction, but abnormalities in periodically performed tests may serve as a warning of serious toxicity (134).

Idarubicin is an anthracycline antibiotic and is a potent bone marrow suppressant. Deaths due to bleeding have occurred during periods of severe myelosuppression.

Doxorubicin HCL (ADR) is an anthracycline antibiotic. Myelosuppression occurs in up to 84% of patients. Persistent, severe myelosuppression may result in hemorrhagic complications.

Mitoxantrone is an antineoplastic antibiotic given in combination with cytosine arabinoside for Acute Nonlymphocytic Leukemia. Induction with this drug causes severe myelosuppression with bleeding complications (in up to 37%), including GI bleeding and petechiae/ecchymosis (134).

Dactinomycin (actinomycin-D, ACT) is an antimammalian antibiotic thought to be a vitamin K antagonist and as such is associated with impaired production of the vitamin K-dependent clotting factors.

2. Alkylating Agents/Nitrogen Mustards (134)

Mechlorethamine HCL induces a severe thrombocytopenia which may lead to bleeding from the gums or the GI tract. Transient petechiae and subcutaneous hemorrhages may also be seen; these disappear with return to a normal platelet count. Use extreme caution when exceeding the average recommended dose; hemorrhagic diathesis with subsequent delayed bleeding may develop. Death may follow. Treat with blood product transfusions.

Melphalan is an alkylating agent inducing thrombocytopenia secondary to severe bone marrow suppression. Bleeding may occur.

Cyclophosphamide, an alkylating agent, interacts with the anticoagulants to increase the anticoagulant effect.

The nitrosoureas *Lomustine* (CCNU) and *Carmustine* (BCNU) cause severe bone marrow suppression, notably thrombocytopenia, which may contribute to bleeding complications. A major toxicity is delayed bone marrow suppression, up to 6 weeks after a dose, and is dose related. Bone marrow toxicity is cumulative.

Thiotepa dosages within and minimally above the recommended therapeutic doses have been associated with potentially life-threatening hematopoietic toxicity. The toxic effect is dose related. Death from hemorrhage has occurred as a result of the hematopoietic depression. Thiotepa is dialyzable, so treatment options include dialysis and transfusions.

Busulfan can induce dose-related severe bone marrow hypoplasia. Treatment options may include support with transfusions, discontinuing the drug, or reducing the dosage.

Carboplatin bone marrow suppression is dose related and cumulative, and may be severe, resulting in significant bleeding and drug-related death.

3. Antimetabolites (38)

Methotrexate (MTX) induces bone marrow depression and thrombocytopenia which has been associated with hemorrhage. Unexpectedly severe and sometimes fatal marrow suppression and GI toxicity have occurred with concomitant administration of MTX and a NSAID. Administer concomitantly with extreme caution, if at all. MTX also causes acute and chronic liver toxicity, thereby causing decreased hepatic synthesis of coagulation factors.

Fluorouracil (5-FU) and *Floxuridine* are highly toxic drugs with a narrow margin of safety. GI ulceration and bleeding, thrombocytopenia, and hemorrhage are complications of therapy. GI hemorrhage and death have occurred.

Cytarabine (ARA-C), *mercaptopurine* (6-MP), and *thioquanine* induce thrombocytopenia which may cause life-threatening bleeding. Treatment is supportive therapy with platelet transfusions.

4. *Hormones (134)*

Testolactone (an androgen) and *Bicalutamide* (antiandrogen) can displace coumarin anticoagulants from their protein-binding sites, thus increasing the anticoagulant effect.

Topotecan HCL, a topoisomerase inhibitor, can induce a grade 4 thrombocytopenia (<25,000 mm^3), but does not usually cause serious bleeding episodes.

Tamoxifen, an antiestrogen, has been only rarely associated with hemorrhagic episodes in patients with significant thrombocytopenia, but it is uncertain if the episodes are due to Tamoxifen therapy. When given in combination with anticoagulants, the hypoprothrombinemic effect is increased.

5. *Miscellaneous Antineoplastic Drugs (134)*

Asparaginase hydrolyzes asparagine into aspartic acid, and is usually associated with thrombotic complications secondary to alterations of levels of plasma proteins necessary for fibrinolytic response (proteins C and S, and AT-III). In addition to hypofibrinogenemia, other clotting factors depressed are factors V and VIII, and sometimes factors VII and IX. Complications of bleeding is rare, but intracranial hemorrhage and fatal bleeding associated with low fibrinogen levels have been reported.

Pegaspargase (PEG-L-asparaginase) is associated with a higher-than-usual risk for bleeding problems, especially when given concomitantly with aspirin, NSAIDs, and other drugs that have anticoagulant properties. Adverse reactions of pegaspargase (in the absence of other drugs) include hypofibrinogenemia, prolonged PT and aPTT, decreased AT-III, thrombosis, DIC, and clinical hemorrhage which may be fatal.

Podophyllotoxin and its derivatives are mitotic inhibitors, and may cause severe myelosuppression with resulting bleeding. This drug may further prolong the PT in patients on Warfarin.

Interferon alfa-2a is associated with GI hemorrhage during therapy; infrequently, the GI hemorrhage is severe or fatal. In CML patients treated with interferon alfa-2a, a severe life-threatening leukopenia and thrombocytopenia were seen in 27% of patients. Retinal hemorrhages have been observed rarely in patients being treated with interferon alfa-2b after use of the drug for several months (134).

Aldesleukin (interleukin-2, IL-2) has caused GI bleeding, ulceration, and perforation, sometimes requiring surgery.

Adverse reactions of *Paclitaxel* in clinical trials included 14% bleeding; most hemorrhagic episodes were localized.

Tretinoin (APL) is associated with a fairly high incidence of GI hemorrhages.

Gemcitabine HCL is associated with usually mild hemorrhages.

The leukopenia and thrombocytopenia due to *decarbazine* may be severe enough to cause death.

E. Antibiotics

It has been estimated that greater than one-third of hospitalized patients receive antibiotic therapy, and the incidence of antibiotic usage increases with age. Antimicrobial agents are administered therapeutically or prophylactically, and in general, cephalosporins represent the most common antibiotic prescribed for both regimens (152).

Bleeding episodes and coagulopathies have long been recognized as untoward side effects of antimicrobials and are reported with increasing frequency. The actual incidence of acquired bleeding disorders associated with antibiotic therapy is not known with certainty, and the causes are multifactorial. Reported cases frequently occur in patients with complicating clinical conditions that alone may lead to bleeding and abnormal hemostasis (152,153).

A dose- and duration-dependent inhibition of platelet function and prolongation of the bleeding time has been demonstrated with many *penicillins* and *cephalosporins* that share the beta-lactam structure (60,61). Platelet function becomes depressed and remains abnormal for several days after the antibiotic is discontinued. The effect can generally be avoided by limiting the dosage (of cephalosporins) to 4 g/day. These antibiotics inhibit platelet surface-receptor functions, presumably through a lipophilic association with the plasma membrane. Concomitant therapy with parenteral *penicillin and heparin* carries an increased risk of bleeding due to additive effects (see Table 9).

High-dose intermittent and/or resumption of interrupted *Rifampin* therapy can cause thrombocytopenia; this is reversible if the drug is discontinued as soon as purpura occurs. Cerebral hemorrhage and fatalities have occurred when Rifampin administration has continued or resumed after the appearance of purpura.

Serious bleeding associated with antibiotic-induced platelet dysfunction has been reported in severely ill patients, but it is difficult to determine if the platelet abnormality was the primary cause of bleeding. The frequency of bleeding complication with *moxolactam* is greater than with other beta-lactam antibiotics, but moxolactam also inhibits the synthesis of vitamin K-dependent proteins, so bleeding may also be related to reduced levels of factors II, VII, IX, and X.

As stated earlier, vitamin K plays an essential, obligatory role in the synthesis of procoagulant factors II, VII, IX, and X, and also anticoagulant proteins C and S. The posttranslational gamma-carboxylation of these proteins produced in the liver is necessary for the proteins to be functionally active (Fig. 1). Gamma-carboxylation is hindered by either depletion of vitamin K or inhibition of the enzyme epoxide reductase. The decarboxylated nonfunctional coagulation factors II, VII, IX, and X are unable to bind calcium and interact with phospholipid membranes. Functional vitamin K is derived from either dietary sources or enteric organisms.

1. Incidence, Mechanism, and Manifestations

The frequency of clinically detectable bleeding in patients on antimicrobial therapy varies with different antibiotic categories, underlying clinical conditions, and concomitant drug therapies. The bleeding onset typically occurs about a week after initiation of antibiotic therapy, and common sites include the GI tract, surgical wounds, GU tract, and the respiratory system. Coagulopathy in the absence of frank bleeding is seen frequently in hospitalized, frequently elderly patients on antimicrobial therapy, usually caused by vitamin K deficiency or antagonism with resultant modest prolongation of the PT. This condition is frequently misdiagnosed as DIC in very ill patients, but quickly corrects with vitamin K therapy. Mechanisms of antibiotic-associated hematologic disorders are summarized in Table 11.

An important source of vitamin K is produced by Gram-negative enteric organisms, and

Table 11 Mechanisms of Antibiotic-Associated Coagulopathies

1. Reduction of vitamin K-producing enteric organisms
2. Inhibition of vitamin K-dependent gamma-carboxylation
3. Development of circulating anticoagulants
4. Inhibition of fibrin formation and polymerization
5. Synergism with hepatotoxic medications
6. Synergism or antagonism with oral anticoagulant agents

Source: Adapted from Acquired Coagulopathies Secondary to Antimicrobial Therapy. ASCP Check Sample No. TH 90-1 (TH-67).

this is especially important in hospitalized patients who do not have adequate intake, poor appetite, or are unable to eat. Susceptible patients frequently receive broad-spectrum antibiotics including penicillin, cephalosporins, and others which have activity against many enteric organisms, reducing the populations of the vitamin K-producing enteric flora (18,152).

Decreased excretion and metabolism of drugs and thus elevated concentrations of the available antibiotic reaching the GI tract, as in renal and hepatic failure, are contributory factors in antibiotic-induced hypoprothrombinemia caused by decreased enteric organisms. Especially observe patients with renal impairment, in whom excretion of the drugs *Ticarcillin*, *Mezlocillin*, and *Piperacillin* is delayed, for prolonged bleeding manifestations.

A coumarin-like effect is seen in cephalosporins that display the molecular attachment N-methylthiotetrazole (MTT) or a similar substitution (*Cefamandole*, *Cefbuperazone*, *Cefmenoxime*, *Cefmetazole*, *Cefonicid*, *Cefoperazone*, *Cefotetan*, *Cefpiramide*, *Moxalactam*, *Ceftriaxone*, *Cefazolin*, and *Cefazedone*) (152). This substitution inhibits gamma-carboxylation of coagulation proteins, producing the coumarin-like effect. Clinically significant bleeding episodes may be seen most commonly in patients with underlying diseases such as sepsis, cancer, intraabdominal infections, or renal and/or hepatic failure. Bleeding may be serious or even fatal in these debilitated patients. Hypoprothrombinemia associated with MTT cephalosporins is rare in patients without complicating disease. Remember that these cephalosporins also may cause platelet dysfunction; use with caution in patients with thrombocytopenia or concomitant use of high-dose heparin, oral anticoagulants, aspirin, or other drugs that affect hemostasis.

Antibiotics have been associated with the development of circulating anticoagulants. Most anticoagulants are immunoglobulins of the IgG class, and these coagulation inhibitors may function as specific, nonspecific, or global inhibitors. Plasma mixing studies that demonstrate a lack of correction or incomplete correction are consistent with the presence of an inhibitor. *Streptomycin* and *aminoglycosides* are associated with factor V inhibitors, and *PCN*, *Ticarcillin*, *Carbenicillin*, *Cephalonidin*, and *Cephalothin* are associated with factor VIII inhibitors. The nonspecific lupus anticoagulant is associated with *PCN* and *Quinidine* therapy (152).

The beta-lactam antibiotics affect the conversion of fibrinogen to fibrin and the polymerization of fibrin monomers. In this case, the aPTT, PT, and TT may be prolonged. Clinical bleeding is most commonly seen in patients with renal failure.

The risk of bleeding in patients on antibiotics is increased when oral anticoagulants are added to the patient's drug therapy regimen (Table 10). Etiologies include vitamin K deficiency, displacement of coumadin by the antibiotic on plasma albumin-binding sites, gamma-carboxylation impairment, or unknown mechanisms. A decrease in the oral anticoagulants effect may be due to enhanced hepatic metabolism induced by some antibiotics.

2. *Laboratory Evaluation of Antibiotic-Associated Bleeding Disorders*

Laboratory evaluation of patients on antibiotic therapy with a hematologic complication should be preceded by baseline studies and initiated with a CBC, platelet count, PT, aPTT, and fibrinogen. Consider a vitamin K deficiency if the PT is prolonged. Consider a factor VIII inhibitor or lupus anticoagulant if the aPTT is prolonged. If both the PT and aPTT are prolonged, rule out DIC and vitamin K deficiency. The bleeding time will help to evaluate the clinical significance of a possible platelet dysfunction associated with penicillins and cephalosporins.

Treatment options according to the type and severity of the specific problem are:

Stop the offending antibiotic and choose an alternative.
Initiate vitamin K therapy if there is no clinically significant bleeding.
Use FFP and vitamin K for clinically significant bleeding.

Use cryoprecipitate if fibrinogen levels are decreased <100 mg/dL.
Use pooled platelets if there is defective platelet function.

Remember that bleeding associated with decreased factors II, VII, IX, and X can be prevented. Give susceptible patients who receive offending antibiotics (especially *Moxolactam*) 10 mg of vitamin K per week prophylactically.

In summary, the acquired bleeding disorders related to medications are common complications of therapy, and are seen in all medical specialties. Unexpected bleeding episodes can lead to significant morbidity and mortality, so physicians must be familiar with the causes, and be able to quickly diagnose and manage patients who present with these hemorrhagic disorders. Keep in mind the numerous drugs which may affect platelets in some manner, and because antibiotics are one of the more common forms of drug therapy, be aware of the offending or potentially offending drugs. Use laboratory diagnostic and monitoring tests which are useful in sorting out the etiologies of encountered coagulopathies.

Case Study 8

A 38-year-old woman presented to the local emergency room with abdominal pain, nausea, vomiting, and possible fever of 3 days duration. History and physical exam were consistent with acute pelvic inflammatory disease. The patient was begun on outpatient antimicrobial therapy consisting of Ceftriaxone and Doxycycline. The patient continued to do poorly, and nausea, vomiting, fever, and chills persisted. She was hospitalized and the antimicrobial regimen was changed to ampicillin, gentamicin, and Cleocin. Three days after hospitalization the patient was afebrile, but remained anorexic, and was noted to have "heme" positive emesis and melena.

Initial Laboratory Studies.

WBC 18,000 mm^3 (3500–10,000 mm^3)
Hematocrit 37% (39–45%)
Platelet count 203,000 mm^3 (150,000–400,000 mm^3)
Prothrombin time 25 sec (10.3–13.3 sec)
aPTT 38 sec (24–36.8 sec)
Fibrinogen 560 mg/dL (170–400 mg/dL)

Questions.

1. *What is the likely diagnosis, and what additional testing would be useful in confirming your impression?* After ruling out DIC, consider Ceftriaxone-induced coumadin effect. Cefriaxone with its MTT substitution has a coumadin effect because it inhibits gamma-carboxylation of coagulation proteins (seen commonly in patients with intraabdominal infections). These cephalosporins also may cause platelet dysfunction. A low plasma factor VII level will confirm your suspicions of a vitamin K deficiency, and a bleeding time will be helpful in evaluating platelet dysfunction associated with cephalosporins and penicillins.
2. *What choices would you consider in management?* Management may include stopping the offending antibiotic and choosing an alternative. Fresh frozen plasma and vitamin K should be used in a patient with clinically significant bleeding.

Case Study 9

A 56-year-old woman who had mitral valve replacement 10 years ago has been on long-term oral anticoagulant (coumadin, 7.5 mg/day) related to her mechanical artificial cardiac valve.

She presented to her local physician for routine follow-up. She has had no problems with unusual bleeding or bruising.

Laboratory Studies.

Hematocrit 34% (39–46%)	Prothrombin time 46 sec (10.4–13.6 sec)
aPTT 57 sec (24–37 sec)	INR 4.0 [for mechanical valve (2.5–3.5)]

Careful questioning of the patient revealed that 2 weeks prior she was visiting her daughter in another state when she developed mild gastritis and signs and symptoms of peptic ulcer disease. Her daughter's local physician had given her "stomach medicine," identified by the pharmacist as Tagamet, which she had been taking every 12 hr for 2 weeks.

Questions.

1. *What is the most likely explanation for the increase in the INR, and what additional test would be appropriate?* Tagamet and Coumadin occupy the same binding sites on albumin. The addition of Tagament to her daily medication displaced coumadin from its protein-binding sites, making more coumadin available for its anticoagulant effect. The prothrombin time and INR increase. With a marked warfarin effect, factor IX may also be reduced, prolonging the aPTT. A stool heme test for blood would be important to rule out active GI bleeding with the low hematocrit. You should follow the hematocrit at 24-hr intervals to assure that it is stable.
2. *What management options should be considered?* Management may include stopping the Tagamet and choosing an alternative H2 blocker that does not compete with coumadin for binding sites. Reduce coumadin dosage temporarily or skip a dose or two until the PT or INR return to a therapeutic range.

NOTE ADDED IN PROOF

Since this manuscript was prepared, the pharmacological management of bleeding associated with portal hypertension has been reviewed in a very comprehensive manner by Lebrec (155). Tranexamic acid has been used successfully for gastric bleeding due to vascular ectasia in cirrhosis by McCormick (156). Aggressive treatment with antibiotics at the time of initial gastrointestinal bleeding in cirrhosis has reduced rebleeding and morbidity (157,158).

Clopidorgrel is a potent inhibitor of ADP platelet aggregation and is used in the management of myocardial infarction and stroke (159,160). It may also have a role in thrombin generation in the platelet-dependent situation, and therefore may also have an anticoagulant effect on hemostasis (161).

REFERENCES

1. Clark R, Rake M, Flute P, Williams. Coagulation abnormalities in acute liver failure: pathogenic and therapeutic implications. Scand J Gastroent 1973; 8:63–70.
2. Cooper R. Hemolytic syndromes and red cell membrane abnormalities in liver disease. Semin Hematol 1980; 17:103–112.
3. Cowan D. Effect of alcoholism on hemostasis. Semin Hematol 1980; 17:137–147.
4. Kelly D. Summerfield, hemostatis I liver disease. Semin Liver Dis 1987; 7:182–191.
5. Lindenbaums J. Hematologic complications of alcohol abuse. Semin Liver Dis 1987; 7:769–781.

6. Zetterman RK. Modern approach to alcoholic liver disease. Scand J Gastroenterol 27(suppl) 1992; 192:55–62.
7. Zimmerman J, Meroz Y, Siguencia J, et al. Upper gastrointestinal hemorrhage: comparison of the causes and prognosis is primary and secondary bleeders. Scand J Gastroenterol 1994; 29:795–797.
8. Chopra S, Griffin P. Laboratory tests and diagnostic procedures in evolution of liver disease. Am J Med 1985; 79:221–230.
9. Merican I, Sprengers D, McCormic PA, et al. Diurnal pattern of variceal bleeding in cirrhotic patients. J Heptol 1993; 19:15–22.
10. Gostout CJ, Viggiano TR, Balm RK. Acute gastrointestinal bleeding from portal hypertensive gastropathy: prevalence and clinical features. Am J Gastroenterol 1993; 88:2030–2033.
11. Brewer TG. Treatment of acute gastroesophageal variceal hemorrhage. Med Clin N Am 1993; 77: 993–1013.
12. Perez E, Tanaka M, Gandara D. Conjugated estrogen for platelet dysfunction associated with liver disease (letter). N Engl J Med 1988; 318:1543.
13. Shimodaria S, Ishida F, Ichikawa N, et al. Serum thrombopoietin (c-Mpl ligand) levels in patients with liver cirrhosis. Thromb Hemostas 1996; 76:545–548.
14. Bick RL. Laboratory evaluation of platelet dysfunction. Clin Lab Med 1995; 15:1–38.
15. Greaves M, Nakielay R, Hampton K, et al. Bleeding times in patients with hepatic cirrhosis (letter). Br Med J 1990; 301:442.
16. Rock W. Laboratory assessment of coagulation disorders in liver disease. Clin Lab Med 1984; 4: 419–442.
17. Rubin M, Weston M, Longley P, et al. Platelet function in chronic liver disease: relationship to disease severity. Dig Dis Sci 1979; 24:197–202.
18. Mammen EF. Coagulation abnormalities in liver disease. Hematol/Oncol Clin N Am 1992(6): 1247–1257.
19. Mannucci P, Vincent V, Vianello L, et al. Controlled trial of Desmopressin in liver cirrhosis and other conditions associated with a prolonged bleeding time. N Engl J Med 1986; 67:1148–1153.
20. Mannucci PM, Frachi F, Dioguardi N. Correction of abnormal coagulation in chronic liver disease by combined use of fresh frozen plasma and prothrombin complex concentrates. Lancet 1976; 542–545.
21. Friedman E, Sussman I. Plasma use for coagulopathy of liver disease (abstr). Blood 1986(suppl); 68:1064.
22. Harrison CR, Polesky HF. College of American Pathologists Conference XXV on current transfusion medicine practice and issues: concluding remarks and recommendations. Arch Pathol Lab Med 1994; 118:462–464.
23. Harrison CR, Sawyer PR. Special Issues in Transfusion Medicine, Selected Topics in Transfusion Medicine, Clinics in Lab Med, 12. Philadelphia: Saunders, 1992:743–751.
24. Harvey MP, Greenfield TP, Sugrue ME, et al. Massive blood transfusion in a tertiary referral hospital: clinical outcomes and haemostatic complications. Med J Austral 1995; 163:356–359.
25. Francis R, Feinstein D. Clinical significance of accelerated fibrinolysis in the upper gastrointestinal tract. Scand J Gastroenterol 1987; 22(suppl):19–21.
26. Isacson S. Fibrinolysis in the upper gastrointestinal tract. Scand J Gastroenterol 1987(suppl 137); 22:19–21.
27. Fourrier F, Chopin C, Huart J, et al. Double-blind, placebo-controlled trial of antithrombin III concentrates in septic shock with disseminated intravascular coagulation. Chest 1993; 104:882–888.
28. Ewaga H, Keeffe EB, Dort J. Liver transplantation for uncontrollable variceal bleeding. Am J Gastroenterol 1994; 89:1823–2033.
29. McNicol PL, Liu G, Harley ID, et al. Patterns of coagulopathy during liver transplantation: experience with the first 75 cases using thrombelastography. Anaesth Intensiv Care 1994; 22:659–665.
30. Tygstrup N, Ranek L. Assessment of prognosis in fulminant hepatic failure. Semin Liver Dis 1986; 6:127–137.
31. Watanabe A, Shiota T, Higashi T. Multiple organ failure in patients with fulminant hepatitis and in post-operative patients with liver cirrhosis. J Med 1992; 23:117–125.

32. Ewe K. Bleeding after liver biopsy does not correlate with indices of peripheral coagulation. Dig Dis Sci 1981; 26:388–393.
33. MacMathuna P, Vlavinos P, Westaby D, et al. Pathophysiology of portal hypertension. Dig Dis 1992; 10(suppl 1):3–15.
34. McCormick RP, Dick R, Burroughs AK. Review article: the transjugular intrahepatic portosystemic shunt (TIPS) in the treatment of portal hypertension. Aliment Pharmacol Ther 1994; 8: 273–282.
35. Orloff MJ, Orloff MS, Rambotti M. Treatment of bleeding esophagogastric varices due to extrahepatic portal hypertension: results of portal-systemic shunts during 35 years. J Ped Surg 1994; 29: 142–154.
36. Plevris JN, Elliot R, Mills PR, et al. Effect of propranolol on prevention of first variceal bleed and survival in patients with chronic liver disease. Aliment Pharmacol Ther 1994; 8:63–70.
37. Rikkers LF, Jin G. Emergency shunt: role in the present management of variceal bleeding. Arch Surg 1995; 130:472–477.
38. Terblanche J. Portal hypertension management. Surg Endosc 1993; 7:472–478.
39. Van Hoek B, Lindor KD, Mintaugh PA, et al. The role of portosystemic shunts for variceal bleeding in the liver transplant. Arch Surg 1994; 129:683–688.
40. Boks AL, Brommer EJP, Schalm SW, et al. Hemostasis and fibrinolysis in severe liver failure and their relation to hemorrhage. Hepatology 1986; 6:79–86.
41. Jalan R, Grose R, Dillon JF. Gastric mucosal bleeding in cirrhosis. Gastrointest Endosc 1994; 40: 599–602.
42. Lee H, Hawker FH, Selby W, et al. Intensive care treatment of patients with bleeding esophageal varices: results, predictors of mortality, and predictors of the adult respiratory distress syndrome. Crit Care Med 1992; 20:1555–1563.
43. Bismuth H, Houssin D, Mazmanion G. Postoperative liver insufficiency: prevention and management world. J Surg 1983; 7:505–510.
44. Koller F. Theory and experience behind the use of coagulation tests in diagnosis and prognosis of liver disease. Scand J Gastroenterol 1973(suppl); 19:51–61.
45. Veltkamp J, Kreuning. J. The diagnostic value of coagulation studies in chronic liver disease. Scand J Gastroenterol 1973(suppl); 19:93–95.
46. Cordova L, Violi F, Alessandri C, et al. Pekallikrein and factor VII as prognostic indexes of liver failure. Am J Clin Pathol 1986; 85:579–582.
47. Orlando M, Casalbore P, Camagna A, Laura R, Tardella L, Hassan H. Factor VII in liver cirrhosis. Hemostasis 1982; 11:73–78.
48. Violi F, Basill S, Ferro D, et al. Association between high values of D-dimer and tissue-plasminogen activator activity and first gastrointestinal bleeding in cirrhotic patients. Thromb Hemostas 1996; 76:117–183.
49. Denison H, Kaezynski J, Wallerstedt S. Paracetomal medication and alcohol abuse: a dangerous combination for liver and kidney. Scand J Gastroenterol 1987; 22:701–704.
50. Abu-Elmagd KM, Aly MA, Fathy OM, et al. Ten years of experience with patients with chronic active liver disease variceal bleeding: ablative versus selective decompressive therapy. Surgery 1993; 114:868–881.
51. Aldersley MA, O'Grady JG. Hepatic disorders: features and appropriate management. Drugs 1995; 49:83–102.
52. Bernuau J, Rueff B, Benhomou J. Fulminant and subfulminant liver failure: definitions and causes. Semin Liver Dis 1986; 6:97–106.
53. Bertoglia E, Belmonte P, Vertolli U, Azzurro M, Martines D. Bleeding in cirrhotic patients: a precipitating factor due to intravascular coagulation or to hepatic failure. Hemostasis 1983; 13: 328–334.
54. Burroughs AK. The natural history of varices. J Hepatol 1993(suppl 2); 17:s10–s13.
55. Forster J, Delcore R, Payne KM, et al. The role of transjugular intrahepatic portosystemic shunts in the management of patients with end-stage liver disease. Am J Surg 1994; 168:592–597.

56. Johansen K, Helton WS. Portal hypertension and bleeding in esophageal varices. Ann Vascular Surg 1992; 6:553–561.
57. Printice C. Acquired coagulation disorders. Clin Haematol 1985; 14:413–442.
58. Wilson DE. Gastrointestinal bleeding in patients with chronic liver disease: a review. J Assoc Acad Minor Physicians 1994; 5:50–58.
59. Heyman SN, Brezis M. Acute renal failure in glomerular bleeding: a puzzling phenomenon. Nephrol Dial Transplant: Editorial Comments 1995; 10:591–593.
60. Zimmerman SW, Moorthy AV, Dreher WH, et al, Prospective trial of warfarin and dipyridamole in patients with membranoproliferative pyleonephritis, Am J Med 1983; 55:920–925.
61. George JN, Shattil SJ. The clinical importance of acquired abnormalities of platelet function. N Engl J Med 1991; 324:27–39.
62. Alexopoulos E, Tambakoudis P, Sakellariou G, et al. Acute renal failure in pregnancy. Renal Failure 1993; 15:609–613.
63. Siebels M, Andrassy K, Waldherr R, Rite E. Hemolytic uremic syndrome complicating postinfectious glomerulonephritis in the adult. Am J Kidney Dis 1995; 25:336–336.
64. Dacie JU, Lewis SM. Practical Hematology. London Churchill Livingston, 1995:353.
65. Hofman M, Monroe DM, Roberts HR. Platelet activation in platelets with thrombotic thrombocytopenic purpura. Am J Hematol 1993; 42:182–185.
66. Sibai BM, Kustermann L, Valasco J. Current understanding of severe preeclampsia, pregnancy associated hemolytic uremic syndrome, thrombotic thrombocytopenic purpura, hemolysis, elevated liver enzymes, and low platelet syndrome, and postpartum acute renal failure: different clinical syndromes or just different names? (review). Curr Opin Nephrol Hypertension 1994; 3:436–445.
67. Conlon PJ, Howell DN, Macik G, et al. The renal manifestations and outcome of thrombotic thrombocytopenic purpura/hemolytic syndrome in adults. Nephrol Dialysis, Transplant 1995; 10: 1189–1193.
68. Hayward CP, Sutton DM, Carter WH Jr, et al. Treatment outcomes in patients with adult thrombotic thrombocytopenic purpura-hemolytic uremic syndrome. Arch Intern Med 1994; 154:982–987.
69. Mokrzycki MH, Kaplan AA. Therapeutic plasma exchange: complications and management. Am J Kidney Dis 1994; 23:817–827.
70. Akmal M, Sawelson S, Karubian F, et al. The prevalence and significance of occult blood loss in patients with predialysis advanced chronic renal failure (CFR), or receiving dialytic therapy. Clin Nephrol 1994; 42:198–202.
71. Hemostatic Disorders and the Blood Bank. Technical Workshop, American Association of Blood Banks, Arlington Virginia, 1984.
72. Horowitz HI, Stein IM, Cohen BD, et al. Further studies on the platelet-inhibitory effect of quanidinosuecinic acid and its role in uremic bleeding. Am J Med 1970; 49:336–345.
73. Rabiner SF, Molinas F. The role of phenol and phenolic acids on the thrombocytopathy and defective platelet aggregation of platelets in renal failure. Am J Med 1970; 49:346–351.
74. Benigni A, Boccardo P, Galbusera M, et al. Reversible activation defect of the platelet glycoprotein IIb-IIIa complex in patients with uremia. Am J Kidney Dis 1993; 22:668–676.
75. Beumer S, Ijsseldijk MJW, De Groot PG, Sixma JJ. Platelet adhesion to fibronectin in flow: dependence on surface concentration and shear rate, role of platelet membrane glycoproteins GP IIb/IIIa and VLA-5, and inhibition by heparin. Blood 1994; 84:3724–3733.
76. Gawaz MP, Dobos G, Spath M. Impaired function of platelet membrane glycoprotein IIb-IIIa in end-stage renal disease. J Am Soc Nephrol 1994; 5:36–46.
77. Sreedhara R, Itagaki I, Hakim RM. Uremic patients have decreased shear-induced platelet aggregation mediated by decreased availability of glycoprotein IIb-IIIa receptors. Am J Kidney Dis 1996; 27:355–364.
78. Slazus W. Increased production of prostacyclin after injury to the microvasculature in uraemic patients. S Afr Med J 1992; 81:315–317.
79. Remuzzi G. Bleeding in renal failure (a review). Lancet 1988; 1:1205–1208.

80. Remuzzi G, Benigni A, Dodesini P, et al. Parathyroid hormone inhibits human platelet function. Lancet 1981; 2:1321–1323.
81. Alvarez L, Puleo J, Balint JA. Investigation of gastrointestinal bleeding in patients with end stage renal disease. Am J Gastroenterol 1993; 88:30–33.
82. Mezzano D, Tagle R, Panes O, et al. Hemostatic disorder of uremia: the platelet defect, main determinant of the prolonged bleeding time, is correlated with indices of activation of coagulation and fibrinolysis. Thromb Hemost 1996; 76:321.
83. Richardson JD, Lordon RE. Gastrointestinal bleeding caused by angiodysplasia: a difficult problem with chronic renal failure receiving hemodialysis therapy. Am Surgeon 1993; 59:636.
84. Mannucci PM, Remuzzi G, Pusineri F, et al. Deamino-8-arginine vasopressin shortens the bleeding time in Uremia. N Engl J Med 1983; 308:8–12.
85. Breddin HK, Radziwon P, Boczkowska-Radziwon B. Laboratory monitoring of new antithrombotic drugs. Clin Lab Med 1994; 14(4):825–846.
86. Bronner M, Marion B, Cunningham J, et al. Estrogen progesterone therapy for bleeding gastrointestinal telangiectasias in chronic renal failure. Ann Intern Med 1986; 105:271–274.
87. Liu YK, Kosfeld RE, Marcum SG. Treatment of uraemic bleeding with conjugated oestrogen. Lancet 1984; 2:887–889.
88. Sloand JA, Schiff MJ. Beneficial effect of low dose transderman estrogen on bleeding time and clinical bleeding in uremia. Am J Kidney Dis 1995; 26:22–26.
89. Carvalho AC. Acquired platelet dysfunction in patients with uremia. Hematol/Oncol Clin N Am 1990; 4:129–143.
90. Kellerman PS. Perioperative care of the renal patient; review article. Arch Intern Med 1994; 154: 1674–1688.
91. Saito H. Alterations of Hemostasis in Renal Disease. In: Forbes C, ed. Disorders of Hemostasis. Philadelphia: Saunders, 1986:443–456.
92. Schreiber S, Korzets A, Powsner E, et al. Surgery in chronic dialysis Patients. Isr J Med Sci 1995; 31:479–483.
93. Zachee P, Vermylen J, Boogaerts MA. Hematologic aspects of end-stage renal failure. Ann Hematol 1994; 69:33–40.
94. Adcock DM, Marlar A. Uremia a cause of bleeding, ASCP check sample. Thromb Hemos 1989; 11:1–10.
95. Safar P. Resuscitation in hemorrhagic shock, coma, and cardiac arrest. In: Adams Cowley R, Trump BF, eds. Pathophysiology of Shock, Anoxia, and Ischemia. Baltimore: Williams & Wilkins, 1982:429–430.
96. Scadden DT. Hematologic disorders and growth factor support in HIV infection. In: Krown SE, Von Roenn, JH, eds. Hematology and Oncologic Aspects of HIV Infection, Hematol/Oncol Clin N Am 10. Philadelphia: Saunders, 1996:1149–1161.
97. Bone RC. Modulators of coagulation: a critical appraisal of their role in sepsis. Arch Intern Med 1992; 153:1381–1389.
98. Philippe J, Offner F, Declerck PJ, et al. Fibrinolysis and coagulation in patients with infectious disease and sepsis. Thromb Haemost 1991; 65:291–295.
99. Matuschak GM. Sepsis: complications and multiple systems organ failure. Contemp Intern Med July/August 1992; 92–115.
100. Fein AM, Niederman MS. New approaches to the management of sepsis. Contemp Intern Med July/August 1992; 35–51.
101. Wuillemin WA, Fijnvandraat K, Derkx BHF, et al. Activation of the intrinsic pathway of coagulation in children with meningococcal septic shock. Thromb Haemost 1995; 74:1436–1441.
102. Ratnoff OD. Disseminated intravascular coagulation. In: Ratnoff OD, Forbes CD, eds. Disorders of Bleeding. Philadelphia: Saunders, 1996:256–295.
103. Warrell RP, Kenpin SJ. Treatment of severe coagulopathy in the Kasabod-Merrit syndrome with aminocaproic acid and cryoprecipitate. N Engl J Med 1985; 313:309–311.
104. Bick RL. Coagulation abnormalities in malignancy: a review. Semin Thromb Hemost 1992; 18: 353–372.

105. Bona RD, Sivijee KY, Hickey AM. The efficacy and safety of oral anticoagulation in patients with cancer. Thromb Haemost 1995; 74:1055–1058.
106. Falange A, Barbui T, Rickles FR. Guidelines for clotting studies in cancer patients. Thromb Haemost 1993; 70:540–542.
107. Goad KE, Gralnick HR. Coagulation disorders in cancer. In Hematologic Complications of Cancer, Hematol/Oncol Clin N Am 10. Philadelphia: Saunders, 1996:451–484.
108. Goldsmith GH. Hemostatic disorders associated with neoplasia. In: Ratnoff OD, Forbes CD, eds. Disorders of Hemostasis. Philadelphia: Saunders, 1991:352–368.
109. Iversen LH, Okholm M, Thorlacius-Ussing O. Pre- and postoperative state of coagulation and fibrinolysis in plasma of patients with benign and malignant colorectal disease—a preliminary study. Thromb Haemost 1996; 76:523–528.
110. Markman M. Common complications and emergencies associated with cancer and its therapy. Cleveland Clin J Med 1994; 61:105–114.
111. Vishney ML, Blades EW, Creger RJ, et al. Role of upper endoscopy in evaluation of upper gastrointestinal symptoms in patients undergoing bone marrow transplantation. Cancer Invest 1994; 12: 384–389.
112. Haire WD, Ruby EI, Gordon BG, et al. Multiple organ dysfunction syndrome in bone marrow transplantation. JAMA 1995; 274:1289–1295.
113. Hasegawa D. Coagulation abnormalities in acute leukemia. Lab Med 1986; 17:388–393.
114. McCauley DL. Therapy review: treatment of adult leukemia. Clin Pharm 1992; 11:767–796.
115. Kunkel LA. Acquired circulating anticoagulants in malignancy. Semin Thromb Hemost 1992; 18: 416–423.
116. Rizk SN, Ryan JJ. Clinicopathologic review of 92 cases of Colon Cancer. S Dakota J Med 1994; 47:89–93.
117. Bouvry P, Recloux P. Acquired hemophilia (review). Haematologica 1994; 79:550–556.
118. Vivaldi PM, Savino M, Mazzon C, Rubertelli M. A hemorrhagic syndrome of the elderly patient caused by anti-factor VIII antibodies. Haematologica 1993; 78:245–248.
119. Rapaport SI, Zivelin A, Minow RA, et al. Clinical significance of antibodies to bovine and human bovine and factor V of surgical use of bovine thrombin. Am J Clin Pathol 1992; 97:84–91.
120. Spero JA. Bovine thrombin induced inhibitor of factor V and bleeding risk in postoperative neurosurgical patients. J Neurosurg 1993; 78:817–820.
121. Carroll JF, Moskowitz KA, Edwards NM. Immunologic assessment of patients treated with bovine fibrin as a hemostatic agent. Thromb Haemost 1996; 76:925–931.
122. Bajaj SP, Rapaport SI, Barclay S, Herbst KD. Acquired hypoprothrombinemia due to nonneutralizing antibodies to prothrombin: mechanism and management. Blood 1985; 65:1538–1543.
123. Exmer T. Diagnostic methodologies for circulating anticoagulants. Thromb Haemost 1995; 74: 338–344.
124. La Spada AR, Skalhegg BS, Henderson R, et al. Brief report: fatal hemorrhage in a patient with an acquired inhibitor of human thrombin. N Engl J Med 1995; 333:494–497.
125. Glaspy JA. Disturbances in hemostasis in patients with B-cell malignancies. Semin Thromb Hemost 1992; 18:440–448.
126. Jakway JL. Acquired von Willebrand's disease in malignancy. Semin Thromb Hemost 1992; 18: 434–439.
127. Ginsberg SS, Clyne LP, McPhedran P, et al. Successful childbirth by a patient with congenital factor XI deficiency and an acquired inhibitor. 1993; 84:172–174.
128. Matsunaga AT, Shafer FE. An acquired inhibitor to factor X in a pediatric patient with extensive burns. J Ped Hematol/Oncol 1996; 18:223–236.
129. Ortel TL, Quinn-Allen MA, Charles LA, et al. Characterization of an acquired inhibitor to coagulation factor V. J Clin Invest 1992; 90:2340–2347.
130. Rosing J, Bevers E, Comfurius P. Impaired factor X and prothrombin activation associated with decreased phospholipid exposure in platelets from a patient with a bleeding disorder. Blood 65: 1557–1561.
131. Tosetto A, Rodeghiero F, Gatto E, et al. An acquired hemorrhagiac disorder of fibrin crosslinking

due to IgG antibodies to FXIII, successfully treated with FXIII replacement and cyclophosphamide. Am J Hematol 1995; 48:34–39.
132. Jensen R, Ens GE. Antiplatelet therapy. Clin Hemost Rev. 1992; 6(3):1–16.
133. Jensen R, Ens GE. Platelet activation markers. Clin Hemost Rev 1992; 6(9):1–10.
134. Olin BR, Hebel SK, Hagemann RC, eds. Drug Facts and Comparisons 1996.
135. Reubinoff BE, Eldor A, Laufer N, et al. Maternal hemorrhagic complications following prophylactic low-dose aspirin and dipyridamole therapy. Gynecol Obstet Invest 1992; 33:241–243.
136. Kakkar R, Feldges A, Mehdorn M, et al. Prophylaxis of venous thromboembolism. World J Surg 1990; 14:670–678.
137. Claes Y, Hemelijck J, Geruen M, et al. Influence of hydroxethyl starch on coagulation in patients during the perioperative period. Anesth Analg 1992; 75:24–30.
138. Nevelsteen A, Mortelmans L, Van de Cruys A, Merckx E, Verhaeghe R. Effect of ticlopidine on blood loss, platelet turnover and platelet deposition on prosthetic surfaces in patients undergoing aorta-femoral bypass grafting. Thromb Res 1991; 64:363–369.
139. Capra R, Marciano N, Fiene F, et al. Cerebral hemorrhage and thrombotic thrombocytopenic purpura during ticlopidine treatment: case report. Acta Neurol Belg 1992; 92:83–87.
140. Carlson JA, Maesner JE. Fatal neutropenia and thrombocytopenia associated with Ticlopidine. Ann Pharmacother 1994; 28:1236–1238.
141. Elias M, Reichman N, Flatau E. Bone marrow aplasia associated with Ticlopidine therapy. Am J Hematol 1993; 44:289–291.
142. Ono K, Kurohara K, Yoshihara M, et al. Agranulocytosis caused by Ticlopidine and its mechanism. Am J Hematol 1991; 37:239–242.
143. Hirsh J, Dalen JE, Deykin D, et al. Oral anticoagulants: mechanism of action, clinical effectiveness and optimal therapeutic range. Chest 1992; 2(suppl):3125–3265.
144. Genewein U, Haeberli A, Straub PW, Beer JH. Rebound after cessation of oral anticoagulant therapy: the biochemical evidence. Br J Haematol 1996; 92:479–485.
145. Warkentin TE, Kelton JG. Heparin-induced thrombocytopenia. In: Coller BS, ed. Progress in Hemostasis and Thrombosis. Philadelphia: Saunders, 1991:1–27.
146. Azrin MA, Mitchel JF, Fram DB, et al. Decreased platelet deposition and smooth muscle cell proliferation after intramural heparin delivery with hydrogel-coated balloons. Circulation 1994; 90:433–441.
147. Samama MM. Contemporary laboratory monitoring of low molecular weight heparins. Clin Lab Med 1995; 15:114–123.
148. Matsuo T, Kario K, Chikahira Y, Nakao K, Yamada T. Treatment of heparin-induced thrombocytopenia by use of argatroban, a synthetic thrombin inhibitor. Br J Haematol 1992; 82:627–629.
148B. Breddin HK, Radziwon P, Boczkowska-Radziwon B. Laboratory monitoring of new antithrombotic drugs. In Bick R, ed. Clinics in Laboratory Medicine, Thrombosis and Hemostasis for the Clinical Laboratory: Part I, Philadelphia: WB Saunders, 1994:825–846.
149. Stein B, Fuster V. Clinical pharmacology of platelet inhibitors. In: Fuster V, Verstraete M, eds. Thrombosis in Cardiovascular Disorders. Philadelphia: Saunders, 1992:99–116.
150. Mackie MJ, Douglas AS. Drug-induced disorders of coagulation. In: Ratnoff OD, Forbes CD, eds. Disorders of Hemostasis, 2d ed. Philadelphia: Saunders, 1991:493–511.
151. Jensen R, Ens GE. Chemotherapy and hemostasis. Clin Hemost Rev 1992; 6(12):1–12.
152. Hicks MJ, Adcock DM, Marlar RA. Acquired coagulopathies secondary to antimicrobial therapy. In ASCP Check Sample, Thrombosis and Hemostasis, 1989; No. TH 90-1 (TH-67):1–11.
153. Cohen H, Scott S, Mackie I, Shearer M, Box R, Karron S, Machin S. The development of hypoprothrombinaemia following antibiotic therapy in malnourished patients with low sodium vitamin K levels. Br J Haematol 1988; 68:66.
154. Corriveau DM, Fritsma GA. Hemostasis and Thrombosis: In the Clinical Laboratory. New York: Lippincott, 1988.
155. Lebrec, D. Pharmacological treatment of portal hypertension; present and future. J of Hepatology 1998; 28:896–907.

156. McCormick PA, Ooi H, Crosbie O. Tranexamic acid for severe, bleeding gastric antral vascular ectasis in cirrhosis. Gut 1998; 43:750–752.
157. Bernard B, Cadranel JF, Valla D, Escolano S, Jarlier V, et al. Prognostic significance of baterial infection in bleeding cirrhotic patients: A prospective study. Gastroenterology 1995; 108:1828–1834.
158. Goulis J, Armonis A, Patch D, Sabin C, Greenslade L, et al. Bacterial infection is independently associated with failure to control bleeding in cirrhotic patients with gastrointestinal hemorrhage. Hepatology 1998; 27:1207–1212.
159. Herbert JM, Frehel D, Bernat A. Bardorc A, Savi P, et al. Clopidogrel hydrogenosulfate. Drugs of the Future 1993; 18:107–112.
160. CAPRIE Steering Committee. A random, blinded, trial of clopidogrel versus aspirin in patients at risk of ischemic events (CAPRIE). Lancet 1996; 348:1329–1339.
161. Herault JP, Dol F, Gaich C, Bernat A, Herbert, JM. Effect of clopidogrel on thrombin generation in platelet-rich plasma in the rat. Thrombo Haemost 1999; 81:957–960.

31

Acquired Bleeding Disorders Associated with the Character of the Surgery

William A. Rock, Jr.
University of Mississippi Medical Center, Jackson, Mississippi

Robert F. Baugh
Medtronic Blood Management, Parker, Colorado

I. INTRODUCTION

The changing clinical scene presents some significant problems in diagnosing both hemorrhagic and thrombotic complications associated with modern-day surgical and interventional procedures. These high-risk procedures for bleeding are by their very nature the cause of the bleeding. This should not suggest in any manner that the surgical procedure is unnecessary or unwarranted, but rather that inherent in the procedure is a greater likelihood of bleeding. These complications include defects in hemostasis by virtue of the surgical procedure or defects from devices employed as an essential aspect of the surgical technique or procedure. These new ways of performing surgery not only require constant vigilance for changing techniques, devices, and drug usage, but also continual contact with physicians in their environment.

These are areas in which the practice of medicine is still somewhat of an art. In addition, there is a likelihood that unique and specialized variances of standard procedures have evolved which are not based on fact, but rather on personal and anecdotal experience. One of the main things to understand is that some aspects of surgery are not characterized by any established standard procedure. This holds even within the same institution, where different clinical teams perform procedures differently. Thus it is not unusual to find predicaments associated with a team, rather than the institution. Two major surgical procedures are discussed in this chapter, cardiopulmonary bypass and trauma with massive blood transfusion. In addition, information is provided on a select list of procedures noted to have unique conditions for bleeding, such as orthopedic surgery, urological surgery, and neurosurgery. Laboratory testing for these procedures is similar, with some specific testing required for the assessment of the unique aspects of that surgery. However, some basic concepts should guide the requesting of coagulation tests. These concepts include: (a) complete preoperative history for diseases and bleeding tendencies; (b) careful history of medications; (c) presurgical baseline coagulation studies including CBC/platelet count, PT, aPTT, and fibrinogen for assessing the bleeding risk associated with a positive history of bleeding problems. This information can be used to determine the need for requesting specialized coagulation analysis, for monitoring and evaluating the significance of coagulation changes that occur during and after surgery, and establish their relationship to clinical bleeding. An added benefit is documentation currently required for hospital blood utilization programs.

II. CARDIOPULMONARY BYPASS AND VASCULAR SURGERY

A. Introduction

Cardiopulmonary bypass (CPB) surgery is the bypass of the patient's complete diluted and heparinized blood volume though an extracorporeal pumping system. The blood is received from the body via a venous line, chilled to 25–28°C, oxygenated, and filtered before being returned to the patient via an arterial line. Since the late 1980s, when the transmission of viral contaminants in the general blood supply became a major issue, cardiovascular surgery has been challenged to limit postsurgical blood loss. Until that time, a high level of blood usage was a common event in cardiovascular surgery. In the ensuing years a number of changes in bypass procedures, equipment, techniques, and the introduction of new drugs have allowed the issue of blood loss and blood product usage to be addressed directly. The challenges are now even more complex. The reduced blood product usage must be achieved in a cost-conscious environment, and the reduction must not be accompanied by a substantial increase in patient bleeding or thrombotic risk. CPB surgery has been challenged to provide a stable postsurgical patient whose hemostatic mechanisms have been altered by the procedure. The patient should be hypocoagulable during the bypass procedure, but not to the extent that blood loss and blood product usage become a major issue postoperatively. If the coagulation is not carefully limited, deep vein thrombosis, stroke, and myocardial infarction are significant risks.

B. Activation of Coagulation During Surgery

Cardiopulmonary bypass surgery produces an observable activation of coagulation. This surgery requires total circulation anticoagulation with heparin, and the entire bypass procedure is one of the few medical areas where STAT coagulation testing has been performed on a routine basis (1). However, the very nature of today's bypass surgery has minimized the obvious appearance of the postsurgical complications of coagulation activation, such as a consumption of clotting factors and activation of the fibrinolytic system. The minimization occurs with heparin, clear prime dilution, hypothermia, dilution with washed red cell salvage, and extracorporeal circulation, all of which help mask the activation of the coagulation system.

1. Surgery and Contact Activation

One of the striking things about cardiopulmonary bypass surgery is the apparent systemic activation of coagulation that occurs when a surgical maneuver is performed. Every event, from the placing of cannulae and catheters to the harvesting of graft vessels, is accompanied by a measurable systemic activation. This appears to be "contact activation." It is measurable by clotting tests that are affected by contact activation, and there does not appear to be any immediate downregulation of this systemic activation. The insertion of a heart catheter will over at least 15–30 min result in the shortening of the activated clotting time. This is noticed, but very rarely is it commented on, nor is there much speculation as to the source of the systemic activation (1). The source is surgical tissue damage, yet this contact activation is more likely to be attributed to the extracorporeal circuit. The usual reason for considering contact activation in cardiovascular (CV) surgery has been the action of pumping blood through the extracorporeal circuit. This provides a significant amount of surface area for the generation of contact activation. A significant amount of work has gone into neutralizing the components of the circuit. Pumps have been redesigned, circuits have had bioactive coatings applied, bubbler oxygenators have been replaced with membrane oxygenators, and numerous other modifications have been made in attempts to reduce the perceived activation induced by the components of the extracorporeal circuit (2,3).

One of the major sources of clotting during cardiopulmonary bypass surgery is the release of tissue factor which activates the extrinsic system. However, it is possible that some other protease or trigger is released during surgery which activates the contact system. Aprotinin,* which is a serine protease inhibitor, appears to inhibit the "systemic contact activation" phenomenon seen in CV surgery (4–11). Furthermore, aprotinin has been used as an anticoagulant in orthopedic surgery, where the results have been similar to heparin with respect to the prevention of postsurgical DVT and excessive bleeding (12). Orthopedic surgery involves no extracorporeal circulation, yet aprotinin appears to provide the same benefits. Either tissue factor-medicated coagulation is linked to systemic contact activation by kallikrein, or some kallikrein-like protease is being released during surgical tissue damage.

2. Platelet Activation

The activation and subsequent destruction of platelets during cardiopulmonary bypass surgery is almost a foregone conclusion. Platelet activation, coupled with the other excesses of extracorporeal circulation and surgery, leads to decreased platelet number and function postsurgically. This postsurgical platelet dysfunction is thought to be the primary reason for excessive blood loss in CV surgery. Although this almost seems intuitive, it should be remembered that not all patients who undergo cardiopulmonary bypass surgery develop a platelet defect that is significant clinically. Why some patients develop the platelet dysfunction and others do not may be a result of a series of occurrences which, when present in a specific patient, result in bleeding. The activation of platelets during bypass occurs through several different mechanisms: (a) the surface and nature of the extracorporeal circuit, (b) thrombin that is generated by the surgery, and (c) the anticoagulant heparin. Although heparin as an activator of platelets is recognized as an inducer of thrombocytopenia and the white clot syndrome (13–17), its producing the consumption of platelets during bypass surgery is somewhat controversial. This is obviously contradictory, because there is other evidence that the levels of heparin used in bypass surgery have a protective effect on platelets (18–23). This may be one of the variables that predisposes one and not another patient to the risk of bleeding from platelet dysfunction as a result of bypass surgery.

3. Pathologic and Hypercoagulable Activation

Pathological activation of coagulation may be associated with a genetic or acquired defect (see Chapter 33 by Fairweather). Under the acquired hypercoagulable states, one of the most common would be associated with a cardiovascular event, such as an acute myocardial infarction, a failed interventional cardiology procedure, trauma, or a triggered immune response. In cardiopulmonary bypass surgery the hypercoagulable patient is usually not a surprise, however, he or she can present major management problems. Since the primary method of monitoring heparinization during bypass is the activated clotting time (ACT), this type of patient is usually characterized by failure to prolong the ACT with heparin or an extremely short activated clotting time. Dosing heparin based on the activated clotting time can take into account the

---

*Aprotinin is a serine protease inhibitor. Current forms of aprotinin are natural products isolated from bovine lung tissue. Aprotinin has the ability to irreversibly inhibit a number of different types of serine proteases. In general these are all based on the structure of trypsin, the protease of the digestive system. In coagulation and fibrinolysis, aprotinin has a concentration-dependent ability to inhibit most of the coagulation and fibrinolytic proteases. The current form of aprotinin is marketed as Trasylol. Aprotinin is an excellent inhibitor of both plasmin and kallikrein. Its ability to inhibit other coagulation or fibrinolytic proteases requires too high a concentration of aprotinin for it to be considered clinically relevant as an anticoagulant for inhibiting such proteases as factor VIIa or thrombin (4,5).

activated state of the patient provided the heparin dose and effect are determined or assessed before going on bypass. Since the activated clotting time responds to hypercoagulable states by getting shorter, it pays to know the performance limitations of the activated clotting time that is being used (24–27).

For example, one shortcoming of the activated clotting time for managing heparin on bypass is its sensitivity to the various alterations of the coagulation system that result from contact activation, such as a factor XII deficiency (28,29). These changes can present difficulties in managing heparin anticoagulation unless the surgical team is equipped with methods other than the activated clotting time to identify their presence. In addition, contact activation is also adversely affected by diseases that produce the lupus anticoagulant and the administration of antiplatelet medications. Each affects the activated clotting time by artificially extending the test so that the *essential relationship* between the clotting time and the circulating heparin concentration is missing. Several cases have been reported in the literature in which an activated clotting time has been extremely extended, even though no heparin has been given (28,29). It is very difficult in the operating room to determine the exact cause of this phenomenon. The actual situation is one of deficient anticoagulation despite the prolongation of the activated clotting time. To deal with this potential quirk in the activated clotting time, you should dose and reverse heparin using a standard protocol, or use protamine titration to monitor the actual circulating heparin concentrations.

C. Inhibition of Coagulation

Cardiopulmonary surgery presents several mechanisms for inhibition of coagulation, including (a) dilution of all clotting elements, (b) heparin, (c) hypothermia, and (d) the mechanical destruction or consumption of clotting factors and platelets.

Comparatively speaking, the use of heparin in bypass surgery gives blood heparin levels that are an order of 10 magnitudes higher than those generally encountered in other medical uses of heparin. The only exception to this is in interventional cardiology, where the use of heparin approaches the blood levels encountered in cardiac catherizations or other invasive procedures requiring heparin.

1. Heparin

Heparin is a mixture of polysaccharides and has been the anticoagulant of choice in most surgical situations in which thrombosis is a major concern. Used properly, heparin either outperforms, performs equivalently to a new anticoagulant, or the new anticoagulant is only slightly better at a significantly higher cost (30–32). One of the problems with heparin has been its heterogeneous nature. It is isolated from two distinct biological sources, beef lung and porcine mucosal tissues. The resulting products are not the same, even though clinically they are treated the same. This situation has been compounded by the introduction of the "low-molecular-weight heparins," in which unfractionated heparins are depolymerized by a variety of different methods (33). This leads to a wide number of different types of low-molecular-weight heparins that either do or do not share most of the properties of the unfractionated heparins.*

*Low-molecular-weight heparins are characterized by having more anti-Xa activity than anti-IIa activity. [Anti-Xa activity is a measure of the inhibitory effect of a patient's circulating heparin (both high- and low-molecular-weight forms) level on Xa as measured by the release of a chromophore in a chromogenic assay. With IIa assay, the measurement is for the amount of thrombin available after high-molecular-weight heparin inhibition of the conversion of prothrombin to thrombin.] There is a significant difference in the catalytic process of thrombin inhibition and the inhibition of the other clotting proteases by heparin. In the inhibition of factor Xa (as well as the rest of the clotting proteases other than thrombin), all that is required is that heparin binds to antithrombin III.

The use of heparin can be broken down into three areas: (a) prophylactic, in which modest doses of heparin are administered in a purely preventative fashion; (b) therapeutic, which is the administration of heparin for an underlying thrombotic condition, either pathologic or induced; and (c) device-oriented use. There are ranges of heparinization associated with each of these uses. Prophylactic uses look at peak whole blood levels of less than 0.2 units/mL, therapeutic uses from 0.2 to almost 1.5 units/mL, and device-oriented uses cover a range from about 1.5 to 10 units/mL. There are no standardized methodologies for using heparin in any of the above areas, and there are innumerable difficulties in using the common tests for monitoring the heparinization. Although there are published recommendations, these recommendations are usually looked at in terms of minimizing heparin use rather than optimizing its use. The nature of the data used to generate the recommendations do not take into account such known variables as the lack of standardized tests, reagents, or instruments, so the utility of any of the recommendations for dosage during cardiopulmonary bypass is open to practical questions of reproducibility (34).

It is not uncommon for the CV surgeon not to know the type of heparin being used. Two types of heparin are used, and there are a number of different suppliers, so it is difficult for the surgeon to be absolutely assured that the quality of the heparin remains consistent. Thus it is common for clinicians not to know either the type or brand of heparin being used. In addition, there are two different methodologies for classifying the activity of heparins. One is the USP, which comes from the U.S. Pharmacopoeia; the other is the WHO, or World Health Organization system. The USP unit of heparin is about 10–12% more potent than the WHO unit of heparin (referred to as an International Unit or I.U.) This difference in labeling causes some confusion when trying to interpret clinical papers. Frequently a paper that originates in the United States will refer to the heparin dosage as I.U.s, which is incorrect. Clinically, this has meant that in countries where the WHO standard is in place, the doses of heparin are less than in the United States, and this holds across all clinical areas.

2. *Hypothermia*

Hypothermia (28–32°C) is used in CV surgery to slow down biologic processes and reduce oxygen demand. These processes of course include coagulation, and this has frequently been used as an argument to reduce the amount of heparin that is used. The problem with this argument is that decreasing the temperature does slow down chemical reactions, but it does not inhibit coagulation. In fact the argument is moot; not only are the reactions that generate thrombin slowed down, the reactions that inhibit thrombin are also slowed down. In recent years the use of hypothermia has been challenged, since several studies have suggested a link between hypothermia and postsurgical blood loss (35–39). However, some types of activated clotting times do not adequately warm the sample to a standardized temperature, so the results are affected by the degree of hypothermia. This results in a variability in the activated clotting time that is related to the temperature of the sample and the efficiency with which temperature control is maintained in performing the test. The testing systems are not at hypothermic body temperatures at the time of collection. Therefore, the in-vitro testing of coagulation does not accurately reflect the in-vivo state of coagulation.

3. *Inhibition of Platelet Function*

The use of platelet inhibitors in cardiovascular surgery has been looked at briefly, but the results did not initially suggest any benefit. The introduction of platelet inhibitors which work through the IIb-IIIa binding site on the platelet membrane may change this. Results have suggested that vessel patency may improve if the inhibitors are used postsurgically. Whether there is any direct benefit to using these inhibitors during surgery has not yet been established.

The use of the inhibitors may occur in an indirect fashion. Failures in interventional cardiology frequently wind up in cardiovascular surgery, and the inhibitors are finding more and more use in interventional cardiology. These platelet inhibitors have potent effects and have the capability of producing serious bleeding when coupled with the use of heparin.

The impact of a platelet inhibitor during bypass surgery was noted several years ago by Moorehead (40). The use of an antiplatelet drug sent activated clotting time values to infinity (as best could be determined). What this was demonstrating is that an activated clotting time is highly influenced by the presence and activity of platelets when measuring the effect of heparin. Does this have some significance to the in-vivo action of heparin? Certain types of activated clotting times are capable of using any type of blood sample. It can be shown that their response to heparin is highly dependent on the presence of platelets. With platelets in the blood sample, the activated clotting time can track the effect of heparin up to and sometimes exceeding 10 units of heparin/mL of whole blood (Fig. 1). If the platelets are removed from the blood sample, the activated clotting time is limited to about 1.5 units of heparin/mL of whole blood. It may well be that the in-vitro response to heparin mimics the in-vivo response

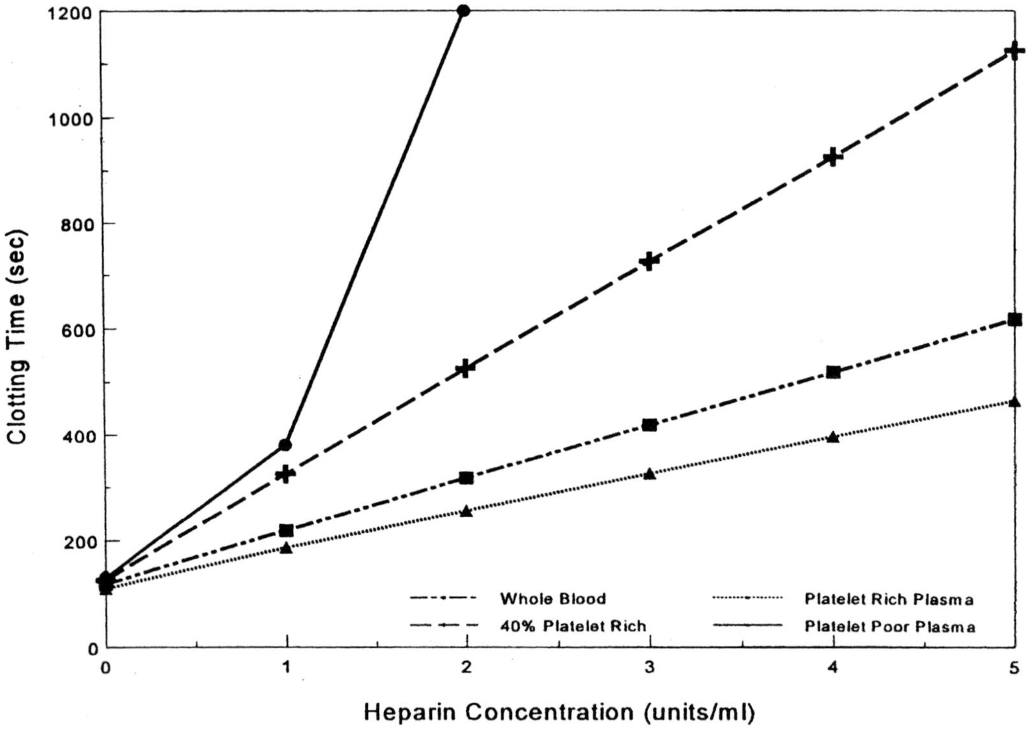

Figure 1 Platelet impact on heparinized activated clotting times. Blood was drawn from a single donor into 0.5 unit of heparin/mL. The blood was centrifuged to produce platelet-rich plasma (PRP) and platelet-poor plasma (PPP). The whole blood, PRP, a mixture of 40% PRP + 60% PPP, and PPP were titrated with heparin to give the concentrations indicated in the figure. The activated clotting time was determined on each at each heparin level. The higher the platelet content, the lower the activated clotting time. The PPP becomes nonlinear with respect to clotting time when an activated clotting time is used.

and that in the presence of drugs that alter the activity of platelets, significantly less heparin is required to achieve the same level of anticoagulation.

4. Other Methods of Anticoagulation

There are clinical situations when the use of heparin is contraindicated in bypass surgery. The most frequent is heparin-induced thrombocytopenia. In this condition, which is an immune response, the presence of heparin can be lethal. This type of patient appears more frequently than in the past. This is probably related to the number of patients who are now experiencing repeat exposures to high-dose heparin regimes. The following is a short list of some methods that have been used to anticoagulate patients without the use of unfractionated pharmaceutical heparin.

a. Defibrination. Defibrination of whole blood using ancrod, a snake enzyme that produces fibrin monomers that cannot polymerize into a fibrin matrix, has been used as an alternative method of achieving an anticoagulant state for bypass. Although the method has been used successfully, the patient is at extreme risk for postsurgical blood loss, and the management of such patients can only be achieved using transfusion therapy (13,41–43).

b. Thrombin Inhibitors. Thrombin inhibitors generally involve direct inhibitors such as recombinant hirudin, hirulog (a modified, engineered variant of hirudin), or synthetic inhibitors such as argatroban. Each has its drawbacks, but all are presently available under a compassionate use basis when heparin is contraindicated. Part of the problem in using these types of inhibitors is that clinical protocols must be modified and there is frequently very little data available on what types of tests should be used to monitor the status of the anticoagulation. Heparin is not consumed in the inhibition of thrombin; it is a catalyst of the inhibition, whereas the direct thrombin inhibitors available are consumed. This is a distinct difference. The system of heparin–antithrombin-III–thrombin is more clinically forgiving in the control of a thrombosis-prone patient. This, coupled with mechanisms for reversing the anticoagulant activity without threatening any other aspect of normal coagulation, a modest half-life, and additional physiologic mechanisms that do not involve thrombin, gives a clinician a much more forgiving system than does direct, high-affinity thrombin inhibitors (30–32,44–47).

c. Nonthrombin Inhibitors of Coagulation. In recent years the most significant impact on postcardiopulmonary bypass surgical blood loss has been the introduction of drugs that have an impact on either contact activation or fibrinolysis. The first of these drugs was aprotinin (Trasylol). Aprotinin is a serine protease inhibitor that blocks the activity of a number of different serine proteases. It is a particularly effective inhibitor of trypsin, plasmin, and kallikrein. Aprotinin, to be effective (4,6,7,10,48–51), must be present during the surgery and while on bypass. The effect is most noticeable at what are called high dose levels, and the impact on postsurgical blood loss appears to be dose dependent. The best explanation of its mechanisms of action revolves around its ability to inhibit kallikrein, with a secondary impact on the inhibition of plasmin. Aprotinin dosed at the conclusion of bypass does not appear to have any major impact on postsurgical blood loss.

Aprotinin is an anticoagulant, but its mechanism of action is such that it does not effectively inhibit thrombin generated by surgery. In CV surgery, it must be used with a drug that can block thrombin, in this case, heparin. However, since heparin is normally monitored with an activated clotting time, and aprotinin inhibits kallikrein, the heparin must be followed in some other manner. The impact of both aprotinin and heparin on activated clotting time are not additive and depend to some extent on the type of activator being used in the activated clotting time test (52–55). If aprotinin is being used, an independent method for monitoring heparin should be considered. There have been several instances of lethal thromboses developing in cases where aprotinin was used, but heparin was followed only using an activated clotting time.

An interesting side effect of the use of aprotinin relates to its ability to inhibit plasmin. The active enzyme plasmin is one of the naturally occurring methods by which protamine sulfate (which is used to neutralize heparin) is degraded in blood. Protamine sulfate is a good substrate for plasmin. Thus, if aprotinin is present, the half-life of protamine sulfate is extended. The use of aprotinin has caused some rather "strange" observations. A dramatic change in patient response to heparin was reported following cardiopulmonary bypass using aprotinin (56). This change was not seen in a control set of patients. The result was that patients treated with aprotinin had an excess of protamine for a longer period of time postsurgically than did the control patient group without aprotinin. If the patients were then later tested for an in-vivo response to heparin, the aprotinin-treated group, having more plasma protamine sulfate present, appeared to be heparin resistant, whereas before the surgery their heparin responses were normal. The increased requirements for heparin if reheparinization was required was due to "titrating" the remaining protamine.

d. Inhibitors of Fibrinolysis. The primary drugs with significant antifibrinolytic activity are epsilon-aminocaproic acid (Amicar) and tranexamic acid (Cyklokapron) (57–59). Neither drug is as effective as aprotinin, but the cost differential pushes a number of clinical sites to use the less effective drugs. With the introduction of the above drugs, combined with a number of other attempts to reduce postsurgical blood loss, the chance of seeing post-CV thrombotic patients has increased (60–62).

D. Coagulation-Related Problems in CV Surgery

Although individual genetic or acquired coagulopathies are occurring more frequently within the patient population undergoing coronary artery grafting, they represent only a small group. Most of the problems are induced by the procedure.

1. Bleeding

In determining the reasons for excessive postsurgical blood loss, it is important to understand the number of variables associated with CV surgery. These can vary considerably, and each has an influence on postsurgical blood loss.

a. Defining "Bleeding." The definition of bleeding has been one of the major difficulties in cardiopulmonary bypass surgery. The most difficult aspect is differentiating surgical bleeding and bleeding from an inadequate coagulation system. This is more difficult because the patient has been anticoagulated during surgery and must be adequately reversed postoperatively, and the bypass surgery damages the coagulation system in an unpredictable way for each patient. The rapid recognition of whatever single or multiple mechanisms are operating is the challenge of the team working to reduce the bleeding problem. Whether specific factor deficiencies (V, VII) and/or demonstrable platelet or accelerated fibrinolysis is the cause of bleeding (63,64), the abnormalities are difficult to diagnose. Numerous decision trees regarding this issue have been published. Extremely simple decision trees have been shown to positively impact blood product usage (65–72).

Our approach has included good medical and surgical history, followed by preoperative, extensive intraoperative and postoperative coagulation testing with readily available tests. Transfusion of blood components and specific medications to reduce bleeding are based on a history of preoperative medication as in aspirin use, surgical bleeding as in microvascular oozing, and coagulation testing demonstrating thrombocytopenia and/or hypofibrinogenemia (see Tables 1 and 2). The definitions we use are as follows:

Table 1 Medication with Value in Reducing Bleeding in Cardiopulmonary Bypass Surgery

Antifibrinolytic agents: epsilon-aminocaproic acid (Amicar, Lederle); tranexamic acid (Cyklokapron, Kabi-Pharmacia)
Neutralize contact activation: aprotinin (Trasylol, Bayer)
Improve platelet function: desmopressin acetate (DDAVP, Rhone-Poulenc Rorer)

Intraoperative bleeding: surgical assessment; continued oozing, cardiac cavity continues to fill with blood, and individual assessment by the surgeon. Other assessments include difficulty maintaining blood pressure off bypass, low intraoperative hematocrit, and excessive extracardiac (pericardial) suction volume returned to pump volume.

Postoperative bleeding as measured by chest tube drainage: >200 mL/hr for 2 hr, >300 mL/hr for 1 hr, continued bleeding >150 mL/hr with no gradual decline over 5 hr, and various combinations of the above depending on experience and preference.

b. Surgical. In cardiopulmonary bypass surgery, bleeding is commonly assumed to be the result of a complication or difficulty in surgical technique. As with everything else, this is a gray area. When does the size of a lesion in the vascular system or the quality of the vascular tissues become so defective that normal coagulation cannot plug the tear? There is also a region in this gray area in which the blood loss is addressed by applying a number of different approaches, one being surgical. The costs of correcting surgical bleeding (sometimes referred

Table 2 Standard Operating Protocol for Coagulation Monitoring in Cardiopulmonary Bypass Surgery[a]

1. Preoperative laboratory testing ordered by the surgeon
   a. CBC (Hct, platelet count)
   b. Prothrombin time, aPTT
   c. Fibrinogen, clot retraction
2. Intraoperative laboratory testing (30 min; on pump, warm-up; 30 min before coming off pump) drawn by the perfusionist during the pump run
   a. CBC (Hct, platelet count)
   b. Fibrinogen, clot retraction
   c. ACT, heparin assay/adequacy
3. Postoperative laboratory testing (20 min post-protamine) obtained by anesthesia, (recovery/SICU) when patient settled, obtained by nursing staff
   a. CBC (Hct, platelet count)
   b. Prothrombin time, a PTT
   c. Fibrinogen, clot retraction
   d. ACT, heparin assay/reversal

[a]Tubes required: 1 lavender, 2 blue, 1 red-top tube (volume = 15 mL per set).
In pediatric cases, use pediatric collection tubes if desired.

to as "mechanical bleeding") are high. It requires taking the patient back to surgery to correct the problem. Therefore the sooner all other reasons for excessive blood loss have been ruled out, the sooner the decision for reoperation can be made, the problem corrected, and the costs limited. This is just one reason for the use of STAT coagulation tests. If they are used properly and knowledgeably, the economic impact can be favorable (73,74).

c. Heparin Rebound. Heparin rebound is the "reappearance" of heparin after it has been demonstrated that there is no heparin present. Cardiopulmonary bypass surgery is the only place where "heparin rebound" has been described, and there are many hypotheses to explain this phenomenon. The explanations include: (a) blood products given back to the patient from the pumping system contain heparin; (b) although initially neutralized with protamine sulfate, the subsequent breakdown or the disassociation of protamine sulfate releases heparin from the protamine:heparin complex back into circulation. The proteolytic breakdown of protamine sulfate appears to be related only to beef lung heparin and not to porcine heparin (75–78).

d. Inadequate Neutralization of Heparin. Under normal circumstances, inadequate neutralization of heparin occurs only if a mistake has been made, such as a miscalculation of the protamine dose, obstruction or diversion of the i.v. infusing the protamine doses, or a delay in giving the full dose. In the reversal phase of systemic heparinization in cardiopulmonary bypass surgery, everyone is apprehensive as to when clots will form, documenting that heparin has been reversed. This process takes approximately 15–20 min after all the protamine sulfate has been infused. Sometimes an apparent initial failure to adequately reverse heparin is actually impatience.

Most protocols for reversing heparin either automatically determine the correct amount of protamine or overdose protamine. Overdosing protamine has many hypothetical problems, but to date there is not much solid experimental data on the physiologic effects of overdosing protamine. Another reason for overdosing protamine has been in response to what is considered excessive bleeding, even though there has been no specific test to indicate that additional protamine is required. This knee-jerk reaction, which automatically associates blood loss with the presence of heparin, has frequently misdiagnosed a modest bleeding problem and turned the event into a major bleeding problem. The existence of a number of STAT coagulation tests which measure both the functional activity and the amount of heparin present can rule out whether or not additional protamine is required; however, even in the presence of this evidence, it is still not uncommon for additional protamine to be administered if the bleeding is considered to be excessive (79).

e. Dilution. Dilution of the patient's circulating whole blood occurs with every cardiopulmonary bypass procedure to some degree. The dilutional effect occurs in the red cells (hematocrit), platelets, and all the plasma clotting factors. This is a function of the volume of the extracorporeal circuit, the size of the patient, and the methods employed for managing patient blood volumes during bypass. A dilution of 50% is not uncommon, and as the size of the patient decreases, the dilution effect becomes more pronounced. In pediatric bypass surgery, dilution can reach more than 70%, the thresholds or triggers for bleeding in pediatric bypass surgery are obviously not the same as for adults. However, in very small infants, dilution can be significant and the cause for bleeding (80–83).

f. Platelet Dysfunction. Platelet dysfunction has been accepted as one of the main causes for excessive postsurgical bleeding in cardiopulmonary bypass patients. Although the presence of "platelet dysfunction" has been characterized by various methods (84–87) to exist postoperatively, the difficulty is that although it is present, the patient does not always bleed. With progress in identifying multiple causes for postoperative bleeding, it has been more difficult to find a single or all-encompassing reason for excessive bleeding. Even though a number of studies have shown that postsurgical platelet function is not the primary reason for postsurgical blood loss, it has nevertheless become the favorite "cause" for bleeding (5,88–92). As we know by now, there are a number of reasons why a patient can bleed, and the best approach is to treat the specific reason or reasons, rather than using a shotgun approach. With the advent of STAT tests for platelet counts and platelet function, platelet therapy will have supporting testing as with fresh frozen plasma and cryoprecipitate. In patients known to have received aspirin preoperatively, DDAVP (desmopressin acetate) has demonstrated value in improving platelet function and reducing chest tube drainage (60,93,94). Desmopressin acetate causes the endothelial storage granules (Weibel-Palade bodies) to release stored von Willebrand factor. von Willebrand factor binds platelets to the subendothelium.

g. Disseminated Intravascular Coagulation. Blood loss in the immediate postsurgical period due to classic disseminated intravascular coagulation (DIC) is relatively rare, but a condition very similar to DIC can exist if there has been inadequate heparinization during bypass surgery. This condition leads to the generation of both thrombin and plasmin during bypass, which can contribute to the lowering of clotting factors such that the patient appears to be in DIC. This condition can look like DIC, but once bypass and the surgery is concluded, the process stops. The condition can be corrected with specific blood component replacement therapy. Classic DIC is often generated by a septic condition (see below), and unless the causes of the sepsis are controlled, blood component therapy will have little impact on bleeding.

h. Salvaged Blood Products Returned to the Patient's Circulation. Salvaged blood products in CV surgery cover a broad range of practices. This varies from the reinfusion of scavenged blood from the surgical field directly or washed, or defibrinated blood from the chest tubes, to the presequestration of whole blood preoperatively. Excessive use of washed red blood cells contributes to the dilutional coagulopathy, since it returns no clotting factors to the patient. If salvaged products contain active proteases, thrombi, and/or tissue fragments, readministration to the patient can create increased fibrinolysis and or intravascular thrombosis (95,96).

i. Fibrinolysis. Twenty-five years ago postsurgical fibrinolysis was considered a major reason for excessive postsurgical blood loss in cardiopulmonary bypass patients. The trauma of older types of tubing, less sophisticated techniques, bubble oxygenators, and using whole blood in the entire bypass circuit created an environment that is not seen today. The use of antifibrinolytics during and following bypass in specific cases has also reduced the incidence of postoperative fibrinolysis. However, controlled clinical studies frequently fail to identify fibrinolysis postoperatively, or as a routine cause of postsurgical blood loss.

Under-anticoagulation will contribute to the generation of plasmin during bypass. Activation of coagulation is linked to fibrinolysis, and thus inadequate heparinization may lead to a postsurgical fibrinolytic state (23,92,97–101).

j. Protamine-Induced Blood Loss It has been postulated for years that excess protamine may play a role in postsurgical blood loss (102–106). Although it can be shown experimentally that protamine can affect the activity of thrombin and platelets, the clinical data are not clear. Practically, protamine has been routinely overdosed for years, without any major difficulties. Immediately after administration of protamine, it can be shown that platelets are relatively nonfunctional; however, the function returns without any intervention in the space of 20–30 min after protamine administration is ceased. One of the more common problems with protamine has always been the methods by which it is administered. Although following the package insert would require more than an hour in most CV cases to reverse heparin, in practice protamine administration for heparin reversal varies anywhere from 10 min to approximately 20 min. Rapid reversal may be accompanied by shock and respiratory collapse. There have been no studies looking at the methods for administering protamine, and how they affect short-term patient outcome.

2. Thrombosis

Systemic thrombosis in a properly heparinized bypass system has generally not been a major concern in bypass surgery. It has become a problem as efforts have been more aggressive to limit postsurgical blood product usage, but this may be related to a failure to maintain an adequate level of anticoagulation. The level of anticoagulation will become even more critical as various procedures in cardiovascular surgery move to "minimally invasive" techniques. Determining the appropriate level of anticoagulation (and possibly antiplatelet therapy) for the newer techniques will have a significant bearing on the clinical acceptance of these techniques as patient outcomes are evaluated (107–111).

a. Insufficient Anticoagulation. Before the introduction of the antifibrinolytic drugs such as aprotinin, insufficient anticoagulation in bypass surgery was only a sporadic event. Although the activated clotting time (ACT) is a standard in bypass surgery, it is not a standardized test and it does not accurately reflect heparin anticoagulation during extracorporeal circulation. This has always been true, but with the introduction of new drugs that can affect the ACT, the ACT has done an even poorer job of determining the level of anticoagulation. The emotional impact of the use of an anticoagulant is difficult to overcome even in the face of heparin assays that clearly indicate that heparin is not a problem. It is not unusual in this clinical setting to demonstrate that no heparin is present in a bleeding patient, yet protamine sulfate will be prescribed. This mind set continues to produce heparin protocols that minimize the use of heparin, rather than optimize its use, so there will continue to be situations in which under-anticoagulation leads to thrombotic complications.

E. Intervention and Correction of the Causes of Bleeding in Cardiopulmonary Bypass Surgery

This discussion outlines the common causes for postoperative bleeding, their mechanisms, early laboratory detection using a standard coagulation protocol, and management options (112). The preoperative, intraoperative and postoperative sources of coagulation information are obtained through the use of a standard protocol (see Form No. 1 and Table 2). The form defines specific times for specimen collection.* The critical values for these coagulation parameters are as follows:

---

*Blood collection tubes are prepacked, labeled, and grouped together as packed to be placed in the operating room or other site as required. These include: 2 adult Na citrate (blue top), 1 EDTA (lavender top), and 1 red-top tube; see Fig. 2.

Preoperative coagulation profile: Obtained by surgeon; CBC, PT, aPTT, fibrinogen, clot retraction

Intraoperative coagulation profiles: Obtained by perfusionist from pump; CBC, fibrinogen, clot retraction, heparin level, ACT

- *Thirty-minute profile*: After approximately 30 min on the pump; note that in a short pump run the 30-min and the warm-up are the same sample.
- *Warm-up profile*: Approximately 30 min before coming off the pump

Postoperative profiles: Obtained by anesthesiologist from patient when off pump, and by nurse in recovery; CBC, PT, aPTT, fibrinogen, clot retraction, heparin assay, ACT

- *Post-protamine sulfate profile*: Approximately 20 min after all protamine sulfate is infused
- *Recovery/postsurgical intensive care profiles*: When the patient is settled into the SICU, and repeated as often as required

Form No. 1 CARDIOPULMONARY COAGULATION PROFILE

Hospital No.____________ Ward________________ Name________________________________

Age______ DOB___________ Race___________ Sex__________ CPB No.________________

Diagnosis____ Date of Surgery______________

CPB Profile	Pre-op Date: Time:	30 min on Date: Time:	Warm up Date: Time:	POST PS Date: Time:	Recovery Date: Time:
1. CBC					
WBC	$x10^9/1$	$x10^9/1$	$x10^9/1$	$x10^9/1$	$x10^9/1$
HGB	gm/dl	gm/dl	gm/dl	gm/dl	gm/dl
HCT	%	%	%	%	%
MCV	fl	fl	fl	fl	fl
Smear					
2. Platelet CT	$x10^9/1$	$x10^9/1$	$x10^9/1$	$x10^9/1$	$x10^9/1$
3. Clot Retraction	hr	hr	hr	hr	hr
4. PT	sec			sec	sec
5. APTT	sec			sec	sec
6. Fibrinogen	mg/dl	mg/dl	mg/dl	mg/dl	mg/dl
7. Heparin assay		units/ml	units/ml	units/ml	units/ml

Comments:

Operating Room Extension: ________
Recovery Room Extension: ________

Staff:

Name: ________________
Office Phone: ____________
Pager: ________________

Resident:

Name: ____________________________
Beeper: ____________________________

62

Form 1

Hematocrit < 20% for any profile
Platelet count less than 100,000 mm^3 for any profile
Prothrombin time > 17 sec for post-protamine or recovery profile
aPTT > 50 sec for post-protamine or recovery profile
Fibrinogen < 100 mg/dL for any profile

1. Preoperative Causes for Excessive Postoperative Bleeding as Recognized in the Past History

The complexity and gravity of the existing heart disease may result in difficult surgery, a long pump run, and possible preoperative or postoperative aortic assist balloon pumping. *Mechanism of coagulopathy*: The increased time results in increased trauma to the coagulation system, with destruction of platelets, loss of clotting factors, consumption of clotting factors, and platelet defect. Examples include double or triple valve replacement with coronary bypass surgery, reoperation for valve or coronary artery bypass, and poor ejection fraction preoperatively, resulting in difficulty weaning patient from the pump upon completion of the surgery. *Management*: Intraoperative and postoperative identification of deficits, and specific replacement with component therapy. Anticipate platelet function defect after 3-hr pump run.

Some medications may also cause excessive bleeding postoperatively: antiplatelet therapy

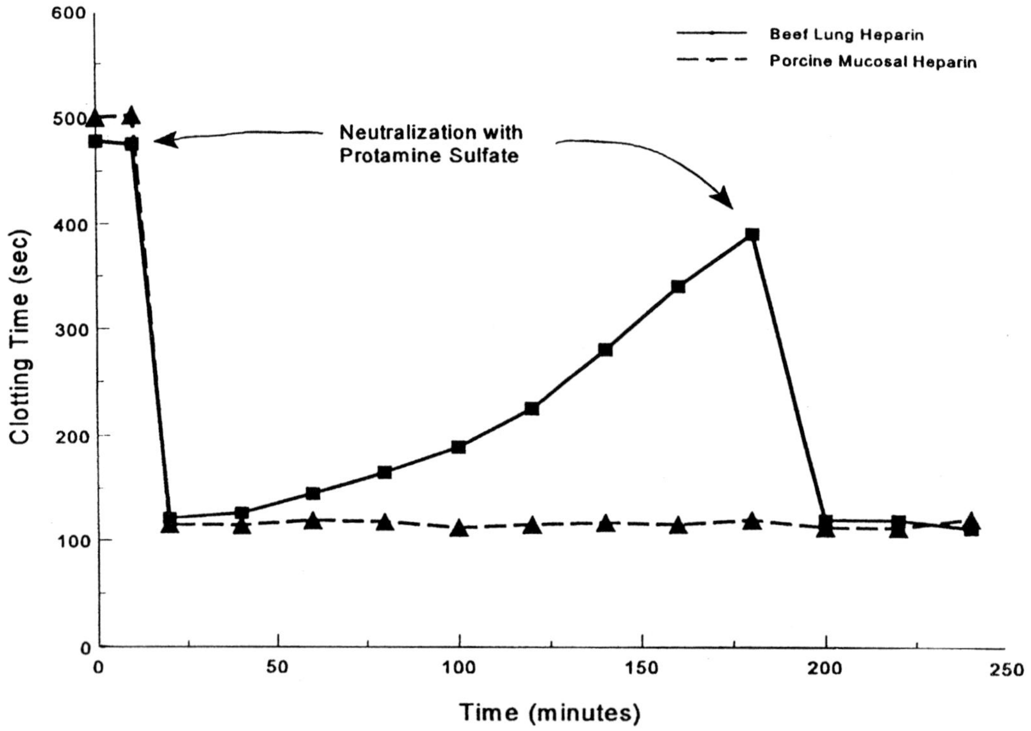

Figure 2 Heparin rebound in vitro. Single-donor whole blood was collected into citrate. Beef lung and porcine mucosal heparins were added to give a final concentration of 4 units/mL. The activated clotting time was determined, and protamine sulfate was added to neutralize the heparin. The samples were then placed in a water bath at 37°C and the activated clotting times determined at the times indicated. At 180 min, the "rebound heparin" present in the beef lung sample was reneutralized with enough protamine to neutralize 3 units/mL heparin.

(aspirin, NSAID = platelet dysfunction), anticoagulation (coumarin = factor II, VII, IX, X deficiency), antifibrinolytic therapy (TPA, streptokinase = fibrinogen deficiency and clot lysis). *Mechanism of coagulopathy*: Anticipate absence of complete and functional clotting system for the items mentioned. *Management*: Identify deficit with intraoperative and postoperative testing and replace. In emergency situations, such as replacing an aortic valve while fully anticoagulated, correction of the clotting factor deficit while on the pump with fresh frozen plasma would be indicated. For the aspirin defect, platelet transfusions as well as DDAVP, 0.3 μg/kg body weight in 50 mL normal saline over 30 min, repeat in 12 or 24 hr if indicated. With systemic fibrinolysis, treatment with tranexamic acid or epsilon-aminocaproic acid to stop the fibrinolysis and then correction with cryoprecipitate when fibrinogen documented below 100–150 mg/dL.

Other diseases that may lead to excessive bleeding are renal failure with acquired platelet defect, liver failure, alcoholic cirrhosis, post-hepatitis; acute or chronic (not a good candidate for surgery) congenital coagulation defects (Example, von Willebrand's disease). Correct the specific defect preoperatively and throughout surgery and postoperatively for an extended period of time. Vitamin K deficiency can be corrected with vitamin K, but it is most important to determine why the patient is vitamin K deficient. *Management*: In an emergency, correction of identified deficiency at once. For those conditions for which surgery is planned, correction and a maintenance program should be initiated.

Prophylaxis: Several medications may be utilized intraoperatively to reduce loss of clotting substances through consumption or lysis and improve function: DDAVP improves platelet function, Aprotinin reduces contact activation during surgery, vitamin K therapy corrects deficit, cryoprecipitate corrects fibrinogen deficit and improves platelet function with von Willebrand factor, and tranexamic acid or epsilon-aminocaproic acid stop fibrinolysis whatever the mechanism.

2. *Intraoperative Causes for Excessive Postoperative Bleeding*

Surgical problems such as technical difficulties, failed suture lines, "redo" procedures, valve versus coronary bypass surgery are all possible causes for excessive postoperative bleeding. *Mechanism*: Surgical hemostasis is not achieved as rapidly as desired, resulting in longer-than-anticipated surgery, more blood loss, and more trauma to the coagulation system. *Management*: Intraoperative assessment with aggressive deficit replacement immediately after heparin reversal, while in the operating room. Medications such as DDAVP and epsilon-aminocaproic acid should also be considered.

Some problems are intrinsic to the bypass system: excessive dilution, inadequate heparinization, long pump run, cardiotomy suction with suctioned fibrin clot and debris into the pump volume, added clear volume, acidosis, type of oxygenator (membrane versus bubble). *Mechanism*: Deficiency in multiple coagulation components or substances due to increased consumption, dilution, or fibrinolysis. *Management*: Identify deficiencies and if possible define the mechanism. Replace with specific components for specific deficits.

3. *Postoperative Causes for Excessive Postoperative Bleeding*

Incomplete heparin neutralization. *Mechanism*: Inadequate heparin monitoring due to method or calculations results in insufficient protamine sulfate administered. *Management*: Add protamine sulfate.

Hypothermia: continued cold body temperature < 37°C. *Mechanism*: Warm-up insufficient, patient unable to warm up. *Management*: More aggressive postoperative warming, such as heater and blankets.

Multiple organ system failure. *Mechanism*: Acidosis, heart failure, preoperative organ failure. *Management*: Difficult or impossible; go back on bypass to allow the heart to rest, and time for insertion of aortic balloon assist pump.

Aortic balloon assist pump. *Mechanism*: Continued trauma to coagulation system and heparin effect on coagulation and platelets. *Management*: The only genuine means to stop this effect is to take off the assist pump, which is not possible; therefore, support is designed to buy time until the patient is off the assist pump. Give platelets and fresh frozen plasma when coagulation studies demonstrate deficiency, and with increased clinical bleeding associated with protracted time such as > 12 hr on the assist pump.

Heparin-induced thrombocytopenia. *Mechanism*: Heparin initiates immune destruction of circulating platelets. Usually seen immediately postoperatively, when platelets fail to increase, yet all other parameters are correcting. *Management*: Eliminate all possible sources of heparin, such as keep open intravenous lines, and be absolutely confident of heparin reversal. Interestingly, these cases do not always have bleeding despite low values. They most often clot well, and platelet infusions may or may not be indicated. Platelet infusions are contraindicated while heparin is still present.

Case Study History 1

This is the case of a 55-year-old woman who underwent mitral valve replacement for mitral valve stenosis, and single coronary vessel bypass.

Personal or family history of bleeding problems, or disorders: *Negative.*

History of other disease: *Negative.*

Previous surgery: Mitral valve commisurotomy, hysterectomy, teeth extraction with bleeding problems.

Denies passing blood in urine, stool, or hemoptysis. Denies aspirin use within last week. Currently using antihistamine, digoxin, bumetanide, insulin.

Coagulation Studies

Pre-op	Warm-up	Post-protamine	Recovery	4-hr repeat
Hct 42.1%	22.2%	25.8	28.0	34.1
WBC 9.9 mm^3	5.8	12.4	18.7	14.0
Platelet count 278 mm^3	29	75	105	91
PT 11.2 sec		14.7	13.9	12.6
aPTT 26.9 sec		36.0	34.2	32.7
Fibrinogen 480 mg/dL	155	170	165	200
Heparin assay	3.0 u/mL WB	0.0		
Pump time			80 min	
Chest tube drainage		200 mL/2 hr, then < 100 mL/hr		
PEEP			5 in recovery	
Therapy			None	

Questions

1. What is the dilution effect on these values at 30 min and warm-up, and what is their significance? The dilution effect is seen immediately after the pump prime has mixed with the patient's blood volume.

2. Why the prolonged prothrombin time? In normal unusual cases, losses in factors V and VII are common and do not reflect a consumption problem. (63) (Note that the PT and aPTT corrected with postoperative diruresis and blood volume concentration.)

Case Study 2

This is a case of a 68-year-old woman who underwent three-vessel coronary artery bypass surgery. She had an angiogram one week before surgery.

Personal and family history of bleeding problems or disorder: *Negative*.
History of other diseases: Renal stones, chronic obstructive pulmonary disease.
Previous surgery: Hysterectomy, cholecystectomy, intestine resection for adhesions and obstruction without bleeding problems.
Denies passing blood in stool, or hemoptysis. History of blood in urine with renal stones. Denies aspirin use within last week. Current medications: nefedipine, theophylline, dipyridamole, nitroglycerin.

Coagulation Studies

	Pre-op	Warm-up	Post-protamine	Recovery	4 hr	6 hr
HCT	38%	19.6	25.6	35.8	30.7	26.8
WBC	6,400 mm^3	1.8	4.5	3.2	5.9	5.6
Platelet count	317,000 mm^3	15	21	26	18	53
PT	11.6 sec		16.8	15.7	15.1	14.0
aPTT	26.2 sec		85.0	52.5	41.9	36.7
Fibrinogen	310 mg/dL	100	130	130	110	140
Heparin assay		3.5 u/mL WB	0.0			
Pump time				75 min		
Chest tube drainage				450 mL/2 ln	100 ml/1 ln	
PEEP				10 in recovery		
Therapy				50 mg PS (10 units platelets)	50 mg PS (10 units platelets)	

Comments

1. Notice the dilution on bypass of hematocrit and fibrinogen, but the platelet count is disproportionally decreased. This suggests unusual loss of platelets on bypass compared to the other parameters. An idiosyncratic response is possible, but consumption is unlikely as fibrinogen is not decreased proportionally. Heparin-induced thrombocytopenia should also be considered.
2. The postoperative prolonged PT and aPTT suggest inadequate heparin reversal or consumption. However, the fibrinogen is increasing, and the PT and aPTT have shortened significantly with the postoperative diuresis. Extraordinary loss of clotting factors during the pump run is a possibility. The heparin assay was zero initially, suggesting no residual heparin immediate postoperatively. Rebound heparin is a possibility, and

an additional trial of protamine sulfate (50 mg) should be tried. *Note*: Postoperative studies confirmed heparin-induced thrombocytopenia.

III. ACQUIRED BLEEDING AS A RESULT OF MANAGEMENT WITH MASSIVE BLOOD TRANSFUSION IN TRAUMA

The nature or kind of trauma, the location of the trauma, and what treatment if any has been given to the patient is important in assessing the significance of all coagulation studies before, during, and after surgery. In major trauma, massive blood and fluid replacement results in the predicament where the transfusion of large volumes of packed red cells, clear fluid replacement, and plasma expanders such as Hespan or dextran contribute to continued bleeding. Recognition of the impact of this massive fluid transfusion, its assessment, and its correction will contribute to the resolution of the bleeding. Also, known congenital or acquired causes for intrinsic deficiencies in coagulation are usually not identified initially in the trauma patient, but will certainly represent a potential for catastrophic bleeding if left unknown. Whatever history can be obtained should obviously be obtained as soon as possible (see Table 3).

A. Recognizing the Varied Causes for Excessive Bleeding Prior to Surgery from Major Trauma

The nature of the trauma, as in tissue destruction in a gunshot wound, or a motor vehicle accident involving the head, chest, abdomen, extremities, or all locations together, attest to the volume of tissue disruption and potential for blood loss. Extensive tissue damage will produce extensive raw surfaces for consumption of clotting factors and platelets, a mechanism for foreign debris or fluids to enter the circulation, as well as provide a large surface for continued weeping of blood in addition to disruption of major vessels. Repair of major tissue damage will also require more time and more blood replacement. The time from injury to volume replacement at the trauma site, and the time from the site to the hospital, will all contribute to blood loss and dilution with fluids.

History of diseases such as hemophilia, von Willebrand's disease, or chronic renal failure

Table 3 Mechanisms for Failure of Blood and Component Replacement in Massive Blood Transfusions

Preexisting clotting defects/diseases and medications
Loss of coagulation substances through wound/trauma site
Dilution of coagulation substances via fluid/colloid/blood/blood component/volume expander or replacement
Defective patient response due to shock on liver (protein synthesis and release), bone marrow (platelet production), capillary damage with loss of intravascular fluids
Trauma-induced fibrinogen/fibrin consumption (DIC) and uncontrolled secondary fibrinolysis
Loss of coagulation modulators or inhibitors, e.g., AT-III, protein C, protein S, α-2-antiplasmin, plasminogen
Adverse reaction to blood transfusion: acute hemolysis, shock, renal failure

Source: Modified after Ref. 113.

Table 4 A Working Checklist of Questions to Ask or Examine When Managing the Trauma Patient with Significant Bleeding

Trauma and the patient:
Type of trauma and time to hospital from site of injury
Variables affecting support decisions in direct observation before and during surgery:
Estimated blood loss
Extent of tissue damage
Patient's change in status over time under observation.
Significance of physiologic changes due to trauma:
Vasoconstriction
Stress response
Decision criteria to be used for transfusion of blood or blood components:
Normal values versus essential values for hemostasis
Vital signs: blood pressure, pulse, respiration
External signs: site of trauma, damage observed
What problems does blood or blood components solve or cause?
What blood/components cannot do

will certainly contribute to catastrophic bleeding. However, diseases such as arthritis, diabetes mellitus, and/or hypertension, with the effects of their required medications, are less obvious. Certainly the use of aspirin on platelet function, extensive vessel disease seen in diabetes, and high blood pressure or medication-induced hypotension will affect the loss of blood through all sizes of blood vessels (see Tables 4 and 5).

B. The Trauma Patient with Catastrophic Bleeding

The trauma patient will frequently present to the hospital with inadequate or incomplete history as to the cause of the massive bleeding, requiring the emergency room physician and surgeon to interpret the patient's history, make decisions, and order blood tests. The laboratory can facilitate the ordering of blood tests particularly in this stressful environment by developing user-friendly coagulation special profiles. These are developed with the user physicians (as in emergency room and trauma surgeons) in mind, as well as the clinical pathologist who uses this information to advise the surgeon (see Table 5).

Table 5 Routine Hematology/Coagulation Tests Profile for Trauma Patients (Prepackaged, 1 lavender 3.5-mL, 1 blue 4.5-mL tube, volume = 8 mL)

CBC
Platelet count
Prothrombin time
aPTT
Fibrinogen

The type of trauma—auto accident, gunshot wound, etc.—will have a direct effect on the coagulation results. In addition, a 4- to 8-hr delay from the time of injury will further alter the coagulation results. Baseline studies are essential regardless of when the patient arrives, but knowing the time delay will help in interpreting the coagulation results. A known or unknown underlying clinical disorder may further compromise the patient. Such diseases as liver cirrhosis, chronic renal failure (114), chronic obstructive lung disease, peripheral vascular or cardiovascular disease, as well as medication use such as aspirin, will increase the likelihood of more severe bleeding from trauma, more severe consequences from excessive bleeding, and more difficult replacement of coagulation components. Recent work by Bickell (115) demonstrated that rapid replacement of fluids just to maintain blood pressure with surgery to follow was more likely to produce a coagulopathy than providing the fluid replacement immediately before surgery is initiated. This partially conflicts with what Hewson (116), Ordog (117), and Wilson (118) have reported about hypotension and shock-induced coagulopathy. However, hypotension may not be as detrimental for short periods of time than was thought in the past. Blood and fluid replacement can wait until surgery is underway with good results (115). In addition, a coagulation panel of laboratory tests (see Table 5) available on a STAT basis will readily facilitate the rapid assessment of the hematologic and coagulation status of the patient at almost any time. This same coagulation profile can be repeated hourly or every 2 hr as needed to follow the patient.

Once at the hospital, a clinical decision is made as to estimated blood loss in concert with the laboratory results. Sources of error include vasoconstriction resulting in near-normal coagulation values, followed by dilution with isotonic fluid or colloids. This change can occur within 1 or 2 hr, suggesting increased blood loss. A marked amount of tissue damage will also result in consumption of platelets and clotting factors at the trauma site, as well as loss through the lacerated vessels. This will alter the lab values over time. Loss of clotting factors may exceed RBC loss over time. In addition, the transfusion of only packed red blood cells, and or large volumes of fresh frozen plasma or fluids without platelet infusions, will increase the risk for bleeding from a plasma clotting or platelet defect, the so-called washout coagulopathy (see Tables 6 and 7).

Hypothermia from the infusion of previously refrigerated blood and blood components, room-temperature fluids, and the exposure of the trauma wound and surgical wound to room-air temperature cools the body significantly. The coagulation system works at 37°C, not 34°C. The clinical correlation of bleeding and coagulation studies is made more difficult still because all the plasma samples for the PT, aPTT, and fibrinogen are warmed to 37°C before the tests are performed. Therefore, the coagulation parameters will not reflect how the coagulation system is working in the body in these particularly hypothermic situations. Warming the body with warmer i.v. fluids and external body warming as soon as possible will contribute significantly to good hemostasis (see Tables 6 and 7) (119,120).

C. The Surgeon's Approach to the Trauma Patient

The surgeon and emergency room physician will more than likely use the Advanced Trauma Life Support program developed by The American College of Surgeons as reported by Trunkey (121). The distinctive aspect of this program is that all activities are performed *simultaneously*: assessment, resuscitation, complete physical examination, diagnostic procedures, and life-saving surgery. Under resuscitation, the prevention of shock and assessment for blood loss will involve obtaining a blood sample and giving replacement fluids including blood and blood components. For those of us not in the trauma facility, the urgency of this approach is not

Table 6 Complications of Massive Transfusion Related to Blood/Component Replacement Therapy

Difficulty	Etiology	Consequence	Prevention
1. Citrate toxicity, rare	Impaired liver function, large transfused volume of bank blood	Cardiac dysfunction, hypotension	IV calcium, adequate hepatic function, reduce hypothermia
2. Acidosis (metabolic)	Poor tissue perfusion	Circulatory failure	Maintain perfusion, bicarbonate
3. Elevated potassium	Volume banked blood, renal failure	Toxicity, cardiac dysfunction	"fresher blood"
4. Elevated ammonia, jaundice	Volume banked blood, hypothermia, liver shock	Toxicity	"fresher blood," maintain blood pressure
5. Decreased 2,3-DPG	Banked blood	Poor oxygen release	"fresher blood," added 2,3-DPG
6. Hypothermia	Infusion of cold blood and fluids, cold operating room	Cardiac dysfunction, poor clot formation, decreased citrate clearance, hypotension	Blood/fluid warming

Table 7 Changes in Coagulation Parameters Resulting from Massive Blood Transfusion

Difficulty	Etiology	Consequence	Prevention
1. Prolongation of prothrombin time (>14 sec), aPTT (45 sec)	Dilution by fluid, plasma expanders, and packed RBC	Obstacle to accurate differentiation of patient's coagulation status from increased utilization, blood loss, or dilution; bleeding	Same-time monitoring of PT, aPTT, and blood Tx followed by appropriate FFP
2. Thrombocytopenia (<60,000 mm^3)	Dilution	Bleeding	Monitor, platelet Tx
3. Microemboli	Failure to filter blood and components	Acute pulmonary insufficiency	Microfilters (20–40 μm)
4. Circulation overload	Excessive blood or fluid infusion	Heart failure, hypertension	Monitor volume of infusions
5. Multisystem failure of lungs, liver, kidney ARDS, sepsis	Shock, acute hypoxia, acidosis, hypertension, tissue thromboplastin release	Total body system failure	Maintenance of blood volume, blood pressure, and perfusion of all organs, as well as oxygen needs
6. Suppression of host immune defenses	Blood transfusion	Infection	Early recognition, prophylaxis, and antibiotic therapy

Table 8 Protocol Driven Critical Points or Triggers of Coagulation Parameter Changes and Blood Replacement Volumes Dictating Massive Blood Replacement, by Different Authors

Counts et al., 1979 (122)	
Decreased platelet count	<100,000 mm^3
	(18 units of blood transfused, or 1.5–2 × blood volume
Prolonged PT /aPTT	>1.5 of control
Murray et al., 1987 (123)	
Decreased platelet count	<100,000 mm^3
Prolonged PT	Factor V < 30% or ≥1.5 × control
Prolonged aPTT	Factor VIII < 30% or ≥1.5 × control
Decreased fibrinogen	<75 mg/dL
Ciraverella et al., 1987 (124) (recognition of microvascular bleeding)	
Decreased platelet count	≤50,000 mm^3
Prolonged PT	Factor V < 30% or ≥1.8 × control
Prlonged aPTT	Factor VIII < 30% or ≥1.8 × control
Decreased fibrinogen	≤75 mg/dL
Leslie, 1991 (125)	
Decreased platelet count	<50,000 mm^3, after 12 units packed red blood cells
Prolonged PT	>1.5 × mean normal PT or after 12 units packed RBC
Prolonged aPTT	>1.5 × mean normal aPTT or after 12 units packed RBC

always apparent. Immediate assessment, often based on clinical experience alone, creates for the distant observer a nonscientific appearance. To reconcile the potential for this problem to dominate any discussion, we have chosen to make each trauma situation an opportunity for growth and education. Each trauma is different, with unique demands. A simplified, rote approach does not provide what is needed. To begin an approach we need a working definition: Massive Blood Transfusion in Trauma; (a) one half blood volume at one time (5-6 units blood for a 70-kg victim), or (b) total blood volume replaced in 24 hr (10–12 units packed red blood cells). The basis for transfusion is based on need, and the need is sometimes criteria based and sometimes based on clinical experience (see Table 8).

The transfusion of blood and blood components should be planned according to useful and scientifically accurate goals. This is not always easy, for there are different personal preferences for the surgeon, anesthesiologist, and clinical pathologist that will affect the choices. We prefer the assessment of the patient as a continuous process designed to quickly identify deficits, and correct them appropriately. This assessment is based on the development of accurate and *practical* trigger points. Dangerously abnormal test levels of hematology and coagulation parameters will predict or suggest increased risk for more bleeding and low tissue oxygenation damage. In addition, the washing and reperfusing of shed blood may add an additional source for an acquired coagulation deficit and risk for bleeding. A consensus among all participants (surgeon, anesthesiologist, clinical pathologist) in defining coagulation triggers is therefore an important aspect of the decision-making process. The following are blood and blood components transfusion triggers we recommend, modified from Sherman (126).

Hematocrit < 20–24%, transfuse 2 units PRBC, reevaluate.
Platelet count < 90,000 mm^3 if bleeding, transfuse 1 apheresed or 6–10 units platelets.
Platelet count < 60,000 mm^3 if not bleeding, as for preceding, re-evaluate.

Prothrombin time > 1.4 times upper limit of reference range, e.g., >16 sec, transfuse 2 units of fresh frozen plasma, reevaluate.
Activated PTT > 5 sec over upper limit of reference range, e.g., > 45 sec, transfuse 2 units fresh frozen plasma, reevaluate.
In neurosurgery, periorbital surgery, or surgery in the glottal areas, keep platelet count ≥ 100,000 mm^3.

The short-term goals of blood transfusion should be to maintain blood pressure and hematocrit to assure oxygenation to all body systems. In surgery for a large traumatic wound, loss of blood will continue until surgical repair is essentially complete. The use of platelets is often of no hemostatic value until the surgical repair process approaches completion. The appropriate time for platelet transfusions may be 2–4 hr into the surgery. This approach also helps in reducing the loss of a limited platelet resource and reducing exposure to different blood donors. Fresh frozen plasma and packed red blood cell units are needed, however, to replace red cells and plasma lost, reduce dilution of clotting factors, and maintain tissue oxygenation. Crystalloid does not adequately replace massive loss of plasma. The system of continuous monitoring and replacement to achieve short-term goals and then later long-term goals has the advantage of continuous correction and overall reduction of blood replacement (see Table 9). At the point when the decision has been made to massively transfuse blood into the patient, we must recognize the effect this blood will have on laboratory tests (see Table 7). These changes in laboratory results are also important, obviously, because the changes can affect our decisions about additional blood or component transfusions. Experiences with the changes observed and their significance have varied over the years. Personal experience based on laboratory testing is our only way out of this forest of ideas and suggestions.

The decision to transfuse blood and blood components is made by the treating physician based on the total compilation of the history, clinical signs and symptoms, laboratory studies, and personal experience. The laboratory test results are (1) part of the initial decision-making process, and (2) when performed at regular intervals, permit better decisions in blood utiliza-

Table 9 Checklist of Questions for the Coagulation Laboratory to Ask in Support of the Trauma Patient

Baseline studies on first entry into your system: The dynamics of coagulation values that change over time; catch-up versus maintenance support.	
What constitutes a dangerous coagulation laboratory result, and does the result mean you initiate blood/component transfusions?	
What are your short term coagulation goals?	
Hematocrit > 20–24%	aPTT < 45 sec
Platelet count > Not applicable	PT < 16 sec
Fibrinogen > 100 mg/dL	
What are your long-term coagulation goals?	
Hematocrit > 24%	aPTT < 40 sec
Platelet count > 100,000 mm^3	PT < 14 sec
Fibrinogen > 150 mg/dL	
Monitoring the coagulation status of the trauma patient: Baseline values, changes over time, replacement therapy, initial goals, ultimate goals, success or failure and why?	
Bleeding problems associated with specific kinds of trauma: head, shock; chest, abdomen/pelvis, extremities, hidden blood in spaces and tissue	

tion (see Table 8). With proper coagulation support, correction for defects can be made during the surgical procedure with more efficient use of component therapy, and fewer complications due to massive blood replacement. Initial baseline studies and periodic studies at 1- and 2-hr intervals until stable is a good start toward this goal. Obviously, the faster and more completely the patient's hemostasis is corrected (resuscitation, surgical correction, treatment of the coagulopathy, and achievement of normothermia), the more successful the result will be.

Case Study 3

A 19-year-old man presents to the hospital Emergency Department via ambulance with the following history.

The man was shot by a single bullet through the chest and upper abdomen. He was rushed to a local hospital, where he received one unit of O-negative blood and "several"?? liters of fluid. On arrival at the hospital, the patient was alert, with low normal blood pressure and rapid pulse. The bullet on examination appeared to have gone through the lower lobe of the left lung, the lower segments of the right lobe of the liver, and was lodged in the wall of the right abdominal wall. The initial laboratory studies were as follows, followed by emergency surgery.

Time	Hct	Platelet count	PT	aPTT	Fibrinogen	Glucose	K^+	Na^+
0919	19.7%	258	15.8	34.2	566	134		
1044	20.4						5.9	143
1100	*Surgery* (5 hr), given 8 P-RBC and 2 FFP							
1105						358	4.0	153
1150	19.3		21.6	99.2		295	3.5	154
1230						241	3.5	153
1241	17.3							
1320						189	3.9	150
1336	31.9							
1442						143	4.1	152
1500	23.1					133	4.1	152
1600	*Out of surgery*; 4 P-RBC, 4 FFP, 10 plt conc infusions began							
	Bleeding present and clinically unrelated to the surgical wound							
1652	21.0	67	18.7	60.8		143	4.3	146
1739	26.0	47	16.2	46.0	86			
1826						136	4.6	150
1915						121	5.2	148
2030	30.2						4.4	
2200						120	4.4	149
2300	31.7	104	14.2	33.3	155			
	Correction achieved 6 hr after surgery completed							
2349						120	4.3	148
0145	33.3					122	4.3	146
0500	32.4	101	14.2	31.3		125	4.3	143
0600						122	4.2	146
0643						122	4.3	145
0500	31.4	124	14.4	33.1		133	435	140

Question 1. *Can the transfusion of blood products be improved*? The patient developed a dilutional coagulopathy during surgery. Attempts at correction were made after surgery rather than during surgery. Awareness of the deficits could have been made during surgery with regular monitoring. Replacement with fresh frozen plasma and/or cryoprecipitate during surgery would have reduced loss of blood due to the acquired coagulopathy from blood loss and fluid and packed red cell replacements. Platelets could have been transfused once surgical hemostasis appeared to be achieved. *Note*: In a patient over 50 to 60 years of age, there can be greater intolerance of dilution with greater risk for consequences of low organ perfusion such as organ failure or stroke.

IV. ACQUIRED BLEEDING ASSOCIATED WITH NEUROSURGERY

Any assessment of bleeding related to a neurosurgical procedure should reflect two kinds of risk: first, the risk for bleeding before surgery in the patient with intracranial or spinal cord lesions who has diseases, is on medication or suffers trauma that results in bleeding; second, the risk for bleeding that is a consequence of those aspects of surgery that are unique to neurosurgery.

Knowing the cause of bleeding events is essential to correcting the deficits in coagulation before surgery if possible, and supporting coagulation needs during surgery. Intrinsic to neurosurgery is the close proximity of life-threatening nerve pathways to surgical sites, and the disastrous effect of seemingly minuscule accumulations of blood or fluid on the nerve pathways. Postoperatively, the bone-enclosed structures make the rapid accumulation of blood or fluid unable to escape easily, resulting in unacceptable pressures on brain and spinal cord tissues. In the vast majority of neurosurgical cases, the operative procedure will not begin unless the surgeon is confident the patient has an adequate coagulation system.

A. Risk Factors Associated with Disease, Medication, and Trauma

Risk factors include systemic diseases such as hypertension, vessel disruption from atherosclerotic defects, aneurysms in the elderly with rebleeding from vasospasm (127), mycotic aneurysms, and arteriovenous malformations with a higher risk for bleeding during pregnancy (128–130). Congenital bleeding disorders such as hemophilia with and without an inhibitor (131,132), antithrombotic medications such as aspirin (133), anticoagulants such as heparin or coumadin (134–136), plasma expanders such as dextran or Hespan (137), and fibrinolytic agents such as tPA or streptokinase (138) all place the patient at increased risk for excessive and inappropriate bleeding during and after surgery. Drugs such as cocaine and amphetamines increase cerebral blood flow and bleeding (139). Trauma resulting in release of brain tissue into the wound results in consumption, and the catecholamine surge is associated with DIC (140–143). Increased local fibrinolysis with bleeding is identified in chronic subdural hemorrhages (144). Both DIC-like syndromes and thrombotic syndromes can be seen with tumors before, during, and after resection (145–147).

B. Preoperative, Intraoperative, and Postoperative Monitoring

Preoperative base line coagulation studies assess the significance of history, as in the use of medication or disease processes, identify unsuspected causes of bleeding or thrombosis (very rare), and provide a baseline with which to evaluate the changes that will occur as the result of surgery or other therapy.

Intraoperative coagulation studies determine or correlate with the clinical observation of excessive bleeding. They also provide for timely correction of deficits identified before bleeding becomes a serious complication.

Postoperative coagulation studies establish the coagulation situation in order to assess the risk for postoperative bleeding, and determine whether observed bleeding is of coagulation origin or vascular origin. This permits more timely correction of the coagulation deficits with blood components or a return to surgery. In the vast majority of neurosurgical cases there will be a postoperative moderate acute-phase hypercoagulable response resulting in an increased risk for thrombosis. In addition to the platelet count and fibrinogen, a factor VIII screen will be helpful in documenting the risk for thrombosis and the justification for anticoagulation therapy or pneumatic boots.

C. Practical Coagulation Studies for Neurosurgery

The following tests* can be performed before, during, and after surgery in most general hospitals where neurosurgery is performed: CBC, platelet count, prothrombin time, aPTT, fibrinogen. The use of this baseline panel assumes: (1) the preoperative history is negative for medication or disease as a cause for bleeding or thrombosis, and (2) the type, complexity, and risk of the neurosurgical procedure dictates that a superior coagulation status be obtained if possible.

In head trauma, the risk for a DIC syndrome adds to the need for monitoring. Tests such as D-dimer and FDP are usually positive in most neurosurgical procedures and therefore do not add information if performed in trauma.

D. Neurosurgical Procedures with an Increased Risk for Bleeding

1. *Spinal Cord Surgery*

Surgical exposure of the spinal cord requires removal of large portions of vascular bone. This surgical technique allows local consumption (thrombosis) and lysis of thrombi, and the entry of these products into systemic circulation. The local DIC becomes a systemic DIC, and all the serious complications of DIC such as continued bleeding may occur. Fortunately, this is a self-limiting process, and when surgery is completed and the wound closed, the underlying cause is no longer present. Replacement with blood components directed at specific deficits will usually correct the bleeding (150,151).

Baseline preoperative coagulation laboratory values are important in assessing the changes in coagulation as a consequence of surgery. Excessive blood loss in this kind of surgery may also result in a dilutional coagulopathy if the losses are not adequately replaced during surgery. Baseline studies provide a benchmark for assessing these losses and the need for replacement component therapy.

2. *Exploratory Intracranial Brain Surgery*

Removing large portions of skull may result in *increased blood loss* due to the very vascular quality of the scalp and bone. Manipulation and surgical removal of portions of the cerebral

---

*The bleeding time has value in assessing the effects of uremia on platelet function and the response to DDAVP and cryoprecipitate. In addition, the bleeding time is of value in screening for congenital platelet defects. However, the bleeding time is generally a poor predictor of surgical bleeding (148,149).

cortex or cerebellum can result in tearing of small and medium-sized vessels, resulting in a surprisingly large volume of blood over a 3- to 4-hr surgical procedure. When the blood loss approaches the patient's blood volume, a *dilutional coagulopathy* may result if appropriate blood components are not used (152–154).

Surgical exposure to clip a vessel break or other mechanical cause for bleeding will require an *intact coagulation system*. Directions often stated include:

Hematocrit > 24%
Platelet count > 100,000 mm^3
Normal prothrombin time and aPTT

The procedures most likely to have blood loss through vessel breaks include:

Intracranial exploration for vascular defects; clipping an aneurysm
Subdural, epidural, subarachnoid hemorrhage evacuation
Sterotatic brain biopsy
Intracranial surgery for primary or secondary tumors made worse by the vascular nature of the tumor or infiltration of adjacent blood vessels

There are no guidelines for coagulation minimal values specific for neurosurgery developed through clinical trials. It is unlikely that guidelines will be tested in a controlled human clinical trial. Remember that the very confined nature of the spinal cord and cerebral cortex within their bony structures makes *any* bleeding hazardous.

E. Methods Often Used to Control and Reduce Intraoperative and Postoperative Bleeding

General guidelines include:

Maintain platelet count > 100,000 mm^3
Maintain prothrombin time and aPTT within reference range
Maintain fibrinogen > 100 mg/dL
Induced hypotension, 90 mmHg systolic
Head elevation
Antifibrinolytics such as tranexamic acid or epsilon-aminocaproic acid

Specific corrective actions to be taken when bleeding is clinically significant include the following. In warfarin reversal, administer vitamin K, fresh frozen plasma, and bypass concentrates such as Autoplex or FEIBA. In fibrinolysis reversal, stop the fibrinolytic agent and heparin, and give protamine sulfate to reverse the heparin. Give epsilon-aminocaproic acid or tranexamic acid to stop systemic fibrinolysis, and cryoprecipitate and/or fresh frozen plasma to replace fibrinogen. With documented antiplatelet medication, stop the medication, and give platelet transfusions and DDAVP. With an intraoperative or postoperative dilutional coagulopathy, give continuous support during the procedure directed by specific laboratory-defined deficits. Sterotatic brain biopsy with the use of bovine topical thrombin may result in thrombin and factor V antibodies. These acquired antibodies are rare but clinically very significant, with difficult management. Overcoming the antibody may require extensive platelet concentrates, fresh frozen plasma, intravenous immunoglobulin, and possibly plasmapheresis in more severe cases (155–157).

V. ACQUIRED BLEEDING ASSOCIATED WITH ORTHOPEDIC SURGERY

Acquired bleeding related to orthopedic surgery is associated with two obvious types of procedures, elective and traumatic repair. Bleeding in each of these groups is related primarily to the particular mechanics of the surgery and the location of the arterial or venous blood vessels to the bony structures.

A. Elective Orthopedic Surgery with Increased Risk for Bleeding

Vertebral fusion for scoliosis. *Mechanism*: This is usually a lengthy operative procedure ranging from 3 to 4 1/2 hr, with large areas of decortication of bone. The long exposure of blood to tissue thromboplastin at the wound site results in a consumptive coagulopathy or DIC. This results in the progressive loss of platelets and clotting proteins (150,151,158,159). *Management*: After visual assessment of blood loss, and vital signs, intraoperative coagulation studies can quantify the loss of platelets and clotting proteins. Specific correction should be made intraoperatively with fresh frozen plasma, cryoprecipitate, and/or platelet concentrates as defined by the intraoperative laboratory assessment. Delay of the coagulation assessment can result in significant dilutional coagulopathy unknown to the surgeon.

B. Orthopedic Surgical Repair of a Traumatic Fracture

Fractured hip with hip replacement and fractured femur. *Mechanism*: Multiple vessels are torn (femoral artery and/or vein) and lacerated with the fracture. These vessels are not compressible, resulting in massive blood loss into the surrounding tissues. Visual inspection may not indicate the significance of this blood loss. Until surgery is underway with good vital sign measurement, hematology and coagulation testing are the most rapid and efficient means to detect the blood volume loss. *Management*: Surgical intervention with specific replacement of blood and blood components dictated by preoperative and intraoperative assessment. Extensive fluid replacement may also contribute to a postoperative hemodilution coagulopathy if not detected intraoperatively.

VI. ACQUIRED BLEEDING ASSOCIATED WITH UROLOGICAL SURGERY

Excessive bleeding in urological surgery is frequently confined to prostate surgery. Occasionally, renal surgery or renal trauma can result in life-threatening hemorrhage. In both cases the operative site which is actively bleeding forms clots which are in turn lysed by the urokinase in urine. Urokinase is a potent plasminogen activator, which converts plasminogen to plasmin, the active enzyme. Bleeding continues as all clots are lysed. The use of epsilon-aminocaproic acid or tranexamic acid blocks the activation of plasminogen. This use is not without controversy (160). Nonetheless, the antifibrinolytic agents have been useful in stopping or slowing the blood loss in prostate surgery (161–164).

In prostate surgery, the preoperative use of aspirin, and a urinary tract infection, contributes significantly to the risk of bleeding postoperatively (165–167). The use of aspirin is often a hidden factor, since many patients and surgeons do not readily recognize aspirin as a medication with a risk for bleeding. The use of aspirin has increased, particularly in the prevention of myocardial infarction and stroke in the age range of patients who have prostate surgery.

REFERENCES

1. Gravlee GP, Whitaker CL, Mark LJ, Rogers AT, Royster RL, Harrison GA. Baseline activated coagulation time should be measured after surgical incision. Anesth Analg 1990; 71:549–553.
2. Mottaghy K, Oedekoven B, Poppel K, et al. Heparin-coated versus non-coated surfaces for extracorporeal circulation. Int J Artif Organs 1991; 14:721–728.
3. Taylor CA. Anticoagulation and heparin-bonded surfaces: treating the patient or the pump? Proc Am Acad Cardiovasc Perf 1992; 13:140–142.
4. Bidstrup BP, Royston D, Sapsford RN, Taylor KM. Reduction in blood loss and blood use after cardiopulmonary bypass with high dose aprotinin (Trasylol). J Thorac Cardiovasc Surg 1989; 97: 364–372.
5. Colman RW. Platelet and neutrophil activation in cardiopulmonary bypass. Ann Thorac Surg 1990; 49:32–34.
6. Dietrich W, Barankay A, Dilthey G, et al. Reduction of homologous blood requirement in cardiac surgery by intraoperative aprotinin application—clinical experience in 152 cardiac surgical patients. Thorac Cardiovasc Surgeon 1989; 37:92–98.
7. Lemmer JH Jr, Stanford W, Bonny SL, et al. Aprotinin for coronary bypass operations: efficacy, safety, and influence on early saphenous vein graft patency: a multicenter, randomized, double-blind, placebo-controlled study. J Thorac Cardiovasc Surg 1994; 107:543–553.
8. Moulton MJ, Creswell LL, Mackey ME, et al. Reexploration for bleeding is a risk factor for adverse outcomes after cardiac operations. J Thorac Cardiovasc Surg 1996; 111(5):1037–1046.
9. van der Meer J, Hillege HL, Ascoop CAPL, et al. Aprotinin in aortocoronary bypass surgery: increased risk of vein-graft occlusion and myocardial infarction: supportive evidence from a retrospective study. Thromb Haemost 1996; 75:1–3.
10. Wachtfogel YT, Kucich U, Hack CE, et al. Aprotinin inhibits the contact, neutrophil, and platelet activation systems during simulated extracorporeal perfusion. J Thorac Cardiovasc Surg 1993; 106:1–10.
11. Murkin JM, Lux J, Shannon N, et al. Aprotinin significantly decreases bleeding and transfusion requirements in patients receiving aspirin and undergoing cardiac operations. J Thorac Cardiovasc Surg, 1994; 107:554–561.
12. Murkin JM, Shannon NA, Bourne RB, et al. Aprotinin decreases blood loss in patients undergoing revision or bilateral total hip arthroplasty. Anesth Analg 1995; 80(2):343–348.
13. Teasdale SJ, Zulys VJ, Mycyk T, Baird RJ, Glynn MFX. Ancrod anticoagulation for cardiopulmonary bypass in heparin-induced thrombocytopenia and thrombosis. Ann Thorac Surg 1989; 48: 712–713.
14. Warkentin TE, Kelton JG. Heparin-induced thrombocytopenia. In: Coller BS, ed. Progress in Hemostasis and Thrombosis. Philadelphia: Saunders, 1991:1–27.
15. Singer RL, Mannion JD, Bauer TL, et al. Complications from heparin induced thrombocytopeniain patients undergoing cardiopulmonary bypass. Chest 1993; 104:1436–1440.
16. AbuRahma AF, Boland JP, Witsberger T. Diagnostic and therapeutic strategies of white clot syndrome. Am J Surg 1991; 162:175–179.
17. Samuels LE, Shektman A, Amron G, et al. Heparin-induced thrombocytopenia; a spectrum of hemorrhage and thrombosis. Case presentations. Vasc Surg 1992; 26:596–604.
18. John LCH, Rees GM, Kovacs IB. Effect of heparin on in vitro platelet reactivity in cardiac surgical patients—a comparative assessment by whole blood platelet aggregometry and haemostatometry. Thromb Res 1992; 66:649–656.

19. John LCH, Rees GM, Kovacs IB. Inhibition of platelet function by heparin: an etiologic factor in postbypass hemorrhage. J Thorac Cardiovasc Surg 1993; 105:816–822.
20. Rohrer MJ, Kestin AS, Ellis PA, et al. High-dose heparin suppresses platelet alpha granule secretion. J Vasc Surg 1992; 15:1000–1009.
21. Azrin MA, Mitchel JF, Fram DB, et al. Decreased platelet deposition and smooth muscle cell proliferation after intramural heparin delivery with hydrogel-coated balloons. Circulation 1994; 90:433–441.
22. Beumer S, Ijsseldijk MJW, DeGroot PG, et al. Platelet adhesion to fibronectin in flow: dependence on surgace concentration and shear rate, role of platelet membrane glycoproteins GP Iib/IIIa and VLA-5, and inhibition by heparin. Blood 1994; 84:3724–3733.
23. Khuri SF, Valeri CR, Loscalzo J, et al. Heparin causes platelet dysfunction and induces fibrinolysis before cardiopulmonary bypass. Ann Thorac Surg J 1995; 60:1008–1014.
24. Bowers J, Ferguson JJ. The use of the activated clotting time in anticoagulation monitoring of intravascular procedures. Texas Heart Inst J 1993; 20:258–263.
25. Exposito RA, Cullifort AT, Colvin SB, et al. The role of the activated clotting time in heparin administration and neutralization for cardiopulmonary bypass. J. Thorac Cardiovasc Surg 1982; 85:174–185.
26. Ferguson JJ. All ACT's are not created equal. Texas Heart Inst J 1992; 19:1–3.
27. Nath FC, Muller DWM, Rosenschein U, et al. Heparin monitoring during coronary intervention: activated clotting time versus activated partial thromboplastin time. Can J Cardiol 1993; 9:797–801.
28. Doherty DC, Ortel TL, De Bruijn N, Greenberg CS, Van Trigt P III. "Heparin-free" cardiopulmonary bypass: first reported use of heparinoid (Org 10172) to provide anticoagulation for cardiopulmonary bypass. Anesthesiology 1990; 73:562–565.
29. Salmenpera M, Rasi V, Mattila S. Cardiopulmonary bypass in a patient with factor XII deficiency. Anesthesiology 1991; 75:539–541.
30. Walenga JM, Bakhos M, Messmore HL, Fareed J, Pifarre R. Potential use of recombinant hirudin as an anticoagulant in a cardiopulmonary bypass model. Ann Thorac Surg 1991; 51:271–277.
31. Koza MJ, Walenga JM, Fareed J, Pifarre R. A new approach in monitoring recombinant hirudin during cardiopulmonary bypass. Semin Thromb Hemost 1993; 19(suppl 1):90–96.
32. Carteaux JP, Gast A, Tschopp TB, Roux S. Activated clotting time as an appropriate test to compare heparin and direct thrombin inhibitors such as hirudin or Ro 46-6240 in experimental arterial thrombosis. Circulation 1995; 91:1568–1574.
33. Samama MM. Contemporary laboratory monitoring of low molecular weight heparins. Clin Lab Med 1995; 15(1):119–123.
34. Despotis GJ, Joist JH, Hogue CW, et al. More effective suppression of hemostatic system activation in patients undergoing cardiac surgery by heparin dosing based on heparin blood concentrations rather than ACT. Thromb Haemost 1996; 76:902–908.
35. Cohen JA, Frederickson EL, Kaplain JA. Plasma heparin activity and antagonism during cardiopulmonary bypass with hypothermia. Anesth Analg 1977; 56:564–568.
36. Kopriva CJ, Sreenivasan N, Stefansson S, Farrell DT, Shaffer WB, Geha AS. Hypothermia can cause errors in activated coagulation time (abstr). Anesthesiology 1980; 63:S85.
37. Patt A, McCroskey BL, Moore EE. Hypothermia-induced coagulopathies in trauma. Vasc Trauma 1988; 68:775–785.
38. Rohrer MG, Natale AM. Effect of hypothermia on the coagulation cascade. Crit Care Med 1992; 20:1402–1405.
39. Michelson AD, MacGregor H, Barnard MR, Kestin AS, Rohrer MJ, Valeri CR. Reversible inhibition of human platelet activation by hypothermia in vivo and in vitro. Thromb Haemost 1994; 71: 633–640.
40. Moorehead MT, Westengard JC, Bull BS. Platelet involvement in the activated coagulation time of heparinized blood. Anesth Analg 1984; 63:394–398.

41. Zulys VJ, Teasdale SJ, Michel ER, et al. Ancrod (Arvin) as an alternative to heparin anticoagulation for cardiopulmonary bypass. Anesthesiology 1989; 71:870–877.
42. O-Yurvati AH, Laub GW, Southgate TJ, McGrath LB. Heparinless cardiopulmonary bypass with ancrod. Ann Thorac Surg 1994; 57:1656–1658.
43. Spiekermann BF, Lake CL, Rich GF, Humphries JE. Normal activated clotting time despite adequate anticoagulation with ancrod in a patient with heparin-associated thrombocytopenia and thrombosis undergoing cardiopulmonary bypass. Anesthesiology 1994; 80:686–688.
44. Bush LR. Argatroban, a selective, potent thrombin inhibitor. Cardiovasc Drug Rev 1991; 9:247–263.
45. Imura Y, Stassen J-M, Collen D. Comparative antithrombotic effects of heparin, recombinant hirudin and argatroban in a hamster femoral vein platelet-rich mural thrombosis model. J Pharmacol Exp Ther 1992; 261:895–898.
46. Matsuo T, Kario K, Chikahira Y, et al. Treatment of heparin induced thrombocytopenia by use of argatroban, a synthetic thrombin inhibitor. Br J Haematol 1992; 82:627–629.
47. Wendel HP, Heller W, Gallimore MJ. Influence of heparin, heparin plus aprotinin and hirudin on contact activation in a cardiopulmonary bypass model. Immunopharmacology 1996; 32:57–61.
48. Dietrich W, Spannagl M, Jochum M, et al. Influence of high-dose aprotinin treatment on blood loss and coagulation patterns in patients undergoing myocardial revascularization. Anesthesiology 1990; 73:1119–1126.
49. Terrel MR, Walenga JM, Koza MJ. Efficacy of aprotinin with various anticoagulant agents in cardiopulmonary bypass. Ann Thorac Surg 1996; 62:506–511.
50. Van Oeveren W, Harder MP, Roozendaal KJ, Eijsman L, Wildevuur CRH. Aprotinin protects platelets against the initial effect of cardiopulmonary bypass. J Thorac Cardiovasc Surg 1990; 99: 788–797.
51. Havel M, Grabenwoger F, Schneider J, et al. Aprotinin does not decrease early graft patency after coronary artery bypass grafting despite reducing postoperative bleeding and use of donated blood. J Thorac Cardiovasc Surg 1994; 107:807–810.
52. Hunt BJ, Segal HC, Yacoub M. Guidelines for monitoring heparin by the activated clotting time when aprotinin is used during cardiopulmonary bypass. J Thorac Cardiovasc Surg 1992; 104: 211–212.
53. Wang J-S, Lin C-Y, Hung W-T, et al. In vitro effects of aprotinin on activated clotting time measured with different activators. J Thorac Cardiovasc Surg 1992; 104:1135–1140.
54. Wang J-S, Lin C-Y, Hung W-T, et al. Monitoring heparin-induced anticoagulation with kaolin-activated clotting time in cardiac surgical patients treated with aprotinin. Anesthesiology 1992; 77: 1080–1084.
55. Despotis GJ, Filos KS, Levine V, et al. Aprotinin prolongs activated and nonactivated whole blood clotting time and potentiates the effect of heparin in vitro. Anesth Analg 1996; 82:1126–1131.
56. Baily CR, Fisher AR, Wielogorski AK. Reheparinisation requirements after cardiopulmonary bypass in patients treated with aprotinin. Br Heart J 1994; 72:442–445.
57. Horrow JC, Hlavacek J, Strong MD, et al. Prophylactic tranexamic acid decreases bleeding after cardiac operations. J Thorac Cardiovasc Surg 1990; 99:70–74.
58. Vander Salm TJ, Kaur S, Lancey RA, et al. Reduction of bleeding after heart operations through the prophylactic use of epsilon-aminocaproic acid. J Thorac Cardiovasc Surg 1996; 112(4):1098–1107.
59. Menzies St. A, Hartley JA, Hitchcock ER, et al. The effect of tranexamic acid on bleeding time and haemostasis. Neurochirurgia 1991; 34:141–143.
60. Horrow JC, Van Riper DF, Strong MD, Brodsky I, Parmet JL. Hemostatic effects of tranexamic acid and desmopressin during cardiac surgery. Circulation 1991; 84:2063–2070.
61. Cosgrove DM III, Heric B, Lytle BW, et al. Aprotinin therapy for reoperative myocardial revascularization: a placebo-controlled study. Ann Thorac Surg 1992; 54:1031–1038.
62. Milne AA, Drummond GB, Paterson DA, Murphy WG, Ruckley CV. Disseminated intravascular

coagulation after aortic aneurysm repair, intraoperative salvage autotransfusion, and aprotinin. Lancet 1994; 334:470–471.
63. Milam JD, Austin SF, Martin RF, et al. Alterations of coagulation and selected clinical chemistry parameters in patients undergoing open heart surgery without transfusions. Am J Clin Pathol 1981; 76:155–162.
64. Mammen EF, Koets MH, Washington BC, et al. Hemostasis changes during cardiopulmonary bypass surgery. Semin Thromb Hemost 1985; 11:281–292.
65. Spence RK, Alexander JB, DelRossi AJ, et al. Transfusion guidelines for cardiovascular surgery: lessons learned from operations in Jehovah's Witnesses. J Vasc Surg 1992; 16:825–831.
66. Goodnough LT, Johnston MFM, Ramsey G, et al. Guidelines for transfusion support in patients undergoing coronary artery bypass grafting. Ann Thorac Surg 1990; 50:675–683.
67. Goodnough LT, Soegiarso RW, Geha AS. Blood lost and blood transfused in coronary artery bypass graft operation as implications for blood transfusion and blood conservation strategies. J Am Coll Surgeons 1993; 177:345–351.
68. Goodnough LT, Wida Soegiarso R, Birkmeyer JD, Gilbert Welch H. Economic impact of inappropriate blood transfusions in coronary artery bypass graft surgery. Am J Med 1993; 94:509–514.
69. Harrison CR, Polesky HF. College of American Pathologists Conference XXV on current transfusion medicine practices and issues: concluding remarks and recommendations. Arch Pathol Lab Med; 118:462–464.
70. Schmidt PJ. Introducing new tests before transfusion: who shall decide? Arch Pathol Lab Med 1994; 118:454–456.
71. Shulman IA, Lohr K, Derdiarian AK, Picukaric JM. Monitoring transfusionist practices: a strategy for improving transfusion safety. Transfusion 1994; 34:11–15.
72. Surgenor DM, Churchill WH, Wallace EL, et al. Determinants of red cell, platelet, plasma, and cryoprecipitate transfusions during coronary artery bypass graft surgery: The Collaborative Hospital Transfusion Study. Transfusion 1996; 36:521–532.
73. Despotis JE, Grishaber JE, Goodnough LT. The effect of an intraoperative treatment algorithm on physician's transfusion practice in cardiac surgery. Transfusion 1994; 34:290–296.
74. Spiess BD. Cardiac anesthesia risk management. Hemorrhage, coagulation and transfusion: a risk benefit analysis (review). J Cardiothor Vasc Anesth 1994; 8:19–22.
75. Pifarre R, Babka R, Sullivan HJ, et al. Management of postoperative heparin rebound following cardiopulmonary bypass. J Thorac Cardiovasc Surg 1981; 81:378–381.
76. Shanberge JN, Murato M, Quattrociocchi-Longe T, van Neste L. Heparin-protamine complexes in the production of heparin rebound and other complications of extracorporeal bypass procedures. Am J Clin Pathol 1987; 87:210–217.
77. Salmenpera MT, Levy JH, Curling PE. Evaluation of a new heparinase activated clotting time to assess heparin rebound following cardiac surgery (abstr). 13th Annual Meeting, Soc Cardiovascular Anesth 1990.
78. Martin P, Horkay F, Grupta NK, Gebitekin C, Walker DR. Heparin rebound phenomenon—much ado about nothing? Blood Coag Fibrinol 1992; 3:187–191.
79. Hobbhahn J, Conzen PF, Habazettl H, Gutmann R, Kellermann W, Peter K. Heparin reversal by protamine in humans—complement, prostaglandins, blood cells, and hemodynamics. J Appl Physiol 1991; 71:1415–1421.
80. Chan AKC, Leaker M, Burrows FA, et al. Coagulation and fibrinolytic profile of paediatric patients undergoing cardiopulmonary bypass. Thromb Haemost 1997; 77:270–277.
81. Guay J, Rivard GE. Mediastinal bleeding after cardiopulmonary bypass in pediatric patients. Ann Thorac Surg 1996; 62(6):1955–1960.
82. Chambers LA, Cohen DM, Davis JT. Transfusion patterns in pediatric open heart surgery. Transfusion 1996; 36:150–154.
83. Petaja J, Lundstrom U, Leijala M. Bleeding and use of blood products after heart operations in infants. J Thorac Cardiovasc Surg 1995; 109:524–529.

84. Harker LA, Malpass TW, Bronson HE, Hessell EA, Slichter SJ. Mechanism of abnormal bleeding in patients undergoing cardiopulmonary bypass: acquired transient platelet dysfunction associated with selective alpha granule release. Blood 1980; 56:824–834.
85. Nevelsteen A, Mortelmans L, Van de Cruys A, et al. Effect of ticlopidine on blood loss, platelet turnover and platelet deposition on prosthetic surfacars in patients undergoing aorto-femoral bypass grafting. Thromb Res 1991; 64:363–369.
86. Beurling-Harburg C. Coagulation and platelet function during cardiopulmonary bypass surgery. Amsect 1978; 10:164–169.
87. McKenna R, Bachman R, Whittaker B, Gibson JR, Weinberg M. The hemostatic mechanisms after open heart surgery. II. Frequency of abnormal platelet functions during and after extracorporeal circulation. J Thor Cardiovasc Surg 1975; 70:298–308.
88. Rinder CS, Bohnert J, Rinder HM, Mitchell J, Ault K, Hillman R. Platelet activation and aggregation during cardiopulmonary bypass. Anesthesiology 1991; 75:388–393.
89. Kestin AS, Valeri CR, Khuri SF, et al. The platelet function defect of cardiopulmonary bypass. Blood 1993; 82:107–117.
90. Ferraris VA, Rodriguez E, Ferraris SP, et al. Platelet aggregation abnormalities after cardiopulmonary bypass. Blood 1994; 83:299–300.
91. Uthoff K, Zehr KJ, Geerling R, Herskowitz A, Cameron DE, Reitz BA. Inhibition of platelet adhesion during cardiopulmonary bypass reduces postoperative bleeding. Circulation 1994; 90: 269–274.
92. Bertolino G, Locatelli A, Noris P, et al. Platelet composition and function in patients undergoing cardiopulmonary bypass for heart surgery. Haematologica 1996; 81:116–120.
93. Salzman EW, Weinstein MJ, Weintraub RM, et al. Treatment with desmopression acetate to reduce blood loss after cardiac surgery. N Engl J Med 1986; 314:1402–1406.
94. Cattaneo M, Harris AS, Stromberg U, et al. The effect of desmopressin on reducing blood loss in cardiac surgery—a metal-analysis of double-blind, placebo-controlled trials. Thromb Haemost 1995; 74:1064–1070.
95. Dietrich W, Barankay A, Wendt P, et al. Fibrinolysis caused by cardio-pulmonary bypass and shed mediastinal blood retransfusion—is it of clinical relevance. Adv Exp Med Biol 1988; 240: 405–410.
96. Griffith LD, Billman GF, Daily PO, Lane TA. Apparent coagulopathy caused by shed mediastinal blood and its prevention by washing of the infusate. Ann Thorac Surg 1989; 47:400–406.
97. Edmunds LH, Ellison N, Coleman R, et al. Platelet function during cardiac operation. Comparison of membrane and bubble oxygenators. I. Thorac Cardiovasc Surg 1982; 83:805–812.
98. Paramo JA, Rifon J, Llorens R, Cesares J, Paloma MJ, Rocha E. Intra- and postoperative fibrinolysis in patients undergoing cardiopulmonary bypass surgery. Haemostasis 1991; 21:58–64.
99. Banos G, De La Pena A, Izaguirre R. The vascular plasminogen activator as a source of the fibrinolytic potential observed during cardiopulmonary bypass. Thromb Res 1992; 67:579–588.
100. Chandler W. The effects of cardiopulmonary bypass on fibrin formation and lysis: is a normal fibrinolytic response essential? J Cardiovasc Pharmacol 1996; 27:S63–S68.
101. Burman JF, Chung HI, Lane DA, Philippou H, Adami A, Lincoln JCR. Role of factor XII in thrombin generation and fibrinolysis during cardiopulmonary bypass. Lancet 1994; 344:1192–1193.
102. Kirklin JK, Chenoweth DE, Naftel DC, et al. Effects of protamine administration after cardiopulmonary bypass on complement, blood elements, and the hemodynamic state. Ann Thorac Surg 1986; 41:193–199.
103. Weiler JM, Gellhaus MA, Carter JG, et al. A prospective study of the risk of an immediate adverse reaction to protamine sulfate during cardiopulmonary bypass surgery. J Allergy Clin Immunol 1990; 85:713–719.
104. Ovrum E, Lindberg H, Holen EA, et al. Systemic and pulmonary circulatory effects of protamine following cardiopulmonary bypass in man. Scand J Thorac Cardiovasc Surg 1991; 25:19–24.

105. Ovrum E, Lindberg H, Holen EA, Abdelnoor M. Hemodynamic effects of intraaortic versus intravenous protamine administration after cardiopulmonary bypass in man. Scand J Thorac Cardiovasc Surg 1992; 26:113–118.
106. Metz S. Administration of protamine rather than heparin in a patient undergoing normothermic cardiopulmonary bypass. Anesthesiology 1994; 80:691–694.
107. Bucx JJJ, De Scheerder I, Beatt K, et al. The importance of adequate anticoagulation to prevent early thrombosis after stenting of stenosed venous bypass grafts. Am Heart J 1991; 121:1389–1396.
108. Reis SE, Polak JF, Hirsch DR, et al. Frequency of deep venous thrombosis in asymptomatic patients with coronary artery bypass grafts. Am Heart J 1991; 122:478–482.
109. Qiao J-H, Walts AE, Fishbein MC. The severity of atherosclerosis at sites of plaque rupture with occlusive thrombosis in saphenous vein coronary artery bypass grafts. Am Heart J 1991; 122: 955–958.
110. Bick RL, Ismail Y, Baker WF Jr. Coagulation abnormalities in patients with precocious coronary artery thrombosis and patients failing coronary artery bypass grafting and percutaneous transcoronary angioplasty. Semin Thromb Hemost 1993; 19:412–417.
111. Eritsland J, Gjonnes G, Sandset PM, Seljeflot I, Arnesen H. Activated protein C resistance and graft occlusion after coronary artery bypass surgery. Thromb Res 1995; 79:223–226.
112. Rock WA, Pearce CW, Weichert RF, Johnson W. Indicators for increased risk for excessive bleeding after cardiopulmonary bypass surgery (abstr). Thromb Hemos 1987; 58:71.
113. Beal RW, Isbister JP. The storage and use of whole blood: management of acute haemorrhage. In: Blood component therapy in clinical practice. London: Blackwell Scientific, 1985:11–24.
114. Cachecho R, Millham FH, Wedel SK. Management of the trauma patient with pre-existing renal disease (review). Crit Care Clin 1994; 10:523–536.
115. Bickell WH, Wall MJ, Pepe PE, et al. Immediate versus delayed fluid resuscitation for hypotensive patients with penetrating torso injuries. N Engl J Med 1994; 331:1105–1109.
116. Hewson JR, Neame PB, Kumar N, et al. Coagulopathy related to dilution and hypotension during massive transfusion. Crit Care Med 1985; 13:387–391.
117. Ordog GJ, Wasserberger J, Balasubramanium S. Coagulation abnormalities in traumatic shock. Ann Emerg Med 1985; 14:650–655.
118. Wilson RF, Dulchavsky SA, Soullier G, et al. Problems with 20 or more blood transfusions in 24 hours. Presented at the 29th Annual Meeting of the Midwest Surgical Association, August 17–20, 1986, MacKinac Island, MI.
119. Luna GK, Maier RV, Pavlin EG, et al. Incidence and effect of hypothermia in seriously injured patients. J Trauma 1987; 27:1014–1018.
120. Patt A, McCroskey BL, Moore EE. Vascular trauma: hypothermia-induced coagulopathies in trauma. Surg Clin N Am 1988; 68:775–785.
121. Trunkey D. Initial treatment of patients with extensive trauma; review. N Engl J Med 1991; 324: 1259–1263.
122. Counts RB, Haisch C, Simon TL, et al. Hemostasis in massively transfused trauma patients. Ann Surg 1979; 190:91–99.
123. Murray DJ, Olsomn J, Strauss R, Tinker JH. Coagulation changes during packed red cell replacement of major blood loss. Anesthesiology 1988; 89:839–845.
124. Ciaverella D, Reed RL, Counts RB, et al. Coagulopathy related to dilution and hypotension during massive transfusion. Crit Care Med 1985; 13:387–391.
125. Leslie SD, Toy P. Laboratory hemostatic abnormalities in massively transfused patients given red blood cells and crystalloid. Am J Clin Pathol 1991; 96:770–773.
126. Sherman LA. Management of bleeding following massive transfusion or post-coronary bypass. In Polesky HF, Walker RH, eds. Safety in Transfusion Practices, CAP Conference/Aspen 1980. Skokie, IL: College of American Pathologists, 1982:257–281.
127. Mori K, Arai H, Nakajima K, et al. Hemorheological and hemodynamic analysis of hypervolemic

hemodilution therapy for cerebral vasospasm after aneurysmal subarachnoid hemorrhage. Stroke 1995; 26:1620–1626.

128. Monobe T, Kawai S, Takemura K, et al. Aspiration and drainage for brain abscess causing massive bleeding from abscess capsule: case report (in Japanese). No Shinkei Geka—Neurol Surg 1994; 22:363–365.
129. Sinson G, Philips MF, Flamm ES. Intraoperative endovascular surgery for cerebral aneurysms. J Neurosurg 1996; 84:63–70.
130. Forster DMC, Kunkler IH, Hartland P. Risk of cerebral bleeding from arteriovenous malformations in pregnancy: the Sheffield experience. Sterotact Funct Neurosurg 1993; 61(suppl):20–22.
131. Bouvry P, Recloux P. Acquired hemophilia. Haematologica 1994; 79:550–556.
132. Majumdar G, Savidge GF. Recombinant factor VIIa for intracranial haemorrhage in a Jehovah's Witness with severe haemophilia A and factor VIII inhibitors. Blood Coag Fibrinol 1993; 4:1031–1033.
133. Reymond M, Marbet G, Radü EW, et al. Aspirin as a risk factor for hemorrhage in patients with head injuries. Neurosurg Rev 1992; 15:21–25.
134. Diamond T, Gray WJ, Chee CP, et al. Subdural haematoma associated with long term oral anticoagulation. Br J Neurosurg 1988; 2:351–356.
135. Nagano N, Tabata H, Hashimoto K. Anticoagulant-related intracerebral hemorrhage in patients with prosthetic heart valves—report of two cases. Neurol Med Chir (Tokyo) 1991; 31:743–745.
136. Landefeld S, Beyth R. Anticoagulant-related bleeding: clinical epidemiology, prediction and prevention. Am J Med 1993; 95:315–328.
137. Claes Y, Hemelrijck J, Gerven M, et al. Influence of hydroxyethyl starch on coagulation in patients during the perioperative period. Anesth Analg 1992; 75:24–30.
138. Eleff S, Borel C, Bell W, et al. Acute management of intracranial hemorrhage in patients receiving thrombolytic therapy: case reports. Neurosurgery 1990; 26:867–869.
139. Aggarwal SK, Williams V, Levine SR, et al. Cocaine-associated intracranial hemorrhage: absence of vasculitis in 14 cases (review). Neurology 1996; 46:1741–1743.
140. White RJ, Likavec MJ. The diagnosis and initial management of head injury. New Engl J Med 1992; 327:1507–1511.
141. Olson J, Kaufman H, Moake J, et al. The incidence and significance of hemostatic abnormalities in patients with head injuries. Neurosurgery 1989; 24:825–832.
142. Miller J, Pattisapu J. Disseminated intravascular coagulation associated with spinal cord laceration: a case report. J Trauma 1989; 29:178–179.
143. Kearney TJ, Bentt L, Grode M, et al. Coagulopathy and catecholamines in severe head injury. J Trauma 1992; 32(5):608–611.
144. Weir B, Gordon P. Factors affecting coagulation: fibrinolysis in chronic subdural fluid collections. J Neurosurg 1983; 58:242–245.
145. Cochrane DD, Gustavsson B, Poskitt KP, et al. The surgical and natural morbidity of aggressive resection for posterior fossa tumors in childhood. Ped Neurosurg 1994; 20:19–29.
146. Di Rocco C, Iannelli A, Tancredi A. Patterns of failure in surgical therapy of medulloblastomas. J Neurosurg Sci 1995; 39:1–6.
147. Sawaya R, Rambo WM Jr, Hammoud MA, et al. Advances in surgery for brain tumors (review). Neurol Clin 1995; 13:757–771.
148. Rodgers RPC, Levin J. A critical reappraisal of the bleeding time. Semin Thromb Hemost 1990; 16:1–20.
149. Gerwitz AS, Miller ML, Keys TF. The clinical usefulness of peroperative bleeding time. Arch Pathol Lab Med 1996; 120:353–356.
150. Mayer PJ, Gehlsen JA. Coagulopathies associated with major spinal surgery. Clin Orthoped 1989; 83:245–250.
151. Suk SL, Kim IK, Lee CK, et al. A study on platelet function in idiopathic scoliosis. Orthopedics 1991; 66A:194–198.

152. Touho H, Hirakawa K, Hino A, et al. Relationship between abnormalities of coagulation and fibrinolysis and postoperative intracranial hemorrhage in head injury. Neurosurgery 1986; 19:523–531.
153. Narayan RK. Development of guidelines for the management of severe head injury. J Neurotrauma 1995; 12:907–912.
154. Solomon RA, Mayer SA, Tarmey JJ. Relationship between the volume of crainotomies for cerebral aneurysm performed at New York state hospitals and in-hospital mortality. Stroke 1996; 27:13–17.
155. Chimowitz M, Barnett G, Palmer J. Treatment of intractable arterial hemorrhage during stereotactic brain biopsy with thrombin. J Neurosurg 1991; 74:301–303.
156. Spero J. Bovine thrombin-induced inhibitor of factor V and bleeding risk in postoperative neurosurgical patients. J Neurosurg 1993; 78:817–820.
157. Banninger H, Hardegger T, Tobler A, et al. Fibrin glue in surgery: frequent development of inhibitors of bovine thrombin and human factor V. Br J Haematol 1993; 85:528–532.
158. Boettcher WG. Total hip arthoplastic in the elderly. Morbidity, mortality, and cost effectiveness. Clin Orthoped 1992; 272:30–35.
159. An HS, Mikhal WE, Jackson WT, et al. Effects of hypotension anesthesia, nonsteroidal antiinflammatory drugs, and polymethylmethacrylate on bleeding in total hip arthroplasty patients. J Arthroplasty 1991; 6:245–251.
160. Sherry S, Fletcher AP, Alkjaersig N, et al. ε-Aminocaproic acid, a potent anti-fibrinolytic agent. Trans Assoc Am Physicians 1959; 72:62–67.
161. McNicol CP, Fletcher AP, Alkjaersig N, et al. Impairment of hemostasis in the urinary tract: the role of urokinase. J Lab Clin Med 1961; 58:34–38.
162. McNicol CP, Fletcher AP, Alkjaersig N. The use of epsilon aminocaproic acid, a potent inhibitor of fibrinolytic activity in the management of postoperative hematuria. J Urol 1961; 86:829–836.
163. Sack E, Spaet TH, Gentile RL, et al. Reduction of postprostatectomy bleeding by epsilon aminocaproic acid. N Engl J Med 1963; 266:541–545.
164. Haygood TA, Atkins R, Kennedy JA, et al. Aminocaproic acid treatment of prolonged hematuria following renal biopsy. Arch Intern Med 1971; 127:478–483.
165. Watson CJE, Deane AM, Doyle PT, Bullock KN. Identifiable factors in post-prostatectomy haemorrhage: the role of aspirin. Br J Urol 1990; 66:85–87.
166. Thurston AV, Briant SL. Aspirin and post-prostatectomy haemorrhage. Br J Urol 1993; 71:574–576.
167. Zhu JP, Davidson MB, Meyhoff HH. Aspirin, a silent risk factor in urology. Scand J Urol Nephrol 1995; 29:369–374.

32

Anticoagulation

Louis M. Fink
University of Arkansas for Medical Sciences and Little Rock Veterans Administration Medical Center, Little Rock, Arkansas

Nicole A. Massoll and Alex A. Pappas
University of Arkansas for Medical Sciences, Little Rock, Arkansas

I. INTRODUCTION

Arterial and venous thromboses with or without embolization are well recognized as leading causes of mortality and morbidity in the United States (1,2). The significance of thrombosis is best realized by the fact that an estimated 25–40% of the population will die of thrombosis or hypercoaguability, and approximately 25% of first thrombotic events are fatal. Efforts to reduce the effects of hypercoaguability and subsequent thrombosis have lead to the discovery and development of many thrombotic inhibitors. These inhibitors inhibit or deplete components of either the coagulation cascade or platelets. Antithrombotic drugs and devices that can be used prophylactically and therapeutically are listed categorically in Table 1. As our understanding of the biochemistry and cellular mechanisms of thrombosis advances, a new generation of antithrombotic agents is beginning to emerge.

A variety of synthetic antithrombotic agents which were originally discovered in hematophagous animals (e.g., leeches, ticks, or vampire bats) have been sequenced and cloned (3). Achieving antithrombotic action without hemorrhagic complications is a persistent clinical dilemma. An ideal anticoagulant, which is not yet available, would have the properties listed in Table 2. Although many clinical situations require anticoagulation, the indications for anticoagulation can be broadly categorized into the general groups listed in Table 3.

The selection of which anticoagulant therapy to use is determined by either the nature of the precipitating thrombotic event(s) or the need for specific prophylaxis. The desired onset, intensity, duration, and route of administration of anticoagulant therapy must also be considered. The patient's response to a specific anticoagulant, the possible development of drug resistance, compliance or unexpected complications, and cost are further factors in selecting or adjusting anticoagulants and their dosage.

Appropriate anticoagulant dosage and administration regimens for specific anticoagulants are constantly being developed and revised. Therapies combining various anticoagulants and adjunct medication are undergoing clinical trials, and the use of anticoagulants with thrombolytic agents is now common (4). Anticoagulants are often used in clinical practice, and there has been an impetus to standardize the optimal laboratory monitoring for specific conditions

Table 1 Methods to Prevent Thrombosis or Embolization

A. Coagulation factor inhibition or depletion
  - Oral anticoagulants
  - Heparin
  - Low-molecular-weight heparin(s) and heparinoids
  - Antithrombins
  - Anti Xa agents
  - Agents in development, including recombinant protein C, thrombomodulin tissue factor pathway inhibitor, and mutated thrombin with anticoagulant activity

B. Platelet activation inhibitors
  - Aspirin, thromboxane antagonists, and thromboxane receptor blockers
  - Antibodies directed against platelet proteins
  - Peptide analogs and nonpeptide platelet receptor inhibitors

C. Physical devices
  - Intravenous filters
  - Compression devices (pumps, stockings)

Table 2 Ideal Theoretical Anticoagulant

1. Few side effects (bleeding)
2. Rapid onset
3. Controllable duration of activity
4. No adverse drug interactions
5. Easily reversibility
6. Requires no/or minimal monitoring
7. Easy administration by either oral or injection route, allowing optimal patient compliance
8. Inexpensive

Table 3 Clinical Situations in Which Anticoagulation May Be Used

1. Veno-occlusive disease (prophyllasis and treatment)
2. Arterial thrombosis and embolism
3. Post-angioplasty
4. Atrial fibrillation
5. Cardiac valve prosthesis
6. Dialysis
7. Extracorporeal perfusion
8. Stroke prevention/TIAA
9. Unstable angina/myocardial infarction

and therapeutic effects. These consensus reports are published periodically by the American Society for Thoracic Medicine in the journal Chest (5). The appropriate cost-effective selection of anticoagulant therapy may have a significant effect on the morbidity and mortality of thrombotic disorders. For example, the use of low-molecular-weight heparins (LMWHs) in the treatment of venous thromboembolic (TE) disease may be undertaken without extensive laboratory monitoring in an outpatient setting. More effective prophylaxis with anticoagulation therapy during and after certain orthopedic procedures may decrease the total cost of postsurgical complications and extended or additional hospitalizations (6,7). Some of the newest antithrombotic agents are in experimental clinical trials and can only be used in limited therapeutic situations. The most common anticoagulant agents in use today are the various heparin preparations, including LMWHs, the oral anticoagulant warfarin, and antiplatelet agents such as aspirin or dipyridamole.

This review will discuss some of the characteristics of selected anticoagulants, the mechanism of action, the dosage, therapeutic monitoring, and complications associated with the therapy. This review is not intended to be encyclopedic; however, new drugs that in our opinion will become part of the armamentarium in preventing thromboembolic disease will be discussed. Brief illustrative cases will be presented that will further elucidate specific clinical problems.

II. HEPARIN AND LOW-MOLECULAR-WEIGHT HEPARIN

A. General

The anticoagulant effect of the heparin mucopolysaccharide was first described in the 1920s, and by 1940 heparin was in widespread use for the treatment of thromboembolic diseases (8–10). Subsequent studies have shown that antithrombin III (AT-III) and heparin cofactor II (HC_0F-II) interact with heparin to inhibit various coagulation enzymes. Heparin is commonly used as an antithrombotic, and it will probably continue to be a major drug in the prophylaxis and treatment of thrombosis. Heparin has a narrow therapeutic index (11,12). Because of heparin's narrow therapeutic index, there has been extensive research into developing more efficacious and safer compounds such as LMWHs and heparinoid compounds (see Table 4) (12–14).

Most heparin produced in the United States is from either porcine intestinal mucosa or bovine lung. Heparin, sometimes referred to as "native heparin" or "unfractionated heparin (UFH)," is an unbranched polysaccharide composed of repeating disaccharide units of uronate and hexosamine joined by a 1–4 glycosidic linkage. The N-acetyl glucosamine of heparin is variably modified to have N-sulpho groups. The second position of the iduronate and the sixth position of the glucosamine have variable O-sulphono groups.

Unfractionated (native) heparins have a molecular weight in the range of 10–50 kD. A variety of chemical, enzymatic, and physical methods have been used to generate LMWHs,

Table 4 LMWH Advantageous over Unfractionated Heparin

1. LMWH has less plasma protein and cellular binding, and a longer half-life and thus can be given subcutaneously in one or two doses per day
2. Does not routinely require laboratory monitoring and can be easily used in outpatient treatment regimes
3. Less likely to cause HIT
4. Causes less osteoporosis

which range in molecular weight from 4 to 6 kD. LMWHs have the same basic glycosaminoglycan backbone as UFH, with alternating uronic acid and d-glucosamine residues. Currently, increasing numbers of commercial preparations of LMWH (Enoxaparin [Rhone-Poulenc, Paris, France], and Fragmin [Kabi Pharmacia, Stockholm, Sweden]) are available for use in the United States, and more are now in clinical trials (12–14).

B. Mechanism of Action and Metabolism

The mechanism by which native heparin or a LMWH acts as an anticoagulant is related to the interaction of heparin or LMWH with antithrombin. The binding and activation of antithrombin occurs through a unique high-affinity pentasaccharide referred to as the anti-Xa binding site. Binding of either UFH or LMWH to antithrombin initiates a conformational change in antithrombin that amplifies the interaction with thrombin and Xa (14). The physical chemical properties of the heparin or heparinoid may markedly influence the activity of antithrombins. Low-molecular-weight heparin facilitates antithrombin inhibition of factor Xa relatively more than it inhibits factor IIa (14). This differential binding of LMWH and UFH to AT and alteration of the actions of AT may explain why UFH causes greater prolongation on the activated partial thromboplastin time (aPTT) than does LMWH. Since LMWH does not effect the aPTT with therapeutic dosages, it is best monitored using a factor Xa inhibition assay (15).

All heparins, including LMWHs, initiate the release of tissue factor pathway inhibitor (TFPI) via endothelial cells (13). The TFPI induction may partially explain why in-vitro addition of heparin to plasma does not exactly recapitulate the in-vivo effects of heparin and why direct addition of heparin to plasma has not been adopted for testing standardization.

Heparin is removed initially from the circulation by the reticuloendothelial system (RES). When the RES system is saturated, the kidneys excrete heparin. The half-life ($T_{1/2}$) for UFH is $1–1_{1/2}$ hr. As the heparin dose is increased, the $T_{1/2}$ becomes longer. $T_{1/2}$ for LMWH is 4–6 hr after subcutaneous injection; its availability is greater than 90%, versus 30% for UFH, and it is thus more available for inhibition of serine esterases. Probably, as the cost of LMWHs decreases, they will become more widely used.

C. Dosage

Unfractionated heparin can be administered subcutaneously (SC) or intravenously (IV). Usually an IV loading dose of 5000–10,000 units is followed by continuous IV administration (see Tables 5 and 6). Subcutaneous administration of UFH has been used effectively for prophylactic heparinization in high-risk settings, such as abdominal or orthopedic surgery. Heparin's anticoagulant effect is monitored clinically using the aPTT. A "therapeutic range" is usually 1.5–1.7 times (×) the median of the respective laboratory's normal aPTT range. Using the patient's initial aPTT is preferable to using the laboratory's "normal" control values. A typical protocol for heparin treatment and monitoring after venous thromboembolism (VTE) is shown in Table 5. The treatment of VTE with heparin is dependent on many clinical variables. Heparin dosage is titrated appropriately using the aPTT, and a sample protocol is shown in Table 6 (16). Attaining a therapeutic level of anticoagulation within the first 24 hr after a presumptive diagnosis of TE may markedly limit the subsequent propagation of the thrombus and embolism (17). The proposed dose for enoxaprin for treatment of an acute deep venous thrombosis (DVT) is 1 mg/kg subcutaneous every 12 hr (17,18).

D. Monitoring Treatment

The incidence of bleeding complications from continuous IV unfractionated heparin therapy varies from 5% to 12% (19). Bleeding is more common with pulsed dosage than from continu-

Table 5 Protocol for the Treatment of Venous Thromboembolism with Intravenous Unfractionated Heparin

1. Initial intravenous heparin bolus: weight base doses of 80 units UFH per kilogram.
2. Continuous intravenous heparin infusion: 16–18 units/kg/hr.
3. The aPTT is performed in all patients as outlined below:
   (a) 6 hr after commencing heparin; the heparin dose is then adjusted according to the nomogram shown.
   (b) 6 hr after implementing the first dosage adjustment.
   (c) The aPTT is then performed as indicated by nomogram for the first 24 hr of therapy.
   (d) Thereafter, the aPTT is performed once daily unless the patient is subtherapeutic, in which case, the aPTT should be repeated 4 hr after increasing the heparin dose.
4. Extreme caution or no haparinization should be used in the following patients:
   (a) Patients who have undergone surgery within the previous 2 weeks.
   (b) Patients with a previous history of peptic ulcer disease, gastrointestinal bleeding, or genitourinary bleeding.
   (c) Patients with recent stroke (i.e., thrombotic stroke within 2 weeks previously).
   (d) Patients with a platelet count $<150 \times 10^9$ per liter.
   (e) Patients with miscellaneous reasons for a high risk of bleeding (e.g., invasive line, hepatic failure, etc.).

ous IV therapy or with concomitant thrombolytic therapy. Protocols which attempt to maximize anticoagulation without excessive bleeding have been developed (see Table 6). However, it is important to note that the risk of bleeding does not correlate with the aPTT value (20). Treatment protocols using subcutaneous LMWH have been developed which minimize bleeding risk and do not require any monitoring (21). There appears to be some evidence that bleeding complications are less likely with LMWH because of its reduced platelet binding and reduced endothelial cell interaction (14).

Table 6 Intravenous Heparin Dose-Titration Using the aPTT for Patients with Venous Thromboembolism[a]

	IV infusion		
aPTT (sec)	Rate change (ml/hr)[b]	Dosage change (units/24 hr)	Additional action
≤45	+6	+5760	Repeat aPTT in 4–6 hr
46–54	+3	+2880	Repeat aPTT in 4–6 hr
55–85	0	0	None[c]
			Stop heparin for 1 hr
			Repeat aPTT 4–6 hr after restarting heparin
86–110	−3	−2800	Stop heparin for 1 hr
>110	−6	−5760	Repeat aPTT 4–6 hr after restarting heparin

[a]Using Actin-FS thromboplastin aPTT reagent (Dade).
[b]Heparin concentration 20,000 units in 500 mL = 40 U/mL.
[c]During the first 24 hr, repeat aPTT in 4–6 hr. Thereafter, the aPTT is done once daily, unless subtherapeutic (16).
Source: Used with permission from Hull R, Raskob G, Rosenbloom D, et al. Optimal therapeutic level of heparin therapy in patients with venous thrombosis. Arch Intern Med 1992; 152:1589–1595. Copyright © 1992, American Medical Association.

Several laboratory methods are used to monitor heparin therapy. These tests include the aPTT, the activated clotting time (ACT), the thrombin time (TT), and the factor Xa inactivation test or HEP (R) test (22–24). These various tests are not equivalent, nor do they correlate well with each other. All of these tests have different analytical sensitivities to the various types and preparation of heparin or heparinoid used and may perform differently depending upon their respective plasma concentrations. Presently, there is no internationally accepted analytical standard for heparin measurements.

The aPTT is the most common laboratory test used to monitor the effects of UFH. There are a variety of aPTT reagent preparations, some of which are designed to be more sensitive to heparin and some of which are more sensitive to coagulation inhibitors such as the lupus anticoagulants (LAS). Thus, one cannot assume that a given degree of prolongation of the aPTT during heparin therapy translates into a specific level of anticoagulation. The selection of the specific reagents for the aPTT needs to be guided by each laboratory's clinical practice. Clinicians and laboratorians, in concert, must determine the appropriate target range for heparin therapy. Issues to be considered in establishing the therapeutic range of the aPTT include: (a) whether the control value is the mean of a normal range for the aPTT; (b) whether the upper limit of the normal range; or (c) whether the patient's initial aPTT is used in the calculation of the therapeutic target values.

Heparin can be measured "directly" by using factor Xa inhibition. The factor Xa inhibition assay can be used to establish the therapeutic heparin range that correlates with the aPTT. The chromogenic factor Xa assays with and without protamine can be used to calculate the plasma heparin level. The therapeutic range for heparin (using an anti Xa inhibition assay without protamine titration) is between 0.3 and 0.7 U/mL and with protamine titration is 0.2–0.4 U/mL (24). The suggested therapeutic range for each LMWH preparation will vary depending on the type of LMWH or heparinoid used. Laboratories monitoring LMWH need to establish a calibration (dose–response) curve for the particular heparin being used (15,25).

The ACT is frequently used before and during extracorporeal circulation (ECC) to guide and monitor heparin therapy. Some perfusionists require that the ACT be 500 sec before ECC, to ensure that no microthrombi interfere with the ECC filtration apparatus. Some ECC teams will accept an ACT in the range of 300–500 sec. Antithrombin (AT) may be decreased in patients who have been on heparin infusion, leading to an inappropriately "low" ACT response to heparin. In some of these cases of "heparin resistance," additional heparin may not prolong the ACT because of a decrease in the patient's plasma AT. In these same cases, subsequent AT administration may lead to "supraheparinization" and excessive bleeding. A factor Xa inhibition test may be useful in deciding whether additional heparin is warranted in such cases. During cardiopulmonary bypass, the heparin level is usually maintained between 4 and 5 u/mL.

A baseline aPTT and platelet count should be obtained prior to heparin therapy initiation for VTE. Most patients will achieve therapeutic anticoagulant levels rapidly with an initial IV loading dose of 5000 U and with subsequent IV infusions of 1000 U/hr. Some patients will fail to prolong their aPTT, a so-called heparin resistance. In clinical practice, true heparin resistance probably is rare and should not be considered unless the patient does not respond to at least 50,000 U of heparin per day. The following should be considered when there is a suboptimal response in the aPTT after confirming proper dosage and administration:

1. Increased factor VIII (acute-phase reactant) levels, which may give a "shortened" pretherapy aPTT
2. An assessment of obesity, since early on in therapy the heparin may be sequestered into adipose tissue

3. Release of inhibitors such as platelet factor IV from platelets
4. Heparin-induced thrombocytopenia (HIT)
5. ATIII deficiency (which is often considered, but is only a very rare cause of heparin resistance)

In certain situations, "direct" measurement of heparin levels using a Xa inhibition assay may be preferable to monitoring heparin with the aPTT or ACT. Such situations include:

1. Low molecular-weight heparin therapy (if monitoring is indicated)
2. The presence of LAS (where the initial aPTT is elevated prior to the therapy)
3. Factor XII, prekallirein, and high-molecular-weight kininogen deficiency
4. When the initial pretherapy aPTT is "shortened" due to increased levels of FVIII
5. Inadequate response to heparin as measured by the ACT
6. Suspicion of inadequate heparin in the infusion fluid (an ATIII source such as plasma must be included in assays for heparin in IV solutions)

In view of the drawbacks of the aPTT and the expanded use of LMWH, direct heparin assays might replace the aPTT for routine monitoring of heparin therapy.

E. Heparin Reversal

Although heparin has a relatively short $T_{1/2}$ (1½ hr), more rapid reversal may be necessary after ECC or in cases where a heparin overdose has occurred. Heparin can be neutralized by protamine sulfate. For acute heparin reversal, the usual therapeutic dose is 1.3 mg of protamine sulfate for each 100 U of UFH in the patient's plasma (26,27). The dose of protamine necessary for reversal of LMWH varies with the specific preparations of LMWH. The amount of protamine necessary for heparin reversal can be determined by adding varying amounts of protamine to the thrombin time assay, by titration of the ACT with varying protamine concentrations, or by using the Xa inhibition assay (to determine the plasma heparin concentration).

Rarely, excessive bleeding post-ECC may be related to failure of heparin reversal with protamine. Excessive protamine may inhibit coagulation. The ACT can also remain prolonged if aprotinin, an agent administered in cardiopulmonary bypass to decrease transfusion requirements, is given. After protamine reversal, there may be a heparin rebound because tissue heparin reenters the circulation from tissues (27). Rapid protamine administration may induce hypotension. When protamine cannot be given or causes an adverse reaction, heparin reversal can be accomplished by waiting for the heparin to be eliminated or by treatment with platelet concentrates with inactivators of heparin.

F. Heparin-Induced Thrombocytopenia

Heparin-induced thrombocytopenia (HIT) is a complication of heparin therapy which may result in thrombosis and potentially life-threatening sequelae. Almost 5% of patients treated with heparin will have some decrease in their platelet count. Most clinicians are not concerned unless the platelet count decreases to below 100,000/μL or greater than 50% of the patient's preheparin therapy platelet count. When platelet decreases are of this magnitude, discontinuation of heparin must be considered and alternative anticoagulant therapy must be evaluated, since morbidity is in excess of 50% and mortality as high as 15%. Severe thrombocytopenia occurs most frequently with bovine heparin, less so with porcine heparin, and even less with LMWH (28). The thrombosis in HIT may be either venous or arterial (28,29).

HIT is thought to be due to the development of immunoglobulin (lgG) which reacts with a complex of heparin, platelet factor 4 (PF4), and the Fc:RII receptors of platelets. This lgG-Heparin-PF4-Fc:RII complex is thought to cause platelet aggregation and injury to vascular endothelial cells, which may lead to thrombosis (30,31). In patients with no past history of heparin exposure, HIT usually develops after 5 days of heparin therapy. Apparent subclinical heparin flushes of indwelling catheters may be enough to initiate HIT (32).

The "gold standard" laboratory test for HIT has been the uptake and subsequent heparin-stimulated release of labeled serotonin by platelets (33,34). The sensitivity and specificity of platelet aggregation studies for HIT are extremely variable. The differences may be due to the number and selection of the donor's platelet pool used for the platelet aggregation. There is a difference of opinion as to whether the same lot number of heparin that the patient received is necessary for the in-vitro testing and whether high concentrations of heparin add specificity to the test (34). An ELISA test for IgG binding to a PF4–heparin complex shows promise in excluding HIT, but additional clinical studies are needed to evaluate this methodology (35,36). Other conditions that present with acute thrombocytopenia, such as disseminated intravascular coagulation (DIC), thrombotic thrombocytopenia purpura (TTP), and immune thrombocytopenia purpura (ITP), need to be ruled out before discontinuing heparin. A rise in platelet count after discontinuation of heparin therapy is very supportive for the diagnosis of HIT (37). A rise in platelets may be seen as early as 24 hr after heparin is discontinued.

Alternatives to heparin must be considered in patients with HIT. Low-molecular-weight heparin may not be a suitable alternative since both unfractionated and LMWH share epitopes. Substitution with a heparinoid such as Danasproid seems to be effective in some cases. Often, Danasproid does not cross-react with the patient's IgG, but it can cross-react in the in-vitro test assay. Previous treatment regimens for HIT included dextrans and defibrinogenation with ancrod. Recombinant hirulog or thrombin inhibitors are now being used for treatment in patients with HIT. The newest drug approved for anticoagulation in heparin-sensitive patients is Refludan (Hoeschst Roussel), a thrombin inhibitor (see below for therapy and monitoring) (38, 39). The initiation of warfarin therapy in acute HIT is contraindicated, since subsequent purpura fulminans may occur. The complications of HIT have been the basis of litigation. Platelet counts after the initiation of heparin should be monitored.

III. ORAL ANTICOAGULATION

A. General

Spoiled hay, which was linked to a hemorrhagic disorder in cattle, was found to contain 3,3′-methylene-bis-4-hydroxycoumarin, which is a vitamin K antagonist. The chemical structure of warfarin is remarkably similar to vitamin K (40). Coumarin (warfarin) usage as an anticoagulant in patients began in the 1940s. Warfarin continues to be the major anticoagulant used clinically, even with the development of newer anticoagulants (41).

Warfarin blocks vitamin K synthesis by inhibiting both the vitamin K reductase and the vitamin K epoxide reductase enzymes. This enzyme inhibition results in a failure of vitamin K-dependent carboxylase to participate in the gamma (γ)-carboxylation of factors II (prothrombin), VII, IX, X, and proteins C and S. Gamma carboxylation is also needed for fetal bone growth. The lack of γ-carboxylation of glutamic acid (GLa) in these coagulation factors results in the production of biologically inactive molecules (42–44).

The relative rate of decrease in the plasma coagulation factors affected by warfarin is related to the rate of synthesis and the plasma $T_{1/2}$ of the respective factor. The loss of procoagulant activity with warfarin anticoagulation begins with factor VII, protein C, followed by IX,

X, II. Because factor VII has the shortest $T_{1/2}$, the prothrombin time (PT) becomes prolonged before the aPTT does. The PT may be prolonged before the maximal anticoagulant effect of warfarin becomes clinically apparent. A normal person with a normal diet and hepatic function given a typical single 10-mg oral dose of warfarin will begin to prolong the PT in about 6–10 hr, and anticoagulation will become effective in 20–24 hr. The plasma $T_{1/2}$ of warfarin, is about 36–42 hr. Warfarin quantitation is rarely performed but may be indicated in rare cases where there has been toxic ingestion or in when all other causes of warfarin resistance have truly been excluded.

B. Indications and Contraindications

Anticoagulation with warfarin is used extensively in patients with DVT with or without pulmonary embolism (PE). Warfarin therapy is initiated concomitantly or shortly after starting heparin therapy. Warfarin therapy for VTE is monitored with the PT; the therapeutic range for most patients using the INR is 2.0–2.5 (43,44). Patients are often treated for up to 6 months after the initial episode of thrombosis. Patients with a recurrence of DVT or TE, or with a diagnosis of either a hereditary thrombophilia or an acquired hypercoaguable state (e.g., antiphospholipid syndrome), may require longer therapy (43–46). Prevention of the reoccurrence of thromboses in patients with antiphospholipid antibodies or lupus anticoagulants (LAS) may require more intensive anticoagulation.

Atrial fibrillation has a significant association with embolic stroke. Anticoagulation has been found to markedly reduce the risk of embolization. Oral anticoagulation reduces the risk of stroke by approximately 70%. The risk of stroke from atrial fibrillation increases markedly with increasing age. Recent congestive heart failure, hypertension, diabetes, an enlarged atrium, or previous thromboembolic events further increase the risk of embolization. In most patients treated with atrial fibrillation, the suggested therapeutic INR is 2.0–3.0. Because of the increased risk of bleeding in the very elderly (>80 years), aspirin may be used in this elderly group. Initiation of therapy in patients with stroke is not clear, but some clinicians wait for several days before initiating anticoagulation. The duration of anticoagulant therapy for stroke has not been firmly established (47–50).

Prosthetic heart valves are prone to developing thrombi and thromboemboli. The thrombosis may be due to atrial dilation, fibrillation-induced stasis, or the presence of valvular thrombogenic materials. Bioprosthetic heart valves are better endothelialized and thus are less prone to generating thrombi than mechanical valves. After prosthetic valve placement, there is a need for intense anticoagulation. The INR needed for prevention of embolization from bioprosthetic valves is lower (INR 2.0–3.0) than that needed for mechanical valves (INR 2.5–4.9), with the caged ball or caged disk valves requiring higher warfarin treatment than other mechanical valves. The prevention of systemic embolization in patients with artificial heart valves is more effective using a combination of warfarin and aspirin. Although the risk of bleeding is increased using this combination therapy, it should be considered where there is a very high risk for embolization or arterial reocculsion (51,52).

The use of warfarin in patients with peptic ulcer disease and in other conditions which predispose to bleeding, or in patients with hereditary bleeding disorders such as hemophilia, is either contraindicated or is done with great trepidation (19). Warfarin is a potential teratogen because it can cross the placenta and retard fetal bone growth which requires γ-carboxylation. If TE is a problem during pregnancy, other anticoagulants such as heparin or LMWH should be considered. High-dose, long-term therapy with heparin during pregnancy may occasionally produce heparin-associated osteoporosis (53).

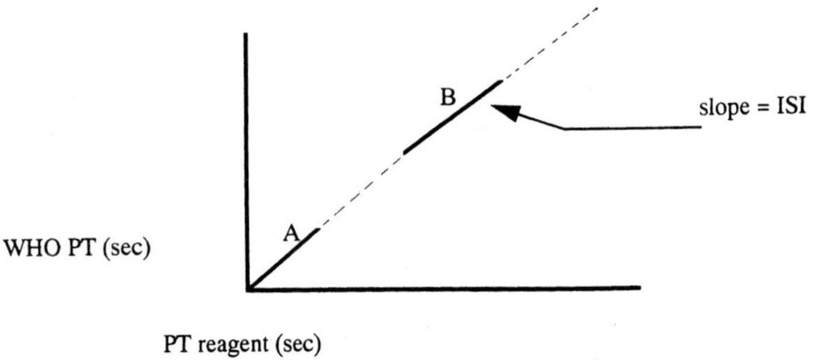

Figure 1 Generation of the International Standardized Index (ISI). A comparison of the PT using WHO thromboplastin and a commercial thromboplastin is shown for (A) unanticoagulated samples from normal controls and (B) samples from patients on stable warfarin therapy. The slope of the best-fit line is the ISI.

C. Initiation and Maintenance of Warfarin Therapy

For the treatment of an acute episode of DVT or PE, warfarin should be initiated during heparin therapy and should be maintained until the desired warfarin therapeutic effect is achieved. Thrombosis related to protein C deficiency can be precipitated by warfarin (54). Concomitant heparin therapy prevents catastrophic purpura fulminans in undiagnosed protein C deficient patients who are initially receiving warfarin. Thrombosis occurs in the skin's small vessels in patients with warfarin-induced skin necrosis. Warfarin anticoagulation is usually effective within 24 hr but may take up to several days. Warfarin's anticoagulant effect is estimated by the PT prolongation. The initiation of warfarin anticoagulant during thrombotic episodes may be unstable as evidenced by erratic PT measurements, and it may take up to several weeks to establish a constant therapeutic regimen.

In the PT, which is a functional assay, calcium is added to the patient's citrated plasma and clotting is activated by tissue factor (thromboplastin) in the presence of lipids. Thromboplastin (tissue factor) activates factor VII, which in turn activates factors IX and X. Activated factor X in turn activates prothrombin (factor II) to form thrombin. Thrombin then cleaves fibrinogen and allows fibrin to form. The rate of fibrin formation is monitored using either optical or mechanical methods.

Because different preparations of thromboplastin can give different PT values on the same sample, a strategy was developed to provide some uniformity in PT results. This system allows various laboratories to calculate a corrected prothrombin ratio, which is called the international normalized ratio (INR) (44,55–58). The INR is defined by the formula below.

$$\left[\frac{\text{Patient's PT (sec)}}{\text{mean of normal PT range (sec)}}\right]^{\text{ISI}}$$

The International Standardized Index (ISI) is the slope of the best-fit curve obtained from comparing the test thromboplastin with a World Health Organization (WHO) standard of human brain thromboplastin on a series of patients not on warfarin and patients on stable warfarin therapy (see Fig. 1).

The normal range (uncoagulated patients) for the PT for most thromboplastins is very similar, but the PT values obtained from patients on warfarin therapy may differ markedly. These ISI differences are due to PT reagent sensitivities and to plasma factor VII levels. Table 7 illustrates how the ISI effects the INR. For example, if reagent A has an ISI of 1.0 and reagent B an ISI of 2.0, and the PT in seconds is 22 in a laboratory with a normal range of 10–12 sec, with reagent A the INR is $(22/11)^1$ or 2, while reagent B with the same PT of 22 has an INR of $(22/11)^2$ or 4. Failure to consider the INR makes it much more difficult to compare PT results from different laboratories. Most laboratories surveyed by the College of American Pathologists (CAP) are reporting the PT as the INR. There are important differences in the INR determinations even when low-ISI recombinant tissue factor preparations are used (59). There are still variances between laboratories even when the same lots of a thromboplastin are used; these may be due to instrument differences. The College of American Pathologists Conference XXXI on Laboratory Monitoring of Anticoagulant Therapy recommends thromboplastins with a manual ISI between 0.9 and 1.7 and that laboratories should use reagent/instrument combinations for when the ISI has been established. The use of 3.2% sodium citrate in the collection tube is the suggested anticoagulant for the PT. Guidelines for clinical use of the INR for oral anticoagulant therapy have been published (44,60–64).

The most common complication of warfarin therapy is hemorrhage (3–5%) (19, 60). Gastrointestinal hemorrhage is the most frequent site of blood loss, but urogenital, retroperitoneal, and CNS hemorrhages may occur. The risk for hemorrhage is greatest when there is a previous bleeding history (particularly during the first month of anticoagulation) and in patients with the greatest prolongation of the PT. Good control of the warfarin therapy by monitoring the PT and adjusting the warfarin dosage can reduce the frequency of hemorrhagic complications (55–57,61–64). Once stable warfarin anticoagulation is attained, then heparin may be discontinued; however, there should not be any intermittent periods of inadequate anticoagulation because of the risk of purpura fulminans, as discussed previously.

Criteria for the initiation or induction of warfarin anticoagulation are not as well established as the criteria for stable anticoagulation. Some investigators find that PT reagent preparations of thromboplastin with low ISI values (≈1.00) may make laboratory monitoring more appropriate during induction of the anticoagulation (54). Some PT reagents have included chemicals that bind heparin so that any potential heparin effect is not observed. Such reagent

Table 7 The International Normalized Ratio

\ ISI PT(s)[a]	*A* 1.00	*B* 2.00	*C* 3.00
11	1.00	1.00	1.00
14	1.27	1.61	2.05
18	1.64	2.69	4.41
22	2.00	4.00	8.00
30	2.73	7.45	20.35

A comparison of the INRs with different thromboplatin reagents (A, B, C) and different PT value in seconds. Most thromboplastin reagents have an ISI between 1 and 3; the recombinant tissue factor reagents may have ISI values close to 1.00.

[a]The PT for the mean of the normal range was 11 sec in this hypothetical laboratory.

formulations make it easier to detect when the warfarin effect occurs even if heparin is present (65).

The typical initial dose of warfarin is 5–10 mg/day, and the dosage is usually adjusted by 2.5-mg increments or decrements, or by altering the dosage schedule. In an average-sized adult a dose of 5 mg/day will prolong the baseline PT about 1.5 times "normal" in about 36–48 hr (63).

A frequently encountered clinical situation is when a patient who is either being initiated or maintained on warfarin has significant unexpected increases or decreases in the PT. These unexpected PT changes can be a result of increases or decreases of dietary vitamin K, which decreases or increases the warfarin effect respectively (see Table 8) (44,66). The marked PT variations often seen in patients receiving multiple drugs is often due to drug interactions, which can enhance or decrease warfarin metabolism (see Table 8) (44,66–68). A variety of antimicrobial agents have been associated with hypoprothrombinemia which may enhance warfarin anticoagulation (68). Failure of the PT to prolong after "appropriate" warfarin dosage is often misinterpreted as "warfarin resistance." True warfarin resistance is rare, and low PT responses to seemingly appropriate doses of warfarin are usually related to altered vitamin K metabolism as described previously. True resistance to warfarin is most likely due to an autosomal-dominant mutant form of vitamin K reductase that displays either a decreased warfarin affinity or an increased vitamin K affinity. Current recommendations for oral anticoagulation therapy in patients with familiar warfarin resistance are to continue increasing until a therapeutic response is achieved. This could be 30 mg to over 600 mg daily (69). Acquired resistance is usually from drug interactions, decreased warfarin absorption, or a high-vitamin K diet (may be seen in patients treated with hyperalimentation regimes).

D. Warfarin Reversal

A frequent problem that needs to be solved is what to do with a patient who has an elevated INR. The factors that need to be considered include the following: (a) Is the patient bleeding? (B) Is the reversal for an acute or for an elective problem? (C) Why is the patient being treated with warfarin? (D) How high is the INR? (E) What is the hepatic function capacity, and what other medical problems may affect the course of treatment chosen? (F) Is the patient an outpatient or an inpatient? (G) What type of coumarin was used?

General guidelines for warfarin reversal must be used within the context of the patient's clinical status (44,62,70,71). If there is no bleeding, if rapid correction is not needed for surgery, and if the INR is <6, several doses of warfarin may be omitted. If the INR is between 6 and 10, there is no bleeding, and rapid reversal is needed, the patient may be treated with 1–2 mg of vitamin K_1. An additional 0.5 mg of vitamin K can be given at 24 hr if reversal has not been achieved. If the INR is greater than 10, 3 mg of vitamin K can be given at 6-hr intervals until the therapeutic range is attained. If the INR is greater than 20 or there is bleeding, 10 mg of vitamin K and FFP should be given. The vitamin K may be given again after 12 hr. When there is an immediate need and IV administration is chosen over SC or oral vitamin K administration, the vitamin K should be diluted and given over 20–30 min IV. If FFP is used without vitamin K treatment, the patient should be checked for a possible rebound elevation in the PT at 12–24 hr post-infusion. Active prothrombin complexes can be used if the above approaches do not work. Vigorous therapy for the bleeding should be undertaken (e.g., anti-ulcer treatment).

In certain situations the INR may be lowered from the usual recommended level and it is possible to switch to heparin while reversing the warfarin. The warfarin may be restarted when

Table 8 Drug and Food Interactions with Warfarin by Level of Supporting Evidence and Direction of Interaction[a]

Level of evidence	Protentiation	Inhibition	No effect
I	Alcohol (if concomitant liver disease) amiodarone (anabolic steroids, cimetidine,[b] clofibrate, cotrimoxazole erythromycin, fluconazole, isoniazid [600 mg daily] metronidazole) miconazole, omeprazole, **phenylbutazone**, piroxicam, propafenone, propranolol,[b] **sulfinpyrazone (biphasic with later inhibition)**	Barbiturates, carbamazepine, chlordiazepoxide, cholestyramine, **griseofulvin**, nafcillin, rifampin, sucralfate, high vitamin K content foods/ enteral feeds, intravenous lipids, large amounts of avocado, phenytoin, estrogens, colestipol, spironolactone	Alcohol, antacids, atenolol, bumetadine, enoxacin, famotidine, fluoxetine, ketorolac, metoprolol, naproxen, nizatidine, psyllium, ranitidine[c]
II	Acetaminophen, chloral hydrate ciprofloxacin, dextropropoxyphene, disulfiram, itraconazole, quinidine, phenytoin (biphasic with later inhibition), tamoxifen, tetracycline, flu vaccine	Dicloxacillin	Ibuprofen, ketoconazole
III	Acetylsalicylic acid, disopyramide, fluorouracil, ifosfhamide, ketoprofen, lovastatin, metozalone, moricizine, nalidixic acid, norfloxacin, ofloxacin, propoxyphene, sulindac, tolmetin, topical salicylates	Azathiprine, cyclosporine, etretinate, trazodone	
IV	Cefamandole, cefazolin, gemfibrozil, heparin, indomethacin, sulfisoxazole		Diltiazem, tobacco, vancomycin

[a]Drugs that are in bold type are those that have supporting level I evidence from both patients and volunteers.
[b]In a small number of volunteer subjects, an inhibitory drug interaction occurred.
[c]Level II evidence of potentiation in patients.

the patient is stable. Careful monitoring of the PT and aPTT will help to assess the effectiveness of the titration of the anticoagulants; however, the patient's clinical status must always be considered in developing the planned therapy.

The pharmacology of coumarin-like compounds used as rodentacides is very different than from that used in human anticoagulant therapy. These rodentacides may have potent effects on humans, and antidotal therapy may require extensive vitamin K and FFP.

Some patients on warfarin who require oral or dental surgery may sustain significant amounts of bleeding. Aminocaproic acid (Amicar) can be administered prior to a dental or oral surgical procedure in order to reduce the amount of hemorrhage without reversing the global coumadin effect (72). Amicar's effect may be allowing less fibrinolysis and more clot stabilization.

IV. DIRECT INHIBITORS OF COAGULATION PROTEINS

A. Antithrombins and Factor Xa Inhibitors

Thrombin inactivation by heparin is neither specific, efficient, nor devoid of side effects. Direct inhibitors of thrombin can be classified according to source, structure, and type of interaction. Some of these agents are directed against the catalytic site of thrombin, while others bind the exosites of thrombin, thus conferring specificity to the molecules for thrombin. In addition, some are reversible inhibitors while others are irreversible. There appears to be a steric hindrance to heparin binding when thrombin is bound to fibrin. Many naturally occurring and synthetic antithrombins have been isolated, synthesized, and are currently undergoing clinical trials. Recombinant hirudin (cloned from *Hirudo medicinalis*, the medicinal leech) forms a tight complex with thrombin, thus inhibiting the formation of fibrin from fibrinogen. Hirudin, which can be administered subcutaneously, is extremely effective at blocking coagulation in vivo and has been reported to reduce platelet deposition after arterial injury. Hirudin has been used in the treatment of patients with unstable angina or acute myocardial infarction and management of postoperative venous thrombosis after hip or knee surgery (73,74). Several peptide reagents mimicking hirudin have been developed, such as Hirugen and Hirulog. Hirulog, for example, is a bifunctional antithrombin peptide which blocks both thrombin-mediated platelet activation and thrombin cleavage of fibrinogen. Argipidine (argatroban), also a hirudin analog, has anticoagulant effects without inhibiting platelets. Argatroban is being tested for use when heparin cannot be used, such as in HIT. A variety of modified peptides, such as D-Phe-Pro-Arg CH_2Cl (P PACK), which inactivate thrombin have been tested for their anticoagulant effects; some of these can be administered orally. The bleeding effects and optimal dosage of these agents are being actively studied. Possible, selected preparation will be advantageous in various specific clinical situations requiring anticoagulation.

Direct thrombin inhibitors have certain advantages over heparin in that they may only react with thrombin and do not have major interactions with other plasma proteins, vessels, platelets, or platelet factor 4. These direct thrombin inhibitors are not dependent on AT-III and do not release endogenous TFPI. Because of their LMW, these agents may be able to inhibit the thrombin contained in the thrombus and control further enlargement of the thrombus (74–76).

B. Dosage and Monitoring

Revasc (Revasc Norartis, Basal, Switzerland) has been compared with both UFH and LMWH in the prophylaxis of DVT after total hip replacement. In these studies, 15 mg b.i.d. of Revasc provided better outcome than heparin or encxaparin. Thrombin inhibitors and hirudin have an extremely short $T_{1/2}$ of about 30–40 min. Molecular engineering of prothrombin molecules has resulted in variants that can complex with hirudin to neutralize its anticoagulant effects. All of the antithrombin agents produce anticoagulant effect in such global tests as PT and aPTT. The mechanism of action of each of these agents is different; therefore differences in their prolongation of the clot-based assays may not be an indication of their anticoagulant/autothrombotic potency. A new clot-based assay known as the ecarin clotting time has been developed recently for the specific monitoring of antithrombin agents. Ecarin represents snake venom that converts prothrombin to meizothrombin, eventually producing a clotting end point. Each thrombin inhibitor has its own distinct anticoagulant effect in this assay. In addition, ELISA-based assays have also been developed for absolute drug concentrations (74).

Direct inhibitors of factor Xa include a peptide isolated from the soft tick *Ornithodoros moubata* which has been prepared in a recombinant form and is a 60-amino acid polypeptide, and antistatin isolated from the Mexican leech *Haementeria officinalis*, which is 119 amino acids. These inhibitors have not been used as widely as the hirudin analogs in clinical trials (73).

V. ANTIPLATELET TREATMENTS

A. Aspirin

Arterial thromboses are currently best treated with drugs which inhibit platelet function. Platelet inhibitors seem to reduce the occurrence of vascular occlusion after coronary angioplasties, may prevent myocardial infarction, and may prevent stroke after a TIA (77,78). Extensive research is in progress to develop antiplatelet drugs which do not prolong the bleeding time and hence decrease the risk for bleeding. The oldest therapeutic antiplatelet drug is aspirin. Aspirin inhibits cyclooxygenase, which blocks synthesis of the prostaglandins thromboxane A_2 and prostacyclin. Thromboxane A_2 is a potent vasoconstrictor and platelet activator (79). Prostacylin is an inhibitor of platelet function. Low-dose aspirin inhibits thromboxane A_2 synthesis but spares prostacyclin. Most clinicians prescribe daily low-dose aspirin in the range of 75–100 mg. Even at these lower doses there is still a 2–3% risk of major bleeding. This risk for bleeding has to be evaluated in the context of the reduction in arterial disease (80).

Aspirin, 325 mg every other day, seems to also prevent platelet hyperreactivity and has been prescribed in males over the age of 50 to prevent myocardial infarction or secondarily to patients who have had a myocardial infarction (81). At low doses, aspirin does not seem to alter the development of atherosclerotic lesions following vascular injury; however, it may inhibit plaque formation when doses of 900 mg/day are used (82). Aspirin may prevent acute coronary occlusion after angioplasty and prevent early saphenous vein graft occlusion. Controversy exists on the dosage or even benefit of aspirin in the prevention and treatment of ischemic cerebrovascular disease (83–85). Because the major risk of gastrointestinal bleeding appears to be related to the aspirin dose, preparations have been developed to attempt to avoid high-dose aspirin. These have included controlled-release preparations which cause acetylation of platelet cyclooxygenase but do not interfere with prostacyclin production. Another formulation is transdermal and selectively inhibits platelet cyclooxygenase, providing an enhanced antithrombotic effect and possibly avoiding gastrointestinal hemorrhage in some patients (85).

Currently, effective laboratory testing or monitoring of aspirin therapy that correlates well with thrombotic disease outcomes do not exist. The platelet inhibition in patients treated with aspirin is irreversible. Effective platelet function can be restored only by production of, or treatment with, unmodified platelets (platelet concentrates). The risk for bleeding in patients is in part dependent upon the aspirin dose and the patient's age (86). Mild bleeding may include skin bruising, epistaxis, or melana in about 1–2% of patients, and severe GI and CNS bleeding may also occur in about 1–2% of patients (87). The risk for bleeding must be weighed against the development of arterial TE in selected patients. Perhaps a reduction in the dose of aspirin will allow a reduction in the risk of TE without an associated increased risk of bleeding.

Dipyridamole is a phosphodiesterase inhibitor which has been used to inhibit platelet function in combination with oral anticoagulants and aspirin (87). Combinations of antiplatelet and oral anticoagulant therapy have been tried in cases where there are combinations of venous and arterial thromboembolic disorders. There has been a continued impetus to develop new platelet inhibitors, because of the bleeding risk associated with aspirin therapy.

B. Ticlopidine

Ticlopidine is a thienopyridine derivative which irreversibly inhibits platelets by inhibiting the adenosine diphosphate (ADP)-induced activation of the platelet fibrinogen receptors. Since ticlopidine works by a different mechanism than aspirin when the two drugs are given in combination, there may be a synergistic effect. Ticlopidine has been observed to produce less gastric irritation and gastrointestinal hemorrhage than aspirin, but diarrhea, nausea, and GI discomfort are not uncommon side effects and ticlopidine should not be given to patients with hepatic impairment. Severe reversible neutropenia occurs in 1% of patients on ticlopidine, which necessitates periodic monitoring of the leukocyte count. Ticlopidine use is contraindicated during pregnancy (88). Thrombocytopenic purpura TTP has been observed in a few patients treated with ticlopidine.

Ticlopidine or ticlopidine in combination with aspirin seems to be useful for preventing strokes or preventing further stroke damage in patients with completed strokes (89). Ticlopidine has been reported to reduce intermittent claudication due to peripheral vascular disease, prevent coronary bypass graft occlusion, and reduce the progression of diabetic retinopathy (77,88). The side effects of ticlopidine have caused a decrease in the use of this drug. Clopidogrel, a derivative of ticlopidine, is a more potent inhibitor of platelet activation and may be more effective than aspirin in preventing vascular occlusions.

C. Peptides and Antibodies

Recently, much has been learned about the mechanism of platelet adhesion, aggregation, and activation. Platelet adhesion involves interaction of the von Willebrand factor (vWF) ligand with platelet glycoprotein Ib. Inhibition of platelet adhesion by monoclonal antibodies (MoAb) against vWF, by selected peptides or by treatment with aurin tricarbozylic acid has been demonstrated experimentally (90–92). Several antibodies against platelet membrane proteins have been produced.

Platelet aggregation can be blocked with MoAbs to the platelet GpIIb/IIIa glycoprotein receptor. Most clinical experience has been with a MoAb against the GPIIb/IIIa receptor (c7E3, abciximab, ReoPro), which is a recombinant chimeric Fab containing mouse variable regions and human constant regions. This GPIIb/IIIa receptor antibody also inhibits well as the α_vB_3 vitronectrin receptor. This MoAB blocks platelet aggregation in vitro (93). In studies of patients undergoing angioplasty or atheroectomy, where c7E3 Fab was added to the treatment, there was a 4.5% decrease in adverse outcomes (94,95). There was a significant reduction in the incidence of death and acute myocardial ischemia. Restenosis was apparent at 30 days and was sustained at the 6-month and 3-year follow-up (96). Treatment with this antibody (administered along with heparin and aspirin) caused an increase in bleeding, which has lead to new study protocols in which the heparin dosage has been decreased. With this new regimen, acute coronary syndrome and unstable angina have a reduction of risk of death and probability of MI of 32% (86). In order to get this reduction in restenosis, the antibody needed to be present for at least 16 hr after the angioplasty. The effect of c7E3 Fab on decreasing restenosis may be due to decreased platelet deposition, decreased thrombin, or inhibition of the α_vB_3 vitronection receptor on endothelial or neointimal cells. This antibody has been used successfully in several thousand patients undergoing coronary angioplasties and is now being tested for use with thrombolytic agents, as a treatment for acute myocardial infarction (95). Some patients have developed profound thrombocytopenia.

Studies on the sequence of the binding sites of various integrins have revealed the nature of a RGD (Arg-Gly-Asp)-binding site leading to the isolation or production of natural or synthetic peptide and nonpeptide agonists and disintegrins (73,97,98). A variety of naturally occurring cysteine-rich polypeptides from snake venom inhibit the binding of fibrinogen to GPIIb/IIIa receptor and abolish platelet functions. This group of polypeptides includes trigramin, bitistatin, echistatin, kistrin, and applaggin. Barbourin isolated from the pygmy rattlesnake has a substitution of a lysine to make a KGD, instead of an RGD, inhibitory sequence. This KGD inhibitor is more specific for glycoprotein IIb/IIIa. These peptides are inhibitory; however, they can cause thrombocytopenia and are immunogenic. Synthetic peptides, some of which are linear and some cyclic in molecular structure, have been developed which act as competitive and specific inhibitors of platelet GPIIb/IIIa binding with its natural ligands. Eptifibate integrilin is an injectable agent used for patients with acute coronary syndrome, especially those undergoing PTCA or elective angioplasty. Integrilin prevents the binding of fibrinogen to the platelet. Because of their relatively low molecular weight, they do not remain in the blood and are thus relatively short-acting and reversible. Some of these peptides are being developed in forms that are active when administered orally. Nonpeptide inhibitors of GPIIb/IIIa, such as xemlofiban, tyrafiban, (MK-383) and lamifiban (44-98833) are being tested (73).

VI. PHYSICAL DEVICES

A. Vena Caval Filters

A variety of intravenous filtration devices to prevent pulmonary TE have been tested (99–103). These filtration devices have been designed so that they can be introduced intravenously and subsequently expanded and anchored in the vena cava, where it is hoped that they will filter out thrombi without impeding blood flow. Visualization of the vena cava by angiography should be done to identify the optimal site for filter placement. For example, if the thrombus extends beyond the renal veins, the filter should be placed in a suprarenal location (104). Vena caval size is used to determine which size and type of filter is best suited for a particular patient. The Greenfield filter is conical and appears to be less efficient in trapping thrombi than the “bird’s nest” filter. The Greenfield filter appears to have been more successful in cases where there are contraindications or serious complications from anticoagulation. Indications for placement of inferior vena caval filters include: failure to respond to anticoagulation, a contraindication or serious complication after anticoagulant therapy, or after an acute massive pulmonary embolus (101). Prophylactic filter placement may be indicated in multiorgan trauma victims or patients undergoing orthopedic procedures who have a number of risk factors for TE.

Vena caval filters in and of themselves may cause further thrombosis and embolism, and with obstruction may cause severe venous stasis and even gangrene of the lower extremities (102). Some patients will need anticoagulant therapy even after filter placement. Patients who develop sepsis will need antibiotic therapy and possibly removal of the infected filter. In situations where there is a high risk for venous thromboembolism, prophylactic placement of filters in the vena cava may be necessary (103).

B. External Compression Devices

External compression devices to reduce lower-extremity blood stasis can be accomplished by graduated compression stockings or intermittent pneumatic compression. Meta-analysis of 11 studies with 1752 patients on the postoperative use of thigh-length compression stockings after moderate-risk surgery shows a risk reduction for venous thromboembolism of 68% ($p < .001$). The benefits of compression stockings in orthopedic surgery, high-risk surgery, and in combination with anticoagulation were not as conclusive. The benefit of knee-high graduated stockings is not as well documented as for thigh-high stockings (105).

Intermittent pneumatic compression (IPC) of the legs has been used on patients undergoing total hip or total knee replacement. The studies on IPC suggest that there is an increase in fibrinolytic activity and that there is a reduction in postoperative DVT (106,107). In a study comparing IPC and warfarin for the prevention of DVT post-total hip replacement, it was found that anticoagulation was more effective than IPC (108).

VII. POINT-OF-CARE TESTING

The coagulation tests that are most often considered for point-of-care (POC) settings are the activated clotting time (ACT), activated partial prothrombin time (aPTT), and prothrombin time (PT). The ACT has been used for many years in the POC setting in cardiac surgery, renal dialysis, and coronary care units to monitor high heparin doses. The ACT has long been clinically accepted because it is relatively easy to perform and produces an immediate result. The aPTT does not lend itself to POC as does the ACT, although whole-blood aPTT POC testing is available but should not be considered equivalent to plasma aPTT results (64). At present, there are no reference reagents or standard procedures to evaluate POC instruments. Many hospitals choose to restrict the aPTT test to the central laboratory setting.

Instruments are currently being marketed in response to the need for monitoring warfarin therapy in outpatient settings. At present, all coagulation testing done at POC sites should be carefully monitored to ensure the integrity of each program. Perhaps clinical correlations for establishment of reference of therapeutic ranges need to be developed which are independent of the central laboratory, rather than attempting to cross-check two different instruments and technologies.

CASE STUDIES

Heparin-Induced Thrombocytopenia (HIT)

A 64-year-old Caucasian male was brought to the hospital because of crescendo angina. Emergency angiography was performed, and treatment with tissue plasminogen activator (TPA) and heparin failed to open the LAD coronary artery. Coronary artery bypass surgery with placement of venous grafts was performed. Six years previously the patient had had cardiac surgery anastamosing his internal mammary artery with his LAD coronary. The operation went well but on the fifth postoperative day the patient's left foot became cold and pulseless. An astute intern noticed that the patient's platelet count was 200,000/μL, but upon admission the patient's platelet count had been 410,000/μL. The patient was no longer on heparin therapy according to the order sheet and nursing notes. Further investigation revealed that heparin flushes were used for an indwelling catheter in the patient's arm. Special testing showed that platelet aggregation occurred when exogenous heparin and patient serum were added to platelet pool. An ELISA test for a platelet factor 4 heparin IgG complex was positive. When heparin was discontinued, the platelet count rose to 350,000. Circulation to the foot could not be restored and the foot had to be amputated.

Discussion

This case illustrates the need for monitoring the platelet count when patients are treated with heparin. Another salient point is the relative platelet decrease of greater than 50% even though platelet count was still within the normal range. In most cases the platelet count is below 100,000/μL. Small amounts of heparin used to flush catheters may be enough to resensitize patients previous immunized to heparin. It is often difficult to find the heparin sources, since heparin rinses may not be recorded or possibly not recognized as being potent enough to induce HIT. When HIT is considered, warnings should be at the patient's bedside as well as in the chart. In addition to the laboratory test described above for HIT, the rise in the platelet count after discontinuing the heparin clinically confirms the diagnosis. Failure to recognize and appropriately treat HIT can lead to extreme morbidity or even mortality.

If anticoagulation therapy is required after HIT is diagnosed, direct thrombin or platelet inhibitors should be considered. The newest drug of choice is Refludan. Refludan (leupirudin [rDNA] for injection) should not be given if the baseline aPTT is greater than 2.5 × baseline (median for the laboratory's normal aPTT range), or if there is a history or evidence of bleeding. The loading dose is 0.4 mg/kg and the maintenance is 0.15 mg/kg per hour. The aPTT should be measured in 4 hr and at least once daily. The target range aPTT for this should be 1.5–2.5x. The short $T_{1/2}$ in patients with normal renal function allows dosage modification by stopping the infusion. There is no available antidote. Refludan can be used with concomitant thrombolytic therapy (109). Other therapies that have been tried include IV immunoglobulin or plasmapheresis. Warfarin therapy is contraindicated.

Heparin Resistance

A 300-lb, 5′10″ 58-year-old white male presented to the ER with mild shortness of breath and pain in the right shoulder with deep inspiration. There was no history of trauma, but the patient had been driving a truck almost continuously for the past 8 hr. There was no history of hemoptysis or cough. There was a history of a brief treatment with corticosteroids one week prior to this admission for an acute "asthmatic attack." The patient had no other health problems. The patient had smoked one package of cigarettes per day for the past 25 years. There was no contributory family history. His right calf was almost 2 in. greater in circumference than his left calf and was painful to mild palpation. The patient had a normal CBC. The BP was 150/92 with a pulse of 77 and respirations of 32. The EKG showed mild left ventricular hypertrophy (LVH) with prominent p waves. The chest x-ray showed mild flattening of the diaphragm, hyperaeration, mild cardiomegaly, and prominence of the right pulmonary artery. A V/Q scan was positive, with a prominent area of low profusion in the right upper lung. The arterial blood gases revealed a PO_2 of 70 mmHg, a PCO_2 of 49 mmHG, and a PH of 7.34. The PT and aPTT were 10.5 and 21 sec. The D-dimer assay was positive.

The diagnosis of thrombophlebitis and PE was made and the patient was started on heparin. An IV bolus injection of 5000 U of porcine heparin was administered, followed by an IV infusion of 700 U/hr. The aPTT at 2 hr was 30 sec (aPTT normal range is 22–37 sec). The IV dose of heparin was then raised to 1,000 U/hr, and at 4 hr the aPTT was 34 sec. The next morning (15 hr after admission) the patient's aPTT was 37 sec. An AT-III was found to be 80 U/dL (normal range 90–127%). The heparin concentration measured using an Xa inhibition assay was found to be subtherapeutic. The heparin dose was then raised to 1500 U/hr and 2 hr later the aPTT was 49 and the heparin was 0.6 U/mL. The ratio of pre-heparin aPTT to post-heparin aPTT was 1.58. The patient was switched to warfarin and treated for 3 months. There was resolution of the PE and the patient had an uneventful recovery.

Discussion

There are at least 50,000 deaths a year due to PE. Autopsy studies indicate that PE is probably underdiagnosed clinically. The diagnoses may be unclear in some cases, and the treatment with anticoagulation may be delayed. Recently it has become evident that adequate anticoagulation during the first day of treatment for DVT is very important in preventing thrombus extension and embolization. The problem of "heparin resistance" seems to be perceived by clinicians when the aPTT response is not appropriate for a given heparin regimen.

Analysis of our consultations for so-called heparin resistance reveals that in most cases the patients are not receiving enough heparin. In adults, the patient should be receiving at least 2,000 units of heparin per hour for at least 24 hr before heparin resistance is considered. Heparin inhibitors may be released during the thrombotic process. Not infrequently the patient has very high levels of coagulation factors, such as factor VIII, which may make their pretherapy aPTT short, as occurred in the patient described above. In this patient, the factor VIII level was 250 with a aPTT of 22 sec (this is the lower limit, normal for the aPTT of an adult male population).

The ratio of pre-heparin aPTT to post-heparin treatment aPTT is 1.58 if the mid-normal aPTT is used and is 1.75 if the initial aPTT is used as the denominator. In this case, the heparin level is probably more valuable in determining the target zone for heparin therapy, since the initial aPTT was abnormally short due to the high factor VIII. The high factor VIII may have been induced by the recent treatment with corticosteroids. There is also some speculation that patients with a short aPTT may have a proclivity for hypercoagulation. The AT-III was measured to exclude heparin resistance due to decreased AT-III. The AT-III was at the low end of the normal range but was sufficient for heparinization. A decrease in the AT-III may occur after heparin treatment because AT-III is cleared at an increased rate. Markedly decreased AT-III is a rare cause of heparin resistance.

When a patient truly shows some resistance to heparinization and the clinician elects to try to overcome this "resistance," greater doses of heparin with monitoring should be more frequent with measurements of the aPTT or heparin. If there are heparin inhibitors such as PF4 in the plasma, there may be a heparin level at which there is saturation of the inhibitors. Dosage beyond this saturation may lead to marked unexpected increases in the heparin anticoagulation and a concomitant increase in the risk of bleeding complications. A similar risk of such supraheparinization may occur by supplying an AT-III. Some of these problems will be eliminated when newer anticoagulants, which are independent of AT-III and are not inhibited by platelet factor 4, are available for clinical use.

Warfarin–Induced Purpura Fulminans

A 19-year-old male developed a reddish-blue skin discoloration of approximately 20 cm in diameter over his thighs and groin. The lesions were flat and nonpurpuric. The lesions appeared about 10 hr after the initiation of warfarin therapy (5 mg) for a suspected thrombosis of the femoral and popliteal veins in his right leg. This was his second episode of deep venous thrombosis. The INR was 1.4. Further investigation revealed that he had a family history of thrombophilia. His sister had a pulmonary embolus at age 24, two first cousins had died shortly after birth with subcutaneous hemorrhages, two other adolescent first cousins had been found to have protein C deficiency after having deep venous thromboses with pulmonary emboli. The patient was found to have a low protein C.

The patient was immediately started on heparin and given 4 units of FFP. He then received heparin and coumadin concomitantly for 3 days. When the PT increased and the INR became

2.5, the heparin was discontinued. The patient continued on long-term warfarin therapy. His INR was kept above 2.5.

Discussion

Warfarin-induced skin necrosis is a complication of anticoagulant therapy which is described above. It occurs in patients who have protein C or S deficiency. Most cases can be avoided if heparinization is started either before or concurrently with warfarin therapy. In the above case, heparin was begun and fresh frozen plasma was given to supply plasma anticoagulant proteins. The measurement of protein C and other anticoagulant proteins is not interpretable in this case, since the plasma concentrations of these proteins are decreased after thrombosis. The measurement of protein C and S after the initiation of warfarin is very difficult to evaluate, since these proteins require γ-carboxylation in order to function.

In patients who have heredity thrombophilia, the warfarin therapy should not be allowed to vacillate to nadirs where there is inadequate anticoagulation. If warfarin therapy is to be decreased, the patient should be anticoagulated with heparin or a direct thrombin inhibitor to prevent purpura fulminans.

REFERENCES

1. Alpert JS, Dalen JE. Epidemiology and natural history of venous thromboembolism. Progress in Cardiovascular Diseases 1994; 36:417–422.
2. Bick RL. Therapy for venous thrombosis: guidelines for a competent and cost-effective approach. Clin Appl Thromb/Hemost 1999; 5(1):2–9.
3. Markwardt F. Inventory of coagulation inhibitors from animals feeding on blood. Thromb Haemost 1994; 72:477–480.
4. Carins JA, Fuster V, Gore J, Kennedy JW. Coronary thrombolysis. Chest 1995; 401S–423S.
5. McIntyre KM. Medicolegal implications of consensus statements. Chest 1995; 108:502S.
6. Hull RD, Raskob GE, Pineo GF, et al. Subcutaneous low-molecular-weight heparin compared with continuous intravenous heparin in the treatment of proximal-vein thrombosis. N Engl J Med 1992; 326:975–982.
7. Levine M, Gent M, Hirsh J, et al. A comparison of low-molecular weight administration primarily at home with fractionated heparin administered in the hospital for deep venous thrombosis. N Engl J Med 1996; 334:677–681.
8. Howell WH. Heparin as an anticoagulant. Am J Physiol 1923; 63:434.
9. Tollefsen DM, Blinder MA. Heparin. In: Hoffman R, Benz EJ Jr, Shattil SJ, et al., eds. Hematology, Basic Principles and Practice. 2d ed. New York: Churchill Livingstone, 1995:1802–1813.
10. Goldhaber S. Pulmonary Embolism. N Eng J Med 1998; 33:93–101.
11. Rosenberg RD, Bauer KA. The heparin-antithrombin system: a natural anticoagulant mechanism. In: Colman RW, Hirsh J, Marder V, Salzman EW, eds. Hemostasis and Thrombosis: Basic Principles and Clinical Practice. 3d ed. Philadelphia: Lippincott, 1994:837–860.
12. Barrowcliffe RW, Thomas DP. Heparin and low molecular weight heparin. In: Bloom AL, Forbes CD, Thomas DP, Tuddenham EGD, eds. Haemostasis and Thrombosis. 3d ed. New York: Churchill Livingstone, 1994:1417–1438.
13. Fareed J, Hoppensteadt DA, Walenga JM. Current perspectives in low molecular weight heparin. Semin Thromb Haemost 1993; 195S:1–11.
14. Hirsh J, Granger CB. Unfractionated and low molecular weight heparin. In: Verstraete M, Fuster V, Topol EJ, eds. Cardiovascular Thrombosis: Thrombocardiology and Thromboneurology. 2d ed. Philadelphia: Lippincott-Raven, 1998:189-219.
15. Laposata M, Green D, Van Cott EM, et al. College of American Pathologists Conference XXXI on Laboratory Monitoring of Anticoagulant Therapy: The Clinical Use and Monitoring of Low-

Molecular-Weight Heparin, Danaparoid, Hirudin and Related Compounds and Argatroban. Arch Pathol Lab Med 1998; 122:782–799.
16. Hull RD, Raskob GE, Rosenbloom D, et al. Optimal therapeutic level of heparin therapy in patients with venous thrombosis. Arch Intern Med 1992; 152:1589–1595.
17. Hull RD, Pineo GF, Raskob GE. Heparin treatment of venous thrombo-embolism. In: Hull R, Pieno GF, eds. Disorders of Thrombosis. Philadelphia: Saunders, 1996:298–303.
18. Hull RD, Pineo GF, Valentine KA. Treatment and prevention of venous thromboembolism. Semin Thromb Hemost 1998; 24:21–31.
19. Levine MN, Raskob G, Landefield S, Hirsh J. Hemorrhagic complications of anticoagulant treatment. Chest 1995; 108:276S–290S.
20. Hyers TM, Hull RD, Weg JG. Antithrombotic therapy for venous thromboembolic disease. Chest 1995; 108:335S–351S.
21. Lassen MR, Borris LC. Prevention in orthopedic surgery and trauma. In: Hull R, Pieno GF, eds. Disorders of Thrombosis. Philadelphia: Saunders, 1996:209–215.
22. Kitchen S, Preston FE. The therapeutic range for heparin therapy: relationship between six activated partial thromboplastin time reagents and two heparin assays. Thromb Haemost 1996; 75: 734–739.
23. Bick RA. Laboratory monitoring. Disorders of thrombosis and hemostasis. In: Johnson KD, ed. Chicago: ASCP Press 1992; 296–305.
24. Brill-Edwards P, Ginsberg S, Johnston M, Hirsh J. Establishing a therapeutic range for heparin therapy. Ann Intern Med 1993; 119:104–109.
25. Boneu B. Low molecular weight heparin therapy: is monitoring needed? Thromb Hemost 1994; 72:330.
26. Salzman EW, Hirsh J, Marder V. Clinical use of heparin. In: Colman RW, Hirsh J, Marder V, Salzman EW, eds. Hemostasis and Thrombosis: Basic Principles and Clinical Practice. 3d ed. Philadelphia: Lippincott, 1994:1584–1591.
27. Kitchens CS. Surgery and hemostasis: the influence of one on the other. In: Ratnoff OD, Forbes CD, eds. Disorders of Hemostasis. 3d ed. Philadelphia: Saunders, 1996:356–382.
28. Warkentin TE, Levine MN, Hirsh J, et al. Heparin-induced thrombocytopenia in patients treated with low-molecular-weight heparin or unfractionated heparin. N Engl J Med 1995; 332:1330–1335.
29. Aster RH. Heparin-induced thrombocytopenia and thrombosis. N Engl J Med 1995; 332:1374–1376.
30. Visentin GP, Aster RH. Heparin-induced thrombocytopenia and thrombosis. Curr Opin Hematol 1995; 2:351–357.
31. Brieger DB, Mak KH, Kottke-Marchant, et al. Heparin induced thrombocytopenia. J Am Coll Cardiol 1998; 31:1449–1459.
32. Laster J, Elfrink R, Silver D. Reexposure to heparin of patients with heparin-associated antibodies. J Vasc Surg 1989; 9:677–682.
33. Kelton JG, Warkentin TF. Heparin-induced thrombocytopenia. Diagnosis, natural history and treatment options. Postgrad Med J 1998; 103:169–171, 175–178.
34. Isenhart GE, Brandt JT. Platelet aggregation studies for the diagnosis of heparin-induced thrombocytopenia. Am J Clin Pathol 1993; 99:324–330.
35. Arepally G, Reynolds C, Tomaski A, et al. Comparison of PF4/heparin ELISA assay with the C-serotonin release assay in the diagnosis of heparin-induced thrombocytopenia. Am J Clin Pathol 1995; 104:648–654.
36. Amiral J, Bridey F, Wolf M, et al. Antibodies to macromolecular platelet factor 4-heparin complexes in heparin-induced thrombocytopenia: a study of 44 cases. Thromb Haemost 1995; 73: 21–28.
37. Cola C, Ansell J. Heparin-induced thrombocytopenia and arterial thrombosis: alternative therapies. Am Heart J 1990; 119:368–374.
38. Warkentin TE, Chong BH, Greinacher A. Heparin induced thrombocytopenia towards consensus. Thromb Haemost 1998; 79:1–7.

39. Hass S, Walenga J, Jeske W, et al. Heparin induced thrombocytopenia: clinical considerations of alternative anticoagulation with various glycosaminoglycans and thrombin inhibitors. Clin Appl Throm/Hemost 1999; 5:52–59.
40. Link KP. The discovery of dicumoral and its sequels. Circulation 1959; 19:97–107.
41. Hirsh J. Oral anticoagulant drugs. N Engl J Med 1991; 324:1865–1875.
42. Hirsh J, Ginsberg JS, Marder VJ. Anticoagulant therapy with coumarin agents. In: Colman RW, Hirsh J, Marder V, Salzman EW, eds. Hemostasis and Thrombosis: Basic Principles and Clinical Practice. 3d ed. Philadelphia: Lippincott, 1994:1567–1583.
43. Becker RC, Ansell J. Oral anticoagulants (antithrombotic agents) for cardiovascular disorders. In: Hull R, Pieno GF, eds. Disorders of Thrombosis. Philadelphia: Saunders, 1996:75–87.
44. Hirsh J, Dalen JE, Deykin D, Poller L, Bussey H. Oral anticoagulants: mechanism of action, clinical effectiveness, and optimal therapeutic range. Chest 1995; 108:231S–246S.
45. Schulman S, Rhedin A-S, Lindmarker P, et al. A comparison of six weeks with six months of oral anticoagulant therapy after a first episode of venous thromboembolism. N Engl J Med 1995; 332: 1661–1665.
46. Hirsh J. The optimal duration of anticoagulant therapy for venous thrombosis. N Engl J Med 1995; 332;1710–1711.
47. Hylek EM, Skates SJ, Sheehan MA, Singer DE. An analysis of the lowest effective intensity of prophylactic anticoagulation for patients with nonhreumatic atrial fibrillation. N Engl J Med 1996; 335:540–546.
48. Albers GW. Atrial fibrillation and stroke. Arch Intern Med 1994; 154:1443–1448.
49. Atrial Fibrillation Investigators. Risk factors for stroke and efficacy of antithrombotic therapy in atrial fibrillation. Arch Intern Med 1994; 154:1449–1457.
50. Laupacis A, Albers GW, Dalen JE, et al. Antithrombotic therapy in atrial fibrillation. Chest 1995; 108:352S–359S.
51. Stein PD, Grandison D, Hua TA, et al. Therapeutic level of oral anticoagulation with warfarin in patients with mechanical prosthetic heart valves: review of literature and recommendations based on international normalized ratio. Postgrad Med J 1994; 70:S72–S83.
52. Stein PD, Alpert JS, Copeland J, et al. Antithrombotic therapy in patients with mechanical and biological prosthetic heart valves. Chest 1995; 108:371S–379S.
53. Dizon-Townson D, Branch W. Anticoagulant treatment during pregnancy. Semin Thromb Hemost 1998; 24:55–62.
54. Comp PC. Coumarin-induced skin necrosis. Incidence, mechanisms, management and avoidance. Drug Safety 1993; 8:128–135.
55. Litin SC, Gastineau DA. Current concepts in anticoagulant therapy. Mayo Clin Proc 1995; 70: 266–272.
56. Andrews TC, Peterson DW, Doeppenschmidt D, et al. Complications of warfarin therapy monitored by the International Normalized Ratio versus the prothrombin time ratio. Clin Cardiol 1995; 18:80–82.
57. Lassen JF, Brandslund I, Antonsen S. International normalized ratio for prothrombin times in patients taking oral anticoagulants: critical difference and probability of significant change in consecutive measurements. Clin Chem 1995; 41:444–447.
58. Bick R. Oral anticoagulants in thromboembolic disease. Lab Med 1995; 26:188–193.
59. Kitchen S, Jennings I, Woods TAL, Walker ID, Preston FE. Two recombinant tissue factor reagents compared to conventional thromboplastins for determination of international normalized ratio: a thirty-three-laboratory collaborative study. Thromb Haemost 1996; 6:372–376.
60. van der Meer FJM, Rosendaal RF, Vandenbroucke JP, Briët E. Assessment of a bleeding risk index in two cohorts of patients treated with oral anticoagulants. Thromb Haemost 1996; 76:12–16.
61. Brigden ML. Oral anticoagulant therapy: newer indications and an improved method of monitoring. Postgrad Med J 1992; 91:285–288, 293–296.
62. Hirsh J, Poller L. The International Normalized Ratio. Arch Intern Med 1994; 154:282–288.
63. Peterson CE, Kwaan HC. Current concepts of warfarin therapy. Arch Intern Med 1986; 146: 581–584.

64. Fairweather RB, Ansellj, van den Besselaar AM, et al. College of American Pathologists Conference XXXI on Laboratory Monitoring of Anticoagulant Therapy: Laboratory Monitoring of Oral Anticoagulant Therapy. Arch Pathol Lab Med 1998; 122:768–781.
65. Marlar R, Fink LM, Joist JH. Pulmonary embolism. N Engl J Med 1998; 339:1556–1557.
66. Wells PS, Holbrook AM, Crowther NR, Hirsh J. Interactions of warfarin with drugs and food. Ann Intern Med 1994; 121:676–683.
67. Buckely NA, Dawson AH. Drug interactions with warfarin. Med J Australia 1992; 157:479–483.
68. Shevchuk YM, Conly JM. Antibiotic-associated hypoprothrombinemia: a review of prospective studies, 1996–1988. Rev Infect Dis 1990; 12:1109–1126.
69. Hulse M. Warfarin resistance: diagnosis and therapeutic alternatives. Pharmacotherapy 1996; 16: 1009–1017.
70. Shetty HGM, Backhouse G, Bentley DP, Routledge PA. Effective reversal of warfarin-induced excessive anticoagulation with low does vitamin K_1. Thromb Haemost 1992; 67:13–15.
71. Ansell JE. Oral anticoagulants for the treatment of venous thromboembolism. In: Hull R, Pieno GF, eds. Disorders of Thrombosis. Philadelphia: Saunders, 1996:311–320.
72. Weibert RT. Oral anticoagulant therapy in patients undergoing dental surgery. Clin Pharm 1992; 11:857–864.
73. Weitz JI, Califf RM, Ginsberg JS, Hirsh J, Théroux P. New antithrombotics. Chest 1995; 108: 471S–485S.
74. Fareed J. Antithrombin agents as anticoagulants and antithrombotics: implications in drug development. Clin Appl Thromb/Hemost 1998; 4:227–237.
75. Tcheng JE. Enhancing safety and outcomes with the newer antithrombotic and antiplatelet agents. Am Heart J 1995; 130:673–679.
76. Harker LA, Hanson SR, Kelly AB. Antithrombotic benefits and hemorrhagic risks of direct thrombin antagonists. Thromb Haemost 1995; 74L:464–472.
77. Goodnight SH. Antiplatelet therapy with aspirin: from clinical trials to practice. Thromb Haemost 1995; 74:401–405.
78. Goodnight SH. Antiplatelet therapy in cardiovascular disease. In: Hull R, Pieno GF, eds. Disorders of Thrombosis. Philadelphia: Saunders, 1996:31–43.
79. Kearon C, Hirsh J. Optimal dose for starting and maintaining low-dose aspirin. Arch Intern Med 1993; 153:700–702.
80. Patrono C. Aspirin as an antiplatelet drug. N Engl J Med 1994; 330:1287–1294.
81. Willard JE, Lange RA, Hillis LD. The use of aspirin in ischemic heart disease. N Engl J Med 1992; 327:175–181.
82. Ranke C, Hecker H, Creutzig A, Alexander K. Dose-dependent effect of aspirin on carotid atherosclerosis. Circulation 1993; 87:1873–1879.
83. Patrono C, Roth GJ. Aspirin in ischemic cerebrovascular disease. How strong is the case for a different dosing regimen? Stroke 1996; 27:756–760.
84. Barnett HJM, Kaste M, Meldrum H, Eliszíw M. Aspirin dose in stroke prevention. Stroke 1996; 27:588–592.
85. Hart RG, Harrison MJG. Aspirin wars: the optimal dose of aspirin to prevent stroke. Stroke 1996; 27:585–587.
86. Thēroux P. Antiplatelet therapy: do the new platelet inhibitors add significantly to the clinical benefits of aspirin? Am Heart J 1997; 134:562–570.
87. Hirsh J, Dalen JE, Fuster V, Harker LB, Patrono C, Roth G. Aspirin and other platelet-active drugs: the relationship among dose, effectiveness, and side effects. Chest 1995; 108:247S–257S.
88. Sharis PJ, Cannon CP, Loscalgzo J. The antiplatelet effects of ticlopidine and clopidogrel. Ann Intern Med 1998; 129:394–405.
89. Albers GW. Role of ticlopidine for prevention of stroke. Stroke 1992; 23:912–916.
90. Coller BS, Peerschke EI, Scudder LE, Sullivan CA. Studies with a murine monoclonal antibody that abolishes ristocetin-induced binding of von Willebrand Factor to platelets: additional evidence in support of GPIb as platelet receptor for von Willebrand factor. Blood 1983; 61:99–111.
91. South V, Searfoss GH, French S, et al. Identification of novel peptide antagonist for von Wille-

brand factor binding to the platelet glycoprotein Ib receptor from a phage epitope library. Thromb Haemost 1995; 73:144–150.
92. Azzam K, Cissé-Thiam M, Drouet L. The antithrombotic effect of aurin tricarboxylic acid in the guinea pig is not solely due to its interaction with the von Willebrand factor-GPIb axis. Thromb Haemost 1996; 75:203–210.
93. Coller BS. Blockade of platelet GPIIb/IIIa receptors as an antithrombotic strategy. Circulation 1995; 92:2373–2380.
94. Ferguson JJ, Kereiakes DJ, Adgey AA, et al. Safe use of platelet GPIIb/IIIa inhibitors. Am Heart J 1998; 135:577–589.
95. The EPIC Investigators. Use of a monoclonal antibody directed against the platelet glycoprotein IIb/IIIa receptor in high-risk coronary angioplasty. N Engl J Med 1994; 330:956–961.
96. Adgey AA. An overview of the results of clinical trials with glycoprotein inhibitors. Am Heart J 1998; 135:543–555.
97. Coutré S, Leung L. Novel antithrombotic therapeutics targeted against platelet glycoprotein IIb/IIIa. Annu Rev Med 1995; 46:257–265.
98. Frishman WH, Burns B, Atac B, et al. Novel antiplatelet therapies for treatment of patients with ischemic heart disease: inhibitors of the platelet glycoprotein IIb/IIIa integrin receptor. Am Heart J 1995; 130:877–892.
99. Alexander JJ, Yuhas JP, Piotrowski JJ. Is the increasing use of prophylactic percutaneous IVC filters justified? Am J Surg 1994; 168:102–106.
100. Schwarz RE, Maurer AM, Conlon KC, Burt M. Inferior vena cava filters in cancer patients: indications and outcome. J Clin Oncol 1996; 14:652–657.
101. Elliott G, Eklof B. Vena Caval Filters. In: Hull R, Pieno GF, eds. Disorders of Thrombosis. Philadelphia: Saunders, 1996:329–335.
102. Athanasoulis CA. Complications of vena cava filters. Radiology 1993; 188:614–615.
103. Becker DM, Philbrick JT, Selby JB. Inferior vena cava filters: indications, safety, effectiveness. Arch Intern Med 1992; 152:1985–1994.
104. Greenfield LJ, Proctor MC. Suprarenal filter placement. J Vasc Surg 1998; 28:432–438.
105. Wells PS, Lensing AWA, Hirsh J. Graduated compression stockings in the prevention of postoperative venous thromboembolism. Arch Intern Med 1994; 154:67–71.
106. Comerota AJ, Chouhan V, Harada RN, et al. The fibrinolytic effects of intermittent pneumatic compression: mechanism of enhance fibrinolysis. Ann Surg 1997; 226:306–313.
107. Jackson MR. Diagnosis and management of venous thrombosis in the surgical patient. Semin Thromb Hemost 1998; 24:67–76.
108. Francis CW, Pellegrini VD, Marder VJ. Comparison of warfarin and external pneumatic compression in prevention of venous thrombosis after total hip replacement. JAMA 1992; 267:2911–2915.
109. Refludan (lepiradin[rDNA]) for injection. 1998 product monograph. Hoechst Marion Roussel, Inc., Kansas City, MO.

33

Hereditary and Acquired Causes of a Hypercoagulable State

Robert B. Fairweather
Dartmouth Hitchcock Medical Center, Lebanon, New Hampshire

I. INTRODUCTION

Thromboembolic disease is one of the leading causes of hospitalization, leading to significant morbidity and mortality in many developed countries. Our knowledge of the hereditary and acquired risk factors for thrombosis has grown significantly over the last few decades. This chapter discusses the more common causes of a hypercoagulable state associated with intrinsic circulating plasma factors and genetic polymorphisms, omitting from the discussion atherosclerotic vascular disease, other vasculopathies, and anatomic defects.

Hereditary causes of a hypercoagulable state have been termed juvenile thrombophilia, which describes a group of disorders characterized by a tendency to thromboembolism which characteristically occurs without apparent cause before age 45 and tends to recur. Acquired thrombophilia, associated with an underlying clinical condition, is more diverse in age and clinical presentation. I will briefly review the mechanisms and pathogenesis of the thrombophilic disorders, consider the importance of clinical and family history in guiding an appropriate laboratory evaluation, discuss the pertinent aspects and interpretation of laboratory testing, and provide some insight into the management of clotting problems. For a more in-depth discussion of individual aspects the reader is referred to recent reviews (1–4).

II. HEREDITARY CAUSES OF THROMBOPHILIA

Depending upon patient selection criteria, current estimates are that approximately 50–60% of thromboembolic events can be related to hereditary factors (Table 1). Venous thrombosis is clearly associated with defects in both the antithrombin and protein C anticoagulant pathways. There are reported associations of antithrombin III, protein C, and protein S deficiency with arterial thrombosis (5,6), but others have disputed this (7). To date, the weight of evidence is that APC resistance due to factor V Leiden plays no significant role in arterial vascular diseases (8). Hyperhomocysteinemia has also been linked to both arterial and venous disease (9,10). Lastly, the most recently reported risk factor is a mutation in the 3′-untranslated region of the prothrombin gene, which appears to date to be associated primarily with venous disease (11).

Table 1 Incidence (%) of Inherited Defects in the General Population and Associated with Thrombophilia in Selected Patients

Defect	Incidence (%) in the general population	Incidence (%) in selected patients	Venous or arterial
AT deficiency	0.02–0.17	0.5–4.9	V, A(?)
PC deficiency	0.14–0.5	1.4–8.6	V, A(?)
PS deficiency	—	1.4–7.5	V, A(?)
APC resistance	3.6–6	10–64	V
Hyperhomocysteinemia	4–10	10–25	V and A
Prothrombin G20210A	1–2	5–20	V

Adapted from Ref. 2.

A. Antithrombin (AT) Deficiency

Antithrombin (AT, formerly antithrombin III) is a 60-kD glycoprotein, synthesized in the liver, with a plasma concentration of approximately 2.3 μM and a half-life of 2–3 days. It is a member of the family of serine protease inhibitors, and it inactivates thrombin, and factors Xa, lXa, Xla, and Xlla, by formation of covalently bonded, inactive complexes. The inhibitory activity of AT is increased over 1000-fold by prior formation of a reversible complex with heparin and a variety of heparinoid glycosaminoglycans at a lysine-rich binding domain of the AT molecule.

Two general types of AT deficiency can be distinguished by phenotype and general molecular lesions. Type I AT deficiency is the result of reduced synthesis of biologically normal protein demonstrating both decreased levels of circulating antigen and functional activity. This has been shown to be the result of mutant alleles with whole or partial deletions, short insertions, or missense mutations leading to premature stop codons (12). Type II AT deficiency, caused by discrete molecular defects in the protein, shows decreased functional activity but normal antigenic levels, and is generally the result of missense mutations giving rise to single amino acid substitution at critical functional sites. In both types affected individuals are heterozygous, with AT activity in the 30–70% range. The homozygous state is extremely rare and appears to be incompatible with life.

A number of examples of functional AT deficiency due to decreased heparin binding have been reported (13). These generally show much milder thrombotic consequences. Heterozygous patients frequently come to attention when they enter consanguineous unions and product homozygous children, occasionally with severe thrombotic disease.

B. Protein C (PC) Deficiency

PC is a vitamin K-dependent glycoprotein, synthesized in the liver, having a plasma concentration of approximately 50 nM and a half-life of 6–8 hr, the shortest of all of the vitamin K-dependent factors. For PC to exert its anticoagulant effect, it requires activation by thrombin, in a reaction which is accelerated by formation of a ternary complex with the endothelial membrane surface protein thrombomodulin. The resultant activated protein C (APC) inactivates factor Va by initial cleavage at Arg-506 of the factor V molecule. Factor VIIIa is also believed to be inactivated in a similar manner. The principal cofactor of APC is protein S, which acts by enhancing the binding of APC and factor Va or VIIIa to phospholipid surfaces.

As with AT, two phenotypes of PC deficiency have been described; type I, with decreased activity and antigenic levels; and type II, with decreased activity but normal antigenic levels. The molecular mechanisms are similar to those of AT deficiencies, and the majority of affected individuals are heterozygotes (12).

Homozygous PC deficiency is rare (estimated frequency less than 1:160,000). Affected individuals with immeasurable PC levels usually present shortly after birth with widespread thrombosis of small cutaneous and subcutaneous vessels resulting in a necrotic disorder, neonatal purpura fulminans. A similar phenomenon, warfarin-induced skin necrosis, may occur in heterozygous PC-deficient patients during initiation of warfarin therapy. This is believed to be due to the rapid fall in PC levels occurring before the protective anticoagulant effect of decreased vitamin K-dependent procoagulant factors can occur. However, this phenomenon is generally not seen when warfarin is started in patients who are receiving heparin anticoagulation concurrently.

Unlike AT, there appears to be a higher frequency of PC deficiency without thrombosis found in healthy individuals (14). In a detailed study of 184 members of a large kindred with type II PC deficiency, Bovill et al. (15) found thromboembolic disease in only 13 of 46 (28%) family members with PC deficiency (age 48 ± 18 years). A second mutation in the PC gene was subsequently found in the kindred, primarily in those with thrombosis (16).

C. Protein S (PS) Deficiency

PS is a vitamin K-dependent glycoprotein, synthesized in the liver, with a plasma half-life of approximately 42 hr. PS is present in plasma in two states, as a free form and as a 1:1, noncovalent complex with C4b-binding protein (C4bBP). The total concentration of PS is approximately 300 nM, with the amount of free PS (approximately 120 nM) determined by the excess of total PS over the concentration of C4bBP. Thus, free PS, which is the only active form, represents about 40% of the total PS in normal plasma.

The frequency of PS deficiency in thrombophilic patients is roughly equal to that of PC deficiency (Table 1); the frequency in the general population is not well documented. Phenotypically the types of PS deficiency correspond to those of PC. However, there is a hereditary variant of type I, sometimes referred to as type III, with low activity (free form) but essentially normal total antigenic levels. This is the result of increased constitutive expression of C4bBP (17). Less is known about the genetics of PS, due to technical difficulties related to the presence of a nonexpressed pseudogene (12). Unlike PC, no kindreds have been found which are completely free from thrombotic disease. As with AT and PC deficiencies, homozygous PS deficiency is very rare, and presents clinically as neonatal purpura fulminans.

D. Resistance to Activated Protein C (APC Resistance) and Factor V Leiden

In a 1993 landmark paper, Dahlback, et al. (18) reported the phenomenon of APC resistance. The index case involved a middle-aged man with a history of recurrent thrombotic events starting at age 19, without an identified inherited defect. The authors observed that when APC was added to normal plasma, the activated partial thromboplastin time (APTT) was prolonged, as would be expected due to inactivation of factors Va and VIIIa. However, plasma from their patient failed to show the expected prolongation, which they termed APC resistance. Furthermore, of 19 family members tested, 14 showed similar resistance, a finding that was highly correlated with clinical thrombosis. Data from two other unrelated families showed a similar correlation. The authors were able to rule out inhibitors, and noted that mixing studies with normal plasma corrected the defect. On the basis of these findings they postulated an inherited defect or deficiency in either a hitherto unrecognized APC cofactor or a defect in the cleavage of factor Va or VIIIa.

Subsequent studies identified factor V in normal plasma as the protein which corrected APC resistance. Linkage analysis in two families, from Holland and Sweden, showed DNA polymorphisms near the factor V gene on chromosome 1 which segregated with the defect (19,20). DNA analysis in these families, and subsequently in many others, has demonstrated APC resistance to be associated in greater than 90% of cases with a unique single-point mutation (G1691A) of the factor V gene. This gives rise to substitution of glutamine for arginine at position 506 of the factor V molecule (FV R506Q), which is the site of primary cleavage of factor Va by APC. The mutation is commonly referred to as factor V Leiden, after the city in Holland where the mutation was identified. The significance of APC resistance in patients who lack factor V Leiden is unclear, but may be explained by nonspecificity of the simple functional assay (See Section V.b). This is one of the simplest yet elegant examples relating a gene defect detected by molecular techniques to its protein-related biologic effect.

Following the above reports, numerous studies have revealed the presence of these defects in anywhere from 20% to 60% of patients with histories of venous thromboembolic disease, the frequency depending upon patient selection criteria. Matched controls generally have a prevalence of 3–6%, giving an apparent relative risk of 5–10-fold associated with the heterozygous mutation, and 50–100-fold for the homozygous state (21). As confirmed by well over 50 reports in the literature, the factor V Leiden mutation is the most common genetic defect in venous thrombosis patients described to date. Of note, although some reports suggest an association between APC resistance and arterial thrombosis, to date there is little conclusive evidence supporting this association, with the exception of female smokers under age 50 (22).

Although the heterozygous mutation is considered by many to be the most frequently encountered defect associated with venous thromboembolic disease, others have questioned its relative importance as an isolated risk factor, especially when compared to heterozygous antithrombin III, protein C, and protein S deficiency (4,23). Heterozygotes for factor V Leiden appear to have lower rates of thrombosis as a function of age, whereas homozygotes have about the same rates as do heterozygotes with these other deficiencies. Furthermore, heterozygous factor V Leiden appears to be present in 3–6% of the Caucasian population, most of whom may never experience a spontaneous venous thrombotic event. The mutation is virtually absent in black Africans, native North Americans, and Asian populations (24), and appears to be due to a single genetic origin arising in Caucasians 21,000–34,000 years ago (25).

A very interesting anecdotal observation of increased thrombosis associated with heterozygous factor V Leiden was made during a strike of French public transportation workers (26). Two of seven hospital workers with factor V Leiden who sat for long periods in traffic developed deep venous thrombosis, whereas five unaffected carriers of the mutation either walked to work or were occupied elsewhere. This is characteristic of the generally held belief that most thrombotic events associated with heterozygous factor V Leiden occur secondary to circumstantial factors such as long periods of immobilization.

In addition to circumstantial risk, what appears to be emerging from the literature is a gene–gene interaction or "multiple hit" hypothesis of inherited thrombophilia, in which inherited defects in two (or more) molecules or pathways are involved (27). Within many kindreds with identified genetic defects in one factor (e.g., protein C deficiency), there is widespread variation in the incidence and age of onset of thrombotic disease. The occurrence of a second mutation, (e.g., factor V Leiden) leading to an expected increase of thrombosis has been identified in several studies of affected kindreds (28,29). Therefore, it is important, in individuals and families with a documented strong clinical history of thrombophilia, to search for more than one potential inherited defect. Preservation of plasma and DNA from these cases is also invaluable for retrospective testing, as new factors and mutations are identified.

E. Hereditary Thrombophilia Caused by Hyperhomocysteinemia

Homocysteine (Hcy) is a sulfhydryl-containing amino acid, an intermediary metabolite derived from methionine and involved in several key transmethylation reactions. It is metabolized by a transulfuration pathway to cystathionine and cysteine, or by two transmethylation routes to methionine (Fig. 1). Severe homozygous forms of hyperhomocysteinemia are well known (30). In these cases plasma levels are markedly increased (>100 μM) resulting in urinary excretion, from which the name of the disorder, homocystinuria, derives. Clinically, these patients present in early childhood and eventually develop severe mental retardation, ectopic lens, skeletal abnormalities, and, importantly, premature arterial vascular disease and venous thromboembolism. The disorder is rare, with an estimated frequency of 1:200,000, and is most commonly due to a defect in the CBS enzyme (Fig. 1, step 1).

Over the past decade numerous case-control and cross-sectional studies and two prospective studies have clearly shown an independent association of arteriovascular and venous thromboembolic disease with mild to moderate hyperhomocysteinemia (9,31). Fasting Hcy levels in affected patients are either in the upper normal range or mildly to moderately elevated. This magnitude of elevation in Hcy may be due to a hereditary defect in one of the enzymes shown in Fig. 1, or acquired deficiencies of one or more of the three vitamin cofactors required

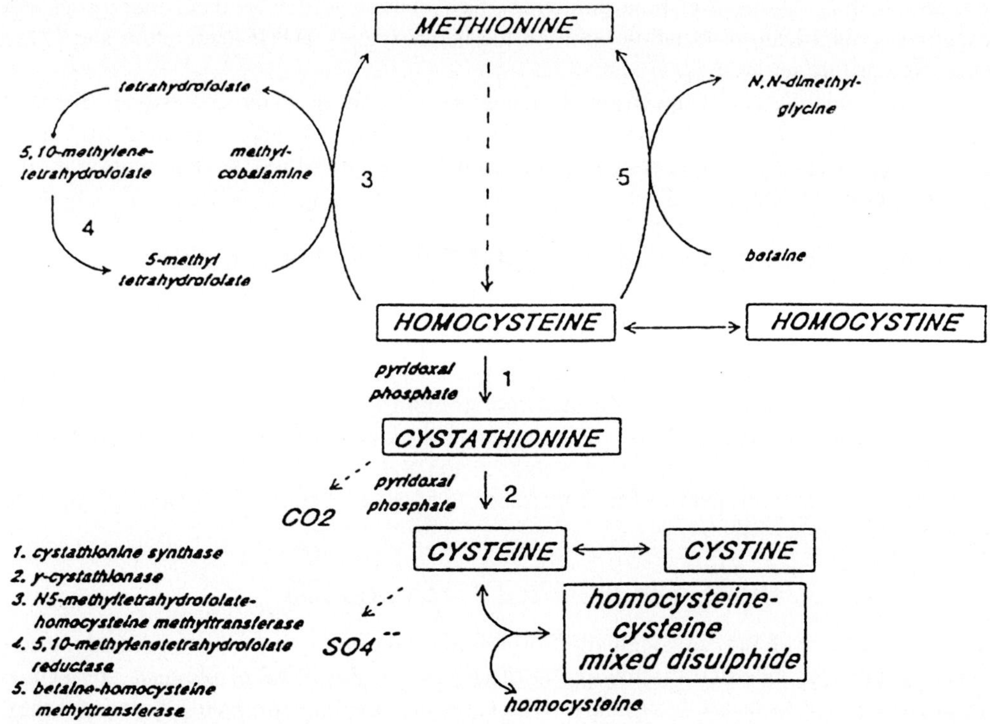

Figure 1 Metabolism of homocysteine (95).

by these enzymes (vitamins B_6, B_{12}, or folate). Selhub et al. (32), in a study of an elderly cohort of participants from the Framingham Study, demonstrated a strong association between Hcy concentration and folate levels, and weaker associations with vitamins B_6 and B_{12} levels. Rasmussen et al. (33) determined age- and gender-specific reference ranges for total Hcy.

Recently, several molecular assays have been reported which identify the more common genetic mutations in enzymes of the homocysteine pathway. The most common cause of an inherited predisposition to mild hyperhomocysteinemia is believed to be the presence of a polymorphism in the gene for the enzyme 5,10-methylenetetrahydrofolate reductase, MTHFR (C677T) (34). This translates to an alanine-to-valine amino acid substitution and results in a thermolabile form of the enzyme with 38% enzyme activity in the homozygous form and 65% in the heterozygous form versus 100% in the wild type (35). The homozygous and heterozygous forms of this mutation occur in the 10–12% and 40–45% of the North American Caucasian population, respectively. A mutation, T833C, in the CBS gene, is found in as high as 1.4% of the general population, and an association with thromboembolic disease has been suggested (30).

As might be expected, individuals with the homozygous MTHFR C677T mutation have higher mean fasting Hcy levels than those with the wild type, but the effect is related to body folate stores. In a study of 365 participants in the National Heart, Lung, and Blood Institute (NHLBI) Family Heart Study, Jacques et al. (36) found that, among individuals with lower plasma folate (<15.4 nmol/L), those with the homozygous MTHFR mutant genotype had fasting Hcy levels significantly higher than individuals with either the wild-type or heterozygous genotype. A difference between genotypes was not seen among individuals with folate levels above 15.4 nmol/L, nor was there any difference in the change in Hcy levels after standard methionine loading among the three genotypes (see Section V.E). To date, there does not appear to be a significant association between the heterozygous MTHFR mutation and either elevated Hcy or thrombotic risk.

The pathogenic effects of hyperhomocysteinemia are only partially understood. Elevated Hcy appears to have a direct effect on vascular endothelium, perhaps mediated by excess production of hydrogen peroxide, resulting in endothelial desquamation, smooth muscle proliferation, and intimal thickening (37).

F. Prothrombin Mutation G20210A and Elevated Prothrombin

This mutation is the most recently described potential risk factor for venous thrombosis (11). The mutation in the 3′-untranslated region of the gene was found in 18% of patients with venous thrombophilia, but in only 1% of controls. Furthermore, an association was found between the 20210 A allele and an elevated prothrombin level, which is a risk factor itself. Multiple subsequent reports (38) have confirmed this mutation as a risk factor for venous thrombotic disease, but of less importance than factor V Leiden (39). Like factor V Leiden, this mutation appears to be confined to Caucasians, and appears similarly to have arisen from a single genetic origin (40).

G. Other Associations with Inherited Thrombophilia

Several other tests involving anticoagulant, fibrinolytic, and other systems have been advocated as screening tests for inherited thrombophilia (Table 2). Since several of the tests are technically demanding and there are few family studies, mostly involving "private" mutations, they are not generally included as part of an initial thrombophilia screening (41). These tests should be considered when more common causes have been ruled out and there is a compelling

Table 2 Less Well Established Associations with Inherited Thrombophilia

Dysfibrinogenemia
Factor XII deficiency
Plasminogen deficiency
Elevated plasminogen activator inhibitor, type 1
Tissue plasminogen activator deficiency
Heparin cofactor II deficiency
Tissue factor pathway inhibitor deficiency
Lipoprotein (a)
Abnormal thrombomodulin
Histidine-rich glycoprotein increase

clinical and family history of inherited thrombophilia. In the future, the importance of these factors may very well increase in light of our understanding of the multiple-hit hypothesis of thrombophilia.

III. ACQUIRED CAUSES OF THROMBOPHILIA

The more common causes of acquired thrombophilia are listed in Table 3. These acquired states may be the sole cause of thrombosis, or may frequently combine with an inherited defect to result in thrombosis. I will discuss three of these in more detail, and leave the reader to consult references for the others.

A. Antibodies Directed Against Phospholipids

Antibodies directed against a variety of negatively charged phospholipids are found in the plasma of some patients with a history of thrombosis. These antiphospholipid antibodies (APAs) are heterogenous and are detected in the laboratory by either of two different assays: lupus anticoagulant (LA) clotting-based tests, or anticardiolipin antibody (ACA) immunologic assays (See Sections VI.G and VI.H). Because of the heterogeneous nature of these antibodies, the two methods show concordant results in only about 50–60% of cases. In the remainder

Table 3 Common Causes of Acquired Thrombophilia

Antiphospholipid antibodies
Malignancy
Acquired PS deficiency
Nephrotic syndrome
Myeloproliferative disorders
Hyperlipidemias
Diabetes mellitus
Paroxysmal nocturnal hemoglobinuria
Postoperative state
Vasculitis
Heparin-induced Thrombocytopenia
Obesity

only one of the tests is positive (42). APAs are frequently associated with arterial thrombosis (≈30% of cases), in addition to venous sites (≈70%).

APAs may occur in a variety of clinical circumstances. They are commonly seen as transient phenomena following infections and in this setting do not appear to be a thrombotic risk factor. They are detected in association with numerous medications (especially procainamide, quinidine, phenytoin, hydralazine, and chlorpromazine), and in this setting may be associated with thrombosis. APAs are common in connective tissue diseases, especially SLE, and are linked to recurrent spontaneous abortion and thrombocytopenia as well as arterial and venous thrombosis (43). Lastly, APAs in high titer with one or more of the triad of recurrent spontaneous abortion, thrombocytopenia, or thrombosis in the absence of underlying disease constitute the so-called primary antiphospholipid antibody syndrome (44).

The pathogenesis of thrombosis in APA syndromes is not well understood, and several mechanisms have been proposed. Phospholipids are poor antigens, and several investigators have show that APAs require the presence of a serum protein, beta-2-glycoprotein I (apolipoprotein H), to bind to anticardiolipin (45). Beta-2-glycoprotein I, as well as prothrombin, have been demonstrated as protein cofactors in the formation and binding of APAs to phospholipids in various LA tests. Other proteins have been implicated as cofactors in APA syndromes including protein C, protein S, high-molecular-weight kininogen, platelet-activating factor, and factor X (46). Protein cofactors are believed to undergo conformational change when bound to phospholipids, giving rise to a neoantigen which elicits formation of APAs. Interaction of these proteins and phospholipids and subsequent APA binding on endothelial surfaces or sites of endothelial damage could result in abnormal triggering of hemostasis or inhibition of anticoagulant control mechanisms such as the protein C pathway.

B. Malignancy and Venous Thrombosis

Patients with cancer are prone to the development of venous thromboembolism, as was first noted over 130 years ago by Trousseau (47). A variety of mediators and procoagulant mechanisms may be involved, including excess tissue factor, platelet-activating factor, tissue necrosis factor, and other cytokines. The occurrence of a deep vein thrombosis (DVT) or other venous thromboemboli in older patients should raise clinical suspicion of an occult malignancy. Although there is no consensus on the extent of workup that should be pursued, at minimum a thorough physical exam and chest x-ray, fecal occult blood, and pelvic exam in female patients should be performed. In our experience between 5% and 15% of patients over the age of 50, with no other demonstrated inherited thrombophilic risk factors, have eventually proven to have an occult malignancy as the underlying cause of an unprovoked DVT or pulmonary embolus.

C. Acquired Deficiencies of AT, PC, and PS

The liver is the site of synthesis of these anticoagulant proteins, and decreased levels have been reported in patients with liver disease. However, there appears to be a compensatory decrease in procoagulant factors in liver disease, with the end result that these patients do not generally show increased thromboembolic complications.

AT levels are often decreased in consumptive situations such as DIC or acute thrombosis. Administration of heparin can result in decreased AT levels. AT is a low-molecular-weight protein that tends to be readily lost in nephrotic syndrome and protein-losing enteropathy.

There are very few specific conditions which lead to a decrease in PC. However, it should be noted that there can be a nonspecific decrease in PC in acutely ill, hospitalized patients with a variety of clinical conditions (48).

Protein S can be significantly decreased in a number of clinical settings. The most notable is during pregnancy or oral contraceptive use, where both total and free levels can decrease to as low as 40% of normal levels (49). This may play a role in the increase incidence of thrombosis during pregnancy. Decreased levels of PS have been observed in diabetes mellitus, HIV infection, liver disease, and acute inflammatory states.

IV. IMPORTANCE OF CLINICAL AND FAMILY HISTORY

A thorough and specific patient clinical history and family history of thrombosis is the compass which guides the appropriate laboratory evaluation and management of thrombotic disease. Patient age at the time of the initial event is of paramount importance. Thromboembolic disease before puberty is exceedingly rare, and in the absence of an underlying anatomic or clinical disorder should evoke an extensive evaluation (50). Thromboembolic disease between puberty and age 45 should also raise the level of suspicion of an inherited defect. In patients over age 45, APC resistance, the prothrombin gene mutation, and acquired causes, especially occult malignancy, should be focal points. Female gender increases the likelihood of an antiphospholipid antibody syndrome. Patients of Native American, black African, or Asian ancestry are unlikely to manifest factor V Leiden, or the prothrombin gene mutation.

Arterial thrombosis increases the importance of APAs and Hcy, particularly in premature stroke. On the other hand, venous thrombosis can result from almost any defect. Thrombosis of uncommon sites such as cerebral, retinal, upper-extremity, or visceral veins is unusual and attention should be directed to an anatomic or inherited etiology, whereas thrombosis of the lower-extremity superficial or deep veins is commonplace and attributable to a broad range of causes.

Recurrent thrombosis, especially at a different site, is very significant clinically. In general this should increase efforts at finding an underlying cause, and is of paramount importance in guiding therapy. It should be noted that one of the most significant risk factors for recurrent DVT is a prior event at or proximal to the recurrence. This is often the result of the "postphlebotic syndrome" in which there is incomplete resolution of the original thrombus, usually with scarring and fibrosis of venous valves leading to venous stasis.

A thorough personal clinical history should include questions designed to elicit circumstantial risk factors. Information on general health status, level of activity, weight, periods of immobilization (e.g., surgery, bedrest, long trips), pregnancy, liver disease, valvular heart disease and atrial fibrillation, smoking, and medications (especially heparin, warfarin, and hormones) are vital in the evaluation of thromboembolism. A family history should include specific questions about venous thromboembolism, premature arterial vascular disease, and ages of occurrence.

Finally, the level of certainty of the diagnosis of thromboembolism is important. Was the DVT confirmed by Doppler ultrasound or just clinical presentation? Was the PE confirmed by high-probability VQ scan or pulmonary angiography, or an intermediate or low-probability VQ scan and clinical presentation? Was the cerebral event characterized by persistence of symptoms and imaging or transient ischemic symptoms? It is not cost-effective to embark on a lengthy and expensive workup to find that there was not a documented thrombosis in the first place.

V. SELECTION OF LABORATORY TESTS

At our institution we have developed an interactive, sequential algorithm for the laboratory evaluation of thromophilia. Clinicians order a "thrombosis screen" at the time of admission, or preferably as an outpatient, and all specimens that may be required are drawn, generally prior to the initiation of any therapy. A platelet count, prothrombin time, activated partial thromboplastin time, fibrinogen, and thrombin time are performed immediately. Aliquots of plasma are snap-frozen after double centrifugation, and serum and leukocytes are set aside for any subsequent immunologic or DNA testing.

A pathologist then contacts the ordering physician to gather the clinical and family history. Based upon the clinical history, a level of suspicion (high, moderate, or low) is assigned and a sequential testing strategy is devised in discussion with the clinician, to maximize the likelihood of a significant finding and minimize the cost. The initial evaluation of all venous events includes a screen for APC resistance, and other tests of high likelihood given the clinical history. After the initial testing is completed, the clinician is again contacted, the findings discussed, and further testing, if any, is decided upon. Since it usually takes several days to this point, there is often additional clinical or family information available which may alter or refocus the evaluation. When all appropriate testing has been completed, the results, interpretation, and suggestions for follow-up testing and management are included in a formal consultative report. Other algorithms have been published (51).

It is important to note in considering the initial evaluation that specimens from patients who are acutely ill with a recent thrombus may often show physiologic reactive changes in levels of AT, PC, PS, fibrinogen and FVIII which may make interpretation of test results equivocal. We may recommend that some testing be deferred until the patient can return as an outpatient. This may be several months later, when oral anticoagulation can be stopped for at least 7 days or alternative anticoagulation substituted, such as subcutaneous LMW heparin (2). It is also extremely important to emphasize that marginally low quantitative test results do not necessarily equate to a diagnosis of a deficiency or defect. Such results should always be repeated, and confirmed in first-degree relatives or by molecular methods, before a confirmed diagnosis is made. The consequences of an inaccurate diagnosis on a patient's future healthcare coverage are extremely important.

VI. MEASUREMENT AND INTERPRETATION OF LABORATORY TESTS

A. AT Deficiency

The preferred screening method for AT deficiency (as well as PC and PS deficiency) should measure functional activity rather than antigenic levels, which could miss some type II deficiencies. The most commonly employed methods utilize a test system containing excess factor Xa (or thrombin), heparin, and test plasma as the source of the AT to be measured. The residual factor Xa (or thrombin) activity is measured in an amidolytic assay using a specific, synthetic, chromogenic peptide substrate. To detect defects in the heparin-binding interaction with AT, a similar assay is run in the absence of heparin (progressive antithrombin activity assay). AT with defective heparin binding will show decreased activity with heparin, but normal activity in the progressive antithrombin activity assay.

Activity is usually reported as percent of normal or U/mL (1 mL of normal plasma by definition contains 1.0 U of AT activity). The adult normal range is generally 80–120% (0.8–1.2 U/mL). There is no gender difference. Children reach adult levels by 90–180 days of age

Table 4 Effect of Clinical Conditions and Medications on Antithrombin (AT) Activity (53)

Clinical condition/drug	Effect on AT activity
Recent thrombosis	Decreased
Nephrotic syndrome	Decreased
Protein-losing enteropathy	Decreased
Disseminated intravascular coagulation	Decreased
Postsurgery	Decreased
Liver disease	Decreased
Heparin therapy	Decreased
Estrogen (oral contraceptives)	Decreased
L-Asparaginase	Decreased
Warfarin	Increased

(52). In interpreting the results of AT functional activity, clinical factors and certain medications need to be considered (Table 4) (53). Note that warfarin can raise the AT activity into the normal range in individuals with hereditary deficiency (54).

AT deficiency detected by a screening functional assay should be repeated, and antigenic levels and progressive antithrombin activity measured to type classify the deficiency. If repeat testing is abnormal, a presumptive diagnosis can be made. Confirmation of a hereditary link should be made by testing first-degree relatives and possibly by molecular methods, if available.

B. PC Deficiency

Screening tests for PC deficiency generally employ snake venom activator to generate activated PC (APC) from the test plasma. The APC may be measured by its amidolytic activity on a synthetic substrate or by mixing with protein C-deficient plasma and utilizing an APTT-based clotting endpoint. The latter method is preferred since it tests the interaction of APC with PS and phospholipid, in addition to the PC proteolytic active site, which is the only function measured by an amidolytic method. Activity is generally reported as percent of normal, with the adult reference range reached at 6–10 years of age (55). In adults, levels appear to increase with age by about 4% per decade (56).

In interpreting the results of PC functional activity, clinical factors and certain medications need to be considered (Table 5). Concurrent acute illness may lower levels. In a study of 3165 hospitalized patients, Miletich found that 12% had below-normal PC levels although none went on to develop thrombosis (14). This reemphasizes the desirability of testing in the outpatient setting.

C. PS Deficiency

As with the other anticoagulants, a functional screening assay is preferred. Several plasma-based clotting endpoint methods are commercially available. These generally involve addition of APC or snake venom PC activators to the test system, and measurement of PS activity in patient plasma diluted in PS-deficient plasma by a clotting endpoint. However, it has been shown that falsely low PS activity can be found in systems in which patient plasma is not diluted sufficiently (57, 58). This discrepancy is found in patients who carry the factor V

Table 5 Effect of Clinical Conditions and Medications on Protein C (PC) Activity (48)

Clinical condition/drug	Effect on PC activity
Recent thrombosis	Decreased
Acute illness	Decreased
Liver disease	Decreased
Disseminated intravascular coagulation	Decreased
Warfarin	Markedly decreased
L-Asparaginase	Decreased
Estrogen (oral contraceptives)	Increased
Danazol	Increased

Leiden mutation and is due to APC resistance prolonging the clotting time despite normal PS levels. Methods which add exogenous FVa or purify free PS by immunoadsorption before testing are minimally affected (59). Before interpreting PS levels, one should look at the APC resistance status and run the PS assay at at least two dilutions to look for the effect of inhibitors which could give rise to false PS activity. Because of these problems, some have suggested using free and total PS antigenic assays as screening methods (2). Most immunoassays for free PS utilize precipitation or immunoadsorption to separate free from bound forms. Recently a direct assay using a new monoclonal Ab specific for the free form has been described (60).

PS activity is generally reported as percent of normal. There is a significant gender bias (61). Males have higher total and free levels than age-matched females who are not taking oral contraceptives, who in turn have higher levels than women on oral contraceptives. For instance, free PS levels were found to be 109% ± 20%, 90% ± 20%, and 86% ± 17% (mean ± SD), respectively, for these three populations. Adult levels are achieved by 6–9 months. In interpreting PS measurements, clinical conditions and medications generally show a greater effect than with AT and PC (Table 6) (62). Total and free PS levels are significantly decreased during pregnancy and the postpartum period (mean 38%), such that testing during this time is not recommended (46). Acute inflammation increases C4bBP without much change in total PS, resulting in decreased free PS.

Table 6 Conditions and Medications Affecting Protein S (PS) (62)

Clinical condition/drug	Effect on PS activity
Pregnancy	Markedly decreased
Acute inflammation	Decreased (free)
Liver disease	Decreased
Diabetes mellitus	Decreased
Oral contraceptives	Decreased
Warfarin	Markedly decreased

D. Resistance to APC

The most widely used screening test for APC resistance is an APTT-based method. The common approach is to measure the ratio of the APTT with and without added APC. A ratio below an established cutoff is considered resistant. However, using the factor V Leiden mutation as the "gold standard," this screening test can show both false positive and false negative results. Several factors contributing to this discrepancy have been identified.

Platelets contain high levels of factor V, and activation of platelets during plasma preparation or the use of frozen-thawed plasma can result in false positive results (63). Preparation of platelet-poor plasma by double centrifugation and performance of the test (normal reference and patients) using all fresh or all frozen-thawed plasmas are recommended.

Elevated levels of factor VIII, an acute-phase reactant, can lower the APC ratio (64). Interestingly, although APC inactivates factor VIIIa in vitro, no mutation of this molecule similar to factor V Leiden has been reported to date. It is possible that APC inactivation of factor VIIIa may not be as important physiologically.

The APC ratio is lower in women than in men (65), especially during pregnancy (66). This may be due to lower free protein S levels, or other hormonal or pregnancy associated alterations in the coagulation system. Surprisingly, protein S-deficient subjects do not generally show APC resistance, which has been ascribed to the fact that protein S is a relatively weak cofactor in vitro (67).

Patients taking oral anticoagulants cannot be screened reliably with the APTT-based test, as the APC ratio is falsely elevated. Lastly, patients on heparin and patients with the lupus anticoagulant cannot be screened by the APTT-based method either, since the specimens may fail to clot or show lower ratios due to a prolonged "baseline" APTT without APC (68).

Several modifications have been proposed to circumvent some of these problems with the APTT-based method. One simple method is to normalize the APC ratio by dividing the patient ratio by the ratio of a pooled normal plasma. This was proposed to control for day-to-day method and instrument variation, and to allow comparison of results between laboratories. A normalized APC ratio of 1.0 is expected. In a study of 894 individuals (422 patients with thrombophilia and 472 controls) (69), individuals with a normalized APC ratio > 0.70 were all normal genetically, 86 of 88 with a normalized APC ratio between 0.50 and 0.70 were heterozygous for factor V Leiden (2 were normal), and 8 of 9 with a normalized APC ratio < 0.50 were homozygous for factor V Leiden with 1 of the 9 heterozygous. With careful control of preanalytical variables, the >0.70 cutoff gave a sensitivity of 100% and specificity of 99.7% for the presence of factor V Leiden mutation.

Alternate plasma clot-based screening tests have been proposed, employing patient plasma diluted to varying degrees in factor V-deficient plasma, sometimes with the addition of a heparin neutralizer (70). This isolates the test to the patient factor V, and compensates for any excess or deficiency of other coagulation factors or inhibitors. Patients taking oral anticoagulants, those with lupus anticoagulants, and heparinized specimens may be tested.

The PCR based DNA assay for factor V Leiden relies on relatively straightforward molecular biology techniques (19). Primers flanking the G-to-A mutation at nucleotide 1691 are used to amplify a 267-base pair fragment, which is then digested with the restriction endonuclease MnlI. The wild-type factor V fragment is cleaved at two sites by the restriction enzyme to yield three fragments of 163, 67, and 37 base pairs. The mutation abolishes one of the endonuclease cleavage sites, resulting in a single cleavage to yield fragments of 200 an 67 base pairs. Interpretation of the electrophoresis gels is straightforward and readily allows identification of wild-type and heterozygous and homozygous mutants. Newer, more rapid, and less expensive PCR heteroduplex techniques are now in use to look for point mutations in multiple genes at one time (71).

E. Hyperhomocysteinemia

Hcy is present in plasma in the free form, as the oxidized disulfide, homocystine, and as a mixed disulfide with cysteine (see Fig. 1). All of these forms may be bound to plasma proteins to a variable degree. Analysis of total Hcy is accomplished by reduction of all disulfide forms, chemical derivatization to a stable sulfide, and separation and quantitation by HPLC, stable isotope dilution, or GC-MS (72). Immunoassays are under development (73). Reference ranges vary from one laboratory to another, and are attributable to patient preparation (e.g., fasting specimen), sample collection, assay methodology, and choice of a reference population.

Some individuals with normal fasting Hcy levels will show an abnormally increased response to methionine. After an overnight fast and drawing of a preloading blood specimen, the patient is given a standardized oral methionine load (0.1 g/kg body weight, in fruit juice), and a postloading specimen is drawn 4–8 hr after. Peak plasma levels appear to be achieved in most individuals at 6 hr (74). As with fasting levels, the reference range after methionine loading is not well established, and published reports vary as to the time of sampling. Therefore, except for markedly elevated pre- or postload Hcy levels, the interpretation of borderline results presents a problem.

The MTHFR C677T mutation is detected by standard PCR-based techniques (34). The association between Hcy and folate has been discussed (see Section II.E).

F. Prothrombin Mutation G20210A and Elevated Prothrombin

As discussed in Section II.F, this mutation in the 3′-untranslated region of the prothrombin gene is associated with increased prothrombin levels and risk of venous thrombosis. The PCR based DNA analysis is straightforward (11). In our laboratory we currently perform PCR multiplexed, restriction enzyme digestion for this mutation, factor V Leiden, and MTHFR C677T together.

G. Lupus Anticoagulant (LA)

Until recently, there was little consensus regarding the laboratory diagnosis of LA. The Scientific and Standardisation Committee of the ISTH (75) has proposed four criteria for the diagnosis. These are: (1) prolongation of a phospholipid-dependent clotting assay, (2) evidence of inhibition demonstrated by mixing studies, (3) evidence of phospholipid dependence, and (4) lack of specific inhibition of any one coagulation factor. The committee made several more specific recommendations concerning preanalytical conditions and test performance. Among these, two deserve mention. First, both patient and normal plasma used in LA testing should be as platelet-free as possible (platelet counts less than 10×10^9L) to avoid neutralization of antibody by phospholipid derived from platelets. Second, two or more screening tests should be employed in ruling out LA, at least one of which should be based on a low phospholipid concentration (e.g., dRVVT, KCT, dAPTT). There have been attempts to quantitate LA, but no recognized system is currently available. A flow chart, adapted from the committee recommendations, is presented in Fig. 2. The reader is referred to this source for more specific details (75).

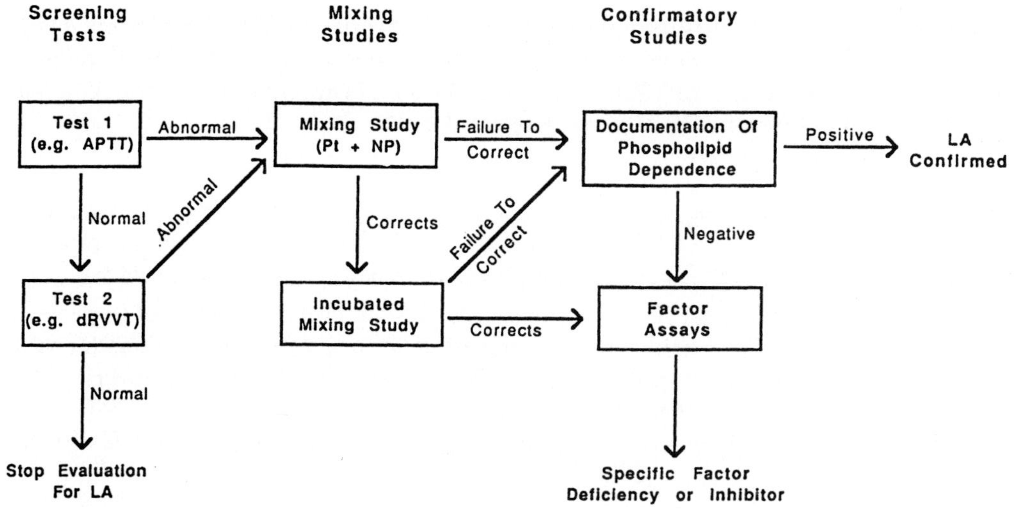

Figure 2 Flow diagram for the evaluation of lupus anticoagulant (see Section VI.G).

H. Anticardiolipin Antibodies (ACA)

ELISA methods for detection of ACA were introduced in 1983, but there is considerable variability of results between laboratories (76). Although other phospholipids such as phosphatidylserine, phosphatidylethanoamine, and phosphatidic acid may play a role in the development and pathogenesis of the antiphospholipid antibody syndromes, the vast majority of ELISA assays in use today use cardiolipin. These assays utilize a range of experimental variables (buffer, added serum, etc). Several international workshops have identified sources of error and have attempted to standardize the assays (77). Isotype-specific (IgG, IgM) reference sera are available, and a scheme for quantitating antibody concentration based upon these reference sera has been proposed. Results are calculated as GPL or MPL units (1 unit representing the binding activity of 1 μg/mL of affinity purified IgG or IgM ACA, respectively). International collaborative studies have shown good performance in identifying strongly positive and negative IgG and IgM antibody titers, but poor correlation at moderate or low levels (76). A semiquatitative scheme of reporting titer results (high, intermediate, or negative) is suggested. In many cases of low or intermediate titer, the antibodies often prove to be transient and of questionable clinical significance. The role of beta-2-glycoprotein I as a serum "cofactor" in these assays has been described (78). Newer ELISA assays are emerging which employ this "cofactor" only, bound to irradiated polystyrene microtiter plates (79). These assays may have increased specificity in predicting thrombosis.

I. Testing for Less Common Causes of Inherited Thrombophilia

In our laboratory we perform a thrombin time on all thrombosis screen cases. We do this to look for the presence of unsuspected heparin contamination and as a general screen for some cases of dysfibrinogenemia. Dysfibrinogenemias leading to thrombosis due to fibrinolysis resistance may show abnormalities in thrombin time as a result of structural changes in the fibrinogen molecule.

Deficiency of factor XII has been suggested as a possible risk factor for thrombosis related to its involvement in the generation of kallikrein and subsequent activation of the fibrinolytic pathway (80). Our screening APTT is sensitive to factor XII levels below about 55%, and serves as a signal to perform a FXII assay in selected cases.

Commercially available assays for plasminogen are available, and plasminogen deficiency has been reported to be a cause of inherited thrombophilia. We rarely perform plasminogen testing, except in compelling cases of thrombophilia in which other more common defects are not identified.

Deficiency of t-PA and elevated levels of its principal inhibitor (PAI-1) have been reported as rare causes of thrombophilia. Assays for these analytes are available, but careful specimen acquisition and handling are required to avoid preanalytical error. We reserve testing for these defects also to compelling cases of thrombophilia without other more common defects.

Assays for some of the other uncommon abnormalities listed in Table 2 are available commercially or from speciality referral laboratories, and may be indicated in selected patients.

VII. MANAGEMENT

The guiding principles in the management of thrombophilia are clinical history and clinical circumstances, combined with laboratory identification of a defect or risk factor. For discussion, management will be divided into: (a) primary prophylaxis for an asymptomatic individual with an inherited risk, (b) secondary prophylaxis for an individual with an identified risk and a previous thrombotic episode, and (c) acute event management. Management options in hyperhomocysteinemia will be discussed separately. Unfortunately, there are no controlled, randomized clinical trials of anticoagulation dealing with the various inherited and acquired causes of thrombophilia. The following discussion is based upon small series and the author's experience. The recommendations suggested must be considered tentative and await larger multicenter trials. They must be considered as general guidelines and are not a substitute for good clinical judgment.

A. Primary Prophylaxis

Except for severe homozygous deficiencies which present at birth, asymptomatic individuals with inherited defects in AT, PC , or PS should not be considered for long-term primary prophylaxis (81,82). However, prophylaxis should be instituted during surgery and prolonged immobilization, and should be considered during pregnancy and the puerperium (7). Subcutaneous, unfractionated heparin, 5000 IU, t.i.d., has been generally recommended in PC and PS deficiencies (83). A more intense regimen may be required in AT deficiency (84).

Prophylaxis for individuals who are heterozygous for factor V Leiden or prothrombin G20210A is controversial, with very little data available for guidance. Because of the high frequency of the mutation in asymptomatic Caucasians and the lower clinical risk associated with this defect, prophylaxis may make sense only in the perioperative period or during extended immobilization. Therapy during pregnancy or the puerperium may not be justified based on risk–benefit considerations. However, use of oral contraceptives in women with heterozygous factor V Leiden should be considered carefully. Vanderbroucke et al. (85) have shown a 35-fold increase in risk of venous thrombosis in oral contraceptive users with heterozygous factor V Leiden compared with nonusers with the factor V wild type. Carriers of the mutation taking oral contraceptives have about a 9-fold higher risk compared with wild-type oral contraceptive users. Recommendation regarding universal screening for factor V Leiden before instituting oral contraceptives awaits study. We recommend screening if there is any question of a family history of pregnancy- or oral contraceptive-associated venous thrombosis.

B. Secondary Prophylaxis

The central question in dealing with a patient who has had a first thrombotic event and who has a proven inherited thrombophilic defect is what should be the long-term management. There are no prospective studies that can answer this. The risks and benefits of life-long or long-term (>6 months) anticoagulation therapy must be weighed on an individual basis. Factors that need to be taken into account include patient age, patient reliability and compliance, site and severity of the thrombotic event, and other inherited and acquired risk factors for thrombosis (86). If the first event occurred in connection with circumstantial risk factors and only a single inherited risk factor has been identified, then long-term therapy is generally not recommended. On the other hand, if the patient has more than one inherited defect, if the first event was life-threatening, or if high-risk circumstances are sustained, then long-term or life-long oral anticoagulation may be considered. If thrombosis is recurrent, particularly in a new location, then life-long oral anticoagulation should be offered.

The recommendation of the Committee on Antithrombotic Therapy of the American College of Chest Physicians and the NHLBI for the intensity of oral anticoagulation therapy for all clinical indications except mechanical prosthetic heart valves is an INR range of 2.0–3.0 (87). Lower INR levels do not appear to provide adequate protection from recurrence. On the other hand, two retrospective studies have shown that an INR range greater than 3.0 provides more effective prophylaxis against recurrent DVT in patients with APA syndromes (88, 89).

C. Acute Thrombosis

The general management of acute venous thrombosis is similar with or without an hereditary defect. Standard therapy consists of heparin (unfractionated), administered either by continuous intravenous infusion or subcutaneously with dose adjusted to maintain the APTT ratio within the range 1.5–2.5. Oral anticoagulation is started within the first or second day, with a target INR of 2–3 generally achieved by day 5–6, at which time the heparin is discontinued. Oral anticoagulation should be continued for 3–6 months (90, 91).

Recently, two prospective, randomized studies have compared low-molecular-weight heparin administered at home by subcutaneous injection to unfractionated heparin administered intravenously in the hospital for the treatment of proximal deep venous thrombosis (92, 93). There was no significant difference in the effectiveness and safety between the two modes of treatment. However, as expected, the outpatient regimen was significantly less costly.

Thrombolytic therapy may be indicated for significant pulmonary embolism or thrombosis at other critical venous or arterial sites. AT concentrates are available and approved for replacement therapy in AT deficiency, but are probably no more effective than standard anticoagulation (94). The use of AT concentrates may be warranted in life-threatening thrombosis or in cases of marked heparin resistance where there is no APTT response to large doses of heparin (>60,000 U/day) and plasma heparin levels are adequate (> 0.3 U/mL) and AT levels are decreased, generally below 50–60%.

D. Treatment of Hyperhomocysteinemia

One of the primary benefits of diagnosing mild hyperhomocysteinemia or a genetic mutation in one of the Hcy pathway enzymes is the low cost and safety of administering vitamin supplements: B_6, B_{12}, and folate. Numerous studies have shown that these therapies can lower mildly elevated Hcy (9, 32), but whether this has an affect on thrombotic risk remains to be proven. Several large studies are underway to answer this question. A strategy advocated by some is administration of these vitamins without any testing, predicated on the low cost, safety, and probable Hcy-lowering effect. In most studies, the recommended daily dose of vitamin supplements are: 1 mg folic acid, 100 mg pyridoxine, and 0.4 μg cobalamin (2).

REFERENCES

1. Comp PC. Congenital and acquired hypercoagulabe states. In: Hull R, Pineo GF, eds., Disorders of Thrombosis, Philadelphia: Saunders, 1996: 339–347.
2. DeStefano V, Finazzi G, Mannucci PM. Inherited thrombophilia: pathogenesis, clinical syndromes, and management. Blood 1996; 87:3531–3544.
3. Green KB, Silverstein RL. Hypercoagulability in cancer. Hematol/Oncol Clin 1996; 10: 499–530.
4. Martinelli I, Mannucci PM, DeStefano V, et al. Different risks of thrombosis in four coagulation defects associated with inherited thromphilia: a study of 150 families. Blood 1998; 92:2353–2358.
5. Allaart CF, Aronson DC, Ruys T, et al. Hereditary protein S deficiency in young adults with arterial occlusive disease. Thromb Haemost 1990; 64:206–210.
6. Meade TW, Cooper J, Miller GJ, Howarth DJ, Stirling Y. Antithrombin III and arterial disease. Lancet 1991; 338:850–851.
7. DeStefano V, Leone G, Mastrangelo S, et al. Clinical manifestations and management of inherited thrombophilia: retrospective analysis and follow-up after diagnosis of 238 patients with congenital deficiency of antithrombin III, protein C, protein S. Thromb Haemost 1994; 72:352–358.
8. Price DT, Ridker PM. Factor V Leiden mutation and the risks for thromboembolic disease: a clinical perspective. Ann Intern Med 1997; 127:895–903.
9. Malinov MR. Homocyst(e)ine and arterial occlusive diseases. J Intern Med 1994; 236:603–617.
10. den Heijer M, Koster T, Blom HJ, et al. Hyperhomocysteinemia as a risk factor for deep-vein thrombosis. N Engl J Med 1996; 334:759–762.
11. Poort SR, Rosendaal FR, Reitsma PH, Bertina RM. A common genetic variation in the 3′-untranslated region of the prothrombin gene is associated with elevated plasma prothrombin levels and an increase in venous thrombosis. Blood 1996; 88:3698–3703.
12. Aiach M, Gandrille S, Emmerich J. A review of mutations causing deficiencies of antithrombin, protein C, and protein S. Thromb Haemost 1995; 74:81–89.
13. Lane DA, Olds RJ, Boisclair M, et al. Antithrombin III Mutation Database: first update. Thromb Haemost 1993; 70:361–367.
14. Meletich JP, Sherman L, Broze G. Absence of thrombosis in subjects with heterozygous protein C deficiency. N Engl J Med. 1987; 317:991–996.
15. Bovill EG, Bauer KA, Dickerman JD, Callas P, West B. The clinical spectrum of heterozygous protein C deficiency in a large New England kindred. Blood 1989; 73:712–717.
16. Tomczak JA, Andro RA, Sobel HG, Bovill EG, Long GL. Genetic analysis of a large kindred exhibiting type I protein C deficiency and associated thrombosis. Thromb Res 1994; 74:243–254.
17. Zoller B, DeFrutos PG, Dahlback B. Evaluation of the relationship between protein S and C4b-binding protein isoforms in hereditary protein S deficiency demonstrating type I and type III deficiencies to be phenotypic variants of the same genetic disease. Blood 1995; 85:3524–3531.
18. Dahlback B, Carlsson M, Svensson PJ. Familial thrombophilia due to a previously unrecognized mechanism characterized by poor anticoagulant response to activated protein C: prediction of a cofactor to activated protein C. Proc Natl Acad Sci USA 1993; 90:1004–1008.
19. Bertina RM, Koeleman PC, Koster T, et al. Mutation in blood coagulation factor V associated with resistance to activated protein C. Nature 1994; 369:64–67.
20. Zoller B, Dahlback B. Linkage between inherited resistance to activated protein C and factor V gene mutation in venous thrombosis. Lancet 1994; 343:1536–1538.

21. Koster T, Rosendaal FR, deRonde H, Briet E, Vandenbroucke JP, Bertina RM. Venous thrombosis due to poor anticoagulant response to activated protein C: Leiden thrombophilia study. Lancet 1993; 342:1503–1506.
22. Rosendaal FR, Siscovick DS, Schwartz SM, et al. Factor V Leiden (resistance to activated protein C) increases the risk of myocardial infarction in young women. Blood 1997; 89:2817–2821.
23. Desmarais S, de Moerloose P, Reber G, Minazio P, Perrier A, Bounameaux HR. Resistance to activated protein C in an unselected population of patients with pulmonary embolism. Lancet 1996; 347:1374–1375.
24. Rees DC, Cox M, Clegg JB. World distribution of factor V Leiden. Lancet 1995; 346:1133–1134.
25. Zivelin A, Griffin JH, Xu X, et al. A single genetic origin for a common Caucasian risk factor for venous thrombosis. Blood 1997; 89:397–402.
26. Eschwege V, Robert A. Strikes in French public transport and resistance to activated protein C (letter). Lancet 1996; 347:206.
27. Miletich JP, Prescott SM, White R, Majerus PW, Bovill EG. Inherited predisposition to thrombosis. Cell 1993;72:477–480.
28. Brenner B, Zivelin A, Lanir N, Greengard JS, Griffin JH, Seligsohn U. Hederitary thrombophilia is a multigenic disease: increased thrombotic risk due to combined hereditary heterozygous protein C deficiency and activated protein C resistance (abstr). Thromb Haemost 1995; 73:942.
29. Zoller SB, de Frutos PG, Dahlback B. Resistance to activated protein C as an additional risk factor in hereditary deficiency of protein S (abstr). Thromb Haemost 1995; 73:1360.
30. Mudd SH, Levy HL, Skovby F. Disorders of transulfuration. In: Scriver CR, Beaudet AL, Slyl WS, Valle D, eds.: The Metabolic Basis of Inherited Disease. New York: McGraw-Hill, 1989:693.
31. D'Angelo A, Selhub J. Homocysteine and thrombotic disease. Blood 1997; 90:1–11.
32. Selhub J, Jacques PF, Wilson PWF, Rush D, Rosenberg IH. Vitamin status and intake as primary determinants of homocysteinemia in an elderly population. JAMA 1993; 270:2693–2698.
33. Rasmussen K, Moller J, Lyngbak M, Pedersen AMH, Dybkjaer L. Age- and gender-specific reference intervals for total homocysteine and methylmalonic acid in plasma before and after vitamin supplementation. Clin Chem 1996;42:630–636.
34. Frosst P, Blom HJ, Milos R, et al. A candidate genetic risk factor for vascular disease: a common mutation in methylenetetrahydrofolate reductase. Nature Genet 1995; 10:111–113.
35. Kang SS, Wong P, Susmano A, Sora J, Norusis M, Ruggie N. Thermolabile methylenetetrahydrofolate reductase: and inherited risk factor for coronary artery disease. Am J Hum Genet 1991; 48: 536–545.
36. Jacques PF, Bostom AG, Williams RR, et al. Relation between folate status, a common mutation in methylenetetrahydrofolate reductase, and plasma homocysteine concentrations. Circulation 1996; 93:7–9.
37. Starkebaum G, Harlan JM. Endothelial cell injury due to copper-catalyzed hydrogen peroxide generation from homocysteine. J Clin Invest 1986; 77:1370–1376.
38. Cumming AM, Keeney S, Salden A, et al. The prothrombin gene G20210A variant: prevalence in a U.K. anticoagulant clinic population. Br J Haematol 1997; 98:353–355.
39. van der Meer FJM, Koster T, Vandenbroucke JP, Briet E, Rosendaal FR. The Leiden Thrombophilia Study (LETS). Thromb Haemost 1997;78:631–635.
40. Zivelin A, Rosenberg N, Faier S, et al. A single genetic origin for the common prothrombotic G20210A polymorphism in the prothrombin gene. Blood 1998; 92:1119–1124.
41. de Moerloose P. Bounameaux HR, Mannucci PM. Screening tests for thrombophilic patients? Which tests, for which patient, by whom, when, and why? Semin Thromb Hemost 1998; 24:321–327.
42. Triplett DA. Antiphospholipid antibodies and thrombosis. A consequence, coincidence, or cause? Arch Pathol Lab Med 1993;117:78–88.
43. Alareon-Segovia D. Clinical manifestations of the antiphospholipid syndromes. J Rheumatol 1992; 19:1778–1781.
44. Asherson RA. A primary antiphospholipid syndrome? J Rheumatol 1988; 15:1742–1746.

45. Triplett DA. Protean clinical presentation of antiphospholipid-protein antibodies (APA). Thromb Haemost 1995; 74:329–337.
46. Esmon NL, Smirnov MD, Esmon CT. Thrombogenic mechanisms of antiphospholipid antibodies. Thromb Haemost 1997; 78:79–82.
47. Trousseau A. Phlegmasia alba dolens. In: Lectures in Clinical Medicine, delivered at the Hotel-Dieu, Paris. New Sydenham Society, 1872.
48. Meletich JP. Laboratory diagnosis of protein C deficiency. Semin Thromb Hemost 1990; 16:169–176.
49. Comp PC, Thurnau GR, Welsh J, Esmon CT. Functional and immunologic protein S levels are decreased during pregnancy. Blood 1986; 68:881–885.
50. Andrew M. Developmental hemostasis: relevance to thromboembolic complications in pediatric patients. Thromb Haemost 1995; 74:415–425.
51. Adcock DM, Fink L, Marlar RA. A laboratory approach to the evaluation of hereditary hypercoagulability. Am J Clin Pathol 1997; 108:434–449.
52. Andrew M, Paes B, Milner R, et al. Development of the human coagulation system in the full-term infant. Blood 1987; 70:165–172.
53. Buller HR, Cate JW. Acquired antithrombin III deficiency: laboratory diagnosis, incidence, clinical implications, and treatment with antithrombin III concentrate. Am J Med 1989; 887(3B): 44S–48S.
54. Marciniak E, Farley C, Disimone P. Familial thrombosis due to antithrombin III deficiency. Blood 1974; 43:219–223.
55. Andrew M, Vegh P, Johnston M, Bowker J, Ofosu F, Mitchell L. Maturation of the hemostatic system during childhood. Blood 1992; 80:1998–2005.
56. Tait RC, Walker ID, Islam SIA, et al. Age related changes in protein C activity in healthy males. Thromb Haemost 1991; 65:326–327.
57. Boyer-Neumann C, Bertina RM Tripodi A, et al. Comparison of functional assays for protein S: European Collaborative Study of Patients with Congenital and Acquired Deficiency. Thromb Haemost 1993; 70:946–950.
58. Faioni EM, Franchi F, Asti D, Sacchi E, Bernardi F, Mannucci PM. Resistance to activated protein C in nine thrombolic families; interference in a protein S functional assay. Thromb Haemost 1993; 70:1067–1071.
59. Faioni EM, Boyer-Neumann C, Franchi F, Wolf M, Meyer D, Mannucci PM. Another protein S functional assay is sensitive to resistance to activated protein C. Thromb Haemost 1994; 72: 643–651.
60. DeStefano Wolf M, Boyer-Neumann C, Peynaud-Deboyle E, Marfaring-Koka A, Amiral J, Meyer D. Clinical applications of a direct assay of free protein S antigen using monoclonal antibodies. A study of 59 cases. Blood Coagul Fibrinol 1994; 5:880–884.
61. Boerger LM, Morris PC, Thurnau GR, Esmon CT, Comp PC. Oral contraceptives and gender affect protein S status. Blood 1987; 69:692–694.
62. Comp PC. Laboratory evaluation of protein S status. Semin Thromb Hemost 1990; 16:177–181.
63. Shizuka R, Kanda T, Amagai H, Kobayashi I. False-positive activated protein C sensitivity ratio caused by freezing and by contamination of plasma with platelets (letter). Thromb Res 1995; 78: 189–190.
64. Rao AK, Elliott D, Stadnicki A, DeLa Cadena R. High levels of plasma factor VIIIC impair anticoagulant response to activated protein C (abstr). Thromb Haemost 1995; 73:1126.
65. Henkens CMA, Bom VJJ, Seinen AJ, van der Meer J. Sensitivity to activated protein C: influence of oral contraceptives and sex. Thromb Haemost 1995; 73: 402–404.
66. Cumming AM, Tait RC, Fildes S, Yoong A, Keeney S, Hay CRM. Development of resistance to activated protein C during pregnancy. Br J Haematol 1995; 90:725–727.
67. Svensson PJ, Dahlback B. Resistance to activated protein C as a basis for venous thrombosis. N Engl J Med 1994; 330:517–522.
68. deRonde H, Bertina RM. Laboratory diagnosis of APC-resistance: a critical evaluation of the test and the development of diagnostic criteria. Thromb Haemost 1995; 72:880–886.

69. Bertina RM, Reitsma PH, Rosendaal FR, Vandenbroucke JP. Resistance to activated protein C and factor V Leiden as risk factors for venous thrombosis. Thromb Haemost 1995; 74:449–453.
70. Strobl FJ, Hoffman S, Huber S, Williams EC, Voelkerding KV. Activated protein C resistance assay performance. Improvement by sample dilution with factor V-deficient plasma. Arch Pathol Lab Med 1998; 122:430–433.
71. Bowen DJ, Bowley S, John M, Collins PW. Factor V Leiden, the prothrombin 3′-untranslated region variant and thermolabile methylenetetrahydrofolate reductase: a single genetic test genotypes all three loci —determination of frequencies in the S. Wales population of the UK. Thromb Haemost 1998; 79:949–954.
72. Ueland PM, Refsum H, Stabler SP, Malinow MR, Andersson A, Allen RH. Total homocysteine in plasma or serum: methods and clinical applications. Clin Chem 1993; 39:1764–1769.
73. Shipchandler MT, Moore EG. Rapid, fully automated measurement of plasma homocysteine with the Abbott IMX analyzer. Clin Chem 1995; 41:991–994.
74. Franken DG, Boers GHJ, Blom HJ, Trijbels JM, Kloppenborg WC. Treatment of mild hyperhomocysteinemia in vascular disease patients. Arterioscler Thromb 1994; 14:465–470.
75. Brandt JT, Triplett DA, Alving B, Scharrer I. Criteria for the diagnosis of lupus anticoagulants: an update (on behalf of the Subcommittee on Lupus Anticoagulant. Antiphospholipid Antibody of the Scientific and Standardisation Committee of the ISTH). Thromb Haemost 1995; 74:1185–1190.
76. Triplett DA. Antiphospholipid-protein antibodies: laboratory detection and clinical relevance. Thomb Res 1995; 78:1–31.
77. Harris EN, Pierangeli S, Birch D. Anticardiopilin Wet Workshop report. Am J Clin Pathol 1994; 101:616–624.
78. McNeil HP, Simpson RJ, Chesterman CN, Krilis SA. Anti-phospholipid antibodies are directed against a complex antigen that includes a lipid-binding inhibitor of coagulation: beta-2-glycoprotein I (apolipoprotein H). Proc Natl Acad Sci USA 1990; 87:4120–4124.
79. Kell LB, Galazka M, El-Kadi H, Erickson E, DeBari V. Binding of beta 2-glycoprotein I to activated polystyreene and its recognition by human IgG autoantibodies. Biotechnol Appl Biochem 1995; 22:305–313.
80. Lammele B, Wuillemin WA, Huber I, et al. Thromboenbolism and bleeding tendency in congenital factor XII deficiency: a study of 74 subjects from 14 Swiss families. Thromb Haemost 1991; 65: 117–121.
81. Rosendaal FR, Heijboer H, Briet E, et al. Mortality in inherited antithrombin III deficiency 1830 to 1989. Lancet 1991; 337:260–263.
82. Allart CF, Rosendaal FR, Noteboom WMP, Briet E. No excess mortality in heterozygotes for hereditary protein C deficiency type I—1820 to 1993. Thromb Haemost 1995; 73:1252–1256.
83. Pabinger I, Kyrle PA, Heistinger M, Eichinger S, Wittmann E, Lechner K. The risk of thromboembolism in asymptomatic patients with protein C and protein S deficiency: a prospective cohort study. Thromb Haemost 1994; 71:441–446.
84. DeStefano V, Leone G, DeCarolis S, et al. Management of pregnancy in women with antithrombin III congenital defect: report of four cases. Thromb Haemost 1988; 59:193–197.
85. Vanderbroucke JP, Koster T, Briet E, Reitsma PH, Bertine RM, Rosendaal FR. Increased risk of venous thrombosis in oral-contraceptive users who are carriers of factor V Leiden mutation. Lancet 1994; 344:1453–1457.
86. Bauer KA. Management of patients with hereditary defects predisposing to thrombosis including pregnant women. Thromb Haemost 1995; 74:94–100.
87. Hirsch J, Dalenm JE, Deykin D, Poller L, Bussey H. Oral anticoagulants: mechanism of action, clinical effectiveness, and optimal therapeutic range. Chest 1995; 108 (suppl):231S–245S.
88. Khamashta MA, Cuadrado MJ, Mujic F, Taub NA, Hunt BJ, Hughes GVR. The management of thrombosis in the antiphospholipid-antibody syndrome. N Engl J Med 1995; 332:993–997.
89. Rosove MH, Brewer PMC. Antiphospholipid thrombosis: clinical course after the first thrombotic event in 70 patients. Ann Intern Med 1992; 117:303–308.
90. Schulman S, Rhedin As, Lindmarker P. A comparison of six weeks with six months of oral antico-

agulant therapy after a first episode of venous thromboembolism. Duration of Anticoagulation Trial Study Group. N Engl J Med 1995; 332:1661–1665.
91. Levine MN, Hirsh J, Gent M, et al. Optimal duration of oral anticoagulant therapy: a randomized trial comparing four weeks with three months of warfarin in patients with proximal deep vein thrombosis. Thromb Haemost 1995; 74:606–611.
92. Levine M, Gent M, Hirsh J, et al. A comparison of low-molecular weight heparin administered primarily at home with unfractionated heparin administered in the hospital for proximal deep-vein thrombosis. N Engl J Med 1996: 334:677–681.
93. Koopman MMW, Prandoni P, Piovella F, et al., for the Tasman Study Group. Treatment of venous thrombosis with intravenous unfractionated heparin administered in the hospital as compared with subcutaneous low-molecular-weight heparin administered at home. N Engl J Med 1996; 334:682–687.
94. Schulman S, Tengborn L. Treatment of venous thromboembolism in patients with congenital deficiency of antithrombin III. Thromb Haemost 1992; 68:634–638.
95. Boers GHJ. Hyperhomocysteinemia as a risk factor for arterial and venous disease. A review of evidence and relevance. Thromb Haemost 1997; 78:520–522.

34

Quality Control and Quality Assurance in Hematology

Bradley E. Copeland*
University of Cincinnati Medical Center, Cincinnati, Ohio

DEFINITIONS

Quality control in the laboratory is the frequent periodic monitoring of precision and accuracy in equipment, technique, or testing.

Quality assurance is the process by which the most desirable and feasible level of quality is created and maintained.

Continual assurance, *high dependability*, and *long-term comparability of data* are all concepts which describe the patient's need for careful and exact laboratory diagnosis followed by a physician or team of physicians.

BENEFITS

The ultimate benefit of such a program is quality, which eventuates in the least morbidity and lowest mortality in the population.

The divisions of quality assurance are listed in Table 1:

1. Prevention of error by careful preparation.
2. Assessment of the work product to keep it at a constant level of excellence and error-free.
3. Corrective action: when errors are detected they must be corrected before erroneous data reach the patient record.

SOURCES OF ERROR

Quality is undermined by several types of error in the hematology laboratory:

1. *Clerical errors* include blood procurement from the wrong patient, mislabelled or interchanged specimens, recording or transcription mistakes.
2. *Sampling errors* are related to improper anticoagulation, inappropriate preservation, hemolysis, or artifacts due to delay in plasma separation.

---

*Former Chairman of the Commission on World Standards, World Association of Pathologists.

Table 1 Divisions of Quality Assurance

Prevention of error	Assessment of error	Corrective action for error
Choice of methods	Using standards	Equipment and controls, troubleshooting
Education, orientation of personnel	Reviewing and surveying of results	Recalibrating instruments
Reporting results	Using replicate or duplicate samples	Repeating tests
Handling specimens	Comparing replicate results with other laboratories	
Maintenance of instruments	Proficiency testing	
Calibration of instruments		
Evaluation of reagents, controls, and instruments		
Direct observation of performance of tests		
Development and retention of quality control charts		

3. *Technical errors* are of two types:
   a. Systematic or constant error usually due to poor-quality reagents and standards. These errors are corrected by replacement of faulty solutions, and by recalibration using new standards.
   b. Indeterminate error or inherent error which is the sum total of many minor fluctuations which is measured as the usual day-to-day standard deviation. It can be minimized by following three basic rules:
      1. Pay attention to detail
      2. Pay attention to detail
      3. *Pay attention to detail!*

Accuracy, *Precision*, and *Reliability*: These words are essential to effective quality control.

Accuracy of a test result is the nearness to the true value.

Precision of a test result is the ability to reproduce that result. Precision may be possible without accuracy, but accuracy is *not* possible without precision.

Reliability of a method involves both accuracy and precision. If a method maintains accuracy and precision over a long period of time under difficult conditions, i.e., change of regents, instruments, and technicians, then the method is considered reliable.

A practical analogy is presented in Figure 1. Accuracy, precision, and reliability can best be explained by an analogy: A VISIT TO A RIFLE RANGE. Hunters A and B were taught the correct procedure for loading, handling, sighting, and firing their rifles at targets. A beginner was also allowed to shoot on the range but was not given instruction in the proper technique of handling his rifle. All three hunters shot 10 rounds. Their results are depicted in Figure 1. The beginner, hunter C, showed a widely scattered pattern. Hunter A showed precision of technique, but was not accurate in hitting the bull's-eye. Hunter B, however, demonstrated both precision and accuracy by hitting 10 bull's eyes. Subsequently, the beginner was taught the technique of sighting and firing his rifle, and Hunter A adjusted his sights so that he was able to shoot repeated bull's eyes. All three were thus able to utilize the technique and repro-

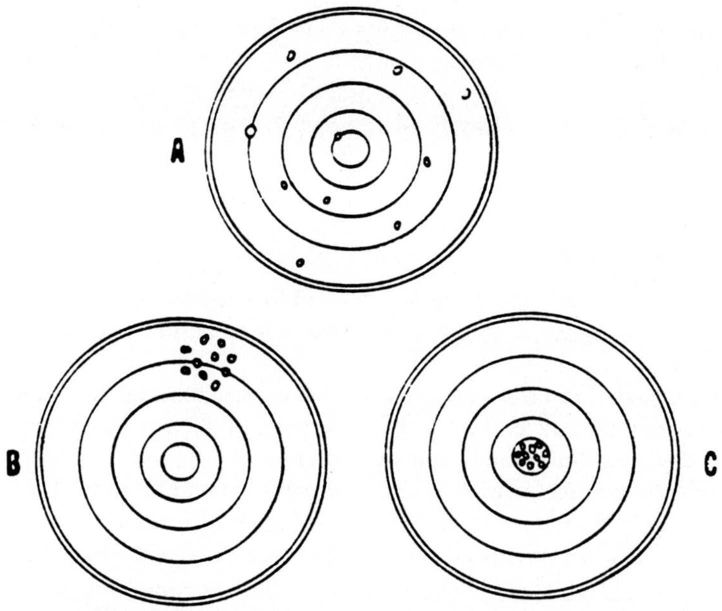

Figure 1 A visit to a rifle range: An analogy to accuracy and precision.

duce bull's eyes over many months of varied weather conditions. This result, or reproducibility of accuracy and precision over a long period of time under varied conditions, demonstrates the reliability of the technique or method they were taught.

Quality control techniques that are *visual* and not *mathematical*:

1. Preparation of a thin blood film and its evaluation.
2. Staining of a blood film and its evaluation.
3. Overall microscopic evaluation of a blood film for diagnostic purposes.

The above three visual steps are an indispensable part of the Hematology Quality Control System.

It is my opinion that the training of all physicians should include proficiency in the skill of making, staining, and microscopic examination of a blood film. This skill should be developed in medical school. Unfortunately, medical schools have given up the teaching of such skills. With the advent of modern hematology analyzers, these skills will still be less required in future hematology laboratories.

METHODS FOR DETECTING ERROR

The basic elements needed in the establishment of a test method to ensure accuracy, precision, and reliability are:

1. Standardization
2. Calibration
3. Controls

The most important individual in the hematologic quality control process is the attending physician at the bedside who evaluates each laboratory test as to whether it is consistent with the working diagnosis or whether it needs to be repeated in order to verify its significance.

It is at the moment when the laboratory's ability to respond to the request for prompt verification within minutes or hours that the quality assurance program becomes most effective and important to the patient.

Reliability, Precision, and Accuracy

The most important aspects of the measurement of human whole-blood constituents are constancy and internal consistency of the reported measurements over a long period of time: in a word, dependability or reliability.

As a physician uses measurements from his own office laboratory or a hospital laboratory or a commercial laboratory, the results must be kept at an even level of accuracy and precision—i.e., consistency day to day, month to month, and year to year.

To treat a patient the physician uses the consistent levels of precision and accuracy (1) to predict the existence of disease, and (2) to judge the efficiency or failure of treatment.

A physician's confidence in a laboratory depends on months or years of reliability. Even a single episode of a shift or a trend which gives falsely high or falsely low values can lead to misdiagnosis and excess treatment or no treatment when needed. Upon having had such an experience the physician's confidence is destroyed for at least a period of months until his or her confidence in the laboratory can be strengthened and reinforced. Until confidence is reestablished, the response to a significant lab value change is, "We'd better check that value before we act on it." Therefore, quality control and quality assurance are cornerstones of the physician-laboratory relationship.

THREE REQUIREMENTS FOR HEMATOLOGY LABORATORY CERTIFICATION

Between 1950 and 1980 the College of American Pathologists set up a voluntary program for inspection and accreditation of medical laboratories. In 1988 the Congress coopted this voluntary program into federal law as the Clinical Laboratory Improvement Act 1988 (CLIA) so that all laboratories would be required to bring themselves up to the CAP standards. The major emphasis in the CAP hematology program is quality control (Fig. 2).

Question: Is there a document for the design and evaluation of the laboratory quality control program?

College of American Pathologists™

Commission on Laboratory Accreditation

Inspection Checklist

HEMATOLOGY

College of American Pathologists • Laboratory Accreditation Program • 325 Waukegan Road • Northfield, Illinois 60093-2750

QUALITY CONTROL 1996.2 EDITION

Figure 2 Masthead: CAP Commission on Laboratory Accreditation Inspection Checklist, Hematology.

Answer: The quality control program in hematology must be under active surveillance by the hematology supervisor (for a physician's office laboratory; read, "the physician") with a documented review at least weekly. Secondary review should occur at least monthly by the pathologist, (physician), and laboratory section director or designee. Using the monthly summary prepared by the manufacturer from submitted data.

The QC program must include system design and evaluation of patient identification and preparation of the patient for specimen collection as well as accurate and careful identification of the specimen and its preservation during transportation to the laboratory. The processing must be under complete QC. Accurate result reporting is all-important; as mentioned above, it must be on time and clearly legible. A log of reported failure in the system must be kept, and each failure must be followed up and documented.

REQUIREMENTS FOR CAP ACCREDITATION

Internal Quality Control

A complete system of calibrators and daily quality control samples and the decision criteria related to day-to-day control must be in place. This is available from every automated hematology instrument manufacturer per FDA rules.

External Quality Control

The performance of tests on unknown samples must be carried out with results submitted to a central agency for evaluation. A passing grade of 80% is required. Twenty to 25 samples per year are submitted.

Reference Intervals

Also called "normal values," reference intervals are required. These must be determined on the laboratory's own instruments when operating "in control."

PRACTICAL INTERNAL QUALITY CONTROL GUIDELINES (FIG. 3)

Three controls are a feasible set of controls to run on each daily shift. The automated hematology instrument will be installed by the manufacturer so that the initial calibration and QC can

CELL-DYN® Quality Control Report

Customer Information

Customer ID#: [redacted]
ADAMS COUNTY HOSPITAL (R 4,5,6)
210 W WILSON DR

WEST UNION, OH 45693

Attn: [redacted] / HEMATOLOGY LAB

Statistical Group

Class of Instrument using :CELL-DYN 1600
Material :CELL-DYN 16
Low Lot# :L16461
Normal Lot# :N16461
High Lot# :H16461

Report Information

Report for the month of March, 1997

Labs reporting for this month :476
Labs reporting cumulative :1522
Days cumulative :90
Date Printed :04/17/97

Abnormal Low Lot#:L16461

This Month's Results

Parameter	Assay Mean	Your Mean	Group Mean	Your SD	Your CV	Group SD	Group CV	S.D.I.	Outside 2 S.D.I.
WBC	2.30	2.38	2.37	0.04	1.84	0.10	4.18	+0.05	
RBC	2.50	2.50	2.51	0.03	1.19	0.05	1.93	-0.23	
→ HGB	7.10	6.98	7.05	0.13	1.86	0.13	1.91	-0.58	
HCT	20.8	20.8	20.9	0.26	1.26	0.51	2.44	-0.24	

Cumulative Results

Your Mean	Group Mean	Your SD	Your CV	Group SD	Group CV	S.D.I.	Outside 2 S.D.I.
2.37	2.37	0.07	2.75	0.10	4.12	-0.06	
2.49	2.51	0.03	1.25	0.05	1.91	-0.34	
→ 7.01	7.05	0.10	1.48	0.14	1.94	-0.28	
20.5	20.8	0.37	1.79	0.51	2.44	-0.50	

Figure 3 CELL-DYN monthly quality control report (March 1997).

be instituted without delay. The limits for the three levels of daily control samples are set as follows. Each commercial control material has an assigned manufacturer's average and two SD limits. For example, low Hgb, 6.3 ± 0.3; normal, 12.6 ± 0.4; high, 14.9 ± 0.5 g/dL.

The user laboratory runs each level of controls daily for a 10-day check period. This establishes for the individual user laboratory a target mean value and a set of ±2 SD limits. At this point, patient samples may be run since the system is in control. The daily control record should have the signature of the technologists and the decision statement "in control" or "out of control." All control data must be recorded.

Figure 3 shows an example of the monthly QC report that is returned to the user. The month of March 1997 being evaluated is reported in the left box, "This Month's Results." The right box shows the "Cumulative Results" averages.

Note: Each individual laboratory is a member of a group of the in group laboratories using the same control lot. Note that in Figure 3 there are 476 laboratories.

MONTHLY EVALUATION

Monthly Average Comparison

The difference between the March 1997 monthly Hb mean value 6.98 g/dL (left box, line 3, column 2) and your cumulative results mean 7.01 (right box, line 3, column 1) is −0.03 g Hb/dL. Rule: ASCP Rapid Method. The maximum allowable change between monthly values is 1 Cumulative Results usual SD: here it is 0.10 g Hb/dL (Fig. 3; right Cumulative Results box, line 3, column 3). In the example for March 1997 there was "no statistically significant change" in the monthly average Hb concentration. The change of 0.03 g/dL between March 1997 average and your cumulative average is less than your Cumulative Results SD 0.10 g/dL. See Cumulative Results box (right) line 3, column 3. Therefore, the system is stable.

Monthly SD Comparison

Current March 1997 monthly SD is 0.13 (see Fig. 3; This Month's Results, left box, line 3, column 4). The cumulative average SD is 0.10 (see Fig. 3; cumulative box, line 3, column 3). *Rule:* ASCP Rapid Method. For there to be a real difference between the monthly SD and the cumulative SD requires that the monthly SD value be 50% greater than cumulative SD value. Here the difference is 0.13 to 0.10* = +0.03 or a +30% change, which is not statistically significant, i.e., <50% increase. The system is "in control" from the SD standpoint.

Figure 4 Levey-Jennings graph of quality control daily values. The graph shows another way to demonstrate the quality control process. The midpoint is the average, and the daily values from left to right are successive daily control values. The system is in control as long as the daily value is ±2 SD. Each day a dot is added representing the QC for that day.

EXTERNAL QUALITY CONTROL

A certified hematology laboratory must participate in the analysis of unknown specimens designed to test the proficiency of each certified laboratory. Table 2 shows a report from a typical external quality control challenge. This external quality control program was distributed and evaluated by the American Academy of Family Physicians in conjunction with the College of American Pathologists. It was approved by Health Care Finance Administration (HCFA) for the certification program by (CLIA Law 1988).

Samples are distributed three times a year. Each test kit consists of five blood samples

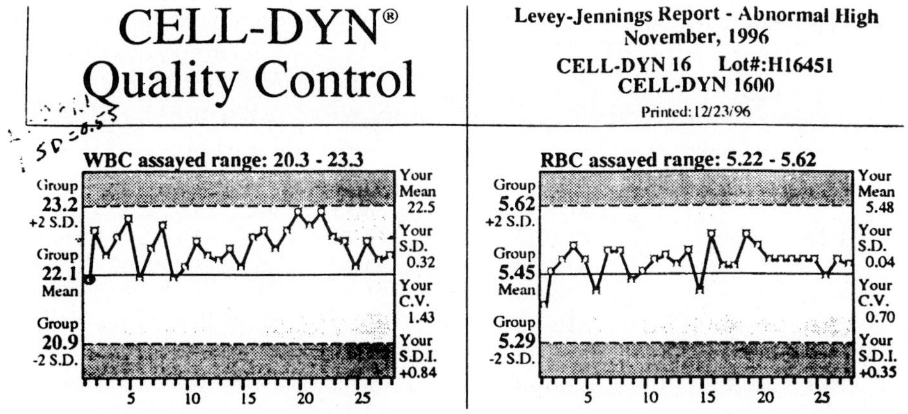

Figure 4 CELL-DYN monthly quality control, Levey-Jennings report, Nov. 1996.

(Table 2) for complete blood count. (See Table 2 for an example of External Quality Control.) Results must be found to be within ±2 SD intervals of the entire group of participants. In order to maintain accreditation a score of 80% must be achieved.

Note that the standard deviation interval column 7 (Table 2) values are all <1.0. This means that the "medical laboratory" values are accurate within 1 SD from the mean of all the participating laboratories. See below for the calculation of the SDI index.

3. Reference Intervals (Normal Values) 95% limits

Each accredited laboratory must have a normal reference interval established for each test performed by the laboratory. Each laboratory must analyze a representative group of normals (for example, 15 women and 15 men) using the instruments in the laboratory itself. It is reasonable to assume good health if the subject (1) is ambulatory, (2) comes to work, and (3) is not obviously sick.

There are two acceptable methods for the expression of the 95% reference interval: (1) parametric (2) nonparametric.

Assume that we have collected data from 30 individuals. "Parametric" refers to the bell-shaped distribution curve. This method emphasizes the values at either extreme and is overly sensitive to outliers.

The mean ±2 SD of the 30 subjects constitutes a valid parametric 95% reference interval. *Note:* Most of PC calculators have an automatic SD button. Since the SD calculation is automatically done, there is no need for a separate section on how to make the calculation.

The nonparametric method avoids the problem of outliers and emphasizes values closer to the mean. Example: arrange the 30 values in ascending order of concentration. The approximate 95% nonparametric methods limits are at the second and 29th values. Note that 2/30 are 7% and represent the number of values excluded by the 95% limits. So for this example, we have a 93% reference interval. For medical decision making there is no practical difference between the 93% and 95% reference intervals. Therefore, either method is an approximation and is acceptable.

Table 2 External Quality Control (Example)

Constituent—unit of measure your reported methods		Specimen number	Your result	Target group statistics Mean	S.D.	C.V.	#Labs	Your SDI
Hematocrit (QBC)	percent	XH6-11	30.1	31.49	1.13	3.6	110	−1.0
QBC autoread (CAP STD)		XH6-12	38.3	38.95	1.39	3.6	103	−0.5
HCFA score:	100%	XH6-13	28.0	28.76	1.06	3.7	111	−0.7
		XH7-14	34.6	34.77	1.06	3.0	107	−0.2
		XH8-15	35.2	35.68	1.11	3.1	106	−0.4
White cell count (QBC)	thousand/UL	XH6-11	9.1	9.19	.87	9.5	114	−0.1
QBC autoread (CAP STD)		XH6-12	15.6	14.61	2.04	13.9	87	+0.5
HCFA score:	100%	XH6-13	8.4	8.93	.80	9.0	113	−0.7
		XH6-14	13.7	13.27	1.35	10.1	107	+0.3
		XH6-15	15.6	15.63	1.20	7.7	97	+0.0
Platelet count (QBC)	thousand/UL	XH6-11	226	254.7	38.9	15.3	110	−0.7
QBC autoread (CAP STD)		XH6-12	148	163.0	40.6	24.9	85	−0.4
HCFA score:	100%	XH6-13	359	350.2	37.1	10.6	110	+0.2
		XH6-14	138	140.9	28.0	19.9	105	−0.1
		XH6-15	142	137.4	25.1	18.3	96	+0.2
Hemoglobin (QBC)	G/DL	XH6-11	10.6	10.17	.40	3.7	112	−0.2
QBC autoread (CAP STD)		XH6-12	13.2	13.14	.48	3.7	103	+0.1
HCFA score:	100%	XH6-13	9.7	9.80	.36	3.8	110	0.3
		XH6-14	11.7	11.91	.37	3.1	110	−0.6
		XH6-15	12.1	12.15	.32	2.7	106	−0.2
Granulocyte %	percent	XH6-11	51	49.4	11.7	23.6	114	+0.1
QBC autoread (CAP STD)		XH6-12	37	42.0	8.2	19.6	88	0.6
		XH6-13	61	52.3	13.2	25.2	113	+0.7
		XH6-14	34	41.1	7.3	17.7	108	−1.0
		XH6-15	35	38.5	3.6	9.3	97	−1.0
Lymph/mono %	percent	XH6-11	49	50.5	11.7	23.1	115	0.1
QBC autoread (CAP STD)		XH6-12	63	58.0	8.2	14.2	88	+0.6
		XH6-13	39	47.6	13.2	27.7	114	−0.7
		XH6-14	66	59.0	7.3	12.3	107	+1.0
		XH6-15	65	61.5	3.6	5.8	97	+1.0

In hematology tests there are certain specific differences between the sexes; for example, Hb and Hct values for males are higher than for females and require separate reference intervals. Tables 3 and 4 show an extensive series of data from ambulatory healthy individuals with a broad range of gender and age by decade distribution. These age and gender groups can be used by the individual laboratory to predict values for all gender-age groups by inserting the local laboratory reference interval, usually the third decade (20 to 30 years), into the Table 3 or 4. This interpolation step allows the estimation of instrument bias. For example, using Table 3 if the local laboratory mean value for third-decade hemoglobin, male, is 15.2 g/dL, the difference would be −0.5 g/dL, which would predict that all other male decade averages need to be increased by +0.5 g/dL to correspond with the Fernald Medical Monitoring Program reference intervals. Decade 4 would be 16.1; decade 5 16.0; and decade 6 15.8. Thus the within-laboratory third-decade values can be used to approximate the entire range of age values.

Table 3 Hematology Means and Standard Deviations (Healthy SW Ohio Nondiabetic Female)

	Decade:	3 (20–30)	4 (30–40)	5 (40–50)	6 (50–60)	7 (60–70)	8 (70–80)
Variable:	Study:	T	T	T	T	T W	T
Hemoglob	Mean	13.7	13.7	13.5	13.8	14.0	13.8
	STD Dev	0.9	1.0	1.2	1.0	0.9	1.0
Hemocrit	Mean	39.5	39.6	39.2	39.9	40.7	40.1
	STD Dev	2.5	2.8	3.1	2.8	2.6	2.7
MCV	Mean	88.3	88.6	88.2	88.7	89.8	88.7
	STD Dev	4.6	4.5	5.6	4.3	3.8	4.9
Platelet	Mean	286.2	282.5	288.1	284.6	282.3	276.3
	STD Dev	62.6	63.9	63.6	58.5	63.0	54.0
WBC	Mean	6.7	6.6	6.4	6.2	6.3	6.1
	STD Dev	2.2	1.9	1.8	1.7	1.9	1.2
MCH	Mean	30.6	30.6	30.4	30.6	31.0	30.6
	STD Dev	1.9	1.8	2.3	1.6	1.4	1.9
MCHC	Mean	34.6	34.6	34.4	34.5	34.5	34.4
	STD Dev	0.7	0.7	0.8	0.6	0.6	0.8
RDW	Mean	12.6	12.8	13.0	12.9	13.0	13.2
	STD Dev	0.8	0.9	1.1	0.7	1.2	0.8
RBC	Mean	4.5	4.5	4.4	4.5	4.5	4.5
	STD Dev	0.3	0.3	0.3	0.3	0.3	0.4
GRPRCNT	Mean	59.9	61.6	61.5	59.2	59.3	59.8
	STD Dev	8.9	8.6	8.5	8.6	10.5	8.0
LYPRCNT	Mean	32.8	30.8	30.9	33.4	32.3	33.1
	STD Dev	7.9	7.7	7.2	7.6	8.5	7.6
GRNUM	Mean	4.1	4.1	4.0	3.8	3.8	3.7
	STD Dev	1.7	1.4	1.4	1.3	1.6	1.0
LYNUM	Mean	2.1	2.0	1.9	2.1	2.0	2.0
	STD Dev	0.6	0.6	0.5	0.6	0.6	0.5

USEFUL TERMS

Standard Deviation Interval (SDI)

See Figure 3, Cumulative Results, second box.

Your mean = 7.01; group mean = 7.05; SD group 0.14:

$$\frac{7.01 - 7.05}{0.14} = \frac{-0.04}{0.14} = -0.28$$

This indicates the degree to which the individual laboratory's average value approaches the average value of the group of laboratories in the pool as a whole. This is a test of accuracy. The example from Figure 3 shows that the hemoglobin test is very accurate.

The group average is accepted as the true accurate average value. The acceptable SDI is found between +1.99 and −1.99, with a preferred ratio between +1.0 and −1.0. Any ratio >2.0 requires immediate attention because of inaccuracy. Our example at −0.28 is very close to the mean for the entire population. A quick scan of the SDI column shows how good these measurements are:

Table 4 Hematology Means and Standard Deviations (Healthy SW Ohio Nondiabetic Male) (Copeland et al. 1999)

Variable:	Decade: / Study:	3 (20–30) T	4 (30–40) T	5 (40–50) T	6 (50–60) T	7 (60–70) T W	8 (70–80) T
Hemoglob	Mean	15.7	15.6	15.5	15.3	15.1	15.0
	STD Dev	0.8	0.8	1.0	0.9	1.1	1.2
Hemocrit	Mean	45.1	45.0	44.7	44.2	43.6	43.6
	STD Dev	2.6	2.4	2.8	2.8	3.2	3.5
MCV	Mean	88.2	88.3	89.3	89.6	90.1	90.5
	STD Dev	3.5	3.6	4.4	4.1	4.3	5.5
Platelet	Mean	262.1	259.7	261.5	257.8	257.6	251.9
	STD Dev	59.3	55.5	53.1	57.2	67.1	58.1
WBC	Mean	6.5	6.6	6.5	6.3	6.4	6.9
	STD Dev	1.7	1.9	2.0	1.6	1.5	1.8
MCH	Mean	30.6	30.6	30.9	31.0	31.1	31.1
	STD Dev	1.4	1.3	1.6	1.5	1.7	2.0
MCHC	Mean	34.7	34.6	34.6	34.5	34.5	34.3
	STD Dev	0.6	0.6	0.6	0.6	0.7	0.7
RDW	Mean	12.5	12.7	12.7	12.8	13.1	13.2
	STD Dev	0.5	0.9	0.6	0.6	1.0	0.9
RBC	Mean	5.1	5.1	5.0	4.9	4.8	4.8
	STD Dev	0.3	0.3	0.3	0.3	0.4	0.4
GRPRCNT	Mean	57.9	59.6	60.7	60.3	60.6	61.1
	STD Dev	8.0	8.4	8.4	7.2	9.0	12.0
LYPRCNT	Mean	34.2	32.6	31.6	32.4	30.9	30.0
	STD Dev	8.0	7.4	7.4	6.7	7.8	7.4
GRNUM	Mean	3.8	4.0	4.0	3.8	3.9	4.3
	STD Dev	1.2	1.5	1.6	1.3	1.3	1.5
LYNUM	Mean	2.2	2.1	2.0	2.0	2.0	2.0
	STD Dev	0.7	0.6	0.5	0.5	0.5	0.6

Coefficient of Variation of a Method

Example: Figure 3.

$$\frac{\text{Your SD } 0.10}{\text{Your mean } 7.01} \times 100 = 1.4\% \text{ CV}$$

This tells how reproducible the method is and allows comparison of precision between methods.

The term CV may be used to determine and compare the inherent variability of methods representing different modalities—i.e., particle counting of suspended cells, chemical concentration, etc. The method with the lowest CV is considered the best. This is a measure of precision. A reliable set of automated hematology instruments have been marketed with excellent standards and quality control materials (Table 5).

Table 5 Major Instruments for Automated CBC Analysis

Manufacturer	Instrument for large lab	Instrument for physician office lab
Abbot	Cell Dyn 4000	Cell Dyn 1700, 3200
Coulter	Coulter Gens	Max M
Technicon	H-3	N/A
Sysmex	NE9000	K1000
Becton Dickinson	N/A	QCB

CONCLUSIONS

1. The patient and the physician must be the focus of all quality control and quality assurance efforts in the hematology laboratory.

2. At present we have accurate hemoglobin recalibration every 6 months and daily quality control on every shift in 100% of U.S. laboratories. This means that every patient in the United States has hemoglobin measurements traceable to the single international reference standard via the NCCLS standard. Hence, hemoglobin measurements made during the life of a U.S. citizen are comparable over time and geographic location. This is a significant achievement resulting from the efforts of many individuals and national groups.

3. Every medical student should acquire two skills: preparation of a thin blood film, and evaluation of a stained blood film.

This is not currently required by the National Board of Medical Examiners, which leads to the assumption by students that practical skills are not important. This is a significant waste of an important learning opportunity.

BIBLIOGRAPHY

Cell Dyn Quality Control Manual. Chicago: Abbott Laboratories, 1997.

College of American Pathologists. Criteria for Inspection and Accreditation 1996. Chicago: CAP, 1996.

Copeland BE. Quality control. In: Kaplan, Pesce, eds. Clinical Chemistry. 2nd ed. St. Louis: Mosby, 1988.

Copeland BE. Workshop Manual on Quality Control. Chicago: American Society of Clinical Pathologists, 1956.

Copeland BE, Pesce AJ, Horn P. Unpublished data, SW Ohio. Department of Pathology and Laboratory Predisease, University of Cincinatti Medical School.

Clinical Laboratory Improvement Act, 1967 revision. Fed Reg 1988.

National Committee for Clinical Laboratory Standards. Reference and Selected Procedures for the Quantitative Determination of Hemoglobin in Blood. 2nd ed. Approved Std NCCLS document H15-A2. NCCLS, 771 East Lancaster Avenue, Villanova, PA: NCCLS, 1994.

NCCLS Performance Goals for Internal Quality Control of Multichannel Hematology Analyzers Approved Std H26A, Vol 16, No. 12, Dec. 1996 (ISBN 1-56238-312-4).

NCCLS. Procedure for Determining Packed Cell Volume by the Microhematocrit Method 2nd ed. Approved Std NCCLS Document H7-A2 Vol 13, No. 9, August 1993 (ISBN 1-56238-199-7).

Schumacher HR, Garvin DF, Triplett DA. Introduction to Laboratory Hematology and Hematopathology. New York, Alan R. Liss, 1984: 577–593.

Modern Diagnostic Hematology. Philadelphia: Williams and Williams, 1984.

Wones R. Fernald medical monitoring program: protocol for ongoing monitoring assay. p. 4–10, June 1996. Dept. of Internal Medicine, University of Cincinnati, Cincinnati, Ohio.

CASE HISTORY

A clinician complained to the laboratory director of a hospital laboratory that the hospital laboratory hemoglobin values were always low. "My patient hemoglobin values are always lower in the hospital than in my private laboratory, which is approved by the American Association of Family Practitioners."

They compared hemoglobin quality control methods and found that they were using the same company product for semiannual calibration and the same daily quality control samples.

The pathologist demonstrated his laboratory's success on the External Quality Control survey from the College of American Pathology (CAP). The clinician showed the pathology results of several successful completions of the AAFP surveys in his office laboratory. It was decided to study the next five patients together. The preadmission afternoon values from the private laboratory were compared with the hospital studies from the samples drawn next morning in the hospital. When the data were reviewed together it became clear that neither laboratory instrument was biased. It was also seen that the clinician was correct that the morning Hb values for his patients were consistently low, as shown here:

Hemoglobin (g/dL)	Time	Patient		
		A	B	C
Physician's office laboratory	3:00 PM	14	16	15
Hospital laboratory	6:00 AM	13	15	14
		−1.0	−1.0	−1.0

The pathologist proposed that this was an example of the shift of plasma water into the extracellular fluid space during the day in the ambulatory erect position concentrating the formed elements and the return of the extracellular fluid to the vascular compartment in the period of sleep in recumbent position lowering the concentration of formed elements. After reviewing the collected data the clinician agreed that the change in extracellular fluid was a logical explanation.

Index

Note: A page reference followed by t *or* f *indicates an entry found within a table or figure (legend), respectively.*